Senior Editors

Bruce G. Wolff, MD, FASCRS
Professor of Surgery, Mayo Clinic College of Medicine, Chairman, Division of Colon and Rectal Surgery, Mayo Clinic Foundation, Rochester, MN, USA

James W. Fleshman, MD, FASCRS
Professor of Surgery, Chief, Section of Colorectal Surgery, Washington University School of Medicine, St. Louis, MO, USA

David E. Beck, MD, FASCRS
Chairman, Department of Colon and Rectal Surgery, Ochsner Clinic Foundation, New Orleans, LA, USA

John H. Pemberton, MD, FASCRS
Professor of Surgery, Mayo Clinic College of Medicine, Consultant, Colon and Rectal Surgery, Mayo Clinic and Mayo Foundation, Rochester, MN, USA

Steven D. Wexner, MD, FASCRS
Chief of Staff, Cleveland Clinic Florida, Weston, FL, USA

Associate Editors

James M. Church, BSc, MBChB, MMed Sci, FASCRS
Victor W. Fazio Chair of Colorectal Surgery, Department of Colorectal Surgery, Cleveland Clinic Foundation, Cleveland, OH, USA

Julio Garcia-Aguilar MD, PhD, FASCRS
Professor of Surgery, Chief, Section of Colon and Rectal Surgery, Department of Surgery, University of California, San Francisco, San Francisco, CA, USA

Patricia L. Roberts, MD, FASCRS
Chair, Department of Colon and Rectal Surgery, Lahey Clinic, Associate Professor of Surgery, Tufts University School of Medicine, Boston, MA, Department of Colon and Rectal Surgery, Lahey Clinic, Burlington, MA, USA

Theodore J. Saclarides, MD, FASCRS
Professor of Surgery, Head, Section of Colon and Rectal Surgery, Rush University Medical Center, Chicago, IL, USA

Michael J. Stamos, MD, FASCRS
Professor of Surgery, Chief, Division of Colon and Rectal Surgery, Department of Surgery, University of California, Irvine Medical Center, Orange, CA, USA

The ASCRS Textbook of
Colon and Rectal Surgery

The ASCRS Textbook of Colon and Rectal Surgery

Senior Editors

Bruce G. Wolff, MD, FASCRS
James W. Fleshman, MD, FASCRS
David E. Beck, MD, FASCRS
John H. Pemberton, MD, FASCRS
Steven D. Wexner, MD, FASCRS

Associate Editors

James M. Church, BSc, MBChB, MMed Sci, FASCRS
Julio Garcia-Aguilar MD, PhD, FASCRS
Patricia L. Roberts, MD, FASCRS
Theodore J. Saclarides, MD, FASCRS
Michael J. Stamos, MD, FASCRS

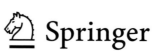 Springer

Library of Congress Control Number: 2006923505

ISBN-13: 978-0387-24846-2

Printed on acid-free paper.

© 2007 Springer Science+Business Media, LLC

9 8 7 6 5 4 3 2

springer.com

Foreword

This text was developed under the aegis of the American Society of Colon and Rectal Surgeons (ASCRS). It represents an attempt to cover the field of colon and rectal surgery with input from expert surgeons who have, in one way or another, shown special interest or expertise in specific areas of the specialty.

The book will hopefully serve as a source of useful information and perhaps even guidance to surgeons whose practice is confined to the specialty of colon and rectal surgery, and also to general surgeons, surgery residents, and medical students with an interest in surgery.

The finished product represents significant efforts from authors who have taken time from their busy schedules to set into writing their often unique perspectives. I know for certain that no author of any chapter in this book has a light schedule, but that fact validates each author's selection for authorship.

Special acknowledgment is due the editors, Bruce Wolff, David Beck, John Pemberton, and Steven Wexner. This project simply would not have come together without their efforts on many levels.

Finally, Jim Fleshman must be singled out for special recognition. The idea of an ASCRS-sponsored text began with Jim—an idea that he advocated, developed, nurtured, and forced until it became realized in the substance you now hold.

Robert Fry, MD
Emilie and Roland deHellebranth
Professor of Surgery
Chief, Division of Colon and Rectal Surgery
The Hospital of the University of Pennsylvania

Preface

The ASCRS Textbook was conceived as a means of providing state of the art information to residents in training and fully trained surgeons seeking recertification. The textbook also supports the mission of the American Society of Colon and Rectal Surgeons (ASCRS) to be the world's authority on colon and rectal disease. The combination of junior and senior authors selected from the membership of the ASCRS for each chapter will provide a comprehensive summary of each topic and allow the touch of experience to focus and temper the material. This approach should provide the reader with a very open-minded, evidence-based approach to all aspects of colorectal disease.

The Editorial Committee of the book has been designed to be a rotating group of experts selected by the ASCRS Executive Council. It has been my distinct pleasure and honor to work with this edition's editors and associate editors. They have sacrificed time and energy with patience to achieve what I believe to be the next gold standard in accumulated knowledge regarding the entire breadth of colorectal surgery. The idea for the book was originally Dr. Bruce Wolff's. The table of contents was intentionally based on the Core Curriculum established by the Association of Program Directors in Colon and Rectal Surgery. The Practice Parameters developed by the ASCRS Standards Committee have been incorporated into the appropriate chapters. The proceeds from the textbook and related publications will be utilized by the ASCRS Executive Council to sponsor the Research and Education Foundation of the society. This is truly an ASCRS effort.

As future editions continue the effort started with this first edition, I hope the fellows and members of ASCRS and trainees at all levels realize that this is the definitive source of knowledge in colon and rectal surgery. I am honored to have been a small part of such a monumental achievement. Dr. Robert Fry, as President of the ASCRS at the time of the textbook's inception, is to be congratulated for looking to the future and seeing the potential of such a project. I must also thank my wife Linda for her support during this effort and my administrative staff (Liz Nordike at Washington University and Beth Campbell, Laura Gillan D. Zerega, and Paula Callaghan at Springer) for all their effort toward completing the book.

James W. Fleshman, MD, FASCRS
August 2006

Contents

Foreword by *Robert Fry* vii

Preface ix

Contributors xv

1 **Anatomy and Embryology of the Colon, Rectum, and Anus** 1
   José Marcio Neves Jorge and Angelita Habr-Gama

2 **Physiology: Colonic** 23
   Tracy L. Hull

3 **Anal Physiology** 33
   Susan M. Parker and John A. Coller

4 **Physiologic Testing** 40
   Lee E. Smith and Garnet J. Blatchford

5 **Diagnostic Evaluations—Endoscopy: Rigid, Flexible Complications** 57
   Santhat Nivatvongs and Kenneth A. Forde

6 **Diagnostic Evaluations—Radiology, Nuclear Scans, PET,
   CT Colography** 69
   Matthew G. Mutch, Elisa H. Birnbaum, and Christine O. Menias

7 **Endoluminal Ultrasound** 101
   Donald G. Kim and W. Douglas Wong

8 **Preoperative Management—Risk Assessment, Medical Evaluation,
   and Bowel Preparation** 116
   Conor P. Delaney and John M. MacKeigan

9 **Postoperative Management: Pain and Anesthetic, Fluids and Diet** 130
   Tracey D. Arnell and Robert W. Beart, Jr.

10 **Postoperative Complications** 141
   David W. Dietz and H. Randolph Bailey

11 **Benign Anorectal: Hemorrhoids** 156
   José R. Cintron and Herand Abcarian

12   **Benign Anorectal: Anal Fissure** **178**
       Sharon L. Dykes and Robert D. Madoff

13   **Benign Anorectal: Abscess and Fistula** **192**
       Carol-Ann Vasilevsky and Philip H. Gordon

14   **Benign Anorectal: Rectovaginal Fistulas** **215**
       Ann C. Lowry and Barton Hoexter

15   **Pilonidal Disease and Hidradenitis Suppurativa** **228**
       Jeffery M. Nelson and Richard P. Billingham

16   **Perianal Dermatology and Pruritus Ani** **240**
       Charles O. Finne

17   **Sexually Transmitted Diseases** **256**
       Charles B. Whitlow and Lester Gottesman

18   **Benign Colon: Diverticular Disease** **269**
       Alan G. Thorson and Stanley M. Goldberg

19   **Colonic Volvulus** **286**
       Michael D. Hellinger and Randolph M. Steinhagen

20   **Lower Gastrointestinal Hemorrhage** **299**
       Frank G. Opelka, J. Byron Gathright, Jr., and David E. Beck

21   **Endometriosis** **308**
       Michael J. Snyder and Steven J. Stryker

22   **Colon and Rectal Trauma and Rectal Foreign Bodies** **322**
       Demetrios Demetriades and Ali Salim

23   **Colorectal Cancer: Epidemiology, Etiology, and Molecular Basis** **335**
       Nancy N. Baxter and Jose G. Guillem

24   **Screening for Colorectal Neoplasms** **353**
       Thomas E. Read and Philip F. Caushaj

25   **Polyps** **362**
       Marcus J. Burnstein and Terry C. Hicks

26   **Polyposis Syndromes** **373**
       Robin K. S. Phillips and Susan K. Clark

27   **Colon Cancer Evaluation and Staging** **385**
       Eric G. Weiss and Ian Lavery

28   **Surgical Management of Colon Cancer** **395**
       Anthony J. Senagore and Robert Fry

29   **The Preoperative Staging of Rectal Cancer** **405**
       Jonathan E. Efron and Juan J. Nogueras

30   **Surgical Treatment of Rectal Cancer** **413**
Ronald Bleday and Julio Garcia-Aguilar

31   **Adjuvant Therapy for Colorectal Cancer** **437**
Judith L. Trudel and Lars A. Påhlman

32   **Colorectal Cancer Surveillance** **446**
Brett T. Gemlo and David A. Rothenberger

33   **Management of Locally Advanced and Recurrent Rectal Cancer** **450**
Robert R. Cima and Heidi Nelson

34   **Colorectal Cancer: Metastatic (Palliation)** **462**
Michael D'Angelica, Kamran Idrees, Philip B. Paty, and Leslie H. Blumgart

35   **Anal Cancer** **482**
Mark Lane Welton and Madhulika G. Varma

36   **Presacral Tumors** **501**
Eric J. Dozois, David J. Jacofsky, and Roger R. Dozois

37   **Miscellaneous Neoplasms** **515**
Richard Devine and Marc Brand

38   **Hereditary Nonpolyposis Colon Cancer** **525**
Lawrence C. Rusin and Susan Galandiuk

39   **Inflammatory Bowel Disease: Diagnosis and Evaluation** **543**
Walter A. Koltun

40   **Medical Management of Inflammatory Bowel Disease** **555**
Stephen B. Hanauer, Wee-Chian Lim, and Miles Sparrow

41   **Surgical Management of Ulcerative Colitis** **567**
Phillip R. Fleshner and David J. Schoetz, Jr.

42   **Surgery for Crohn's Disease** **584**
Scott A. Strong

43   **Less-common Benign Disorders of the Colon and Rectum** **601**
Walter E. Longo and Gregory C. Oliver

44   **Intestinal Stomas** **622**
Bruce A. Orkin and Peter A. Cataldo

45   **Stoma Complications** **643**
Neil Hyman and Richard Nelson

46   **Incontinence** **653**
Cornelius G. Baeten and Han C. Kuijpers

47   **Rectal Prolapse** **665**
Anthony M. Vernava, III and David E. Beck

48 **Constipation** 678
    Amanda Metcalf and Howard Michael Ross

49 **Pelvic Floor Disorders** 687
    Frank J. Harford and Linda Brubaker

50 **Laparoscopy** 693
    Peter W. Marcello and Tonia Young-Fadok

51 **Pediatric: Hirschsprung's, Anorectal Malformations,
    and Other Conditions** 713
    Alberto Peña and Marc Sher

52 **Healthcare Economics** 727
    David A. Margolin and Lester Rosen

53 **Ethical and Legal Considerations** 735
    *Ira J. Kodner, Mark Siegler, Daniel M. Freeman,
    and William T. Choctaw*

54 **Critically Reviewing the Literature for Improving Clinical Practice** 764
    Clifford Y. Ko and Robin McLeod

55 **Surgical Education: A Time for Change** 779
    Clifford L. Simmang and Richard K. Reznick

56 **Legal Considerations** 786
    Michael J. Meehan

Index 795

Contributors

Herand Abcarian, MD
Turi Josefsen Professor and Head, Department of Surgery, University of Illinois at Chicago Medical Center, Chicago,
IL, USA

Tracey D. Arnell, MD
Assistant Professor, Department of Surgery, Division of General Surgery, Section of Colon and Rectal Surgery, Columbia University New York-Presbyterian Hospital Columbia Campus, New York, NY, USA

Cornelius G. Baeten, PhD
Professor, Department of Surgery, University Hospital Maastricht, Maastricht, The Netherlands

H. Randolph Bailey, MD
Clinical Professor, Department of Surgery, University of Texas Health Science Center, Houston, Houston, TX, USA

Nancy N. Baxter, MD, PhD
Assistant Professor, Department of Surgery, University of Minnesota, Fairview–University Medical Center, Minneapolis, MN, USA

Robert W. Beart, Jr., MD
Professor and Chairman, Department of Colorectal Surgery, University of Southern California, Keck School of Medicine, Los Angeles, CA, USA

David E. Beck, MD
Chairman, Department of Colon and Rectal Surgery, Ochsner Clinic Foundation, New Orleans, LA, USA

Richard P. Billingham, MD
Clinical Professor, Department of Surgery, University of Washington, Seattle, WA, USA

Elisa H. Birnbaum, MD
Department of Colon and Rectal Surgery Washington University School of Medicine, St. Louis, MO, USA

Garnet J. Blatchford, MD
Clinical Assistant Professor, Department of Surgery, Creighton University Omaha, NE, USA

Ronald Bleday, MD
Associate Professor, Department of Surgery, Brigham and Women's Hospital, Boston, MA, USA

Leslie H. Blumgart, MD
Professor, Department of Surgery, Hepatobiliary Service, Weill Medical College of Cornell
University, Memorial Sloan-Kettering Cancer Center, New York, NY, USA

Marc Brand, MD
Assistant Professor, Department of Surgery, Director, Colorectal Surgical Research,
Director, Sandra Rosenberg Registry for Hereditary and Familial Colon Cancer, Department
of General Surgery, Section of Colorectal Surgery, Rush University Medical Center,
Chicago, IL, USA

Linda Brubaker, MD
Professor, Departments of Obstetrics and Gynecology and Urology, Loyola University Medical
Center, Maywood, IL, USA

Marcus J. Burnstein, MD, MSc
Associate Professor, Department of Surgery, University of Toronto, St. Michael's Hospital,
Toronto, Ontario, Canada

Peter A. Cataldo, MD
Associate Professor, Department of Colon and Rectal Surgery/General Surgery,
University of Vermont College of Medicine, Fletcher Allen Health Care, South
Burlington, VT, USA

Philip F. Caushaj, MD
Chair, Department of Surgery, Western Pennsylvania Hospital, Clinical Campus of Temple
University School of Medicine, Professor and Vice Chair, Department of Surgery, Temple
University School of Medicine, Adjunct Professor of Surgery, University of Pittsburgh School
of Medicine, Clinical Professor of Surgery, Lake Erie College of Osteopathic Medicine,
Pittsburgh, PA, USA

William T. Choctaw, MD, JD
Clinical Faculty, Chief of Surgery, University of Southern California Keck School of
Medicine, Citrus Valley Medical Center, St, Covina, CA, USA

James M. Church, BSc, MBChB, MMed Sci
Victor W. Fazio Chair of Colorectal Surgery, Department of Colorectal Surgery, Cleveland
Clinic Foundation, Cleveland, OH, USA

Robert R. Cima, MD
Assistant Professor, Department of Surgery, Division of Colon and Rectal Surgery, Mayo
Clinic College of Medicine, Mayo Clinic, Rochester, Rochester, MN, USA

José R. Cintron, MD
Associate Professor, Department of Surgery, University of Illinois at Chicago Medical Center,
Chicago, IL, USA

Susan K. Clark, MD
Consultant Colorectal Surgeon, Royal London Hospital, Center for Academic Surgery,
Whitechapel, London, UK

John A. Coller, MD
Senior Staff, Colon and Rectal Surgeon, Lahey Clinic; Assistant Clinical Professor,
Department of Surgery, Tufts University School of Medicine, Department of Colon and Rectal
Surgery, Burlington, MA, USA

Michael D'Angelica, MD
Assistant Professor, Assistant Attending, Department of Surgery, Hepatobiliary Division,
Cornell University, Weill Medical College, Memorial Sloan-Kettering Cancer Center, New
York, NY, USA

Conor P. Delaney, MD, PhD
Staff Surgeon, Department of Colorectal Surgery and Minimally Invasive Surgery, Cleveland
Clinic Foundation, Cleveland, OH, USA

Demetrios Demetriades, MD PhD
Professor, Department of Surgery, Director, Division of Trauma/SICU, University of Southern
California, Los Angeles County and University of Southern California Trauma Center, Sierra
Madre, CA, USA

Richard Devine, MD
Professor, Department of Colon and Rectal Surgery, Mayo Clinic, Rochester, MN, USA

David W. Dietz, MD
Assistant Professor, Section of Colon and Rectal Surgery, Washington University School of
Medicine, Barnes-Jewish Hospital, St. Louis, MO, USA

Eric J. Dozois, MD
Assistant Professor, Department of Colon and Rectal Surgery, Mayo Medical Schook, Mayo
Clinic; Saint Marys Hospital, Rochester, MN, USA

Roger R. Dozois, MD
Professor (Emeritus), Division of Colon and Rectal Surgery, Mayo Medical School, Rochester,
MN, USA

Sharon L. Dykes, MD
Adjunct Instructor, Department of Surgery, University of Minnesota, St. Paul, MN, USA

Jonathan E. Efron, MD
Cleveland Clinic Florida, Naples, FL, USA

Charles O. Finne, MD
Adjunct Professor, Division of Colon and Rectal Surgery, University of Minnesota,
Minneapolis, MN, USA

James W. Fleshman, MD
Professor of Surgery, Chief, Section of Colorectal Surgery, Washington University School of
Medicine, St. Louis, MO, USA

Phillip R. Fleshner, MD
Program Director, Colorectal Surgery Residency, Division of Colorectal Surgery, Cedars-Sinai
Medical Center, Associate Clinical Professor of Clinical Surgery, UCLA School of Medicine,
Los Angeles, CA, USA

Kenneth A. Forde, MD
José M. Ferrer Professor, Department of Surgery, Columbia University College of Physicians
and Surgeons, New York Presbyterian Hospital, New York, NY, USA

Daniel M. Freeman, AB, JD
3224 Brooklawn Court, Chevy Chase, MD, USA

Robert Fry, MD
Emilie and Roland deHellebranth, Professor, Chief, Division of Colon and Rectal Surgery, University of Pennsylvania, Philadelphia, PA, USA

Susan Galandiuk, MD
Professor, Department of Surgery, University of Louisville School of Medicine, Louisville, KY, USA

Julio Garcia-Aguilar, MD, PhD
Professor of Surgery, Chief, Section of Colorectal Surgery, Department of Surgery, University of California, San Francisco, CA, USA

J. Byron Gathright, Jr., MD
Professor (Clinical), Department of Surgery; Emeritus Chairman, Department of Colon and Rectal Surgery, Ochsner Clinic Foundation, New Orleans, LA, USA

Brett T. Gemlo, MD
Assistant Adjunct Professor, Department of Surgery, University of Minnesota, St. Paul, MN, USA

Stanley M. Goldberg, MD
Clinical Professor, Department of Surgery, Division of Colorectal Surgery, University of Minnesota, Abbott Northwestern and Fairview Southdale, Minneapolis, MN, USA

Philip H. Gordon, MD
Professor, Department of Surgery and Oncology, McGill University, Montreal, Quebec, Canada

Lester Gottesman, MD
Associate Professor, Department of Colon and Rectal Surgery, Columbia University, St. Luke's Roosevelt Hospital Center, New York, NY, USA

Jose G. Guillem
Memorial Sloan Kettering Cancer Center, New York, NY, USA

Angelita Habr-Gama, MD
Professor, Department of Gastroenterology–Discipline of Coloproctology, University of São Paulo Medical School, Hospital Das Clínicas, São Paulo, Brazil

Stephen B. Hanauer, MD
Professor, Departments of Medicine and Clinical Pharmacology, Section of Gastroenterology, University of Chicago, Chicago, IL, USA

Frank J. Harford
Professor, Department of Surgery, Loyola University Medical Center, Maywood, IL, USA

Michael D. Hellinger, MD
Associate Professor, Department of Clinical Surgery, Chief, Division of Colon and Rectal Surgery, DeWitt Daughtry Family Department of Surgery, University of Miami, Miller School of Medicine, University of Miami, Sylvester Comprehensive Cancer Center, Miami, FL, USA

Terry C. Hicks, MD
Ochsner Clinic, New Orleans, LA, USA

Barton Hoexter, MD
1000 Northern Boulevard, Great Neck, NY, USA

Tracy L. Hull, MD
Staff Colorectal Surgeon, Department of Colon and Rectal Surgery, Cleveland Clinic
Foundation, Cleveland, OH, USA

Neil Hyman, MD
Professor, Department of Surgery; Chief, Division of General Surgery, University of Vermont
College of Medicine, Fletcher Allen Healthcare, Burlington, VT, USA

Kamran Idrees, MD
Colorectal Clinical Fellow, Department of Colorectal Surgery Service, Memorial Sloan-
Kettering Cancer Center, New York, NY, USA

David J. Jacofsky, MD
Assistant Professor, Department of Orthopedics, Mayo Clinic School of Medicine, Rochester,
MN, USA

José Marcio Neves Jorge, MD
Associate Professor, Department of Gastroenterology, Division of Coloproctology, University
of São Paulo Medical School, Hospital Das Clínicas, São Paulo, Brazil

Donald G. Kim, MD
Staff Colon and Rectal Surgeon, Ferguson Clinic, Grand Rapids, MI, USA

Clifford Y. Ko, MD, MS
Associate Professor, Department of Surgery, UCLA School of Medicine, West Los Angeles
VA Medical Center, Los Angeles, CA, USA

Ira J. Kodner, MD
Solon and Bettie Gershman Professor, Department of Colon and Rectal Surgery, Washington
University in St. Louis, Barnes-Jewish Hospital, St. Louis, MO, USA

Walter A. Koltun, MD
Peter and Marshia Carlino Chair in IBD, Professor of Surgery, Chief, Division of Colon and
Rectal Surgery, Pennsylvania State University, Milton S. Hershey Medical Center, Hershey,
PA, USA

Han C. Kuijpers, MD, PhD
Department of Gastrointestinal Surgery, Gelderse Vallei Ziekenhuis, Gelderland, The
Netherlands

Ian Lavery, MD
Cleveland Clinic, Cleveland, OH, USA

Wee-Chian Lim, MBBS, M.Med(Int. Med.), MRCP(UK)
Consultant, Department of Gastroenterology, Tan Tock Seng Hospital, Singapore

Walter E. Longo, MD
Professor, Department of Surgery, Chief, Section of Gastrointestinal Surgery, Director of
Colon and Rectal Surgery, Program Director in Surgery, Yale University, New Haven,
CT, USA

Ann C. Lowry, MD
Adjunct Professor and Program Director, Department of Surgery, Division of Colon
and Rectal Surgery, University of Minnesota, St. Paul, MN, USA

John M. MacKeigan, MD
Associate Clinical Professor, Department of Surgery, Michigan State University School of
Human Medicine, Spectrum, St. Mary's and Metropolitan Hospital, Grand Rapids, MI, USA

Robert D. Madoff, MD
Adjunct Professor, Department of Surgery, University of Minnesota, St. Paul, MN, USA

Peter W. Marcello, MD
Assistant Professor of Surgery, Tufts University School of Medicine, Boston, MA; CRS
Department, Lahey Clinic, Burlington, MA, USA

David A. Margolin, MD
Department Colon and Rectal Surgery, Ochsner Main Campus, New Orleans, LA, USA

Robin McLeod, MD
Professor, Department of Surgery and Health Policy, Management and Evaluation,
University of Toronto; Head, Division of General Surgery, Mount Sinai Hospital, Toronto,
Ontario, Canada

Michael J. Meehan, AB, JD
Assistant Secretary and Associate Counsel, Cleveland Clinic Foundation, Office of General
Counsel, Lyndhurst, OH, USA

Christine O. Menias, MD
Assistant Program Director, Co-Director of Body Computed Tomography, Department of
Diagnostic Radiology, Washington University, St. Louis, MO, USA

Amanda Metcalf, MD
Professor, Department of Surgery, University of Iowa, Iowa City, IA, USA

Matthew G. Mutch, MD
Assistant Professor, Department of Surgery, Section of Colon and Rectal Surgery, Washington
University School of Medicine, Barnes-Jewish Hospital, St. Louis, MO, USA

Heidi Nelson, MD
Professor, Department of Surgery, Mayo Medical School, Mayo Clinic College of Medicine;
Chair, Division of Colon and Rectal Surgery, Mayo Clinic–Rochester, Rochester, MN, USA

Jeffery M. Nelson, MD
General Surgery Clinic, Walter Reed Army Medical Center, Washington, DC, USA

Richard Nelson, MD
Consultant Surgeon, Department of General Surgery, Northern General Hospital,
Sheffield, UK

Santhat Nivatvongs, MD
Professor, Department of Surgery, Mayo Medical School, Mayo Clinic, Rochester,
MN, USA

Juan J. Nogueras, MD
Cleveland Clinic Florida, Weston, FL, USA

Gregory C. Oliver, MD
Associate Clinical Professor, Department of Colon and Rectal Surgery, Robert Wood Johnson
Medical School, University of Medicine and Dentistry of New Jersey, Edison, NJ, USA

Frank G. Opelka, MD
Associate Dean of Health Care Quality and Safety, Professor of Surgery, Louisiana State HSC,
New Orleans, LA, USA

Bruce A. Orkin, MD
Professor of Surgery, Division of Colon and Rectal Surgery, George Washington University,
Washington, DC, USA

Lars A. Påhlman, PhD, MD
Professor, Department of Surgical Sciences, Section of Surgery, Uppsala University, Uppsala,
Sweden

Susan M. Parker, MD
606 24 Avenue South, Minneapolis, MN, USA

Philip B. Paty, MD
Associate Professor and Associate Attending, Department of Surgery, Weill Medical
College of Cornell University, Memorial Sloan-Kettering Cancer Center, New York,
NY, USA

John H. Pemberton, MD
Professor of Surgery, Mayo Clinic College of Medicine, Consultant, Colon and Rectal Surgery,
Mayo Clinic and Mayo Foundation, Rochester, MN, USA

Alberto Peña, MD
Professor, Department of Surgery, Division of Pediatric Surgery, Albert Einstein
College of Medicine, Schneider Children's Hospital, NSLIJ Health System,
New Hyde Park, NY, USA

Robin K. S. Phillips, MBBS, MS
Professor, Department of Colorectal Surgery, Imperial College, London, St. Mark's Hospital,
Harrow, UK

Thomas E. Read, MD
Chief, Division of Colon and Rectal Surgery, Western Pennsylvania Hospital, Clinical Campus
of Temple University School of Medicine; Associate Professor, Department of Surgery,
Temple University School of Medicine, Pittsburgh, PA, USA

Richard K. Reznick, MD, MEd
Professor and Chair, Department of Surgery, University of Toronto, Toronto, Ontario, Canada

Patricia L. Roberts, MD
Chair, Department of Colon and Rectal Surgery, Lahey Clinic, Associate Professor of Surgery,
Tufts University School of Medicine, Boston MA; Department of Colon and Rectal Surgery,
Lahey Clinic, Burlington, MA, USA

Lester Rosen, MD
Professor, Department of Colon and Rectal Surgery, Pennsylvania State University, Hershey
Medical Center, Allentown, PA, USA

Howard Michael Ross, MD
Assistant Professor, Department of Surgery, Director, Surgery Student Education, Director, Laparoscopic Colon and Rectal Surgery, University of Pennsylvania School of Medicine, Philadelphia, PA, USA

David A. Rothenberger, MD
Professor, Department of Surgery, University of Minnesota Cancer Center, Minneapolis, MN, USA

Lawrence C. Rusin, MD
Senior Staff, Lahey Clinic, Assistant Clinical Professor, Department of Colon and Rectal Surgery, Tufts School of Medicine, Burlington, MA, USA

Theodore Saclarides, MD
Professor of Surgery, Head, Section of Colon and Rectal Surgery, Rush University Medical Center, Chicago, IL, USA

Ali Salim, MD
Assistant Professor, Department of Surgery, University of Southern California Keck School of Medicine, Los Angeles, CA, USA

David J. Schoetz, Jr., MD
Chairman Emeritus, Professor, Department of Surgery, Tufts University School of Medicine; Department of Colon and Rectal Surgery, Lahey Clinic, Burlington, MA, USA

Anthony J. Senagore, MD
Professor and Chairman, Department of Surgery, Medical University of Ohio, Toledo, OH, USA

Mark Sher, MD
Assistant Clinical Professor, Department of Colon and Rectal Surgery, Albert Einstein College of Medicine, Long Island Jewish Medical Center, New Hyde Park, NY, USA

Mark Siegler, MD
Lindy Bergman Distinguished Service Professor, Department of Medicine and Surgery, University of Chicago, Chicago, IL, USA

Clifford L. Simmang, MD, MS
Medical Center of Plano, Plano, TX, USA

Lee E. Smith, MD
Professor, Department of Surgery, Georgetown University, Washington Hospital Center, Washington, DC, USA

Michael J. Snyder, MD
Program Director, Department of Colon and Rectal Surgery, University of Texas Medical School at Houston, Houston, TX, USA

Miles Sparrow, MB.BS
Inflammatory Bowel Disease Fellow, Department of Gastroenterology, Mount Sinai School of Medicine, New York, NY, USA

Michael J. Stamos, MD
Professor of Surgery, Chief, Division of Colon and Rectal Surgery, Department of Surgery, University of California, Irvine School of Medicine, Orange, CA, USA

Randolph M. Steinhagen, MD
Associate Professor, Department of Surgery, Division of Colon and Rectal Surgery, Mount Sinai School of Medicine, New York, NY, USA

Scott A. Strong, MD
Staff Surgeon, Department of Colorectal Surgery, The Cleveland Clinic Foundation, Cleveland, OH, USA

Steven J. Stryker, MD
Professor, Department of Clinical Surgery, Northwestern University, The Feinberg School of Medicine, Chicago, IL, USA

Alan G. Thorson, MD
Clinical Associate Professor, Department of Surgery, Program Director, Section of Colon and Rectal Surgery, Creighton University School of Medicine; Clinical Associate Professor, Department of Surgery, University of Nebraska College of Medicine, Omaha, NE, USA

Judith L. Trudel, MD, MSc, MHPE
Adjunct Associate Professor, Department of Surgery, University of Minnesota, St. Paul, MN, USA

Madhulika G. Varma, MD
Assistant Professor, Department of Surgery, University of California, San Francisco, San Francisco, CA, USA

Carol A. Vasilevsky, MDCM
Assistant Professor, Departments of Surgery and Oncology, McGill University, Montreal, Quebec, Canada

Anthony M. Vernava, III, MD
Vice Chairman of Clinical Affairs, Professor, Department of Colorectal Surgery, University of Rochester Medical Center, Rochester, NY, USA

Eric Weiss, MD
Director of Surgical Endoscopy, Residency Program Director, Cleveland Clinic Florida, Department of Colorectal Surgery, Weston, FL, USA

Mark Lane Welton, MD
Associate Professor, Chief, Department of Colon and Rectal Surgery, Stanford University, Stanford, CA, USA

Steven D. Wexner, MD
Professor, Department of Surgery, Ohio State University Health Sciences Center; Clinical Professor, Department of Surgery, University of Florida College of Medicine; Professor of Biomedical Sciences, Charles E. Schmitt College of Science at Florida Atlantic University; and Chairman and Chief of Staff, Department of Colorectal Surgery, 21st Century Oncology Chair in Colorectal Surgery, Chief of Staff, Cleveland Clinic Florida, Weston, FL, USA

Charles B. Whitlow, MD
Ochsner Clinic Foundation, Department of Colon and Rectal Surgery, New Orleans, LA, USA

Bruce G. Wolff, MD
Professor of Surgery, Mayo Clinic College of Medicine, Chairman, Division of Colon and Rectal Surgery, Mayo Clinic Foundation, Rochester, MN, USA

W. Douglas Wong, MD
Associate Professor, Department of Surgery, Cornell University Medical Center;
Chief, Co-rectal Service, Department of Surgery, Memorial Sloan-Kettering Cancer Center,
New York, NY, USA

Tonia M. Young-Fadok, MD, MS
Associate Professor, Department of Surgery, Mayo Clinic College of Medicine; Chair, Division
of Colon and Rectal Surgery, Mayo Clinic Arizona, Scottsdale, AZ, USA

1
Anatomy and Embryology of the Colon, Rectum, and Anus

José Marcio Neves Jorge and Angelita Habr-Gama

Although much of our fundamental understanding of the anatomy of the colon, rectum, and anus comes from the efforts of researchers of the 19th and early 20th centuries, comprehensive observations of this region had been made as early as 1543 by Andreas Vesalius through anatomic dissections.[1] However, anatomy of this region, especially that of the rectum and anal canal, is so intrinsically related to its physiology that much can be appreciated only in the living. Thus, it is a region in which the surgeon has an advantage over the anatomist through in vivo dissection, physiologic investigation, and endoscopic examination. However, anatomy of the pelvis is also challenging to the surgeon: the pelvis is a narrow space, packed with intestinal, urologic, gynecologic, vascular, and neural structures, all confined within a rigid and deep osseous-muscular cage. Therefore, detailed anatomy of this region is difficult to learn in the setting of an operating room and it demands not only observations in vivo, but historical reviews, anatomy laboratory studies, including dissections of humans and animals, with in-depth descriptions and drawings and sometimes associated with physiologic evaluation. Based on these studies, some controversial concepts of the anatomy, especially of the rectum and anal canal, have been actually changed.[2–8] In addition, virtual reality models have been designed to improve visualization of three-dimensional structures and more properly teach anatomy, pathology, and surgery of the anorectum and pelvic floor.[9]

Anatomy

Anus and Rectum

Anal Canal Structure, Anus, and Anal Verge

The anal canal is anatomically peculiar and has a complex physiology, which accounts for its crucial role in continence and, in addition, its susceptibility to a variety of diseases. The anus or anal orifice is an anteroposterior cutaneous slit, that along with the anal canal remains virtually closed at rest, as a result of tonic circumferential contraction of the sphincters

and the presence of anal cushions. The edge of the anal orifice, the anal verge or margin (anocutaneous line of Hilton), marks the lowermost edge of the anal canal and is sometimes the level of reference for measurements taken during sigmoidoscopy. Others favor the dentate line as a landmark because it is more precise. The difference between the anal verge and the dentate line is usually 1–2 cm. The epithelium distal to the anal verge acquires hair follicles, glands, including apocrine glands, and other features of normal skin, and is the source of perianal hidradenitis suppurativa, inflammation of the apocrine glands.

Anatomic Versus Surgical Anal Canal

Two definitions are found describing the anal canal (Figure 1-1). The "anatomic" or "embryologic" anal canal is only 2.0 cm long, extending from the anal verge to the dentate line, the level that corresponds to the proctodeal membrane. The "surgical" or "functional" anal canal is longer, extending for approximately 4.0 cm (in men) from the anal verge to the anorectal ring (levator ani). This "long anal canal" concept was first introduced by Milligan and Morgan[10] and has been considered, despite not being proximally marked by any apparent epithelial or developmental boundary, useful both as a physiologic and surgical parameter. The anorectal ring is at the level of the distal end of the ampullary part of the rectum and forms the anorectal angle, and the beginning of a region of higher intraluminal pressure. Therefore, this definition correlates with digital, manometric, and sonographic examinations.

Anatomic Relations of the Anal Canal

Posteriorly, the anal canal is related to the coccyx and anteriorly to the perineal body and the lowest part of the posterior vaginal wall in the female, and to the urethra in the male. The ischium and the ischiorectal fossa are situated on either side. The fossa ischiorectal contains fat and the inferior rectal vessels and nerves, which cross it to enter the wall of the anal canal.

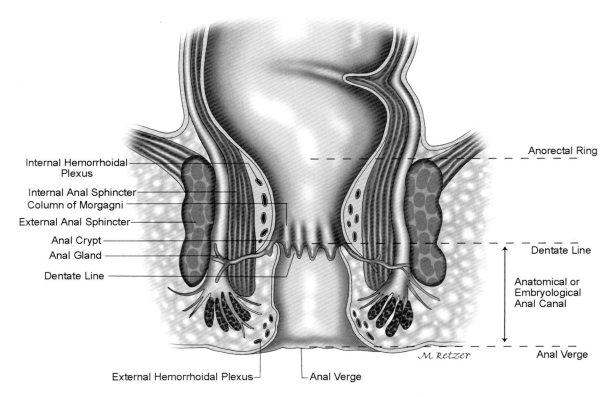

Internal Hemorrhoidal Plexus

Internal Anal Sphincter
Column of Morgagni

External Anal Sphincter

Anal Crypt
Anal Gland

Dentate Line

Anorectal Ring

Dentate Line

Anatomical or
Embryological
Anal Canal

Anal Verge

M. Retzer

External Hemorrhoidal Plexus   Anal Verge

FIGURE 1-1. Anal canal.

Muscles of the Anal Canal

The muscular component of the mechanism of continence can be stratified into three functional groups: lateral compression from the pubococcygeus, circumferential closure from the internal and external anal sphincter, and angulation from the puborectalis (Figure 1-2). The internal and external anal sphincters, and the conjoined longitudinal are intrinsically related to the anal canal, and will be addressed here.

Internal Anal Sphincter

The internal anal sphincter represents the distal 2.5- to 4.0-cm condensation of the circular muscle layer of the rectum. As a consequence of both intrinsic myogenic and extrinsic autonomic neurogenic properties, the internal anal sphincter is a smooth muscle in a state of continuous maximal contraction, and represents a natural barrier to the involuntary loss of stool and gas.

The lower rounded edge of the internal anal sphincter can be felt on physical examination, about 1.2 cm distal to the dentate line. The groove between the internal and external anal sphincter, the intersphincteric sulcus, can be visualized or easily palpated. Endosonographically, the internal anal sphincter is a 2- to 3-mm-thick circular band and shows a uniform hypoechogenicity.

External Anal Sphincter

The external anal sphincter is the elliptical cylinder of striated muscle that envelops the entire length of the inner tube of smooth muscle, but it ends slightly more distal than the internal anal sphincter. The external anal sphincter was initially described as encompassing three divisions: subcutaneous, superficial, and deep.[10] Goligher et al.[11] described the external anal sphincter as a simple, continuous sheet that forms, along with the puborectalis and levator ani, one funnel-shaped skeletal muscle. The deepest part of the external anal sphincter is intimately related to the puborectalis muscle, which can actually be considered a component of both the levator ani and the external anal sphincter muscle complexes. Others considered the external anal sphincter as being subdivided into two parts, deep (deep sphincter and puborectalis) and superficial (subcutaneous and superficial sphincter).[6,12,13] Shafik[14] proposed the three U-shaped loop system, but clinical experience has not supported this schema. The external anal sphincter is more likely to be one muscle unit, attached by the anococcygeal ligament posteriorly to the coccyx, and anteriorly to the perineal body, not divided into layers or laminae. Nevertheless, differences in the arrangement of the external anal sphincter have been described between the sexes.[15] In the male, the upper half of the external anal sphincter is enveloped anteriorly by the conjoined longitudinal muscle, whereas the lower half is crossed by it. In the female, the

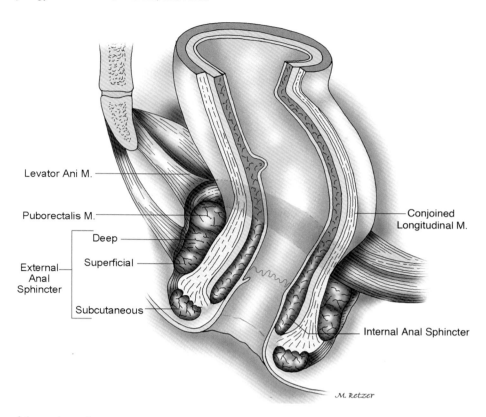

FIGURE 1-2. Muscles of the anal canal.

entire external anal sphincter is encapsulated by a mixture of fibers derived from both longitudinal and internal anal sphincter muscles.

Endosonographically, the puborectalis and the external anal sphincter, despite their mixed linear echogenicity, are both predominantly hyperechogenic, with a mean thickness of 6 mm (range, 5–8 mm). Distinction is made by position, shape, and topography. Recently, both anal endosonography and endocoil magnetic resonance imaging have been used to detail the anal sphincter complex in living, healthy subjects.[16–19] These tests provide a three-dimensional mapping of the anal sphincter; they help to study the differences in the arrangement of the external anal sphincter between the sexes and uncover sphincter disruption or defect during vaginal deliveries. In addition, there is some degree of "anatomical asymmetry" of the external anal sphincter, which accounts for both radial and longitudinal "functional asymmetry" observed during anal manometry.[20]

The automatic continence mechanism is formed by the resting tone, maintained by the internal anal sphincter, magnified by voluntary, reflex, and resting external anal sphincter contractile activities. In response to conditions of threatened incontinence, such as increased intraabdominal pressure and rectal distension, the external anal sphincter and puborectalis reflexively and voluntarily contract further to prevent fecal leakage. Because of muscular fatigue, maximal voluntary contraction of the external anal sphincter can be sustained for only 30–60 seconds. However, the external anal sphincter and the pelvic floor muscles, unlike other skeletal muscles, which are usually inactive at rest, maintain unconscious resting electrical tone through a reflex arc at the cauda equina level. Histologic studies have shown that the external anal sphincter, puborectalis, and levator ani muscles have a predominance of type I fibers, which are a peculiarity of skeletal muscles connecting tonic contractile activity.[21]

Conjoined Longitudinal Muscle

Whereas the inner circular layer of the rectum gives rise to the internal anal sphincter, the outer longitudinal layer, at the level of the anorectal ring, mixes with fibers of the levator ani muscle to form the conjoined longitudinal muscle. This muscle descends between the internal and external anal sphincter, and ultimately some of its fibers, referred to as the *corrugator cutis ani muscle*, traverse the lowermost part of the external anal sphincter to insert into the perianal skin. Some of these fibers may enter the fat of the ischiorectal fossa.[22] Other sources for the striated component of the conjoined longitudinal muscle include the puborectalis and deep external anal sphincter, the pubococcygeus and top loop of the external anal sphincter, and the lower fibers of the puborectalis.[7,23,24] In its descending course, the conjoined longitudinal muscle may give rise to medial extensions that cross the internal anal sphincter to contribute the smooth muscle of the submucosa (*musculus canalis ani, sustentator tunicae mucosae, Treitz muscle, musculus submucosae ani*).[25]

Possible functions of the conjoined longitudinal muscle include attaching the anorectum to the pelvis and acting as a skeleton that supports and binds the internal and external sphincter complex together.[22] Haas and Fox[26] consider that the meshwork formed by the conjoined longitudinal muscle may minimize functional deterioration of the sphincters after surgical division and act as a support to prevent hemorrhoidal and rectal prolapse. In addition, the conjoined longitudinal muscle and its extensions to the intersphincteric plane divide the adjacent tissues into subspaces and may actually have a role in the septation of thrombosed external hemorrhoids and containment of sepsis.[7] Finally, Shafik[23] ascribes to the conjoined longitudinal muscle the action of shortening and widening of the anal canal as well as eversion of the anal orifice, and proposed the term *evertor ani muscle*. This is controversial. In addition to this primary function during defecation, a limited role in anal continence, specifically a potentialization effect in maintaining an anal seal, has also been proposed.[23]

Epithelium of the Anal Canal

The lining of the anal canal consists of an upper mucosal (endoderm) and a lower cutaneous (ectoderm) segment (Figure 1-1). The dentate (pectinate) line is the "saw-toothed" junction between these two distinct origins of venous and lymphatic drainage, nerve supply, and epithelial lining. Above this level, the intestine is innervated by the sympathetic and parasympathetic systems, with venous, arterial, and lymphatic drainage to and from the hypogastric vessels. Distal to the dentate line, the anal canal is innervated by the somatic nervous system, with blood supply and drainage from the inferior hemorrhoidal system. These differences are important when the classification and treatment of hemorrhoids are considered.

The pectinate or dentate line corresponds to a line of anal valves that represent remnants of the proctodeal membrane. Above each valve, there is a little pocket known as an anal sinus or crypt. These crypts are connected to a variable number of glands, in average 6 (range, 3–12).[27,28] The anal glands first described by Chiari[29] in 1878 are more concentrated in the posterior quadrants. More than one gland may open into the same crypt, whereas half the crypts have no communication. The anal gland ducts, in an outward and downward route, enter the submucosa; two-thirds enter the internal anal sphincter, and half of them terminate in the intersphincteric plane.[28] Obstruction of these ducts, presumably by accumulation of foreign material in the crypts, may lead to perianal abscesses and fistulas.[30] Cephalad to the dentate line, 8–14 longitudinal folds, known as the rectal columns (columns of Morgagni), have their bases connected in pairs to each valve at the dentate line. At the lower end of the columns are the

anal papillae. The mucosa in the area of the columns consists of several layers of cuboidal cells and has a deep purple color because of the underlying internal hemorrhoidal plexus. This 0.5- to 1.0-cm strip of mucosa above the dentate line is known as the anal transition or cloacogenic zone. Cephalad to this area, the epithelium changes to a single layer of columnar cells and macroscopically acquires the characteristic pink color of the rectal mucosa.

The cutaneous part of the anal canal consists of modified squamous epithelium that is thin, smooth, pale, stretched, and devoid of hair and glands. The terms pecten and pecten band have been used to define this segment.[31] However, as pointed out by Goligher, the round band of fibrous tissue called pecten band, which is divided in the case of anal fissure (pectenotomy), probably represents the spastic internal anal sphincter.[11,32]

Rectum

Both proximal and distal limits of the rectum are controversial: the rectosigmoid junction is considered to be at the level of the third sacral vertebra by anatomists but at the sacral promontory by surgeons, and likewise, the distal limit is regarded to be the muscular anorectal ring by surgeons and the dentate line by anatomists. The rectum measures 12–15 cm in length and has three lateral curves: the upper and lower are convex to the right and the middle is convex to the left. These curves correspond intraluminally to the folds or valves of Houston. The two left-sided folds are usually noted at 7–8 cm and at 12–13 cm, respectively, and the one on the right is generally at 9–11 cm. The middle valve (Kohlrausch's plica) is the most consistent in presence and location and corresponds to the level of the anterior peritoneal reflection. Although the rectal valves do not contain all muscle wall layers from a clinical point of view, they are a good location for performing a rectal biopsies, because they are readily accessible with minimal risk for perforation.[13,33] The valves of Houston must be negotiated during proctosigmoidoscopy; they are absent after mobilization of the rectum, and this is attributed to the 5-cm length gained after complete surgical dissection. The rectal mucosa is smooth, pink, and transparent, which allows visualization of small and large submucosal vessels. This characteristic "vascular pattern" disappears in inflammatory conditions and in melanosis coli.

The rectum is characterized by its wide, easily distensible lumen, and the absence of taeniae, epiploic appendices, haustra, or a well-defined mesentery. The prefix "meso," in gross anatomy, refers to two layers of peritoneum that suspend an organ. Normally the rectum is not suspended but entirely extraperitoneal on its posterior aspect, and closely applied to the sacral hollow. Consequently, the term "mesorectum" is anatomically inaccurate. An exception, however, is that a peritonealized mesorectum may be noted in patients with procidentia. But, the word "mesorectum" has gained widespread popularity among surgeons to address the perirectal areolar tissue, which is thicker posteriorly, containing terminal branches of the inferior mesenteric artery and enclosed by the fascia propria.[34,35] The "mesorectum" may be a metastatic site for a rectal cancer and is removed during surgery for rectal cancer without neurologic sequelae, because no functionally significant nerves pass through it.

The upper third of the rectum is anteriorly and laterally invested by peritoneum; the middle third is covered by peritoneum on its anterior aspect only. Finally, the lower third of the rectum is entirely extraperitoneal, because the anterior peritoneal reflection occurs at 9.0–7.0 cm from the anal verge in men and at 7.5–5.0 cm from the anal verge in women.

Anatomic Relations of the Rectum

The rectum occupies the sacral concavity and ends 2–3 cm anteroinferiorly from the tip of the coccyx. At this point, it angulates backward sharply to pass through the levators and becomes the anal canal. Anteriorly, in women, the rectum is closely related to the uterine cervix and posterior vaginal wall; in men, it lies behind the bladder, vas deferens, seminal vesicles, and prostate. Posterior to the rectum lie the median sacral vessels and the roots of the sacral nerve plexus.

Fascial Relationships of the Rectum

The parietal endopelvic fascia lines the walls and floor of the pelvis and continues on the internal organs as a visceral pelvic fascia (Figure 1-3A and B). Thus, the *fascia propria of the rectum* is an extension of the pelvic fascia, enclosing the rectum, fat, nerves, and the blood and lymphatic vessels. It is more evident in the posterior and lateral extraperitoneal aspects of the rectum.

The *lateral ligaments or stalks of the rectum* are distal condensations of the pelvic fascia that form a roughly triangular structure with a base on the lateral pelvic wall and an apex attached to the lateral aspect of the rectum.[32] Still a subject of misconception, the lateral stalks are comprised essentially of connective tissue and nerves, and the middle rectal artery does not traverse them. Branches, however, course through in approximately 25% of cases.[36] Consequently, division of the lateral stalks during rectal mobilization is associated with a 25% risk for bleeding. Although the lateral stalks do not contain important structures, the middle rectal artery and the pelvic plexus are both closely related, running, at different angles, underneath it.[37] One theoretical concern in ligation of the stalks is leaving behind lateral mesorectal tissue, which may limit adequate lateral or mesorectal margins during cancer surgery.[34,35,38]

The *presacral fascia* is a thickened part of the parietal endopelvic fascia that covers the concavity of the sacrum and coccyx, nerves, the middle sacral artery, and presacral veins. Operative dissection deep to the presacral fascia may cause troublesome bleeding from the underlying presacral veins. Presacral hemorrhage occurs as frequently as 4.6% to 7.0% of resections for rectal neoplasms, and despite its venous nature, can be life threatening.[39–41] This is a consequence of two factors: the difficulty in securing control because of retraction of the vascular stump into the sacral foramen and the high hydrostatic pressure of the presacral venous system. The presacral veins are avalvular and communicate via basivertebral veins with the internal vertebral venous system. The adventitia of the basivertebral veins adheres firmly to the sacral periosteum at the level of the ostia of the sacral foramina,

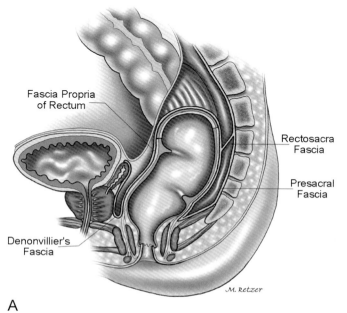

A

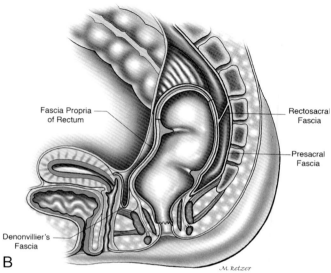

B

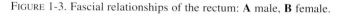

FIGURE 1-3. Fascial relationships of the rectum: **A** male, **B** female.

mainly at the level of S3-4. With the patient in the lithotomy position, the presacral veins can attain hydrostatic pressures of 17–23 cm H$_2$O, two to three times the normal pressure of the inferior vena cava.[40]

The *rectosacral fascia* is an anteroinferiorly directed thick fascial reflection from the presacral fascia at the S-4 level to the fascia propria of the rectum just above the anorectal ring.[42] The rectosacral fascia, classically known as the fascia of Waldeyer, is an important landmark during posterior rectal dissection.[2,42]

The *visceral pelvic fascia of Denonvilliers* is a tough fascial investment that separates the extraperitoneal rectum anteriorly from the prostate and seminal vesicles or vagina.[43] Therefore, three structures lie between the anterior rectal wall and the seminal vesicles and prostate: anterior mesorectum, fascia propria of the rectum, and Denonvilliers' fascia. A consensus has generally been reached about the anatomy of the plane of posterior and lateral rectal dissection, but anteriorly, the matter is more controversial. The anterior plane of rectal dissection may not necessarily follow the same plane of posterior and lateral dissection, and the use of the terms close rectal, mesorectal, and extramesorectal have been recently suggested to describe the available anterior planes.[44] The close rectal or perimuscular plane lies inside the fascia propria of the rectum and therefore it is more difficult and bloody than the mesorectal plane. The mesorectal plane represents the continuation of the same plane of posterior and lateral dissection of the rectum. This is a natural anatomic plane and consequently more appropriate for most rectal cancers. Finally, the extramesorectal plane involves resection of the Denonvilliers' fascia, with exposure of prostate and seminal vesicles, and is associated with high risk of mixed parasympathetic and sympathetic injury because of damage of the periprostatic plexus.

Urogenital Considerations

Identification of the ureters is advisable to avoid injury to their abdominal or pelvic portions during colorectal operations. On both sides, the ureters rest on the psoas muscle in their inferomedial course; they are crossed obliquely by the spermatic vessels anteriorly and the genitofemoral nerve posteriorly. In its pelvic portion, the ureter crosses the pelvic brim in front of or a little lateral to the bifurcation of the common iliac artery, and descends abruptly between the peritoneum and the internal iliac artery. Before entering the bladder in the male, the vas deferens crosses lateromedially on its superior aspect. In the female, as the ureter traverses the posterior layer of the broad ligament and the parametrium close to the side of the neck of the uterus and upper part of the vagina, it is enveloped by the vesical and vaginal venous plexuses and is crossed above and lateromedially by the uterine artery.

Arterial Supply of the Rectum and Anal Canal

The superior hemorrhoidal artery is the continuation of the inferior mesenteric artery, once it crosses the left iliac vessels.

The artery descends in the sigmoid mesocolon to the level of S-3 and then to the posterior aspect of the rectum. In 80% of cases, it bifurcates into right, usually wider, and left terminal branches; multiple branches are present in 17%.[45] These divisions, once within the submucosa of the rectum, run straight downward to supply the lower rectum and the anal canal. Approximately five branches reach the level of the rectal columns, and condense in capillary plexuses, mostly at the right posterior, right anterior, and left lateral positions, corresponding to the location of the major internal hemorrhoidal groups.

The superior and inferior hemorrhoidal arteries represent the major blood supply to the anorectum. In addition, it is also supplied by the internal iliac arteries.

The contribution of the middle hemorrhoidal artery varies with the size of the superior hemorrhoidal artery; this may explain its controversial anatomy. Some authors report absence of the middle hemorrhoidal artery in 40% to 88%[46,47] whereas others identify it in 94% to 100% of specimens.[45] It originates more frequently from the anterior division of the internal iliac or the pudendal arteries, and reaches the rectum. The middle hemorrhoidal artery reaches the lower third of the rectum anterolaterally, close to the level of the pelvic floor and deep to the levator fascia. It therefore does not run in the lateral ligaments, which are inclined posterolaterally.[2] The middle hemorrhoidal artery is more prone to be injured during low anterior resection, when anterolateral dissection of the rectum is performed close to the pelvic floor and the prostate and seminal vesicles or upper part of the vagina are being separated.[37] The anorectum has a profuse intramural anastomotic network, which probably accounts for the fact that division of both superior and middle hemorrhoidal arteries does not result in necrosis of the rectum.

The paired inferior hemorrhoidal arteries are branches of the internal pudendal artery, which in turn is a branch of the internal iliac artery. The inferior hemorrhoidal artery arises within the pudendal canal and is throughout its course entirely extrapelvic. It traverses the obturator fascia, the ischiorectal fossa, and the external anal sphincter to reach the submucosa of the anal canal, ultimately ascending in this plane. Klosterhalfen et al.[4] performed postmortem angiographic, manual, and histologic evaluations and demonstrated that in 85% of cases the posterior commissure was less well perfused than were the other sections of the anal canal. In addition, the blood supply could be jeopardized by contusion of the vessels passing vertically through the muscle fibers of the internal anal sphincter with increased sphincter tone. The resulting decreased blood supply could lead to ischemia at the posterior commissure, in a pathogenetic model of primary anal fissure.

Venous Drainage and Lymphatic Drainage of the Rectum and Anal Canal

The anorectum also drains, via middle and inferior hemorrhoidal veins, to the internal iliac vein and then to the inferior vena cava. Although it is still a controversial subject, the presence of communications among these three venous systems may explain the lack of correlation between portal hypertension and hemorrhoids.[48] The paired inferior and middle hemorrhoidal veins and the single superior hemorrhoidal vein originate from three anorectal arteriovenous plexuses. The external hemorrhoidal plexus, situated subcutaneously around the anal canal below the dentate line, constitutes when dilated the external hemorrhoids. The internal hemorrhoidal plexus is situated submucosally, around the upper anal canal and above the dentate line. The internal hemorrhoids originate from this plexus. The perirectal or perimuscular rectal plexus drains to the middle and inferior hemorrhoidal veins.

Lymph from the upper two-thirds of the rectum drains exclusively upward to the inferior mesenteric nodes and then to the paraaortic nodes. Lymphatic drainage from the lower third of the rectum occurs not only cephalad, along the superior hemorrhoidal and inferior mesentery arteries, but also laterally, along the middle hemorrhoidal vessels to the internal iliac nodes. Studies using lymphoscintigraphy have failed to demonstrate communications between inferior mesenteric and internal iliac lymphatics.[49] In the anal canal, the dentate line is the landmark for two different systems of lymphatic drainage: above, to the inferior mesenteric and internal iliac nodes, and below, along the inferior rectal lymphatics to the superficial inguinal nodes, or less frequently along the inferior hemorrhoidal artery. In the female, drainage at 5 cm above the anal verge in the lymphatic may also spread to the posterior vaginal wall, uterus, cervix, broad ligament, fallopian tubes, ovaries, and cul-de-sac, and at 10 cm above the anal verge, spread seems to occur only to the broad ligament and cul-de-sac.[50]

Innervation of the Rectum and Anal Canal

Innervation of the Rectum

The sympathetic supply of the rectum and the left colon arises from L-1, L-2, and L-3 (Figure 1-4A and B). Preganglionic fibers, via lumbar sympathetic nerves, synapse in the preaortic plexus, and the postganglionic fibers follow the branches of the inferior mesenteric artery and superior rectal artery to the left colon and upper rectum. The lower rectum is innervated by the presacral nerves, which are formed by fusion of the aortic plexus and lumbar splanchnic nerves. Just below the sacral promontory, the presacral nerves form the hypogastric plexus (or superior hypogastric plexus). Two main hypogastric nerves, on either side of the rectum, carry sympathetic innervation from the hypogastric plexus to the pelvic plexus. The pelvic plexus lies on the lateral side of the pelvis at the level of the lower third of the rectum, adjacent to the lateral stalks.

The parasympathetic fibers to the rectum and anal canal emerge through the sacral foramen and are called the nervi erigentes (S-2, S-3, and S-4). They pass laterally, forward, and upward to join the sympathetic hypogastric nerves at the pelvic plexus. From the pelvic plexus, combined postganglionic parasympathetic and sympathetic fibers are distributed to the left colon and upper rectum via the inferior mesenteric plexus, and directly to the lower rectum and upper anal canal. The periprostatic plexus, a subdivision of the pelvic plexus situated on Denonvilliers' fascia, supplies the prostate, seminal vesicles, corpora cavernosa, vas deferens, urethra, ejaculatory ducts, and bulbourethral glands. Sexual function is regulated by cerebrospinal, sympathetic, and parasympathetic components. Erection of the penis is mediated by both parasympathetic (arteriolar vasodilatation) and sympathetic inflow (inhibition of vasoconstriction).

All pelvic nerves lie in the plane between the peritoneum and the endopelvic fascia and are in danger of injury during rectal dissection. Permanent bladder paresis occurs in 7% to 59% of patients after abdominoperineal resection of the rectum[51]; the incidence of impotence is reported to range from 15% to 45%, and that of ejaculatory dysfunction from 32% to 42%.[52] The overall incidence of sexual dysfunction after proctectomy has been reported to reach 100% when wide dissection is performed for malignant disease[53–55]; however, this kind of procedure is unnecessary and these rates are much lower for benign conditions, such as inflammatory bowel disease (0% to 6%).[53,54,56,57] Dissections performed for benign conditions are undertaken closer to the bowel wall, thus reducing the possibility of nerve injury.[58]

Trauma to the autonomic nerves may occur at several points. During high ligation of the inferior mesenteric artery, close to the aorta, the sympathetic preaortic nerves may be injured. Division of both superior hypogastric plexus and hypogastric nerves may occur also during dissection at the level of the sacral promontory or in the presacral region. In such circumstances, sympathetic denervation with intact nervi erigentes results in retrograde ejaculation and bladder dysfunction. The nervi erigentes are located in the posterolateral aspect of the pelvis, and at the point of fusion with the sympathetic nerves are closely related to the middle hemorrhoidal artery. Injury to these nerves will completely abolish erectile function.[56] The pelvic plexus may be damaged either by excessive traction on the rectum, particularly laterally, or during division of the lateral stalks when this is performed close to the lateral pelvic wall. Finally, dissection near the seminal vesicles and prostate may damage the periprostatic plexus, leading to a mixed parasympathetic and sympathetic injury. This can result in erectile impotence as well as a flaccid, neurogenic bladder. Sexual complications after rectal surgery are readily evident in men but are probably underdiagnosed in women.[59]

Anal Canal

The internal anal sphincter is supplied by sympathetic (L-5) and parasympathetic nerves (S-2, S-3, and S-4) following the same route as the nerves to the rectum. The external anal sphincter is innervated on each side by the inferior rectal branch of the pudendal nerve (S-2 and S-3) and by the perineal branch of S-4. Despite the fact that the puborectalis and

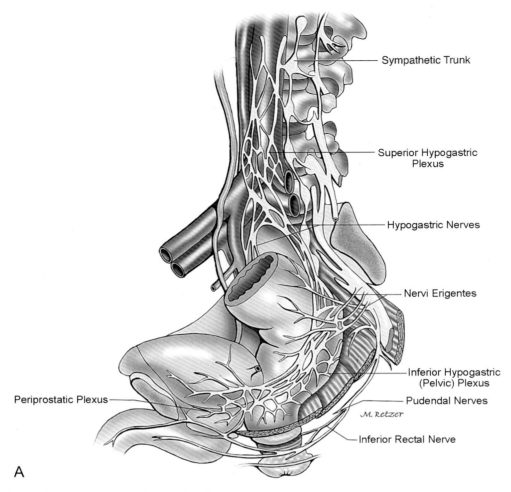

Sympathetic Trunk

Superior Hypogastric
Plexus

Hypogastric Nerves

Nervi Erigentes

Inferior Hypogastric
(Pelvic) Plexus

Pudendal Nerves

Inferior Rectal Nerve

Periprostatic Plexus

M. Retzer

A

FIGURE 1-4. **A, B** Innervation of the colon, rectum, and anal canal.

external anal sphincter have somewhat different innervations, these muscles seem to act as an indivisible unit.[14] After unilateral transection of a pudendal nerve, external anal sphincter function is still preserved because of the crossover of the fibers at the spinal cord level.

Anal sensation is carried in the inferior rectal branch of the pudendal nerve and is thought to have a role in maintenance of anal continence. The upper anal canal contains a rich profusion of both free and organized sensory nerve endings, especially in the vicinity of the anal valves.[60] Organized nerve endings include Meissner's corpuscles (touch), Krause's bulbs (cold), Golgi-Mazzoni bodies (pressure), and genital corpuscles (friction).

Anorectal Spaces

The potential spaces of clinical significance in close relation to the anal canal and rectum include: ischiorectal, perianal, intersphincteric, submucosal, superficial postanal, deep postanal, supralevator, and retrorectal spaces (Figure 1-5A and B).

The ischiorectal fossa is subdivided by a thin horizontal fascia into two spaces: the perianal and ischiorectal. The ischiorectal space comprises the upper two-thirds of the ischiorectal fossa. It is pyramid-shaped, situated on both sides between the anal canal and the lower part of the rectum medially, and the side wall of the pelvis laterally.[61] The apex is at the origin of the levator ani muscle from the obturator fascia; the base is the perianal space. Anteriorly, the fossa is bounded by the urogenital diaphragm and transversus perinei muscle. Posterior to the ischiorectal fossa is the sacrotuberous ligament and the inferior border of the gluteus maximus. On the superolateral wall, the pudendal nerve and the internal pudendal vessels run in the pudendal canal (Alcock's canal). The ischiorectal fossa contains fat and the inferior rectal vessels and nerves.

The perianal space surrounds the lower part of the anal canal and contains the external hemorrhoidal plexus, the subcutaneous part of the external anal sphincter, the lowest part of the internal anal sphincter, and fibers of the longitudinal muscle. This space is the typical site of anal hematomas,

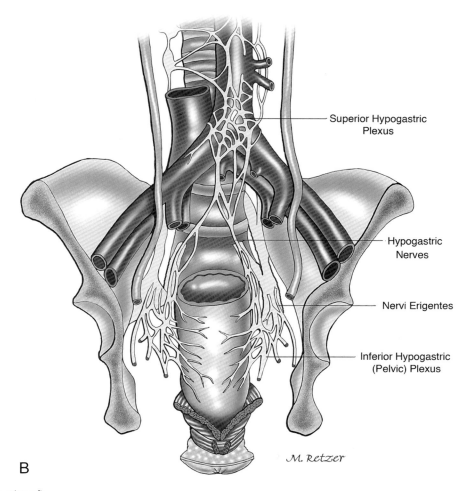

Superior Hypogastric Plexus

Hypogastric Nerves

Nervi Erigentes

Inferior Hypogastric (Pelvic) Plexus

M. Retzer

B

FIGURE 1-4. **A, B** (*Continued*)

perianal abscesses, and anal fistula tracts. The perianal space is continuous with the subcutaneous fat of the buttocks laterally and extends into the intersphincteric space medially. The intersphincteric space is a potential space between the internal and external anal sphincters. It is important in the genesis of perianal abscess, because most of the anal glands end in this space. The submucous space is situated between the internal anal sphincter and the mucocutaneous lining of the anal canal. This space contains the internal hemorrhoidal plexus and the muscularis submucosae ani. Above, it is continuous with the submucous layer of the rectum, and, inferiorly, it ends at the level of the dentate line.

The superficial postanal space is interposed between the anococcygeal ligament and the skin. The deep postanal space, also known as the retro-sphincteric space of Courtney, is situated between the anococcygeal ligament and the anococcygeal raphe. Both postanal spaces communicate posteriorly with the ischiorectal fossa and are the sites of horseshoe abscesses.

The supralevator spaces are situated between the peritoneum superiorly and the levator ani inferiorly. Medially, these bilat-

eral spaces are limited by the rectum, and laterally by the obturator fascia. Supralevator abscesses may occur as a result of upward extension of a cryptoglandular infection or develop from a pelvic origin. The retrorectal space is located between the fascia propria of the rectum anteriorly and the presacral fascia posteriorly. Laterally are the lateral rectal ligaments and inferiorly the rectosacral ligament, and above the space is continuous with the retroperitoneum. The retrorectal space is a site for embryologic remnants and rare presacral tumors.

Pelvic floor musculature

The muscles within the pelvis can be divided into three categories: 1) the anal sphincter complex; 2) pelvic floor muscles; and 3) muscles that line the sidewalls of the osseous pelvis.[61] Muscles in this last category form the external boundary of the pelvis and include the obturator internus and piriform. These muscles, compared with the other two groups, lack clinical relevance to anorectal diseases; however, they provide an open communication for pelvic infection to reach extrapelvic spaces. For example, infection from the deep

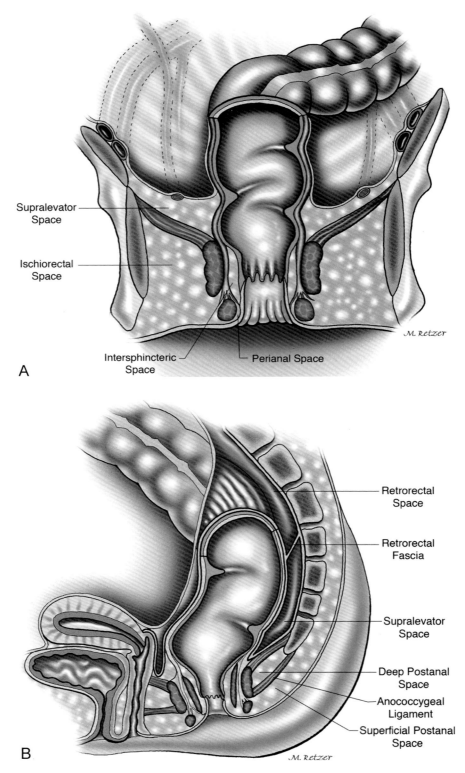

FIGURE 1-5. Para-anal and pararectal spaces. **A** Frontal view. **B** Lateral view.

rom posterior midline glands, can
internus fascia and reach the

elvic floor muscles, based on phy-
om two embryonic cloaca groups,
l lateral compressor.[62] The sphinc-
nost all animals. In mammals, this
tral (urogenital) and dorsal (anal)
, the latter form the external anal
pressor or pelvicaudal group con-
is to the caudal end of the vertebral
e differentiated and subdivided into
tments only in reptiles and mam-
lateral compartment is the ischio-
dial, pelvicaudal compartment, the
ccygeus. In addition, most primates
roup of muscle fibers close to the
pelvicaudal muscle, which attaches
rectum to the pubis. In humans, the fibers are more distinct and known as the puborectalis muscle.

Levator Ani

The levator ani muscle, or pelvic diaphragm, is the major
component of the pelvic floor. It is a pair of broad, symmetric sheets composed of three striated muscles: ileococcygeus, pubococcygeus, and puborectalis (Figure 1-6A and
B). A variable fourth component, the ischiococcygeus or
coccygeus, is rudimentary in humans and represented by
only a few muscle fibers on the surface of the sacrospinous
ligament. The levator ani is supplied by sacral roots on its
pelvic surface (S-2, S-3, and S-4) and by the perineal branch
of the pudendal nerve on its inferior surface. The puborectalis muscle receives additional innervation from the inferior
rectal nerves.

The ileococcygeus muscles arise from the ischial spine and
posterior part of the obturator fascia and course inferiorly and
medially to insert into the lateral aspects of S-3 and S-4, the
coccyx, and the anococcygeal raphe. The pubococcygeus
arises from the posterior aspect of the pubis and the anterior
part of the obturator fascia; it runs dorsally alongside the
anorectal junction to decussate with fibers of the opposite side
at the anococcygeal raphe and insert into the anterior surface
of the fourth sacral and first coccygeal segments.

The pelvic floor is "incomplete" in the midline where the
lower rectum, urethra, and either the dorsal vein of the penis
in men, or the vagina in women, pass through it. This defect
is called the levator hiatus and consists of an elliptic space situated between the two pubococcygeus muscles. The hiatal
ligament, originating from the pelvic fascia, keeps the intrahi-
atal viscera together and prevents their constriction during
contraction of the levator ani. A possible (but controversial)
dilator function has been attributed to the anococcygeal raphe
because of its crisscross arrangement.[14]

The puborectalis muscle is a strong, U-shaped loop of striated muscle that slings the anorectal junction to the posterior
aspect of the pubis (Figure 1-7). The puborectalis is the most
medial portion of the levator ani muscle. It is situated immediately cephalad to the deep component of the external
sphincter. Because the junction between the two muscles is
indistinct and they have similar innervation (pudendal
nerve), the puborectalis has been regarded by some authors
as a part of the external anal sphincter and not of the levator
ani complex.[14,15] Anatomic and phylogenetic studies suggest
that the puborectalis may be a part of the levator ani[63] or
of the external anal sphincter.[24,62] Embryologically, the puborectalis has a common primordium with the ileococcygeus
and pubococcygeus muscles, and it is never connected with
the external anal sphincter during the different stages of
development.[6] In addition, neurophysiologic studies have
implied that the innervation of these muscles may not be the
same, because stimulation of the sacral nerves results in electromyographic activity in the ipsilateral puborectalis muscle
but not in the external anal sphincter.[64] Currently, because of
this controversy, the puborectalis has been considered to
belong to both muscular groups, the external anal sphincter
and the levator ani.[65]

The Anorectal Ring and the Anorectal Angle

Two anatomic structures of the junction of the rectum and
anal canal are related to the puborectalis muscle: the anorectal ring and the anorectal angle. The anorectal ring, a term
coined by Milligan and Morgan,[10] is a strong muscular ring
that represents the upper end of the sphincter, more precisely
the puborectalis, and the upper border of the internal anal
sphincter, around the anorectal junction. Despite its lack of
embryologic significance, it is an easily recognized boundary
of the anal canal appreciated on physical examination, and it
is of clinical relevance, because division of this structure during surgery for abscesses or fistula inevitably results in fecal
incontinence.

The anorectal angle is thought to be the result of the
anatomic configuration of the U-shaped sling of puborectalis
muscle around the anorectal junction. Whereas the anal
sphincters are responsible for closure of the anal canal to
retain gas and liquid stool, the puborectalis muscle and the
anorectal angle are designed to maintain gross fecal continence. Different theories have been postulated to explain the
importance of the puborectalis and the anorectal angle in the
maintenance of fecal continence. Parks et al.[66] opined that
increasing intraabdominal pressure forces the anterior rectal
wall down into the upper anal canal, occluding it by a type of
flap valve mechanism that creates an effective seal.
Subsequently, it has been demonstrated that the flap mechanism does not occur. Instead, a continuous sphincteric occlu-
sion-like activity that is attributed to the puborectalis is
noted.[67,68]

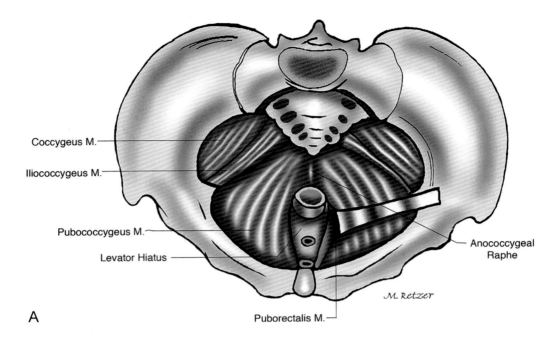

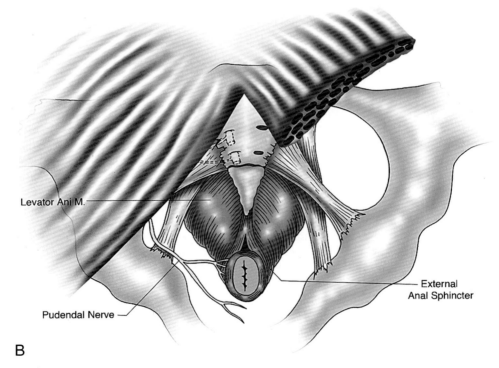

FIGURE 1-6. Levator ani muscle. **A** Superior. **B** Inferior surface.

Colon

General Considerations

The colon is a capacious tube that roughly surrounds the loops of small intestine as an arch. Named from the Greek *koluein* ("to retard"), the colon is variable in length, averaging approximately 150 cm, which corresponds to one-quarter the length of the small intestine. Its diameter can be substantially augmented by distension, it gradually decreases from 7.5 cm at the cecum to 2.5 cm at the sigmoid. In humans, the colon is described to be somewhere between the short, straight type with a rudimentary cecum, such as that of the carnivores, and

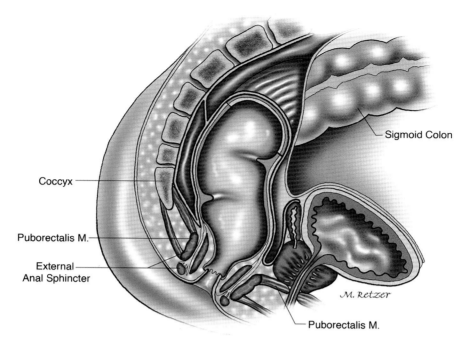

FIGURE 1-7. The anteriorly directed pull of the puborectalis contributes to the angulation between the rectum and anal canal, the anorectal angle.

a long sacculated colon with a capacious cecum, such as that of the herbivores.

Anatomic differences between the small and large intestines include position, caliber, degree of fixation, and, in the colon, the presence of three distinct characteristics: the taeniae coli, the haustra, and the appendices epiploicae. The three taeniae coli, anterior (taenia libera), posteromedial (taenia mesocolica), and posterolateral (taenia omentalis), represent bands of the outer longitudinal coat of muscle that traverse the colon from the base of the appendix to the rectosigmoid junction, where they merge. The muscular longitudinal layer is actually a complete coat around the colon, although it is considerably thicker at the taeniae.[69] The haustra or haustral sacculations are outpouchings of bowel wall between the taeniae; they are caused by the relative shortness of the taeniae, about one-sixth shorter than the length of the bowel wall.[13] The haustra are separated by the plicae semilunares or crescentic folds of the bowel wall, which give the colon its characteristic radiographic appearance when filled with air or barium. The appendices epiploicae are small appendages of fat that protrude from the serosal aspect of the colon.

Cecum

The cecum is the sacculated segment (Latin *caecus*, "blind") of the large bowel that projects downward as a 6- to 8-cm blind pouch below the entrance of the ileum. Usually situated in the right iliac fossa, the cecum is almost entirely, or at least in its lower half, invested with peritoneum. However, its mobility is usually limited by a small mesocecum. The ileum terminates in the posteromedial aspect of the cecum; the angulation between these two structures is maintained by the superior and inferior ileocecal ligaments. These ligaments, along with the mesentery of the appendix, form three pericecal recesses or fossae: superior ileocecal, inferior ileocecal, and retrocecal. Viewed from the cecal lumen, the ileocecal junction is represented by a narrow, transversely situated, slit-like opening known as the ileocecal valve or the valve de Bauhin. At either end, the two prominent semilunar lips of the valve fuse and continue as a single frenulum of mucosa. A circular sphincter, the ileocecal sphincter, originates from a slight thickening of the muscular layer of the terminal ileum. A competent ileocecal valve is related to the critical closed-loop type of colonic obstruction. However, ileocecal competence is not always demonstrated on barium enema studies. Instead of preventing reflux of colonic contents into the ileum, the ileocecal valve regulates ileal emptying. The ileocecal sphincter seems to relax in response to the entrance of food into the stomach.[70] As in the gastroesophageal junction, extrasphincteric factors such as the ileocecal angulation apparently have a role in the prevention of reflux from the colon to the ileum.[71]

Appendix

The vermiform appendix is an elongated diverticulum that arises from the posteromedial aspect of the cecum about 3.0 cm below the ileocecal junction. Its length varies from 2 to 20 cm (mean, 8–10 cm), and it is approximately 5 mm in diameter. The appendix, because of its great mobility, may occupy a variety of positions, possibly at different times in the same individual. It has been estimated that in 85% to 95% of cases, the appendix lies posteromedial on the cecum toward the ileum, but other positions include retrocecal, pelvic, subcecal, pre-ileal and retroileal.[72–74] The confluence of the three taeniae is a useful guide in locating the base of the appendix. The mesoappendix, a triangular fold attached to the posterior leaf of the mesentery of the terminal ileum, usually contains the appendicular vessels close to its free edge.

Ascending Colon

The ascending colon is approximately 15 cm long. It ascends, from the level of the ileocecal junction to the right colic or hepatic flexure, laterally to the psoas muscle and anteriorly to the iliacus, the quadratus lumborum, and the lower pole of the right kidney. The ascending colon is covered with peritoneum anteriorly and on both sides. In addition, fragile adhesions between the right abdominal wall and its anterior aspect, known as Jackson's membrane, may be present. Like the descending colon on its posterior surface, the ascending colon is devoid of peritoneum, which is instead replaced by an areolar tissue (fascia of Toldt) resulting from an embryologic process of fusion or coalescence of the mesentery to the posterior parietal peritoneum. In the lateral peritoneal reflection, this process is represented by the white line of Toldt, which is more evident at the descending-sigmoid junction. This line serves as a guide for the surgeon when the ascending, descending, or sigmoid colon is mobilized. At the visceral surface of the right lobe of the liver and lateral to the gallbladder, the ascending colon turns sharply medially and slightly caudad and ventrally to form the right colic (hepatic) flexure. This flexure is supported by the nephrocolic ligament and lies immediately ventral to the lower part of the right kidney and over the descending duodenum.

Transverse Colon

The transverse colon is approximately 45 cm long, the longest segment of the large bowel. It crosses the abdomen, with an inferior curve immediately caudad to the greater curvature of the stomach. The transverse colon is relatively fixed at each flexure, and, in between, it is suspended by a 10- to 15-cm-wide area which provides variable mobility; the nadir of the transverse colon may reach the hypogastrium. The transverse colon is completely invested with peritoneum, but the greater omentum is fused on its anterosuperior aspect. The left colic or splenic flexure is situated beneath the lower angle of the spleen and firmly attached to the diaphragm by the phrenocolic ligament, which also forms a shelf to support the spleen. Because of the risk for hemorrhage, mobilization of the splenic flexure should be approached with great care, preceded by dissection upward along the descending colon and medially to laterally along the transverse colon toward the splenic flexure. This flexure, when compared with the hepatic flexure, is more acute, higher, and more deeply situated.

Descending Colon

The descending colon courses downward from the splenic flexure to the brim of the true pelvis, a distance of approximately 25 cm.[32] Similarly to the ascending colon, the descending colon is covered by peritoneum only on its anterior and lateral aspects. Posteriorly, it rests directly against the left kidney and the quadratus lumborum and transversus abdominis muscles. However, the descending colon is narrower and more dorsally situated than the ascending colon.

Sigmoid Colon

The sigmoid colon is commonly a 35- to 40-cm-long, mobile, omega-shaped loop completely invested by peritoneum; however, it varies greatly in length and configuration. The mesosigmoid is attached to the pelvic walls in an inverted V shape, resting in a recess known as the intersigmoid fossa. The left ureter lies immediately underneath this fossa and is crossed on its anterior surface by the spermatic, left colic, and sigmoid vessels. Both the anatomy and function of the rectosigmoid junction have been matters of substantial controversy. As early as 1833, it was postulated that the sigmoid could have a role in continence as the fecal reservoir, based on the observation that the rectum is usually emptied and contracted.[74] Since then, a thickening of the circular muscular layer between the rectum and sigmoid has been described and diversely termed the sphincter ani tertius, rectosigmoid sphincter, and pylorus sigmoidorectalis, and it has probably been mistaken for one of the transverse folds of the rectum.[75–79] The rectosigmoid junction has been frequently regarded by surgeons as an indistinct zone, a region comprising the last 5–8 cm of sigmoid and the uppermost 5 cm of the rectum.[32,80] However, others have considered it a clearly defined segment, because it is the narrowest portion of the large intestine; in fact, it is usually characterized endoscopically as a narrow and sharply angulated segment.[81] According to a study in human cadavers, the rectosigmoid junction, macroscopically identified as the point where the taenia libera and the taenia omentalis fuse to form a single anterior taenia and where both haustra and mesocolon terminate, is situated 6–7 cm below the sacral promontory.[5] With microdissection, this segment is characterized by conspicuous strands of longitudinal muscle fibers and the presence of curved interconnecting fibers between the longitudinal and circular muscle layers, resulting in a delicate syncytium of smooth muscle that allows synergistic interplay between the two layers. The rectosigmoid does not fit the anatomic definition of a sphincter as "a band of thickened circular muscle that closes the lumen by contraction and of a longitudinal muscle that dilates it"; however, this segment may be regarded as a functional sphincter because mechanisms of active dilation and passive "kinking" occlusion do exist.[81]

Blood Supply

The superior and inferior mesenteric arteries nourish the entire large intestine, and the limit between the two territories is the junction between the proximal two-thirds and the distal third of the transverse colon. This represents the embryologic division between the midgut and the hindgut. The superior mesenteric artery originates from the aorta behind the superior border of the pancreas at L-1 and supplies the cecum, appendix, ascending colon, and most of the transverse colon. After passing behind the neck of the pancreas and anteromedial to the uncinate process, the superior mesenteric artery crosses the third part of the duodenum and continues downward and to the right along the base of the mesentery. From its left side arises a series of 12–20 jejunal and ileal branches. From its right side arises the colic branches: middle, right, and ileocolic arteries. The ileocolic, the most constant of these vessels, bifurcates into a superior or ascending branch, which communicates with the descending branch of the right colic artery, and an inferior or descending branch, which gives off the anterior cecal, posterior cecal, and appendicular and ileal divisions.[82] The right colic artery may also arise from the ileocolic or middle colic arteries and is absent in 2% to 18% of specimens.[45,82,83] It supplies the ascending colon and hepatic flexure through its ascending and descending branches, both of them joining with neighboring vessels to contribute to the marginal artery. The middle colic artery is the highest of the three colic branches of the superior mesenteric artery, arising close to the inferior border of the pancreas. Its right branch supplies the right transverse colon and hepatic flexure, anastomosing with the ascending branch of the right colic artery. Its left branch supplies the distal half of the transverse colon. Anatomic variations of this artery include absence in 4% to 20% of cases and the presence of an accessory middle colic artery in 10%; the middle colic artery can be the main supply to the splenic flexure in about 33% of cases.[82,84]

The inferior mesenteric artery originates from the left anterior surface of the aorta, 3–4 cm above its bifurcation at the level of L2-3, and runs downward and to the left to enter the pelvis. Within the abdomen, the inferior mesenteric artery branches into the left colic artery and two to six sigmoidal arteries. After crossing the left common iliac artery, it acquires the name superior hemorrhoidal artery (superior rectal artery). The left colic artery, the highest branch of the inferior mesenteric artery, bifurcates into an ascending branch, which runs upward to the splenic flexure to contribute to the arcade of

Riolan, and a descending branch, which supplies most of the descending colon. The sigmoidal arteries form arcades within the sigmoid mesocolon, resembling the small-bowel vasculature, and anastomose with branches of the left colic artery proximally, and with the superior hemorrhoidal artery distally. The marginal artery terminates within the arcade of sigmoidal arteries. The superior hemorrhoidal artery is the continuation of the inferior mesenteric artery, once it crosses the left iliac vessels. The artery descends in the sigmoid mesocolon to the level of S-3 and then to the posterior aspect of the rectum. In 80% of cases, it bifurcates into right and left terminal branches; multiple branches are present in 17%.[45] These divisions, once within the submucosa of the rectum, run straight downward to supply the lower rectum and the anal canal.

The venous drainage of the large intestine basically follows its arterial supply. Blood from the right colon, via the superior mesenteric vein, and from left colon and rectum, via the inferior mesenteric vein, reaches the intrahepatic capillary bed through the portal vein.

Collateral Circulation

The anatomy of the mesenteric circulation is still a matter of controversy, and this may in part be related to the inherent confusion of the use of eponyms. The central anastomotic artery connecting all colonic mesenteric branches, first described by Haller[85] in 1786, later became known as the marginal artery of Drummond, because this author was the first to demonstrate its surgical significance (1913).[86,87] Subsequently, discontinuity of the marginal artery has been shown at the lower ascending colon, and especially at the left colic flexure and the sigmoid colon. This potential hypovascularity is a source of concern during colonic resection. The splenic flexure comprises the watershed between midgut and hindgut supplies (Griffiths' critical point); this anastomosis is of variable magnitude, and it may be absent in about 50% of cases.[88] For this reason, ischemic colitis usually affects or is most severe near the splenic flexure.[89,90] Another potential area of discontinuity of the marginal artery is the Sudeck's critical point, situated between the lowest sigmoid and the superior hemorrhoidal arteries; however, surgical experience and radiological studies have both demonstrated adequate communications between these vessels.[91] There is also a collateral network involving middle hemorrhoidal, internal iliac, and external iliac arteries which could potentially prevent gangrene of the pelvis and even the lower extremities in case of occlusion of the distal aorta.[92,93]

The term arc of Riolan was vaguely defined as the communication between superior and inferior mesenteric arteries in the author's original work. Later, the eponym marginal artery of Drummond confused the subject.[94] In 1964, Moskowitz et al.[95] proposed another term, meandering mesenteric artery, and differentiated it from the marginal artery of Drummond. The meandering mesenteric artery is a thick and tortuous vessel that makes a crucial communication between the middle colic artery and the ascending branch of the left colic artery, especially in advanced atherosclerotic disease.[94] The presence of the meandering mesenteric artery indicates severe stenosis of either the superior mesenteric artery (retrograde flow) or inferior mesenteric artery (antegrade flow).

Lymphatic Drainage

The submucous and subserous layers of the colon and rectum have a rich network of lymphatic plexuses, which drain into an extramural system of lymph channels and follow their vascular supply.[50] Colorectal lymph nodes are classically divided into four groups: epiploic, paracolic, intermediate, and principal.[96] The epiploic group lies on the bowel wall under the peritoneum and in the appendices epiploicae; they are more numerous in the sigmoid and are known in the rectum as the nodules of Gerota. The lymphatic drainage from all parts of the colon follows its vascular supply. The paracolic nodes are situated along the marginal artery and on the arcades; they are considered to have the most numerous filters. The intermediate nodes are situated on the primary colic vessels, and the main or principal nodes on the superior and inferior mesenteric vessels. The lymph then drains to the cisterna chyli via the paraaortic chain of nodes. Colorectal carcinoma staging systems are based on the neoplastic involvement of these various lymph node groups.

Innervation

The sympathetic and parasympathetic components of the autonomic innervation of the large intestine closely follow the blood supply. The sympathetic supply of the right colon originates from the lower six thoracic segments. These thoracic splanchnic nerves reach the celiac, preaortic, and superior mesenteric ganglia, where they synapse. The postganglionic fibers then course along the superior mesenteric artery to the small bowel and right colon. The parasympathetic supply comes from the right (posterior) vagus nerve and celiac plexus. The fibers travel along the superior mesenteric artery, and finally synapse with cells in the autonomic plexuses within the bowel wall. The sympathetic supply of the left colon and rectum arises from L-1, L-2, and L-3. Preganglionic fibers, via lumbar sympathetic nerves, synapse in the preaortic plexus, and the postganglionic fibers follow the branches of the inferior mesenteric artery and superior rectal artery to the left colon and upper rectum.

Embryology

Anus and Rectum

The distal colon, rectum, and the anal canal above the dentate line are all derived from the hindgut. Therefore, this segment is supplied by the hindgut (inferior mesenteric) artery, with corresponding venous and lymphatic drainage. Its parasym-

pathetic outflow comes from S-2, S-3, and S-4 via splanchnic nerves.

The dentate line marks the fusion between endodermal and ectodermal tubes, where the terminal portion of the hindgut or cloaca fuses with the proctodeum, an ingrowth from the anal pit. The cloaca originates at the portion of the rectum below the pubococcygeal line, whereas the hindgut originates above it.

Before the fifth week of development, the intestinal and urogenital tracts terminate in conjunction with the cloaca. During the sixth to eighth weeks of fetal life, the urorectal septum or fold of Tourneux migrates caudally and divides the cloacal closing plate into an anterior urogenital plate and a posterior anal plate (Figure 1-8). Any slight posterior shift in the position of the septum during its descent will reduce the size of the anal opening, giving rise to anorectal defects.

The cloacal part of the anal canal, which has both endodermal and ectodermal elements, forms the anal transitional zone after breakdown of the anal membrane.[73] During the 10th week, the anal tubercles, a pair of ectodermal swellings around the proctodeal pit, fuse dorsally to form a horseshoe-shaped structure and anteriorly to create the perineal body. The cloacal sphincter is separated by the perineal body into urogenital and anal portions (external anal sphincter). The internal anal sphincter is formed later (6th to 12th week) from enlarging fibers of the circular layer of the rectum.[6,97]

In the female, the fused Müllerian ducts that will form the uterus and vagina move downward to reach the urogenital sinus about the sixteenth week. In the male, the site of the urogenital membrane will be obliterated by fusion of the genital folds and the sinus will become incorporated into the urethra. The sphincters apparently migrate during their development; the external sphincter grows cephalad and the internal sphincter moves caudally. Concomitantly, the longitudinal muscle descends into the intersphincteric plane.[6]

Anorectal Malformations

The anorectal malformations can be traced to developmental arrest at various stages of normal maturation. The Duhamel's theory of "syndrome of caudal regression" is supported by the high incidence of spinal, sacral, and lower limb defects associated with these anomalies.[98] In fact, associated anomalies, most frequently skeleton and urinary defects, may occur in up to 70%.[99] Digestive tract, particularly tracheoesophageal fistula or esophageal stenosis, cardiac, and abdominal wall defects may also occur in patients with anorectal anomalies. There is evidence for familial occurrence of anorectal defects; the estimated risk in a family of a second occurrence of some form of imperforate anus is up to 50 times the normal chance.[100]

The proposed classification systems for the congenital malformations of the anorectal region are usually either incomplete or complex. The most comprehensive system has been proposed by Gough[101] and Santulli,[102] and takes into consideration whether the rectum terminates above (anorectal defects) or below (anal defects) the puborectalis sling (Table 1-1).

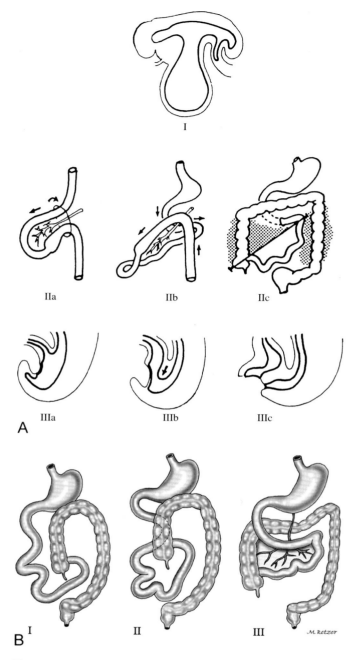

TABLE 1-1. Classification of anorectal malformations

A. Anal defects ("low" defects)
  1. Anal stenosis
  2. Membranous atresia (rare)
  3. Anal agenesis
    a. Without fistula
    b. With fistula (ectopic anus)
B. Anorectal defects ("high" defects)
  1. Anorectal agenesis
    a. Without fistula
    b. With fistula
  2. Rectal atresia ("high" atresia)
C. Persistent cloaca
  1. Rectal duplication
  2. Developmental cysts

Anal Defects

Anal Stenosis

Some degree of stricture of the rectum is present in 25% to 39% of infants, and only about 25% of these will show some degree of disordered evacuation, but spontaneous dilation occurs between 3 and 6 months of age in the vast majority of patients.[103] Although stenosis has been attributed to excessive fusion of the anal tubercles, probably the cause is a posterior shift in the position of the urorectal septum during its descent at the sixth week of fetal life.[101]

Membranous Atresia

This defect, also known as "covered anus" is very rare. It is characterized by presence of a thin membrane of skin between the blind end of the anal canal and the surface. Most cases occur in males and probably represent excessive posterior closure of the urogenital folds.[101]

Anal Agenesis

The rectum extends below the puborectalis and ends, either blindly, or more often, in an ectopic opening or fistula to the perineum anteriorly, to the vulva, or urethra. Regardless of the location of the ectopic orifice, the sphincter is present at the normal site.

Anorectal Defects

Anorectal Agenesis

Anorectal agenesis more often affects males and represents the most common type of "imperforate anus." The rectum ends well above the surface, the anus is represented by a dimple, and the anal sphincter is usually normal. This malformation is the result of excessive obliteration of the embryonic tailgut and the adjacent dorsal portion of the cloaca. The descending urorectal septum reaches the dorsal wall of the diminished cloaca, leaving a blindly ending colon above and an isolated rectal membrane below.

FIGURE 1-8. **A** Embryology of the large intestine. I. Sagittal section of early embryo with the primitive tube at the third week of development. II. Normal development of intestine. IIa: Midgut loop within the umbilical cord (physiologic herniation); IIb: midgut rotation and return to the abdomen; IIc: rotation complete with wide retroperitoneal fixation of small bowel mesentery as well as ascending and descending colon. III. Development of the anus and rectum. IIIa: The hindgut, tailgut, and the allantois form the cloaca; IIIb: at the sixth week, the urogenital septum grows to separate the hindgut posteriorally and the allantois anteriorly; IIIc: the rectum with the persistent anal membrane has been separated from the urogenital structures. **B** Malformations of the digestive systems. I, Nonrotation; II, incomplete rotation; III, reversed rotation.

In most cases, there is a fistula or fibrous remnant connecting the rectal ending to the urethra or vagina. Fistulae represent areas in the septum where the lateral ridges have joined but failed to unite, although the more caudal union is complete. High fistulae, vaginal and urethral, with anorectal agenesis originate as early as the sixth or seventh week, whereas low fistulae (perineal) of anal ectopia originate in the eighth or ninth week of fetal life.

Rectal Atresia or "High Atresia"

Although considered clinically as an anorectal defect, embryologically this is the most caudal type of atresia of the large intestine. The rectum and anal canal are separated from each other by an atretic portion.

Persistent Cloaca

This is a rare condition that occurs only in female infants. It results from the total failure of the urorectal septum to descend, and therefore occurs at a very early stage of development (10-mm stage).

Colon and Small Bowel

The primitive gut tube develops from the endodermal roof of the yolk sac. At first, the primitive intestine is a straight tube suspended in a sagittal plane on a common mesentery. At the beginning of the third week of development, it can be divided into three regions: the foregut in the head fold, the hindgut with its ventral allantoic outgrowth in the smaller tail fold, and, between these two portions, the midgut, which at this stage opens ventrally into the yolk sac (Figure 1-8). The normal embryologic process of rotation of the intestinal tract includes three stages, as outlined below.

First Stage: Physiologic Herniation of the Primitive Digestive Tube

The first stage of rotation begins between the sixth and eighth weeks of intrauterine life, when the primitive intestinal tube elongates on its mesenteric around the superior mesenteric artery and bulges through the umbilical cord as a temporary physiologic herniation. This intraumbilical loop moves, at the eighth week of embryologic development, counterclockwise 90° from the sagittal to the horizontal plane. The anomalies of this stage are rare and include situs inversus, inverted duodenum, and extroversion of the cloaca.

Second Stage: Return of the Midgut to the Abdomen

The second stage of gut rotation occurs at the 10th week of intrauterine life. During this stage, the midgut loop returns to the peritoneal cavity from the umbilical herniation, and simultaneously rotates 180° counterclockwise around the pedicle formed by the mesenteric root. The prearterial segment of the midgut or duodenojejunal loop returns first to the abdomen, as the gut rotates counterclockwise. The duodenum comes to lie behind the superior mesenteric artery. The postarterial segment or cecocolic loop also reduces and comes to lie in front of the superior mesenteric artery. Anomalies of the second stage are relatively more common than the ones originated from the first stage and include nonrotation, malrotation, reversed rotation, internal hernia, and omphalocele.

Third Stage: Fixation of the Midgut

The third stage of gut rotation starts after return of the gut to the peritoneal cavity and ends at birth. The cecum, initially in the upper abdomen, descends, migrating to the right lower quadrant, as counterclockwise rotation continues to 270°. After completion of the sequential rotation of the gastrointestinal tract, in the latter weeks of the first trimester, the process of fixation initiates. Gradually, fusion of parts of the primitive mesentery occurs, with fixation of the duodenum, and the ascending and descending parts of the colon to the posterior abdominal wall in their final position. Anomalies of this stage are common and include mobile cecum, subhepatic or undescended cecum, hyperdescent of the cecum, and persistent colonic mesentery.

The midgut progresses below the major pancreatic papilla to form the small intestine, the ascending colon, and the proximal two-thirds of the transverse colon. This segment is supplied by the midgut (superior mesenteric) artery, with corresponding venous and lymphatic drainage.

The neuroenteric ganglion cells migrate from the neural crest to the upper end of the alimentary tract and then follow vagal fibers caudad. The sympathetic innervation of the midgut and likewise the hindgut originates from T-8 to L-2, via splanchnic nerves and the autonomic abdominopelvic plexuses. The parasympathetic outflow to the midgut is derived from the 10th cranial nerve (vagus) with preganglionic cell bodies in the brain stem.

The distal colon (distal third of the transverse colon), the rectum, and the anal canal above the dentate line are all derived from the hindgut. Therefore, this segment is supplied by the hindgut (inferior mesenteric) artery, with corresponding venous and lymphatic drainage. Its parasympathetic outflow comes from S-2, S-3, and S-4 via splanchnic nerves.

Abnormalities of Rotation

Nonrotation

In this condition, the midgut loop returns to the peritoneal cavity without the process of rotation, and, consequently, the entire small bowel locates on the right side of the abdomen, and the left colon is on the left side. This condition may be entirely asymptomatic and constitute a finding at laparotomies. However, it may complicate with volvulus affecting the entire small bowel. The twist of the entire midgut loop on its pedicle can occur, usually at the level of the duodenojejunal junction and the midtransverse colon, because of the defective fixation of the mesenteric root.

Malrotation

In malrotation, the cecum fails to complete the 360° rotation around the superior mesenteric, and does not complete the migration process. As a result of this failure in the migration process, the malrotated cecum locates in the right upper quadrant and is fixed by lateral bands or adhesions. These bands can overlie the distal part of the duodenum and cause extrinsic compression.

Reversed Rotation

In this condition, the midgut rotates clockwise instead of counterclockwise; consequently, the transverse colon locates posteriorly and the duodenum anteriorly, in relation to the mesenteric artery.

Omphalocele

Omphalocele is the retention of the midgut in the umbilical sac as a result of failure of the gut to return to the peritoneal cavity.

Incomplete Attachment of Cecum and Mesentery

In normal conditions, the cecum is almost entirely, or at least in its lower half, invested with peritoneum. However, its mobility is usually limited by a small mesocecum. In approximately 5% of individuals, the peritoneal covering is absent posteriorly; it then rests directly on the iliacus and psoas major muscles.[32] Alternatively, an abnormally mobile cecum-ascending colon, resulting from an anomaly of fixation, can be found in 10% to 22% of individuals.[104] In this case, a long mesentery is present, and the cecum may assume varied positions. This lack of fixation may predispose to the development of volvulus.

Internal Hernias Around Ligament of Treitz

Both internal hernias and congenital obstructive bands or adhesions are causes of congenital bowel obstruction, and result from an anomaly during the process of fixation. This failure may occur when the fusion of mesothelial layers is incomplete or if it occurs between structures that are abnormally rotated. Retroperitoneal hernias can occur in any intraperitoneal fossae, particularly paraduodenal, paracecal, and intersigmoid. The most common internal hernias resulting from abnormal fixation of the colon are right and left paraduodenal hernias.[103]

Other Congenital Malformations of the Colon and Small Intestine

Proximal Colon Duplications

Duplication of the colon comprises three general groups of congenital abnormalities: mesenteric cysts, diverticula, and long colon duplication.[105]

Mesenteric cysts, similarly to the duplication cysts found at the retroperitoneum and the mediastinum, are lined by intestinal epithelium and a variable amount of smooth muscle. These cysts lie in the mesentery of the colon or behind the rectum, may be separable or inseparable from the bowel wall, and usually present, as the size increases, either as a palpable mass or intestinal obstruction. Diverticula are blind ending pouches of variable lengths and arise either from the mesenteric or the antimesenteric border of the bowel. They may have heterotopic gastric mucosa or pancreatic-type tissue. Long colon duplication or tubular duplication of the colon is the rarest form of duplication. Almost invariably, the two parts lie parallel, sharing a common wall throughout most of their length; frequently it involves the entire colon and rectum. Often, there is an association of pelvic genitourinary anomalies.

Meckel's Diverticulum

Meckel's diverticulum is a remnant of the vitelline or omphalomesenteric duct, arising from the antimesenteric border of the terminal ileum, usually within 50 cm of the ileocecal valve.[73] Associated abnormalities include persistence of a fibrous band connecting the diverticulum to the umbilicus or a patent omphalomesenteric duct, presence of ectopic mucosa or aberrant pancreatic tissue (in more than half of asymptomatic diverticula), and herniation of the diverticulum in an indirect inguinal hernia (Littré's hernia).

In most people, Meckel's diverticulum is asymptomatic, and according to autopsy series, it exists in 1% to 3% of the general population.[106] Surgical complications are more frequent in infants and children and include hemorrhage from ectopic gastric mucosa, intestinal obstruction resulting from associated congenital bands or ileocolic intussusception, diverticulitis, perforation, and umbilical discharge from a patent omphalomesenteric duct.

Atresia of the Colon

Colonic atresia is a rare cause of intestinal obstruction; it represents only 5% of all forms of gastrointestinal atresia. It is probably caused by a vascular accident occurring during intrauterine life.[104] Colonic atresia can be classified in three basic types: 1) incomplete occlusion of the lumen by a membranous diaphragm; 2) proximal end distal colonic segments that end blindly and are joined by a cord-like remnant of the bowel; and 3) complete separation of the proximal anal distal blind segments with absence of a segment of megacolon.[107] Colonic atresia may be variable in length and can occur at any site in the colon, and its association with Hirschsprung's disease has been reported.[104]

Hirschsprung's Disease

Congenital megacolon is one of the most distressing of nonlethal anomalies, and was promptly attached to Hirschsprung's name after his description of autopsies of two infants who died from this condition in 1888.[108] However, it was recognized as early as 1825 in adults, and, in 1829, in infants.[109] This disease results from the absence of ganglion cells in the myenteric plexus of the colon caused by interruption of migration of neuroenteric cells from the neural crest before they reach the rectum. The physiologic obstruction, more insidious than an anatomic atresia, results in proximal dilation and hypertrophy of the colon above. The extent of the aganglionosis is variable. The internal anal sphincter is involved in all cases, and the entire rectum in most cases. The disease is more common in males and its severity is related to the length of the aganglionic segment. Although most patients reach surgery before they are a year old, many are older, and a few reach adulthood.

References

1. Vesalii Bruxellensis Andreae, de Humani corporis fabrica. De Recti intestini musculis. 1st ed. 1543:228.
2. Church JM, Raudkivi PJ, Hill GL. The surgical anatomy of the rectum—a review with particular relevance to the hazards of rectal mobilisation. Int J Colorectal Dis 1987;2:158–166.
3. Shafik A. A concept of the anatomy of the anal sphincter mechanism and the physiology of defecation. Dis Colon Rectum 1987;30:970-982.
4. Klosterhalfen B, Vogel P, Rixen H, Mitterman C. Topography of the inferior rectal artery. A possible cause of chronic, primary anal fissure. Dis Colon Rectum 1989;32:43–52.
5. Stoss F. Investigations of the muscular architecture of the rectosigmoid junction in humans. Dis Colon Rectum 1990;33:378–383.
6. Levi AC, Borghi F, Garavoglia M. Development of the anal canal muscles. Dis Colon Rectum 1991;34:262–266.
7. Lunniss PJ, Phillips RKS. Anatomy and function of the anal longitudinal muscle. Br J Surg 1992;79:882–884.
8. Tjandra JJ, Milsom JW, Stolfi VM, et al. Endoluminal ultrasound defines anatomy of the anal canal and pelvic floor. Dis Colon Rectum 1992;35:465–470.
9. Dobson HD, Pearl RK, Orsay CP, et al. Virtual reality: new method of teaching anorectal and pelvic floor anatomy. Dis Colon Rectum 2003;46:349–352.
10. Milligan ETC, Morgan CN. Surgical anatomy of the anal canal: with special reference to anorectal fistulae. Lancet 1934;2:1150–1156.
11. Goligher JC, Leacock AG, Brossy JJ. The surgical anatomy of the anal canal. Br J Surg 1955;43:51–61.
12. Garavoglia M, Borghi F, Levi AC. Arrangement of the anal striated musculature. Dis Colon Rectum 1993;36:10–15.
13. Nivatvongs S, Gordon PH. Surgical anatomy. In: Gordon PH, Nivatvongs S, eds. Principle and Practice of Surgery for the Colon, Rectum and Anus. St. Louis: Quality Medical Publishing; 1992:3–37.
14. Shafik A. A new concept of the anatomy of the anal sphincter mechanism and the physiology of defecation. II. Anatomy of the levator ani muscle with special reference to puborectalis. Invest Urol 1975;12:175–182.
15. Oh C, Kark AE. Anatomy of the external anal sphincter. Br J Surg 1972;59:717–723.
16. Bollard RC, Gardiner A, Lindow S, Phillips K, Duthie GS. Normal female anal sphincter: difficulties in interpretation explained. Dis Colon Rectum 2002;45:171–175.
17. Fritsch H, Brenner E, Lienemann A, Ludwikowski B. Anal sphincter complex: reinterpreted morphology and its clinical relevance. Dis Colon Rectum 2002;45:188–194.
18. Morren GL, Beets-Tan RGH, van Engelshoven JMA. Anatomy of the anal canal and perianal structures as defined by phased-array magnetic resonance imaging. Br J Surg 2001;88:1506–1512.
19. Williams AB, Bartram CI, Halligan S, Marshall MM, Nicholls RJ, Kmiot WA. Endosonographic anatomy of the normal anal compared with endocoil magnetic resonance imaging. Dis Colon Rectum 2002;45:176–183.
20. Jorge JMN, Habr-Gama A. The value of sphincter asymmetry index in anal incontinence. Int J Colorectal Dis 2000;15:303–310.
21. Swash M. Histopathology of pelvic floor muscles in pelvic floor disorders. In: Henry MM, Swash M, eds. Coloproctology and the Pelvic Floor. London: Butterworth-Heinemann; 1992:173–183.
22. Courtney H. Anatomy of the pelvic diaphragm and anorectal musculature as related to sphincter preservation in anorectal surgery. Am J Surg 1950;79:155–173.
23. Shafik A. A new concept of the anatomy of the anal sphincter mechanism and the physiology of defecation. III. The longitudinal anal muscle: anatomy and role in sphincter mechanism. Invest Urol 1976;13:271–277.
24. Lawson JON. Pelvic anatomy. II. Anal canal and associated sphincters. Ann R Coll Surg Engl 1974;54:288–300.
25. Roux C. Contribution to the knowledge of the anal muscles in man. Arch Mikr Anat 1881;19:721–723.
26. Haas PA, Fox TA. The importance of the perianal connective tissue in the surgical anatomy and function of the anus. Dis Colon Rectum 1977;20:303–313.
27. Gordon PH. Anorectal anatomy and physiology. Gastroenterol Clin North Am 2001;30:1–13.
28. Lilius HG. Investigation of human fetal anal ducts and intramuscular glands and a clinical study of 150 patients. Acta Chir Scand (Suppl) 1968;383:1–88.
29. Chiari H. Über die Nalen Divertik Fel der Rectum-schleimhaut und Ihre Beziehung zu den anal fisteln. Wien Med Press 1878;19:1482.
30. Parks AG. Pathogenesis and treatment of fistula-in-ano. BMJ 1961;1:463–469.
31. Abel AL. The pecten band: pectenosis and pectenectomy. Lancet 1932;1:714–718.
32. Goligher J. Surgery of the Anus, Rectum and Colon. London: Bailliére Tindall; 1984:1–47.
33. Abramson DJ. The valves of Houston in adults. Am J Surg 1978;136:334–336.
34. Cawthorn SJ, Parums DV, Gibbs NM, et al. Extent of mesorectal spread and involvement of lateral resection margin as prognostic factors after surgery for rectal cancer. Lancet 1990;335:1055–1059.
35. Heald RJ, Husband EM, Ryall RD. The mesorectum in rectal cancer surgery—the clue to pelvic recurrence? Br J Surg 1982;69:613–616.
36. Boxall TA, Smart PJG, Griffiths JD. The blood-supply of the distal segment of the rectum in anterior resection. Br J Surg 1963;50:399–404.

37. Nano M, Dal Corso HM, Lanfranco G, Ferronato M, Hornung JP. Contribution to the surgical anatomy of the ligaments of the rectum. Dis Colon Rectum 2000;43:1592–1598.

38. Quirke P, Durdey P, Dixon MF, Williams NS. Local recurrence of rectal adenocarcinoma due to inadequate surgical resection. Histopathological study of lateral tumour spread and surgical excision. Lancet 1986;1:996–998.

39. Jorge JMN, Habr-Gama A, Souza AS Jr, Kiss DR, Nahas P, Pinotti HW. Rectal surgery complicated by massive presacral hemorrhage. Arq Bras Circ Dig 1990;5:92–95.

40. Wang Q, Shi W, Zhao Y, Zhou W, He Z. New concepts in severe presacral hemorrhage during proctectomy. Arch Surg 1985;120:1013–1020.

41. Zama N, Fazio VW, Jagelman DG, Lavery IC, Weakley FL, Church JM. Efficacy of pelvic packing in maintaining hemostasis after rectal excision for cancer. Dis Colon Rectum 1988;31:923–928.

42. Crapp AR, Cuthbertson AM. William Waldeyer and the rectosacral fascia. Surg Gynecol Obstet 1974;138:252–256.

43. Tobin CE, Benjamin JA. Anatomical and surgical restudy of Denonvilliers' fascia. Surg Gynecol Obstet 1945;80: 373–388.

44. Lindsey I, Guy RJ, Warren BF, Mortensen NJ. Anatomy of Denonvilliers' fascia and pelvic nerves, impotence, and implications for the colorectal surgeon. Br J Surg 2000;87: 1288–1299.

45. Michels NA, Siddharth P, Kornblith PL, Park WW. The variant blood supply to the small and large intestines: its importance in regional resections. A new anatomic study based on four hundred dissections with a complete review of the literature. J Int Coll Surg 1963;39:127–170.

46. Ayoub SF. Arterial supply of the human rectum. Acta Anat 1978;100:317–327.

47. Didio LJA, Diaz-Franco C, Schemainda R, Bezerra AJC. Morphology of the middle rectal arteries: a study of 30 cadaveric dissections. Surg Radiol Anat 1986;8:229–236.

48. Bernstein WC. What are hemorrhoids and what is their relationship to the portal venous system? Dis Colon Rectum 1983;26:829–834.

49. Miscusi G, Masoni L, Dell'Anna A, Montori A. Normal lymphatic drainage of the rectum and the anal canal revealed by lymphoscintigraphy. Coloproctology 1987;9:171–174.

50. Block IR, Enquist IF. Studies pertaining to local spread of carcinoma of the rectum in females. Surg Gynecol Obstet 1961;112:41–46.

51. Gerstenberg TC, Nielsen ML, Clausen S, Blaabjerg J, Lindenberg J. Bladder function after abdominoperineal resection of the rectum for anorectal cancer. Am J Surg 1980;91:81–86.

52. Orkin BA. Rectal carcinoma: treatment. In: Beck DE, Wexner SD, eds. Fundamentals of Anorectal Surgery. New York: McGraw-Hill; 1992:260–369.

53. Balslev I, Harling H. Sexual dysfunction following operation for carcinoma of the rectum. Dis Colon Rectum 1983;26:785.

54. Danzi M, Ferulano GP, Abate S, Califano G. Male sexual function after abdominoperineal resection for rectal cancer. Dis Colon Rectum 1983;26:665–668.

55. Weinstein M, Roberts M. Sexual potency following surgery for rectal carcinoma. A follow-up of 44 patients. Ann Surg 1977;185:295–300.

56. Bauer JJ, Gerlent IM, Salky B, Kreel I. Sexual dysfunction following proctectomy for benign disease of the colon and rectum. Ann Surg 1983;197:363–367.

57. Walsh PC, Schlegel PN. Radical pelvic surgery with preservation of sexual function. Ann Surg 1988;208:391–400.

58. Lee ECG, Dowling BL. Perimuscular excision of the rectum for Crohn's disease and ulcerative colitis. A conservative technique. Br J Surg 1972;59:29–32.

59. Metcalf AM, Dozois RR, Kelly KA. Sexual function in women after proctocolectomy. Ann Surg 1986;204:624–627.

60. Duthie HL, Gairns FW. Sensory nerve endings and sensation in the anal region in man. Br J Surg 1960;47:585–595.

61. Kaiser AM, Ortega AE. Anorectal anatomy. Surg Clin North Am 2002;82:1125–1138.

62. Wendell-Smith CP. Studies on the morphology of the pelvic floor [Ph.D. thesis]. University of London; 1967.

63. Paramore RH. The Hunterian lectures on the evolution of the pelvic floor in non-mammalian vertebrates and pronograde mammals. Lancet 1910;1:1393–1399, 1459–1467.

64. Percy JP, Swash M, Neill ME, Parks AG. Electrophysiological study of motor nerve supply of pelvic floor. Lancet 1981;1:16–17.

65. Russell KP. Anatomy of the pelvic floor, rectum and anal canal. In: Smith LE, ed. Practical Guide to Anorectal Testing. New York: Igaku-Shoin Medical Publishers; 1991:744–747.

66. Parks AG, Porter NH, Hardcastle J. The syndrome of the descending perineum. Proc R Soc Med 1966;59:477–482.

67. Bannister JJ, Gibbons C, Read NW. Preservation of faecal continence during rises in intra-abdominal pressure: is there a role for the flap valve? Gut 1987;28:1242–1245.

68. Bartolo DCC, Roe AM, Locke-Edmunds JC, Virjee J, Mortensen NJ. Flap-valve theory of anorectal continence. Br J Surg 1986;73:1012–1014.

69. Fraser ID, Condon RE, Schulte WJ, Decosse JJ, Cowles VE. Longitudinal muscle of muscularis externa in human and non-human primate colon. Arch Surg 1981;116:61–63.

70. Guyton AC, ed. Textbook of Medical Physiology. Philadelphia: WB Saunders; 1986:754–769.

71. Kumar D, Phillips SF. The contribution of external ligamentous attachments to function of the ileocecal junction. Dis Colon Rectum 1987;30:410–416.

72. Wakeley CPG. The position of the vermiform appendix as ascertained by an analysis of 10,000 cases. J Anat 1983;67: 277–283.

73. Skandalakis JE, Gray SW, Ricketts R. The colon and rectum. In: Skandalakis JE, Gray SW, eds. Embryology for Surgeons. The Embryological Basis for the Treatment of Congenital Anomalies. Baltimore: Williams & Wilkins; 1994:242–281.

74. O'Beirne J, ed. New Views of the Process of Defecation and Their Application to the Pathology and Treatment of Diseases of the Stomach, Bowels and Other Organs. Dublin: Hodges and Smith; 1833.

75. Hyrtl J. Handbuch der topographischen Anatomie und ihrer praktisch medicinisch-chirurgischen Anwendungen. II. Band, 4. Aufl. Wien: Braumüller; 1860.

76. Mayo WJ. A study of the rectosigmoid. Surg Gynecol Obstet 1917;25:616–621.

77. Cantlie J. The sigmoid flexure in health and disease. J Trop Med Hyg 1915;18:1–7.

78. Otis WJ. Some observations on the structure of the rectum. J Anat Physiol 1898;32:59–63.

79. Balli R. The sphincters of the colon. Radiology 1939;33: 372–376.

80. Ewing MR. The significance of the level of the peritoneal reflection in the surgery of rectal cancer. Br J Surg 1952;39:495–500.

81. Stelzner F. Die Verschlubsysteme am Magen-Darm-Kanal und ihre chirurgische Bedeutung. Acta Chir Austriaca 1987;19: 565–569.

82. Sonneland J, Anson BJ, Beaton LE. Surgical anatomy of the arterial supply to the colon from the superior mesenteric artery based upon a study of 600 specimens. Surg Gynecol Obstet 1958;106:385–398.

83. Steward JA, Rankin FW. Blood supply of the large intestine. Its surgical considerations. Arch Surg 1933;26:843–891.

84. Griffiths JD. Surgical anatomy of the blood supply of the distal colon. Ann R Coll Surg Engl 1956;19:241–256.

85. Haller A. The large intestine. In: Cullen W, ed. First Lines of Physiology. A reprint of the 1786 edition (Sources of Science 32). New York: Johnson Reprint Corporation; 1966: 139–140.

86. Drummond H. Some points relating to the surgical anatomy of the arterial supply of the large intestine. Proc R Soc Med (Proctology) 1913;7:185–193.

87. Drummond H. The arterial supply of the rectum and pelvic colon. Br J Surg 1914;1:677–685.

88. Meyers CB. Griffiths' point: critical anastomosis at the splenic flexure. Am J Roentgenol 1976;126:77.

89. Landreneau RJ, Fry WJ. The right colon as a target organ of non-occlusive mesenteric ischemia. Arch Surg 1990;125: 591–594.

90. Longo WE, Ballantyne GH, Gursberg RJ. Ischemic colitis: patterns and prognosis. Dis Colon Rectum 1992;35:726–730.

91. Sudeck P. Über die Gefassversorgung des Mastdarmes in Hinsicht auf die Operative Gangran. Munch Med Wochenschr 1907;54:1314.

92. Griffiths JD. Extramural and intramural blood supply of the colon. BMJ 1961;1:322–326.

93. Lindstrom BL. The value of the collateral circulation from the inferior mesenteric artery in obliteration of the lower abdominal aorta. Acta Chir Scand 1950;1:677–685.

94. Fisher DF, Fry WI. Collateral mesenteric circulation. Surg Gynecol Obstet 1987;164:487–492.

95. Moskowitz M, Zimmerman H, Felson H. The meandering mesenteric artery of the colon. AJR 1964;92:1088–1099.

96. Jameson JK, Dobson JF. The lymphatics of the colon. Proc R Soc Med 1909;2:149–172.

97. Nobles VP. The development of the human anal canal. J Anat 1984;138:575.

98. Duhamel B. From the mermaid to anal imperforation: The syndrome of caudal regression. Arch Dis Child 1961;36:152–155.

99. Moore TC, Lawrence EA. Congenital malformations of rectum and anus. II. Associated anomalies encountered in a series of 120 cases. Surg Gynecol Obstet 1952;95:281.

100. Anderson RC, Reed SC. The likelihood of congenital malformations. J Lancet 1954;74:175–179.

101. Gough MH. Congenital abnormalities of the anus and rectum. Arch Dis Child 1961;36:146–151.

102. Santulli TV, Schullinger JN, Amoury RA. Malformations of the anus and rectum. Surg clin North Am 1965;45:1253–1271.

103. Brown SS, Schoen AH. Congenital anorectal stricture. J Pediatr 1950;36:746–750.

104. Romolo JL. Congenital lesions: intussusception and volvulus. In: Zuidema GD, ed. Shackelford's surgery of the alimentary tract. Philadelphia: WB Saunders; 1991:45–51.

105. McPherson AG, Trapnell JE, Airth GR. Duplication of the colon. Br J Surg 1969;56:138.

106. Benson CD. Surgical implications of Meckel's diverticulum. In: Ravitch MM, Welch KJ, Benson CD, et al., eds. Pediatric Surgery. 3rd ed. Chicago: Year Book Medical Publishers; 1979:955.

107. Louw JH. Investigations into the etiology and congenital atresia of the colon. Dis Colon Rectum 1964;7:471.

108. Hirschsprung H. Fälle von angeborener Pylorusstenose beobachtet bei Säulingen. Jahrb Kinderh 1888;27:61–69.

109. Finney JMT. Congenital idiopathic dilatation of the colon. Surg Gynecol Obstet 1908:624–643.

2
Physiology: Colonic

Tracy L. Hull

The human colon is a dynamic organ that performs many functions including absorption of water and electrolytes, salvage of nutrients not absorbed in the small intestine, and transport of luminal contents. It is not an essential organ because life can be sustained after its removal. However, it has a major role in maintaining the health of the human body. Understanding the physiologic principles of its function is essential when treating diseases affecting it—both surgically and medically.

Embryology

To understand the colon, embryology is an important starting point. The midgut begins just distal to the entrance of the bile duct into the duodenum and ends at the junction of the proximal two-thirds of the transverse colon with its distal one-third. Over the entire length, the midgut is supplied by the superior mesenteric artery. The distal third of the transverse colon, the descending colon, the sigmoid, the rectum, and the upper part of the anal canal are derived from the hindgut. The inferior mesenteric artery supplies the hindgut.[1]

The epithelial lining (mucosa) is derived from endodermal tissue. The muscular and peritoneal components are of mesodermal origin surrounding the endoderm.[1] The primitive intestinal loops normally rotate 270 degrees counterclockwise around an axis formed by the superior mesenteric artery. Bowel loops are herniated outside the abdominal cavity. At the end of the third month, the loops return into the abdominal cavity and complete the rotation. The cecum normally rotates down to the right lower quadrant when the process is complete. The appendix begins as a bulge on the cecum at about the sixth week of intrauterine life. As the cecum grows, this bulge lags behind the elongation of the remaining portion of the cecum, forming the appendix.[2]

Innervation

The innervation to the colon comes from two sources—one from outside (extrinsic) and the other inside (intrinsic). The extrinsic component comes from the autonomic nervous system and affects both motor and sensory functions. Parasympathetic fibers reach the proximal colon through the posterior vagal trunk running with the arterial blood supply (along the ileocolic and middle colic branches of the superior mesenteric artery). The distal colon receives parasympathetic fibers from the sacral parasympathetic nerves (S2-4) through the pelvic plexus. These pelvic splanchnic (splanchnic means visceral) nerves give off discrete branches, which run under the peritoneum and into the sigmoid mesocolon toward the left colonic flexure.[3] The parasympathetic nerves are predominantly excitatory for the colon's motor component via the neurotransmitter acetylcholine and tachykinins, such as substance P. The parasympathetic nerves also convey visceral sensory function.[4]

Sympathetic input is inhibitory to colonic peristalsis (excitatory to sphincters and inhibitory to nonsphincteric muscle).[4] The effector cells originate from the thoracic and lumbar sections of the spinal cord. The thoracic splanchnic (visceral nerves) are divided into the greater (T4 to T10), lesser (T9 to T11), and least (T11 to L1). The lumbar input is L2-3.[3,5] As they emerge via anterior spinal nerve roots they merge into paired paravertebral ganglia, which are located along the medial margin of the psoas muscle in the retroperitoneum. The nerve fiber enters these ganglia as a white ramus and does one of the following: 1) travels up or down the trunk to synapse at another level and supply a segment without its own sympathetic input (i.e., above T1 and below L2); 2) synapses in the ganglion and exits as a gray ramus to supply viscera; 3) passes through the ganglion to a "prevertebral" ganglion such as the celiac plexus where it synapses; or 4) synapses in the ganglion and rejoins its own segmental nerve as a gray ramus.[5] Most preganglionic fibers serving the colon pass through to synapse in a prevertebral ganglia (number 3 above).[6] They form a plexus around the superior and inferior mesenteric arteries where there are perivascular ganglia. Here they synapse and follow the arteries which supply the gut.[7] The inhibition in tone to the colon from sympathetic input is believed to be mediated in part from alpha-2 adrenergic receptors.[8] In one study in humans, alpha-2 agonists (clonidine) have been found to reduce colonic tone, whereas the alpha-2 antagonist (yohimbine) increased the tone.[9] Alpha-1 agonist and beta-2 agonist did not affect tone.[9] However, more research is needed. In other studies, beta-1, beta-2, and beta-3 adrenoceptors detected on the human colon were tested in vitro. Agonists relaxed the colon.[10]

The intrinsic innervation is called the enteric nervous system. The enteric nervous system has the unique ability to mediate reflex behavior independent of input from the brain or spinal cord.[11] It does this through an abundance of different types of neurons within the walls of the intestinal tract. It has neuronal plexuses in the myenteric and submucosal/mucosal layers. The myenteric plexus regulates smooth muscle function. The submucosal plexus modulates mucosal ion transport and absorptive functions. There is substantial diversity within the enteric nervous system and all the modulators and transmitters of the central nervous system are found in the enteric nervous system.[11] The amine and peptide neurotransmitters currently believed to be important are acetylcholine, opioids, norepinephrine, serotonin, somatostatin, cholecystokinin, substance P, vasoactive intestinal polypeptide, neuropeptide Y,[4] and nitric oxide.[12] Control of colonic motor function via the enteric nervous system remains poorly understood at this time.

Colonic Function

Salvage, Metabolism, and Storage

Even though the majority of our food undergoes digestion in the stomach and small intestine, the colon still has a major role in digestion. It processes certain starches and proteins, which are resistant to digestion and absorption in the foregut.[13] The large quantity of heterogeneous bacteria in the colon is responsible for fermentation—the process by which these starches and proteins are broken down and energy is produced. There are more than 400 different species of bacteria, the majority of which are anaerobes.[14] The bacteria feed upon mucous, residual proteins, and primarily complex carbohydrates that enter the colon.[15] During fermentation of complex carbohydrates, short-chain fatty acids (SCFAs) are produced. More than 95% of SCFAs are produced and absorbed within the colon.[14,16] The principle ones are acetate, propionate, and butyrate. This process for the most part occurs in the right and proximal transverse colon. Protein residue, which reaches the colon is also fermented by anaerobic bacteria.[17] Proteins are fermented in the left colon. Proteins are broken down into SCFAs, branched chain fatty acids, and ammonia, amines, phenols, and indoles. Part of these metabolites become a nitrogen source for bacterial growth.[17,18] These products are either passed in feces or absorbed. Thus, the colon salvages and actively processes carbohydrates and proteins that reach the cecum. Dietary fat is probably not absorbed to any degree in the colon.[14]

The colonic mucosa is unable to nourish itself from the bloodstream.[19] Therefore, the nutrient requirements are met from the luminal contents. Butyrate (produced in the least amount) is important as the primary energy source for the colonocyte.[13] Butyrate may also have a major role in cell proliferation and differentiation[20,21] as well as being important in absorption of water and salt from the colon. Regarding the other SCFAs produced, propionate combines with the other 3 carbon compounds in the liver for gluconeogenesis. Acetate is the most abundantly produced SCFA. It is used by the liver to synthesize longer-chain fatty acids[13] and as an energy source for muscle.[15]

The proximal colon differs from the distal colon in many functions. Besides being derived from different embryologic origins, the proximal colon is more saccular and the distal more tubular.[22] SCFAs are principally derived in the proximal colon and proteins degraded in the distal colon. When considering storage, the two parts also differ. The proximal colon acts as a reservoir and the distal colonic segments mainly act as a conduit.[23] When confronted with large amounts of fluid, the fluid seems to move quickly into the transverse colon with the solid material catching up later.[24,25] Even after right colon resection, the transverse colon can adapt to store colonic contents nearly as efficiently as the right colon.[26] In addition, the haustral segmentation of the colon facilitates mixing, retention of luminal material, and formation of solid stool.[4]

Transport of Electrolytes

The colon is extremely efficient at conserving sodium and water.[4] Normally the colon is presented 1–2 L of water daily.[15] It efficiently absorbs 90% such that approximately 100–150 mL of fluid is eliminated in the stool. When challenged, it can increase the absorption to 5–6 L daily.[27,28] Therefore, when the ileal flow of fluid and electrolytes exceeds the capacity of the colon, diarrhea will result.

Additionally, the colon is important in the recovery of salts. Under normal conditions, the colon absorbs sodium and chloride and secretes bicarbonate and potassium. Sodium is actively absorbed against a concentration and electrical gradient. This concept is extremely important for the colon's ability to conserve sodium. The average concentration of sodium in the chyme which enters the colon is 130–140 mmol/L. Stool has approximately 40 mmol/L.[17] As long as the luminal sodium content is more than 25 mmol/L, there is a linear relationship between luminal concentration and the amount of sodium absorbed.[29] However, when the luminal concentration of sodium is less than 25 mmol/L, sodium is secreted.

Aldosterone is secreted by the adrenal gland in response to sodium depletion and dehydration. Aldosterone enhances fluid and sodium absorption in the colon. (This is in contrast to angiotensin, which also participates in fluid balance but via the small intestine.)[29,30] SCFAs produced in the colon are the principle anions. They also stimulate sodium absorption.[15]

Chloride is exchanged for bicarbonate, which is secreted into the lumen to neutralize organic acids that are produced.[15] This occurs at the luminal border of the mucosal cells.[17] Potassium movement, overall, is believed to be passive as a result of the active absorption of sodium. There is evidence that active potassium secretion occurs in the distal colon.[31] This secretion combined with potassium in bacteria and colonic mucous in stool may explain the relatively high concentration of potassium, 50–90 mmol/L, in stool.[32,33] Additionally, the colon secretes urea into the lumen. The urea is metabolized to ammonia. The majority is absorbed passively.[17]

Similar to differences in salvage of food components that enter the colon, there exist qualitative differences in several ion transport processes between different segments of colon.[34,35] Absorption of water and salt occurs primarily in the ascending and transverse colon.[17,36] Active transport of sodium creates an osmotic gradient and the water passively follows. Additionally, there is a difference in the functional nature of the mucosal cells. The surface cells in the colon seem to be responsible for absorption whereas the crypt cells are involved with fluid secretion.[30]

Colonic Motility

Methodology for Determining Motility

Even though altered motility is thought to have a major role in some gastrointestinal disorders, it is surprising how little is known about colonic motility. This is because of the difficulty and inaccessibility of the proximal colon for direct study. Interestingly, stool frequency has been shown to correlate poorly with colorectal transit time.[37] Early studies used barium but lacked the ability to give precise measurement of colonic motility.[7]

Marker

Radiopaque markers orally ingested and followed sequentially through the intestinal tract via plain X-rays is one of the first methods used to actually measure transit time.[38] This test is still used frequently to evaluate patients with severe constipation looking for slow transit through the colon. Variations in the protocol exist. Patients stop taking all laxatives 48 hours before the ingestion of the markers. One method calls for a capsule with 24 markers to be ingested and an X-ray obtained on day 5. This reflects the transit time of the entire gut. On day 5, 80% (17) of the markers should be expelled.

With sequential abdominal X-rays, markers can be localized to specific regions of the colon: right, left, and pelvis. One protocol asks patients to take one capsule with 20 markers and abdominal X-rays are taken every other day until all markers are passed. In an effort to decrease radiation exposure, patients ingest 84 markers on three successive days. (Some protocols call for markers to be different shapes on each of the 3 days.) Then one X-ray is obtained on day 4.[39]

Total colonic transit time is 30.7 (SD 3.0) hours for men and 38.3 (SD 2.9) hours for women.[7]

Scintigraphy

Some centers favor colonic scintigraphy to study colonic transit. Patients refrain from taking laxatives or opiates 24 hours before the test. They remain on their normal diet throughout the study. Typically, a capsule coated with pH-sensitive polymer containing ^{111}In-labeled radioisotope is ingested. The coating dissolves in the distal ileum and the radioactive material passes into the colon.[23] Alternately, the patient will ingest the ^{111}In-labeled material with water and serial images will be obtained with the gamma camera at specified hours (this varies but can be as frequent as twice daily or daily).[40] Segmental transit is usually calculated for the right, left, and rectosigmoid regions of the colon. Results are expressed as the percentage of the total amount of isotope ingested in each segment or the geometric center of the isotope mass at any given time point.[40] For clinical use, the total percentage retained compared with normal data seems to be the most convenient reporting system.

Recording Techniques of Colonic Motility

Most techniques that record colonic motility using some form of colonic manometry still remain in the researcher's domain and have not been assimilated into the clinical armamentarium for the caregiver. Difficulty in accessing the colon is the obvious obstacle. However, significant information is being obtained from these types of studies in the research domain. Typically, a flexible catheter is placed into the colon. It is either a solid-state manometry catheter or a water-perfused system. It is argued that the water-perfused system increases the amount of fluid in the colon and may alter results. However, solid-state manometry catheters are fragile, expensive, and sensitive to corrosive damage from colonic irritants.[41] The catheter is placed in the colon using one of several ways: it can be placed via the nasal-oral route and the position confirmed with fluoroscopy. The goal is to position the catheter so right colonic information can be obtained.

Alternately, it can be placed with a colonoscope using two methods. The catheter can be grasped with a biopsy forceps, which has been passed through the port of the colonoscope. It is then pulled along in a piggyback manner with the colonoscope. The scope is advanced via the anus and positioned in the colon usually as far as the transverse colon and then released. The colonoscope is carefully withdrawn in an effort to avoid displacing the catheter. The other method uses a guidewire threaded through a colonoscope. The guidewire remains as the scope is withdrawn. Then the catheter is threaded over the guidewire using fluoroscopic guidance. Initial studies asked patients to prep the entire colon. Because this is not physiologic, unprepped colons are more frequently used today (some still use enemas before colonoscopy). Retained stool can then hamper retrograde placement of the catheter. Minimal air is insufflated via the colonoscope and as much air as possible is aspirated with removal of the colonoscope. Usually, the transverse colon is the most proximal point examined and fluoroscopy may be used to verify the proximal point. Using the direct placement technique, the proximal transverse colon is usually reached in all subjects and the probe remains in place in more than 80% of cases.[41–44]

Frequently, with prolonged data collection, the subject keeps a diary and has some method to mark events on the data (such as eating and passing flatus). In an effort to gain more data regarding colonic tone (which cannot be measured from manometry), a barostat was developed. It uses a compliant bag maintained at a constant pressure in contact with the colonic wall. Changes of volume in the bag reflect tone in the colonic segment, which can be measured.[45,46]

Myoelectrical signals from the colon are studied in the research setting by placing electrodes intraoperatively on the serosal surface of the colon, or intraluminally through scopes. This modality documents electrical signals in the colon, which initiate muscular activity.[47,48]

Peristalsis

Peristalsis is the waves of alternate contraction and relaxation of the muscles of the intestinal tube, which propels contents. Using transit studies, scintigraphy, and especially ambulatory colonic manometry, information has been learned about motor and pressure activity in humans that leads to peristalsis. Unfortunately, it is difficult to precisely define colonic contractions, pressure waves, and electrical events because no standard terminology or definitions exist. There is also no standardized way that the measurements are obtained. It is also difficult to study the colon because of the inaccessibility of the proximal portion. In contrast to the small intestine where contents are quickly propelled forward, the colon needs prolonged observation to be correctly studied.

In an effort to standardize observations, Bassotti and colleagues[49,50] have proposed a classification system, which encompasses previous observations. Contractile events are divided as: 1) segmental contractions that are either single contractions or bursts of contractions, either rhythmic or arrhythmic contractions; 2) propagated contractions—low-amplitude propagated contraction (LAPC) (long spike bursts) and high-amplitude propagated contraction (HAPC) (migrating long spike bursts).[50]

HAPCs have also been referred to in the past as large bowel peristalsis, giant migrating contractions, and migrating long spike bursts.[50] HAPC is thought to be the equivalent of mass movement.[42,51,52] The main function of HAPCs is to move large amounts of colonic contents toward the anus.[49,53] They occur approximately five times daily. More than 95% of HAPCs propagate toward the anus (not retrograde).[50] They usually occur upon awakening, during the day, and after meals.[50] They are usually associated with abdominal sensation and defecatory stimulation (or defecation).[50]

Less is known regarding LAPCs. They occur in all normal volunteers and are strongly related to meals and sleep–wake cycles. They may also be related to the passage of flatus.[54] The mechanism regulating LAPCs and HAPCs remains unknown.

Single segmental contractions also have been referred to as electrical response activity, contractile electrical complex, and short-duration contractions. Bursts of segmental contractions have been referred to as long-duration contractions, continuous electrical response activity, and short spike bursts.[50] The majority of the colonic motility is represented by segmental contractions. This allows slow transit and the opportunity for the luminal contents to maximally come in contact with the mucosal surface.

The colon in humans differs from the small intestines and colons of other mammals in that there is no cyclic motility.[49] Combining what is seen with contrast fluoroscopy with what is known myoelectrically, haustra appear as ring-like segmenting contractions. They are static and partially occluding. With peristalsis, the haustra disappear as concentric waves of contraction spread distally along the now unsegmented colon. This seems to correspond to the descriptions of mass movement when contents in the right colon could be propelled distally into the left colon in seconds.[23]

Cellular Basis for Motility

Cells important for movement in the colon include the circular muscle, longitudinal muscle, and interstitial cells of Cajal (ICC). Electrical activity is associated with mechanical activity. Electrical activity, which generates motility patterns in the human colon, is poorly understood.[55] All electrical activity in the human colon is dependent on stimulation by stretch or chemical mediation. Critical volumes of distention are needed for propulsion. Fiber may augment this degree of stretch.

ICC are the pacemaker cells of the gut that have a central role in regulation of intestinal motility.[56] These are mesenchymal cells, which form a three-dimensional network, placed between and in smooth muscle layers.[57] They are also in close association with elements of the enteric nervous system.[58] They are electrically active and create ion currents for pacemaker function. ICC in the submucosal layer (of the circular smooth muscle) initiate slow waves in the colon. There is also an additional pacemaker in the colon in the septa separating individual circular muscle bundles.[55,57,59] It is difficult to determine the exact role of ICC in spreading the waves, but slow waves appear to spread along the long axis and around the circumference of the colon with the ICC representing a basal pathway.[57,60] Slow waves of circular and longitudinal muscle cells are in phase, which indicates that a link must exist between these layers.[57]

Characteristics of Colonic Motility in Health

Using 24-hour manometry, it has been found that the colon is continually active. There is a well-established circadian rhythm with marked diminution of pressure activity at night.[41,61] Immediately after waking, there is a threefold increase in colonic pressure activity. This may account for bowel patterns in some individuals who move their bowels after awakening in the morning. Colonic pressure activity also increases after meals, which in one study lasted for up to 2 hours after a meal.[41] Propagating pressure waves (probably HAPCs) were seen intermittently throughout the day and especially after meals or after waking. There was also regional differences in pressure activity. During the day, the transverse to descending colon had more pressure activity than the rectosigmoid colon. Even though activity decreased at night, the rectosigmoid region was the most active. Women had less activity in the transverse/descending colon compared with men.[41] One other factor from this study was that even though scintigraphic studies have shown retrograde movement of radiotransducers, this type of wave occurred infrequently and usually after a meal or during the morning waking response.[41]

Stress can influence gut function. One study[62] found that psychological stress induced prolonged propagated contractions without appreciable autonomic response. These contractions propagated across several areas of the colon. The motor activity persisted after the stressor ceased. Physical stress induced simultaneous contractions defined as pressure waves occurring simultaneously in several areas of the colon. The motor activity ceased immediately after the activity stopped. In another study, it was found that acute physical exercise increased LAPCs and HAPCs.[63]

The right colon and transverse colon are major sites of storage of solid stool. Solid residue remains in the right colon for extended periods allowing for mixing.[23] There is also considerable variability among individuals as far as right colon transit.[23] After eating, the proximal colon has an immediate increase in tonic contraction.[22,64] There is also increased tone in the distal colon, but this is less pronounced than the one on the right.[22,64] Therefore, well before the ingested food reaches the colon, there is an increase in colonic motility and tone. This is known as the gastrocolic reflex.[64] The mediator of this response is unknown and neither a stomach nor intact nervous system is required for it to occur.[65] Cholecystokinin (CCK) is a well-known colonic stimulator increasing colonic spike activity in a dose-dependent manner. It has been postulated to be the mediator of this postprandial colonic activity.[17] However, CCK antagonists do not block the gastrocolic response[66] and CCK infusion that maximally stimulates the pancreatic exocrine secretion and gallbladder contraction has no effect on motor function or transit in a prepared colon.[67]

Defecation and Colonic Sensation

The process of defecation seems to involve the entire colon. It has been shown to begin up to an hour before stool elimination—a preexpulsive phase. It is characterized by increased propagating and nonpropagating activity in the entire colon

and is largely unperceived.[68] This early component may result in stool contents being propelled into the distal colon and stimulating distal colonic afferent nerves. However, scintigraphic studies have also shown that the right colon can also be emptied during one episode of defecation. This could be associated with a total colonic propulsive activity that in some manner is associated with defecation.[23,69–71] A second component begins approximately 15 minutes before stool expulsion. Propagating sequences during this time are associated with an increasing sensation of an urge to defecate. Even though several studies have shown that caudally propagating HAPCs occur in close temporal association with defecation,[72,73] not all HAPCs end in defecation and defecation is not always preceded by HAPCs.[49] However, it does appear that usually at least one very high amplitude HAPC occurs with the sensation of the urge to defecate.[68]

Colonic sensation is complicated and poorly understood. The colon has no specialized sensory end organs. There are naked nerve endings within the wall and Pacinian corpuscles in the mesentery. Afferent fibers reach the central nervous system via sympathetic and parasympathetic pathways. Parasympathetic fibers convey nonconscious sensory information to the brainstem.[4,64] Pain from abdominal viscera is almost exclusively conducted through the sympathetic afferents to the spinal cord via the dorsal root ganglia. The afferent neuron can mediate conscious perception of visceral events by synapsing in the dorsal portion of the spinal cord and then exiting back to the viscera, ascending within the spinothalamic or spinoreticular tract toward the thalamus or reticular formation of the brain, or ascending directly to higher sensory centers of the brain.[4]

Modulation of visceral sensation occurs through several methods. The first allows for enteroenteric reflexes that are mediated in the spinal cord to alter smooth muscle tone thereby increasing or decreasing the activation of the nerve endings in the gut or mesentery.[74] Another method involves direct central modulation of pain. This can occur through the descending noradrenergic and serotonergic pathways from the brainstem. These project in the dorsal horn and can modify the actual afferent input.[4] This is the suspected mechanism by which wounded soldiers in the midst of battle will feel no pain.[75] A further method explains "referred pain." To initially understand this phenomena, it is recognized that somatic afferent nerves enter the same dorsal portion of the spinal cord as the visceral nerves. There is a wide overlap over multiple spinal lamina and some changes may occur in the ascending projection of the visceral stimuli. The dorsal horn may function as a "gate" controlling central transmission or changing excitability of the neuron. When the overlap of input appears more recognized by higher central brain forces from somatic input, referred pain may occur. The input is actually occurring in the visceral structure, but is perceived to be from the somatic structure.[4,75] It is of note that when pain is referred it is usually to a structure that developed from the same embryonic dermatome.[75] And lastly, visceral sensation can relay information via collaterals to the reticular formation and thalamus. This can induce changes in affect, appetite, pulse, and blood pressure through autonomic, hypothalamic, and limbic system connections.[4,76]

Disturbances in Colonic Physiology

Physiology of Constipation

Constipation refers to stools that are infrequent or hard to pass (or both). Arbitrary definitions have been used. Individuals with constipation are an incredibly heterogeneous group. Distinct subtypes of constipation occur and require different treatment modalities, but even within these subtypes there can be wide variability in the clinical presentation and pathophysiologic etiology. There may be dietary, pharmacologic, systemic, or local causes. Many people have constipation caused by dietary and lifestyle neglect. Two primary functions of the colon, solidifying chyme into stool and laxation, are interdependent on adequate dietary fiber. Dietary fiber "normalizes" large bowel function.[77,78] Recommendations for adequate fiber intake ranges from 20 to 35 g per day for adults.[79] Fiber is generally soluble or insoluble and seems to improve stool weight by different mechanisms. Oat bran, which is soluble, seems to increase stool weight by providing rapidly fermenting soluble fiber to the proximal colon. This allows for bacterial growth which is sustained until excretion. It seems that the increase in stool mass is from higher bacterial content and increased excretion of lipid and fat.[80] Insoluble fiber such as wheat bran increases stool weight by increasing dietary fiber (undigested plant material) in the stool. Wheat bran also increases fat excretion, but not to the extent of oat bran.[80] Interestingly, fiber intake in the United States is low. One explanation is that to achieve 15 g of fiber intake daily, 11 servings of refined grains and 5 servings of fruit and vegetables are needed for individuals consuming 1500–2000 kcal daily.[77]

Additionally, constipation may be seen more frequently in sedentary people. In fact, abdominal cramps and diarrhea are reported more frequently in runners.[81,82] Acute graded exercise has been shown to actually decrease phasic colonic motor activity. However, after the exercise, there was an increase in the number and amplitude of propagated pressure waves. It is believed that this post-exercise pattern may increase the propagating activity and propel stool.[43]

Idiopathic slow transit constipation involves a measurable delayed movement of material through the colon. These patients are not helped (in fact may be made worse) with increased dietary fiber. They seem to have altered colonic motor response to eating and impaired or decreased HAPCs of the colon.[50,64] This leads to reduced or absent colonic propulsive activity.[83,84] Abnormalities in the neuronal network are suspected and recently a pan-colonic decrease in the ICC has been shown.[56] As with other areas of colonic study, this one also needs much more investigation.

Irritable bowel syndrome (IBS) can manifest with multiple forms. It usually is characterized as altered bowel habits and pain directly related to the altered bowel habits. In one form, constipation can be the predominant feature. This may encompass about 30% of the IBS population and traditionally overwhelmingly affects women. This group of patients can show an overlap with those having slow transit constipation, but may have a normal transit study.[85] Pharmaceutical companies have targeted drugs that affect metabolism of serotonin, which seems to be involved in the regulation of motility, sensitivity, and intestinal secretions. The specific 5-hydroxytryptamine (5-HT)4 receptor is involved in intrinsic sensory reflexes within the gut. Tegaserod is a 5-HT4[86] agonist that has been approved by the Food and Drug Administration (FDA) (July 2002) for treatment of this group of patients.[87] Additionally, cholecystokinin-1 antagonists are in trials for treatment of patients with constipation-predominant IBS.[87]

Obstructed Defecation

Obstructed defecation usually results from abnormalities in pelvic function versus colonic function. Typically this problem is associated with failure of the puborectalis to relax with defecation, rectocele, perineal descent, or other pelvic- and rectal-associated issues. Failure of the rectum to evacuate may lead to marker studies which also show marker collection in the left colon.[88] This may also be associated with colonic total inertia.[89]

A colonic source, which is a variant in obstructed defecation, is a sigmoidocele. Although rare, the sigmoid is seen to migrate into the pelvis with defecation and obstruct evacuation of stool. This form can be relieved and treated with a sigmoid resection, but the clinician should be aware of other pelvic floor abnormalities.

Ogilvie's Syndrome

Ogilvie's syndrome was described initially in 1948. It is also known as acute colonic pseudoobstruction. The pathophysiology is not clearly understood. Based on evidence from pharmacologic studies, it seems that Ogilvie's original hypothesis is as correct as the current facts; namely, there seems to be an imbalance of autonomic innervation to the gut. The parasympathetic nerves, which are responsible for stimulating gut motility, have decreased function or input and the sympathetic nerves, which are inhibitory, increase their input.[90] Because of the law of Laplace, the cecum can be the site of extreme dilatation (it requires the smallest amount of pressure to increase in size and therefore increase the wall tension). Treatment has focused on ruling out a distal obstruction with a Gastrografin enema and if needed colonoscopic decompression. However, pharmacologic treatment with neostigmine has been successful.[91] This drug is a cholinesterase inhibitor that allows more available acetylcholine for neurotransmission in the parasympathetic system (excitatory) to promote contractility.[92]

Irritable Bowel Syndrome

As stated above, IBS is characterized by altered bowel habits associated with pain. Besides the constipation-predominant type described above, there can be a diarrhea-predominant type and a mixed type. The pathophysiology of IBS has received extensive study, but it remains unclear. Abnormal motility, visceral hypersensitivity, inflammation, abnormalities in extrinsic autonomic innervation, abnormal brain–gut interaction, and the role of psychosocial factors have been investigated. If IBS is found in men it tends to be more diarrhea-predominant type. Treatment is based on the nature and severity of symptoms. Education, reassurance, and dietary modification (elimination of foods that aggravate the problem) are the first steps. For those who do not respond, medication is considered. Antispasmodics (anticholinergic) medication is considered for those with pain and bloating that is especially aggravated by meals. Usually, antispasmodics and anticholinergic agents are considered on an as-needed basis. Low-dose tricyclic antidepressants may be considered when the pain is more constant and perhaps disabling.[86]

Considering specific types, no good pharmacologic research is available for the mixed-type IBS patients. However, for the diarrhea prone, 5-HT3 antagonists have been found to be effective. Alosetron was initially FDA approved (March 2000) only to be withdrawn after some patients suffered ischemic colitis and even death.[87] In June 2002, it was reapproved with restrictions that require the prescriber to demonstrate educational understanding regarding the drug. Additional drugs are also undergoing trials.[87]

Implications of Colonic Physiology for the Surgeon

Why is colonic physiology important for the surgeon? Recognizing the innervation and differences in embryologic development may be important in colon resections when considering nerve preservation, blood flow, and resection margins. Colonic motility is poorly understood. However, as knowledge is gained through research, the surgeon will be asked to evaluate and use pharmaceutical products to reduce ileus and treat other conditions.

Resection of all or a portion of the colon can have profound ramifications for the patient. It is the surgeon's responsibility to understand the physiologic possibilities, recognize, and manage the outcome. For instance, this may be important for patients with a new ileostomy who may need counseling regarding fluids and increased salt intake to compensate for the colon, which has been resected.

Disorders or colonic motility are numerous in the human species. Surgeons will be consulted regarding surgical intervention. Knowledge of basic physiology will prepare the surgeon to make decisions regarding which patients are appropriate for medical treatment and the treatments available. Surgical intervention will then be reserved for appropriate patients.

In the colon, many metabolic processes can be influenced by food components. Prebiotics are "non-digestible food ingredients that beneficially affect the host by selectively stimulating the growth and/or activity of one or a limited number of bacteria in the colon, that can improve the host health."[93] The most common area has been stimulation of the growth of lactic acid–producing bacteria. This growth changes the colonic environment and may reduce the ability of carcinogens to form or lead to cancer.[18] Probiotics are "a live microbial feed supplement which beneficially affects the host by improving its intestinal microfloral balance."[94] With increasing resistant bacteria in our hospitals, the World Heath Organization has recommended trying to combat this problem by using microbial interference therapy or nonpathogens to eliminate pathogens.[19] Work is underway with probiotics in this manner in an effort to reduce potentially pathogenic microorganisms. Currently, probiotics may be used in cases of disturbed microbial balance, such as antibiotic-associated diarrhea, to lessen the risk and duration. In the future, pre- and probiotics may become important supplements administered to patients to promote health and prevent complications from illness.

Conclusion

In conclusion, the colon is a mysterious organ. It salvages water and electrolytes, which have passed through the small intestine. It produces SCFAs, which nourish its mucosa and provide substrate for energy. It propels its contents slowly toward the anus, continuously mixing them and exposing them to the luminal surface. Its ultimate task is to store stool until it is socially acceptable to eliminate.

References

1. Langman J. Digestive system. In: Langmen J, ed. Medical Embryology. 4th ed. Baltimore: Williams & Wilkins; 1982: 212–233.
2. Cobb RA, Williamson RCN. Embryology and developmental abnormalities of the large intestine. In: Phillips SF, Pemberton JH, Shorter RG, eds. The Large Intestine: Physiology, Pathophysiology, and Disease. New York: Raven Press; 1991:3–12.
3. Woodburne RT. The abdomen. In: Woodburne RT, ed. Essentials of Human Anatomy. 6th ed. New York: Oxford University Press; 1978:363–464.
4. Camilleri M, Ford MJ. Review article: colonic sensorimotor physiology in health, and its alteration in constipation and diarrhoeal disorders. Aliment Pharmacol Ther 1998;12:287–302.
5. Anderson JE. Grant's Atlas of Anatomy. 7th ed. Baltimore: Williams & Wilkins; 1978.
6. Nivatvongs S, Gordon PH. Surgical anatomy. In: Gordon PH, Nivatvongs S, eds. Principles and Practice of Surgery for the Colon, Rectum, and Anus. St. Louis: Quality Medical Publishing; 1992:3–37.

7. Keighley MRB, Williams NS. Anatomy and physiology investigations. In: Keighley MRB, Williams NS, eds. Surgery of the Anus, Rectum, and Colon. 2nd ed. London: WB Saunders; 1999:1–48.

8. Gillis RA, Dias Souza J, Hicks KA, et al. Inhibitory control of proximal colonic motility by the sympathetic nervous system. Am J Physiol 1987;253:G531–539.

9. Bharucha AE, Camilleri M, Zinsmeister AR, Hanson RB. Adrenergic modulation of human colonic motor and sensory function. Am J Physiol 1997;273:G997–1005.

10. Manara L, Croci T, Aureggi G, et al. Functional assessment of B adrenoceptor subtypes in human colonic circular and longitudinal (taenia coli) smooth muscle. Gut 2000;47:337–342.

11. Tack J, Vanden Berghe P. Neuropeptides and colonic motility: it's all in the little brain. Gastroenterology 2000;119:257–260.

12. Mitolo-Chieppa D, Mansi G, Rinaldi R, et al. Cholinergic stimulation and nonadrenergic, noncholinergic relaxation of human colonic circular muscle in idiopathic chronic constipation. Dig Dis Sci 1998;43:2719–2726.

13. Rombeau JL. Rethinking the human colon: a dynamic metabolic organ. Contemp Surg 2003;59:450–452.

14. Nordgaard I. Colon as a digestive organ: the importance of colonic support for energy absorption as small bowel failure proceeds. Danish Med Bull 1998;45:135–156.

15. Christl SU, Scheppach W. Metabolic consequences of total colectomy. Scan J Gastoenterol 1997;32(suppl 222):20–24.

16. Topping DL, Clifton PM. Short-chain fatty acids and human colonic function: roles of resistant starch and nonstarch polysaccharides. Physiol Rev 2001;81:1031–1064.

17. Schouten WR, Gordon PH. Physiology. In: Gordon PH, Nivatvongs S, eds. Principles and Practice of Surgery for the Colon, Rectum, and Anus. St. Louis: Quality Medical Publishing; 1992:39–79.

18. Priebe MG, Vonk RJ, Sun X, He T, Harmsen HJM, Welling GW. The physiology of colonic metabolism. Possibilities for interventions with pre- and probiotics. Eur J Nutr 2002;41(suppl):1101–1108.

19. Bengmark S. Colonic food: pre- and probiotics. Am J Gastroenterol 2000;95(suppl):S5–S7.

20. Mortensen PB, Clausen MR. Short-chain fatty acids in the human colon: relation to gastrointestinal health and disease. Scand J Gastroenterol 1996;216(suppl):132–148.

21. Litvak DA, Evers BM, Hwang KO, Hellmich MR, Ko TC, Townsend CM Jr. Butyrate-induced differentiation of Caco-2 cells is associated with apoptosis and early induction of p21Waf1/Cip1 and p27Kip1. Surgery 1998;124:161–169.

22. Jouet P, Coffin B, Lemann M, et al. Tonic and phasic motor activity in the proximal and distal colon of healthy humans. Am J Physiol 1998;274:G459–G464.

23. Proano M, Camilleri M, Phillips SF, Brown ML, Thomforde GM. Transit of solids through the human colon: regional quantification in the unprepared bowel. Am J Physiol 1990;258:G856–G862.

24. Hammer J, Phillips SF. Fluid loading of the human colon: effects of segmental transit and stool composition. Gastroenterology 1993;7:543–551.

25. Kamath PS, Phillips SF, O'Connor MK, Brown ML, Zinsmeister AR. Colonic capacitance and transit in man: modulation by luminal contents and drugs. Gut 1990;31:443–449.

26. Fich A, Steadman CJ, Phillips SF, et al. Ileocolic transit does not change after right hemicolectomy. Gastroenterology 1992;103:794–799.

27. Phillips SF, Giller J. The contribution of the colon to electrolyte and water conservation in man. J Lab Clin Med 1973;81:733–746.

28. Debongnie JC, Phillips SF. Capacity of the human colon to absorb fluid. Gastroenterology 1978;74:698–703.

29. Binder HJ, Sandle GI, Rajendran VM. Colonic fluid and electrolyte transport in health and disease. In: Phillips SF, Pemberton JH, Shorter RG, eds. The Large Intestine: Physiology, Pathophysiology, and Disease. New York: Raven Press; 1991:141–168.

30. Cooke HJ. Regulation of colonic transport by the autonomic nervous system. In: Phillips SF, Pemberton JH, Shorter RG, eds. The Large Intestine: Physiology, Pathophysiology, and Disease. New York: Raven Press; 1991:169–179.

31. Hawker PC, Mashiter KE, Turnberg LA. Mechanisms of transport of Na, Cl, and K in the human colon. Gastroenterology 1978;74:1241–1247.

32. Giller J, Phillips SF. Electrolyte absorption and secretion in the human colon. Am J Dig Dis 1972;17:1003–1011.

33. Binder HJ, Sandle GI. Electrolyte absorption and secretion in mammalian colon. In: Johnson LR, ed. Physiology of the Gastrointestinal Tract. 2nd ed. New York: Raven Press; 1987:1398–1418.

34. Sellin JH, DeSoignie R. Ion transport in the human colon in vitro. Gastroenterology 1987;93:441–448.

35. Hubel KA, Renquist KS, Shirazi S. Ion transport in human cecum, transverse colon and sigmoid colon in vitro: baseline and response to electrical stimulation of intrinsic nerves. Gastroenterology 1987;92:501–507.

36. Devroede GJ, Phillips SF, Code CF, Lund JF. Regional differences in rates of insorption of sodium and water from the human large intestine. Can J Physiol Pharmacol 1971;49:1023–1029.

37. Devroede G. Dietary fiber, bowel habits, and colonic function. Am J Clin Nutr 1978;10(suppl 31):157–160.

38. Hinton JM, Lennard-Jones JE, Young AC. A new method for studying gut transit times using radiopaque markers. Gut 1969;10:842–847.

39. Metcalf AM, Phillips SF, Zinsmeister AR, MacCarty RL, Beart RW, Wolff BG. Simplified assessment of segmental colonic transit. Gastroenterology 1987;92:40–47.

40. Scott SM, Knowles CH, Newell M, Garvie N, Williams NS, Lunniss PJ. Scintigraphic assessment of colonic transit in women with slow-transit constipation arising de novo following pelvic surgery or childbirth. Br J Surg 2001;88:405–411.

41. Rao SSC, Sadeghi P, Beaty J, Kavlock R, Ackerson K. Ambulatory 24-h colonic manometry in healthy humans. Am J Physiol Gastrointest Liver Physiol 2001;280:G629–G639.

42. Bassotti G, Gaburri M. Manometric investigation of high-amplitude propagating contractive activity of human colon. Am J Physiol Gastrointest Liver Physiol 1988;255:G660–G664.

43. Rao SSC, Beaty J, Chamberlain M, Lambert P, Gisolfi C. Effects of acute graded exercise on human colonic motility. Am J Physiol Gastrointest Liver Physiol 1999;276:G1221–G1226.

44. Narducci F, Bassotti G, Gaburri M, Morelli A. Twenty-four hour manometric recordings of colonic motor activity in healthy man. Gut 1987;28:17–25.

45. Steadman CJ, Phillips SF, Camilleri M, et al. Variation of muscle tone in the human colon. Gastroenterology 1991;101: 373–381.

46. Steadman CJ, Phillips SF, Camilleri M, et al. Control of muscle tone in the human colon. Gut 1992;33:541–546.

47. Sarna SK, Otterson MF. Myoelectric and contractile activities. In: Schuster MM, ed. Atlas of Gastrointestinal Motility in Health and Disease. Baltimore: Williams & Wilkins; 1993:3–42.

48. Dapoigny M, Trolese J-F, Bommelaer G, et al. Myoelectric spiking activity of right colon, left colon, and rectosigmoid of healthy humans. Dig Dis Sci 1988;33:1007–1012.

49. Bassotti G, Germani U, Morelli A. Human colonic motility: physiological aspects. Int J Colorect Dis 1995;10:173–180.

50. Bassotti G, Iantorno G, Fiorella S, Bustos-Fernandez L, Bilder C. Colonic motility in man: features in normal subjects and in patients with chronic idiopathic constipation. Am J Gastroenterol 1999;94:1760–1770.

51. Crowell MD, Bassotti G, Cheskin LJ, Schuster MM, Whitehead WE. Method for prolonged ambulatory monitoring of high-amplitude propagated contractions from colon. Am J Physiol 1991;261:G263–G268.

52. Bassotti G, Betti C, Fusaro C, Morelli A. Colonic high-amplitude propagated contractions (mass movements): repeated 24-h studies in healthy volunteers. J Gastrointest Motil 1992;4:187–191.

53. Garcia D, Hita G, Mompean B, et al. Colonic motility: electric and manometric description of mass movement. Dis Colon Rectum 1991;34:577–584.

54. Bassotti G, Clementi M, Antonelli E, Peli MA, Tonini M. Low-amplitude propagated contractile waves: a relevant propulsive mechanism of human colon. Digest Liver Dis 2001;33:36040.

55. Rae MG, Fleming N, McGregor DB, Sanders KM, Keef KD. Control of motility patterns. I. The human colonic circular muscle layer by pacemaker activity. J Physiol 1998;510.1:309–320.

56. Lyford GL, He Cl, Soffer E, et al. Pan-colonic decrease in interstitial cells of Cajal in patients with slow transit constipation. Gut 2002;51:496–501.

57. Camborova P, Hubka P, Sulkova I, Hulin I. The pacemaker activity of interstitial cells of Cajal and gastric electrical activity. Physiol Res 2003;52:275–284.

58. Vanderwinden JM. Role of interstitial cells of Cajal and their relationship with the enteric nervous system. Eur J Morphol 1999;37:250–256.

59. Szurszewski JH. Electrical basis for gastrointestinal motility. In: Johnson LR, ed. Physiology of the Gastrointestinal Tract. New York: Raven Press; 1987:1435–1466.

60. Sanders KM, Stevens R, Burke EP, Ward SM. Slow waves actively propagate at submucosal surface of circular layer in canine colon. Am J Physiol 1990;259:G258–G263.

61. Roarty TP, Suratt PM, Hellmann P, McCallum RW. Colonic motor activity in women during sleep. Sleep 1998;21:285–288.

62. Rao SSC, Hatfield RA, Suls JM, Chamberlain MJ. Psychological and physical stress induce differential effects on human colonic motility. Am J Gastroenterol 1998;93:985–990.

63. Cheskin LJ, Crowell MD, Kamal D, et al. The effects of acute exercise on colonic motility. J Gastrointest Motil 1992;4: 173–177.

64. O'Brien MD, Phillips SF. Colonic motility in health and disease. Gastroenterol Clin North Am 1996;25:147–162.

65. Duthie H-L. Colonic response to eating. Gastroenterology 1978;75:527–529.

66. Niederau C, Faber S, Karaus M. Cholecystokinin's role in regulation of colonic motility in health and in irritable bowel syndrome. Gastroenterology 1992;102:1889–1898.

67. O'Brien MD, Camilleri M, Thomforde GM, Wiste JA, Hanson RB, Zinsmeister AR. Effect of cholecystokinin octapeptide and atropine on human colonic motility, tone, and transit. Dig Dis Sci 1997;42:26–33.

68. Bampton PA, Kinning PG, Kennedy ML, Lubowski DZ, deCarle D, Cook IJ. Spatial and temporal organization of pressure patterns throughout the unprepared colon during spontaneous defecation. Am J Gastroenterol 2000;95:1027–1035.

69. Kamm MA, van der Sup JR, Lennard-Jones JE. Colorectal and anal motility during defecation. Lancet 1992;339:820.

70. Karaus M, Sarna SK. Giant migrating contractions during defecation in the dog colon. Gastroenterology 1987;92:925–933.

71. Lubowski DZ, Meagher AP, Smart RC, et al. Scintigraphic assessment of colonic function during defecation. Int J Colorectal Dis 1995;10:91–93.

72. Hardcastle JD, Mann CV. Study of large bowel peristalsis. Gut 1968;9:512–520.

73. Hardcastle JD, Mann CV. Physical factors in the stimulation of colonic peristalsis. Gut 1970;11:41–46.

74. ParkmanHP, Ma RC, Stapelfeldt WH, Szurszewski JH. Direct and indirect mechanosensory pathways from the colon to the inferior mesenteric ganglion. Am J Physiol 1993;265:G499–G505.

75. Ganong WF. Cutaneous, deep, and visceral sensation. In: Ganong WF, ed. Review of Medical Physiology. 10th ed. Los Altos, CA: Lange Medical Publishers; 1981:97–106.

76. Ganong WF. The reticular activating system, sleep, and the electrical activity of the brain. In: Ganong WF, ed. Review of Medical Physiology. 10th ed. Los Altos, CA: Lange Medical Publishers; 1981:144–153.

77. Haack VS, Chesters JG, Vollendorf NW, Story JA, Marlett JA. Increasing amounts of dietary fiber provided by food normalizes physiologic response of the large bowel without altering calcium balance or fecal steroid excretion. Am J Clin Nutr 1998; 68:615–622.

78. Harvey RF, Pamare EW, Heaton KW. Effects of increased dietary fibre on intestinal transit time. Lancet 1973;1:1278–1280.

79. Pilch SM, ed. Physiological Effects and Health Consequences of Dietary Fiber. Bethesda, MD: Life Sciences Research Office, Federation of American Societies for Experimental Biology; 1987.

80. Chen HL, Haack VS, Janecky CW, Vollendorf NW, Marlett JA. Mechanisms by which wheat bran and oat bran increase stool weight in humans. Am J Clin Nutr 1998;68:711–719.

81. Moses FM. Effect of moderate exercise on the gastrointestinal tract. Sports Med 1990;9:159–172.

82. Riddoch C, Trinick T. Prevalence of running-induced gastrointestinal (GI) disturbances in marathon runners. Br J Sports Med 1998;22:71–74.

83. Krevsky B, Maurer AH, Fisher RS. Patterns of colonic transit in chronic idiopathic constipation. Am J Gastroenterol 1989;84: 127–132.

84. Hutchinson R, Notghi A, Harding LK, et al. Scintigraphic measurement of ileocecal transit in irritable bowel syndrome and chronic idiopathic constipation. Gut 1995;36:585–589.

85. Pemberton JH, Rath DM, Ilstrup DM. Evaluation and surgical treatment of severe chronic constipation. Ann Surg 1991;214: 403–411.

86. Drossman DA, Camilleri M, Mayer EA, Whitehead WE. AGA technical review on irritable bowel syndrome. Gastroenterology 2002;123:2108–2131.

87. IBS: a checkered history. www.ims-global.com. IMS Health. Vol. 28. November 2002.

88. Kuijpers HC, Bleijenberg G, deMorree H. The spastic pelvic floor syndrome. Large bowel outlet obstruction caused by pelvic floor dysfunction: a radiological study. Int J Colorectal Dis 1986;1:44–48.

89. Karlbom U, Pahlman L, Nilsson S, Graf W. Relationship between defecographic findings, rectal emptying and colonic transit time in constipated patients. Gut 1995;36:907–912.

90. Carpenter S, Holmstrom B. Ogilvie syndrome. www.emedicine.com. Updated October 23, 2002.

91. Law N-M, Bharucha AE, Undale AS, Zinsmeister AR. Cholinergic stimulation enhances colonic motor activity, transit, and sensation in humans. Am J Physiol Gastrointest Liver Physiol 2001;281:G1228–G1237.

92. Trevisani GT, Hyman NH, Church JM. Neostigmine: safe and effective treatment for acute colonic pseudo-obstruction. Dis Colon Rectum 2000;43:599–603.

93. Gibson GR, Roberfroid MB. Dietary modulation of the human colonic microbiota: introducing the concept of prebiotics. J Nutr 1995;125:1401–1412.

94. Fuller R. Probiotics in man and animals. J Appl Bacteriol 1989;66:365–378.

3
Anal Physiology

Susan M. Parker and John A. Coller

Normal bowel continence is a complex process that involves the coordinated interaction between multiple different neuronal pathways and the pelvic and perineal musculature.[1] The importance of the anatomic relationships of the pelvic floor in maintaining normal continence has been suggested since the 1950s.[2] Yet the complex series of neural and behavioral-mediated interactions, combined with a lack of an ideal study to take all elements into account, makes complete understanding of anorectal anatomy and physiology's role in preserving continence difficult.[3] Complicating this are multiple other factors that have a role in normal regulation such as systemic disease, emotional effects, bowel motility, stool consistency, evacuation efficiency, pelvic floor stability, and sphincter integrity.[4]

Anorectal physiology testing allows evaluation of the patient with pelvic floor complaints using techniques such as manometry, endoanal ultrasound, electrophysiologic studies, and defecography, all of which help to elucidate anorectal structures and function. A physician with an in-depth knowledge of normal and abnormal anorectal physiology can apply the results in a meaningful way to diagnose and direct therapy. This chapter reviews the current knowledge regarding muscular, neurologic, and mechanical factors.

Pelvic Floor Muscles

The pelvic floor consists of a striated muscular sheet through which viscera pass. This striated muscle, the paired levator ani muscles, is actually subdivided into four muscles defined by the area of attachment on the pubic bone. The attachments span from the pubic bone, along the arcus tendineus (a condensation of the obturator fascia), to the ischial spine. The components of the levator ani are therefore named the pubococcygeus, ileococcygeus, and ischiococcygeus. The pubococcygeus is further subdivided to include the puborectalis. Between the urogenital viscera and the anal canal lies the perineal body. The perineal body consists of the superficial and deep transverse perinei muscles and the ventral extension of the external sphincter muscle to a tendinous intersection with the bulbocavernosus muscle.[5]

The fourth sacral nerve innervates the levator ani muscles. Controversy continues regarding the innervation and origin of the puborectalis muscle. Cadaver studies differ from in vivo stimulation studies as to whether the puborectalis muscle receives innervation only from the sacral nerve or also from the pudendal nerve. Comparative anatomy and histologic studies of fiber typing also support the inclusion of the puborectalis muscle with the sphincter complex and not as a pelvic floor muscle. In addition, electromyographic (EMG) studies of the external anal sphincter (EAS) and puborectalis muscle indicate that the muscles function together with cough and strain.[6]

The rectal smooth muscle consists of an outer muscularis mucosa, inner circular muscle, and outer longitudinal layer. The inner circular muscle forms the valves of Houston proximally and distally extends down into the anal canal becoming the internal anal sphincter (IAS). This is not a simple extension of muscle because there are histologic differences between the upper circular muscle and the IAS. For instance, the IAS is thicker than the circular muscle because of an increased number of smaller muscle cells. The outer longitudinal layer surrounds the sigmoid colon coalescing proximally into thicker bands called taenia coli. This same layer continues down to the anorectal junction where it forms the conjoined longitudinal muscle along with fibers from the pubococcygeus muscle. Distally, this muscle lies in the intersphincteric plane and fibers may fan out and cross both the IAS and EAS muscles. In an ultrasound view of the anal canal, the longitudinal muscle is seen as a narrow hyperechoic line in the intersphincteric space. The terminal fibers extend to skin as the corrugation cutaneous ani muscles.

External Anal Sphincter

Anatomic and sonographic studies indicate that the EAS begins development, along with the puborectalis muscle, at 9–10 weeks' gestation. At 28–30 weeks, it is mature and the anal sphincter then consists of three components: the striated puborectalis muscle, the smooth IAS muscle, and the smooth and striated EAS muscle.[7] Further differentiation of the EAS into two or three components is highly debated. In 1715, Cowper described it as a single muscle. Later, Milligan and Morgan promoted the naming of the components as subcutaneous, superficial, and deep. Recently, Dalley[8] made a convincing point that the three components can only be seen in the exceptionally dissected specimen and, in most cases, the muscle is one continuous mass and should be considered as such.

The EAS is innervated bilaterally by the pudendal nerve arising from S2-S4. Motor neurons arise in the dorsomedial and ventromedial divisions of Onuf's nucleus in the ventral horn of the spinal cord. Crossover of the pudendal innervation was first suggested in studies by Wunderlich and Swash[9] on rhesus monkeys. Hamdy and associates[10] evaluated corticoanal stimulation of humans and found variable crossover which was symmetric in some and either right- or left-sided dominant in others. This has been offered as one possible explanation for the inconsistent relationship between unilateral pudendal neuropathy and fecal incontinence.

Internal Anal Sphincter

The IAS is an involuntary, smooth muscle. It is relatively hypoganglionic.[11] There are nerve fibers expected in an autonomic muscle—cholinergic, adrenergic, and nonadrenergic, noncholinergic fibers. It receives sympathetic innervation via the hypogastric and pelvic plexus. Parasympathetic innervation is from S1, S2, and S3 via the pelvic plexus. There is considerable evidence that the sympathetic innervation is excitatory but conflicting information regarding the parasympathetic effect.[11] The IAS contributes 55% to the anal resting pressure. The myogenic activity contributes 10%, and 45% is attributed to the sympathetic innervation. The remainder of the resting tone is from the hemorrhoidal plexus (15%) and the EAS (30%).[12] Spinal anesthesia decreases rectal tone by 50% and the decreased resting tone seen in diabetic patients may be attributable to an autonomic neuropathy.[13] The IAS has slow waves occurring 6–20 times each minute increasing in frequency toward the distal anal canal. Ultraslow waves occur less than 2 times a minute and are not present in all individuals, occurring in approximately 5%–10% of normal individuals. Ultraslow waves are associated with higher resting pressures, hemorrhoids, and anal fissures.[11] Ultrasound examination of the anal canal shows the hypoechoic IAS ending approximately 10 mm proximal to the most distal portion of the hyperechoic EAS.

The puborectalis muscle, EAS, and IAS muscles are easily viewed with endoanal ultrasound. In the hands of an experienced ultrasonographer, the technique is highly sensitive and specific in identifying internal and external sphincter defects.

Sensory

Anal canal sensation to touch, pinprick, heat, and cold are present from the anal verge to 2.5–15 mm above the anal valves. This sensitive area is thought to help discriminate between flatus and stool but local anesthesia does not obliterate that ability. The rectum is only sensitive to distention. Rectal sensation may be attributable to receptors in the rectal wall but also in the pelvic fascia or surrounding muscle. The sensory pathway for rectal distention is the parasympathetic system via the pelvic plexus to S2, S3, and S4. Below 15 cm, rectal distention is perceived as flatus, but above 15 cm, air distention causes a sensation of abdominal discomfort. Anal canal sensation is via the inferior rectal branch of the pudendal nerve that arises from S2, S3, and S4. This is the first branch of the pudendal nerve and along with the second branch, the perineal nerve, arises from the pudendal nerve in the pudendal canal (Alcock's canal). The remainder of the pudendal nerve continues as the dorsal nerve of the penis or clitoris.[14]

Reflexes

There are a great number of reflexes that end with the name "... anal reflex." The reason for this is, in part, that the EAS is readily accessible and represents a convenient end point for recording during electrophysiologic study. Consequently, there are several ways that one can assess the integrity of neurologic connection through or around the spinal chord.[15]

Cutaneous-anal Reflex

The cutaneous-anal reflex was first described by Rossolimo[16] in 1891 as a brief contraction of the anal sphincter in response to pricking or scratching the perianal skin. This is a spinal reflex that requires intact S4 sensory and motor nerve roots. Both afferent and efferent pathways travel within the pudendal nerve.[16] If a cauda equina lesion is present, this reflex will usually be absent. Henry et al.[17] recorded the latency of the anal reflex in 22 incontinent patients as compared with 33 control subjects. The mean latency was 13.0 versus 8.3 ms, respectively. The mean latency was within normal range in only 3 (14%) of the incontinent patients.[17] However, Bartolo et al.[18] have suggested that latency measurement of the cutaneous-anal reflex may be an inadequate means of demonstrating nerve damage in patients with fecal incontinence. From a practical standpoint, this is a sacral reflex that can be interrogated during physical examination by simply scratching the perianal skin with visualization of contraction of the subcutaneous anal sphincter. The response to perianal scratch fatigues rapidly so it is important to test this as the first part of the sphincter examination.

Cough Reflex

Chan et al.,[19] using intercostal, rectus abdominis, and EAS electrodes, studied the latencies in response to voluntary cough and sniff stimulation. When compared with latencies from transcranial magnetic stimulation, it appeared that the EAS response was consistent with a polysynaptic reflex pathway.[19] The visible contraction of the subcutaneous EAS as a consequence to cough and sniff stimulation is a simple nonintrusive validation of the pathways involved in the anal reflex. This response can also be displayed during anal sphincter manometry. Amarenco et al.[20] demonstrated that the greater the intensity of the cough, the greater was the electromyographic response within the anal sphincter. The reflex is preserved in paraplegic patients with lesions above the lumbar spine but it is lost if the trauma involves the lumbar spine or with cauda equine lesions. The mechanism of the cough–anal reflex contributes to the maintenance of urinary and fecal continence during sudden increases in intraabdominal pressure as might also be seen with laughing, shouting, or heavy lifting.

Bulbocavernosus Reflex

The bulbocavernosus reflex was first described by Bors and Blinn[21] in 1959. The bulbocavernosus reflex is the sensation of pelvic floor contraction elicited by squeezing the glans penis or clitoris.[22] The EAS is used as the end point because it is easily accessed either for visual assessment or by concentric needle EMG recording. The bulbocavernosus reflex latency will be prolonged by various disorders affecting the S2-S4 segments of the spinal chord.

Rectoanal Inhibitory Reflex

The rectoanal inhibitory reflex (RAIR) represents the relaxation of the IAS in response to distension of the rectum. This was first described by Gowers[23] in 1877 and documented by Denny-Brown and Robertson[24] in 1935. It is believed that this permits fecal material or flatus to come into contact with specialized sensory receptors in the upper anal canal.[25] This sampling process, the sampling reflex, creates an awareness of the presence of stool and a sense of the nature of the material present. It is believed that this process of IAS relaxation with content sampling is instrumental in the discrimination of gas from stool and the ability to pass them independently.[25] The degree to which IAS relaxation occurs seems to be related to the volume of rectal distension more so in incontinent patients than in constipated or healthy control patients.[26] Lower thresholds for the RAIR have been found to be associated with favorable response to biofeedback therapy in patients with fecal incontinence for formed stool.[27] The amplitude of sphincter inhibition is roughly proportional to the volume extent of rectal distension.

The RAIR is primarily dependent on intrinsic nerve innervation in that it is preserved even after the rectum has been isolated from extrinsic influences, following transaction of

hypogastric nerves and the presence of spinal chord lesions. The inhibition response is in part controlled by nonadrenergic, noncholinergic mediators.[28] The reflex matures quite early in that it is generally present at birth and has been detected in 81% of premature infants older than 26 weeks postmenstrual age.[29] The reflex is destroyed in Hirschsprung's disease when myenteric ganglion are absent. In addition, the reflex is lost after circumferential myotomy and after generous lateral internal sphincterotomy.[30] Saigusa et al.[31] found that at an average of 23 months following closure of ileostomy after ileal pouch anal anastomosis, only 53% of patients maintained a positive RAIR as compared with 96% preoperatively. The incidence of nocturnal soiling was significantly greater: 72% in those who did not have preserved, or recovered RAIR as compared with 40% who had postoperative preserved RAIR.[31]

The RAIR seems to be nearly abolished in the early postoperative period after low anterior resection for cancer. In a study involving 46 patients, O'Riordain et al.[32] found that the RAIR that had been present in 93% of patients preoperatively was only present in 18% 10 days after low anterior resection. However, at 6–12 months, the RAIR was intact in 21% of patients and this increased to 85% after 2 years.[32] Similarly, van Duijvendijk et al.,[25] in a study of 11 patients, found RAIR present in only 36% of patients after undergoing total mesorectal excision for carcinoma at 4 months after operation. However, 81% of patients had a detectible RAIR at 12 months after surgery. The degree to which IAS relaxation occurs appears to be related to the volume of rectal distension more so in incontinent patients than in constipated or healthy control patients.[33]

Loss of RAIR is often a consequence of restorative proctocolectomy. Saigusa et al.[31] found that the RAIR was present in only 53% of double-stapled ileal pouch anal anastomosis patients at a mean of 23 months after closure of the ileostomy. Preservation of the RAIR correlated with less nocturnal soiling.

The RAIR in children can be elicited even when general anesthetic agents or neuromuscular blockers are used. Glycopyrrolate, an anticholinergic, seems to inhibit RAIR.[34]

Disturbances in the RAIR seem to be involved in the incontinence that is associated with systemic sclerosis. Heyt et al.[35] found that 25 of 35 patients (71.4%) with systemic sclerosis demonstrated an impaired or absent RAIR compared with none of 45 controls. Impaired RAIR was closely correlated with fecal incontinence in that 11 of 13 (84%) of incontinent systemic sclerosis patients exhibited an impaired RAIR.

Rectoanal Excitatory Reflex

The rectoanal excitatory reflex (RAER), or inflation reflex, is the contraction of the EAS in response to rectal distension. Rectal distension sensation is likely transmitted along the S2, S3, and S4 parasympathetic fibers through the pelvic splanchnic nerves.[36] However, on the motor side, a pudendal nerve block abolishes the excitatory reflex suggesting that pudendal neuropathy may interfere with the RAER. Common methodologies for assessing the integrity of the pudendal nerve involve both single fiber density (SFD) of the EAS and pudendal nerve terminal motor latency (PNTML). However, derangement of the distal RAER was shown by Sangwan et al.[37] to compare favorably with these more traditional and discomforting methodologies as an indicator of neuropathic injury to the EAS. It would seem that patients that have both an abnormal PNTML and an abnormal distal RAER do not require further study with SFD.

Mechanical Factors of Continence and Defecation

Anorectal Angle and Flap Valve

As a part of the pelvic floor musculature, the puborectalis arises from the pubic bone and passes horizontally and posteriorly around the rectum as the most medial portion of the levator ani muscle. This forms a U-shaped sling around the rectum near its anatomic junction with the anus, pulling the rectum anteriorly, and giving rise to the so-called anorectal angle. There are differences of opinion as to whether the puborectalis and anorectal angle are truly important in maintaining continence. Unlike the fine control of the external and internal sphincter muscles, the puborectalis sling is believed to be more involved with gross fecal continence.[38] Parks[39] postulated a mechanism by which this takes place. As intra-abdominal pressure is increased—such as with sneezing, coughing, or straining—and the force is transmitted across the anterior wall of the rectum at the anorectal angle. The underlying mucosa is opposed against the upper anal canal, creating a flap-valve mechanism that prevents stool from passing to the lower anal canal and preserving continence. Yet other authors have disputed this flap-valve mechanism and downplayed the role and reliability of measuring the anorectal angle. Bannister et al.,[1] in a study of 29 patients including 14 patients with incontinence, found no evidence of a flap valve in the normal subjects by using manometric measurements during increasing intraabdominal pressures. However, in the incontinent patients, the manometric pressures were consistent with a flap valve. Yet, subjects still had leakage of stool, questioning the contribution to overall continence. Bartolo and colleagues[18] also used manometric and EMG measurements in 13 subjects both at rest and during Valsalva, demonstrating a similar increase in rectal and sphincter pressures and puborectalis EMG recordings. Yet, with concomitant barium studies, the anterior rectal wall separated from the mucosa, allowing contrast to fill the rectum. The authors proposed that the puborectalis functions more like a sphincter rather than contributing to the flap-valve mechanism.

Furthermore, quantifying the anorectal angle and relating that to patient symptoms has resulted in mixed views. Jorgensen and colleagues[40] noted significant interobserver variation in anorectal angle measurements among three interpreters but good intraobserver consistency, suggesting that variation in anorectal angle measurements may be attributable to subjective interpretation of the rectal axis along the curved rectal wall. The authors of another study, assessing the reproducibility of anorectal angle measurement in 43 defecating proctograms, found significant intra- and interobserver variations, and concluded that the anorectal angle is an inaccurate measurement. Jorge and associates[41] measured the anorectal angle during rest, squeeze, and push in 104 consecutive patients and also found highly significant differences in each measurement category.

Reservoir

As an additional part of the continence mechanism, the rectum must be able to function as a temporary storage site for liquid and solid stool. With passage of the fecal stream into the rectum, the pliable rectal walls are able to distend and delay the defecation sequence until an appropriate time. This process relies both on rectal innervation to sense and tolerate the increasing volume of stool (capacity), as well as maintain a relatively low and constant pressure with increases in volume (compliance). Extremes of either of these components can lead to fecal incontinence through decreased accommodation or overflow states. Although decreased compliance has been demonstrated more often in patients with fecal incontinence, it has also been shown to occur as a normal consequence of aging.[42] In addition, Bharucha and associates,[43] in a study of 52 women with fecal incontinence, demonstrated that the rectal capacity was reduced in 25% of women, and these lower volume and pressure thresholds were significantly associated with rectal hypersensitivity and urge fecal incontinence. Furthermore, after low anterior resection for cancer, those patients with resultant lower rectal compliance and lower rectal volume tolerability (capacity) have been associated with higher rates of fecal incontinence.[44]

Normal Defecation

The awareness of the need to defecate occurs in the superior frontal gyrus and anterior cingulate gyrus. The process begins with movement of gas, liquid, or solid contents into the rectum. Distention of the rectum leads to stimulation of pressure receptors located on the puborectalis muscle and in the pelvic floor muscles, which in turn stimulate the RAIR. The IAS relaxes allowing sampling of contents. If defecation is to be deferred, voluntary contraction of the EAS and levator ani muscles occurs and the rectum accommodates with relaxation after an initial increase in pressure. When the anal canal is deemed to have solid contents and a decision to defecate is made, the glottis closes, pelvic floor muscles contract, and diaphragm and abdominal wall muscles contract, all increasing abdominal pressure. The puborectalis muscle relaxes, resulting in straightening of the anorectal angle, and the pelvic floor descends slightly. The EAS relaxes and anal canal contents are evacuated. Upon normal complete evacuation, the pelvic floor rises and sphincters contract once more in a "closing reflex."

Pathologic Conditions

Incontinence

Incontinence is the inability to defer the passage of gas, liquid, or solid stool until a desired time. Numerous alterations in anorectal physiology can lead to incontinence and many patients have more than one deficit. Structural defects in the IAS or EAS muscles occur because of obstetric injury, trauma, or anorectal surgery. The keyhole deformity is a groove in the anal canal allowing the seepage of stool or mucus. Originally described as a complication after the posterior midline fissurectomy or fistulotomy, it can also occur with lateral IAS defects. Intact sphincter muscles with impaired neurologic function, because of pudendal nerve damage or systemic disorders such as diabetes, can also result in incontinence, especially if the impaired sphincter is further stressed by diarrhea or irritable bowel syndrome.

Abnormal rectal sensation can lead to incontinence in two ways. Conditions such as proctitis caused by inflammation or radiation can result in hyperacute sensation. The rectum fails to accommodate and the reservoir function is impaired leading to urgency and frequency stooling. Fragmentation of stools is often described by patients after low anterior resection, particularly if the pelvis has been radiated as in the case of adjuvant therapy for the treatment of rectal cancer. In the case of blunted sensation, because of a large rectocele, megarectum, or neurogenic disorders, the rectum becomes overdistended and overflow incontinence occurs.

The majority of patients with rectal prolapse are incontinent. Chronic stretching of the anal sphincters from full-thickness prolapse leads to a patulous anus through which gas and liquid stool easily leak. A reflex relaxation of the IAS may also occur as the rectal wall descends toward the anal canal. Patients with mucosal prolapse may have seepage of mucus or small amounts of liquid stool. Correction of the prolapse can resolve the incontinence if anal sphincter tone sufficiently returns. Age and duration of prolapse can affect this.

Obstructed Defecation

Suspected Enterocele or Rectocele (Obstructed Defecation)

Patients with symptoms of enterocele or rectocele describe prolonged straining at defecation, with a sensation of partial or complete blockage (frequently a "closed trap door" preventing passage of stool). Defecography can demonstrate the presence of a rectocele or enterocele, suggest the presence of a peritoneocele, and clarify contributing disorders such as a nonrelaxing pelvic floor, rectal intussusception or prolapse, and potentially uterovaginal prolapse.

Rectocele

A rectocele is defined as greater than 2 cm of rectal wall outpouching or bowing while straining, and can precede or accompany rectal intussusception. The rectocele can prevent passage of stool both by obstructing the anal orifice and by acting as a diverticulum to sequester stool. Patients with rectoceles often complain of the need for frequent sequential episodes of defecation, and even for manual compression or splinting of the anterior perineum or posterior vagina in order to completely evacuate. Additionally, patients may experience incontinence with relaxation, leading to reduction of the rectocele and return of the sequestered stool to the lower rectum.

Van Dam and associates[45] investigated the utility of defecography in predicting the outcome of rectocele repair. Rectocele size, barium trapping, intussusception, evacuation, and perineal descent were measured during defecography examinations of 74 consecutive patients with symptomatic rectoceles. The patients then underwent a transanal/transvaginal repair, followed by 6-month-postoperative defecography and reassessment of the five most common presenting symptoms (excessive straining, incomplete evacuation, manual assistance required, sense of fullness, bowel movement less than three times per week). No postoperative defecograms demonstrated a persistent or recurrent rectocele; however, one-third of patients had a poor result based on persistent symptoms. There was no association between defecography measurements and outcome of the repair. Still, the authors concluded that defecography serves three major purposes in the evaluation of a rectocele: preoperative evidence of its presence and size, documentation of additional pelvic floor abnormalities, and an objective assessment of postoperative changes.

An abnormal increase in perineal descent (typically greater than 2 cm) has been described among both incontinent patients and continent patients who strain during defecation.[31,32] These conflicting data underscore the poorly understood relationship between neuropathic pelvic floor damage and symptomatology.

Bartolo and associates[46] evaluated patients with perineal descent using manometric, radiographic, and neurophysiologic studies. When comparing 32 patients with incontinence and increased perineal descent with 21 patients with obstructed defecation and increased perineal descent, the authors found no significant difference in the extent of perineal descent or neuropathic damage to the EAS. Patients who were incontinent had lower manometric pressures (both resting and squeeze pressures) whereas those with obstructed defecation had normal manometric pressures. In a separate study, these authors also found that incontinent patients with increased perineal descent had severe denervation of both the puborectalis and the external sphincter compared with continent patients with increased perineal descent, who had partial denervation of the external sphincter only.[46] Miller and colleagues[47] evaluated sensation in two similar patient groups. Patients who were frankly incontinent actually had less perineal descent than continent patients with descent, but had severely impaired anal sensation.

Berkelmans et al.[48] tried to determine whether women with increased perineal descent and straining at stool were at risk for future development of incontinence. The authors identified 46 women with perineal descent who strained during defecation but were continent. Twenty-four of the 46 were followed after 5 years and 13 of these (54%) had developed fecal incontinence, compared with 3 of 20 (15%) control patients. During their initial evaluation, the patients who previously strained and later developed incontinence had significantly greater perineal descent at rest and less elevation of the pelvic floor during maximal sphincter contraction than the women who strained but did not develop incontinence.

Thus, perineal descent may be a predictor of incontinence among patients with denervation of both the external sphincter and the puborectalis, and in patients with impaired anal sensation. Among patients with constipation, perineal descent and straining at stool may predict future fecal incontinence.

Dyskinetic Puborectalis

Dyskinetic puborectalis, paradoxical puborectalis, nonrelaxing puborectalis, and anismus are terms that describe the absence of normal relaxation of pelvic floor muscles during defecation, resulting in rectal outlet obstruction.[49] Once diagnosed, dyskinetic puborectalis is usually treated with biofeedback and bowel management. Patients who fail conservative treatment have been offered botulism toxin injections into the puborectalis muscle with limited success.[50]

Continence

The dynamic intention of all the aforementioned anatomy and physiology ensures continence. It does not follow that a deficit in any one area ensures incontinence. Continence achieved in patients with an ileoanal pouch is proof the rectum is not essential. An intact and functional puborectalis muscle can provide continence in the patient with pediatric imperforate anus, but incontinence can ensue during adulthood. Even profound deficits do not necessarily lead to incontinence if stool consistency is solid, whereas minor deficits can easily lead to incontinence and gas. To determine and treat abnormal fecal incontinence requires a systematic approach focusing on identifying the specific deficits present, applying appropriate testing to elucidate anal physiology and anatomy, and then directing therapy accordingly.

References

1. Bannister JJ, Gibbons C, Read NW. Preservation of faecal continence during rises in intra-abdominal pressure: is there a role for the flap-valve? Gut 1987;28:1242–1244.
2. Berglas B, Rubin IC. Study of the supportive structures of the uterus by levator myography. Surg Gynecol Obstet 1953;97: 677–692.
3. Cherry DA, Rothenberger DA. Pelvic floor physiology. Surg Clin North Am 1988;68(6):1217–1230.
4. Mavrantonis C, Wexner SD. A clinical approach to fecal incontinence. J Clin Gastroenterol 1998;27(2):108–121.
5. Woodburne RT. Essentials of Human Anatomy. New York: Oxford University Press; 1994.
6. Henry MM, Swash M, eds. Coloproctology and the Pelvic Floor. Oxford: Butterworth-Heinemann; 1992:3–249.
7. Bourdelat D, Muller F, Droulle P, Barbet JP. Anatomical and Sonographical studies of the development of fecal continence and sphincter development in human fetuses. Eur J Pediatr Surg 2001;11:124–130.
8. Dalley AF. The riddle of the sphincters. The morphophysiology of the anorectal mechanism reviewed. Am Surg 1987;53:298–306.
9. Wunderlich M, Swash M. The overlapping innervation of the two sides of the external anal sphincter by the pudendal nerves. J Neurol Sci 1983;59:97–109.
10. Hamdy S, Enck P, Aziz Q, Uengoergil S, Hobson A, Thompson DG. Laterality effects of human pudendal nerve stimulation on corticoanal pathways: evidence for functional asymmetry. Gut 1999;45(1):58–63.
11. Penninckx F, Lestar B, Kerremans R. The internal anal sphincter: mechanisms of control and its roles in maintaining anal continence. Clin Gastroenterol 1992;6:193–213.
12. Lestar B, Penninckx F, Kerremans R. The composition of anal basal pressure: an in vivo and in vitro study in man. Int J Colorectal Dis 1989;4:118–122.
13. Sangwan Y, Solla J. Internal anal sphincter: advances and insights. Dis Colon Rectum 1998;41:1297–1311.
14. Marcio J, Jorge N, Wexner S. Anatomy and physiology of the rectum and anus. Eur J Surg 1997;163:723–731.
15. Uher E, Swash M. Sacral reflexes: physiology and clinical application. Dis Colon Rectum 1998;41:1165–1177.
16. Rossolimo G. Der Analreflex, seine physiologie und pathologie. Neurologisches Centralblatt 1891;4:257–259.
17. Henry MM, Parks AG, Swash M. The anal reflex in idiopathic faecal incontinence: an electrophysiological study. Br J Surg 1980;67:781–783.
18. Bartolo DC, Jarratt JA, Read NW. The cutaneo-anal reflex: a useful index of neuropathy? Br J Surg 1983;70(11): 660–663.
19. Chan CL, Ponsford S, Swash M. The anal reflex elicited by cough and sniff: validation of a neglected clinical sign. J Neurol Neurosurg Psychiatry 2004;75(10):1449–1451.
20. Amarenco G, Ismael SS, Lagauche D, et al. Cough anal reflex: strict relationship between intravesical pressure and pelvic floor muscle electromyographic activity during cough. Urodynamic and electrophysiological study. J Urol 2005;173(1):149–152.
21. Bors E, Blinn K. Bulbocavernosus reflex. J Urol 1959;82: 128–130.
22. Podnar S. Electrodiagnosis of the anorectum: a review of techniques and clinical applications. Tech Coloproctol 2003;7: 71–76.
23. Gowers WR. The automatic action of the sphincter ani. Proc R Soc Lond (Biol) 1877;26:77–84.
24. Denny-Brown D, Robertson EG. An investigation of the nervous control of defecation. Brain 1935;58:256–310.
25. van Duijvendijk P, Slors F, Taat CW, Heisterkamp SH, Obertop H, Boeckxstaens GEE. A prospective evaluation of anorectal

function after total mesorectal excision in patients with a rectal carcinoma. Surgery 2003;133:56–65.

26. Duthie HL, Bennett RC. The relation of sensation in the anal canal to the functional anal sphincter: a possible factor in anal continence. Gut 1963;4:179–182.

27. Chiarioni G, Bassotti G, Stanganini S, Vantini I, Whitehead WE. Sensory retraining is key to biofeedback therapy for formed stool fecal incontinence. Am J Gastroenterol 2002;97(1):109–117.

28. Tomita R, Tanjoh K, Fujisaki S, Fukuzawa M. The role of nitric oxide (NO) in the human internal anal sphincter. J Gastroenterol 2001;36(6):386–391.

29. de Lorijn F, Omari TI, Kok JH, Taminiau AJM, Benninga MA. Maturation of the rectoanal inhibitory reflex in very premature infants. J Pediatr 2003;143:630–633.

30. Lubowski DZ, Nichols RJ, Swash M, Jordan MY. Neural control of internal anal sphincter function. Br J Surg 1987;74:668–670.

31. Saigusa N, Belin BM, Choi HJ, et al. Recovery of the rectoanal inhibitory reflex after restorative proctocolectomy: does it correlate with nocturnal continence? Dis Colon Rectum 2003;46(2):168–172.

32. O'Riordain MG, Molloy RG, Gillen P, Horgan A, Kirwan WO. Rectoanal inhibitory reflex following low stapled anterior resection of the rectum. Dis Colon Rectum 1992;35(9):874–878.

33. Kaur G, Gardiner A, Duthie GS. Rectoanal reflex parameters in incontinence and constipation. Dis Colon Rectum 2002;45(7):928–933.

34. Pfefferkorn MD, Croffie JM, Corkiins MR, Gupta SK, Fitzgerald JF. Impact of sedation and anesthesia on the rectoanal inhibitory reflex in children. J Pediatr Gastroenterol Nutr 2004;38(3):324–327.

35. Heyt GJ, Oh MK, Alemzadeh N, et al. Impaired rectoanal inhibitory response in scleroderma (systemic sclerosis): an association with fecal incontinence. Dig Dis Sci 2004;49(6):1040–1045.

36. Rao SSC. Pathophysiology of adult fecal incontinence. Gastroenterology 2004;126:S14–S22.

37. Sangwan YP, Coller JA, Barrett RC, Murray JJ, Roberts PL, Schoetz DJ Jr. Prospective comparative study of abnormal distal rectoanal excitatory reflex, pudendal nerve terminal motor latency, and single fiber density as markers of pudendal neuropathy. Dis Colon Rectum 1996;39:794–798.

38. Beck DE, Wexner SD. Fundamentals of Anorectal Surgery. 2nd ed. Philadelphia: WB Saunders; 1998:19–20.

39. Parks AG. Anorectal incontinence. Proc R Soc Med 1975;68:681–690.

40. Jorgensen J, Stein P, King DW, Lubowski DZ. The anorectal angle is not a reliable parameter on defaecating proctography. Aust N Z J Surg 1993;63(2):105–108.

41. Jorge JM, Wexner SD, Marchetti F, Rosato GO, Sullivan ML, Jagelman DG. How reliable are currently available methods of measuring the anorectal angle? Dis Colon Rectum 1992;35(4):332–338.

42. Broen PM, Penninckx FM. Relation between anal electrosensitivity and rectal filling sensation and the influence of age. Dis Colon Rectum 2005;48(1):127–133.

43. Bharucha AE, Fletcher JG, Harper CM, et al. Relationship between symptoms and disordered continence mechanisms in women with idiopathic fecal incontinence. Gut 2005;54(4):546–555.

44. Rasmussen O. Anorectal function. Dis Colon Rectum 1994;37(4):386–403.

45. van Dam JH, Ginai AZ, Gosselink MJ, et al. Role of defecography in predicting clinical outcome of rectocele repair. Dis Colon Rectum 1997;40(2):201–207.

46. Bartolo DC, Roe AM, Locke-Edmunds JC, Virjee J, Mortensen NJ. Flap-valve theory of anorectal continence. Br J Surg 1986;73(12):1012–1014.

47. Miller R, Bartolo DC, Cervero F, Mortensen NJ. Differences in anal sensation in continent and incontinent patients with perineal descent. Int J Colorectal Dis 1989;4(1):45–49.

48. Berkelmans I, Heresbach D, Leroi AM, et al. Perineal descent at defecography in women with straining at stool: a lack of specificity or predictive value for future anal incontinence? Eur J Gastroenterol Hepatol 1995;7(1):75–79.

49. Lowry AC, Simmang CL, Boulos P, et al. Consensus statement of definitions for anorectal physiology and rectal cancer: report of the Tripartite Consensus Conference on Definitions for Anorectal Physiology and Rectal Cancer, Washington, DC, May 1, 1999. Dis Colon Rectum 2001;44(7):915–919.

50. Ron Y, Avni Y, Lukovetski A, et al. Botulinum toxin type-A in therapy of patients with anismus. Dis Colon Rectum 2001;44(12):1821–1826.

4
Physiologic Testing

Lee E. Smith and Garnet J. Blatchford

Physiologic testing has been used to assess pelvic floor and anorectal disorders for the past 35 years, but only in the past two decades has this testing become of value for clinical use. These physiologic tests are performed in conjunction with a history, diary of the disorder, physical examination, endoscopy, and often imaging studies. Physiologic tests have provided or confirmed a diagnosis in 75% of patients with constipation, 66% of patients with incontinence, and 42% of patients with chronic anorectal pain according to one study.[1]

The original physiologic testing equipment was homemade, so that all of the studies were based on a specific unit, which was not available anywhere else; thus, the ability to compare studies was almost impossible. In the past two decades equipment has been commercially produced such that reproducible results are possible. Even now a major problem is lack of a good set of normal values for healthy patients of both sexes and of all ages. Physiologic testing includes several tests that complement each other, because there is not a single test that contributes the data necessary to analyze disorders of the pelvic floor. Unfortunately, many patients have diseases or disorders that are of multifactorial pathophysiologies that will give several abnormal results, which then are more difficult to interpret. These tests include manometry, defecography, anal ultrasound, magnetic resonance imaging (MRI), transit time, pudendal nerve terminal motor latency (PNTML), and electromyography (EMG). This chapter describes these tests and their usefulness in evaluating adult diseases and disorders.

Manometry

Manometry is a technique for measuring pressures existing in the rectum and anus, and pressures and reflexes elicited by voluntary actions or by local stimuli. The equipment and techniques vary, but investigators are beginning to use more standardized equipment and methods so that our descriptions of the equipment and techniques can be focused on just a few. To be able to interpret the data, the range of normals by sex and

age is needed. These normal measurements may be obtained from sites using the same system, or studies of your own normal patients.

Indications

First, manometry is used for evaluation of incontinence. A sphincter defect can be located and quantified. Second, constipation, mainly outlet obstruction type, is investigated to determine whether abnormal pressures exist. The loss of the rectoanal inhibitory reflex (RAIR) suggests Hirschsprung's disease. Third, some anorectal pain syndromes are associated with abnormal pressures within the sphincter mechanism. Fourth, the study is conducted to establish a baseline when an anorectal or pelvic floor procedure is contemplated. For example, if biofeedback or a surgical procedure is to be used for incontinence or constipation, a pre- and postprocedure study provides the means to quantify a change.

Equipment

The equipment consists of several essential components: the probe, the transducers, the recorder, and the hydraulic pump for water infusion methods. There are two frequently used methods: the water-perfusion method and the solid-state method. The choice is based on cost and user experience.

Probes

The probes may be water perfusion, solid state, small balloon, or large balloon; they may be either open-tipped or side-opening. The open-tipped and balloon probes have fallen into disfavor. The most popular type is the water-perfusion probe, which is relatively inexpensive, durable, and easy to use.

The water-perfusion catheter probe has side holes through which water is slowly perfused, and pressure resistance of the sphincter is exerted against the holes. The simplest catheters have four holes at the same level on the probe; this circumferential array will show asymmetry within the anal canal. A balloon is attached to the tip, and a central channel in the tube opens into the balloon so that it can be inflated to elicit reflexes or elicit sensations in the rectum. Each of the side holes has an individual channel that can be connected to transducers. The mechanical water pressure is transmitted to the transducer.

The solid-state catheter is expensive and fragile, but it gives the most accurate, reproducible results. The sensors are located at the same level on the catheter, and a balloon, which is inflatable, is attached to the tip. One sensor is located at the tip within the balloon to measure the pressures within the rectum. The sensors are wired to a computer which gives a digital readout and a graph to show the pressure measurements. During this discussion, the terms probe and catheter will be used interchangeably.

Hydraulic Water-Perfusion Machines

The water-perfusion machine is a key part of the water-perfusion method. The water is driven through each of the individual channels in the tube at a chosen rate; the water perfuses through the holes near the tip and thus is exposed to pressure changes.

Transducers

Transducers are an essential part of the water-perfusion system. The water-perfusion catheter has individual channels as described above; each perfusion channel has a side channel that connects to a transducer. The side holes through which water is slowly perfused also transmits pressures back to individual transducers. The mechanical water pressure is changed to electrical signals in the transducer.

Amplifier/Recorder

Many recording devices are available, but at present computerized systems with small amplifiers and recorders are preferable. Software has been designed to give chart, table, and graph printouts. An attached monitor is a useful way to observe the tracings as the procedure is in progress.

Technique of Manometry

Initial Considerations

Usually manometry is performed using either the water-perfusion method or the solid-state microtransducer method. In this section, reference to both will be made. In our laboratory, we first used homemade systems, later the water-perfusion method, and now the solid-state method. Most of the discussion will be based on the solid-state system, but mention of differences between systems will be made when appropriate.

The informed consent form is not necessary in many American and international institutions, but our institutional policy requires that we obtain a signed consent form. The study is performed with focus on the distal 5 cm, which is the

segment that contains the sphincter muscles. It is not possible to separate the puborectalis muscle from the external anal sphincter. However, the internal sphincter and the external sphincter may be analyzed based on the portions of pressure represented by the resting tone and the squeeze pressure.

Preparation

The preparation is a simple small, tap-water enema or commercially prepared enema to empty stool from the rectum and anus before coming for the examination. The patient is placed in the left lateral position with the hips and knees flexed to 90 degrees. A digital examination with a well-lubricated glove is done first to verify that the rectum is empty, sense the direction of the rectal lumen, and recognize any abnormalities. Instructions about what the patient is to expect regarding relaxation, breathing normally, not talking, squeezing on command, and sensing the balloon will make the conduct of the examination quicker and easier for all.

Calibration

Calibration is critical to obtain accurate, reproducible results. The calibration record should be saved with the actual procedure recording to validate the measurements. For the water-perfusion method, the reservoir is filled, and the hydraulic pump is set for a pressure of about 10 psi at a rate of less than 3 mL per minute. A large volume of water introduced may produce an error; so ideally the flow rate should be far less at a rate of 0.2–0.4 mL per minute. The transducers and the perfusion holes in the catheter should be at the same level during calibration and during the procedure, or the baseline must be zeroed again at the beginning. The transducers need to be inspected for the presence of air bubbles which produce error; the bubbles need to be removed.

The solid-state system does not need to be kept at the same level during the procedure. Following the vendors instructions, the zero atmospheric level is the baseline, and usually a high point on the scale of 100 mm Hg is measured.

Resting Pressure

The probe is introduced higher than the 5-cm level and left in place for 5 minutes to permit the temperature to equalize to body temperature and the sphincter mechanism to relax to a baseline. The probe is oriented so that the posterior sensor corresponds to the recording of the posterior aspect of the anus. The recordings are made by either the station pull-through technique or the continuous pull-through technique. Most laboratories use the station pull-through method. The catheter is pulled through at 1-cm intervals, stopping to record the pressure at each increment for 10 seconds. As the sensors enter the sphincter mechanism, the pressure will be seen to increase over the baseline rectal pressure. There is usually a stepwise increase in pressure as the sensors progress distally (Figure 4-1). As the sensor leaves the sphincter mechanism, the pressure will drop to zero.

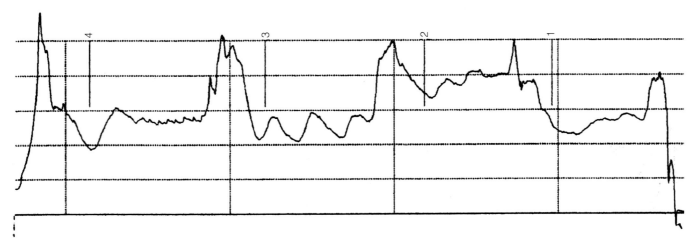

FIGURE 4-1. Normal tracing of resting tone in one quadrant on the manometry probe. The scale is 100 mm Hg. The pressure progressively increases from the 4-cm level to 2-cm level with a small decrease in pressure at the 1-cm level, and then to zero as the probe exits.

In the continuous pull-through method, the probe is pulled through with a small motor at a continuous rate. A curve reflecting the pressure zone is generated. The pressures generated by continuous pull through tend to be higher than those obtained from station pull through.

Squeeze Pressure

The probe is reinserted to at least the 6-cm level and reoriented. The probe is again removed at 1-cm increments. The patient is instructed to squeeze the sphincter muscles as if to stop a bowel movement and hold the squeeze for 3 seconds (Figure 4-2). The patient is also instructed to avoid using accessory muscles, especially the gluteals.

Using the continuous pull-through method, the patient is asked to squeeze and hold the squeeze as a motor pulls the catheter through the sphincter mechanism. The pull through can be performed several times and the results can be averaged.

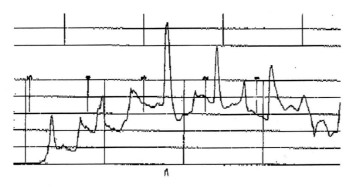

FIGURE 4-2. Normal tracing of voluntary squeeze in one quadrant on the manometry probe. The scale is 100 mm Hg. The squeeze essentially doubles the resting pressure.

Squeeze-Duration Study

The probe is positioned in the site of the highest pressure in the anal canal. The high pressure zone is the length of the anal canal with resting pressures at least 30% higher than rectal pressure.[2] The patient is instructed to squeeze and hold the squeeze for 45 seconds as the recording is made (Figure 4-3). Some investigators perform this maneuver once and others do two or three runs and average the results. This study is also termed sphincter endurance.

Reflexes

The probe is again positioned in the high pressure zone in the anal canal to observe for the RAIR. Then 10 cc of air is injected into the balloon and the pressures are observed for 10 seconds. Then air is inflated into the balloon at 20-, 30-, 40-, 50-, and 60-cc increments (Figure 4-4). The recording normally shows a relaxation from the baseline, which verifies the intact reflex from the stimulated rectal wall to the internal sphincter.

The probe is positioned in the high pressure zone again, and the patient is asked to cough to elicit the "cough reflex." The squeeze pressure increases involuntarily to counteract the increased abdominal pressure. Unfortunately, the artificial situation in the laboratory while lying on the left side on a table interferes with the patient's willingness to make as good efforts as they would in the privacy of their own toilet.

Strain Maneuver

The probe is positioned in the high pressure zone. The patient is instructed to bear down as if to defecate for at least 5 seconds. The pressure is normally reduced for a few seconds similar to the RAIR (Figure 4-5). This maneuver is repeated after a 30-second rest. The result is obtained by averaging the total runs. To appreciate what is happening to the sphincter, the rectal

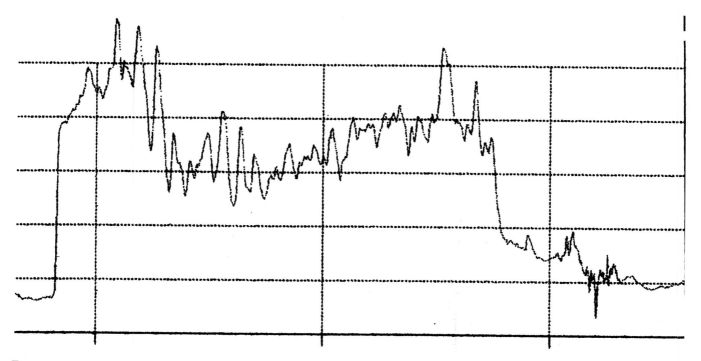

FIGURE 4-3. Normal squeeze duration study in one quadrant on the manometry probe positioned in the highest pressure zone.

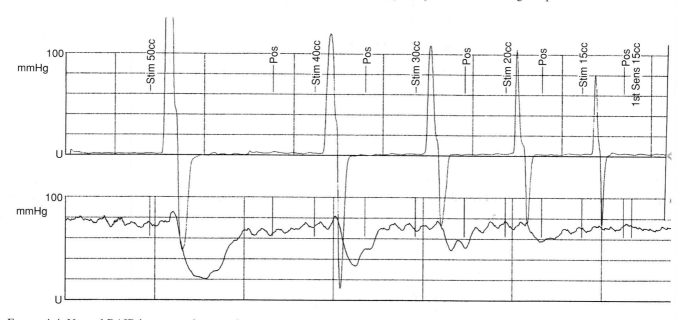

FIGURE 4-4. Normal RAIR in one quadrant on the manometry probe. The scale is 100 mm Hg.

pressure is measured at the same time with the rectal balloon, which corresponds to the increased abdominal pressure.

Rectal Sensation

The balloon is inflated in 10-cc increments until the patient senses the balloon. The first sensation is normally at or before 20-cc inflation. The compliance test can be recorded by continuing the balloon inflation as detailed below.

Compliance

Having recorded the first rectal sensation, the balloon is inflated slowly in 50-cc increments. The patient will feel a point at which there is a strong urge to defecate. This is recorded. At a further point, the patient will experience a discomfort, which is recorded as the maximal tolerated volume. In the normal-sized rectum, this will be 200–250 cc (Figure 4-6).

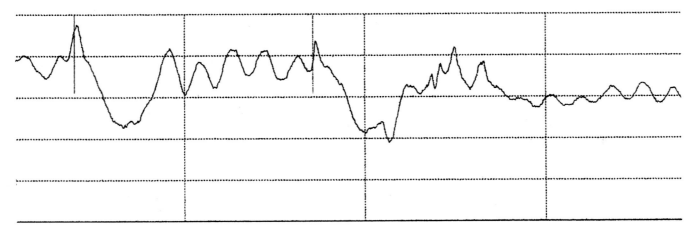

FIGURE 4-5. Normal strain maneuver. A relaxation occurs.

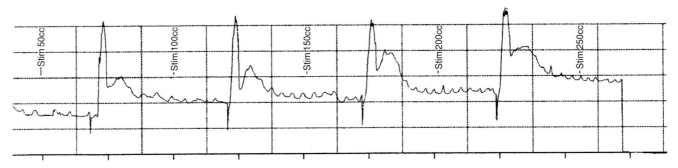

FIGURE 4-6. Normal compliance in one quadrant on the manometry probe. The patient reports the insufflation causing the first sensation, the first urge, and the last tolerable volume.

Other

Ambulatory Anorectal Manometry

To record pressures over a long period of time, a sleeve catheter, which simply records the highest pressure in the anal canal, is fixed in place. The patient then carries a recorder during the decided upon time, perhaps 24 hours. This is generally a research tool at this time.

Vector Manometry

This is best achieved with a probe that contains eight sensors in radial orientation. The probe is drawn through the anal canal, and the pressure profile shows the direction of abnormally decreased pressure. Vector manometry has been generally replaced by anal ultrasound.

Interpretation

Normals

In the anal canal there are subtle differences in the upper, middle, and distal segments.[3] In the upper anus the pressure anteriorly is lower; in the mid anus the pressures are about equal

circumferentially; and in the distal anus the pressure is slightly less posteriorly. Overall, men and young patients have higher pressures. However, there is overlap of normal measurements by sex and age.[4] The resting pressure has contributions from both the internal and external sphincters, with the internal sphincter providing 75%–80% of the total. The squeeze pressure is derived dominantly from the voluntary external sphincter.

Normal values are difficult to verify, because the literature sources are based on small numbers of patients. Some of the values vary, but by combining the totals from several authors, average numbers for practical purposes can be obtained.[5,6] These will be listed in the following sections.

Interpretation of Resting Pressure

The resting pressure is the pressure in the high pressure zone at rest after a period of stabilization.[2] Seventy-five to 80% of the resting pressure is a measure of the internal sphincter tone.[7] For women, the resting pressure is approximately 52 mm Hg (range, 39–65). For men, the resting pressure is approximately 59 mm Hg (range, 47–71). Sometimes a normal patient may have low pressures, but does not have a

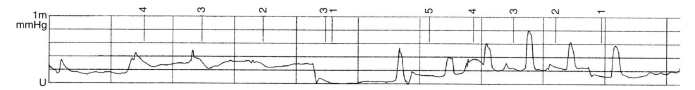

FIGURE 4-7. Low resting and voluntary squeeze pressures in an incontinent patient.

complaint if the stool is well formed. However, a patient may have "normal" pressures, but yet complains of incontinence. These measurements cannot be interpreted alone, but must be analyzed in the context of the history and other measurements. At times, slow waves of 8–12 cycles/minute can be seen on the tracings, but these are not associated with any specific pathology.

Low resting pressures are usually seen in patients who have the chief complaint of incontinence (Figure 4-7).[6,8,9] Patients who have low pressures may not be good candidates for a surgery that will leave them with a poorly formed or liquid stool, such as total colectomy with ileorectal anastomosis or proctocolectomy with ileal pouch to anal anastomosis; these patients might be better served with a permanent ileostomy.

High basal pressures may be associated with anorectal pain. Some patients have spastic sphincters, which may be associated with outlet obstruction. Also, patients with anal fissure have a spastic internal sphincter with high pressure measurements as part of the pathophysiology. These patients may be candidates for lateral internal sphincterotomy. Pharmacologic relaxation may be achieved in lieu of surgery. Relaxation of internal sphincter spasm can be achieved by 10 mg of sublingual nitroglycerine. Topical 0.2% nifedipine or 0.2% nitroglycerine applied to the anoderm relaxes the underlying muscle.[10]

Observation with a longer baseline tracing may show periods in which there is relaxation of the sphincter, even down to the zero level; incontinence might be expected to be a complaint from patients with this finding. However, the opposite can happen with episodes of spasms of high pressure. Some of these patients can be seen to have ultraslow wave activity of 1–2 cycles/minute.

Interpretation of Squeeze Pressure

The maximum voluntary pressure is the highest pressure recorded above the zero baseline at any level of the anal canal during maximum squeeze effort by the patient.[2] The squeeze pressure is the pressure increment above resting pressure after voluntary squeeze contraction and is a calculated value that is the difference between the maximum voluntary pressure and the resting pressure at the same level of the anal canal. The squeeze pressure is mainly a measure of the external sphincter.[11] For women, the squeeze pressure is approximately 128 mm Hg (range, 83–173). For men, the squeeze pressure is approximately 228 mm Hg (range, 190–266). The squeeze

pressure is examined as a total squeeze pressure, which includes the resting pressure plus the squeeze, and as a maximum squeeze pressure, which is the squeeze pressure minus the resting pressure.

A low squeeze pressure may be associated with sphincter injury or nerve damage from surgery, especially anal fistula surgery, obstetric trauma, or other anorectal trauma (Figure 4-7). Sometimes a patient will not cooperate during the test, often because of local pain. At this point, use of an anal ultrasound is appropriate to identify possible sphincter injury.

High squeeze pressure is found in those patients who have pelvic floor spasm (anismus), often associated with anorectal pain. These same patients are unable to relax the sphincter when asked to bear down as if to defecate.

Interpretation of Squeeze Duration

The sphincter duration is the length of time the patient can maintain a squeeze pressure above the resting pressure. The duration of squeeze should be >30 seconds at >50% of maximum squeeze pressure. When patients are unable to maintain a squeeze, they may be incontinent. In this case, there may be too few Type I motor nerves. There is a conversion from a dominantly Type I nerve to Type II nerves as patients grow older. The actual importance for this part of the manometry study is not clear.

Interpretation of Reflex Studies

The RAIR is the transient decrease in resting anal pressure by >25% of basal pressure in response to rapid inflation of a rectal balloon, with subsequent return to baseline.[2] The decrease in pressure during the RAIR test is a measure of the internal sphincter relaxation.[12] The reflex varies with the volume inflated into the balloon, the rate of inflation, and the rectal compliance. This reflex may be present even with central nervous system disorders; however, disease that interferes with the peripheral nerves or ganglion cells of the myenteric plexus or fibrosis of the internal anal sphincter may interfere with a measurable reflex relaxation. Likewise, a megarectum might be associated with a poor reflex, because the balloon does not touch the rectal wall to stimulate the reflex. The presence of a normal RAIR rules out Hirschsprung's disease (Figure 4-8).[13] When the balloon is deflated, a rebound contraction may be seen in patients who have a hypertonicity of the sphincter mechanism. Patients with fissures may also manifest this rebound phenomenon.

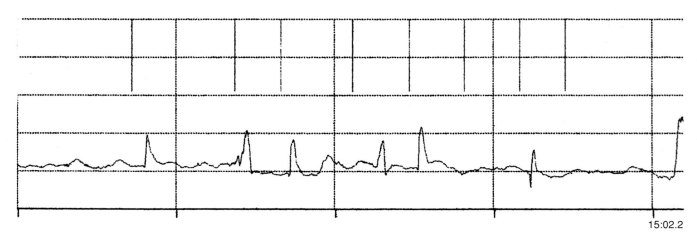

15:02.2

FIGURE 4-8. Absent rectoanal reflex (RAIR), consistent with Hirschsprung's disease. Each spike is an insufflation, but no RAIR follows.

The cough reflex is the pressure increment above resting pressure after a cough, and is a calculated value that is the difference between the maximum pressure recorded during cough and the resting pressure at the same level in the anal canal.[2] The cough reflex, also equated with a Valsalva reflex, is a rectal reflex to counter a sudden abdominal pressure increase. This sacral reflex prevents soiling during abdominal pressure increases. This reflex may be abolished if there is a disruption of nerves in the cauda equina, sacral nerves, pudendal nerves, or peripheral nerves, but is maintained if nerves higher than the sacrum are injured.

Interpretation of Strain Maneuver

The ability to defecate requires both anal relaxation and abdominal compression. As mentioned previously, the patient has difficulty straining and bearing down as if to defecate in this artificial environment. Embarrassment and fear of accidental passage of gas, liquid, or solid stool prevents complete cooperation.

Low abdominal pressures may be seen when there is central nervous system disruption or skeletal muscle disorders that prevent abdominal compression. Very high abdominal compression occurs when the anal sphincter does not relax, permitting high, recurrent pressures to be exerted on the pelvic floor.

The failure for the sphincter to relax appropriately is termed anismus or paradoxical pelvic floor contraction (Figure 4-9).[14] Such outlet obstruction may also interfere with interpretation of a transit time study. The failure to relax has been found in sexually abused patients and in neurologic disorders where inhibitory pathways are ablated.

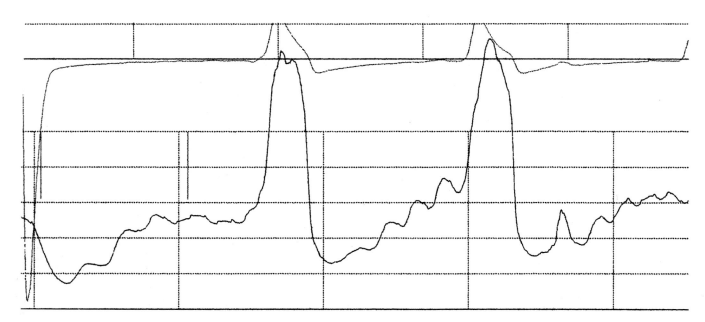

FIGURE 4-9. Paradoxical increase in sphincter pressure during the strain maneuver, rather than a relaxation, is consistent with anismus.

Interpretation of Rectal Sensation

The sensory threshold is the minimum rectal volume perceived by a patient.[2] A normal value for perception of rectal distention is approximately 15-mL (range, 9–25) inflation. Poor or absent sensation portends a poor response to biofeedback. The inability to sense suggests neural impairment, which may be related to a primary or secondary disorder, such as diabetes or amyloidosis. Constipated patients who have severe straining may progressively lose their ability to sense rectal fullness. Hypersensitivity may be evident in patients who have inflammatory bowel diseases, or have irritable bowel syndrome.

Interpretation of Compliance

The urge sensation is the volume associated with the initial urge to defecate.[2] The rate of inflation, fast or slow, the balloon size and shape, and the distance up within the rectum may alter the result. Therefore, the laboratory must standardize their method. The maximum tolerated volume is the volume at which the patient experiences discomfort and an intense desire to defecate.[2] The maximal tolerable volume and pain threshold are reduced in patients who have a fixed, noncompliant rectal wall. For example, patients who have had proctectomy, fibrosis caused by ischemia, or fibrosis caused by inflammatory bowel disease will have lower maximal tolerable volumes and lower pain thresholds. A low tolerable volume may indicate rectal hypersensitivity and irritability. Increased compliance may be found in the megarectum. Decreased compliance caused by rectal reservoir reduction will result in fecal frequency and urgency with possible incontinence.

Defecography

Defecography is a dynamic fluoroscopic examination performed with rectal contrast to study the anatomy and function of the anorectum and pelvic floor during defecation.[2] This procedure may be performed using standard radiology equipment and with relatively low radiation exposure. The specific points to be analyzed may be captured on still radiographs, but cineradiography provides a better look at the potential pathophysiologies that may influence and perhaps interfere with successful and normal evacuations.

Indication

The use of defecography is indicated as part of the evaluation of a patient who has an outlet obstruction type of constipation. There are several mechanical obstructions that may be evident; however, these obstructions must fit symptoms associated, because normal patients have been found to have what appears to be an abnormal finding, which does not result in outlet constipation. This study may be used after a repair for outlet obstruction to compare the efficiency of the defecation process before and after the procedure.

Equipment

The equipment is standard or inexpensive pieces that can be obtained from commercial surgical supply houses or hardware stores.

Table

A standard fluoroscopic table capable of cineradiography, which can be used in the supine or erect positions, is used. Ideally, large radiograms are used, but fluorographic spot films might be substituted.

Videocassette Recorder

Video recordings and spot films are helpful in analyzing the stages of defecation.

Chair and Cushion

A defecography chair, which has a standard-shaped toilet seat, fits onto the footboard of the table. The seated position on a toilet is better accepted by the patient, because the act of defecation is easier, and the staff performing the study find it to be cleaner than defecation while the patient is lying on the radiologic table. For the person analyzing the study, the seated position is more physiologic. A cushion is placed on the toilet seat to raise the patient off the opaque seat, which interferes with imaging the anal area. Films can be made through the cushion filled with water, permitting the best images to the lowest point of perineal descent. If air is used in the cushion, it gives adequate images, and there is a slightly lower radiation dose.

Contrast System

High density, barium paste (Anatrast E-Z-EM, Westbury, NY; or Evacupaste) is introduced into the rectum. These come prepackaged in a caulking tube. This tube fits into a standard caulking gun. Some radiologists place a thinner barium mixture into the rectum first and thus up into the sigmoid colon to better appreciate sigmoidocele. A thin, 240-cc barium contrast similar to that for a small bowel study may be given orally to better elucidate an enterocele. A tampon soaked in barium may be used to outline the vagina. Contrast in the bladder may be used to identify a suspected cystocele. Barium paste may be placed on the perineal skin to better see the lower limits of the perineal descent. More recently, the use of a water-soluble contrast in the peritoneal cavity outlines the depth of the cul-de-sac and structures within it.[15]

Technique

Preparation

The bowel may be studied with or without preparation. Our preference is to use a small enema an hour before the examination to minimize interference with sharp outlines of the rectal wall. Friendly, clear explanations of what the patient is to expect and to do aids in conducting a rapid, complete examination.

Introduction of Contrast

The clinician will have decided which sites require contrast based on the clinical history. The rectum, vagina, bladder, colon, small bowel, perineal skin, and/or peritoneum may be marked with contrast material.

If an enterocele is suspected, the patient should take 240 cc of diluted liquid barium orally 1 hour before the procedure. This use of barium must be used cautiously in the severely constipated, slow transit patient, because barium mixed with stool will harden to rock-like consistency during transit.

The patient is placed on a table with their left lateral side down. Tubing for injection of the contrast material is well lubricated and inserted through the anus into the rectum. The initial rectal contrast introduced is 50 cc of liquid barium to coat the rectal mucosa. To evaluate the sigmoid colon, additional barium may be injected, which will flow upwards. Air may be insufflated to better outline the mucosa. Then 250 cc of the thick barium paste in the caulking tube is inserted into the rectum using a caulking gun. If the bladder is to be evaluated, a urinary catheter is introduced into the bladder, and water-soluble contrast is injected.[16]

If the vagina needs to be seen, a tampon soaked in barium is inserted. If the cul-de-sac of the peritoneal cavity is to be seen, under sterile technique, a needle is inserted into the cavity, and 100 cc of water-soluble contrast is injected. When the patient assumes an upright position, the contrast fluid will descend by gravity into the cul-de-sac. To see the perineal skin level, barium paste may be spread across the skin down the midline, anterior and posterior to the anus.

Imaging

The patient is asked to be seated on the defecography chair (toilet), which is adjacent to the radiography table which has been erected to an upright 90-degree angle. The chair must have a water-filled cushion placed on the toilet seat to elevate the patient above the opaque seat. The patient is oriented so that lateral films can be taken. Video recording and fluoroscopy are begun. A baseline resting spot film is first (Figure 4-10). Second, the patient is asked to squeeze as if to hold a bowel movement tightly while the film is taken (Figure 4-11). Third, forceful straining without evacuating is urged for a spot film (Figure 4-12). Fourth, the patient evacuates as completely as possible with maximal straining. Ideally, this activity is captured on high-resolution videotape, plus a spot film near the end of evacuation. Last, a postevacuation film is taken. Anteroposterior filming may be done if there is a question of a lateral abnormality. The same procedures are performed with the patient facing the fluoroscope sitting in a semi-erect position in order to view the pelvic structures with the legs out of the image. It is important to remember that patients sometimes are quite embarrassed and intimidated by the mechanisms of this study; abnormal defecation dynamics may be nothing more than inability to defecate caused by embarrassment.

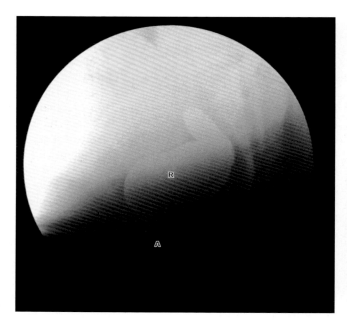

FIGURE 4-10. Defecography. The rectum at rest. R is rectum; A is the margin of the distal anus.

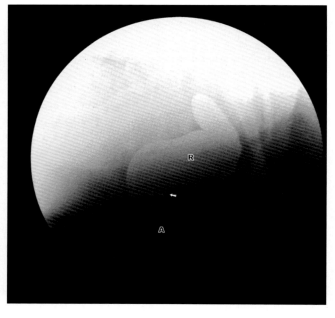

FIGURE 4-11. Defecography. The rectum with a voluntary squeeze. R is the rectum; A is the margin of the distal anus. The arrow shows the angle created by the puborectalis muscle pull.

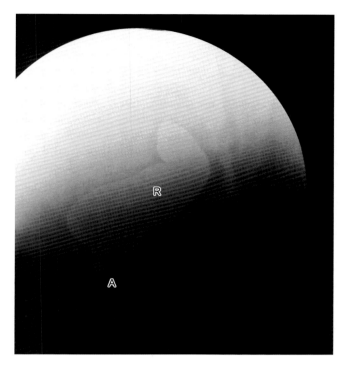

FIGURE 4-12. Defecography. Rectum during bearing down. R is rectum; A is margin of the distal anus. The anorectal angle opens as the puborectalis muscle relaxes.

Interpretation

Nonetheless, measurements and observations must be recorded on a data sheet which is designed to note all of the potential abnormalities. Having the study as cinedefecography allows repeated viewing of points where abnormality is suspected. The patient certainly does not want to do repeated studies. The findings include the anorectal angle, perineal descent, efficiency of emptying, and possibly rectocele, enterocele/sigmoidocele, anismus, and intussusception. There is an overlap of symptomatic and asymptomatic patients, so that the findings must be correlated with the clinical symptoms and signs. The patient at rest serves as the control, and the actions can then be observed. Future defecographies may be compared with this baseline study. This is important when a surgery is performed, and a change can be noted.

Anorectal Angle

The anorectal angle is the proctographic angle between the mid-axial longitudinal axis of the rectum and the anal canal.[2] The videodefecography can be reviewed to see that the puborectalis muscle relaxes appropriately. The anorectal angle decreases during squeezing and increases during defecation and straining. This change shows that the puborectalis muscle is tightening and relaxing.[17] The resting anorectal angle ranges from 90 to 110 degrees.[2] During squeeze, the angle becomes more acute in the range of 75 to 90 degrees. On evacuation, the angle becomes obtuse in the range of 110 to 180 degrees.

Perineal Descent

Perineal descent is the caudad movement of the pelvic floor with straining.[2] A baseline is a line drawn from the tip of the coccyx to the underside of the pubis, the pubococcygeal line. The descent and ascent can be measured from this line. Normally the pelvic floor will rise during squeezing and lower during straining and evacuation.[17–19] The pelvic floor should not rise or fall more than 4 cm from the pubococcygeal line. If there is greater descent, it suggests a decreased muscle tone, which is most often the result of pudendal nerve injury. This finding is usually associated with other mechanical abnormalities.

Anal Canal Length

During maximal evacuation, the length of the anal canal can be measured. The width of the anal canal can be noted to open and close adequately. During maximal strain to evacuate, the width of the anal canal should not exceed 2.5 cm. Wider openings suggest an incompetent muscle and possible incontinence.

Efficiency of Emptying

Normally the rectum should empty completely, but 90% is the lower limit of normal. If an ileal pouch is being examined, 60% evacuation is the lower limit of normal.

Rectocele

The rectocele is the most common finding in defecography. A rectocele is a bulging of the rectum into the posterior wall of the vagina (Figure 4-13).[2] A rectocele is much better defined by defecography than by clinical examination, giving better measurements of the size and adequacy of emptying.[17–19] Generally one that is <3 cm is not of consequence. Yet, even large rectoceles must be associated with outlet obstruction symptoms to be considered pathologic. Most of these patients have found that pressing upon the bulge of the rectocele aids them in evacuation. The best time to recognize a rectocele is during maximal straining to evacuate. The postevacuation film may show barium to be trapped in the rectocele. These bulges may be seen to be most often anterior, but occasionally posterior.

Enterocele/Sigmoidocele

Enterocele is a protrusion of the peritoneum between the rectum and vagina containing small intestine (Figure 4-14).[2] A sigmoidocele (pouch of Douglas descent) is a protrusion of the peritoneum between the rectum and vagina that contains sigmoid colon.[2] During straining is the best time to look for a loop of contrast-filled small bowel or sigmoid colon.[17–19]

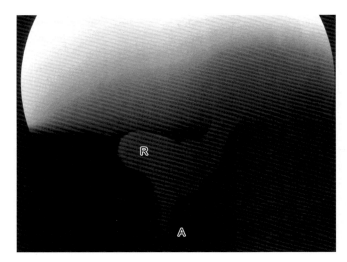

FIGURE 4-13. Defecography. A rectocele. R is the rectocele; A is the margin of the distal anus.

Bowel can be seen to indent the upper rectum or, if a space is present in front of the rectum, to herniate down toward the perineum. It is abnormal for bowel to descend below the upper rectum, and it is abnormal for a space to be present of >2 cm between the rectum and vagina. The postevacuation film may show the abnormal movement of bowel into the deep cul-de-sac. It is not necessary for viscera to enter the space to be abnormal. The best way to detect the depth of the pouch of Douglas is to introduce water-soluble contrast into the peritoneal cavity.[20,21] This finding is suspected in only half of the cases.

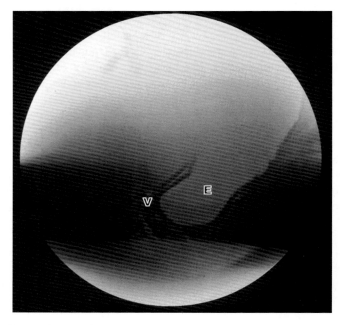

FIGURE 4-14. Defecography. An enterocele. V is the vagina; E is the enterocele descending between the vagina and rectum.

Anismus

Anismus is a nonrelaxing puborectalis or levator muscle complex, which is seen as a fixed anorectal angle with a puborectalis indentation in the face of straining down or evacuation.[17–19,22] Normally the puborectalis relaxes, and the anorectal angle opens up. The patient with anismus complains of severe straining to evacuate, and sometimes pain. If the act of defecation is timed, patients with anismus take >30 seconds to empty, starting when the anal canal begins to open. Normally evacuation takes 10 seconds after the anal canal starts to open. In addition, the anal canal width is narrow.

Intussusception/Prolapse

The rectum may be seen to prolapse or intussuscept during straining or evacuation (Figure 4-15A–C).[17–19] The intussusception or prolapse can be characterized as upper, mid, or lower rectal, and the origin can be described as anterior or posterior. The intussusception usually begins at 6–8 cm above the anus. Generally the upper rectum should remain attached to the sacrum and the retrorectal (presacral) space should not vary. The distal part of the rectum may be in either a vertical or horizontal plane and still be normal. Radiologists have some difficulty deciding whether the enfolding is a full-thickness intussusception or a normal rectal fold. Measurement of the thickness of the enfolding rectal wall will be twice as thick as the rectal wall or a normal fold of the rectum, because it represents two adjacent layers of the wall.[23]

Megarectum

This diagnosis is a combination of a large measurement of the diameter of the rectum and incomplete emptying. The measurement of the width of the rectum at the level of the distal sacrum >9 cm suggests megarectum.

Incontinence

During the procedure, incontinent patients may not be able to hold the barium in the rectum, and it can be seen to run out of the anal canal before the instruction to defecate is given. Incontinence is often associated with other pathology.

Balloon Expulsion Test

The balloon expulsion test measures the ability of the patient to expel a balloon inflated with 50–60 mL of water.[2] Condoms and Foley catheter balloons have been used for this test.[24] Patients with outlet obstruction are not able to pass this balloon readily. The problem is that some patients may pass the balloon, but have undetected outlet obstruction. Conversely, patients with outlet obstruction may call upon compensatory mechanisms to pass the balloon.

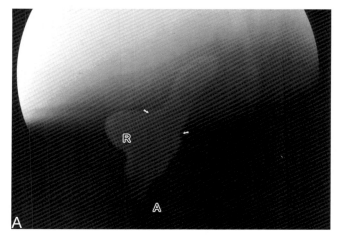

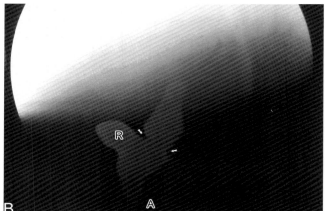

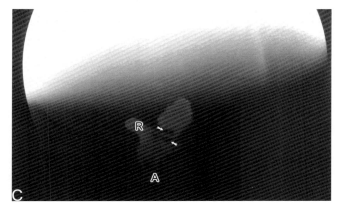

FIGURE 4-15. **A–C** Defecography. Intussusception of the rectum. R is the rectum; A is the margin of the distal anus. The arrows show the progressive infolding of the rectum.

Anal Ultrasound

Anal ultrasound is used to look for anatomic abnormality of the anal sphincters. See the chapter on Endoluminal Ultrasound, to see images of anal ultrasounds. Ultrasound has replaced EMG as the best means to define an injury.

Indication

If a defect in the sphincter mechanism is suspected, ultrasound is the diagnostic technique of choice.[25] It is most useful in the work-up of incontinence. The obstetric injury is readily seen, and the ability to find the defect approaches 100%.

Equipment

The most often used ultrasound machine displays a 360-degree image made possible by a mechanically rotating transducer on a hand probe. The 10-MHz transducer provides the clearest images. The transducer is covered by a plastic cap.[25,26]

Technique

The only preparation is a small enema. Sedation is not necessary. The patient is placed in the left decubitus position. The ultrasound system is assembled, and water is introduced to fill the cap covering the transducer. Air bubbles must be removed, because they cause an artifact. A digital examination is performed to find abnormality, but also to define the direction for insertion of the probe. The probe is introduced blindly to the point where the transducer is in the rectum. Images are made in the upper, middle, and distal anus, which is the distal 4–5 cm.

Interpretation

Bartram[26,27] describes six ultrasonographic layers in the anal canal: 1) a hyperechoic layer that is the interface of the cone with the tissues; 2) a hypoechoic layer that represents the mucosa; 3) a hyperechoic layer that represents the submucosa; 4) a hypoechoic layer that is the internal anal sphincter; 5) a hyperechoic layer that represents the intersphincteric plane and the longitudinal muscle; and 6) a layer of mixed echogenicity representing the external anal sphincter.

In the upper anal canal, the puborectalis muscle is seen to loop around the upper anus. In the middle anus, both the internal and external sphincters may be seen. In the distal anus, the subcutaneous portion of the external sphincter is visualized, but the internal sphincter does not extend this far. The thickness of the internal sphincter stands out in the middle of the anus. The normal adult sphincter is 2–3 mm thick. A neonate may have a sphincter of 1 mm, and in the elderly 3–4 mm thick.

Incontinence

A thin muscle suggests primary degeneration of the internal sphincter. After lateral internal sphincterotomy, a distal defect can be seen in the internal sphincter. Obstetric trauma may extend into the transverse perineus muscle, the external sphincter, or completely down through the internal sphincter. The injury blurs out portions of the normal rings of tissue described above.[28]

Magnetic Resonance Imaging

MRI of pelvic floor function is developing rapidly. Dynamic studies have yielded additional information compared with static examinations alone. Identification of the anal and rectal structures is fairly easy on MRI because the perirectal fat shows a high degree of contrast when compared with the musculature. Indications for MRI examination are primarily sepsis, trauma, congenital abnormalities, and tumor.

There is a significant change in T1 and T2 weighted imaging associated with infection. This change produces high soft tissue contrast and enables abscess and fistulous tracks to be demonstrated. Sensitivity of MRI using the body coil can be as high as 89% in identifying fistulas, but demonstration of site of internal opening and differentiation of various muscle layers is not always possible.[29] In this study, there was concordance between MRI and surgical findings for the primary tract and secondary tracts of 86% and 93%, respectively.

Muscular anatomy is seen so well that MRI has become useful in the evaluation of anal trauma. When compared with endorectal ultrasound, endoanal coil MRI is superior in identifying the outer aspect of the external sphincter muscle. Concordance between MRI and surgical findings has been shown with regard to location of sphincter tears after obstetric trauma.[30] Studies have shown endoanal MRI to be comparable to endoanal ultrasound for identifying defects and/or thinning of the internal sphincter. MRI, however, may also show thinning of the external sphincter and puborectalis, which are not easily seen on endoanal ultrasound. This may represent atrophy in the pelvic musculature. Atrophy may correlate with a poor result after sphincter repair. Determination of atrophy on endoanal MRI may help in predicting the outcome after sphincteroplasty.[31] Atrophy on MRI has been shown to correlate with single fiber needle EMG which confirms denervation at the level of the muscle.[32] However, PNTML may be normal even in the presence of external anal sphincter atrophy. Prolongation of the PNTML reflects damage to only the large heavily myelinated nerve fibers and does not reflect the nerve function at the muscle level.

Congenital abnormalities of the anus and rectum can be delineated by MRI examination.[33] MRI can be used to identify sphincter involvement by rectal tumors. Distance from the distal aspect of the tumor to the levator muscle can be accurately assessed before surgical planning. Because of the length of the endorectal coil, visualization of the musculature of the sphincter up to 2 cm above the levator ani only is seen.[34] Visualization of depth of invasion by tumor can be done by manipulation of contrast with the use of T2 weighted images.

Defecatory problems may also be evaluated by MRI. Dynamic pelvic MRI (or MRI proctography) is now possible since techniques for rapid MRI acquisition have been developed. This allows pelvic floor motion to be visualized in real time during defecation. Generally this does not require addition of contrast although some limitations with motion artifact can be seen. It has been suggested that examination in the supine position (MRI) compared with the study in a seated position (balloon proctography) shows minimal and probably clinically insignificant differences in pelvic organ prolapse between these two techniques.[35] MRI is able to demonstrate peritoneoceles, cystoceles, perineal descent, and prolapse during evacuation. Evidence of obstruction defecation may be seen with the anorectal angle becoming more acute with straining, suggesting paradoxical contraction of the puborectalis.

EMG of the Anal Sphincter

EMG is used primarily in evaluating fecal incontinence. EMG is a means of assessing the motor unit. The integrity of the muscle may be assessed as well as its nerve supply. The integrity of external anal sphincter innervation after sphincter injury can be demonstrated. Sphincter reinnervation secondary to pelvic neuropathy can be demonstrated. EMG may also be used to "map" specific anatomic sphincter defects. This mapping technique has largely been replaced by anal ultrasonography, which is simple, accurate, and painless. Anal EMG may also be used to demonstrate appropriate relaxation and contraction of the anal muscle and can be used in biofeedback therapy.

Concentric Needle EMG

Concentric needle EMG focuses on different motor unit characteristics. A concentric needle electrode will record muscle contractions as motor unit potentials (MUPs). A single MUP is caused by depolarization of the muscle from a single motor unit. Three variables are noted within a MUP: amplitude, duration, and shape. Amplitude is dependent on the number of muscle fibers discharging. The larger the number of fibers, the greater is the amplitude of the MUP. Generally only the fibers lying within 1 mm of the electrode (typically less than 20) contribute to the spike of the MUP. Distance may also influence amplitude to some degree. Duration of the MUP is a result of dispersion of the action potentials originating from the different muscle fibers of a motor unit. Duration of MUPs increases with age. Denervation also causes a prolongation of duration and polyphasic potentials. Shape of the MUP results from summation of the single fiber action potentials in the motor unit. Most normal MUPs are bi- or triphasic. Polyphasic potentials (four or more phases) have been reported in up to 25% of normal external anal sphincter muscles. Polyphasic potentials of short duration occur in myopathic disorders and those with long duration correlate with histologic evidence of regeneration in denervated muscle. Concentric needle EMG can be of particular value in the diagnosis of specific neurologic problems, including conditions of the cone and cauda equina, sacral roots, pudendal nerve, and for differential diagnosis of the various types of multisystemic atrophy.[36] Normal amplitude of the MUP is <600 μV and duration is <6 ms.[37]

Single Fiber EMG

Single fiber EMG electrodes are used because the area of measurement is so small each fiber generates a single spike. In normal circumstances, only a few muscle fibers from a single motor unit are within the recording area of a single fiber electrode. In reinnervated muscle, the numbers of fibers belonging to a single motor unit increase, thereby increasing action potentials are recorded at the electrode. The number of spikes can be recorded from separate potentials and fiber density can be calculated. Fiber density is the measurement of the mean number of muscle fibers innervated by one alpha-motor unit. This is usually an average from numerous separate potentials. Technique of single fiber EMG involves placing a sterilized fine needle (single fiber electrode) with a recording surface of 25 μm into the external anal sphincter just outside the anal verge. Readings are taken in both the left and right lateral areas with 20 needle positions or more done for calculation of fiber density. A value >1.7 is considered abnormal.[38] Criteria for pudendal nerve damage in single fiber EMG are the presence of an increased fiber density, increase of MUP duration and amplitude at rest, decrease of the number of MUPs during maximum contraction, and presence of "jitter and blocking" phenomena.[39]

Surface Electrodes

Surface EMG electrodes are generally used to document anal sphincter activity at rest, strain, and squeeze. Documentation of paradoxical sphincter contraction may improve assessment of patients with defecation disorders. When compared with proctography, both needle EMG and surface EMG have a low positive predictive value, but they have high negative predictive values.[40] Therefore, EMG alone is not optimal for diagnosing the presence of nonrelaxing puborectalis. Surface electrodes avoid the pain of needle EMG.

Biofeedback training is often done using surface electrodes. This may be done for fecal incontinence or for difficulties with evacuation, particularly if paradoxical sphincter contraction is present. A plug electrode may be used within the anal canal or surface electrodes may be placed near the anus in a lateral position. Surface electrodes are easy and painless to apply and therefore well tolerated by patients. They come with self-adhesive or can be secured with tape. They should be placed over the subcutaneous part of the external anal sphincter 1 cm from the anal verge in right and left lateral positions. A grounding electrode is then placed on the patient's buttock. EMG recordings from the external anal sphincter during straining using surface electrodes applied to the skin correlate well with the result from needle electrodes inserted into the muscle.[41] Other studies have shown that the anal plug electrodes correlate well with anal manometry and with wire electrodes during rest, squeezing, and straining. Normal values for surface EMG show short contraction (3-second) amplitude from 8–10 μV, 10-second contraction

amplitude from 8–10 μV, endurance (maintenance of sustained contraction) of 30–40 seconds. Normal patients demonstrated no evidence of paradoxical activity.[37]

Pudendal Nerve Terminal Motor Latency

The pudendal nerve originates from S2, S3, S4 nerve roots and travels along the lateral pelvic wall down to near the ischial spine where it exits the pelvis to supply the external anal sphincter and the periurethral muscles through its terminal perineal branch. Prolongation in the pudendal nerve conduction indicates injury to the pudendal nerve sheath that results in focal demyelination with resultant slowing of conduction. Testing is usually done with a St. Mark's electrode with a stimulating electrode mounted at the fingertip portion and a recording electrode mounted at the finger base portion. The electrode has a constant distance of 50 mm between stimulation of the nerve and recording of the external anal sphincter response. Latency between stimulation and response can then be recorded (Figure 4-16). This latency reflects the myelin function of the peripheral nerve. Therefore, a normal PNTML does not exclude partial damage. However, when unilaterally or bilaterally severely prolonged, PNTML has been shown to affect results after sphincter repair.[39,42,43]

Evaluation of Transit

The time it takes for food to travel through the digestive tract is known as bowel transit time. Gastric emptying, small bowel transit, and colonic transit may be studied. Transit is dependent on diet and varies greatly from person to person. For this reason, a dietary history and bowel evacuation history should be obtained in conjunction with any transit testing. Dietary history can be evaluated for fiber, fat, and calorie intake. Patients who believe they eat a high fiber diet may be shown to have a very modest fiber intake. Stool history will further delineate the extent of the patient's problem. In patients complaining of chronic constipation who believed that they had less than or equal to three stools per week for more than 6 months, a 4-week stool diary revealed that only 49% actually met this criteria. The remaining 51% of patients had, on average, six stools per week.[44] This study also showed that a history of psychiatric illness was five times more frequent among those whose bowel symptoms correlated poorly with objective evidence of constipation.

Colonic Transit

The rate at which fecal residue moves through the colon is important in determining whether the stool is liquid, semi-formed, or hard. Evaluation of constipation and pelvic problems may require determination of colonic transit times in order to assist in treatment. Transit may be measured by radiopaque markers or radionucleotide techniques.

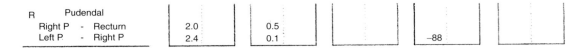

R	Pudendal				
Right P	-	Recturn	2.0	0.5	
Left P	-	Right P	2.4	0.1	−88

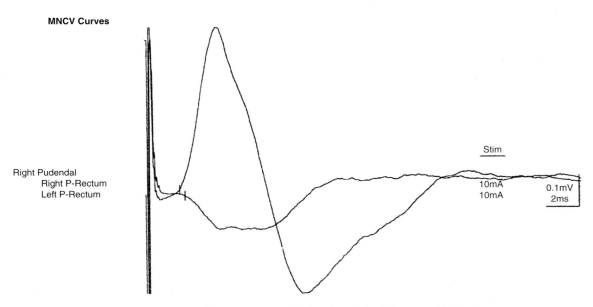

MNCV Curves

Right Pudendal
Right P-Rectum
Left P-Rectum

Stim

10mA   0.1mV
10mA   2ms

FIGURE 4-16. PNTML curves showing a latency of the right nerve of 2.0 msD and the left nerve of 2.4 msD.

Colonic transit is most easily measured by use of a marker test. The patient ingests a capsule containing radiopaque markers, which are then followed through the colon by abdominal radiographs. Markers consist of a capsule containing radiopaque markers, which are commercially available (Sitz-Mark, Konsyl Pharmaceuticals, Fort Worth, TX) or can be individually created by filling gel capsules with small circles cut from radiopaque tubing. In the most simplified colon transit technique, the patient takes one marker tablet which contains 24 markers on day 0. On day 5, a supine abdominal film is taken to determine the number and position of remaining markers. If five or fewer markers are remaining, the patient has normal colonic transit. If more than five markers are present, then the pattern of residual markers is noted. Diffuse scattering throughout the colon would suggest colonic inertia or decreased motility. If the markers are present in the rectosigmoid region, then the presence of pelvic outlet problems should be considered. Segmental transit may be calculated as described by Metcalf et al.[45] On day 0, day 1, and day 2, the patient takes one marker capsule for a total of three capsules. On day 4, an abdominal film is taken. If there are more than a total of 50 markers remaining, transit time is abnormal and an additional abdominal radiograph is taken on day 7 to determine the location and number of residual markers. The abdominal radiograph is divided into the following sections: right colon, left colon, and rectosigmoid. The number

of markers present in each section is counted on both the 4- and 7-day films. A table can then be made with the values (Table 4-1). Average normal transit is 11.3 hours, 11.3 hours, and 12.4 hours for the right, left, and rectosigmoid colon, respectively. Normal total transit averages 35 hours. Segmental colectomy is not indicated for constipation even in the face of markedly abnormal segmental transit time. Stool weight has been shown to correlate with transit time in constipated patients.[44]

Radionuclide Transit

Transit may be measured by radionuclide gamma scintigraphic techniques.[46] Radiographic and scintigraphic methods correlate well. The major advantage of scintigraphy is that 24–48 hours of scanning is needed compared with 5–7 days for marker test completion.

TABLE 4-1. Results of a colon transit study

	Right colon	Left colon	Rectosigmoid	Total
Day-4 film	15	21	16	52
Day-7 film	0	4	14	18
Transit time (h)	15	25	30	70

The theoretical numbers of ingested markers by time and colonic segment. This example shows a right colon transit of 15 h, left colon of 25 h, rectosigmoid of 30 h, and a total colonic transit of 70 h.

Small Bowel Transit

Small intestinal transit should be evaluated before surgical treatment of constipation because the patient may have a global motility problem. Small bowel transit may be measured by breath hydrogen analysis. Hydrogen breath analysis depends on the presence of bacteria in the large intestine to metabolize lactulose. Up to 25% of the population cannot metabolize the sugar because they lack certain bacterial strains in the colon.[47] A meal of lactulose and beans is ingested and hydrogen breath analysis is undertaken. Fermentation of the meal occurs when the substrate reaches the colon. The fermentation process releases hydrogen gas that is absorbed and excreted by the lungs. Time to a 20-ppm increase in hydrogen in the breath correlates with small bowel transit. Some conditions such as low colonic pH, bacterial overgrowth, or antibiotic administration may interfere with the use of this test for small bowel transit.

Small bowel transit may also be determined by scintigraphic techniques. These techniques have the advantage of also measuring gastric emptying. Scintigraphy has a tendency toward slightly shorter transit times, but this is probably not clinically significant. Radiation exposure with scintigraphy is highest for the colon and can be reduced by the administration of laxatives after the procedure. Radiation to the ovaries is less than in a plain abdominal X-ray.

References

1. Wexner SD, Jorge JMN. Colorectal physiological tests: use or abuse of technology? Eur J Surg 1994;160:167–174.
2. Lowry AC, Simmang CL, Boulos P, et al. Report of the tripartite consensus conference on definitions for anorectal physiology and rectal cancer, Washington, D.C., May 1, 1999. Dis Colon Rectum 2001;44(7):915–919.
3. Pedersen IK, Christiansen J. A study of the physiological variation in anal manometry. Br J Surg 1989;76:69–71.
4. Loening-Baucke V, Anuras S. Effects of age and sex on anorectal manometry. Am J Gastroenterol 1991;80:50–53.
5. Hallan RI, Marzouk DEMM, Waldron DJ, et al. Comparison of digital and manometric assessment of anal sphincter function. Br J Surg 1989;76:973–975.
6. Felt Bersma RJF, Klinkenberg-Knol, Meuwissen SGM. Anorectal function investigations in incontinent and continent patients. Dis Colon Rectum 1990;33:479–486.
7. Duthie HL, Watts JM. Contribution of the external anal sphincter to the pressure zone in the anal canal. Gut 1965;17:64–68.
8. McHugh SM, Diamant NE. Effect of age, gender and parity on anal canal pressures. Contribution of impaired anal sphincter function to fecal incontinence. Dig Dis Sci 1987;32:726–736.
9. Rattan S, Chakder S. Role of nitric oxide as a mediator of internal anal sphincter relaxation. Am J Physiol 1992;262:G107–112.
10. Perry RE, Blatchford GJ, Christensen MA, et al. Manometric diagnosis of anal sphincter injuries. Am J Surg 1990;159:112–117.
11. Tjandra JJ, Sharma BRK, McKirdy HC, et al. Anorectal physiological testing in defecatory disorders: a prospective study. Aust N Z J Surg 1994;64:322–326.
12. Bouchoucha M, Faye A, Arsac M, Rocaries F. Anal sphincter response to distension. Int J Colorectal Dis 2001;16:119–125.
13. Tobon F, Reid NCRW, Talbert JL, et al. Nonsurgical test for the diagnosis of Hirschsprung's disease. N Engl J Med 1968;278:188–194.
14. Preston DM, Lennard-Jones JE. Anismus in chronic constipation. Dig Dis Sci 1985;30:413–418.
15. Bremmer S. Peritoneocele: a radiological study with defaecoperitoneography. Acta Radiol Suppl 1998;413:1–33.
16. Maglinte DD, Kelvin FM, Hale DS. Dynamic cystoproctography: a unifying diagnostic approach to pelvic floor and anorectal dysfunction. AJR Am J Roentgenol 1999;169:759–767.
17. Jorge JMN, Habr-Gama A, Wexner S. Clinical applications and techniques of cinedefecography. Am J Surg 2001;182:93–101.
18. Wiersma T, Mulder CJJ, Reeders WAJ. Dynamic rectal examination: its significant clinical value. Endoscopy 1997;29:462–471.
19. Jones HJS, Blake H, Swift RI. A prospective audit of the usefulness of evacuating proctography. Ann R Coll Surg Engl 1998;80:40–45.
20. Halligan S, Bartram C, Hall C, et al. Enterocele revealed by simultaneous evacuation proctography and peritoneography: does "defecation block" exist? AJR Am J Roentgenol 1996;167:461–466.
21. Sentovich SM, Rivela LJ, Thorson AG, et al. Simultaneous dynamic proctography and peritoneography for pelvic floor disorders. Dis Colon Rectum 1995;38:912–915.
22. Halligan S, Malouf A, Bartram C, et al. Predictive value of impaired evacuation at proctography in diagnosing anismus. AJR Am J Roentgenol 2001;177:633–637.
23. Pomerri F, Zuliani M, Mazza C, et al. Defecographic measurements of rectal intussusception and prolapse in patients and in asymptomatic subjects. AJR Am J Roentgenol 2001;176:641–645.
24. Rao SS, Hatfield R, Soffer E. Manometric tests of anorectal function in healthy adults. Am J Gastroenterol 1999;94:773–783.
25. Sentovich SM, Blatchford GJ, Rivela LJ, et al. Diagnosing anal sphincter injury with transanal ultrasound and manometry. Dis Colon Rectum 1997;40:1430–1434.
26. Bartram CI, Burnett SJD. Atlas of Anal Endosonography. Oxford: Butterworth-Heinemann; 1991.
27. Bartram C. Radiologic evaluation of anorectal disorders. Gastroenterol Clin North Am 2001;30:55–75.
28. Sultan AH, Kamm MA, Talbot IC, et al. Anal endosonography for identifying external sphincter defects confirmed histologically. Br J Surg 1994;81(3):463–465.
29. Barker PG, Lunniss PJ, Armstrong P, et al. Magnetic resonance imaging of fistula-in-ano: technique, interpretation and accuracy. Clin Radiol 1994;49:7–13.
30. Fletcher JG, Busse RF, Riederer SJ, et al. Magnetic resonance imaging of anatomic and dynamic defects of the pelvic floor in defecatory disorders. Am J Gastroenterol 2003;98:399–411.
31. Briel JW, Stoker J, Rociu E, et al. External anal sphincter atrophy on endoanal magnetic resonance imaging adversely affects continence after sphincteroplasty. Br J Surg 1999;86:1322–1327.
32. William AB, Bartram CI, Modhwadia D, et al. Endocoil magnetic resonance imaging quantification of external anal sphincter atrophy. Br J Surg 2001;88:853–859.
33. Sato T, Konishi F, Kanazawa K. Variations in motor evoked potential latencies in the anal sphincter system with sacral magnetic stimulation. Dis Colon Rectum 2000;43:966–970.

34. deSouza NM, Hall AS, Puni R, et al. High resolution magnetic resonance imaging of the anal sphincter using a dedicated endoanal coil. Dis Colon Rectum 1996;39:926–934.

35. Fletcher JG, Busse RF, Riederer SJ, et al. Magnetic resonance imaging of anatomic and dynamic defects of the pelvic floor in defecatory disorders. Am J Gastroenterol 2003;98:399–411.

36. Del Rey AP, Entrena BF. Reference values of motor unit potentials (MUPs) of the external anal sphincter muscle. Clin Neurophysiol 2002;113:1832–1839.

37. Ferrara A, Lujan JH, Cebrian J, et al. Clinical, manometric, and EMG characteristics of patients with fecal incontinence. Tech Coloproctol 2001;5:13–18.

38. Osterberg A, Graf W, Eeg-Olofsson KE, et al. Results of neurophysiologic evaluation in fecal incontinence. Dis Colon Rectum 2000;43(9):1256–1261.

39. Jacobs PPM, Scheuer M, Kuijpers JHC, et al. Obstetric fecal incontinence: role of pelvic floor denervation and results of delayed sphincter repair. Dis Colon Rectum 1990;33(6):494–497.

40. Yeh CY, Pikarsky A, Wexner SD, et al. Electromyographic findings of paradoxical puborectalis contraction correlate poorly with cinedefecography. Tech Coloproctol 2003;7:77–81.

41. Lopez A, Nilsson BY, Mellgren A, et al. Electromyography of the external anal sphincter: comparison between needle and surface electrodes. Dis Colon Rectum 1999;42:482–485.

42. Laurberg S, Swash M, Henry MM. Delayed external sphincter repair for obstetric tear. Br J Surg 1998;75:786–788.

43. Wexner SD, Marchetti F, Jagelmen DG. The role of sphincteroplasty for fecal incontinence reevaluated: a prospective physiologic and functional review. Dis Colon Rectum 1991;34:22–30.

44. Ashraf W, Park F, Lof J, et al. An examination of the reliability of reported stool frequency in the diagnosis of idiopathic constipation. Am J Gastroenterol 1996;91:26–32.

45. Metcalf AM, Phillips SF, Zinsmeister AR, et al. Simplified assessment of segmental colonic transit. Gastroenterology 1987; 92:40–47.

46. Charles F, Camilleri M, Phillips SF, Thomforde GM, Forstrom LA. Scintigraphy of the whole gut: clinical evaluation of transit disorders. Mayo Clin Proc 1995;70(2):113–118.

47. Caride VJ, Prokop EK, Troncale FJ, et al. Scintigraphic determination of small intestinal transit time: comparison with the hydrogen breath technique. Gastroenterology 1984;86: 714–720.

5
Diagnostic Evaluations—Endoscopy: Rigid, Flexible Complications

Santhat Nivatvongs and Kenneth A. Forde

The large intestine from cecum to anus can be effectively and accurately examined as part of a complete physical examination. An ultimate diagnosis of large bowel diseases can only be made by direct observation of the abnormalities and, if indicated, a biopsy. Different equipment is designed and used for different purposes.

Anoscopy

Anoscopy is the examination of the anal canal. The lower part of the rectal mucosa, upper anal mucosa, anoderm, dentate line, internal and external hemorrhoids can be seen through this examination.

There are basically two types of anoscopes: beveled type such as the Buie or Hirschman scope (Figure 5-1) and the lighted Welch-Allen scope (Figure 5-2) that uses the same light source as the rigid proctosigmoidoscope. Another type is the side-opening Vernon-David scope with Hirschman handle (Figure 5-3). The Hinkel-James anoscope (Figure 5-4) is much longer than the Vernon-David scope and is suitable for patients with deep buttock cheeks.

Indications

Any anal and perianal diseases or conditions require a full examination of the anal canal. These include anal fissures, anal fistulas, anal Crohn's disease, anal tumors, hemorrhoids, anal condyloma, bright red rectal bleeding, and pruritus ani.

Anoscopy is frequently used in conjunction with colonoscopy, flexible sigmoidoscopy, and rigid proctosigmoidoscopy as part of the examination.

Contraindications

Patients who have severe anal pain such as an acute anal fissure or a perianal or intersphincteric abscess may not tolerate the examination. In general, if a patient can tolerate a digital examination, anoscopy can usually be done. A 2% lidocaine jelly should be used in patients with anal pain. Anal stricture or severe anal stenosis is another contraindication.

Preparation

No preparation is required.

Positioning

A prone jackknife position gives the best exposure. An alternative is a left lateral recumbent position.

Technique

The Vernon-David, which is a side-opening endoscope, gives the best examination. Inspection of the anal area should always precede any other examination and, for this, good lighting is essential. The cheeks of the buttock are gently spread to gain exposure. Skin tags, excoriation, and change in color or thickness of the anal verge and perianal skin can be detected quickly. A scarred, patulous, or irregularly shaped anus may give clues to the cause of anal incontinence. Particularly in multiparous women, the anal verge may be pushed down quite far during straining—a feature of the descending perineum syndrome. When the anal verge is pricked with a needle, the external sphincter visibly contracts because of the anal reflex. It is useful for testing the sensibility of the anal canal, which may be absent in areas of previous scar or defect, or in patients with an underlying neuropathy.

The next step is to do a digital examination. The index finger should be well lubricated with a lubricant jelly, and the finger pressed on the anal aperture to "warn" the patient. Then the finger should be gradually inserted and swept all around the anal canal to detect any mass or induration. In men, the prostate should be felt. In women, the posterior vaginal wall should be pushed anteriorly to detect any evidence of a rectocele. Anal tone, whether tight or loose, can be easily estimated. A stricture or narrowing from scarring or a defect in the internal or external sphincters from a previous

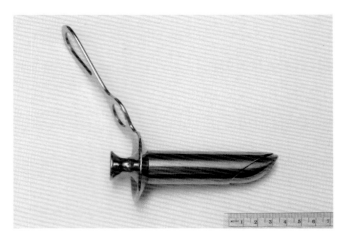

FIGURE 5-1. Buie anoscope.

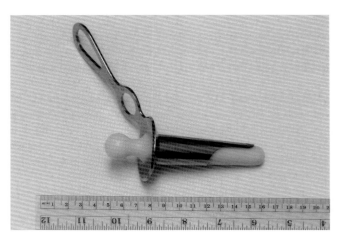

FIGURE 5-3. Vernon-David with Hirschman handle anoscope.

operation can be felt. A fibrous cord or induration in the anal area and the anal canal may indicate a fistulous tract. The external sphincter, puborectalis, and levator ani muscles can also be appreciated by digital examination. When the puborectalis is pulled in the posterior quadrant, the anus will gape but will close immediately when the traction is released. Persistence of the gaping indicates an abnormal reflex pathway in the thoracolumbar region frequently seen in paraplegic patients. The finger should press gently on these muscles for signs of tenderness. When the person with good anal function is asked to contract the muscles, the examiner not only feels the squeeze of the muscle on the examining finger but also feels the finger pulled forward by the puborectalis muscle.

Insertion of the anoscope should always be done with the obturator in place. The obturator is removed during examination and reinserted to rotate the instrument to another area. However, if the beveled type of endoscope is used, the endoscope can be rotated all around without having to reinsert the obturator. If an inverted (jackknife) position is used, the examination table need not be tipped down more than 10–15 degrees. If a left lateral position is used, an assistant needs to pull up the right cheek of the buttock for exposure. During examination, the patient is asked to strain with the anoscope sliding out to detect any prolapse of the rectal mucosa and the anal cushion. Excoriation, metaplastic changes, and friable mucosa indicate a prolapsed hemorrhoid.

A biopsy via an anoscope is not advisable because of its poor exposure. If indicated, a biopsy via a rigid proctosigmoidoscope or a flexible sigmoidoscope is more appropriate.

Complications

Anal tear, especially at the posterior midline, can occur in patients with anal stenosis.

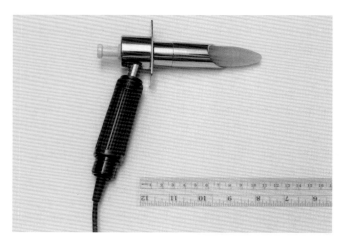

FIGURE 5-2. Lighted Welch-Allen anoscope.

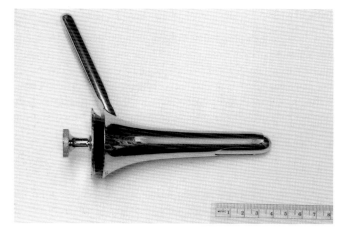

FIGURE 5-4. Hinkel-James anoscope.

Rigid Proctosigmoidoscope

Three sizes of rigid proctosigmoidoscope are available (Figure 5-5). A 19 mm × 25 cm scope is the standard size for a general examination and for polypectomy or electrocoagulation. A 15 mm × 25 cm endoscope is an ideal size for general examination. It is much better tolerated by the patient, causing less spasm of the rectum and, thus, minimal air insufflation, yet enables as adequate an examination as the standard-size endoscope. An 11 mm × 25 cm endoscope should be available for examining the patient who has anal or rectal stricture, such as Crohn's disease. Some physicians and surgeons prefer a disposable standard-size rigid proctosigmoidoscope for routine examination.

Indications

Rigid proctosigmoidoscopy has largely been replaced by flexible sigmoidoscopy. However, rigid proctosigmoidoscopy is still useful in examination of the anorectum. One of its advantages is that any blood clots or stool can easily be washed out. In fact, in a patient who has massive gastrointestinal bleeding, a rigid proctosigmoidoscopy is the first line of examination to rule out the source of bleeding in the anorectum.

A rigid proctosigmoidoscopy is used when an abnormality of the anal canal and rectum is suspected such as nonspecific proctitis, radiation proctitis, anorectal ulcer, anorectal neoplasm, infectious proctitis, and anorectal Crohn's disease. Rigid proctosigmoidoscopy is also useful to identify the precise site and size of rectal neoplasm.

Contraindications

Patients with severe anal pain from an acute fissure, thrombosed external hemorrhoids, and perianal abscess may not allow an examination. The examination should be postponed to some other date. Anal stricture that will not allow the passage of the smallest size rigid proctosigmoidoscope is a contraindication to its use.

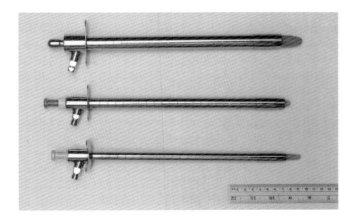

FIGURE 5-5. Rigid proctosigmoidoscope. Top, 19 mm × 25 cm; middle, 15 mm × 25 cm; bottom, 11 mm × 25 cm.

Patients with acute abdomen of any cause, rectal and sigmoid anastomosis less than 2 weeks postoperatively should not have a rigid proctosigmoidoscopy.

Preparation

Two phosphate enemas should be given within 2 hours of the examination. This is not necessary in a patient who has diarrhea or active bleeding. Sedation is unnecessary.

Positioning

A prone jackknife is the position of choice. However, a left lateral position also gives an adequate examination and should be used in conditions such as pregnancy, severe hypertension, retinal detachment or postoperative eye surgery, and some apprehensive patients.

Technique

Although a standard proctosigmoidoscope is 25 cm in length, the average distance that the scope can be passed is 20 cm. In men, the scope can be passed to 21–25 cm half of the time, and in women, it can be passed that distance one-third of the time.[1] Rigid proctosigmoidoscopy is suitable only to examine the rectum and, in some patients, the distal sigmoid colon. The pain experienced from proctosigmoidoscopy is from stretching the mesentery of the rectosigmoid colon when the scope is pushed against the rectal wall, and from the air insufflation. When properly performed, rigid proctosigmoidoscopy should produce no pain or only mild discomfort. Most patients are fearful of the examination because of past bad experience with the procedure or from what they have heard. A few words of reassurance will be helpful.

With the obturator in place and held steady with the right thumb, the well-lubricated rigid proctosigmoidoscope is gently inserted into the anal canal, aiming toward the umbilicus for a distance of about 4–5 cm. Then the endoscope is angled toward the sacrum and advanced another 4–5 cm into the rectum. The obturator is removed and the bowel lumen is negotiated under direct vision. Air insufflation is limited to the amount necessary to open the lumen. When an angle is encountered, the endoscope is withdrawn 3–4 cm and then readvanced. This may be repeated several times to straighten the angulation. If further advancement is unsuccessful, the procedure is terminated at this point. Careful examination is done as the instrument is withdrawn. It is usually necessary to insufflate a small amount of air for good visualization of the lumen. The instrument should be rotated on withdrawal to ensure examination of the entire circumference. The mucosal folds in the rectum (valves of Houston) can be flattened with the tip of the endoscope to see the area behind them.

The length of insertion should be measured from the anal verge without stretching the bowel wall. Some physicians measure it in relation to the dentate line. The appearance of the mucosa and depth of insertion should be accurately described. If a lesion is seen, the size, appearance, location, and level must be recorded. If a biopsy is performed, the location, level, number of biopsies, and whether electrocoagulation is necessary should be noted. During the entire procedure, suction and water irrigation should be available.

Complications

If not careful, the tip of the endoscope can tear the mucosa; a small or moderate amount of bleeding may occur. Abdominal pain and distention can occur from excessive air insufflation.

Perforation from diagnostic rigid proctosigmoidoscopy is extremely rare. Gilbertsen[2] reported an incidence of five perforations in 103,000 examinations. Nelson et al.[3] reported two perforations in more than 16,000 examinations.

Flexible Sigmoidoscopy

The present-day flexible sigmoidoscope is no longer fiberoptic but contains a videochip at the tip of the endoscope. This videochip transmits the image through the processing unit to the monitor. The flexible videosigmoidoscope is 60 cm in functional length (Figure 5-6). The entire sigmoid colon can be reached by the flexible sigmoidoscope in 45%–85% of cases and, in a few, the splenic flexure can also be visualized.[4,5] The discrepancies in success depend on patient selection and the experience of the endoscopist. For selective screening examination, flexible sigmoidoscopy has a 3–6 times greater yield than does rigid proctosigmoidoscopy in detecting colonic and rectal abnormalities, especially neoplasms.[6,7] Because of this higher yield and better exposure, many physicians have discarded rigid proctosigmoidoscopy.

Indications

The role of flexible sigmoidoscopy is difficult to define because it can examine only the sigmoid colon and rectum in most cases. However, it is more convenient to use, and in many cases the entire colon need not be examined.

In acute diarrhea, flexible sigmoidoscopy can be used to rule out *Clostridium difficile* colitis, acute bacterial colitis, amebic colitis, and ischemic colitis particularly after aortic aneurysm repair. Flexible sigmoidoscopy is also an excellent tool to examine bright red rectal bleeding to detect its cause such as nonspecific proctitis, radiation proctitis, anorectal Crohn's disease, rectal ulcer, and also anorectal neoplasm. Flexible sigmoidoscopy is also used for colorectal cancer screening in conjunction with tests for fecal occult blood and to complement a barium enema examination. In this situation, CO_2 may be used for air insufflation if a barium enema is to follow.

Contraindications

Patients with severe anal pain from anal diseases may not tolerate the insertion of the scope. This also applies to anorectal stricture and colorectal anastomosis less than 2 weeks postoperatively. Other contraindications include acute sigmoid diverticulitis, toxic colitis, and patients with an acute abdomen.

Preparation

Bowel preparation with two Fleet enemas given within 2 hours of examination is adequate. The patient may eat normally. Patients with diarrhea do not require the enemas.

Positioning

Left lateral recumbent.

Technique

Sedation is unnecessary. The anal canal is lubricated by digital examination. A well-lubricated flexible sigmoidoscope is then inserted. Advancement of the endoscope is performed under direct vision. Pushing the endoscope through a bend in the bowel is a poor technique. Instead, the endoscope should be withdrawn to straighten the bowel. The key of success is short withdrawal and advancement of the endoscope or a to-and-fro movement, together with rotating the instrument clockwise and/or counterclockwise as needed. Use of air insufflation should be kept to a minimum. The procedure should be completed within 5–10 minutes. If a lesion is detected and proved by biopsy to be a neoplasm, a complete colonic investigation is indicated, ideally by total colonoscopy at some other date. A polyp up to 8 mm in size can be sampled with coagulation (hot) biopsy forceps or biopsied and electrocoagulated. To prevent possible explosion, because of hydrogen or methane gas in the lumen, air should be exchanged in the colon and rectum with repeated insufflation and suction. A larger polyp should be reserved for colonoscopy and polypectomy.

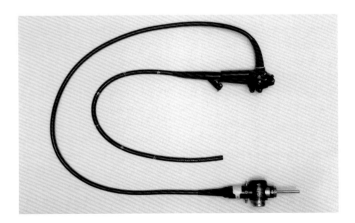

FIGURE 5-6. Flexible videosigmoidoscope.

Complications

Excessive air insufflation can cause acute abdominal distention and abdominal pain. This is best corrected by reinsertion of the endoscope and aspiration of air. Too rough and improper technique can cause perforation and other injuries.

The most common site of perforation in flexible sigmoidoscopy is in the distal sigmoid colon where it is angulated from the relatively fixed rectum at promontory of the sacrum. Complications from flexible sigmoidoscopy are uncommon but can be serious. They can be immediately apparent or delayed. Gatto et al.[8] reported a large population-based cohort that consisted of a random sample of 5% of Medicare beneficiaries living in the region of the United States covered by the Surveillance, Epidemiology, and End Results (SEER) program registries between 1991 and 1998. There were 35,298 flexible sigmoidoscopies performed. The perforation rate within 7 days of the procedure was 0.9 per 1000. Anderson et al.[9] evaluated the 10-year experience between 1987 and 1996 at Mayo Clinic, Scottsdale, AZ. There were 49,501 flexible sigmoidoscopies performed. Two perforations occurred: one of the perforations was in the cecum, likely from excessive air. Another perforation was in the sigmoid colon but was not detected until 17 days later as a pelvic abscess. Both required operation. There was no mortality. Levin et al.[10] analyzed 107,704 individuals who underwent 109,534 flexible sigmoidoscopic screenings as part of Colorectal Cancer Prevention Program from 1994 to 1996 at North California Kaiser Permanente Medical Care Program. There were two perforations, two episodes of diverticulitis requiring operation, two cases of bleeding requiring blood transfusion, and one episode of unexplained colitis. In this study in multivariate models, complications were significantly more common in men than in women (odds ratio, 3.34; confidence interval, 95%).

Ileoscopy

Examination of the small intestine via an ileostomy can be performed using a rigid proctosigmoidoscope or a flexible sigmoidoscope.

Indications

Indications for endoscoping the terminal ileum are few. Most of the time it is to rule out recurrent Crohn's disease or to find an abnormality in patients with high ileostomy output.

Contraindications

Stricture of the stoma.

Preparation

Bowel preparation is not required, but it is helpful if the patient has been on a clear liquid diet for 1 day. Sedation is not required.

Positioning

Supine.

Technique

The examination starts with a digital examination to gently dilate the stoma, which is frequently slightly stenotic. The well-lubricated rigid scope is introduced directly into the ileostomy. The terminal ileum is quite active with frequent spasm. It requires more air insufflation than scoping the rectum. The distance traversed by the endoscope is usually limited to 12–15 cm. In patients with a large para-ileostomy hernia, the endoscope may usually not be passed beyond 10 cm.

Flexible sigmoidoscopy is much easier to perform. The angulation of the small bowel can be straightened by push, pull, and rotation of the scope. A moderate amount of air insufflation is usually required.

Complications

The small bowel has thin walls and requires gentle maneuvering of the endoscope. Perforation can easily occur. If an angle cannot be straightened, the procedure should be terminated.

Pouchoscopy

Kock Pouch or Continent Ileostomy

Indications

Although the ileoanal pouch has almost completely replaced the Kock pouch, there are still many patients with a Kock pouch constructed more than 30 years ago. One of the most common problems that require endoscopy is the extrusion or slippage of the valve causing difficulty or impossibility of intubation to evacuate the stool. The examination is performed to help decompress the obstructed pouch and to place a draining tube. Other indications included Crohn's disease and complication of the pouch with fistulas and high output of the pouch. Both rigid and flexible endoscopes can be used. Church et al.[11] advised using a pediatric flexible endoscope.

Contraindications

Stricture of the stoma.

Preparation

Bowel preparation is unnecessary and sedation is not usually required. If possible, the pouch should be emptied or irrigated just before the examination. It is also preferable if the patient has been on a clear liquid diet for 1 day before the procedure.

Positioning

Supine.

Technique

The endoscope can usually be passed easily into the pouch with inspection of the stoma being performed on insertion or withdrawal. The pouch can be lavaged as necessary.

A general inspection of the pouch is performed noting the mucosal appearance, the pouch size, distensibility, and the status of suture lines. If possible, the afferent loop of ileum should be intubated, especially in patients presenting with pouch inflammation. The endoscope must be retroflexed within the pouch to check valve length and symmetry. A careful search for foreign material should be made, particularly around the base of the valve. If mesh was used to reinforce the nipple valve, a fistula may form at this area. In patients with extrusion of the valve, passing the endoscope will be difficult.

For an obstructed pouch from a slipped valve, Church et al.[11] used a flexible endoscope as an obturator to insert the rigid proctosigmoidoscope. The rigid endoscope is placed over the flexible endoscope, which is itself inserted into the pouch. The rigid endoscope is advanced over the flexible endoscope into the pouch. Now the flexible endoscope can be withdrawn and a drainage catheter inserted to temporarily relieve the obstruction. Surgical repair of the nipple valve is required.

Complications

Perforation can occur, particularly when there is an obstruction of the pouch.

Ileoanal Pouch

Examination of the ileoanal pouch is best performed using a flexible sigmoidoscope although a rigid proctoscope can also be used. Unless there is an anastomotic anal stricture, the examination is usually easy. The endoscope can be used to examine the entire pouch and usually the terminal ileum proximal to the pouch.

Indications

Examination of the pouch is indicated for patients with bleeding from the pouch, diarrhea, recent onset of fecal incontinence, obstructive symptoms, pouchitis, for surveillance follow-up examination to exclude neoplastic changes, and to rule out Crohn's disease.

Contraindications

Severe anal or anastomotic stricture.

Preparation

The patient is prepared by taking clear liquids for 1 day or administered a small enema before the examination. Sedation is not required.

Positioning

Left lateral recumbent.

Technique

The examination starts with a digital examination to evaluate the anal canal and the anal anastomosis. If there is a stricture, it should first be dilated with a finger or with Hegar dilators.

The well-lubricated flexible sigmoidoscope or a colonoscope is introduced into the anal canal. The endoscope is advanced into the pouch. The terminal ileum proximal to the pouch can usually be intubated. The examiner should evaluate the mucosa of the pouch and anal canal for any edema of the mucosa, granularity, mucosal bleeding, contact bleeding, erosion, fibrin exudate, pattern of mucosal ulceration, plaque, and mass. Abnormal mucosa should be biopsied. Only cold biopsy should be performed.

Complications

Tear of the anal canal can occur if there is stricture of the anus or anastomosis. Traumatic injury from the scope may cause moderate bleeding but it usually stops spontaneously. A perforation can occur from the instrumentation or a biopsy.

Colonoscopy

With the many imaging methods available for evaluation and often therapy of colorectal disorders, colonoscopy has emerged as the gold standard for diagnosis. It is also, in some areas, an increasingly frequent option for therapy, be it definitive or palliative.

Indications

Indications for diagnostic colonoscopy include: the evaluation of virtually all symptoms associated with potential benign or malignant, acute, or chronic diseases of the colorectum; for resolution of abnormalities seen on other imaging modalities; for investigating otherwise unexplained symptoms such as anemia; the evaluation of chronic and acute bleeding per annum; for screening and surveillance of patients at high risk for colon adenomas or carcinoma; and localization of nonpalpable lesions at open or laparoscopic operation. It is also increasingly possible to combine diagnostic colonoscopy and other imaging techniques such as ultrasound.

Contraindications

Contraindications to diagnostic colonoscopy may be classified as *absolute* or *relative*. Although colonoscopy is appropriately considered a minimally invasive procedure, there are risks involved that may be avoided, or at least minimized, by careful patient selection and certainly these risks should be discussed before the performance of the procedure.

Absolute contraindications are suspected bowel perforation or recent anastomosis, established peritonitis, and fulminant colitis.

Relative contraindications include suspected ischemia and acute colitis, in either of which instance an experienced examiner may safely perform a limited examination. Active bleeding is a relative contraindication unless the examiner has had significant experience with elective diagnostic colonoscopy and we believe the procedure should not be attempted if one is unprepared to provide, or for the patient to accept, treatment of complications of the procedure.

Preparation

Preparation for colonoscopy, of necessity, should include preparation of the endoscopist, preparation of the patient in general, and of the colon specifically. Several organizations have prepared and published guidelines for credentialing the individual who is permitted to perform colonoscopy in an institutional setting[12] and, in some institutions, Credentials Committees have been established that grant privileges. Although there is some controversy involving required numbers of experiences in training, all recommendations include the following elements: background knowledge of anatomy, physiology, and pathology of the colon as well as familiarity with instruments and accessories used in endoscopy; some formal training; and quality assurance practices. The concept of proctoring has also been addressed by some.[13] Equipment for resuscitation should be available and individuals qualified to perform cardiopulmonary resuscitation should be present in the area where colonoscopy is performed. We cannot overstate the necessity for qualified assistance during the performance of the procedure and for monitoring the patient's condition.

Obtaining informed consent is an opportunity for discussing with the patient elements of the past and present medical history, especially medications and operative procedures, which may expose psychological concerns or the need to modify preparation, add prophylactic antibiotics, or change medication, timing, and dosage. In other words, taking an adequate history and performing pertinent physical examination are important. It is necessary to point out the potential hazards of colonoscopy, noting aspects of the process that might cause discomfort but it is also important to give reassurance that although the risk of complication is low the examiner is prepared for prompt management. The question of the need for antibiotic prophylaxis stems from concern that although diagnostic colonoscopy is a low risk procedure for bacteremia, infection of damaged cardiac valves or implanted prosthesis is a risk. The American Heart Association and the American Society of Colon and Rectal Surgeons have issued joint guidelines recommending antibiotic prophylaxis for patients with certain conditions associated with carditis.[14]

These recommendations include implanted prostheses, primarily orthopedic.

Thorough mechanical preparation of the colon is absolutely essential for efficient, safe, and complete endoscopic examination. In addition, should perforation occur, the empty colon certainly poses less risk of significant peritoneal contamination. There are various forms of mechanical preparation possible but the most thorough and safest current regimen involves the use of polyethylene glycol electrolyte lavage solutions. Other forms of preparation that are sometimes used involve ingestion of a saline cathartic (usually sodium phosphate or magnesium citrate) as well as enemas. With the latter, there is more concern about electrolyte imbalance especially in patients taking diuretic medications chronically or those with renal insufficiency. Some patients after gastrectomy may experience symptoms of dumping after saline cathartic administration.

Monitoring

Although the use of pulse oximetry and intermittent monitoring of blood pressure as well as electrocardiography (if clinically indicated) have now become standard procedures, it is important for the assistant as well as the endoscopist to be aware of any changes in the patient's level of awareness, respiration, and abdominal distention.

Bleeding Prophylaxis

Although bleeding is rarely associated with diagnostic colonoscopy, there are concerns about bleeding at or after colonoscopy, if biopsy or polypectomy are contemplated, and this has led to modification of anticoagulation regimens and cessation of drugs that might alter platelet function. There are no universally accepted guidelines for management of antiplatelet therapy in relation to endoscopy, especially because cessation of these agents may increase the risk of thromboembolism in some of these patients. If a particular patient has a known hematologic disorder (for example, factor V deficiency), precautions should be taken to optimize the coagulation potential by correcting missing or deficient factors as necessary before initiation of the endoscopic procedure.

Technique

For successful passage of the colonoscope to the most proximal desired anatomic region (cecum or anastomosis), it is imperative that a few principles be understood.[15] The examiner must appreciate that the colon is of variable length, that respiratory and peristaltic activity is in progress during the examination, and that some areas of the colon are more fixed (by normal anatomy, previous inflammation, or postoperative change). It is dangerous to proceed with introduction of the endoscope without knowing at all times the location of the lumen.

Before starting the examination, the equipment should be checked to verify that it is in good working order. It should be verified that irrigation, suction, and air insufflation channels are open and that the directional controls are in the unlocked position.

With the patient in the left lateral recumbent position, the examination is initiated by thoroughly inspecting the perianal area for fissures, fistulae, hemorrhoids, condylomata, and rarer conditions such as melanoma, Bowen's disease, extramammary Paget's disease, squamous and anal gland carcinomas. Next, the lubricated gloved right index finger is inserted into the anus and a rectal examination carefully performed, giving especial attention to the surface of the prostate gland in the middle aged and older male patient. With the right index finger still in the rectum, the endoscopist then holds the tip of the instrument in the left hand, places it at right angles to the right index finger, and by effacing the sphincter with gentle pressure of the right index finger, the instrument tip can be gently inserted as the right index finger is withdrawn. The examiner then grasps the head of the instrument in the palm of the left hand, leaving the thumb and index finger free to manipulate the knobs for tip deflection with the former and the air and water insufflation as well as suction buttons with the other. The right hand is placed on the instrument shaft. With the instrument in the rectal ampulla, it is usually necessary to insufflate the lumen with a small amount of air in order to visualize the direction of the lumen.

The main objective on insertion of the instrument is to reach the most proximal point desired in as expeditiously a manner as possible, leaving detailed inspection until the process of withdrawal of the endoscope. However, detection of an abnormality on insertion may require a change in strategy. For example, it may be important to detect, localize, sometimes biopsy, or even remove a small lesion for fear of not being able to find it easily on withdrawal. In some circumstances, therefore, at least localization and biopsy should be performed, even on insertion.

One of the earliest challenges to insertion is advancing the instrument into the descending colon. The unprepared examiner, looking at the stylized cartoons of many an endoscopy record form and even many anatomic and surgical textbooks may not recognize how long the sigmoid colon can be and how easy it may be to insert a considerable length of the instrument into it. Because the sigmoid is usually not fixed, it accepts the instrument so readily that when the acute angle at the junction of the sigmoid and (fixed) descending colon is reached, the unprepared examiner may think that he/she has achieved insertion to the splenic flexure. Attempts at further insertion may be hindered then by the loop created in the sigmoid colon. Most of the time this frustrating situation may be entirely avoided by attempting to keep the sigmoid collapsed and shortened as early as possible. We have found that a clockwise turn with the right hand on the shaft of the instrument and with jiggling of the shaft as well as back and forth motion will often allow the bowel to fall over the instrument,

so to speak, allowing insertion with a less than one-to-one motion. It is this pleating or accordioning of the bowel over the instrument with alternating release that allows for efficient advancement and more than one-to-one motion. As a matter of fact, the recognition of this intermittent intussusception and reduction as part of the normal advancement of the instrument makes it understandable that, in estimating the extent of intubation or the location of a lesion, the least accurate determination is measuring on the shaft of the instrument.

Having entered the descending colon with the sigmoid shortened and "straight," it is usually quite easy to advance to and around the splenic flexure. Difficulty in intubation beyond the splenic flexure is, in our experience, more common when the patient has undergone previous operation within this area with adhesions in the left upper quadrant that may produce fixation. If the endoscopist recognizes the distal transverse colon by endoscopic anatomy or transmitted cardiac apical pulsation that one is in, it is to be recalled that, similar to the sigmoid, the transverse colon is on a long mesentery and is rarely fixed. The hepatic flexure can be more easily reached by keeping the transverse colon as collapsed as possible.

The hepatic is often a more complicated flexure than is the splenic and one may wander a while before entering the distal ascending colon. However, once the latter has been entered and there has been no prior right abdominal operation (for example, cholecystectomy, appendectomy), the cecum is often rapidly reached by application of suction to collapse the bowel over the instrument. It is important to be fully cognizant of the vagaries of endoscopic anatomy in order to confirm cecal intubation—by visualization of the appendiceal orifice and the ileocecal valve. Looking for translumination from the instrument tip through the abdominal wall in the right lower quadrant is, unfortunately, a trap for the unsophisticated endoscopist who uses it to verify cecal entry. It merely points out that the instrument tip is in the right lower quadrant but the endoscopic tip may be in any mobile part of the colon, for example, the transverse colon or even the sigmoid. In fact, the student of anatomy recognizes that the cecum is not always in the right lower quadrant.

There are aids to overcoming obstacles to cecal intubation. A common one is the attempt to keep the sigmoid in a straight position so that on further insertion the tip may progress proximally. Abdominal pressure by an assistant is often used in an attempt to keep the sigmoid from reforming a loop once it has already been straightened. We think it important not to expect or direct the assistant to reduce the loop by compression because this could theoretically lead to injury of the bowel wall. Rather, the sigmoid has to be straightened and then pressure may be used to keep the loop from being re-formed. If one reviews a series of barium enema films or has acquaintance with the position of the omega loop of the sigmoid at abdominal operation, it helps to understand these maneuvers. For those who have the capability of fluoroscopy in their endoscopy units, much can be learned and much assistance provided in this maneuver, especially in the individual's early endoscopic experience. For one, it is humbling to recognize how inaccurate one can be of the extent of insertion or the shape of the bowel with the endoscope inserted. There are two recent developments in endoscopic and related instrumentation that may facilitate overcoming the difficult sigmoid loop, still the most challenging aspect of diagnostic colonoscopy.

One recent development in the design of some colonoscopies is the ability of the endoscopist to vary the stiffness of the endoscope to allow a previously shortened and straightened segment of bowel from re-forming a loop. The assumption is that the endoscopist knows with certainty that the loop has been adequately reduced and that it is safe to insert a now more rigid instrument. Those who have expertise with fluoroscopy know that this can be a fallible assumption. Another development is an extracorporeal magnetic device that can track the course and shape of the endoscope during insertion.[16] If proven accurate, this device could potentially obviate fluoroscopy for localization, reduction of difficult loops, and even allow for safer stiffening of the endoscope using either a variable-stiffness endoscope or the external splinting device introduced by Shinya in the early days of colonoscopy.

Certainly, the external splinting device should never be used without the benefit of fluoroscopic assistance because, with an angulated segment of bowel, it is possible to damage the bowel wall if the mucosa is caught in the space between the edge of the splinting device and the shaft of the instrument. When using the external splinting device, the fluoroscope is used to first verify that the tip of the instrument is just beyond the splenic flexure and acutely angled (Figure 5-7). The deflection knobs are then placed in the locked position and, as the instrument is withdrawn and the sigmoid loop

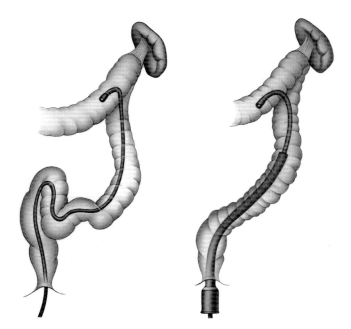

FIGURE 5-7. Use of external splint.

straightened under fluoroscopic control, the external splint is advanced over the endoscope up to, but not beyond, the proximal descending colon.[14] One does not wish to advance it to the splenic flexure where the lienocolic ligament may be vulnerable to avulsion. An assistant has to keep the splinting device fixed at the anus so that the examiner does not insert it further than desired during the remainder of the examination.

External manipulation may also be helpful in two other circumstances. Sometimes the transverse colon, having a long mesentery, may form a loop extending well into the pelvis. Reduction of this loop by withdrawing the instrument and using suction will usually achieve rapid progress into the ascending colon. But one can sometimes keep the loop from re-forming by having an assistant apply pressure from the right abdomen directed to the left upper quadrant (because the transverse colon mesentery is longer on the right and the loop is therefore more prominent in the right portion of the abdomen or pelvis). If the cecum is not fixed (as from prior operation, for example, appendectomy or pelvic surgery), it may be possible with gentle pressure on the abdominal wall to collapse it onto the tip of the instrument, remembering, however, that the cecum is not always in the right lower quadrant. Sometimes placing the patient in the prone position allows easier intubation of the cecum.

On withdrawal of the instrument, one has to be sure that the entire mucosa is visualized. As one withdraws the instrument and the bowel recedes, inspection is accomplished but it requires close attention because one can easily withdraw too rapidly as a previously accordioned segment escapes without the examiner's control. It may be necessary to go back over an area not adequately visualized initially. In this connection, adequate preparation is even more important at this time than on insertion. If liquid material is present but too thick to be aspirated by suction through the instrument channel, one may purposefully change the patient's position to allow the fluid to shift to another area. Withdrawal through the sigmoid colon perforce requires more time and attention because there are more folds and recesses. Although the experienced examiner can usually withdraw very slowly through the anal canal and thus visualize its entire circumference, this is sometimes better if complemented by retroflexing the tip of the instrument in the anal ampulla to visualize the region of the dentate line (if the rectal ampulla is readily distensible). As the endoscope is withdrawn through each segment of the colon, it is useful to decompress each examined segment with suction so that at the conclusion of the examination the abdomen is minimally distended.

Normal Endoscopic Anatomy

Some segments of the colon are more readily recognized than others and one has to be careful not to be overconfident unless a classic appearance is present. On insertion it is important to first recognize the three rectal valves of Houston because the relationship of a lesion to them will have great relevance if surgical intervention is to be contemplated. Diverticula may be seen throughout the intraperitoneal colon but rarely below the peritoneal reflection. The descending colon, being fixed along the white line of Toldt, will often present a long straight "tunnel view." Occasionally the splenic flexure is specifically recognized if there is an external bulging bluish mass indenting the colon, descending with respiration. More common in the sigmoid colon, diverticula may be seen throughout the length of the large intestine. Their orifices may be so wide that they may be mistaken for the bowel lumen. It is therefore safer to back away somewhat and have a longer view to be sure of the location of the lumen. In any one field of view, the diverticulum will of course be at right angles to the lumen (Figure 5-8).

The transverse colon, on insertion, being suspended by the three taenia coli presents the appearance of an equilateral triangle (the so-called "cathedral ceiling" appearance). Quite often, the distal transverse colon can be identified in relation to the proximal because the point of maximal impulse of the heart is transmitted through the diaphragm which overlies the distal transverse colon. Especially in thin patients, the liver casts a broad, flat, bluish-green cast outside the colon but because this may be seen for a variable distance from distal transverse colon to mid-ascending colon, it is not particularly helpful with localization of a lesion, from a surgeon's point of view. At the hepatic flexure, the colon often assumes a spiral configuration which can cause the taenia to so approximate each other as to make the novice assume the cecum has been reached (what one of us has called "the fool's cecum").

The interhaustral folds in the ascending colon are low in profile compared with those in the left colon. The ileocecal valve is usually recognized as an eccentric bulge with a sometimes visible umbilication. Because there is more adipose tissue in it, the appearance is often a yellowish color compared with the pink of the rest of the colon. The ileocecal valve is rarely seen head on but is, of course, more easily recognizable when it is. It is important to intubate proximal to the valve because the true caput of the colon may be at a variable distance form the ileocecal valve. As the three taenia come together at the caput (often appearing like the branches of a tree or a crow's foot), the appendiceal orifice is usually recognized, even in the patient who has undergone previous appendectomy.

Abnormal Findings

Exophytic lesions are the easiest to visualize and recognize at colonoscopy, the most common being adenocarcinoma. All polypoid lesions of the colon may be visualized at colonoscopy and virtually all have distinguishing characteristics. Several are submucosal (lymphoid hyperplasia, stromal tumors, lipomas, carcinoids, endometriomas, hemangiomas, neurofibromas, lymphoma). A few are metastatic from other organs (for example, prostate, pancreas, kidney). The diagnosis of most of these lesions can be made by endoscopic visualization or sampling. Some, being of no clinical consequence, require only recognition (lymphoid, hyperplasia, lipoma).

In addition to lesions that protrude, there are numerous inflammatory or degenerative conditions that have a recognizable endoscopic appearance and many can be safely sampled if necessary. These include the various colitides (bacterial, viral, ulcerative, granulomatous), ischemia, radiation proctopathy (formerly called "proctitis") and melanosis

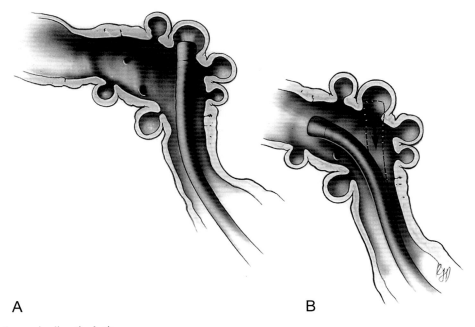

A   B

FIGURE 5-8. Finding lumen in diverticulosis.

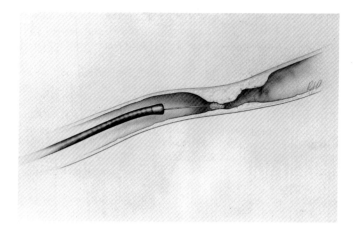

FIGURE 5-9. Cytology through stricture.

coli. Melanosis coli, when marked, may help in visualization of adenomatous tissue because the pigment is not deposited in only normal mucosa. Areas of angiodysplasia (vascular ectasias, arteriovenous malformations) can be recognized on diagnostic colonoscopy but must be distinguished from bruises created from instrumentation or even preparation. The endoscopist has to recognize colonic anatomy disturbed by previous operation and therefore has to be familiar with the variety of intestinal anastomoses performed.

Areas of stenosis and stricture may be encountered secondary to benign conditions (previous resection and anastomosis, diverticulitis, colitis, radiation injury) or malignancy. Other rare findings to be recognized include: colitis cystica profunda, pneumatosis, and Behçet's syndrome. The manner in which the nature of a lesion is established at diagnostic colonoscopy will vary. A tiny sessile lesion (for example, a diminutive polyp) may be removed in its entirety with the biopsy forceps for pathologic examination. A pedunculated lesion suspected of being a benign adenoma may be removed at the time of diagnostic examination by snare polypectomy. A sessile lesion suspected of being a carcinoma or villous adenoma may be biopsied at one or more sites or even partially removed with a snare and cautery to obtain a satisfactory specimen. A stricture may be sampled for possible malignant cells by advancing a cytology brush into the stricture ahead of the colonoscope (Figure 5-9). Malignant cells may thus be harvested even though the stricture cannot be traversed with the endoscope. A lesion that appears vascular and friable may be simply photographed. A submucosal lesion may be exposed by disrupting the overlying mucosa.

Complications

Although colonoscopy is, in general, a safe procedure, it is invasive and adverse events do occur. The most common serious complication of diagnostic colonoscopy is perforation with the reported incidence of 0.03%–0.65% and the mortality of 0.01%–0.02%.[17-19] Other reported complications

include abdominal distension, dehydration, respiratory depression, vasovagal reaction, thrombophlebitis, incarcerated hernia, splenic capsular tear and subcutaneous and/or mediastinal emphysema, and equipment failure.

In diagnostic colonoscopy, perforation may be caused by the instrument itself, traction on a fixed segment of colon, or over-insufflation of a segment, especially a closed loop as may occur in patients with multiple strictures (inflammatory bowel disease) or as a consequence of prior radiation therapy and with hernia incarceration. Impaction of the instrument in a diverticulum with overdistention of the latter has also been a cause of perforation. Adequate training and experience should decrease adverse events to a minimum. Because perforation is related to the use of coagulation ("hot") biopsy forceps and because of the low risk of bleeding from multiple forceps biopsies, use of the hot biopsy technique has declined. Perforation during diagnostic colonoscopy tends to be detected earlier when it is from instrumental causes, whereas perforation from therapeutic procedures is frequently related to thermal injury and is often delayed. Indeed, the management of perforation after colonoscopy is still controversial.[20] Whereas there is universal agreement that perforation with generalized peritonitis demands an operation, some believe that if the onset of symptoms is delayed, signs are localized, and the patient is not septic (even with the demonstration of pneumoperitoneum) that nonoperative management may be followed. An uncommon presentation of a contained perforation may be the presence of retroperitoneal or mediastinal air and even subcutaneous emphysema, which usually resolves without drainage.

Avoidance of perforation during diagnostic colonoscopy, related as it is to training, skill, and experience may be best achieved by the following: avoidance of dehydration and oversedation; discontinuation of the procedure if the preparation is poor; avoiding forceful instrument insertion; recognition of vulnerable bowel (inflammation, ischemia, narrowing, fixation); careful identification and avoidance of diverticular ostia; avoidance of bowing of the instrument; awareness of fixation from pelvic adhesions or tumor extending through and beyond the colon wall; ensuring that abdominal and inguinal hernias remain reduced; avoiding over-insufflation; and looping in the splenic flexure region. There should be constant identification of the location of the lumen with avoidance of "slide by" (sidewise passage of the instrument without direct visualization of the lumen), not attempting colonoscopy during acute bleeding if one has not had adequate experience with routine diagnostic colonoscopy.

If perforation occurs, early diagnosis will ensure more efficient management. Undue and sustained pain (especially shoulder discomfort), absence of liver dullness on percussion, demonstration of pneumoperitoneum on upright chest film, and subcutaneous emphysema all help in making the diagnosis. Signs and symptoms will in general be related to factors such as adequacy of bowel preparation, size of injury, and underlying pathologic state of the colon. For example, the ischemic colon or one involved with active colitis will be more vulnerable to instrumental injury. Surgical intervention is favored by most surgeons for early recognized perforation at diagnostic colonoscopy. There are, however, some patients with either a delayed perforation or one that has remained localized without symptoms or signs of diffuse peritonitis. Nonoperative management but continuing observation of this subset of patients may be entirely satisfactory. With early surgical intervention of a mechanical perforation, if technically feasible, primary closure with or without protective proximal stoma is, of course, the most desirable and usually is feasible. However, the surgeon must use good judgment in assessment of such factors as adequacy of tissue perfusion, degree of spillage, and colon tissue free of inflammation.

References

1. Nivatvongs S, Fryd DS. How far does the proctosigmoidoscope reach? A prospective study of 1000 patients. N Engl J Med 1980; 303:380–382.
2. Gilbertsen VA. Proctosigmoidoscopy and polypectomy in reducing the incidence of rectal cancer. Cancer 1974;34(suppl):936–939.
3. Nelson RL, Abcarian H, Prasad ML. Iatrogenic perforation of the colon and rectum. Dis Colon Rectum 1982;25:305–308.
4. Lehman GA, Buchner DM, Lappas JC. Anatomic extent of fiberoptic sigmoidoscopy. Gastroenterology 1983;84:803–808.
5. Ott DJ, Wu WC, Gelfand DW. Extent of colonic visualization with fiberoptic sigmoidoscope. J Clin Gastroenterol 1982;4:337–341.
6. Marks G, Boggs HW, Castro AF, Gathright JR, Ray JE, Salvati E. Sigmoidoscopic examinations with rigid and flexible fiberoptic sigmoidoscopes in the surgeon's office. A comparative prospective study of effectiveness in 1012 cases. Dis Colon Rectum 1979;22:162–168.
7. Winnan G, Berci G, Parrish J, Talbot TM, Overholt BF, McCallum RW. Superiority of the flexible to the rigid sigmoidoscope in routine proctosigmoidoscopy. N Engl J Med 1980; 302:1011–1012.
8. Gatto NM, Frucht H, Sundararajan V, Jacobson JS, Grann VR, Neugut AI. Risk of perforation after colonoscopy and sigmoidoscopy: a population-based study. J Natl Cancer Inst 2003;95: 230–236.
9. Anderson ML, Pasha TM, Leighton JA. Endoscopic perforation of the colon: Lessons from a 10-year study. Ann J Gastroenterol 2000;95:3418–3422.
10. Levin TR, Conell C, Shapiro JA, Chazan SG, Nadel MR, Selby JV. Complications of screening flexible sigmoidoscopy. Gastroenterology 2002;123:1786–1792.
11. Church JM, Fazio VW, Lavery IC. The role of fiberoptic endoscopy in the management of the continent ileostomy. Gastrointest Endosc 1987;33:203–209.
12. Society of American Gastrointestinal Endoscopic Surgery (SAGES). Granting of privileges for gastrointestinal endoscopy by surgeons. Los Angeles: SAGES; 1992.
13. Society of American Gastrointestinal Endoscopic Surgeons (SAGES) framework for postresidency surgical education and training: a SAGES guideline. Surg Endosc 1994;8:1137–1142.
14. Practice parameters for antibiotic prophylaxis to prevent infective endocarditis or infective prosthesis during colon and rectal endoscopy. Dis Colon Rectum 2000;43:1193.
15. Forde KA, Technique of diagnostic colonoscopy. In: Greene FI, Ponsky JL, eds. Endoscopic Surgery. Philadelphia: Saunders; 1994:219–234.
16. Shah SG, Pearson HJ, Moss S, et al. Magnetic endoscopic imaging: a new technique for localizing colonic lesions. Endoscopy 2002;34:900–904.
17. Ackroyd FW. Complications of flexible endoscopy. In: Greene FL, Ponsky JL, eds. Endoscopic Surgery. Philadelphia: Saunders; 1994:440–441.
18. Korman LY, Overholt BF, Box T, et al. Perforation during colonoscopy in endoscopic ambulatory surgical centers. Gastrointest Endosc 2003;58:554–557.
19. Wexner SD, Forde KA, Sellers G, et al. How well can surgeons perform colonoscopy? Surg Endosc 1998;12:1410–1414.
20. Damore LJ, Rantis PC, Vernava AM, et al. Colonoscopic perforations. Dis Colon Rectum 1996;39:1308–1314.

6
Diagnostic Evaluations—Radiology, Nuclear Scans, PET, CT Colography

Matthew G. Mutch, Elisa H. Birnbaum, and Christine O. Menias

The goal of this text is not to provide the definitive chapter on gastrointestinal (GI) radiology, but rather to provide a sturdy foundation for the techniques, indications, and interpretation of radiologic imaging studies used in everyday colon and rectal surgery practices. Diagnostic radiology is the application of data or image acquisition to our knowledge of anatomy and pathology. Advances in technology have allowed us to diagnose many common diseases at earlier stages as well as identify new pathology previously not detectable with radiologic studies.

Plain Films

The information or picture provided by plain films is the result of differential absorption of the X-rays by the various components of the abdominal wall, bony skeleton, and the intraabdominal contents. In particular, it is the interfaces between the different anatomic planes created by the inherent contrast of the various tissues attributed to the relative fat content of each structure and intraluminal gas of the GI tract that gives the image seen on the film. It is these interfaces that allow for the delineation of the liver edge, renal shadow, psoas shadow and differentiation of the patterns of the stomach, small bowel, and colon. The typical flat plate X-ray uses 60–75 kV to expose each film. This varies depending on the equipment used and the size of the patient. A reciprocating grid and collimation are used to reduce scatter of the radiation and improve tissue contrast.

Controversy exists over the number of views or films needed to adequately examine the abdomen. Classical teaching recommends three views consisting of a supine abdomen, upright or lateral decubitus abdomen, and upright chest. The rationale for these films is as follows[1]: 1) the supine abdomen offers the most detail and contrast of the intraabdominal structures; 2) the upright or decubitus abdominal views allow for a change in intraluminal gas distribution and identification of extraluminal free-air; 3) the upright chest contributes diagnostic information in 20% of cases.[2] However, Mirvis et al.[3]

argued that the upright abdominal view was unnecessary. They reviewed 252 examinations and found that the supine abdominal and upright chest films alone provided the diagnosis 98% of the time. Whether two or three films are obtained is of secondary importance as long as the entire abdomen is viewed and the examination is able to address the clinical scenario in question.

Plain films clearly do not offer as much anatomic detail as the cross-sectional imaging modalities, but they remain highly sensitive and specific when there is suspicion of a bowel obstruction or a perforated viscus.[4] Other useful indications for plain films include longitudinal examination of megacolon, identification of foreign bodies, check positions of drains or catheters, and evaluation of associated skeletal diseases.

Intestinal Obstruction

Small Bowel Obstruction

Investigation of intestinal obstruction, whether it is small versus large bowel or mechanical versus functional, is a common indication for abdominal plain films. The signs and symptoms of a small or large bowel obstruction depends on the location and extent of the obstruction and can include nausea, vomiting, abdominal pain, abdominal distention, and obstipation. Just as the clinical manifestations of the obstruction depend on its location so do its radiographic findings. Duration of symptoms, significant emesis, use of a nasogastric tube, and degree of obstruction also contribute to the radiographic appearance of a bowel obstruction. With regard to small bowel obstruction (SBO), the most common causes in descending order are adhesions, Crohn's disease, neoplasia, and hernia.[5] Abdominal plain films have been shown to be diagnostic in 50%–66% of cases with approximately 20% false-negative rate.[4]

The radiographic diagnosis of an SBO depends on the intraluminal gas pattern projected upon the plain film. A normal gas pattern is defined as small amounts of gas distributed throughout the small and large bowel without bowel distention (<2.5 cm in diameter). An abnormal gas pattern is a variable amount of gas in the presence of one or more loops of dilated small bowel (>2.5 cm in diameter).[6] The mucosal markings of the small bowel, known as the plicae circularis, traverse the entire diameter of the lumen and help to distinguish it from the colon, which has haustral markings that project into the lumen but do not reach the opposite wall. The amount of intraluminal fluid or material also greatly affects the radiographic appearance of the intestinal gas pattern. Air-fluid levels, which are the dependent layering of fluid and air within a dilated loop of intestine when viewed in the upright position, are common radiographic findings of an SBO. A complete or high-grade SBO is characterized by dilated loops of small bowel, air-fluid levels, and absence of colonic gas (Figure 6-1A and B). There can be a single or multiple dilated loops of small bowel, and the dilated bowel loops may also be stacked on top of each other giving it a ladder-like appearance. Generally, the more dilated loops of intestine present, the more distal the obstruction is located. Several factors can confound the radiographic appearance of an SBO. First, a distal bowel obstruction may appear to be more proximal when the distal bowel is filled with fluid and not gas. If the obstruction has been longstanding or the patient has had excessive vomiting, the bowel may be completely filled with fluid and have a complete absence of gas. Clues that support the diagnosis of an SBO in a gasless abdomen are a ground-glass

appearance and loss of solid organ outlines such as the liver edge, renal shadow, and the psoas shadow. These findings are consistent with significant intraabdominal and intraluminal sequestration of fluid. Second, the presence of colonic gas in the setting of dilated small bowel and air-fluid levels is compatible with an early SBO without complete evacuation of distal gas, a partial SBO, or an adynamic ileus. If the diagnosis is uncertain clinically and radiographically, then a follow-up study with either computed tomography (CT) or small bowel contrast study is warranted.

Plain films are not able to reliably differentiate a simple obstruction from a strangulating obstruction. Findings that are considered to be high risk for vascular compromise include complete bowel obstruction, extensive mucosal thickening or edema, pneumatosis, portal venous gas, or a closed loop obstruction. A study of 51 patients with radiographic findings of a complete SBO found 29% of patients had infarcted bowel requiring resection.[7] This highlights the importance of interpreting the radiographic data in the context of the patient's clinical condition.

Large Bowel Obstruction

Colonic obstructions typically present with the same signs and symptoms as an SBO. The most common causes of large bowel obstruction are carcinoma, volvulus, Ogilvie's syndrome, and fecal impaction. Other etiologies include Crohn's

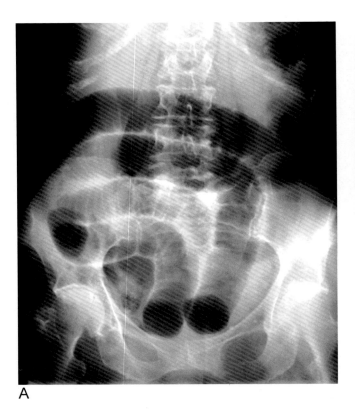

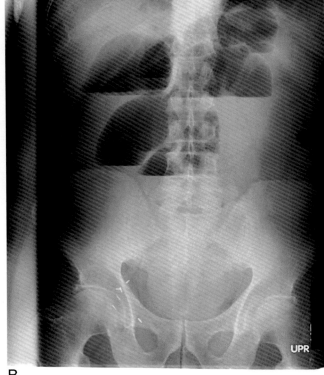

A

B

FIGURE 6-1. **A** Plain film of SBO dilated loops, ladder. **B** SBO air-fluid levels.

disease, diverticulitis, ischemic stricture, anastomotic stricture, and endometriosis.

Cancer

Typically the colon will be distended up to the point of obstruction with a paucity of distal gas. If the ileocecal valve (ICV) is competent, the cecum can be markedly dilated and there may be little dilation of the small bowel (Figure 6-2). With a competent ICV, the entire colon becomes dilated and the cecum has the greatest distensibility. Once the cecal diameter reaches >12 cm, it is generally agreed that the risk of impending perforation is high. However, if the ICV is incompetent, gas can reflux back into the small bowel. As a result, the colon may not be all that dilated and the small bowel may become dilated with air-fluid levels mimicking an SBO (Figure 6-3). In this case, careful review of clinical data is necessary to guide the next diagnostic evaluation.

If a colonic obstruction is suspected, the diagnosis can be confirmed with a water-soluble contrast enema. It is difficult to differentiate the etiology of the obstruction with plain films so a contrast enema can give significant information regarding the cause of the obstruction. Water-soluble contrast is preferred over barium in this situation for several reasons. First, this avoids the risk of barium peritonitis if there is any concern for perforation or compromise in the integrity of the colon wall. Second, by avoiding barium, subsequent radiologic studies are not compromised. Third, if the obstruction is the result of fecal impaction, water-soluble contrast is both diagnostic and therapeutic.

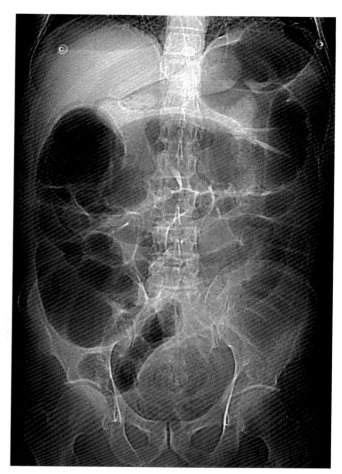

FIGURE 6-3. Large bowel obstruction secondary to sigmoid cancer. Incompetent ICV.

Pseudoobstruction

Dr. Ogilvie first described acute colonic pseudoobstruction in 1948, which is a condition characterized by massive dilation of the colon with no evidence of mechanical obstruction.[6] Radiographically, it is characterized by marked dilation of the cecum, ascending colon, and transverse colon (Figure 6-4). The descending colon and rectum are infrequently dilated. If the diagnosis is in question, it can be confirmed by a water-soluble enema, where there should be free flow of contrast into the cecum with no evidence of obstruction. Once again, in the acute setting, barium should be avoided.

Colonic Volvulus

Plain films are able to diagnose sigmoid volvulus in 75% of the cases. The classic plain film findings include a dilated, U-shaped loop of colon that is projected toward the right upper quadrant. This characteristic finding has also been called the "bent inner tube" sign (Figure 6-5A). The direction the volvulus points depends on the redundancy of the involved segment of sigmoid colon. In the middle of this loop is a vertically oriented white stripe that represents the two

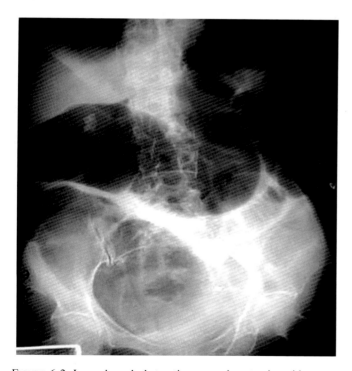

FIGURE 6-2. Large bowel obstruction secondary to sigmoid cancer. Competent ICV.

apposing walls of the obstructed loop of sigmoid colon. It is not uncommon to see dilated colon and even small bowel proximal to the volvulus because it does create a complete obstruction. If the diagnosis cannot be made with plain films, a water-soluble contrast enema will provide the diagnosis. Gentle instillation of contrast will demonstrate a smooth, tapered point of obstruction at the rectosigmoid junction known as a "bird's beak" (Figure 6-5B). If the diagnosis is still in question a CT can be obtained.

The diagnosis of rotational cecal volvulus can be made with plain films 75% of the time. Classically, the medially placed ICV indents the dilated cecum giving it the characteristic "coffee bean" or "kidney" shape (Figure 6-6A). The dilated right colon folds into the left upper quadrant (opposite to sigmoid). Dilated proximal small bowel may obscure the diagnosis. A CT will demonstrate dilated small bowel and cecum centered around the "swirly" mesentery. The "bascule" type volvulus produces a sharp, flat cut off of retrograde contrast as the mobile, redundant cecum flips up medially into the upper abdomen, causing a dilated cecum and small bowel on plain films.

Pneumoperitoneum

The plain film radiograph has been used since the early 1940s to diagnose free air within the peritoneal cavity.[8] The amount of air, patient position, direction of the X-ray projection, and phase of respiration contribute to the sensitivity of detecting pneumoperitoneum. In 1971, Miller and Nelson[9] demonstrated that as little as 1 cc of free air could be detected by upright chest plain film. The upright chest film is the most sensitive view for identifying free air under the diaphragm.[10]

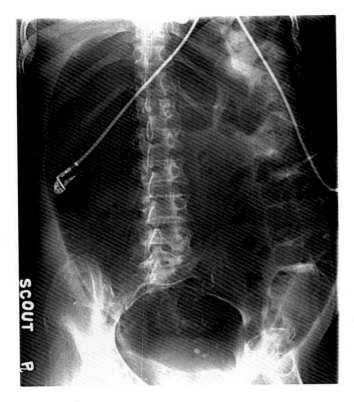

FIGURE 6-4. Ogilvie's syndrome.

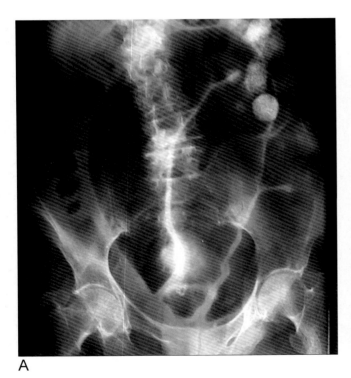

A

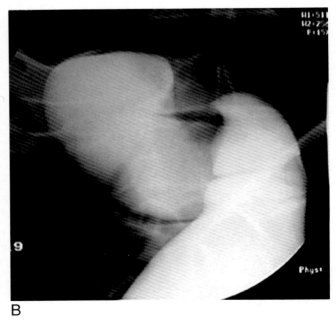

B

FIGURE 6-5. **A** Plain film of sigmoid volvulus. **B** Contrast enema of sigmoid volvulus.

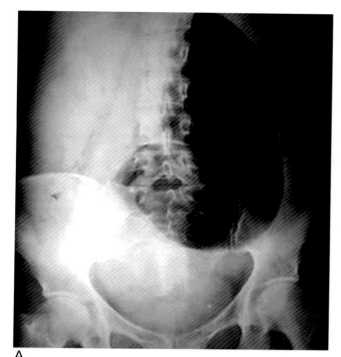

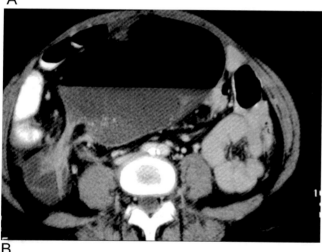

FIGURE 6-6. **A** Plain film of cecal volvulus. **B** CT of cecal volvulus.

In this position, the X-ray beam hits the diaphragm tangentially at its highest point and minimizes the collection of air being obscured by other organs. The left lateral decubitus film is also fairly sensitive for patients who are unable to be transported or stand. Some authors recommend keeping the patient in the left lateral position for 10–15 minutes before shooting the X-ray.[10] This allows adequate time for the air to rise above the lateral edge of the liver. When the plain film is performed during mid-expiration or mid-inspiration the ability to detect small amounts of air is increased.[11]

Intraperitoneal gas can be trapped in many locations such as under the diaphragm, in the lesser sac, under the liver, between the liver and the anterior abdominal wall, between loops of bowel, within the peritoneal ligaments, and in Morison's pouch. The appearance and configuration of the air depends on the shape of the space in which it has accumulated. The most common plain film finding is the accumulation of air under the right hemidiaphragm (Figure 6-7A). The relatively dense liver offers a sharp contrast to the air and the diaphragm. The Rigler sign or double-wall sign, which has been found in 32% of cases of pneumoperitoneum, is created when gas accumulates on both sides of the intestinal wall.[12] Both sides of the wall are visualized as a thin, white stripe. Often, the air trapped between the loops of bowel or leafs of mesentery will appear in a triangular configuration. Gas that has entered the lesser sac appears as an ill-defined lucency just above the lesser curve of the stomach. When air has entered into Morison's pouch, the inferior edge of the liver becomes outlined (Figure 6-7B). If there is any question about the diagnosis, the films should be repeated in another position or a CT should be obtained, which is the most sensitive study to detect free air.

Colitis

The diagnosis of colitis is typically a clinical one, but careful inspection of plain film radiographs can provide a wealth of valuable information. Plain films can give information regarding the condition of the mucosa, extent of colonic involvement, presence of perforation, evidence of bowel infarction, severity of colitis, and presence of associated ileus or obstruction.

When the colon is filled with gas, the gas/mucosa interface gives characteristic patterns associated with colitis. Thumbprinting is a sign for bowel wall and mucosal edema associated with most causes of acute colitis. Bowel wall edema results in thickening of the mucosal or haustral folds so that they appear as thick white lines projecting into the lumen. Also, the angle of the haustral folds becomes blunted and smooth versus the normal sharp angulation of the haustra. The edema also causes the bowel wall to become thick and stiff. As a result, the gas-filled loops tend to lie straight or gently curve and the gas distribution changes little when the patient is in different positions. When two edematous loops are adjacent to each other, the distance between the two lumens is greater than usual. An ominous sign is the presence of massively dilated segment of colon associated with bowel wall thickening and thumbprinting (Figure 6-8). This is diagnostic for toxic megacolon when associated with the clinical findings of leukocytosis, severe abdominal tenderness, and hemodynamic instability. All of these signs are suggestive of bowel wall edema, inflammation, and ischemia, but give little indication as to the underlying cause.

Examining five characteristics can provide considerable data regarding the severity and extent of the Crohn's or ulcerative colitis (UC).[13] First, the extent of solid colonic fecal material gives a general sense of the extent of disease. Solid

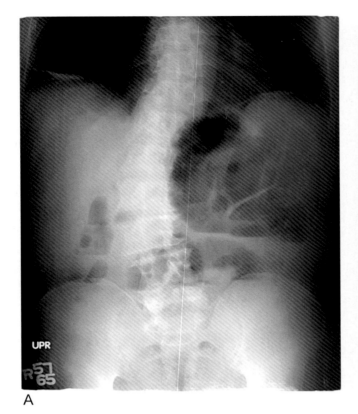

A

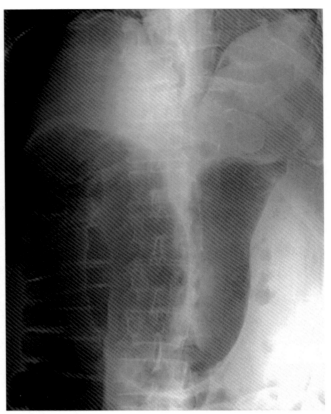

FIGURE 6-8. Plain film of colitis with megacolon.

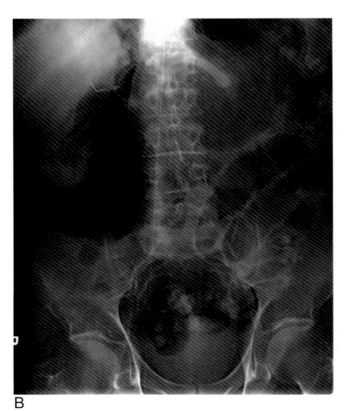

B

FIGURE 6-7. **A** Plain film of intraperitoneal free air under diaphragm. **B** Plain film of free air under liver edge.

stool in the right and transverse colon indicates left-sided colitis, and absence of solid stool anywhere in the colon suggests pancolitis. Second, examining the mucosal contours can help determine which segments of the colon are involved. Normally, the mucosal edge is smooth with sharp, narrow haustral markings. In the presence of active or longstanding inflammatory bowel disease (IBD), the mucosal contours are altered. The mucosal edge becomes blurred and has a granular appearance because of inflammation and ulceration. Depending on the extent of ulceration, the haustral markings may appear thick or be absent all together. Third, the character of the haustral markings provides information regarding the severity of disease. The haustral clefts are normally narrow with sharp angulation from the mucosal edge and are closely spaced. As the colitis progresses, the haustra become thicker, the angulation with the mucosal edge becomes blunted, and they are spaced farther apart. The haustra begin to disappear as the mucosal ulcerations progress. Fourth, the diameter of the colon can indicate the severity and chronicity of the disease. A markedly dilated (>5 cm) colon with thumbprinting and bowel wall edema is concerning for toxic megacolon. At the other end of the spectrum, a chronic, "burned out" colon takes on a tubular, narrowed appearance (Figure 6-9). This is more characteristic of UC than Crohn's disease. Finally, the thickness of the wall becomes thicker

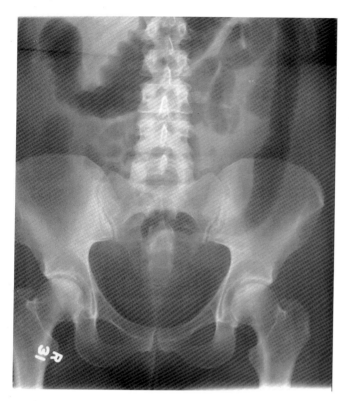

FIGURE 6-9. Plain film of chronic burned out colitis.

over time in patients with IBD. The distribution of the bowel wall thickening provides clues as to the extent of colonic involvement. Plain films are also able to provide information regarding the extraintestinal manifestations of IBD. Abnormalities of the skeletal system such as sacroiliitis, ankylosing spondylitis, and osteopenia secondary to chronic steroid use can be seen.

Another manifestation of colitis is pneumatosis where gas has accumulated within the wall of the intestine. This may be a relatively benign process such as pneumatosis cystoides intestinalis or it may represent the very grave situation of bowel infarction. Pneumatosis has two characteristic radiographic patterns. It may show a bubbly appearance where the gas accumulates within multiple cyst-like sacs in the colonic wall or the pneumatosis may dissect along the axis of the colon wall appearing as thin, linear streaks that are aligned along the axis of the bowel. Other associated findings that are concerning for vascular compromise of the colon include bowel dilatation, thumbprinting of the mucosa, and intraperitoneal free air. As the ischemia progresses to infarction, mucosal integrity is disrupted and gas may find its way into the mesenteric and portal venous systems. This is characterized by thin, branching lucencies within the liver, typically seen near the periphery. In the clinical setting of abdominal pain, known colitis, acidosis, or hemodynamic compromise, no further radiographic studies are needed to define the etiology of the pneumatosis or to indicate the severity of disease.

Contrast Studies

Contrast Enemas

Barium studies of the colon are designed for the detection of mucosal and intramural lesions. With the widespread use and availability of colonoscopy, the role of single or double contrast barium studies has diminished. Despite the direct competition with colonoscopy, barium studies continue to be an important player in the diagnosis of colonic pathology. The advantages of barium as a contrast medium are its ability to coat and adhere to the mucosa. This then allows for the instillation of air as second contrast medium. In air-contrast examinations, the colon is filled with barium. It is drained and then the colon is insufflated with air as a second contrast medium. The barium outlines the mucosal edges and the air distends the colon allowing for maximum visualization of mucosal detail. The indications for a barium study include screening and diagnosis of mucosal disease processes in the elective setting. Its disadvantages are the need for a colon preparation, the inherent characteristics of the medium, and the toxicity when exposed to the peritoneal cavity. The exposure of barium to the peritoneal cavity results in an intense inflammatory response that has a mortality rate of approximately 50%. Therefore, the use of barium should be avoided in urgent situations such as studying the integrity of an anastomosis, evaluating a large bowel obstruction, examining acute colitis, or when there is concern for bowel perforation. In these situations, a water-soluble contrast agent should be used. Water-soluble agents do not coat the mucosa. Instead, the bowel is visualized by passive filling of the lumen with the contrast as a single contrast study. As a result, water-soluble enemas do not provide as much detailed information as barium studies. Indications for a water-soluble study include evaluating the integrity of a colonic anastomosis, evaluating colonic obstruction, the preoperative evaluation of the colon for evidence of gross pathology, delineating colonic fistulas, and therapeutic enema for fecal impaction. The peritoneal cavity tolerates exposure of water-soluble contrast with very little reaction and, therefore, it is the contrast agent of choice in urgent situations.

Cancer and Polyps

The most common reason for ordering an air contrast barium enema is for the screening and diagnosis of neoplastic lesions of the colon and rectum, especially when screening for colorectal cancer in conjunction with flexible sigmoidoscopy, when colonoscopy is not possible.[14] The sensitivity of air contrast barium enema depends on the quality of colonic preparation, the size of lesion, the ability to adequately distend the colon with air, and obtaining multiple views. There are many regimens available for cleansing the colon that range from oral agents such as magnesium citrate and polyethylene glycol to enemas and suppositories.[15] The cleaner the colon, the better the barium is able to coat the mucosa and provide more detailed images.

A barium enema can detect up to 90% of polyps and cancers that are >1 cm in size, but sensitivity decreases to 50% for lesions <1 cm in size.[16,17] Lesions can appear sessile, pedunculated, flat, exophytic, and circumferential. The outline of the mucosal edge helps to differentiate benign versus malignant and intraluminal versus extraluminal processes. The configuration and the location of the lesion within the lumen dictate its radiographic appearance. Specifically, the profile in which the lesion is imaged and the location of the lesion within the lumen relative to retained pools of barium help to create its appearance on film. For example, lesions on the dependent portion of the lumen that sit in a puddle of barium will appear as filling defects. In contrast, lesions that are outlined in barium and are away from pools of barium appear as sessile, pedunculated, flat, or annular outlines that project into the lumen of the colon. When pedunculated lesions are viewed in profile, the stalk and head are easily identified.

Early cancers and polyps are very difficult to differentiate radiographically. The size of the lesion is the most helpful indicator of malignancy, with lesions >2 cm having a 50% chance of invasive cancer.[18,19] Also, the presence of an ulcer is highly suggestive of a malignant lesion. Polyps and early cancers can be sessile, flat, or pedunculated. Tubular adenomas tend to have a more regular, smooth mucosal surface. In contrast, villous lesions have many frondlike projections of the mucosa and barium gets trapped in these projections giving them a very irregular mucosal pattern. Sessile lesions when viewed in face take on a "bowlers hat" appearance that project into the lumen (Figure 6-10). The brim of the hat corresponds to the base of the lesion and the dome of the hat represents the head of the lesion. Depending on the size and complexity of a sessile lesion, the dome may be smooth or multi-lobulated. Pedunculated lesions are recognized by the appearance of their discrete stalk. When viewed obliquely or tangentially, the barium coats the stalk and it is easily identified. If viewed on end, it has the appearance of a "Mexican hat," which consists of two concentric circles where the outer circle represents the head of the lesion and the inner circle corresponds to its base.[20]

As neoplastic lesions grow they tend to occupy greater portions of the circumference wall and lumen of the colon. As a result, it is easier to distinguish the lesions as malignant. The most common appearances of colon cancers found during an air contrast barium enema are annular or semiannular (53%), polypoid (38%), and flat (9%).[21] The size, complexity, and villous component of the lesion all contribute to its ability to retain barium and thus its radiographic appearance. Once again, its position within the lumen may require multiple views to accurately visualize the lesion. Lesions that straddle one-third to half of the circumference of the lumen are called semiannular or saddle lesion (Figure 6-11). When viewed in profile, semiannular cancers appear as convex lines with the margins etched in barium. The smooth outline of normal

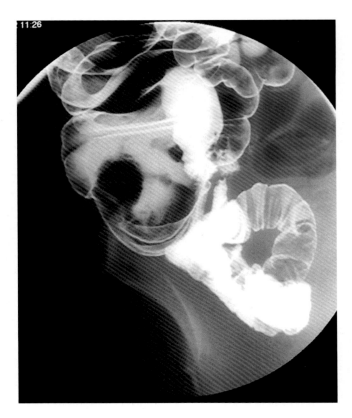

FIGURE 6-10. ACE of polyp or early cancer.

mucosa abruptly transitions into a convexity with complex, irregular borders. Given this characteristic shape, these lesions are often described as saddle lesions. Annular lesions refer to cancers that encompass the entire circumference of the colon's lumen. They are usually found in the sigmoid colon, but can

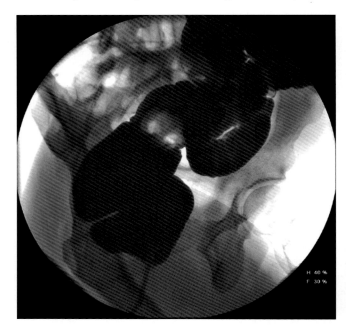

FIGURE 6-11. ACE of semiannular cancer.

occur anywhere within the colon. Annular lesions are characterized as a circumferential narrowing of the lumen of the colon. Characteristic findings implicating a malignant lesion include destruction and irregularity of the overlying mucosa with shelf-like, overhanging borders, and there is a sharp transition from normal mucosa into the annular lesion. Benign strictures from ischemic colitis, diverticulitis, anastomotic strictures, or Crohn's disease, in contrast, tend to have smooth, tapering borders. Malignant strictures are best identified when viewed in profile. If a large bowel obstruction is suspected, barium should be avoided and a water-soluble contrast agent should be used, and only a single column contrast study is needed to define the pathology. Annular lesions in this setting can present as a completely obstructing lesion or a near obstructing lesion, where only a string of contrast may get past the lesion. A completely obstructing lesion will have an abrupt cutoff of contrast at the level of the lesion. There will be shouldering or evidence of mucosal destruction at the point of obstruction. If the lesion permits some contrast to flow past the lesion, a "string sign" may be seen (Figure 6-12). This will be seen as a thin line of contrast extending from the column of contrast at the level of the obstruction. There is an abrupt cutoff of normal mucosa to a shouldering, overhanging lesion. The "string" of contrast will show irregular, destroyed mucosa along the length of the lesion.

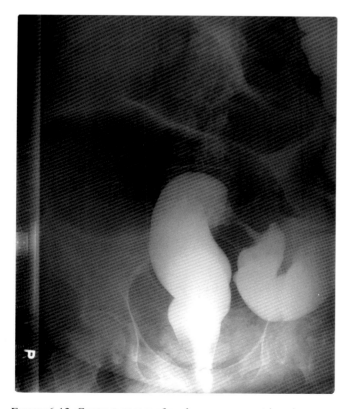

FIGURE 6-12. Contrast enema of apple-core cancer string sign.

Polyposis Syndromes—Familial Adenomatous Polyposis, Peutz-Jeghers, Juvenile Polyposis

It is not possible to distinguish between the sporadic adenomatous polyps and these polyposis syndromes using contrast studies. Confirming the diagnosis of these polyposis syndromes requires histologic examination of the polyps. The polyps can be seen with contrast as previously described in the majority of instances, but contrast studies should only be used if endoscopy is not possible.[22,23]

Ulcerative Colitis

Barium enema is used 1) to confirm the diagnosis of UC and differentiate it from Crohn's disease, 2) to assess the extent and severity of disease, and 3) for surveillance of the disease and its complications. The radiographic appearance of UC seen during barium enema examination depends on the state of the disease process. Changes consistent with acute colitis involve mucosal loss to varying degrees and bowel wall edema. The pattern by which the barium outlines the mucosa depends on the depth and size of ulceration. A granular mucosal pattern is one of the earliest changes seen, which corresponds to the accumulation of inflammatory cells and edema within the mucosa but the mucosa maintains its integrity. When the barium coats the swollen and edematous mucosal edge, it appears fuzzy and indistinct rather than the normal sharp edges. As the inflammatory process progresses, the integrity of the mucosa is broken, leading to the development of ulcers. These ulcerations are shallow, punctate lesions confined to the mucosal layer. They appear as small, dense collections of barium that are on the same plane as the rest of the mucosa. This pattern is known as mucosal stippling (Figure 6-13A). With continued inflammation, the crypt abscesses rupture, exposing the submucosa. The ulcers begin to extend laterally and undermine the adjacent mucosa. These are called collar button ulcers and are characterized by a narrow neck and wide base that extends below the level of the mucosal edge. As the ulcerations enlarge and coalesce, small islands of residual mucosa are left, and as these mucosal islands regenerate in the face of ongoing inflammation, they develop into inflammatory pseudopolyps. Pseudopolyps are irregular projections into the lumen of the bowel (Figure 6-13B). The projections can be round, linear, or have a complex branching pattern that represents mucosal bridging. The depth of ulcerations seen on air contrast enema has been found to correlate reliably with the depth and extent of ulceration seen on histopathologic examination.[24]

The chronic changes of UC are related to the effects of repeated ulceration and regeneration of the colonic mucosa. Over time, the persistent inflammation causes the muscular tone of tenia to relax and muscular hypertrophy of the muscularis mucosa. The changes of the musculature of the colon and the chronic scarring of the mucosa are what lead to the loss of all normal mucosal folds and haustra, narrowing of the bowel lumen, and foreshortening of the colon. Radiographically, this

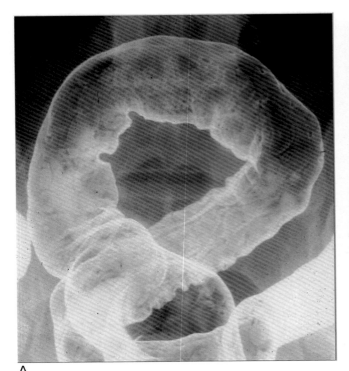

A

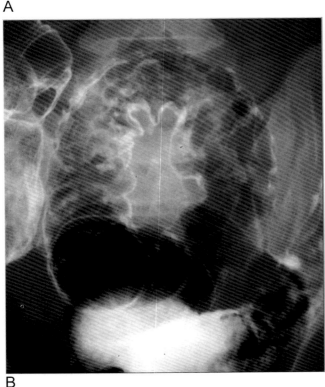

B

FIGURE 6-13. **A** Contrast enema of UC showing stippling ulcers or early colitis. **B** Contrast enema of UC with pseudopolyps.

appears as blunting or complete loss of the haustral markings, a narrow tubular appearance to the colon, and loss of the redundant course of the sigmoid and transverse colon (Figure 6-14). The point of transition from narrowed and flat mucosa

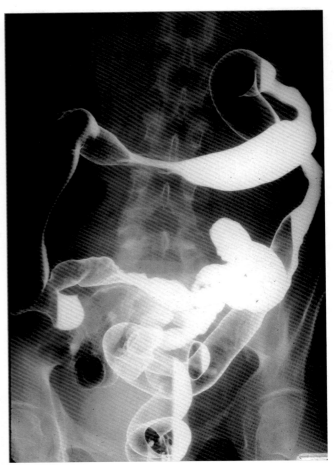

FIGURE 6-14. Contrast enema of chronic UC.

to normal haustral configuration can help determine the extent of the colitis. There may be areas of the colon where the contraction of the bowel wall is worse giving rise to the appearance of symmetric, gentle narrowing resulting in a stricture. The presence of backwash ileitis is also a sign of chronic disease because the ICV has been scarred open. Barium contrast studies are also able to detect other colonic complications of UC such as adenomatous polyps and cancers. These appear as the neoplastic lesions previously described. However, it should be remembered that IBD-associated cancers tend to be more flat and infiltrating and do not always appear as typical neoplasms. Some authors argue that double contrast enemas are able to identify areas of dysplasia,[25] but contrast enemas are not recommended for routine surveillance.

Crohn's Disease

Contrast studies help differentiate Crohn's disease from UC, define the severity and extent of the colitis, and identify complications of the disease. Contrast enemas are better than colonoscopy at identifying and characterizing fistulas, strictures, and the distribution of disease.[26]

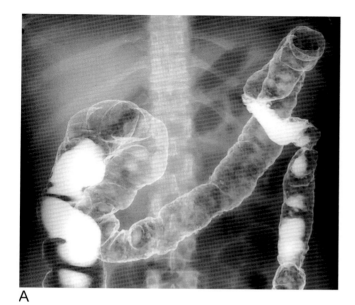

A

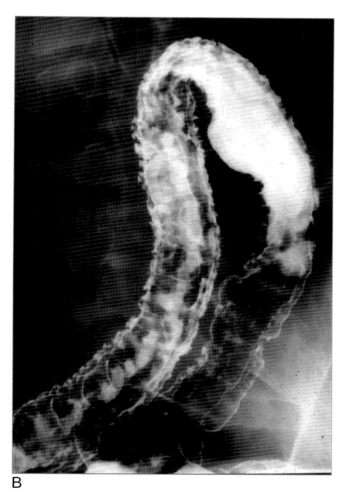

B

FIGURE 6-15. **A** Contrast enema of Crohn's disease showing ulcers. **B** Contrast enema of Crohn's with fissures, and long linear ulcers.

As with UC, the radiographic appearance of Crohn's disease depends on the acuity or chronicity of the disease. Aphthous ulcerations are the earliest mucosal lesions seen in Crohn's disease.[22] Barium accumulates within the lesions and they appear as small, shallow, or punctate collections with a surrounding radiolucent halo (Figure 6-15A). These lesions occur more frequently in the colon than the small intestine, and they help to distinguish Crohn's disease from UC. As the aphthous lesions progress, the ulcerations deepen, widen, and coalesce. The transmural nature of the inflammation allows the ulcerations to extend into the musculature of the bowel wall and even lead to fistulization. The result is deep longitudinal and transverse fissuring with edematous mucosa in between that gives the colon a cobblestone appearance. Barium deposits in the deep fissures and appear as multiple irregular white stripes (Figure 6-15B). The deepest portions of the fissures penetrate beyond the submucosa and the resulting image is one of "rose thorns" extending below the level of the mucosal edge. Once the ulcerations progress through the submucosa, the distinction of Crohn's disease can be made. Also, the identification of skip lesions or areas of normal mucosa in between areas of active colitis distinguish Crohn's disease from UC (Figure 6-16). Severe colitis leads to the development of long, deep linear ulcers typically along the mesenteric border of the colon. These long ulcers are known as "rake" or "bear claw" ulcers. If the ulcerations continue to burrow in the wall of the bowel, a fistula or sinus tract can result. Fistulas can be identified by early filling of the small bowel before opacification of the proximal colon or as irregular projections of contrast outside of the lumen. Another significant feature of Crohn's disease is the development of strictures. Crohn's strictures are a result of transmural fibrosis. Radiographically, the strictures are asymmetric, have irregular borders, and are not circumferential (they are centered on the mesenteric edge) (Figure 6-17). This is in contrast to the strictures associated with UC, which are symmetric, smooth, and circumferential.

Diverticulitis

Air contrast barium enemas are more sensitive than single contrast studies at detecting diverticula because of better colonic distension and mucosal detail. The radiographic appearance of diverticula varies based on their size, number, angle at which they are viewed, amount of barium within the diverticula, and amount of colonic distention. When viewed in profile, they are flask-shaped with an associated neck that point away from the lumen. When filled with barium, they will appear as white projections or a white line outlining the mucosa when the barium has emptied from the diverticula. When viewed en face, they have the appearance of a bowler's hat projecting away from the lumen when they are empty of barium. If filled with barium, they will appear as a white spot or when partially filled, they will appear as a bowler's hat with a white meniscus. Diverticula can be distinguished from polyps and small cancers because they project away from the lumen as compared with neoplasms

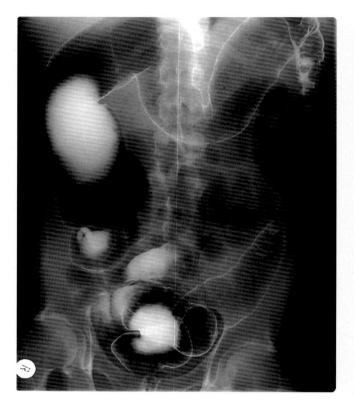

FIGURE 6-16. Contrast enema of Crohn's disease showing skip lesions.

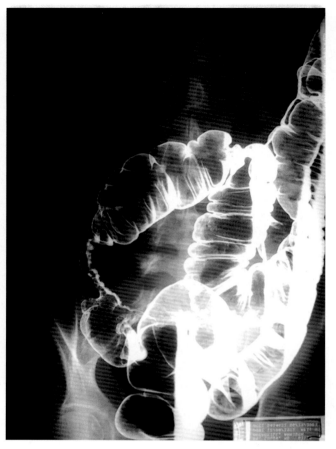

FIGURE 6-17. Contrast enema of Crohn's disease showing a stricture.

that project into the lumen. Other findings associated with diverticulosis include a shortened, narrowed, and spastic sigmoid colon. Hyperelastosis leads to a stiff, thickened, and nondistendible colon that is characteristic of extensive diverticulosis. The combination of a shortened, thickened colon and extensive diverticula can disrupt the symmetric appearance of the haustral clefts, giving the mucosal outline an irregular zigzag appearance (Figures 6-18A and B). This is best seen with single column contrast enemas.

In the acute setting, a water-soluble contrast agent should be used rather than barium to avoid the highly morbid case of barium peritonitis. In acute diverticulitis, the inflammation is pericolonic and contrast studies are unable to directly demonstrate the inflammation. They are able to infer the effects of the pericolonic inflammation on the mucosa. Findings such as narrowing of the sigmoid colon, extrinsic compression, mucosal edema, and spasm in the presence of diverticula are all suggestive of diverticulitis but they lack significant specificity. Contrast enemas are able to demonstrate complications of diverticulitis such as perforation, abscess, fistula, and strictures. Extraluminal leak of contrast is diagnostic of diverticulitis with free perforation, when associated with the appropriate clinical scenario. The contrast can flow freely into the peritoneal cavity, into a contained cavity, or a blind ending sinus. Contrast that flows into the bladder, vagina, or early filling of proximal loops of intestine are all findings consistent with a

fistula. A colovesical fistula is the most common diverticular-associated fistula, but contrast enemas are able to make the diagnosis only 20% of the time.[23] Therefore, a contrast enema should not be the first test used to confirm the diagnosis of a fistula. A pericolonic abscess that impinges on the colon can be seen as a smooth contour defect along one wall of the colon that does not distend with the instillation of contrast material or air.

Stricture formation may occur after a single attack of diverticulitis but more frequently it is the result of recurrent episodes of inflammation. The site of the stricture is at the point of inflammation, which is typically within the sigmoid colon. Benign strictures have a smooth, gentle transition to the stricture with intact mucosa. The radiographic appearance of the stricture and adjacent colon along with the clinical scenario should help to elucidate the cause of the stricture.[27]

Submucosal and Extracolonic Lesions

Lipoma

On double contrast barium enema, lipomas can appear as a submucosal mass or a polypoid lesion. The lesions can have an oval, lobulated, or pear shape and the overlying mucosa is smooth with sharp, well-demarcated borders. Lipomas are soft and pliable, so during fluoroscopic examination, com-

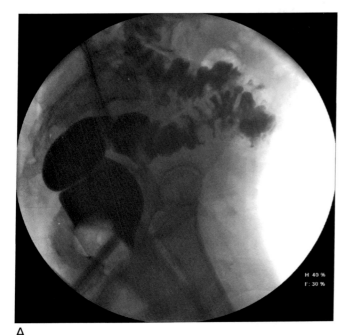

A

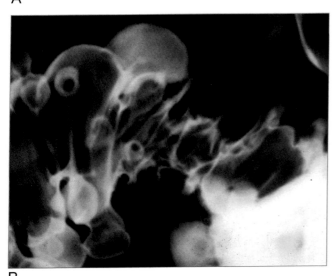

B

FIGURE 6-18. **A** Contrast enema single column showing severe diverticulosis with the sawtooth mucosa. **B** Air contrast enema of severe diverticulosis.

pression can change the configuration of the lesion; this is called the "pillow sign."[28]

Lymphoma

There are three basic radiographic morphologies that primary colonic lymphomas can demonstrate.[29] First, they can appear as discrete polypoid lesions. Typically occurring in the cecum, these lesions can range from 2 to 20 cm in size. In contrast, adenomatous polyps have mucosal irregularities because of their frond-like appendages. These are submucosal lesions, so the overlying mucosa remains intact and smooth with the edges of the lesion being distinct (Figure 6-19). The involved segments tend to be long, with discrete proximal and distal edges, and the overlying mucosa remains intact. The barium may highlight nodular, irregular mucosal edges, but there is no ulceration. This is unlike annular carcinomas, which have short strictures with shouldering and ulcerated mucosa. Second, the mass can infiltrate the mesentery resulting in cavitation of the lesion into the mesentery. On barium enema, this appears similar to the annular lesions, but at some point within the affected segment, there is a nodular projection that is beyond the lumen of the colon. Finally, disseminated lymphoma appears as multiple, long segments of nodular, narrowed colon.

Endometriosis

The findings on barium enema in the patient with endometriosis are consistent with an extracolonic process, because the mucosa remains smooth and intact.[30] Mild involvement will show a short, focal area with bunching of the mucosal folds, which has been termed mucosal pleating. This short segment will also show evidence of extraluminal narrowing. With more extensive involvement with scarring and contracture, stricturing can develop (Figure 6-20). Radiographically, this appears as a short, benign stricture with a sharp transition, mucosal pleating, and intact mucosa.

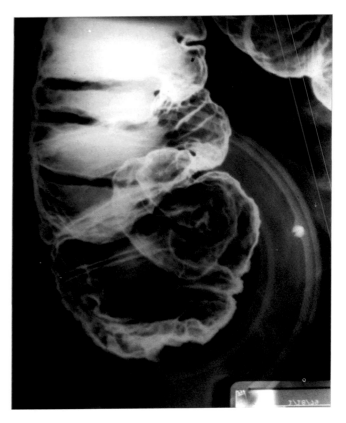

FIGURE 6-19. Contrast enema showing colonic lymphoma.

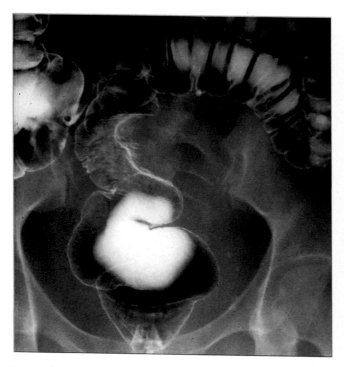

FIGURE 6-20. Contrast enema showing endometriosis.

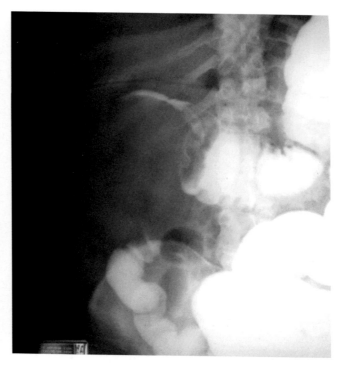

FIGURE 6-21. Contrast enema showing colonic intussusception.

Colonic Intussusception

Intussusception occurs when a proximal segment of bowel (intussusceptum) telescopes into the lumen of the distal bowel (intussuscipiens), much like turning a sock inside out. When viewed in cross-section, there are three rings or six layers across the diameter, which represent walls of the intestine—the outer wall is the distal lumen, the middle ring is the distal wall folded back onto itself, and the inner wall is the proximal intussuscepting wall. Plain films may reveal the pathognomonic "crescent sign." As the intussusceptum telescopes into the intussuscipiens, the distal lumen folds into itself. At this transition, air can get trapped within the lumen, and this is seen as the "crescent sign." Plain films may also show a dilated proximal colon that is decompressed distally. As a result, a contrast enema is often ordered to evaluate a large bowel obstruction. The classic appearance of an intussusception on contrast enema is the spring coil appearance or crescent sign (Figure 6-21). Contrast gets trapped between the lumens of the intussuscipiens and intussusceptum leaving a thin, circular line that encircles the intussuscipiens.

Anastomotic Assessment

Contrast enema studies are frequently used postoperatively to examine a colocolic, colorectal, coloanal, or ileal-anal anastomosis. The studies are used to evaluate for anastomotic leak in a septic patient, before closure of a diverting stoma, or to rule out an anastomotic stricture in patients with defecation difficulties. When testing the integrity of an anastomosis,

a water-soluble contrast agent should be used. Contrast should be allowed to fill the colon under the weight of gravity, with the bag placed no higher than 1 m above the patient. Initially, the flow of contrast should be tightly controlled and increased as the examination permits. As previously mentioned, there is minimal peritoneal toxicity with water-soluble agents, and a single column study provides adequate detail to detect the majority of clinically significant leaks. The expected findings depend on the clinical scenario for ordering the examination. In the early postoperative period when evaluating for an anastomotic leak, water-soluble contrast enema is more sensitive than CT with rectal contrast.[31] Radiographic findings of an anastomotic dehiscence include the extravasation of contrast freely into the peritoneal cavity or into a contained cavity (Figures 6-22A and B). Key findings that influence the management of an early anastomotic leak are the size of the disruption, the containment of the leak, and how well it empties back into the lumen after evacuation. A leak identified before closure of a diverting stoma can be contained within a cavity or be a blind sinus. Typically, delaying the closure of the stoma will give the anastomotic disruption time to heal. There are several views that are important to see before a leak can be excluded. Obtaining anterior-posterior and lateral views of early filling of the lumen, full distention of the colon, and the postevacuation periods are necessary for an adequate study. Early filling may reveal subtle leaks that are either obscured by the distended rectum or empty readily when the bowel is decompressed. Distention of the bowel is necessary to unroll mucosal folds and provide some intraluminal pressure to test

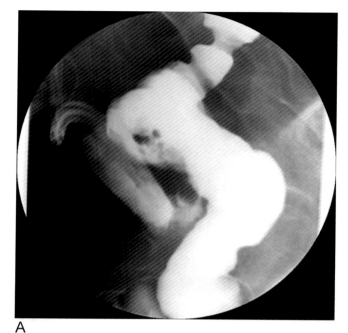

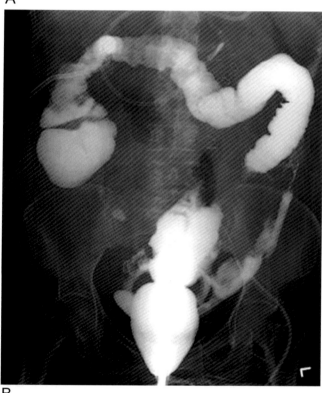

FIGURE 6-22. **A** Contrast enema showing a contained anastomotic leak. **B** Contrast enema showing a free-flowing leak.

the anastomotic integrity. Finally, the postevacuation films are the most important because they identify any residual contrast outside of the lumen, which may be the only finding that a leak is present. The presence of smooth-bordered extraluminal compression at the level of the anastomosis is consistent with an associated abscess. Anastomotic strictures are the result of ischemia or a septic complication of the surgery. Strictures typically occur remotely from surgery, therefore the concern for a leak is low and barium can be used as the contrast agent of choice. Radiographically, they have abrupt, short, symmetric narrowing with intact mucosa.

Small Bowel Series and Enteroclysis

The small bowel represents 75% of the length and 90% of the mucosal surface of the entire GI tract, but the incidence of pathology is much less frequent than that of the upper and lower portions of the intestinal system. Consequently, radiologic studies of the small bowel are often used to finish an examination of the GI tract for the sake of completeness. Indications for small bowel studies include unexplained GI bleeding, evaluation for small bowel tumors, SBO, Crohn's disease, and malabsorption.[32] Examination of the small bowel is challenging for several reasons. First, with the enormous mucosal surface, it is difficult to adequately visualize all segments of the bowel. Second, the multiple overlapping loops of the small bowel can make visualization difficult. Finally, the flow of contrast through the small bowel cannot be controlled. As a result, findings may be missed if the physician is not paying close attention at all times. Nonetheless, small bowel contrast studies have a vital role in the practice of surgeons.

Barium follow-through and enteroclysis are the principle methods for examining the small bowel. During a small bowel follow through (SBFT), the patient drinks a large volume of dilute barium. The radiologist follows the flow of contrast through the small bowel with the use of fluoroscopy and spot films. The pylorus and gastric emptying limit the rate that the contrast enters the small bowel. Various techniques that apply pressure to the abdomen are used to manipulate and flatten out the loops of bowel to improve visualization. The major disadvantages are the inability to completely distend the bowel, and the time and attention required by the patient, radiologist, and radiology staff to perform an adequate examination.[26] During enteroclysis, the contrast and methylcellulose are administered through a small tube passed into the duodenum. This allows for rapid instillation of barium into the small bowel allowing for better distention and visualization. Advantages over SBFT include better filling and distention of the bowel and decreased study time. The major disadvantages are the placement of the nasoduodenal tube, the relatively high radiation dose, and hyperosmotic nature of the methylcellulose. When comparing the diagnostic results between SBFT and enteroclysis, the results are mixed. Regardless of the indication for the examination, the quality of the study depends on the radiologist's preferred technique and their attention to detail during the study.

The technical aspects of the SBFT begin with the oral administration of a 40%–50% barium suspension with a volume of 300–500 mL. The flow of barium, which is limited by pyloric emptying, is then followed under fluoroscopy. The patient and bowel are manipulated and spot images are taken at points of interest or every 15 minutes. Normal transit time for the small bowel can vary widely but is generally defined as 90–120 minutes. Enteroclysis requires nasal or oral intubation of the pylorus so contrast may be rapidly administered to maximize the distention of the small intestine. The catheter is typically 12 French in caliber and can be passed with minimal discomfort to the patient. The catheter is passed under fluoroscopic guidance to ensure its postpyloric position. The contrast is then infused at an initial rate of 75 mL/minute and then is increased as needed and tolerated. Serial images are obtained in the same manner as the SBFT.

Crohn's Disease

Barium studies of the small bowel are essential for staging the severity and extent of bowel involvement in patients with Crohn's disease. Indications for the studies include routine surveillance of known small bowel disease, assessing the severity of disease during a flare, defining the disease distribution for a new diagnosis, preoperative assessment, and to assist in the differentiation between Crohn's disease and UC. The radiographic appearance of Crohn's disease depends on the severity of disease and its distribution. Early or mild Crohn's disease is characterized by thickened, irregular mucosal folds, a coarse villous pattern of the mucosa, and aphthous ulcers (Figure 6-23A). The early edema and inflammation are typically confined to the mucosa, which can be seen as a fine nodularity of the mucosal edge. The edema also causes the villi to swell allowing barium to get trapped between them, producing a fuzzy, ground-glass, or coarse villous pattern. Aphthous ulcerations appear as shallow collections of barium surrounded by a radiolucent halo. As the disease progresses, more of the bowel wall becomes involved and the edema and inflammation extend into the submucosa and muscularis. The plicae circularis is made up of the mucosa and submucosa so submucosal involvement causes these folds to become even thicker and blunted producing the characteristic thumbprinting. Chronic or severe inflammation causes further distortion and disruption of the plicae circularis and enlargement, deepening, and coalescence of the aphthous ulcerations. The ulcers are classically located on the mesenteric border of the lumen, which is fairly specific to Crohn's disease. They enlarge and coalesce taking on various configurations such as stellate or rose thorn shapes and linear or crescent shapes. Continued progression leads to the characteristic deep linear ulcers of Crohn's disease.

Advanced disease is characterized by transmural inflammation that can be seen radiographically as deep, long linear ulcers, sawtoothed nodularity of the mucosa, cobblestoning, severe thickening of the bowel wall, luminal narrowing, and the complications of the disease. Inflammation of the submucosa and subserosa allows for the deep, knife-like clefts to burrow into the bowel wall. These clefts and fissures begin to merge into a longitudinal and transverse network of ulcerations.

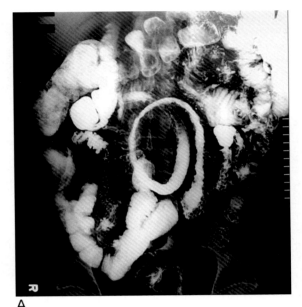

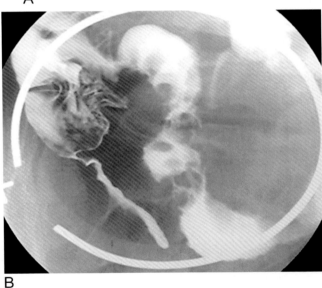

FIGURE 6-23. **A** Small bowel series showing TI Crohn's disease strictures. **B** SBFT showing cobblestoning.

Between the ulcers remain pieces of relatively uninflamed mucosa. This produces a sharp, sawtooth nodularity of the mucosal edge, and ultimately develops a cobblestone pattern (Figure 6-23B). Barium fills the clefts and fissures and does not cling to the relatively spared mucosa in between, which is the basis for the cobblestone pattern. As these islands of residual mucosa attempt to regenerate, they heap up and branch giving rise to pseudopolyps. Once again, the barium does not adhere to these polyps so the cobblestoning becomes more irregular and complex. Transmural inflammation leads to fat creeping and bowel-wall thickening. The thickened bowel wall displaces adjacent loops of intestine so the distance between loops is increased. During the barium study, these loops cannot be compressed or manipulated. The thickening also causes narrowing of the lumen. Radiographically, this can be seen as areas of nondistensible, ulceronodular bowel producing a string sign. The narrowing is caused by reversible edema, spasm, and inflammation or irreversible fibrosis.

Barium studies are more sensitive at identifying fistulas than endoscopy. The fistula tract may be visualized directly or indirectly. Early filling of the colon is highly suggestive of an enterocolic fistula. For example, an ileal-transverse colon fistula will show contrast entering the transverse colon before the right colon fills with contrast. An abscess may be seen as an extraluminal mass or compression of the adjacent loops of intestine.

Small Bowel Obstruction

A complete bowel obstruction is readily apparent based on clinical grounds and easily supported by plain films of the abdomen. However, the diagnosis is not always clear in up to one-third of cases.[33] Subsequent delays in the diagnosis can lead to significant increases in morbidity and mortality. When the diagnosis is uncertain and the clinical circumstances support further testing, contrast studies of the small bowel can be very useful. Specific indications for either SBFT or enteroclysis include equivocal plain films, unclear etiology, early postoperative obstructions, or when preoperative localization of the site of obstruction is important. Dilute barium studies are the most useful because they provide the best mucosal detail and the barium typically does not become inspissated in the small bowel, therefore its use in the setting of a complete or partial SBO is not contraindicated. However, the use of water-soluble agents can be problematic in the setting of a complete SBO because of their hypertonicity, which draws water into the bowel lumen further exacerbating the fluid sequestration caused by the obstruction. Finally, traditional SBFT is the preferred technique for assessing the presence of partial SBO.

Findings consistent with an adhesive obstruction include a smooth, sharp transition point with a straight or curved line that stretches across the bowel (Figure 6-24). This is most apparent when the band is a single, thin adhesion. If multiple adhesions are present, the transition point is not as easily depicted. Typically, adhesions will fix the loop of intestine to the pelvis, retroperitoneum, or abdominal wall so that it does not move with manipulation or respiration. Peritoneal metastasis can also fix the affected loop of intestine to the peritoneal cavity. These two etiologies can often be differentiated. As mentioned, adhesions typically cause smooth transitions that stretch across the entire lumen and the surrounding mucosa appears normal. In contrast, metastasis will cause a desmoplastic reaction in the surrounding bowel so the mucosa at the transition point will appear irregular and tethered. Also, the tumor begins at one edge of lumen and either directly invades the lumen or infiltrates around the bowel circumference. This further exaggerates the mucosa irregularities and

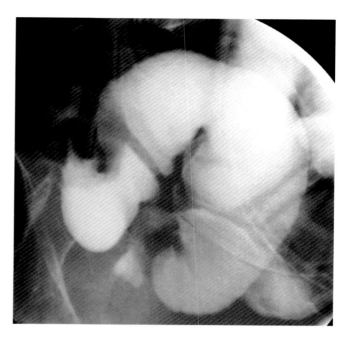

FIGURE 6-24. SBFT showing a simple SBO.

may not completely obstruct the flow of barium into the distal, collapsed bowel. Metastasis can also cause obstruction by external compression of the bowel. This will be seen as an external mass effect and the overlying mucosa, in this case, will appear more normal.

Lesions intrinsic to the small bowel can also be elucidated. Primary adenocarcinomas of the small bowel are more common in the proximal bowel and occur with decreasing frequency more distal along the small intestine. Their findings are very similar to those seen for colon cancers on barium enema. There is mucosal destruction with sharp demarcation between normal mucosa and the lesion. The lesion may be semiannular or annular. Carcinoid tumors typically occur in the terminal ileum and start as submucosal lesions. As they grow, there may be mucosal destruction and tethering toward the center of the abdomen as the mesenteric desmoplastic reaction progresses.

Computed Tomography

CT has become a routine examination to evaluate a wide range of disease processes because it is an easy, fast, and accurate test that provides cross-sectional imaging. The benefit of cross-sectional imaging is the detailed imaging and resolution of the hollow viscus and solid organs. Accurate interpretation requires optimal opacification of the GI tract and vascular structures. The bowel is opacified by administering a water-soluble oral contrast agent. The density of barium interferes with the acquisition of data during the scan and thus should be avoided as a contrast agent. The oral contrast is typically administered 45–60 minutes before scanning to allow the contrast to opacify as much of the bowel as possible. If pelvic or rectal pathology is being evaluated, the contrast may also be administered per rectum at the time the scan is being performed. Intravenous (IV) contrast agents typically are iodinated so it is important to take a thorough history of allergies. It is administered as a bolus at the time of the examination. The reason for the examination dictates the exact timing between when the contrast is administered and when the CT images are acquired (i.e., venous versus arterial phase). The CT scan uses ionizing radiation to acquire the images with 5- to 10-mm collimation. Smaller collimation allows for sharper, more detailed images.

CT scans are usually ordered for the staging of colorectal cancer, evaluation of abdominal complaints, and evaluation of postoperative complications. Once again, having a specific question in mind when ordering the scan will allow the scan to be tailored to the appropriate parameters.

Colorectal Cancer

An abdominal and pelvic CT is the most common method for staging colorectal cancer before definitive surgical resection. The aims of the CT scan are to 1) evaluate the liver for distant metastatic disease, 2) evaluate for regional lymphadenopathy, especially in rectal cancer, where nodes may have been missed during a transrectal ultrasound, and 3) assess for the presence of intraperitoneal disease. CT is also used to follow colorectal cancer patients longitudinally for the development of recurrent disease. It is most effective when used to evaluate patients who have symptoms concerning for recurrent disease or have a rising carcinoembryonic antigen (CEA) level. There are no strong data to support its use in routine surveillance for detecting metastasis in the absence of symptoms or rising CEA.[34]

There are several modalities, such as CT, ultrasound, and magnetic resonance imaging (MRI), available to assess the liver for metastatic disease. All of them have their advantages and disadvantages, but they all have equivalent diagnostic accuracy for the detection of liver metastasis.[27,35] CT images are typically obtained in two phases: the hepatic artery phase (20–25 seconds after the IV contrast is initiated) and the portal venous phase (65–70 seconds after the IV contrast is started). The majority of colorectal metastases are hypovascular and show up as hypodense lesions during the portal venous stage because the majority of metastatic lesions derive their blood supply from the arterial system. During the portal venous phase, contrast enhances the hepatic parenchyma and portal veins and the metastatic lesions do not enhance (Figure 6-25).

CT is able to differentiate many hepatic lesions based on their imaging characteristics and the dynamic effects of contrast on these lesions. Common liver lesions that need to be differentiated from colorectal metastasis include simple cysts, hepatic adenomas, primary liver tumors, hemangiomas, and focal nodular hyperplasia. Colorectal metastases typically are round, well-circumscribed lesions that are fairly homoge-

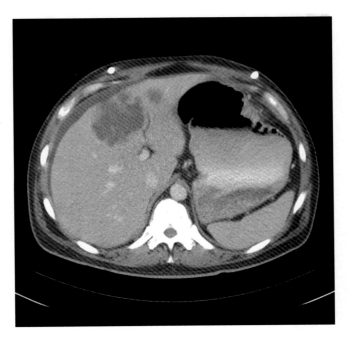

FIGURE 6-25. CT scan showing liver metastasis.

neous in density, which is consistent with solid tissue. As lesions grow they become more irregular in shape and their enhancement becomes more heterogeneous. Central necrosis and calcification may also be present. In contrast, simple cysts have a density consistent with fluid, which is more hypodense than solid tissue, and there is very little change in their enhancement during the various phases of imaging. Hemangiomas can be differentiated from metastatic lesions by the fact that they remain enhanced throughout the portal venous phase. The other hepatic lesions are typically hypervascular so they can be reliably differentiated from metastatic lesions during dual-phase CT imaging. The accuracy of CT for the detection and differentiation of liver lesions is greatest for lesions >1 cm.[36,37] Lesions <1 cm generally do not have the dynamic enhancing properties to be readily differentiated and, as a result, they are named indeterminate lesions.

Other advantages of the CT scans include the ability to detect regional adenopathy and to assess the relationship of the primary tumor to adjacent structures (Figure 6-26). Detecting regional adenopathy is most important for rectal cancer because the presence of adenopathy may influence the surgeon to give neoadjuvant chemoradiation therapy. The CT criteria for pathologic adenopathy are based on size only. Typically, nodes >1 cm in size are concerning for metastatic disease.

Diverticulitis

The most common CT findings associated with diverticulitis are pericolonic/mesenteric inflammation (98%), diverticula (84%), colonic wall thickening (70%), and abscess (47%).[28] Normally, the colonic mesentery and pericolonic tissues are

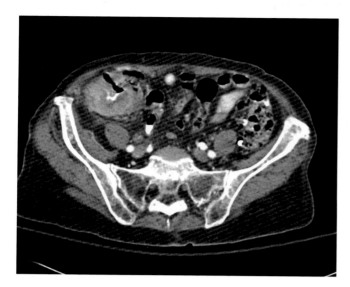

FIGURE 6-26. CT scan showing primary lesion and adenopathy.

hypodense because of the high water content of the surrounding fat and sharp edges between adjacent structures. As the inflammatory process begins, the tissue becomes edematous and more vascular. This causes the pericolonic tissue to become more enhanced and the sharp contrasts between the various tissue plains become hazy, resulting in the so-called "dirty fat." When the inflammatory response is centered on a portion of colon that is thickened (>5 mm), the diagnosis of diverticulitis is confirmed. Often, the inflammatory process can be extensive, producing a phlegmon in the absence of an organized abscess (Figure 6-27). Depending on the size of the perforation, there may be small flecks of extraluminal air within the mesentery or pericolonic tissue or in the upper abdomen above the liver. The inflammatory process is

typically localized around a short segment of the colon, thus if a long segment, several segments, or the entire colon is involved, a different diagnosis should be sought. The presence or absence of diverticula does not impact the radiographic diagnosis. The development of diverticula is associated with hyperelastosis of the colonic wall, which is evident by the thickening of the wall. This leads to decreased compliance and shortening of the involved segment of colon. When the thickness of the colon wall is >5 mm, it is considered abnormal. The wall thickening may be circumferential or just localized to the segment adjacent to the inflammation.

As mentioned, not only does CT allow for confirmation of the diagnosis of diverticulitis, but it can also identify associated complications. Abscess formation is the most common complication of diverticulitis. An abscess appears as a fluid collection typically near the area of diverticulitis (Figure 6-28). Often, oral and IV contrast are needed to distinguish an abscess from adjacent loops of intestine. When the surrounding loops of bowel are able to be opacified with oral contrast and the rim of the abscess is enhanced with IV contrast, the accuracy of diagnosing an abscess is maximized. The presence of air or an air-fluid level within the abscess cavity is also highly suggestive of an abscess.

A colovesical fistula in the most common fistula associated with diverticulitis, and a CT scan is the most sensitive for the detection of such a fistula.[29] Air within a bladder that has not been instrumented is diagnostic for an enterovesical fistula (Figure 6-29). When the wall of the bladder is thickened and in close proximity to the area of sigmoid colon that is thickened and contains diverticula, the etiology is likely related to diverticular disease. If the fistula is large enough, contrast, either administered orally or per rectum, may fill the bladder. Rectal contrast filling the bladder can help distinguish the source of fistula from a terminal ileal fistula associated with Crohn's disease.

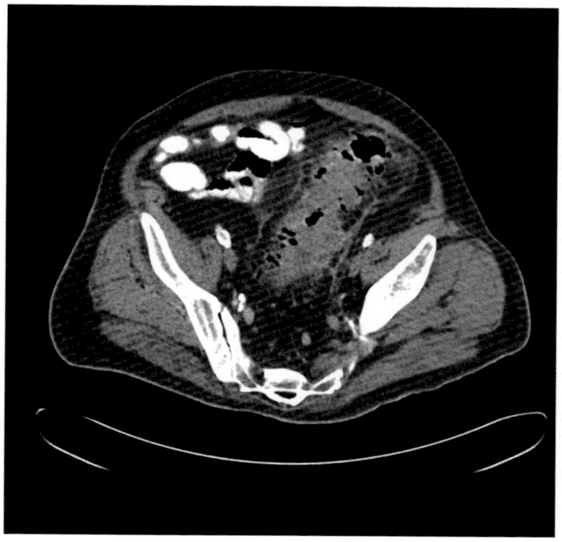

FIGURE 6-27. CT scan showing uncomplicated diverticulitis.

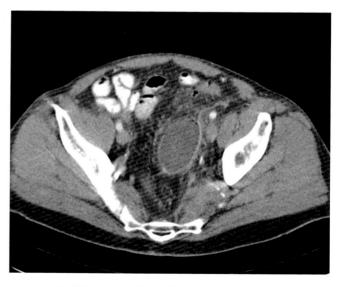

FIGURE 6-28. CT scan showing a diverticular abscess.

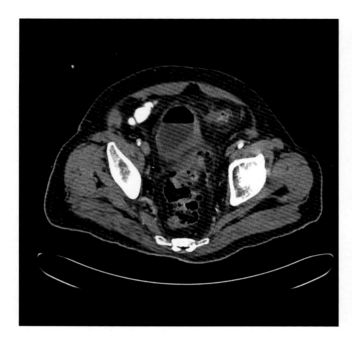

FIGURE 6-29. CT scan demonstrating a colovesical fistula.

Crohn's Disease

The role of CT in the diagnosis and evaluation of Crohn's disease continues to evolve. A CT scan is used in two general situations during the management of Crohn's disease. First, a CT is obtained to evaluate a patient with new onset abdominal pain, and findings consistent with Crohn's disease are incidentally found. Second, a CT scan is obtained to evaluate for complications in a patient that is known to have Crohn's disease. The distribution of the disease greatly impacts the findings seen on CT. The most common findings associated with Crohn's disease are bowel wall thickening, peri-intestinal inflammation, and regional lymphadenopathy. The bowel wall can reach 11–13 mm in thickness, which can be either symmetric or asymmetric. The halo sign, which is a low-attenuation ring caused by submucosal deposition of fat between the enhancing mucosa and bowel musculature, is a common finding associated with Crohn's disease (Figure 6-30A). The transmural nature of the inflammatory process allows it to extend into the mesentery and adjacent structures so there is often an extensive inflammatory response centered on the affected bowel. There are many features that help to distinguish Crohn's disease from other inflammatory diseases of the GI tract. First, Crohn's disease is usually found to involve the terminal ileum and right colon. Second, there may be skip lesions. For example, multiple segments of small bowel and/or colon may be involved (Figure 6-30B). Third, the presence of mesenteric adenopathy suggests Crohn's or UC, but is not specific for IBD. Finally, the presence of complications such as abscess, fistula, or perforation points to a diagnosis of Crohn's disease. Abscesses can be located between intestinal loops, within the mesentery, in the psoas muscle, pelvic sidewall, and subcutaneous tissues (Figure 6-31). Fistulas

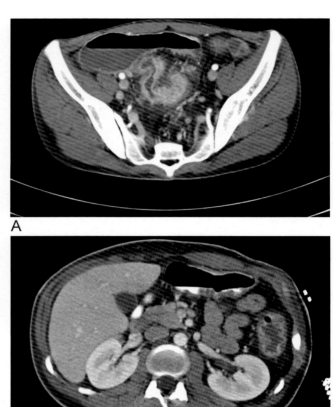

A

B

FIGURE 6-30. **A** CT scan showing Terminal Ileum (TI) Crohn's disease with abscess. **B** CT scan showing Crohn's colitis.

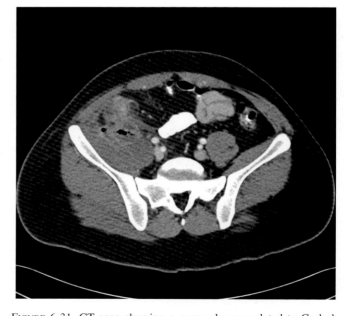

FIGURE 6-31. CT scan showing a psoas abscess related to Crohn's disease.

from the diseased segment of bowel to the bladder, skin, vagina, or normal bowel can also be delineated on CT.

Small Bowel Obstruction

As mentioned above, SBO is a clinical diagnosis based on the signs, symptoms, and clinical condition of the patient. Radiologic studies are obtained to confirm the clinical diagnosis. Typically, the first line investigation is plain films of the abdomen, but their accuracy varies from 46% to 80%.[30] As a result, there is often a delay in the diagnosis, which can lead to an increase in morbidity and mortality. The use of CT in the evaluation of an SBO is expanding and in many cases can eliminate the delay in diagnosis. CT has the advantages of being able to identify the site of obstruction, cause of obstruction, and it can provide information regarding vascular compromise of the bowel. Indications when a CT scan is particularly helpful include 1) a patient with no prior surgery, 2) a patient with equivocal plain films and an uncertain diagnosis, and 3) a patient with known intraabdominal pathology such as Crohn's disease or cancer.

Oral contrast is not always necessary and should be avoided in patients with a high-grade or complete bowel obstruction. The intraluminal fluid often distends the bowel and acts as a natural contrast agent. The low-density intestinal fluid also extenuates the enhancement of the bowel wall after the administration of IV contrast, which can provide information regarding the flow of blood of the bowel.

The diagnostic criteria of an SBO by CT are based on the presence of dilated proximal small bowel (> 2.5 cm) and collapsed distal bowel. When a transition between dilated and collapsed bowel is identified, then the diagnosis is confirmed (Figure 6-32). But when a transition point is not identified, it is difficult to distinguish between an SBO and adynamic ileus. In such cases, one must search for other clues to differentiate the processes. For example, the presence of "small bowel feces," which is gas bubbles mixed within particulate matter, in the dilated bowel is a reliable indicator of an SBO. The presence of other intraabdominal pathology, particularly inflammatory processes, would generally indicate an adynamic ileus. This is a case in which oral contrast may be particularly helpful because if contrast reaches the colon, a complete SBO is not present.

CT can also provide significant information regarding the cause of the obstruction. Once again, the findings must be interpreted in context with the patient's clinical situation. When there is a sharp transition from dilated to decompressed bowel in the absence of other findings, this is highly suggestive of an SBO secondary to adhesions. CT does an excellent job identifying hernias such as inguinal, umbilical, incisional, or more of the atypical types. Often these hernias contain bowel but not all are obstructing. Clues indicating obstruction include dilate bowel going into the hernia and collapsed bowel exiting the hernia, oral contrast proximal to the hernia and no contrast distal to the hernia, and a localized inflammatory process surrounding the hernia, particularly in the subcutaneous tissues (Figure 6-33). Another common extrinsic cause of obstruction is recurrent cancer. A CT scan is often able to demonstrate a mass at the site of obstruction and may also provide evidence of more widespread peritoneal disease. Unexpected causes of obstruction may also be identified such as Crohn's disease, intussusception, or small bowel cancers.

When the affected bowel becomes strangulated, the morbidity and mortality associated with an SBO increase significantly. No test is able to provide definitive proof of strangulated bowel, but CT is able to provide a wealth of

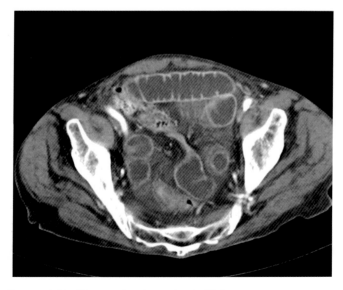

FIGURE 6-32. CT scan showing a simple SBO.

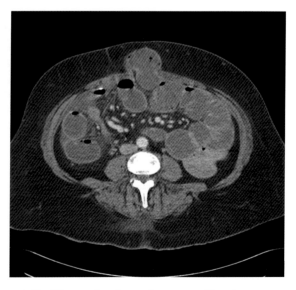

FIGURE 6-33. CT scan showing an incarcerated hernia.

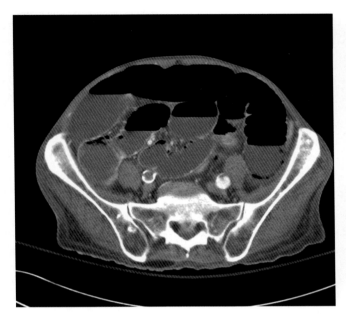

FIGURE 6-34. CT scan of SBO with evidence of ischemia.

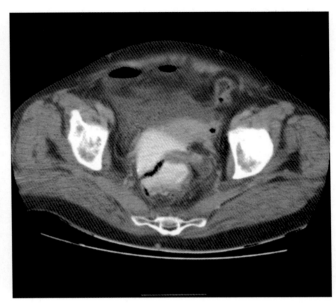

FIGURE 6-35. CT scan of colorectal anastomotic leak.

information that can indicate concern for vascular compromise. Thickened, congested bowel with increased attenuation at the site of obstruction associated with engorgement of the mesenteric vasculature is concerning for strangulation (Figure 6-34). The mesentery may become hazy or the vasculature may be obliterated as the inflammation progresses and it becomes filled with fluid or even blood. Other findings of ischemia include lack of enhancement after IV contrast administration or the presence of ascites. The presence of pneumatosis and portal venous gas are the more ominous signs of intestinal ischemia. Finally, a spiral pattern of engorged mesenteric blood vessels may indicate an internal hernia or rotation of small intestine around fixed adhesions.

Postoperative Evaluation

CT has greatly impacted the postoperative evaluation of the surgical patient. It is typically used to evaluate a patient with abdominal pain, fevers, leukocytosis, or persistent ileus in the postoperative period. The yield of a CT scan is greatest when it is obtained 5 days or more after surgery. Before postoperative day five, it is difficult to differentiate normal postoperative intraperitoneal free air or fluid from air or fluid that represents a leak from a hollow viscus or infected fluid. It usually takes more than 5 days for an abscess to organize into a walled-off, contained collection. Once again, the findings of the CT scan must be interpreted in the context of the clinical condition of the patient. Therefore, the yield will be greatest when the scan can address a specific question.

Findings highly suggestive of an anastomotic leak include an inappropriate volume of free air or fluid in the abdomen. The presence of extraluminal oral contrast confirms a perforation of a hollow viscus. The presence of localized fluid and air around an anastomosis are concerning for a leak but must be taken in context to the postoperative period and the condition of the patient. As mentioned above, water-soluble enemas are more sensitive than a CT with rectal contrast at detecting a colorectal anastomotic leak. However, a CT is often more easily and readily obtained. An abscess is defined as an organized fluid collection with or without air that has an enhancing rim (Figure 6-35). As mentioned above, CT is very good at distinguishing between an ileus and a mechanical bowel obstruction, which is an important distinction in the perioperative period.

Other Colitides

There are a handful of inflammatory processes that affect the colon that have not been addressed. The CT findings are very similar for all inflammatory processes of the colon. However, their clinical presentations are different, so combining the presenting signs and symptoms with the distribution of CT findings will usually lead to the correct diagnosis. This section will briefly address some these remaining processes.

Neutropenic enterocolitis or typhlitis typically occurs in patients who are neutropenic either from cytotoxic chemotherapy or severe immunosuppression. The terminal ileum, cecum, and right colon are most frequently affected. CT is the study of choice for the diagnosis. Circumferential thickening of the terminal ileum, cecum, and variably the right colon are the common CT findings consistent with typhlitis (Figure 6-36). The bowel wall may become so thickened because of edema that a hypodense ring develops between the mucosa and musculature. Complications such as pneumatosis or perforation can also be detected.

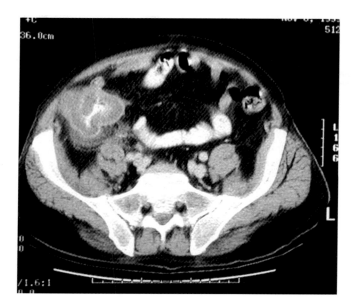

FIGURE 6-36. CT scan of neutropenic enterocolitis.

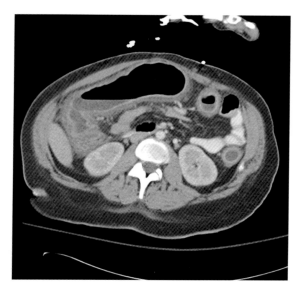

FIGURE 6-38. CT scan of pseudomembranous colitis.

Ischemic colitis is the most common vascular abnormality of the colon. Presenting symptoms include abdominal pain associated with bloody diarrhea. The age of the patient and onset of symptoms will help to differentiate between IBD, infectious colitis, and ischemic colitis. Endoscopy is the gold standard for diagnosing ischemic colitis. CT is much more readily available so it is often the first test ordered. The colitis may be segmental or diffuse, typically occurring in the watershed areas of the right colon, splenic flexure, and rectosigmoid. CT findings consist of thickened, edematous colon in these areas (Figure 6-37). The typical "thumbprinting" in the colonic mucosa can be seen on CT scan as well as plain films. There may be a halo sign of either low attenuation caused by edema or high attenuation caused by hemorrhage within the bowel wall. A pericolonic inflammatory response is often present as well. Thrombus within the colonic

mesenteric vessels may also be seen. Finally, pneumatosis or portal venous gas may be present indicating bowel infarction.

Pseudomembranous colitis resulting from the toxins produced by *Clostridium difficile* can cause profound inflammation of the colon. Computed tomographic findings include nonspecific thickening and edema of the colon and pericolonic inflammation. Generally, the edema and thickening of the colon is greater than that seen with infectious colitis or other inflammatory processes. The presence of pancolitis also tends to suggest pseudomembranous colitis versus other colitides (Figure 6-38). Once again, the CT results must be interpreted in the clinical context of the patient.

Radionuclide Imaging

Radionuclide imaging studies base their imaging on physiology rather than anatomy, and have a wide spectrum of use in clinical medicine. Radiopharmaceuticals and gamma cameras are the mainstay of radionuclide imaging. The specific radionuclides are chosen based on either the biologic properties of the element (i.e., iodine has an affinity for thyroid tissue) or the physical and chemical properties that allow linkage to appropriate compounds. These radiolabeled compounds are given to a patient to localize within a specific organ system (such as the thyroid) or identify the sight of an ongoing physiologic process (as in GI bleeding). The quality of a scan depends on how well the agent targets the organ or the physiologic process. A gamma camera is used to acquire images once the agent is given to the patient. Gamma and X-ray photons are absorbed and converted into flashes of light.[38] The location and intensity of these scintillation events are determined and recorded. Spot images are generally taken in 10-minute intervals and the completed image reflects the

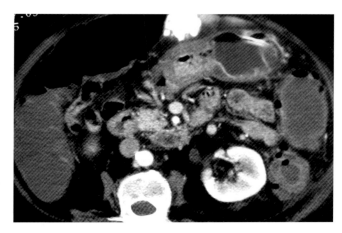

FIGURE 6-37. CT scan of ischemic colitis.

distribution of scintillation events (counts) detected during the acquisition phase. Image quality improves as the number of counts increases.

Radionuclide imaging studies are widely used in the diagnosis of lower GI bleeding. The principle is that the intravascular tracer will be extravasated into the bowel lumen during active bleeding. Concentration of the tracer on the acquired images allows identification of the bleeding sight. Technetium ^{99m}Tc is the radionuclide used in bleeding scans. This radiopharmaceutical can label colloid or red blood cells for scanning purposes. Radiolabeled colloid is readily available, but is metabolized rapidly. Red blood cells take longer to label but clearance of the tagged cells is prolonged and the tracer can remain active up to 24 hours after injection. Most centers prefer to use tagged red blood cells because lower GI bleeds are characteristically intermittent and the opportunity to identify the active bleeding sight lasts only a few minutes with labeled colloid. The preparation for a tagged red blood cell scan requires an aliquot of the patient's blood to be labeled with [99m]Tc. Once labeled, ^{99m}Tc red blood cells are injected back into the patient and the patient is imaged with 10-minute acquisition intervals for approximately 60–120 minutes. Focal areas of increased activity identified within the lumen of the bowel indicate that active bleeding occurred during this acquisition period (Figure 6-39). A positive scan may localize the region of bowel that contains the bleeding site, but may not accurately localize the specific site, if the bleeding is slow or intermittent. The labeled red blood cells remain in circulation as long as the cells are viable and the limiting factor to imaging is the half-life of the [99m]Tc. If no bleeding occurs during the initial acquisition phase, then delayed views can be obtained up to 24 hours later to determine whether active bleeding has occurred. Bleeding scans have greater prognostic value than diagnostic value when the tracer is only seen on delayed images.[39,40] The location of activity seen on delayed images does not reflect the exact bleeding sight but does indicate that active bleeding occurred during this observation period. The accuracy for localizing the actual bleeding site increases if the extravasation of tracer is identified within the first 15–30 minutes.[36] The longer it takes the tracer to accumulate, the less likely the bleeding site will be accurately

identified by angiography. Backwash and washout of blood caused by peristalsis account for some of this inaccuracy.

Bleeding scans are more sensitive than angiograms in the detection of lower GI bleeding. The required rates of bleeding for detection are lower for bleeding scans (0.1–0.2 mL per minute) than for angiograms (0.5 mL per minute).[37,41] The early (within 3 minutes) detection of intraluminal tracer indicates a high likelihood of successful arteriographic localization of the bleeding site. For this reason, some interventional radiologists require a positive scan before performing angiography. The addition of early colonoscopy to the diagnostic algorithm requires a bowel preparation. Cathartics will remove any intraluminal tracer making delayed images worthless. If the patient is hemodynamically unstable and rapidly bleeding, some centers may prefer to go directly to arteriograms because the time involved in pretest preparation for tagged red blood scans may be too lengthy.

A Meckel's scan, although not used as often as the tagged red blood scan, can be useful in the evaluation of patients with occult bleeding with no identifiable colonic source. These scans are generally limited to the evaluation of children and young adults who have complaints of abdominal pain and intestinal bleeding. The abnormal bleeding from a Meckel's diverticulum is caused by the aberrant gastric mucosa that lines the diverticulum. [99]Tc pertechnetate is actively extracted by mucous secreting cells in gastric mucosa.[42,43] Meckel's scans are performed with ^{99m}Tc per pertechnetate as a radiolabel for the detection of ectopic gastric mucosa. Imaging is usually done for approximately 30–60 minutes after injection of the tracer. All views should be obtained early because the tracer is extracted into the stomach and then into lumen of the GI tract. Rapid transit of the tracer through the GI tract will obscure extravasation on later images.

A focus of increased radioactivity outside of the stomach indicates ectopic gastric mucosa (Figure 6-40). Typically, the collection of activity is identified in the right lower quadrant within 10–20 minutes. The sensitivity of the Meckel's scan is 85% and the specificity is 95%.[43]

Arteriography

Arteriography is an invasive procedure performed by specialty trained physicians and is used in the diagnosis and treatment of a variety of colorectal diseases. The arteriogram is performed through a percutaneous approach under sterile conditions. The femoral artery is a preferred puncture sight although axillary and brachial arteries may be used. A guidewire is introduced through the needle and a catheter is introduced over the guidewire. Various catheters and guide wires allow the interventional radiologist to access the vessels in question.

Arteriography is an invasive procedure with an overall mortality of one in 40,000.[44] Complications from the performance of the procedure and manipulation of the wires and catheters

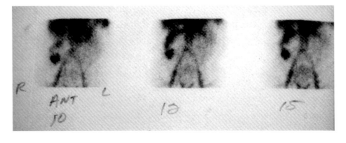

FIGURE 6-39. ^{99m}Tc-tagged red blood cell study shows early blood pool activity within the ascending colon in this patient with bleeding after a recent polypectomy.

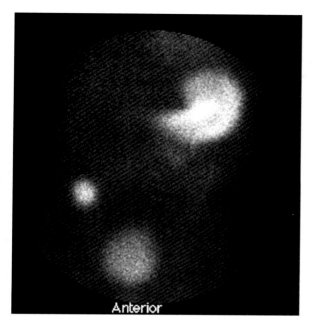

FIGURE 6-40. ^{99m}Tc-pertechnetate scan (Meckel's) shows a discrete focus of increased uptake in the right lower quadrant, with approximately the same intensity as the stomach indicating gastric mucosa is present within this Meckel's diverticulum.

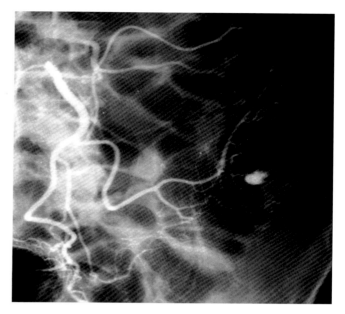

FIGURE 6-41. Mesenteric angiogram shows pooling of contrast in the sigmoid colon in this patient with surgically proven diverticular bleeding.

are more common than reactions to the contrast itself.[45] The most common complications are related to hematomas or pseudoaneurysms at the puncture sight, dissection or embolization secondary to catheter manipulation. Contrast reactions and contrast toxicity (renal failure) occur in <1% of studies done. Experience and technique can minimize many of the complications. Hydration and IV mannitol can reduce the nephrotoxicity. If the patient has allergies to iodine or has had a prior contrast reaction, premedication with methyl prednisolone is done 12 and 2 hours before arteriography.

The arteriogram is a useful diagnostic and therapeutic modality in the treatment of active lower GI bleeding. If a radionuclide scan is performed and localizes the site of bleeding, a selective angiogram can then be performed. For bleeding localized to the left colon on tagged RBC study, the inferior mesenteric artery is selected first. The superior mesenteric artery is selected first for those bleeds that occur in the right colon. If the bleeding site is not identified after injection of both the superior and inferior mesenteric arteries, a celiac run is performed looking for an upper intestinal bleeding source. Active bleeding can be diagnosed by the accumulation of contrast in the arterial phase that persists through the venous phase (Figure 6-41). Bleeding needs to occur at a higher rate for a positive angiogram (0.5 mL per minute) than for nuclear imaging (0.1–0.2 mL per minute). Because lower GI bleeding can be intermittent, the bleeding site is sometimes not identified at the time of the angiogram.

Diverticulosis and vascular ectasias are presumed to be the leading cause of lower GI bleeding in most patients.

Diverticular bleeds appear as a blush of contrast contained within a diverticulum. Vascular ectasias often occur in the right colon and appear as small vascular clusters, a blush in the wall of the colon and early opacification of a draining vein.[46] Arteriovenous malformations are developmental in origin and are often seen in the small bowel. They appear as tortuous, dilated arteries and early prominent veins. Capillary telangiectasias (common in Osler Weber Rendu syndrome) appear as multiple, tiny areas of blush and no arteriovenous shunting. Postpolypectomy bleeding has been diagnosed and treated with angiography. A rapid blush of dye occurs at the site of bleeding and often stops with direct infusion of vasopressin or embolization (Figure 6-42).

Acute mesenteric ischemia is one of the most common intestinal disease processes for which arteriography is used for diagnosis and treatment. Acute mesenteric ischemia can be either nonocclusive or occlusive. Nonocclusive mesenteric ischemia arises from a "low flow" state typically secondary to reduction in mesenteric blood flow from cardiac failure or hypotensive shock. This diagnosis can frequently be made with clinical symptoms and computer tomography images. The typical early angiographic images show diffuse vasoconstriction of mesenteric arterial branches and decreased parenchymal vascularity (Figure 6-43). In the late stage there is increased accumulation of contrast in the bowel wall. Treatment includes volume resuscitation and cardiac support. The diagnostic percutaneous catheter can be used to treat the mesenteric phase of constriction with IV glucagon or intraarterial infusion of the papaverine in an intensive care unit setting.

Occlusive acute mesenteric ischemia is a medical emergency, thus early diagnosis and treatment may prevent bowel

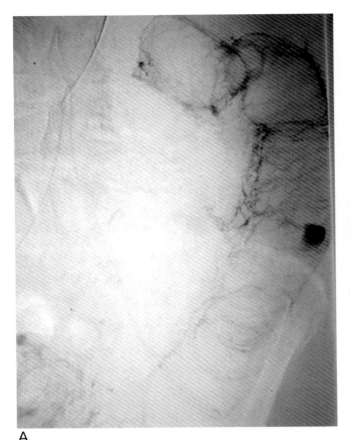

A

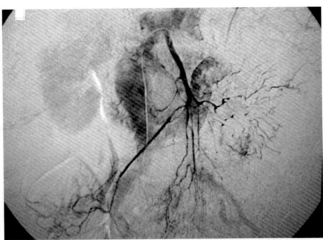

FIGURE 6-43. Mesenteric angiogram shows vasoconstriction and pruning of the superior mesenteric artery and its branches in this patient who presented with mesenteric ischemia secondary to severe hypotension.

necrosis and perforation. These patients typically have severe abdominal pain with nonspecific physical findings.[47] An arteriogram is the most useful diagnostic examination for patients in whom one has a high clinical suspicion of acute occlusive mesenteric ischemia.[48] A catheter is inserted into the aorta and an aortogram is obtained. The celiac and superior mesenteric arteries are catheterized and injected with contrast in order to identify the level of occlusion and document collateral circulation. A superior mesenteric artery embolus typically lodges just proximal or distal to the take off of the middle colic artery and is seen as a meniscus at the site of occlusion and blockage of contrast (Figure 6-44). Atherosclerotic occlusion will often involve the origin of the superior mesenteric artery seen as stenosis or plaque with a trickle of glow beyond (Figure 6-45). Collaterals will develop from the inferior mesenteric artery through the marginal artery. If the inferior mesenteric artery is occluded or absent, the collaterals will develop from the middle or inferior hemorrhoidal arterial branches of the internal iliac artery.[48,49]

CT Colonography

CT colonography is rapidly developing as a noninvasive total colonic examination for the detection of colon polyps and cancers. This technique uses volumetric data acquired by helical CT scanners and workstations which use two- and three-dimensional images to evaluate data. Since 1994, there have been technical improvements in the CT hardware and software allowing better visualization and discrimination of the reconstituted images. The three-dimensional endoluminal imaging is better at evaluation of surface morphology and discriminating between polyps and haustral folds (Figure 6-46).[50] The

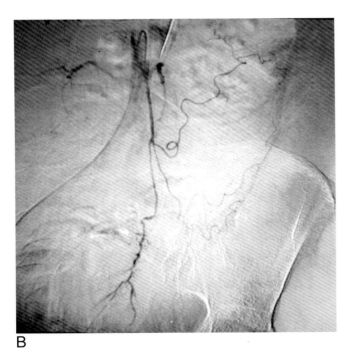

B

FIGURE 6-42. Mesenteric angiogram shows extravasation of contrast **A** indicating an acute bleed that was successfully treated after infusion of pitressin **B**.

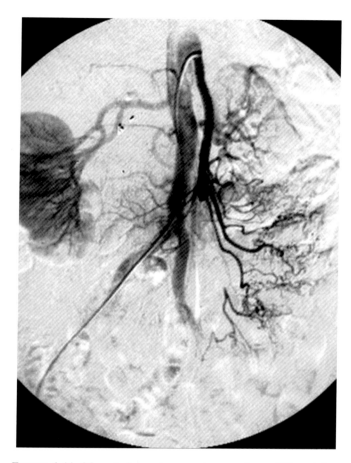

FIGURE 6-44. Mesenteric angiogram shows a large filling defect within the proximal superior mesenteric artery consistent with an embolism in this patient with ischemic bowel.

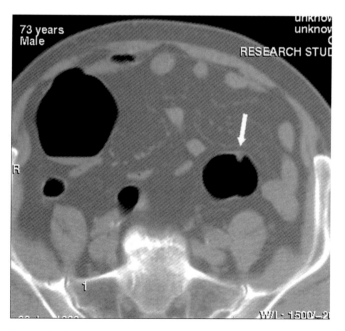

FIGURE 6-45. Axial two-dimensional image from a CT colon study shows a well-defined 6-mm polyp in the sigmoid colon.

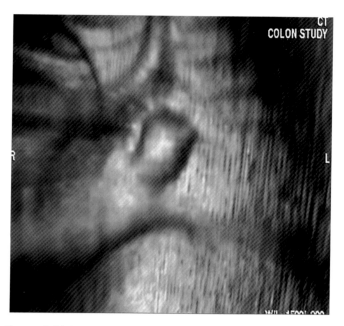

FIGURE 6-46. Three-dimensional image confirms the presence of the polyp in Figure 6-45.

two-dimensional images help in the correlation of images seen on the three-dimensional fly-through.

Image processing and interpretation has improved with newer software and an experienced radiologist can generally complete the examination in <15 minutes.

Although the colon is evaluated in a noninvasive way, a bowel preparation is still required the day before the examination to eliminate formed fecal matter. Air insufflation is done via a small tube placed within the rectum to distend the bowel and to minimize folds within the colonic wall. Insufflation with a handheld bulb, or with a CO_2 insufflator is performed. A CT tomogram is obtained to confirm adequate insufflation in both the prone and supine positions and further air is insufflated as needed. Unlike colonoscopy, IV sedation is not required. Patient satisfaction after colonoscopy and CT colonography are similar because bowel preparation is needed for both tests.[51]

Rapid scanning can be done in a single breath hold. Volumetric data are acquired twice, once with the patient prone and once with the patient supine. The change in position allows any fluid within the bowel lumen to shift, revealing abnormalities within the contralateral wall. Most tests can be completed in <15 minutes. Once the images are acquired, a trained radiologist reviews them at the workstation and the images are recreated in such a way as to give an endoluminal view of the colon similar to that seen on colonoscopy. Several studies have compared CT colonography to colonoscopy for high- and low-risk patients. The sensitivity of this technique per individual patient ranges from 75% to 100% and the specificity ranges from 72% to 100%.[50–54] Both the sensitivity and specificity are dependent on the polyp size. In randomized,

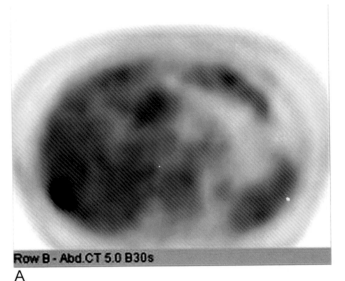

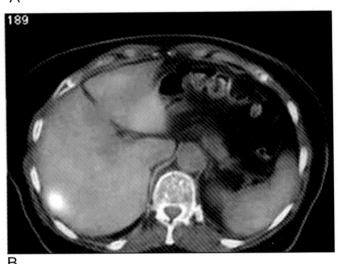

FIGURE 6-47. Axial attenuation corrected PET image **A** and fusion PET CT image **B** show an area of intense FDG uptake in the right hepatic lobe consistent with hepatic metastatic disease in this patient with cecal adenocarcinoma.

controlled trials, the specificity is greater for polyps larger than 1 cm than for polyps larger than 5 mm.[53] The detection of small (< 5 mm) polyps is poor in most studies with sensitivities as low as 11.5%.[54,55] The importance of these small lesions continues to be debated by the medical community. A recent nonrandomized multicenter blinded study comparing CT colonography with colonoscopy found that the sensitivity for CT colonography detecting polyps ≥6 mm was 39% and those ≥10 mm was 55%.[56] This study acknowledged that the accuracy of CT colonography varied between centers and with the experience of the radiologists. Interobserver variability can be significant and is evidence of the steep learning curve.[57]

The main limitation of CT colonography has been distinguishing polypoid tissue from fecal matter and the detection of flat lesions.[55] Acquiring images after a change from the prone to the supine position can frequently unmask hidden polyps and tagging residual stool with subsequent digital subtraction is being evaluated.[58] An added benefit of the technique is the potential for the discovery of incidental extracolonic findings. The dose of radiation used for CT colonography is less than for conventional CT with the result that the scanned images are not the same. Nonetheless, the incidence of clinically important extracolonic findings is approximately 11%.[59]

Whether CT colonography can be used for mass screening of average-risk patients has yet to be determined. Currently, most centers are using CT colonography for those patients who have had incomplete colonoscopies or who cannot undergo colonoscopy for medical reasons. Clinical trials are ongoing as educational efforts and technical improvements are made in an attempt to improve this potential screening technique.

Positron Emission Tomography

Whole body positron emission tomography (PET) was originally developed as a research technique in the 1970s. The clinical use of this technique has evolved over the past several decades. This technique uses [18F] 2-fluoro-2-deoxy-D-glucose (FDG) which is a radiopharmaceutical glucose analog to measure increased glucose uptake and metabolism in rapidly dividing cells. Malignant and other rapidly dividing cells that have a high metabolic rate will take up FDG for use as a glucose substrate. The first metabolite of FDG is FDG-6-phosphate which is not a substrate for glucosephosphate isomerase because of the configuration of FDG. FDG-6-phosphate has a low membrane permeability and thus the labeled substrate accumulates intracellularly.[60] The imaging technique of PET utilizes differences in uptake of FDG in malignant versus benign cells. The intracellular accumulation concentrates the radiopharmaceutical analog, which appears "bright" upon imaging (Figure 6-47).

The performance of a PET scan requires that the patient fast for 4–6 hours before the injection of FDG. A urinary catheter is placed to minimize the effect of the accumulation of tracer in the bladder. Emission scans are then performed with the patient motionless shifting the table between scans to alter the field of view. Older techniques required that a patient remain motionless for approximately 1–2 hours. Newer techniques have reduced the scan per bed position to approximately 2 minutes. Scans are then enhanced through a segmentation calibration and the scattered events outside the body are removed. Attenuation in each area is altered depending on tissue within the region.[61]

FDG PET has been used to evaluate metastatic disease and to improve staging accuracy (Figure 6-48). This technique images the whole body and is more sensitive than CT for the detection of hepatic and extrahepatic colorectal cancer

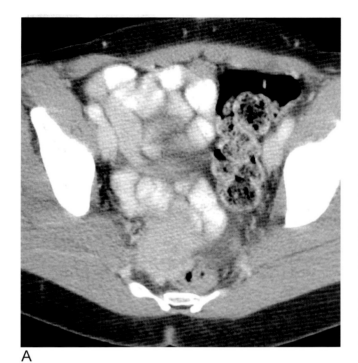

A

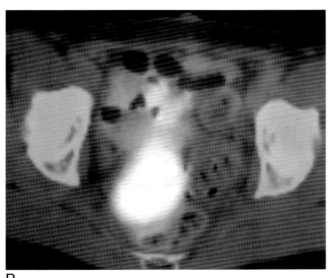

B

FIGURE 6-48. CT scan in a patient who had prior rectal resection for carcinoma shows soft tissue mass in the surgical bed of the perirectal fat **A**. Follow-up PET examination **B** shows intense FDG uptake within this soft tissue mass consistent with recurrence.

metastases and the detection of local recurrence. The reported sensitivities for PET detection of liver metastases range from 89% to 95% and for extrahepatic metastases 87% to 92%.[62–66] The use of FDG PET versus CT or MRI is based on the premise that functional differences in tumor appear before size changes. Postoperative changes, particularly for rectal cancers, are difficult to evaluate using standard modalities. The distinction between tumor and scar is not easily defined with the

current CT and MRI scans. FDG PET is extremely useful in this arena because a positive FDG PET scan in the setting of no inflammation would indicate a local recurrence of a rectal cancer. Furthermore, detection of small extrapelvic metastases is more accurate using FDG PET than CT or MRI. Thus, the use of FDG PET for staging or recurrent cancers may help plan or avoid expensive and possibly more morbid surgical procedures.

False-positive and false-negative tests have been reported to occur in several distinct situations. FDG is not a tumor-specific substance and increased FDG activity is seen in the normal urinary and GI tracts. The cellular glucose metabolism is also increased in inflammation as the increased uptake of FDG can be seen in leukocytes and macrophages. Inflammatory processes such as diverticulitis and pneumonia can lead to false-positive readings thus making it imperative to correlate positive PET findings with the clinical picture and conventional radiologic evaluation.[67,68]

Detection of metastatic disease is dependent on the size and degree of metabolic activity. Limited spatial resolution may lead to false-negative readings for small, <1-cm lesions.[69] Adenocarcinomas with a high mucinous content may result in false-negative readings because of the low cellularity of these cancers. Sensitivity can be as low as 59% for mucinous carcinomas.[70] The combination of CT and FDG PET imaging has reduced some of the inaccuracies and makes the study more readily correlated anatomically.

The routine use of FDG PET for primary cancers is more problematic. Although the risks and radiation doses are low and the technique is noninvasive, the cost per scan is very high. Thus, for primary cancers in which the information would not alter the planned surgical procedure, it is probably not indicated. However, in patients that are poor surgical risk, the findings in FDG PET may help avoid or alter the surgical procedure and might change the goal from a curative to palliative intent. Current CMS (HCFA) recommendations for reimbursed PET imaging in colorectal cancer include 1) evaluation of patients with a question of recurrent disease as indicated by rising CEA, 2) evaluation of resectability, and 3) evaluation of patients with locally advanced disease to determine unresectability on the basis of metastasis when the operation is a large otherwise debilitating procedure.

MRI is a continually evolving field of radiology. The technique was developed in the early 1980s and currently there is a wide range of MRI systems in use. This technique relies on the difference in tissue contrast or signal intensity. High signal intensity appears white on the image whereas low signal intensity is dark. T^1 and T^2 refer to specific tissue properties that describe the way protons behave after being excited by a radiofrequency pulse in a strong magnetic field.[71,72] The specific parameters chosen to acquire an image on an MR magnetic system determine whether an image is T^1 or T^2 weighted. T^1 refers to the longitudinal relaxation rate and T^2 refers to the transverse relaxation rate. Structures containing water appear black on T^1-rated images and structures containing fluid (cysts or gallbladder) are white on T^2-weighted images. Unlike CT scans, iodinated contrast is not used for the performance of these scans. The contrast agents that have been developed can be used in patients with renal insufficiencies, and those with iodinated contrast allergic reaction. The risk from MRI is attributed to the interaction between the strong magnetic field and certain implantable devices such as cardiac pacemakers, cerebral aneurysms clips, and cochlear implants.

The use of MR for intraabdominal bowel anatomy is limited because of the peristaltic action of the bowel wall and motion of the abdominal cavity caused by respirations. MRI has evolved to be better than CT for tissue characterization and evaluation of tissues planes within the pelvis. The layers of the bowel wall can be visualized easily for evaluation of rectal cancers. The muscularis propria is low signal intensity and the submucosa has higher signal intensity.[73,74] The accuracy of MRI for preoperative staging for rectal carcinoma continues to be evaluated. Contrast enhancement improves the correlation with histologic stage.[75] Endorectal MRI is similar to endoluminal ultrasound for determination of tumor depth and nodal staging although some studies have shown ultrasound to be more accurate in determining local invasion.[76,77] Overstaging and interobserver variation make reliable preoperative staging difficult.[75,78] MRI more accurately predicts the circumferential resection margin (Figure 6-49).[79] Several parameters help distinguish pathologic tissues. After pelvic irradiation, the radiation edema or fibrosis can be differentiated from tumor on T^2-weighted images. The fibrosis appears low signal in the T^2 images and enhances slowly. Recurrent tumors have a higher signal and enhance quickly during dynamic gadolinium-enhanced scanning.[80,81] Changes in postradiation normal tissue result in slow tissue enhancement with gadolinium.[80]

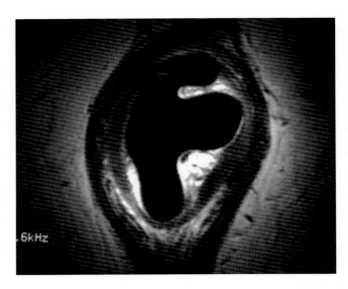

FIGURE 6-50. Endoanal MRI image demonstrates a nondisrupted (normal) signal of the internal and external sphincter.

The anal sphincter and pelvic anatomy have been imaged with MR using an internal coil (Figure 6-50). The internal sphincter has higher signal intensity than the external sphincter. Pelvic muscle morphology, sphincter injuries, and abscesses can be identified. Clinical experience with MR has not been as extensive as with endoluminal ultrasound but comparative studies have been favorable. MRI of the puborectalis is better than endorectal ultrasound and capable of showing atrophy.[82] It remains to be seen what the role of MR will be in the evaluation of fecal incontinence because of variability of scanner capabilities among institutions and limited access to high-performance scanners.

References

1. Flak B, Rowley VA. Acute abdomen: plain film utilization and analysis. Can Assoc Radiol J 1993;44:423–428.
2. Simeone JF, Novelline RA, Ferrucci JT, et al. Comparison of sonography and plain films in the evaluation of the acute abdomen. AJR Am J Roentgenol 1985;144(1):49–52.
3. Mirvis S, Young J, Keramati B, et al. Plain film evaluation of patients with abdominal pain: are three radiographs necessary? AJR Am J Roentgenol 1986;144:501–503.
4. Maglinte D, Heitkamp D, Howard T, et al. Current concepts in imaging of small bowel obstruction. Radiol Clin North Am 2003;41:263–283.
5. Miller G, Boman J, Shier I, et al. Etiology of small bowel obstruction. Am J Surg 2000;180:33–36.
6. Ogilvie H. Large intestine colic due to sympathetic deprivation. Br Med J 1948;2:671–673.
7. Sarr MG, Bulkey GB, Zuidena GD, et al. Preoperative recognition of intestinal strangulation obstruction. Prospective evaluation of diagnostic capability. Am J Surg 1983;145:176–182.
8. Rigler LG. Spontaneous pneumoperitoneum: a roentgenologic sign found in the supine position. Radiology 1941;37:604–607.

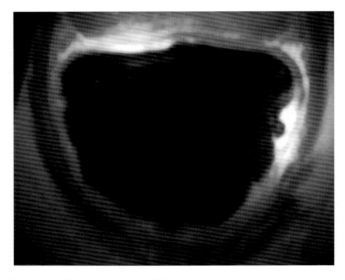

FIGURE 6-49. Endorectal MRI examination shows an ulcerated plaque-like cancer arising from the mucosa and extending to the first muscular layer of the muscularis propria.

9. Miller RE, Nelson SW. The roentgenological demonstration of tiny amounts of free intraperitoneal gas: experimental and clinical studies. AJR Am J Roentgenol 1971;112:487–490.

10. Ly J. The Rigler sign. Radiology 2003;228:706–707.

11. Miller RE, Becker GJ, Slabaugh RA. Detection of pneumoperitoneum: optimum body position and respiratory phase. AJR Am J Roentgenol 1980;135:487–490.

12. Levine MS, Scheiner JD, Rubesin SE, et al. Diagnosis of pneumoperitoneum on supine abdominal radiographs. AJR Am J Roentgenol 1991;156:731–735.

13. Almer S, Bodemar G, Franzen L, et al. Plain X-ray films and air enema films reflect severe mucosal inflammation in acute ulcerative colitis. Digestion 1995;56:528–533.

14. Walsh JM, Terdiman JP. Colorectal cancer screening: clinical applications. JAMA 2003;289:1297–1302.

15. Fork ET, Ekberg O, Nilsson G, et al. Colon cleansing regimens. Gastrointest Radiol 1982;7:383–389.

16. Klabunde CN, Jones E, Brown ML, et al. Colorectal cancer screening with double-contrast barium enema: a national survey of diagnostic radiologists. AJR Am J Roentgenol 2002;179:1419–1427.

17. Winawer SJ, Stewart ET, Zauber AG, et al. A comparison of colonoscopy and double-contrast barium enema from surveillance after polypectomy. New Engl J Med 2000;342:1766–1772.

18. Kronborg O. Colon polyps and cancer. Endoscopy 2004;36:3–7.

19. Yamamoto M, Mine H, Kusumoto H, et al. Polyps with different grades of dysplasia and their distribution in the colorectum. Hepatogastroenterology 2004;51:121–123.

20. Levine MS, Rubesin SE, Laufer I, et al. Diagnosis of colorectal neoplasms at double-contrast barium enema examination. Radiology 2000;216:11–18.

21. McCarthy PA, Rubesin SE, Levine MS, et al. Colon cancer: morphology detected with barium enema versus histologic stage. Radiology 1995;197:683–687.

22. Hizawa K, Iida M, Kohrogi N, et al. Crohn's disease: early recognition and progress of aphthous lesions. Radiology 1994; 190:451–454.

23. Najjar SF, Jamal MK, Savas JF, et al. The spectrum of colovesical fistula and diagnostic paradigm. Am J Surg 2004;188: 617–621.

24. Almer S, Bodemar G, Franzen L, et al. Use of air enema radiology to assess depth of ulceration during acute attacks of ulcerative colitis. Lancet 1996;347:1731–1735.

25. Giardiello FM, Bayless TM. Colorectal cancer and ulcerative colitis. Radiology 1996;199:28–30.

26. Nolan DJ, Traill ZC. The current role of barium examinations of the small intestine. Clin Radiol 1997;52:809–820.

27. Scott DJ, Guthrie JA, Arnold P, et al. Dual phase helical CT versus portal venous phase CT for the detection of colorectal liver metastases: correlation with intra-operative sonography, surgical and pathological findings. Clin Radiol 2001;56:235–242.

28. Larimore T, Rhea J. Computed tomography evaluation of diverticulitis. J Intensive Care Med 2004;19:194–204.

29. Jarrett TW, Vaughan ED Jr. Accuracy of computerized tomography in the diagnosis of colovesical fistula secondary to diverticular disease. J Urol 1995;153:44–46.

30. Furukawa A, Yamasaki M, Takahashi M, et al. CT diagnosis of small bowel obstruction: scanning technique, interpretation and role in the diagnosis. Semin Ultrasound CT MR 2003;24:336–352.

31. ASCRS.

32. Maglinte DDT, Kelvin FM, O'Connor K, et al. Current status of small bowel radiology. Abdom Imaging 1996;21:247–257.

33. Shrake PD, Rex DK, Lappas JC, et al. Radiographic evaluation of suspected SBO. Am J Gastroenterol 1991;86:175–178.

34. Anthony T, Simmang C, Hyman N, et al. Practice parameters for the surveillance and follow-up of patients with colon and rectal cancer. Dis Colon Rectum 2004;47:807–817.

35. Bhattacharjya S, Bhattacharjya T, Bader S, et al. Prospective study of contrast-enhanced computed tomography, computed tomography during arterioportography, and magnetic resonance imaging for staging colorectal liver metastasis for liver resection. Br J Surg 2004;91:1361–1369.

36. Ng DA, Opelka FA, Beck DF, et al. Predictive value of technetium Tc 99-M-labeled red blood cell scintigraphy for positive angiogram in massive lower gastrointestinal bleeding. Dis Colon Rectum 1997;40:471–477.

37. Siddiqui AR, Schanwekcer DS, Wellman HN, et al. Comparison of tech-99-M sulfur colloid and in vitro labeled technetium-99M RBCs in the detection of GI bleeding. Clin Nucl Med 1985; 8:546.

38. Sorenson JA, Phelps ME. Physics in Nuclear Medicine. 2nd ed. Orlando: Grune & Stratton; 1987:298.

39. Winzelberg GG, McKusick KA, Froelich JW, et al. Detection of gastrointestinal bleeding with TC-99m labeled red blood cells. Semin Nucl Med 1982;12:139–146.

40. Jacobson AF, Cerqueira MD. Prognostic significance of late imaging results in technetium-99m-labeled blood cell gastrointestinal bleeding studies with early negative images. J Nucl Med 1992;33:202–207.

41. Alavi A, Dann RW, Baum S, et al. Scintigraphic detection of acute GI bleeding. Radiology 1977;124:753.

42. Sfakianakis GN, Conway JJ. Detection of ectopia gastric mucosa in Meckel's diverticulum and in other aberrations by scintigraphy. I. Pathophysiology and 10 year clinical experience. J Nucl Med 1981;22:647–654.

43. Sfakianakis GN, Conway JJ. Detection of ectopia gastric mucosa in Meckel's diverticulum and in other aberrations by scintigraphy. II. Indications and methods—a 10-year experience. J Nucl Med 1981;22:732–738.

44. Witten DM, Hirsch FD, Hartman GW. Acute reaction to urographic contrast medium: incidence, clinical characteristics and relationship to history of hypersensitivity states. AJR Am J Roentgenol 1973;119:832–840.

45. Hessel SJ, Adams DF, Abrams HL. Complications of angiography. Radiology 1981;138:273.

46. Baum S, Athanasoulis CA, Waltman AC, et al. Angiodysplasia of the right colon: a cause of gastrointestinal bleeding. AJR Am J Roentgenol 1977;129:789.

47. Tomchik FS, Wittenberg J, Ottinger LW. The roentgenographic spectrum of bowel infarction. Radiology 1970;96:249.

48. Flickinger EG, Johnsrude IS, Ogburn NL, Weaver MD, Pories WJ. Local streptokinase infusion for SMA thromboembolism. AJR Am J Roentgenol 1983;140:771–772.

49. Odurny A, Sniderman KW, Colapinto RF. Intestinal angina: percutaneous transluminal angioplasty of the celiac and SMA arteries. Radiology 1988;167:59.

50. Yee J, Akerkar GA, Hung RK, et al. Colorectal neoplasia: performance characteristics of CT colonography for detection in 300 patients. Radiology 2001;219:685.

51. Ristvedt SL, McFarland EG, Weinstock LB. Patient preferences for CT colonography, conventional colonoscopy, and bowel preparation. Am J Gastroenterol 2003;98:578.

52. Fenlon HM, Nunes DP, Schroy PC III, et al. A comparison of virtual and conventional colonoscopy for the detection of colon polyps. N Engl J Med 1999;341:1496–1503.

53. Fletcher JG, Johnson CD, Welch TJ. Optimization of CT colonography technique: prospective trial in 180 patients. Radiology 2000;216:704–711.

54. Pickhardt PF, Choi R, Hwang I, et al. Computed tomography virtual colonoscopy to screen for colorectal neoplasia in asymptomatic adults. N Engl J Med 2003;349:2191.

55. Macari M, Bini E, Jacobs S. Colorectal polyps and cancers in asymptomatic average-risk patients: evaluation with CT colonography. Radiology 2004;230:629.

56. Cotton PB, Durkalski VL, Pineau BC. Computed tomographic colonography (virtual colonoscopy). JAMA 2004;291:1713.

57. Pescatore P, Glucker T, Delarive J, et al. Diagnostic accuracy and interobserver agreements of CT colonography. Gut 2000;47:126.

58. Pickhardt PJ, Jong-Ho RC. Electronic cleansing and stool tagging in CT colonography: advantages and pitfalls with primary three-dimensional evaluation. AJR Am J Roentgenol 2003; 181:799.

59. Hara AK, Johnson CD, MacCarty RL, et al. Incidental extracolonic findings at CT colonography. Radiology 2000;215:353.

60. Pauwels E, McCready VR, Stoot JH, et al. The mechanism of accumulation of turnover localizing radiopharmaceuticals. Am J Nucl Med 1998;25:277.

61. Dobkin J, Xu M, Latifi H, et al. Initial clinical results with segmented transmission images for attenuation correction of whole-body PET [abstract]. J Nucl Med 1995;36:105.

62. Ito K, Kato T, Tadakoro M, et al. Recurrent rectal cancer and scar: differentiation with PET and MR imaging. Radiology 1992;182:549.

63. Beets G, Pennickx F, Schiepers C, et al. Clinical value of whole-body position emission tomography with [18F] fluoro deoxy glucose in recurrent colorectal cancer. Br J Surg 1994;81:1666.

64. Lai DT, Fulham M, Stephen MS, et al. The role of whole body position emission tomography with [18F] fluoro deoxy glucose in identifying operable colorectal cancer metastases and the liver. Arch Surg 1996;131:703.

65. Ogunbiyi OA, Flanagan FL, Dehdashti F, et al. Detection of recurrent and metastatic colorectal cancer: comparison of position emission tomography and computed tomography. Ann Surg Oncol 1997;4:613–620.

66. Whitford MH, Whitford HM, Yee LF, et al. Usefulness of suspected metastatic or recurrent adenocarcinoma of the colon and rectum. Dis Colon Rectum 2000;43:759.

67. Meyer MA. Diffusely increased colonic F-18-FDG uptake in acute enterocolitis. Clin Nucl Med 1995;20:434.

68. Strauss LG. Fluorine-18-deoxyglucose and false positive results: a major problem in the diagnostics of oncological patients. Eur J Nucl Med 1996;23:1409–1415.

69. Flamen P, Stroobants S, Van Cutsem E, et al. Additional value of whole-body positron emission tomography with fluorine-18-2-fluoro-2-deoxy-D-glucose in recurrent colorectal cancer. J Clin Oncol 1999;17:894.

70. Berger KL, Nicholson SA, Dehadastiti F, et al. FDG PET evaluation of mucinous neoplasms: correlation of FDA uptake with histopathologic features. AJR Am J Roentgenol 2000;174;1005.

71. Hendrick RE. The AAPM/RSNA physics tutorial for residents: basic physics of MR imaging: an introduction. Radiographics 1994;14:829.

72. Balter S. An introduction to the physics of magnetic resonance imaging. Radiographics 1987;7:371.

73. Meyenberger C, HuchBoni RA, Bertschinger P, et al. Endoscopic ultrasound and endorectal magnetic resonance imaging: a prospective, comparative study for preoperative staging and follow up of rectal cancer. Endoscopy 1995;270:469.

74. Schnall MD, Furth EE, Rosato EF, Kressel HY. Rectal tumor stage: correlation of endorectal MR imaging and pathologic findings. Radiology 1994;190:709–714.

75. Vogl TJ, Pegios W, Mack MG, et al. Accuracy of staging rectal tumors with contrast-enhanced transrectal MR imaging. AJR Am J Roentgenol 1997;168:1427.

76. Gualdi GF, Casciani E, Guadalaxara A, et al. Local staging of rectal cancer with transrectal ultrasound and endorectal magnetic resonance imaging: comparison with histologic findings. Dis Colon Rectum 2000;43:338.

77. Bipat S, Glas AS, Slors FJ, et al. Rectal cancer: local staging and assessment of lymph node involvement with endoluminal US, CT, and MR imaging—a metaanalysis. Radiology 2004;232:773.

78. Drew PJ, Farouk R, Turnbull LW, et al. Preoperative magnetic resonance staging of rectal cancer with an endorectal coil and dynamic gadolinium enhancement. Br J Surg 1999;86:250.

79. Branagan G, Chave H, Fuller C, et al. Can magnetic resonance imaging predict circumferential margin and TNM stage in rectal cancer? Dis Colon Rectum 2004;47:1317.

80. Hawighorst H, Knapstein PG, Schaeffer U, et al. Pelvic lesions in patients with terminal cervical carcinoma: efficiency of pharmacokinetic analysis of dynamic MR images in distinguishing recurrent tumors from benign conditions. AJR Am J Roentgenol 1996;166:401.

81. Torricelli P, Pecchi A, Luppi G, Romagnoli R. Gadolinium-enhanced MRI with dynamic evaluation in diagnosing the local recurrence of rectal cancer. Abdom Imaging 2003;28:19.

82. Fletcher JG, Busse RF, Riederer SJ, et at. Magnetic resonance imaging of anatomic and dynamic defects of the pelvic floor in defecatory disorders. Am J Gastroenterol 2003;98:399.

7
Endoluminal Ultrasound

Donald G. Kim and W. Douglas Wong

Evaluation of the anal canal and rectum has traditionally relied on digital examination, anoscopy, and rigid or flexible proctosigmoidoscopy. The introduction of imaging methods, particularly endoluminal ultrasonography has brought a greater degree of objectivity to the evaluation of the anorectum.

Endoluminal ultrasound has become the diagnostic procedure of choice in the evaluation of many anorectal disorders. Endorectal ultrasound (ERUS) has evolved into the best imaging modality for accurate staging of rectal neoplasms. The accurate determination of tumor penetration depth and regional lymph node status has become critical to guiding subsequent treatment of rectal malignancies. In addition, endoanal ultrasound (EAUS) has become invaluable in the diagnostic workup of fecal incontinence and anorectal suppurative conditions. This chapter will focus on the use of endoluminal ultrasound in the evaluation of patients with benign and malignant conditions of the anorectum.

History

Endoluminal ultrasound of the rectum was first introduced by Wild and Reid[1] in 1952. They were the first to develop an "echoendo probe," but it was never used clinically. Because of limitations in technology, it was not until 1983 that this type of imaging was introduced into clinical practice by Dragsted and Gammelgaard.[2] They used a Bruel and Kjaer (Type 8901) ultrasound probe with a rigid rotating endosonic probe with 4.5-MHz transducer initially designed for prostatic ultrasound. Thirteen primary rectal cancers were evaluated and invasion was correctly predicted in 11 cases when compared with the final histopathology. Two patients could not be adequately imaged because of stricture. Although successful, they did not define their reporting criteria. In 1985, Hildebrandt and Feifel[3] found that ultrasonography correlated with pathologic finding in 23 of 25 rectal cancers. They proposed a modification of the tumor-node-metastasis (TNM) classification[4] for ultrasound tumor staging (uTNM).[3] The prefix "u" indicated ultrasound staging as opposed to the prefix "p" representing pathologic staging. Similar to Dragsted and Gammelgaard, they also made no reference to the reporting criteria used for degree of invasion. Further refinements of the technique and improvement in the ultrasound equipment have made endoluminal ultrasound routine in the evaluation of patients with anorectal disorders.

Endorectal Ultrasound

As the treatment for rectal cancer has evolved, the importance of accurate preoperative staging of the lesion has become paramount in determining the patient's treatment regimen. Radical surgery, either low anterior or abdominoperineal resection is not always the initial or only therapy available for patients diagnosed with rectal carcinoma. With the development of preoperative neoadjuvant therapies for rectal cancer, accurate staging of these patients' lesions has become increasingly important. In addition, local excision has become an option in highly selected early-stage rectal cancers necessitating accurate preoperative staging.

The goal of preoperatively staging the rectal lesion is an accurate evaluation of the primary tumor, which includes the depth of tumor penetration and an evaluation of regional lymph node disease. ERUS accomplishes these goals using an intraluminal high-frequency sonographic transducer via a handheld rotating probe to accurately image the rectal wall and adjacent structures. For this reason, ERUS has become the preferred method used to stage the patient with rectal cancer.

Equipment and Technique

Equipment used for endoluminal ultrasonography includes a handheld endocavitary probe with rotating transducer which acquires a 360-degree image. Most investigators use a B-K Medical scanner with a rigid handheld Type 1850 rotating probe and a 7- or 10-MHz transducer (B-K Medical,

Wilmington, MA). Transducers of 7 and 10 MHz provide a focal length of 2–5 and 1–4 cm, respectively, rotating a 90-degree scanning plane at four to six cycles per second to obtain a 360-degree radial scan of the rectal wall and surrounding structures. Because of its superior near-image clarity, the 10-MHz transducer is preferred. Rectal imaging requires a latex balloon covering the transducer for acoustic contact. The balloon is instilled with water allowing the ultrasound signals to easily pass through the water to image the rectum. The water instilled distends the rectum allowing the balloon to maintain contact with the rectal wall without separation, preventing any distortion of the image by the interposition of nonconductive air between the probe and the rectal wall.

Patients receive one or two phosphosoda enemas to cleanse the rectum before examination. The procedure is performed with the patient in the left lateral decubitus position without sedation. A digital rectal and proctoscopic examination is performed to assess the tumor size, appearance, location, and distance from the anal verge. Any residual stool or enema effluent that might interfere with the ultrasound is removed. A wide-bore ESI proctoscope (Electrosurgical Instrument Company, Rochester, NY) is inserted into the rectum to examine the rectum and lesion of interest. Optimally, the proctoscope is advanced proximal to the lesion to facilitate complete examination of the tumor by the transducer. The wide-bore ESI proctoscope permits passage of the ultrasound probe through the proctoscope to facilitate positioning of the probe above the lesion. This facilitates complete imaging of the lesion from its most proximal to distal extent as well as the proximal mesorectum, which may harbor involved lymph nodes. This approach is preferred to blind insertion of the ultrasound probe into the rectum. With blind insertion, distortion of the image can occur and the proximal areas of a lesion as well as the adjacent mesorectum will often be missed.

After correct positioning of the wide-bore ESI proctoscope, the ultrasound probe with latex balloon is lubricated and passed through the proctoscope to its full extent. The ultrasound probe is oriented with the stopcock and syringe positioned upright to the patient's right. The proctoscope is slightly withdrawn keeping the ultrasound probe in place to expose the transducer protruding beyond the end of the proctoscope, above the rectal lesion. The latex balloon is filled with 30–60 mL of water providing an optimal acoustic environment surrounding the rotating transducer. Initial preparation of the ultrasound probe includes careful removal of all air bubbles within the latex balloon to minimize acoustic interference. The probe and attached proctoscope are slowly withdrawn together carefully scanning the rectum from proximal to distal. The ultrasonographer observes for alterations of the rectal wall and perirectal tissues to assess depth of invasion and perirectal lymph node involvement. Optimal evaluation often requires several passes back and forth across a lesion. The evaluation of the lesion occurs on the basis of real-time imaging intermittently capturing still images that are representative of the lesion being studied. With the patient and ultrasound posi-

tioned as above, the images obtained are oriented radially similar to a computed tomography scan, looking up from the patient's feet. The patient's right side is oriented to the left of the image, anterior is up, and posterior is down. The studies can also be videotaped for further review.

Image Interpretation

On most ERUS images, a series of five distinct layers can be identified in the rectal wall. They consist of three hyperechoic (white) layers separated by two hypoechoic (black) layers. Beynon and colleagues[5] proposed a five-layer model based on an anatomic study, demonstrating that the five basic layers seen on an ultrasonographic scan of the rectal wall correspond directly to the anatomic layers present in the rectal wall. It is this five-layer model that we continue to use today (Figure 7-1). The five layers from the center to the periphery consist of the following:

First hyperechoic layer: Interface between the balloon and the rectal mucosal surface
Second hypoechoic layer: Mucosa and muscularis mucosa
Third hyperechoic layer: Submucosa
Fourth hypoechoic layer: Muscularis propria
Fifth hyperechoic layer: Interface between the muscularis propria and perirectal fat

Occasionally, a seven-ring model may be visualized when the muscularis propria is observed as two black rings separated by a white ring (Figure 7-2). This model represents the inner circular and outer longitudinal muscle layers as hyperechoic (black) rings separated by a hypoechoic (white) interface.

Assessment of Rectal Neoplasms

Depth of Invasion

As discussed above, ultrasound classification of rectal tumor stage was initially proposed by Hildebrandt and Feifel[3] as a modification of the TNM classification. Ultrasound staging

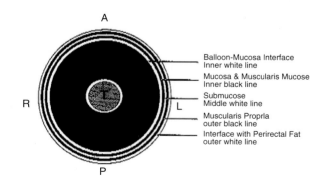

FIGURE 7-1. Five-layer anatomic model of an ERUS scan. Three hyperechoic (white) layers and two hypoechoic (black) layers are visualized. A, anterior; L, left; P, posterior; R, right; T, transducer.

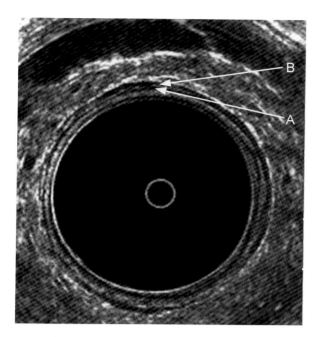

FIGURE 7-2. This endorectal ultrasonography image depicts the typical five layers of the rectal wall. Seven layers are depicted anteriorly, where an interface can be seen between the inner circular (A) and outer longitudinal (B) muscle layers of the muscularis propria.

classification (uTNM) is presented in Table 7-1. The depth of invasion is classified as follows: uT0 lesions are benign, noninvasive lesions confined to the mucosa; uT1 lesions indicate an invasive lesion confined to the mucosa and submucosa; uT2 lesions penetrate but are confined to the muscularis propria; uT3 lesions penetrate the entire bowel wall and invade the perirectal fat; and a uT4 lesions penetrate a contiguous organ (i.e., uterus, vagina, cervix, bladder, prostate, seminal vesicles) or the pelvic sidewall or sacrum.

uT0 Lesions

uT0 lesions are benign, noninvasive lesions confined to the rectal mucosa. Sonographically, the mucosal layer (inner black band) is expanded with an intact submucosa (middle white, hyperechoic line) (Figure 7-3). Benign rectal villous adenomas are classified as uT0 lesions and may be treated with local excision with excellent results. Important in this decision is to accurately exclude any focus of invasion. The accuracy of ERUS is probably highest for T0 lesions. In an

TABLE 7-1. Ultrasound staging classification (uTNM) for rectal cancer

uT0	Noninvasive lesion confined to the mucosa
uT1	Tumor confined to the mucosa and submucosa
uT2	Tumor penetrates into but not through the muscularis propria
uT3	Tumor extends into the perirectal fat
uT4	Tumor involves an adjacent organ
uN0	No evidence of lymph node metastasis
uN1	Evidence of lymph node metastasis

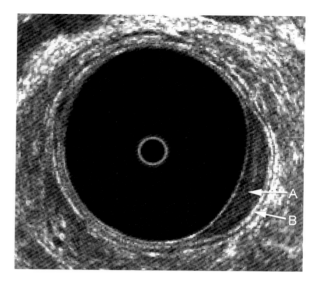

FIGURE 7-3. This image demonstrates a benign uT0 lesion in the left posterolateral aspect of the rectum. There is an expansion of the inner black line that represents the mucosa (A), but the submucosa (B) is seen to be completely intact.

initial study by Deen and colleagues[6] from the University of Minnesota, 47 of 53 lesions (89%) were correctly staged preoperatively. A more recent update reported 129 of 148 patients (87%) were correctly staged preoperatively from that same institution.[7] Pikarsky et al.[8] reported that 25 of 27 patients (96%) were accurately staged a benign lesion when compared with pathologic results. Because of the frequent misdiagnosis of rectal adenomas by biopsy and the subsequent finding of invasive cancer in the final pathologic specimen after transanal excision, Worrell et al.[9] conducted a systematic literature review to assess the utility of ERUS in the assessment of rectal villous adenomas comparing the diagnosis by biopsy alone with diagnosis by a combination of biopsy and ERUS. This metaanalysis revealed that, of 258 biopsy-negative rectal adenomas, 24% had focal carcinoma on final histopathology and that ERUS correctly detected the cancer in 81%.

uT1 Lesions

uT1 lesions are early invasive cancers. uT1 lesions have invaded the mucosa and submucosa without penetrating into the muscularis propria. Sonographically this is characterized by an irregular middle white line (submucosa) without alteration of the outer black line (muscularis propria) (Figure 7-4). Irregularities are indicated by a thickening or stippling of the submucosal layer but there must not be a distinct break in the submucosal layer. A distinct break in the submucosal (middle white line) layer indicates invasion of the muscularis propria, hence a T2 lesion.

Local transanal excision is an acceptable treatment method for selected T1 lesions highlighting the need for accurate staging of these cancers. Criteria for the use of local therapies

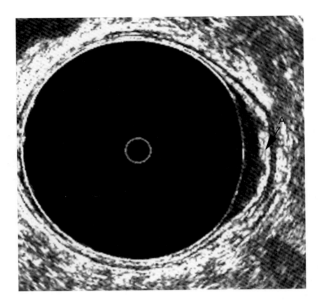

FIGURE 7-4. This image depicts a uT1 cancer in the left lateral wall of the rectum. The middle white line or submucosa is irregular and somewhat thickened (A), but not completely disrupted.

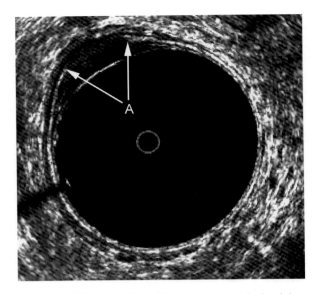

FIGURE 7-5. A uT2 lesion is identified in this image, in the right anterior location. The hallmark of a uT2 lesion, as seen on endorectal ultrasonography, is the distinct break (A) in the submucosa (the middle white line) as seen in this image.

to treat early rectal cancers have been described[10] and include tumor size less than 4 cm, involvement less than one-third of the rectal circumference, location less than 8 cm from the anal verge, well- to moderately well-differentiated histology, absence of lymphatic or vascular invasion, and no involvement of perirectal lymph nodes.

uT2 Lesions

uT2 lesions penetrate into the muscularis propria (second hypoechoic, black line) but are confined to the rectal wall. Sonographically the hallmark finding is a distinct break in the submucosal layer. Characteristically, there is an expansion of the muscularis propria (outer black line) but the interface between the muscularis propria and the perirectal fat (the outermost white line) remains intact. The expansion of the muscularis propria may be variable depending on the degree or invasion. "Early" uT2 lesions may just invade the muscularis propria with minimal expansion of the layer. "Deep" uT2 lesions have significant expansion of the muscularis propria (outer black line) and may appear to scallop the outer aspect of the muscularis propria but preserve the interface with the perirectal fat. An example of a uT2 lesion is illustrated in Figure 7-5.

uT3 Lesions

uT3 lesions penetrate the full thickness of the muscularis propria and into the perirectal fat. Continuous structures are not involved. The sonographic appearance reveals disruption of the submucosa, thickening of the muscularis propria, and disruption of the outer hyperechoic, white line indicating penetration into the perirectal fat (Figure 7-6). The recognition of

perirectal fat invasion is an important determinant in the preoperative evaluation of the rectal cancer patient. Because of the high incidence of lymph node metastases (30%–50%), local therapy cannot be recommended for these patients, who are usually candidates for preoperative radiation and chemotherapy followed by surgery. ERUS obviously has an important role in selecting those patients who will undergo preoperative radiation and chemotherapy.

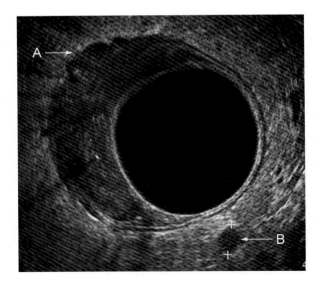

FIGURE 7-6. This image demonstrates a uT3N1 lesion. The tumor disrupts all layers of the rectal wall, with extensions evident into the perirectal fat (A). A lymph node (B) is identified in the left posterior location within the mesorectum.

uT4 Lesions

uT4 lesions are locally invasive into contiguous structures such as the uterus, vagina, cervix, bladder, prostate and seminal vesicles, or involve the pelvic sidewall or sacrum. They are clinically fixed and tethered. Sonographically, there is loss of the normal hyperechoic interface between the tumor and adjacent organ (Figure 7-7). Therapy of a T4 lesion usually requires preoperative radiation and chemotherapy followed by surgical resection of the rectal cancer and involved adjacent organ. The overall prognosis is poor, with less than half of patients resected for cure. Preoperative radiation and chemoradiation therapy can shrink the tumor for increased resectability and decreased local recurrence. ERUS provides the means to preoperatively identify those lesions with T4 involvement to adequately plan the patient's treatment.

Nodal Involvement

Lymph node involvement in rectal cancer is associated with decreased survival rates and increased local recurrence rates. ERUS is able to detect metastatic lymph nodes in the mesorectum. Unfortunately, the accuracy of detecting involved lymph nodes is less than the accuracy in determining the depth of invasion. The accuracy of ERUS in detecting lymph node metastases ranges from 50% to 88%.[11–13] ERUS determination of metastatic lymph nodes is certainly more accurate than clinical (digital) evaluation[14] as well as other imaging modalities including CT[11,15] and conventional magnetic resonance imaging (MRI).[16] However, phased array MRI and endorectal coil MRI are comparable to ERUS in lymph node assessment.

As indicated in Table 7-1, lymph node staging parallels pathologic TNM staging classifying tumors with (uN1) or without (uN0) lymph node involvement. Undetectable or benign-appearing lymph nodes are classified as uN0. Malignant-appearing lymph nodes are classified as uN1. Normal, nonenlarged lymph nodes are usually not detectable by ERUS. Inflamed, enlarged lymph nodes appear hyperechoic with irregular borders. Lymph nodes suspicious for malignancy include larger, round, hypoechoic lymph nodes with an irregular contour. ERUS findings consistent with metastatic lymph nodes are demonstrated in Figure 7-8. Hypoechoic lymph nodes greater than 5 mm are highly suspicious for metastases. Involved lymph nodes are usually found adjacent to the primary tumor or within the proximal mesorectum.

The echogenic pattern and size of imaged lymph nodes have been suggested to be indicators of metastatic nodal disease. Tio and Tytgat[17] were the first to recognize the hypoechoic pattern of malignant lymph nodes using ERUS. Hildebrandt et al.[18] differentiated two main groups of lymph nodes: hypoechoic and hyperechoic lymph nodes. Compared with pathologic findings, hypoechoic lymph nodes represent metastases, whereas hyperechoic lymph nodes are visualized because of nonspecific inflammation. There is no definitive size threshold to determine if an identified lymph node is malignant. Lymph nodes smaller than 5 mm can harbor metastatic disease.[19–21] In a pathology-based study, Herrera-Ornelas et al.[19] found that two-thirds of metastatic lymph nodes from colorectal cancer were smaller than 5 mm in diameter. Katsura and associates[20] found that 18% of nodes

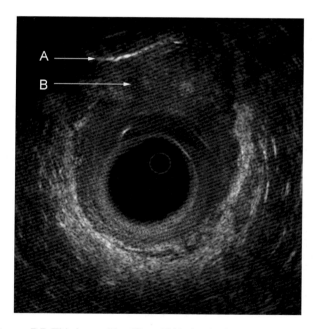

FIGURE 7-7. This image identifies a T4 lesion in the distal rectum and upper anal canal extending to the vagina. The curved white line (A) seen anteriorly represents the examiner's finger in the vagina, and the hypoechoic anterior tumor (B) can be seen to extend into the vagina.

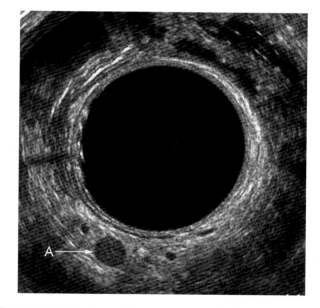

FIGURE 7-8. This image demonstrates a typical metastatic lymph node (A), which is round and hypoechoic.

measuring 4 mm or less on ERUS were involved with metastatic disease. Similarly, Akasu et al.[21] found that approximately 50% of cases of lymph nodes measuring 3–5 mm on ERUS harbored metastases. Sunouchi et al.[22] described a "small spot sign" for lesions at the margin of rectal carcinomas on ERUS measuring 1–3 mm in diameter. The small hypoechoic "spots" correlated with massive venous or lymphatic invasion histologically.

Nodes larger than 5 mm harbored metastatic disease 54% of the time. Sunouchi et al.[23] studying hypoechoic lesions larger than 5 mm on ERUS demonstrated that 68% were metastatic lymph nodes and 20% were tumor deposits. Statistically, the incidence of metastatic disease increases as lymph node size increases.

Overall, four nodal patterns are seen with differing probabilities of being involved with metastatic disease. Nonvisible lymph nodes on ultrasound have a low probability of harboring lymph node metastases. Hyperechoic lymph nodes with nonsharply delineated boundaries are more often benign resulting from inflammatory changes. Hypoechoic lymph nodes larger than 5 mm are highly suggestive of lymph node metastases. Mixed echogenic lymph nodes larger than 5 mm are difficult to classify but should be considered malignant.

Accurate lymph node staging of rectal cancers by ERUS relies on the experience of the examiner. False-positive results may occur because of inflammatory lymph nodes or confusing the cross-sectional appearance of perirectal blood vessels for metastatic lymph nodes. Scanning longitudinally will distinguish between blood vessels and lymph nodes because blood vessels will extend longitudinally, change direction, and/or branch. The sonographic continuity of the hypoechoic vessel over a distance greater than the cross-sectional area is the criterion used to distinguish the two. Three-dimensional imaging can help in making this distinction.

False-negative results are also problematic in interpreting nodal involvement on ERUS. Lymph nodes harboring micrometastases are difficult to detect. Grossly malignant lymph nodes may be present outside the range of the ultrasound probe and remain undetectable. This may be the case of lateral pelvic lymph nodes such as the obturator nodes as well as those within the mesorectum beyond the proximal extent of the rigid probe.

Accuracy of Ultrasound in the Diagnosis of Rectal Cancer

The success of any imaging modality is the result of its diagnostic accuracy. Preoperative therapy for rectal cancer depends on the accurate staging of the primary lesion. The determination of the lesion's depth of invasion (T stage) and lymph node involvement (N stage) are important factors dictating the therapeutic options. ERUS has the ability to determine the depth of tumor invasion and lymph node involvement of rectal cancers. ERUS has been found to be accurate in determining the tumor's depth of invasion within the bowel wall, although ERUS is only moderately accurate in the assessment of lymph node involvement.

The accuracy of ERUS for the staging of rectal cancer has been established from studies comparing preoperative ultrasound staging with the pathologic staging from the operative specimens. The accuracy of ERUS for tumor depth of invasion has been reported in the range of 69%–94% (Table 7-2). Overstaging has been reported in approximately 10% of patients and is believed to be the result of peritumoral inflammation beyond the leading edge of the tumor. Understaging for depth of wall invasion has been reported to be approximately 5% and is considerably more serious than overstaging because inadequate management may result. With overstaging, potentially more aggressive management is recommended than might be required.

Detection of lymph node metastases with ERUS has been less accurate, ranging from 61% to 83% in reported series (Table 7-2). Solomon and McLeod[24] reviewed the literature and pooled raw data were collected from eight published cross-sectional surveys assessing the degree of tumor penetration in 873 patients and lymph node involvement in 571 patients with primary rectal cancer. As previously noted, ERUS was very accurate in determining tumor penetration (kappa = 0.85), but only a moderate correlation was found between ERUS and histopathology for detecting lymph node involvement (kappa = 0.58). Furthermore, the positive predictive value was 74% with a negative predictive value of 84%, indicating only moderate accuracy among the included series.

There is a significant learning curve associated with the performance and interpretation of ERUS. Accuracy rates have been demonstrated to improve significantly with experience.[13] ERUS is highly operator dependent and thus accuracy is dependent on the experience and expertise of the examiner.[7,25]

TABLE 7-2. Accuracy of ERUS in the staging of rectal cancer

Author	Year	n	Accuracy (%) T stage	Accuracy (%) N stage
Hildebrandt and Feifel[3]	1985	25	92	n/a
Romano et al.[84]	1985	23	87	n/a
Hildebrandt et al.[85]	1986	76	88	74
Holdsworth et al.[86]	1988	36	86	61
Beynon et al.[11,87]	1989	100	93	83
Dershaw et al.[88]	1990	32	75	72
Glaser et al.[25]	1990	86	88	79
Glaser et al.[89]	1990	110	94	80
Jochem et al.[90]	1990	50	80	73
Milsom and Graffner[14]	1990	52	83	83
Orrom et al.[13]	1990	77	75	82
Katsura et al.[20]	1992	112	92	n/a
Herzog et al.[91]	1993	118	89	80
Sentovich et al.[92]	1993	24	79	73
Deen et al.[6]	1995	209	82	77
Adams et al.[93]	1999	70	74	83
Garcia-Aguilar et al.[7]	2002	545	69	64
Marusch et al.[94]*	2002	422	63	n/a
Manger and Stroh[95]	2004	357	77	75

Several factors can lead to the misinterpretation of ERUS images.[26] These factors include a lesion in close proximity to the anal verge, improper balloon inflation with associated balloon-wall separation, a nonperpendicular imaging plane, shadowing artifacts caused by air or stool, reverberation artifacts, refraction artifacts, and a transducer gain setting that is too high. Postbiopsy and postsurgical changes, hemorrhage, and bulky or pedunculated tumors can cause changes in the ultrasound image significantly affecting the accuracy of the ERUS interpretation.

The accuracy of ERUS after neoadjuvant therapy is decreased.[27–31] Radiation therapy can significantly downstage tumors and may in fact leave no residual tumor within the pathologic specimen. In fact, up to 24% of patients treated with preoperative radiation therapy have a complete pathologic response with no evidence of residual tumor.[32] Radiation therapy can cause tissue edema and fibrosis of the rectal lesion making ERUS interpretation difficult. One cannot accurately distinguish radiation-induced changes from residual tumor. For these reasons, reevaluation of rectal lesions with ERUS after radiation therapy is inaccurate, unreliable, and not recommended.

Postoperative Follow-up

Local recurrence continues to be a difficult problem in the treatment of rectal cancer. Overall, local recurrence rates have been reported between 4% and 30% after curative rectal cancer surgery. More than 50% of patients will have local recurrence only at the surgical site without distant metastases.[33,34] Even with newer adjuvant therapies available, surgical resection remains the best chance of cure for the patient with isolated local recurrence. Clearly, early detection of local recurrence is important and follow-up programs should be directed at this goal in order to be successful. ERUS may be used in a variety of settings for surveillance purposes after surgery for rectal cancer. When used in combination with a digital rectal examination and endoscopic surveillance, ERUS may significantly improve the sensitivity of detecting recurrent lesions.[35–37] ERUS may improve the ability to diagnose recurrent neoplasm by as much as 30%.[38] In a series studying ERUS as a means to identify local recurrence, overall local recurrence ranged from 11% to 20% with the proportion of local recurrences diagnosed exclusively by ERUS varying from 18% to 35%.[37–39] These ERUS-only recurrences represent only 3.2%–5% of the entire group of patients. The University of Minnesota group presented similar results although the impact on overall survival is unclear.[36]

Although local recurrence occurs intraluminally at the anastomosis, locally recurrent tumor usually occurs from extrarectal tumor that invades through the rectum, often at the level of an anastomosis. Extrarectal tumor not involving the mucosa may be undetectable endoscopically, but can be identified at an early stage with ERUS. Recurrent tumor appears as a circumscribed hypoechoic lesion in the para-anastomotic tissues with all or a portion of the rectal wall

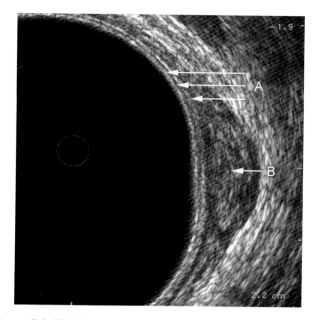

FIGURE 7-9. This image demonstrates a recurrent rectal cancer. It is located in the left lateral rectal wall. Note the intact inner three lines (A) on the ultrasound image, indicating no involvement of the mucosa or submucosa but an obvious abnormality at the level of the muscularis propria (B), representing the recurrence.

intact on the inner, luminal aspect (Figure 7-9). Early postoperative changes, particularly adjacent to the anastomosis, can make the interpretation of the ERUS difficult. Interpretation is aided if a "baseline" ultrasound is obtained soon (3 months) after surgery and compared with subsequent surveillance images. A baseline examination is useful to document postoperative scarring and to evaluate that area for potential changes on serial examinations. Lesions that increase in size on subsequent examinations are more likely to represent recurrent tumor. Because ERUS cannot establish that a lesion is malignant with absolute certainty, a biopsy of suspicious lesions is recommended to confirm recurrent disease. Biopsies may be performed by ultrasound-guided biopsy or computed tomography scan-guided biopsy.

The optimal interval and length of time for serial follow-up ERUS examinations have not been determined. Because most recurrences present within the first 2 years after surgery, more intensive follow-up is justified during this period. Imaging every 3–4 months for the first 2–3 years may be appropriate with less frequent, every 6-month evaluations until 5 years.

Endoanal Ultrasound

EAUS is useful in the evaluation of the anal canal in both benign and malignant disease. The anal sphincter anatomy can be clearly identified detecting abnormalities in the external and/or internal sphincter. EAUS is routinely used in the evaluation of fecal incontinence and may be particularly useful in the evaluation of complex perianal abscesses and fistulas. EAUS is also useful in the evaluation of anal canal neoplasms accurately staging these lesions.

Equipment and Technique

The equipment used for EAUS is similar to that used for ERUS. The same B-K scanner is used with the 1850 rotating probe and 10-MHz transducer (B-K Medical). In place of the latex balloon, a translucent plastic cap (B-K type WA0453) is placed over the transducer to maintain contact with the anal canal. The plastic cap is again filled with water to provide the acoustic medium. There is a pinhole in the apex of the plastic cap that permits the escape of any air through displacement of the space with water.

The examination technique for EAUS is similar to that of ERUS. Patients are examined in the left lateral decubitus position, again usually without sedation. A careful external examination of the perianal area followed by a digital rectal examination is performed. The probe is lubricated with a water-soluble gel and gently inserted into the anal canal until the plastic cap is no longer visible. This will usually ensure that the transducer is at the level of the upper anal canal. The probe is slowly withdrawn to image the full length of the anal canal. Images are typically obtained in the upper, mid, and distal anal canal. In most instances, patients can be reassured that the examination should cause no more discomfort than a digital rectal examination. Certain instances of complex anorectal sepsis may be painful and require examination under anesthesia to adequately image the patient with EAUS.

Image Interpretation

Normal anal canal anatomy is well visualized with EAUS. As with the rectum, the interpretation of these images must be based on a precise definition of normal endosonographic anatomy of the anal canal that correlates well with anatomy. EAUS of the anal canal and pelvic floor have been correlated with cadaveric anatomic dissections.[40] The ultrasonographic anatomy of the anal canal is generally divided into three levels: the upper, mid, and distal anal canal. Each level has a different appearance on EAUS. The upper anal canal is illustrated in Figure 7-10. The puborectalis is an important landmark delineating the upper anal canal. The puborectalis is imaged as a horseshoe-shaped mixed-echogenic structure forming the lateral and posterior portion of the upper anal canal.

The mid anal canal is illustrated in Figure 7-11. Within the mid anal canal, the internal anal sphincter is represented by a hypoechoic band surrounded by the hyperechoic external anal sphincter. Between the transducer and the internal anal sphincter is an additional hyperechoic ring of variable thickness representing the epithelial, hemorrhoidal, and submucosal tissues. Perineal body measurements can be made at the level of the mid anal canal (Figure 7-12). With the probe positioned within the mid anal canal, the right index finger is

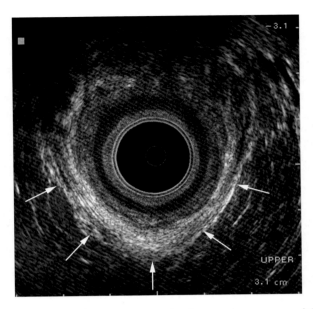

FIGURE 7-10. This image represents the ultrasound appearance of the upper anal canal at the level of the puborectalis, which can be seen as the hyperechoic U-shaped structure seen posteriorly and laterally (arrows) in this image.

placed within the vagina against the rectovaginal septum and ultrasound probe. The distance between the hyperechoic ultrasound reflection of the finger and the inner aspect of the internal anal sphincter may be measured and represents the perineal body thickness. Normal measurements for perineal body thickness range from 10 to 15 mm, with a lower limit of

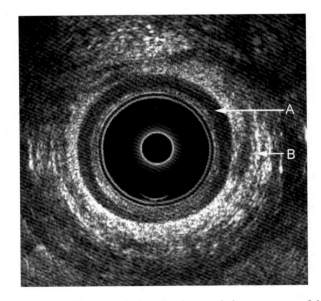

FIGURE 7-11. This image depicts the characteristic appearance of the mid anal canal. The circular hypoechoic structure represents the internal anal sphincter (A), surrounded by the thicker hyperechoic circumferential external anal sphincter (B).

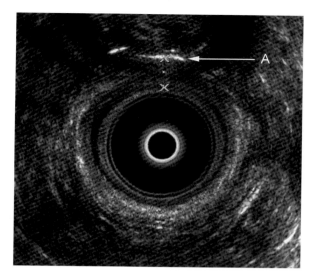

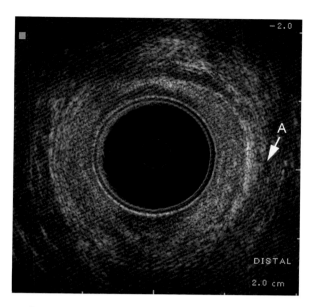

FIGURE 7-12. This image depicts the technique used to measure the anterior perineal body in a female patient. The examiner's finger is placed in the vagina, and the hyperechoic curvilinear structure (A) seen anteriorly delineates the examiner's finger. The two cross-hatches between the examiner's finger and the transducer measure the thickness of the perineal body in this intact sphincter at the mid anal canal level.

FIGURE 7-13. This image represents the distal anal canal below the inferior level of the internal sphincter, where only the hyperechoic circumferential fibers of the superficial external anal sphincter (A) are imaged.

normal considered to be approximately 8 mm. This measurement is useful in the evaluation of women with fecal incontinence from anterior sphincter defects. The examining index finger not only better defines the perineal body, but may accentuate an anterior sphincter defect that may otherwise appear intact.

The distal anal canal is illustrated in Figure 7-13. The distal anal canal is defined as the point where the internal anal sphincter is no longer seen. Only the hyperechoic external anal sphincter and surrounding soft tissues are visualized.

Evaluation of Fecal Incontinence

EAUS has an important role in the evaluation of fecal incontinence, accurately delineating anal sphincter anatomy.[41–43] Causes of anal sphincter defects include obstetric injuries, anorectal surgeries, traumatic injuries, and congenital abnormalities.

Fecal incontinence is eight times more frequent in women,[44] the most common cause being obstetric trauma leading to injury of the anal sphincter muscles or traction neuropathy involving the pudendal nerve.[44–46] Although anal sphincter injury identified during delivery does not lead to significant deterioration in sphincter function immediately, it is suspected to lead to fecal incontinence in approximately 40% of women in long-term follow-up despite primary sphincter repair.[47–49] Anal incontinence is not restricted to patients with recognized third- or fourth-degree obstetric tears. Patients may also develop delayed symptoms of incontinence several years after an unrecognized sphincter injury.[50] The introduction of EAUS

has led to the recognition of unsuspected sphincter defects in asymptomatic, continent women thought to have normal perineums.[51–54] Traumatic sphincter disruption can frequently be associated with a subsequent rectovaginal fistula. These patients may be anally continent but have symptoms of fecal incontinence associated with the fistula. Because these patients may have an unrecognized anal sphincter defect, all patients with rectovaginal fistula should undergo preoperative evaluation for occult sphincter defects by EAUS.[55] Local tissues are inadequate for endorectal advancement flap repairs in patients with anal sphincter defects and these patients should be treated by sphincteroplasty with levatoroplasty.[55] EAUS has become an accurate method to image the anal sphincters identifying anal sphincter defects that result in fecal incontinence.[46,56–58]

EAUS has become the best modality to accurately demonstrate the anatomy of the anal canal as well as anal sphincter defects that contribute to fecal incontinence.[43] Defects in the external anal sphincter usually appear hypoechoic, although some may appear hyperechoic or demonstrate mixed echogenicity. Defects of the internal anal sphincter are represented by the lack of segment of the hypoechoic band of internal sphincter muscle. There is usually associated contralateral thickening of the hypoechoic internal anal sphincter. With complete sphincter disruption, EAUS demonstrates the ends of the internal and external anal sphincter widely separated and bridged with intervening scar tissue of variable echogenicity (Figure 7-14). Many times, complete sphincter disruption is not seen, but attenuation of the sphincter mechanism is noted anteriorly, indicating a significant partial

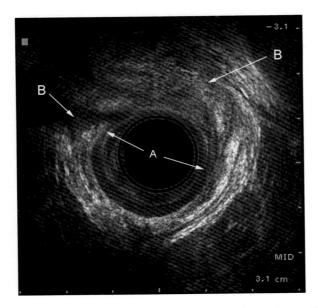

FIGURE 7-14. This image depicts a complete anterior sphincter disruption in a female patient. The hypoechoic internal anal sphincter can be seen completely disrupted in its anterior location (A arrows). Similarly, the hyperechoic external anal sphincter is completely disrupted anteriorly (B arrows).

sphincter defect. An examining digit used to measure the perineal body distance in the mid anal canal can accentuate an anterior sphincter defect, helping to identify a sphincter injury (Figure 7-15).[59]

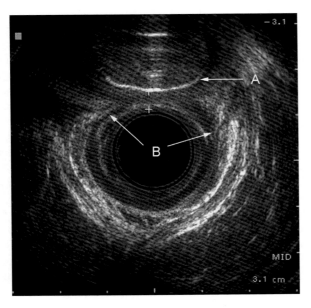

FIGURE 7-15. This image demonstrates the measurement of the anterior perineal body in this patient with an anterior sphincter disruption. The curvilinear hyperechoic structure (A) is the examiner's finger in the vagina. This technique can often accentuate the defect (B) seen in the internal anal sphincter and the external anal sphincter, and documents the decreased thickness of the anterior sphincter and perineal body.

Other causes of anatomic anal sphincter defects include anorectal trauma or surgery and congenital anomalies. Blunt or penetrating trauma to the perineum may involve the sphincter mechanism. Management often includes fecal diversion, and debridement of the associated perineal soft tissues. After the perineal wound has healed, EAUS may be used to assess anal sphincter anatomy to determine if sphincter reconstruction is necessary before colostomy closure.

Patients undergoing anorectal surgery may experience transient minor incontinence in the early postoperative period, which usually resolves spontaneously. Patients who have persistent symptoms of incontinence may warrant evaluation. EAUS provides an objective means to evaluate the anal sphincter mechanism in patients with postoperative fecal incontinence after anorectal surgery such as hemorrhoidectomy, fistulotomy, lateral internal sphincterotomy, or sphincteroplasty.

The surgical correction of congenital anorectal anomalies is based on reconstituting the anatomy of the anorectum. The goal of posterior sagittal anorectoplasty (PSARP) is to place the bowel within the striated muscle complex of the levator ani and external anal sphincter.[60] EAUS has been used to accurately confirm the position of the neo-anus within the anal sphincter complex comparing favorably with MRI.[61] EAUS in fact provided greater detail of the anal muscles than MRI and had better correlation with direct perineal muscle stimulation.[61] Adult patients who present with severe fecal incontinence after previous surgical repair of a congenital anorectal malformation can undergo successful PSARP.[62] Usually, the existing anus is anterior to the sphincteric muscle complex.[62] An EAUS can be performed to help define the relationship of the anus to the sphincteric mechanism.

The identification of localized sphincter defects is important in the evaluation of the incontinent patient, because these defects may be amenable to surgical repair. EAUS can clearly and objectively image the anal sphincter mechanism and has replaced needle electromyography as the procedure of choice for anal sphincter mapping. EAUS is better tolerated and less painful than needle electromyography sphincter mapping. Anorectal manometry and pudendal nerve terminal motor latency testing are complementary but do not definitively correlate with a surgically correctable defect.[46,52,54,63,64] EAUS remains the definitive test that can identify a surgically correctable defect in a symptomatic patient with fecal incontinence.

Evaluation of Perianal Sepsis and Fistula-in-Ano

Typically, the diagnosis of a perianal or perirectal abscess is quite apparent on physical examination and only requires proper identification and prompt drainage. Occasionally, an abscess is strongly suspected on clinical grounds but is not readily identified on physical examination. In these situations, an EAUS may be useful in the evaluation of perianal or perirectal abscesses. EAUS can be helpful to localize an obscure abscess to plan the appropriate surgical intervention.

Often, clinical examination of perianal or perirectal abscesses is quite painful and examination under anesthesia is required. Because the ultrasound equipment is portable, the EAUS examination can be performed in the operating room while the patient is anesthetized. Abscesses appear as hypoechoic areas often surrounded by a hyperechoic border. In patients with perianal Crohn's disease, EAUS may be useful in distinguishing discrete abscesses that require surgical drainage from inflammation that requires medical treatment. The use of EAUS has also been evaluated in patients with ileoanal pouch anastomosis and can be helpful in demonstrating pouch pathology including inflammation, abscesses, and fistulas.[65]

The natural history of a drained perianal/rectal abscess is either complete resolution or fistula formation. The majority of fistulas that occur are simple intersphincteric fistulas that are easily identified and treated by simple unroofing. However, occasionally fistula tracts develop that are extensive and highly complex. These complex fistulas present a diagnostic challenge to even the most experienced colon and rectal surgeon. Use of EAUS can be helpful in identification of fistulous communications in patients with complex and recurrent fistula-in-ano.[66–68] Fistula tracts are generally hypoechoic defects that can be followed to identify direction and extent. The anatomic details of the fistula tract can be delineated in relation to the anal sphincter. The EAUS examination should include the anal canal and distal rectum to search for the presence of high blind tracts. Hydrogen peroxide has been used to enhance the imaging of complex fistula.[69–72] Hydrogen peroxide causes a release of oxygen, accentuating the fistula and appears as a brightly hyperechoic image on the ultrasound image. The technique increases the identification of the internal opening to greater than 90%.[69,72] An example of a fistula-in-ano with hydrogen peroxide enhancement is demonstrated in Figure 7-16. When evaluating an anal fistula with ERUS, it is important to use both the balloon-covered transducer to evaluate the perirectal region to assess for any supralevator extension as well as the plastic cap for evaluation of the anus and surrounding anatomy.

Anal Canal Neoplasms

Endoanal ultrasonography images the normal anal canal and associated pathologies quite well. EAUS can have an important role in the evaluation of benign and malignant anal canal neoplasms. The normal anatomic structures are clearly defined and any changes in the normal anatomy and their relationships with specific anatomic structures are clearly defined. Benign neoplasms such lipomas and leiomyomas can be demonstrated along with their relationship to adjacent anal canal structures. Lesions within the anal canal appear as hypoechoic areas. Tissue diagnosis may be obtained with ultrasound-directed needle biopsies when desired.

Anal canal malignancies are an uncommon cancer in the gastrointestinal tract. Diagnosis requires appropriate clinical

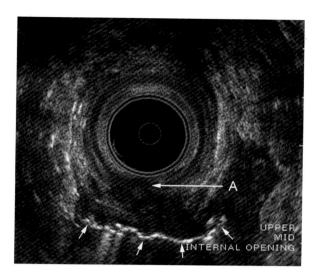

FIGURE 7-16. This image depicts a fistula-in-ano that has been enhanced by the introduction of hydrogen peroxide. The hyperechoic features posteriorly represent the hydrogen peroxide within the fistula tract (short arrows). There is an obvious hypoechoic defect in the internal anal sphincter in the midline posteriorly (A), representing the internal fistula opening. The hypoechoic horseshoe tract can be seen extending toward the patient's left.

evaluation and histologic confirmation by tissue biopsy. Anal canal malignancies evaluated by EAUS include leiomyosarcomas, malignant melanomas, anal canal adenocarcinomas, and squamous cell carcinomas. Squamous cell or epidermoid carcinoma of the anal canal are the most common anal canal malignancy. EAUS can be used in the initial evaluation to stage the lesion as well as in follow-up for patients with squamous cell carcinoma of the anal canal.[73–76] Because squamous cell carcinomas of the anus are primarily treated nonoperatively with combined chemoradiation therapy, it is desirable to have an accurate method of staging to assess response to multimodality therapy. EAUS accurately stages the initial tumor and can be used in follow-up to detect residual tumors as well as early recurrences after treatment. Surgical treatment in the form of abdominoperineal resection is reserved as salvage surgery for those patients who fail standard chemoradiation therapy.

Although clinical (digital) examination is important in the assessment of squamous cell carcinoma of the anus, EAUS is more precise in accurately measuring the actual size and circumferential involvement of the lesion. EAUS staging (uTNM) of anal cancers corresponds to the TNM [UICC (International Union Against Cancer)] staging (Table 7-3).[4] Tumor staging for anal cancer depends primarily on the maximal tumor diameter, which is accurately measured by EAUS. Additionally, the depth of invasion of the lesion can be measured in relationship to the sphincter mechanism. The extent of sphincter involvement can be determined and other staging systems stage these lesions based on depth of invasion.[76,77] One such staging system is depicted in Table 7-4.[77] The eval-

TABLE 7-3. Ultrasound staging classification (uTNM) for anal canal cancer

Primary tumor (T)
Tx	Primary tumor cannot be assessed
T0	No evidence of primary tumor
Tis	Carcinoma in situ
T1	Tumor 2 cm or less in greatest dimension
T2	Tumor more than 2 cm but no more than 5 cm in greatest dimension
T3	Tumor more than 5 cm in greatest dimension
T4	Tumor of any size that invades an adjacent organ(s), e.g., vagina, urethra, bladder (involvement of the sphincter muscle(s) alone is not classified as T4)

Regional lymph nodes (N)
Nx	Regional lymph nodes cannot be assessed
N0	No regional lymph node metastasis
N1	Metastasis in perirectal lymph node(s)
N2	Metastasis in unilateral internal iliac and/or inguinal lymph node(s)
N3	Metastasis in perirectal and inguinal lymph nodes and/or bilateral internal iliac and/or inguinal lymph nodes

Distant metastasis
Mx	Distant metastasis cannot be assessed
M0	No distant metastasis
M1	Distant metastasis

TABLE 7-4. Ultrasound staging classification by depth of invasion (uTNM) for anal canal cancer

uT1	Tumor confined to the submucosa
uT2a	Tumor invades only the internal anal sphincter
uT2b	Tumor penetrates into the external anal sphincter
uT3	Tumor invades through the sphincter complex and into the perianal tissues
uT4	Tumor invades adjacent structures

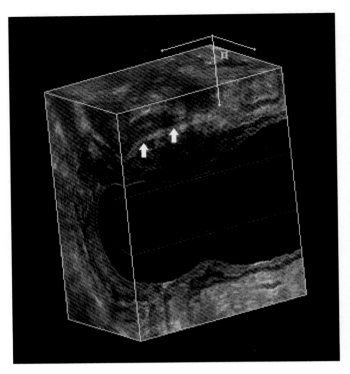

FIGURE 7-17. This three-dimensional ultrasound image demonstrates an anteriorly based rectal cancer that extends full-thickness through the rectal wall (uT3). However, a clear hyperechoic plane can be seen between the prostate gland and the rectal tumor, as depicted by the arrows.

uation of squamous cell carcinomas of the anus should include an evaluation of the rectum with ERUS to determine the presence of metastatic lymph nodes within the mesorectum. The mesorectum as well as the anal canal can also be evaluated in follow-up after treatment. Any suspicious areas detected during follow-up may be biopsied if necessary.

Three-dimensional Ultrasound

Three-dimensional ultrasound allows for multiplanar imaging of both the rectum and the anal canal. This new technology is currently being evaluated to compare its efficacy relative to conventional two-dimensional ultrasound as well as to other modalities such as MRI. Three-dimensional ultrasound can be used to assess anal fistulous tracts, to evaluate anal sphincter injury, as well as to stage both rectal and anal tumors. An example of a three-dimensional ERUS image (3D-ERUS) of a rectal cancer is shown in Figure 7-17.

Hunerbein et al.[78] compared standard two-dimensional ultrasound with 3D-ERUS and endorectal MRI and reported an accuracy for depth of wall invasion by rectal cancer of 84%, 88%, and 91%, respectively. Because of the small sample size, these differences were not statistically significant. However, they believed that the additional scan planes improved the understanding of three-dimensional imaging and facilitated interpretation of the findings. In another small study of 33 patients comparing conventional ERUS to 3D-ERUS, Kim et al.[79] reported no statistically significant differences in the two modalities in determining depth of invasion or lymph node status. However, it is of interest to note that the accuracy of 3D-ERUS was 90.9% for T2 lesions and 84.8% for T3 lesions compared with 84.8% and 75.8% for conventional ultrasound. The accuracy of 3D-ERUS for predicting lymph node status was 84.8% compared with 66.7% for conventional ERUS. They concluded that although there was no statistical advantage, three-dimensional imaging made the visualization of focal lesions and lymph nodes easier.

Three-dimensional EAUS has also been applied to benign anal disorders such as anal sphincter injury and anal fistula assessment. Several comparative studies have been reported evaluating its efficacy and comparing 3D-EAUS with MRI. West et al.[80] reported that 3D-EAUS and endoanal MRI were comparable for detecting external sphincter defects. Gold et al.[81] determined that 3D-EAUS revealed a direct relationship between the length of a sphincter tear and its radial extent. In addition, they demonstrated marked gender differences in anal sphincter configuration using three-dimensional ultrasound imaging. In the evaluation of anal fistula tracts, West et al.[82] reported equivalency between 3D-EAUS and endoanal MRI for the evaluation of anal fistula tracts. In a recent study by Buchanan et al.,[83] 3D-EAUS was found to be very accurate in the assessment of both the internal opening and the primary tract of an anal fistula. They reported an accuracy of 90% in identifying the internal opening and an accuracy of 81% in delineating the primary tract. Three-dimensional EAUS was less accurate (68%) in identifying secondary tracts or extensions. In their study, the use of hydrogen peroxide did not increase the accuracy but in some instances it did make the tract and internal opening more conspicuous.

Summary

Endoluminal ultrasound has been shown to be extremely useful in the evaluation and management of many benign and malignant anorectal conditions. ERUS has become the best imaging technique to accurately stage rectal cancers and anal canal tumors preoperatively. Moreover, ERUS can have a role in the follow-up evaluation of these patients. EAUS is the diagnostic test of choice in the evaluation of fecal incontinence and is used routinely. The EAUS has also been used to help define complex anal fistulas to facilitate their management. The accuracy of diagnosis is operator dependent and improves with experience. Endoluminal ultrasound has made a major contribution to the understanding and management of many anorectal conditions. Three-dimensional ultrasound may prove to be advantageous, but requires further study.

References

1. Wild JJ, Reid JM. Diagnostic use of ultrasound. Br J Phys Med 1956;19(11):248–257.

2. Dragsted J, Gammelgaard J. Endoluminal ultrasonic scanning in the evaluation of rectal cancer: a preliminary report of 13 cases. Gastrointest Radiol 1983;8(4):367–369.

3. Hildebrandt U, Feifel G. Preoperative staging of rectal cancer by intrarectal ultrasound. Dis Colon Rectum 1985;28(1):42–46.

4. Greene FL, et al., ed. AJCC Cancer Staging Manual. 6th ed. New York: Springer; 2002.

5. Beynon J, et al. The endosonic appearances of normal colon and rectum. Dis Colon Rectum 1986;29(12):810–813.

6. Deen KI, Madoff RD, Wong WD. Preoperative staging of rectal neoplasms with endorectal ultrasonography. Semin Colon Rectal Surg 1995;6:78–85.

7. Garcia-Aguilar J, et al. Accuracy of endorectal ultrasonography in preoperative staging of rectal tumors. Dis Colon Rectum 2002;45(1):10–15.

8. Pikarsky A, et al. The use of rectal ultrasound for the correct diagnosis and treatment of rectal villous tumors. Am J Surg 2000;179(4):261–265.

9. Worrell S, et al. Endorectal ultrasound detection of focal carcinoma within rectal adenomas. Am J Surg 2004;187(5):625–629.

10. Kim DG, Madoff RD. Transanal treatment of rectal cancer: ablative methods and open resection. Semin Surg Oncol 1998;15(2):101–113.

11. Beynon J, et al. Preoperative assessment of mesorectal lymph node involvement in rectal cancer. Br J Surg 1989;76(3):276–279.

12. Rifkin MD, Ehrlich SM, Marks G. Staging of rectal carcinoma: prospective comparison of endorectal US and CT. Radiology 1989;170(2):319–322.

13. Orrom WJ, et al. Endorectal ultrasound in the preoperative staging of rectal tumors. A learning experience. Dis Colon Rectum 1990;33(8):654–659.

14. Milsom JW, Graffner H. Intrarectal ultrasonography in rectal cancer staging and in the evaluation of pelvic disease. Clinical uses of intrarectal ultrasound. Ann Surg 1990;212(5):602–606.

15. Pappalardo G, et al. The value of endoluminal ultrasonography and computed tomography in the staging of rectal cancer: a preliminary study. J Surg Oncol 1990;43(4):219–222.

16. Thaler W, et al. Preoperative staging of rectal cancer by endoluminal ultrasound vs. magnetic resonance imaging. Preliminary results of a prospective, comparative study. Dis Colon Rectum 1994;37(12):1189–1193.

17. Tio TL, Tytgat GN. Endoscopic ultrasonography in analysing peri-intestinal lymph node abnormality. Preliminary results of studies in vitro and in vivo. Scand J Gastroenterol Suppl 1986;123:158–163.

18. Hildebrandt U, et al. Endosonography of pararectal lymph nodes. In vitro and in vivo evaluation. Dis Colon Rectum 1990;33(10):863–868.

19. Herrera-Ornelas L, et al. Metastases in small lymph nodes from colon cancer. Arch Surg 1987;122(11):1253–1256.

20. Katsura Y, et al. Endorectal ultrasonography for the assessment of wall invasion and lymph node metastasis in rectal cancer. Dis Colon Rectum 1992;35(4):362–368.

21. Akasu T, et al. Limitations and pitfalls of transrectal ultrasonography for staging of rectal cancer. Dis Colon Rectum 1997;40(10 suppl):S10–15.

22. Sunouchi K, et al. Small spot sign of rectal carcinoma by endorectal ultrasonography: histologic relation and clinical impact on postoperative recurrence. Dis Colon Rectum 1998;41(5):649–653.

23. Sunouchi K, et al. Limitation of endorectal ultrasonography: what does a low lesion more than 5 mm in size correspond to histologically? Dis Colon Rectum 1998;41(6):761–764.

24. Solomon MJ, McLeod R.S. Endoluminal transrectal ultrasonography: accuracy, reliability, and validity. Dis Colon Rectum 1993;36(2):200–205.

25. Glaser F, Schlag P, Herfarth C. Endorectal ultrasonography for the assessment of invasion of rectal tumours and lymph node involvement. Br J Surg 1990;77(8):883–887.

26. Kruskal JB, et al. Pitfalls and sources of error in staging rectal cancer with endorectal US. Radiographics 1997;17(3):609–626.

27. Bernini A, et al. Preoperative adjuvant radiation with chemotherapy for rectal cancer: its impact on stage of disease and the role of endorectal ultrasound. Ann Surg Oncol 1996;3(2):131–135.

28. Fleshman JW, et al. Accuracy of transrectal ultrasound in predicting pathologic stage of rectal cancer before and after preoperative radiation therapy. Dis Colon Rectum 1992;35(9):823–829.

29. Meade PG, et al. Preoperative chemoradiation downstages locally advanced ultrasound-staged rectal cancer. Am J Surg 1995;170(6):609–612; discussion 612–613.

30. Rau B, et al. Accuracy of endorectal ultrasound after preoperative radiochemotherapy in locally advanced rectal cancer. Surg Endosc 1999;13(10):980–984.

31. Williamson PR, et al. Endorectal ultrasound of T3 and T4 rectal cancers after preoperative chemoradiation. Dis Colon Rectum 1996;39(1):45–49.

32. Brown CL, et al. Response to preoperative chemoradiation in stage II and III rectal cancer. Dis Colon Rectum 2003;46(9): 1189–1193.

33. Michelassi F, et al. Local recurrence after curative resection of colorectal adenocarcinoma. Surgery 1990;108(4):787–792; discussion 792–793.

34. Sagar PM, Pemberton JH. Surgical management of locally recurrent rectal cancer. Br J Surg 1996;83(3):293–304.

35. Beynon J, et al. The detection and evaluation of locally recurrent rectal cancer with rectal endosonography. Dis Colon Rectum 1989;32(6):509–517.

36. de Anda EH, et al. Endorectal ultrasound in the follow-up of rectal cancer patients treated by local excision or radical surgery. Dis Colon Rectum 2004;47(6):818–824.

37. Mascagni D, et al. Endoluminal ultrasound for early detection of local recurrence of rectal cancer [see comment]. Br J Surg 1989;76(11):1176–1180.

38. Ramirez JM, et al. Endoluminal ultrasonography in the follow-up of patients with rectal cancer. Br J Surg 1994;81(5):692–694.

39. Rotondano G, et al. Early detection of locally recurrent rectal cancer by endosonography. Br J Radiol 1997;70(834):567–571.

40. Tjandra JJ, et al. Endoluminal ultrasound defines anatomy of the anal canal and pelvic floor. Dis Colon Rectum 1992;35(5): 465–470.

41. Sentovich SM, Wong WD, Blatchford GJ. Accuracy and reliability of transanal ultrasound for anterior anal sphincter injury. Dis Colon Rectum 1998;41(8):1000–1004.

42. Rieger N, Tjandra J, Solomon M. Endoanal and endorectal ultrasound: applications in colorectal surgery. ANZ J Surg 2004; 74(8):671–675.

43. Tjandra JJ, et al. Endoluminal ultrasound is preferable to electromyography in mapping anal sphincteric defects. Dis Colon Rectum 1993;36(7):689–692.

44. Mellgren A, et al. Long-term cost of fecal incontinence secondary to obstetric injuries. Dis Colon Rectum 1999;42(7):857–865; discussion 865–867.

45. Allen RE, et al. Pelvic floor damage and childbirth: a neurophysiological study [see comment]. Br J Obstet Gynaecol 1990; 97(9):770–779.

46. Sultan AH, et al. Anal-sphincter disruption during vaginal delivery [comment]. N Engl J Med 1993;329(26):1905–1911.

47. Poen AC, et al. Third-degree obstetric perineal tear: long-term clinical and functional results after primary repair. Br J Surg 1998;85(10):1433–1438.

48. Sorensen M, et al. Sphincter rupture in childbirth. Br J Surg 1993;80(3):392–394.

49. Tetzschner T, et al. Anal and urinary incontinence in women with obstetric anal sphincter rupture [see comment]. Br J Obstet Gynaecol 1996;103(10):1034–1040.

50. Burnett SJ, et al. Unsuspected sphincter damage following childbirth revealed by anal endosonography. Br J Radiol 1991; 64(759):225–227.

51. Varma A, et al. Obstetric anal sphincter injury: prospective evaluation of incidence [see comment]. Dis Colon Rectum 1999;42(12):1537–1543.

52. Zetterstrom J, et al. Effect of delivery on anal sphincter morphology and function. Dis Colon Rectum 1999;42(10):1253–1260.

53. Sultan AH, Kamm MA, Hudson CN, Bartram CI. Effect of pregnancy on anal sphincter morphology and function. Int J Colorectal Dis 1993;8(4):206–209.

54. Willis S, Faridi A, Schelzig S, et al. Childbirth and incontinence: a prospective study on anal sphincter morphology and function before and early after vaginal delivery. Langenbecks Arch Surg 2002;387(2):101–107.

55. Tsang CB, et al. Anal sphincter integrity and function influences outcome in rectovaginal fistula repair. Dis Colon Rectum 1998;41(9):1141–1146.

56. Deen KI, et al. Anal sphincter defects. Correlation between endoanal ultrasound and surgery. Ann Surg 1993;218(2):201–205.

57. Falk PM, et al. Transanal ultrasound and manometry in the evaluation of fecal incontinence. Dis Colon Rectum 1994;37(5):468–472.

58. Farouk R, Bartolo DC. The use of endoluminal ultrasound in the assessment of patients with faecal incontinence. J R Coll Surg Edinb 1994;39(5):312–318.

59. Zetterstrom JP, et al. Perineal body measurement improves evaluation of anterior sphincter lesions during endoanal ultrasonography. Dis Colon Rectum 1998;41(6):705–713.

60. deVries PA, Pena A. Posterior sagittal anorectoplasty. J Pediatr Surg 1982;17(5):638–643.

61. Jones NM, et al. The value of anal endosonography compared with magnetic resonance imaging following the repair of anorectal malformations. Pediatr Radiol 2003;33(3):183–185.

62. Simmang CL, et al. Posterior sagittal anorectoplasty in adults: secondary repair for persistent incontinence in patients with anorectal malformations. Dis Colon Rectum 1999;42(8): 1022–1027.

63. Gilliland R, et al. Pudendal neuropathy is predictive of failure following anterior overlapping sphincteroplasty. Dis Colon Rectum 1998;41(12):1516–1522.

64. Donnelly V, et al. Obstetric events leading to anal sphincter damage. Obstet Gynecol 1998;92(6):955–961.

65. Solomon MJ, et al. Assessment of peripouch inflammation after ileoanal anastomosis using endoluminal ultrasonography. Dis Colon Rectum 1995;38(2):182–187.

66. Deen KI, et al. Fistulas in ano: endoanal ultrasonographic assessment assists decision making for surgery. Gut 1994;35(3): 391–394.

67. Cataldo PA, Senagore A, Luchtefeld MA. Intrarectal ultrasound in the evaluation of perirectal abscesses. Dis Colon Rectum 1993;36(6):554–558.

68. Law PJ, et al. Anal endosonography in the evaluation of perianal sepsis and fistula in ano. Br J Surg 1989;76(7):752–755.

69. Lengyel AJ, Hurst NG, Williams JG. Pre-operative assessment of anal fistulas using endoanal ultrasound. Colorectal Dis 2002;4(6):436–440.

70. Cheong DM, et al. Anal endosonography for recurrent anal fistulas: image enhancement with hydrogen peroxide. Dis Colon Rectum 1993;36(12):1158–1160.

71. Poen AC, et al. Hydrogen peroxide-enhanced transanal ultrasound in the assessment of fistula-in-ano. Dis Colon Rectum 1998;41(9):1147–1152.

72. Navarro-Luna A, et al. Ultrasound study of anal fistulas with hydrogen peroxide enhancement. Dis Colon Rectum 2004; 47(1):108–114.

73. Goldman S, et al. Transanorectal ultrasonography in the staging of anal epidermoid carcinoma. Int J Colorectal Dis 1991;6(3): 152–157.

74. Herzog U, Boss M, Spichtin HP. Endoanal ultrasonography in the follow-up of anal carcinoma. Surg Endosc 1994;8(10): 1186–1189.

75. Roseau G, et al. Endoscopic ultrasonography in the staging and follow-up of epidermoid carcinoma of the anal canal. Gastrointest Endosc 1994;40(4):447–450.

76. Giovannini M, et al. Anal carcinoma: prognostic value of endorectal ultrasound (ERUS). Results of a prospective multi-center study. Endoscopy 2001;33(3):231–236.

77. Tarantino D, Bernstein MA. Endoanal ultrasound in the staging and management of squamous-cell carcinoma of the anal canal: potential implications of a new ultrasound staging system. Dis Colon Rectum 2002;45(1):16–22.

78. Hunerbein M, et al. Prospective comparison of endorectal ultrasound, three-dimensional endorectal ultrasound, and endorectal MRI in the preoperative evaluation of rectal tumors. Preliminary results. Surg Endosc 2000;14(11):1005–1009.

79. Kim JC, et al. Comparative study of three-dimensional and conventional endorectal ultrasonography used in rectal cancer staging. Surg Endosc 2002;16(9):1280–1285.

80. West RL, Dwarkasing S, Briel JW, et al. Can three-dimensional endoanal ultrasonography detect external anal sphincter atrophy? A comparison with endoanal magnetic resonance imaging. Int J Colorectal Dis 2005;20(4):328–333.

81. Gold DM, et al. Three-dimensional endoanal sonography in assessing anal canal injury. Br J Surg 1999;86(3):365–370.

82. West RL, et al. Hydrogen peroxide-enhanced three-dimensional endoanal ultrasonography and endoanal magnetic resonance imaging in evaluating perianal fistulas: agreement and patient preference. Eur J Gastroenterol Hepatol 2004;16(12):1319–1324.

83. Buchanan GN, et al. Value of hydrogen peroxide enhancement of three-dimensional endoanal ultrasound in fistula-in-ano. Dis Colon Rectum 2005;48(1):141–147.

84. Romano G, et al. Intrarectal ultrasound and computed tomography in the pre- and postoperative assessment of patients with rectal cancer. Br J Surg 1985;72(suppl):S117–119.

85. Hildebrandt U, et al. Endorectal ultrasound: instrumentation and clinical aspects. Int J Colorectal Dis 1986;1(4):203–207.

86. Holdsworth PJ, et al. Endoluminal ultrasound and computed tomography in the staging of rectal cancer. Br J Surg 1988; 75(10):1019–1022.

87. Beynon J. An evaluation of the role of rectal endosonography in rectal cancer. Ann R Coll Surg Engl 1989;71(2):131–139.

88. Dershaw DD. Endorectal sonography for rectal carcinoma. Bull NY Acad Med 1990;68(3):411–419.

89. Glaser F, et al. Influence of endorectal ultrasound on surgical treatment of rectal cancer. Eur J Surg Oncol 1990;16(4):304–311.

90. Jochem RJ, et al. Endorectal ultrasonographic staging of rectal carcinoma. Mayo Clin Proc 1990;65(12):1571–1577.

91. Herzog U, et al. How accurate is endorectal ultrasound in the preoperative staging of rectal cancer? Dis Colon Rectum 1993;36(2):127–134.

92. Sentovich SM, et al. Transrectal ultrasound of rectal tumors. Am J Surg 1993;166(6):638–641; discussion 641–642.

93. Adams DR, et al. Use of preoperative ultrasound staging for treatment of rectal cancer. Dis Colon Rectum 1999;42(2):159–166.

94. Marusch F, et al. Routine use of transrectal ultrasound in rectal carcinoma: results of a prospective multicenter study. Endoscopy 2002;34(5):385–390.

95. Manger T, Stroh C. Accuracy of endorectal ultrasonography in the preoperative staging of rectal cancer. Tech Coloproctol 2004;8(suppl 1):14–15.

8
Preoperative Management—Risk Assessment, Medical Evaluation, and Bowel Preparation

Conor P. Delaney and John M. MacKeigan

Preparation of the patient for surgery is a vital component of optimizing recovery after surgery, and must be individually tailored to the medical status of the patient.[1] Patients who undergo colorectal surgery may present in normal health, such as in a young patient undergoing hemorrhoid surgery, or may present in extreme ill health, such as the octogenarian with multiple medical conditions, who has developed perforated diverticulitis. Preoperative assessment and medical intervention are important components of care, and may account for the difference in perioperative mortality noted after abdominal and colorectal surgery between the United States and some European countries.[2]

Since the initial studies by Tyson and Spaulding in the 1950s, preparation of the bowel before surgery has been considered an essential component of care. More recently, this has become a contentious issue, and metaanalyses have suggested that bowel preparation provides no benefit, and may actually increase the incidence of some complications.

This chapter addresses the issues of medical evaluation and bowel preparation before surgery. These are considered on the background of reviewing some of the more important scoring systems for risk assessment before surgery, which permit comparison among different surgeons, institutions, and care pathways.

Perioperative Risk Assessment Scoring Systems

The risk related to surgery is a function of many factors. Patient-related factors include the underlying disease processes and the patient's physical ability to tolerate the physiologic stress related to the surgical procedure. Increasing amounts of data now show that risk is also affected by the volume of a procedure performed at the medical institution, but perhaps most importantly by the experience, training, and volume of surgery performed by the individual surgeon.

Scoring systems assess the patients' risk for morbidity and mortality as a result of anesthesia and surgery. These systems generally use data acquired during pre-hospital and in-hospital care, and some supplement this with components measuring operative severity. Some classification systems are designed to allow comparison of results between institutions and surgeons, whereas others are designed to distinguish patients who subsequently will have postoperative adverse events from those who will not.[3,4] The influence of each of these factors on overall morbidity and mortality is currently unknown but an ideal risk scoring system would incorporate all of these factors allowing accurate evaluation of surgical risk to the patient.

Thus, a primary aim of a scoring system is the evaluation of therapeutic benefit, i.e., the ratio of the relative harm and the relative benefit that are likely to follow a specific operation for a specific illness, whether in a specific patient, institution, or health system. Parameters that are useful in this evaluation include the natural history of the disease process, and the urgency of a specific procedure. Age may have an influence on operative risk, as many elderly patients require concurrent management of multiple organ degenerative disease. Elderly patients often tolerate operations well but complications poorly, hence prediction of the potential morbidity of an operation is particularly important in this group of patients. Scoring systems also provide a useful means of comparing outcomes from different institutions and patient groups by correcting for different comorbidities. Various scoring systems have been developed in an effort to quantify the risk of a patient from disease or intervention, and systems can be classified as preoperative or physiologic (Table 8-1).

Some scores are useful in predicting outcomes in specific conditions, such as Ranson's for pancreatitis, Child for liver failure, and the Burns index, but they are not of use for the general assessment of patients with other disorders. Some studies have tried to predict risk in a less specific manner, and have suggested that a surgeon's gut feeling upon completion of a major procedure may be a good indicator of subsequent outcome.[5]

TABLE 8-1. Perioperative scoring systems (references in text)

Physiologic scores	Preoperative scores
APACHE (I and II)	ASA grading
E-PASS	Goldman cardiac risk index
ISS/TRISS	Hospital prognostic index
POSSUM	Prognostic nutritional index
P-POSSUM	Pulmonary complication risk
SAPS	
Sepsis score	
Sickness score	
Therapeutic intervention score	

Risk Assessment for Complications from Specific Organ Systems

Some scoring systems define patient characteristics that are associated with increased morbidity and mortality because of involvement of a particular organ system. Scoring systems that have been described to predict the risk of death include those for respiratory,[6] gastrointestinal,[7–10] and cardiovascular disease.[11,12]

Cardiac Risk

Goldman Cardiac Risk[13]

The Goldman risk model is probably the best-accepted model for pure determination of cardiac risk for surgery. Point scores are assigned to each of nine clinical factors and patients are divided into four risk classes based on the total point score (Table 8-2). This is an important score because it reminds clinicians of the major cardiac risk factors in noncardiac surgery. Although the system is easy to use and utilizes relative weighting of risk factors, it was designed in the 1970s, and has not been updated for modern practice in anesthesia, medicine, or surgery. Cardiac risk for patients undergoing noncardiac surgery has also been evaluated by other studies.[11,12]

TABLE 8-2. Goldman cardiac risk index

Cardiac risk event	Points
Myocardial infarction within 6 mo	10
Age >70 y	5
S3 gallop or jugular venous distension	11
Important aortic valve stenosis	3
Rhythm other than sinus, or sinus rhythm and atrial premature contractions on last preoperative electrocardiogram	7
More than five premature ventricular contractions per minute anytime before surgery	7
Poor general medical status	3
Intraperitoneal, intrathoracic, or aortic operation	3
Emergency operation	4

Class	Points	Life-threatening complication risk (%)	Cardiac death risk (%)
I	0–5	0.7	0.2
II	6–12	5	2
III1	3–25	11	2
IV	≥26	22	56

Respiratory Risk

Pulmonary Complication Risk

Findings on respiratory examination, chest X-ray, Goldman's cardiac risk index, and the Charlson comorbidity index have been used for predicting respiratory complications.[6]

Risk Assessment for Postoperative Morbidity and Mortality

American Society of Anesthesiologists Classification

The American Society of Anesthesiologists (ASA) classification system (Table 8-3)[14] was initially developed to alert anesthesiologists to preexisting diseases. Because of the ease of use, and the fact that no tests are required, it has also been used to estimate operative risk.[15,16] ASA class directly correlates with perioperative mortality and morbidity[17–19] and also correlates significantly with perioperative variables such as intraoperative blood loss, duration of postoperative ventilation, and duration of intensive care unit (ICU) stay.[19] The severity of operative procedure, higher ASA class, symptoms of respiratory disease, and malignancy predicted postoperative morbidity in one study.[20]

Disadvantages to using the ASA score are that the score awarded depends on the subjective clinical judgment of the attending anesthesiologist, and that the small numbers of groups available means there can be little meaningful comparison between different surgeons or institutions.

Prognostic Nutritional Index

The prognostic nutritional index (PNI) was devised[21] to predict complication risk based on mortality, and correlates with postoperative sepsis and death. The PNI uses four factors, namely, serum albumin level, serum transferrin level, triceps skinfold thickness, and cutaneous delayed-type hypersensitivity. Serum albumin level, serum transferrin level, and delayed hypersensitivity were the only accurate predictors of postoperative morbidity and mortality. In addition to predicting postoperative morbidity and mortality, PNI can be used for predicting patients who might need nutritional support in the perioperative period. The authors concluded that perioperative nutritional support might reduce operative morbidity and mortality in malnourished patients, although this has not been routinely agreed with in the literature.

TABLE 8-3. ASA classification scheme

I	Normal healthy patient
II	Mild systemic disease
III	Severe, noncapacitating systemic disease
IV	Incapacitating systemic disease, threatening life
V	Moribund, not expected to survive 24 h
E	Emergency

APACHE (Acute Physiology and Chronic Health Evaluation) Scoring Systems

APACHE was initially described in 1981[22] and subsequently replaced in 1985[23] by APACHE II. This score was initially designed primarily for patients in the ICU but has been used for the assessment of patients with severe trauma, abdominal sepsis, postoperative enterocutaneous fistulas, acute pancreatitis, and to predict postoperative outcome.[24] The main disadvantage is that it is not independent of the effects of treatment, thus scoring for emergency patients being admitted to the ICU is best performed before surgical intervention.[25] Other disadvantages are that it is relatively complex and does not take into consideration the nutritional status of the patient or cardiology findings that add to operative risk. APACHE scores also do not take into account the extent of surgery. The APACHE III has been proposed more recently, but it is also very complex for routine use.[26] Several simpler scoring systems have also been developed from the APACHE system. These include SAPS (simplified acute physiology score),[27] which uses 14 of the 34 variables, and SAPS II, which also takes into consideration the urgency of the procedure and any associated chronic medical illness.

POSSUM

The POSSUM (Physiological and Operative Severity Score for enUmeration of Mortality and morbidity) was developed by multivariate discriminant analysis[28] of retrospective and prospective data, primarily to permit surgical audit for assessment of quality of care. It has been suggested that it works independent of geographical factors, and several publications have now come from the United States suggesting that it may also have a role in this health care system.[2,29]

POSSUM calculates expected death and expected morbidity rates based on 12 physiologic variables and six operative variables each of which are scored 1, 2, 4, or 8 (Table 8-4). The major advantage is that it predicts both morbidity and mortality and has successfully been used for a comparative audit of performance among surgical units, hospitals, and countries.[2] Disadvantages include that it does not take into account differences among surgeons, anesthetists, and operating time, all of which may influence outcome. This is because POSSUM was

TABLE 8-4. Parameters for calculation of the POSSUM score

Physiologic parameters	Operative parameters
Age (y)	Operative severity
Cardiac signs/chest X-ray	Multiple procedures
Respiratory signs/chest X-ray	Total blood loss (mL)
Pulse rate	Peritoneal soiling
Systolic blood pressure (mm Hg)	Presence of malignancy
Glasgow coma score	Mode of surgery
Hemoglobin (g/dL)	
White cell count ($\times 10^{12}$/l)	
Urea concentration (mmol/L)	
Na$^+$ and K$^+$ levels (mmol/L)	
Electrocardiogram	

developed as a scoring system for audit, so other factors may need to be considered when using POSSUM for risk assessment of patients for surgery. POSSUM also does not use primary diagnosis as a factor for scoring. Nevertheless, comparison of APACHE II with POSSUM showed that POSSUM is superior in predicting mortality in patients admitted to a high-dependency unit after general surgery.[30]

Portsmouth Modification of POSSUM (P-POSSUM)

One concern with POSSUM has been that it may overpredict mortality and morbidity rates by up to six times with a minimum mortality of 1.1%. P-POSSUM was therefore developed using a different mathematical formula to counter these disadvantages,[31] with the minimum mortality score in P-POSSUM reduced to 0.2%. Whereas some studies found that both scoring systems overpredicted mortality rates for vascular surgery patients,[32,33] others found that P-POSSUM was a better predictor of mortality and morbidity than POSSUM for vascular,[34] gastrointestinal,[35] and laparoscopic colorectal surgery.[36]

Other Scoring Systems

Various other scoring systems have also been developed primarily for assessment of critically ill patients in the ICU and for trauma and sepsis, and these are listed in Table 8-1.[37–45]

Risk Assessment for Colorectal Disease

Preoperative pulmonary and nutritional problems have been significant contributing factors in patients who died from sepsis after colon resection in the elderly. Others have suggested that age, congestive heart failure, hepatic, renal or pulmonary impairment, and extent of involvement by malignancy and postoperative complications were associated with greater mortality after colon surgery. Subsequently, it has been reported that age influenced mortality but not 5-year survival.[46] Ondrula et al.[47] assessed the predictive value of a variety of preoperative risk factors on operative outcomes and defined a colon index that assessed patients' operative risk. More recently, POSSUM was found to allow a realistic comparison of performance of different units performing colorectal resection and also permit comparison of outcome after colorectal resection among different surgeons.[48,49] POSSUM has also been reported in patients undergoing laparoscopic colectomy[29] but even the P-POSSUM overpredicted mortality and morbidity. Further modifications may be required to provide a validated tool for comparisons between laparoscopic and open approaches to colorectal resection.

Preoperative Medical Evaluation

Once a patient has a diagnosis requiring colorectal surgery, most surgeons intuitively categorize them into those needing minimal assessment, or extensive medical evaluation and treatment before surgery. Young patients having minor surgery will require no assessment. Young patients having more significant surgery may require minor evaluation, whereas older patients having minor surgery may require a similar level of evaluation. Older patients, and those with more extensive comorbidities will require assessment and possible treatment before surgery. Few definite guidelines exist as to who requires any exact pattern of assessment, and the benefits of individual tests are described below.

At the Cleveland Clinic, a questionnaire called Health Quest is given to patients who complete this on-line. Based on their answers, a score of 1–5 is generated indicating a level of complexity of medical history that can help stratify patients for level of preoperative assessment.[50] This process is also associated with a reduction in preoperative surgical delay, and increased patient satisfaction.

Evaluation is performed with a combination of history, physical examination, and selected investigations. In a large prospective clinical-epidemiologic study, Arvidsson and colleagues[3] found that a standardized assessment before surgery, by a combination of questionnaires, interview, physical examination, and laboratory screening identified a high proportion of patients who were likely to have an adverse event in the postoperative period.

Preanesthesia Interview

Of the techniques available that are used in preoperative evaluation of patients, namely, history, physical examination, and investigations, history taking is the most efficient and profitable.[3,51] A thorough review of previous medical records including history of anesthesia and surgery helps identify many potential problems that can occur perioperatively. Questionnaires have previously been found to be efficient and reliable for anesthesia preadmission assessment.[52] Thus, a preoperative questionnaire is suitable for patients undergoing daycare surgery, because most of these patients are at low risk.

History taking should include information on the condition for which the procedure is being performed, history of surgical procedures (local procedures that may complicate surgery such as reoperative pelvic surgery, as well as general procedures that may complicate recovery such as prior splenectomy), and prior outcomes with intubation and anesthesia. Special consideration should be given to cardiopulmonary function, allergy, renal and hepatic function, bleeding tendency, and medication use. History of chronic medical conditions of the cardiorespiratory system and medications including dosage is important. In children, history should be focused on other specific factors such as birth history and history of recent infections, especially pneumonia and upper respiratory tract infections. Aspirin and other nonsteroidal anti-inflammatory drugs are best discontinued 1 week before surgery. Other questions should pertain to immunization, smoking, and alcohol and drug use. Cessation of smoking 8 or more weeks before surgery helps optimize the mucociliary apparatus of the patient before surgery. Review of

functional status of the patient, activities of daily living (ADL), and social support are also important, although this primarily relates to longer term recovery, hospital stay, and likely discharge status from hospital, rather than direct perioperative morbidity and mortality.

History taking for cardiac assessment has been reasonably well standardized, and very well reviewed recently by Mukherjee and Eagle.[53] The primary factors to be considered are whether the patient has recent myocardial infarction, decompensated heart failure, unstable angina, symptomatic arrhythmias, or symptomatic valvular heart disease. In general, noninvasive testing is most effective in intermediate-risk patients, whereas invasive evaluation should be considered in those with multiple risk factors and ischemia on preoperative testing, because perioperative beta-blockade may be inadequate.

Formal anesthetic evaluation is also needed for many patients. Similar to the selective levels of medical work-up, not all patients will need to be seen by an anesthesiologist preoperatively. Young, healthy patients with normal anatomy, and no adverse findings in history or examination, may not need any evaluation. Patients having more major surgery should probably all meet the anesthesia service before surgery, for assessment as well as instruction about what will happen around the time of surgery. This may be expediently performed by nurse practitioners. Some patients with complex anesthetic histories or with major perioperative risk factors may require formal anesthetic assessment by a staff anesthesiologist. Usually, such guidelines are institution-specific, but it is recommended that the surgeon and anesthesiologist have a similar plan for assessment, so that unexpected surprises are avoided on the day of surgery.

Physical Examination

A review of preoperative evaluation[54] noted that history and physical examination focusing on risk factors for cardiac, pulmonary, and infectious complications and determination of a patient's functional capacity are important for preoperative evaluation of patients. General indicators of fitness of a patient for surgery include activities of daily living competence (ADL) and general mobility. Specific evaluation for subtle signs of cardiopulmonary dysfunction is important, because these have been shown to correlate strongly with major perioperative complications.[13]

Preoperative Tests

Preoperative tests serve to complement the history and physical examination in assessing the suitability of the patient for surgery. They have been used to assess levels of known disease, detect unsuspected but modifiable conditions that may be treated to reduce risk before surgery, or detect unsuspected conditions that may not be possible to treat, and therefore simply be baseline results before surgery.

Many patients undergoing minor surgery need minimal investigation, even if they have chronic medical conditions. Review of current evidence indicates that routine laboratory tests are rarely helpful except in the monitoring of known disease states. New guidelines have a significant impact on reducing preoperative testing and have not caused an increase in untoward perioperative events.[55,56] Historically, ordering routine preoperative investigations was quite often driven more by personal experience than by scientific evidence.[57] This led to inefficient clinical practice, with healthy patients undergoing useless, time-consuming, costly, and sometimes harmful procedures. A prospective study found that whereas 16% of results were abnormal, only 0.013% caused a change in management for 400 patients undergoing elective surgery.[58] Higher complication rates were significantly associated with the extent of surgery, but not with abnormal preoperative blood results. Other studies have also found that only a small percentage of abnormal preoperative investigations changed management.[59] This is especially true, as a repeat test is an adequate response to most abnormal biochemical results because an abnormal test does not necessarily correlate with pathology. Because reference intervals of most tests take the normal distribution and standard deviation of the population into consideration, cut-off points for normality are set such that patients whose test results exceed the upper 2.5% of healthy individuals or are below the lower 2.5% of healthy individuals are said to have abnormal results. Thus, 5% of patients whose values are outside the reference range do not necessarily have disease and may be normal. The greater the number of tests ordered, the greater the probability of finding a result outside the reference range.

Age, history of chronic heart disease, renal disease, emergency surgery, and type of operation are predictors of the risk of mortality.[60] Fit, young patients undergoing minor and intermediate procedures do not need routine preoperative investigations and in the pediatric age group, a thorough clinical examination has been found to be of greater value than routine laboratory screening. A good history and physical examination have been said to be more important rather than laboratory data in the development of a treatment plan for anesthesia.

Quality cost-effective preoperative preparation of patients undergoing anesthesia and surgical procedures is a central issue in perioperative patient management. Minimizing routine preoperative testing results in better utilization of resources and a greater cost-benefit ratio without adverse effect to the patient. Review of preoperative evaluation of patients found that 60% of the amount spent on preoperative laboratory testing was wasted.[61] False-positive and borderline tests led to further investigation causing reduced efficiency of practice, creating the potential for iatrogenic disease and increasing medicolegal risk. Thus, guidelines for preoperative testing based on best available evidence are important for efficient resource utilization and prevention of undue surgical risk to the patient. Although the general consensus is that screening must be replaced by indicated testing, the danger

identified is that some indicated tests may also be abandoned in the quest for reducing routine investigations.[62] Review of previous tests helps avoid duplication of tests and also helps identify potential problems.

Assessment of Specific Organ Systems

Cardiac Evaluation

The detection of a rhythm other than sinus and the presence of premature atrial contractions and frequent premature ventricular contractions increase the risk of perioperative cardiac events.[13] Yield of electrocardiogram in unselected patients is highly correlated to age but most dysrhythmia can be suspected from physical examination.[63] The American College of Cardiology (ACC) and American Heart Association (AHA) recommendations for preoperative cardiac evaluation consider the magnitude of the particular procedure being performed and patient factors that influence perioperative cardiac risk. History of coronary artery disease, cardiovascular procedures, and symptoms of angina or congestive heart failure are important. Patients without symptoms and with a normal cardiac stress test within 2 years or coronary artery bypass graft in the last 5 years, those who are clinically stable and underwent angioplasty 6 months to 5 years previously do not need any further assessment. Patients who had an angioplasty within 6 months and those having emergency surgery may need cardiac evaluation and angiography. Patients with intermediate risk and poor functional capacity may need stress testing. Assessment of left ventricular function by radionuclide scan or echocardiography is also indicated for patients in whom an impaired left ventricular function is suspected on clinical examination or radiology although the best test remains unclear.[64] Further cardiac evaluation is only needed in patients with definite clinical predictors identified from history, physical examination, electrocardiogram, and functional status along with the risk associated with the operation itself. Cardiac interventions are generally only recommended for patients who would otherwise have benefited regardless of any unplanned noncardiac surgery. These recommendations have been reviewed and summarized by the ACC (www.acc.org/clinical/guidelines/perio/update/fig1.htm) and others.[53,65]

Transfusion and Hematologic Evaluation

Most patients with anemia tolerate operations well unless they have associated disease, and therefore anemia rarely changes management unless operative blood losses are expected to be great. Risk of thromboembolism and bleeding disorders can be assessed by a detailed history and by tests that measure coagulation factors (prothrombin and partial thromboplastin time) and that assess platelet count and function (bleeding time). Measures to reduce the risk of thromboembolism have been well documented and are part of the practice parameters available from the American Society of Colon and Rectal Surgeons[66,67] (see Appendix A).

Blood grouping and cross-matching is obviously critical when planning major surgery in which significant blood losses may occur. An important consideration is to have a routine sample for blood type on file for patients undergoing major surgery, even if transfusion is not expected, and cross-matching would not usually take place. This allows a double level of security when urgent samples are sent if bleeding occurs during surgery. This may help avoid the risk of transfusion reaction if there is concern about errors with sample labeling or source at any time.

Anemic patients who are scheduled for elective surgery may be treated preoperatively by allogenic transfusion but consideration is also given to autologous donation, erythropoietin, intraoperative hemodilution with autotransfusion, or consideration of cell salvage techniques, which are still being evaluated in colorectal surgery. Preoperative autologous donation (PAD) has been criticized recently because of cost-ineffectiveness, large wastage of PAD units, and the potential for leaving patients more anemic after surgery than without PAD.[68] Techniques including acute normovolemic hemodilution and cell salvage may be more efficient; however, investigations into their use continue.[69]

Renal Function Evaluation

When indicated, measurement of serum electrolytes in the preoperative period helps in preventing perioperative problems. This is particularly true for serum potassium, because both hypokalemia and hyperkalemia may lead to cardiac conduction disturbances. Normal renal function is necessary for the excretion of the nondepolarizing muscle relaxants used for anesthesia and surgery. Renal function is also a consideration when choosing postoperative analgesic regimens including nonsteroidal medications such as Ketoralac. Age, hypertension, and diabetes may be indications for preoperative selective renal function testing.

Respiratory Tract Evaluation

Patients with a history of chronic lung disease require careful assessment to minimize problems with anesthesia. In addition, patients with grossly normal lungs may rarely develop respiratory abnormalities secondary to anesthetic agents and operation. Common pulmonary complications after surgery are atelectasis, pneumonia, and bronchitis and predisposing risk factors include cough, dyspnea, smoking, history of lung disease, obesity, and abdominal or thoracic surgery. Cessation of smoking 8 weeks before surgery is beneficial to the patient by allowing recovery of the mucociliary apparatus. Bronchodilators are helpful in patients with asthma and bronchitis. Active pulmonary infection should be treated before surgery when possible. A Global Initiative for Chronic Obstructive Lung Disease (COLD) now recommends optimal treatment for COLD patients, and these treatments may need to be optimized before surgery.

The incidence of abnormalities detected on a routine preoperative chest film is higher in elderly patients but most occur in patients with recognizable risk factors. Preoperative chest X-rays may be of value in ruling out metastases but do not otherwise have a major influence on the decision to operate or on the type of anesthesia, and abandonment of routine ordering of preoperative chest X-rays does not produce adverse patient effects.[70] The Royal College of Radiologists recommended preoperative chest X-rays only for patients with acute respiratory symptoms, possible metastases, those with suspected or established cardiorespiratory disease without a chest X-ray in the preceding 12 months, and recent migrants from endemic countries. Other studies also suggest using specific indications for preoperative testing rather than routine X-rays, culminating in a metaanalysis by Archer and colleagues.[71]

There are no well-established guidelines as to who requires pulmonary function testing. Such candidates may include patients with chronic pulmonary disease, wheezing or dyspnea on exertion, chest wall and spinal deformities, morbid obesity, heavy smokers with persistent cough, thoracic surgery, elderly patients (>70 years of age), and patients who are to undergo upper abdominal surgery. The American College of Chest Physicians criteria recommend preoperative spirometry only in patients undergoing lung resection, those who undergo cardiac and upper abdominal surgery in the presence of a history of smoking and dyspnea, and patients with pulmonary symptoms and uncharacterized disease scheduled for prolonged lower abdominal surgery.

Neurologic System

The prevalence of occult cerebrovascular disease in elderly patients, who constitute a large proportion of patients requiring surgical attention, is a special concern. An asymptomatic carotid bruit indicates the presence of peripheral vascular disease and is an indication for further evaluation by duplex scanning. However, prophylactic endarterectomy is not indicated usually, because the increased risk of a perioperative stroke compared with the unselected population is small.[72] Symptomatic disease that is untreated or undiagnosed before preoperative assessment should be assessed and treated before all but emergency surgery. Patients at high risk may be kept on aspirin products during the time of surgery to minimize their risk of stroke. Some may require endarterectomy before their scheduled surgery, although this is quite rare.

Metabolic and Endocrine System

Assessment for diabetes, thyroid disorders, and other endocrine problems is an integral part of preoperative evaluation. Obesity is now so prevalent that fasting blood glucose in obese patients may pick cases of unexpected diabetes.[73] Pregnancy may dictate reassessment of the indication for surgery, type of procedure being performed, and issues related to anesthesia. Patients on steroids may need extra dosage in the perioperative period. Patients with known diabetes will need careful management of their blood sugar in the per-operative period, with standard recommendations for insulin and oral hypoglycemic use.

Nutritional Assessment and Hepatic Function

Nutritional measurements help in assessing the physiologic status and optimizing function of the patient with regard to immunology, fluid balance, and metabolic response to trauma and surgery. Patients at particular concern for malnutrition are those who have lost more than 10% of their body weight in the previous 6 months, and those with an albumin less than 3 g/dL. Malnourished patients have increased complications after surgery, although nutrition must be supplemented for at least 2 weeks before clinical outcome parameters are improved.[74]

Abnormal liver function may affect hemostatic mechanisms and drug metabolism, but is an unusual clinical problem. Significant liver impairment is detectable on certain standard clinical and laboratory examinations, but is not routinely evaluated biochemically. Hepatitis may pose increased risk to the medical personnel taking care of the patient.

Preoperative Assessment Specific for Colorectal Procedures

For patients undergoing surgery for colorectal disorders, a previous major laparotomy may preclude laparoscopic surgery or indicate an increased risk of conversion to open surgery. Body habitus of the patient, mental status, visual acuity, and the presence of other disorders such as arthritis may determine the decision on whether a stoma is formed and its placement. Assessment of patients' attitudes toward surgery, addressing their concerns, and counseling them regarding what to expect during hospitalization forms an integral part of the preoperative evaluation.

Current Recommendations[1,54]

Tests that need to be performed include hemoglobin for evidence of anemia and as a baseline level for postoperative management. Renal and liver function tests are not routinely indicated but rather in patients with medical conditions or taking medication that would indicate these tests. Preoperative blood glucose determination is obtained in patients 45 years of age or older because current recommendations suggest that all patients older than 45 years ought to be screened; diabetes mellitus also increases perioperative risks. A urine pregnancy test ought to be considered for all women of childbearing age. Coagulation tests are only indicated in patients on anticoagulation, with a family or personal history of bleeding disorder, or those with liver disease. Patients undergoing major surgery with a potential for blood loss should have a type and screen taken for filing in the laboratory, even if transfusion is not expected. This may help minimize the risk of later transfusion reaction.

Electrocardiogram is indicated in male patients older than 40 years of age, females older than 50 years, and those with a history suggestive of cardiac disorders. Chest X-rays are performed on the basis of findings from the medical history or physical examination. As part of preoperative risk assessment, patients found to have medical conditions requiring further specific therapy before surgery should also be considered for more intensive medical supervision. This is important while in the hospital for their surgery, and also as part of their post-discharge follow-up.

Bowel Preparation

The practice of mechanical bowel preparation (MBP) before surgery has undergone major changes over the last century. Mechanical preparation became routine for all surgeons by the start of the 1990s,[75] and this was used in combination with oral or intravenous antibiotic prophylaxis. This practice was thought to offer less risk of anastomotic leak, and to reduce the risk of wound infection, both postulated to be related to the bacterial load of stool. There are approximately 10^9 to 10^{11} anaerobic bacteria and 10^5 to 10^7 aerobic bacteria in the colon, per gram of stool. The normal colonic flora comprises approximately 20 species of aerobic bacteria and more than 50 species of anaerobic bacteria. *Bacteroides fragilis* is the most frequently cultured species, followed by clostridia and peptostreptococci, in postoperative infections in colon and rectal surgery.

Method of Bowel Preparation

The techniques used to mechanically prepare the bowel have changed hugely over the last 25 years. When Goligher reported outcomes in the 1970s, patients were restricted to a liquid diet for 3–5 days, before being given cathartic agents and enemas.[76] Some authors recommended 10 L of crystalloid solution by nasogastric tube while the patient remained on the commode.[77] Others recommended diet restriction for up to 10–14 days. These dietary restrictions were combined with oral aperients such as castor oil, and the use of enemas before surgery. Such protocols were associated with problems of fluid overload, hyponatremia, and nausea and vomiting.

The description of polyethylene glycol (PEG) preparations, which were minimally absorbed and could irrigate the bowel effectively, changed MBP practice. Preparation time was shortened to 1 day by drinking 4 L of a balanced electrolyte solution which would not be absorbed or metabolized.[78] Studies quickly showed that PEG provided better bowel preparation and was more easily tolerated by patients than the traditional 5-day regimes.

Sodium phosphate was then developed and used to clean bowel for colonoscopy. Similarly with this product, patient acceptance was high, because volumes to drink were smaller. Transient phosphatemia was noted but was rarely a significant event.[79] The new solution was quickly used for elective colonic surgery.[80] The preparations were also given at home, so that patients could come to the hospital the morning of surgery. Although this practice adequately cleans bowel, it does mean that patients tend to need more fluid resuscitation in the perioperative period.[81] The lower-volume sodium phosphate preparations are now used routinely by many surgeons, but should be avoided in those with significant history of cardiac or renal dysfunction.

The most recent development is the description of a sodium phosphate pill. This may now be taken as a series of 28–32 pills on two occasions to give an effective preparation, although some concerns remain about hydration and electrolyte issues.[82] This has been reported to give equivalent results at bowel cleansing for colonoscopy[83]; however, many clinicians do not use this form of preparation because of concerns about electrolyte imbalance.[84] Indeed, any sodium phosphate preparation may cause hypocalcemia, hyperphosphatemia, and hypokalemia, leading to increased caution for their use in the elderly and those with renal dysfunction.

Whether to Use an MBP

Over the last decade, several studies have suggested that a mechanical preparation may not be necessary, and these data will be reviewed here. Initial studies included several case series that suggested low anastomotic leak rates could be obtained without bowel preparation.[85,86] These results were reminiscent of the trauma literature suggesting that equally good or better outcomes could be achieved performing repair in unprepared bowel.[87]

These studies have been accompanied by a series of randomized, controlled trials evaluating the presence or absence of MBP, culminating in the recent publication of a Cochrane review on the subject (Table 8-5).[88–94] Of the five randomized trials over the last decade, two showed higher anastomotic leak rates with bowel preparation. The remaining trials showed no difference. Interestingly, some authors suggested that anastomotic leak may be worse in those who received a bowel preparation who had a poor result, leaving the colon loaded with liquid stool. No study showed a worse outcome in control patients (no preparation).

A Cochrane review was performed to analyze all randomized, controlled data and specifically to determine the effect of MBP on morbidity and mortality rates after elective colorectal surgery.[93] Of patients with anastomoses, there were 576 MBP patients and 583 without MBP. There was no difference in anastomotic leak rates for low anterior resection (12.5% versus 12%), or colonic surgery (1.2% versus 6%) in patients with or without MBP. Overall anastomotic leak rates were significantly lower without MBP (5.5% versus 2.9%; $P = .02$). Mortality, peritonitis, reoperation, wound infection, and extraabdominal complications were similar between groups. The results failed to support the hypothesis that MBP reduces complication rates, but because there was no a priori hypothesis that MBP might increase complication rates, this could not be stated.

These data certainly show the safety of performing anastomosis in unprepared bowel in patients undergoing gynecologic or other surgery who have not had MBP and are found to have other pathology. Furthermore, this metaanalysis provides important evidence questioning the routine use of MBP in elective colorectal surgery. Whereas avoidance of bowel preparation may not be possible for laparoscopic approaches for technical reasons, it should be considered for open surgery, perhaps especially when using PEG preparations.[94]

Bowel Preparation in Special Situations

Obviously, patients with acute intestinal or colonic obstruction cannot be given a high-volume or cathartic bowel preparation. Certain other patients are not suitable for bowel preparation. Perhaps the most important example are those with obstructive symptoms, or a chronic partial obstruction. Most surgeons would avoid a bowel preparation in this circumstance, and if necessary perform an on-table lavage before anastomosis. This practice is further supported by the data suggesting that bowel preparation may be unnecessary.

Some surgeons will reserve use of milder preparative agents for patients with chronic partial obstruction, such as that seen in cases of longstanding Crohn's disease. Options here would include prescribing small volumes of magnesium citrate, or managing the patient with older regimes, such as dietary restriction for a longer period of time than overnight.

TABLE 8-5. Randomized, controlled trials and Cochrane report relating to preoperative mechanical bowel preparation (all results as MBP versus no MBP, %)

Author	Year	n	Anastomotic leak	Wound infection	Mortality
Brownson et al.[88]	1992	179	11.9 vs 1.5*	5.8 vs 7.5	0.0 vs 0.0
Burke et al.[89]	1994	169	3.8 vs 4.6	4.9 vs 3.4	2.4 vs 0.0
Santos et al.[90]	1994	149	10.0 vs 5.0*	24.0 vs 10.0	0.0 vs 0.0
Miettinen et al.[91]	2000	267	4.0 vs 2.0	4.0 vs 2.0	0.0 vs 0.0
Zmora et al.[92]	2003	249	4.2 vs 2.3	6.6 vs 10.0	1.7 vs 0.8
Guenga et al.[93]	2003	1159	5.5 vs 2.9	7.4 vs 5.7	0.6 vs 0.0
Slim et al.[94]	2004	1454	5.6 vs 3.2*	7.4 vs 5.7	1.4 vs 0.8

*Significant result.

Prophylactic Antibiotic Usage (See Appendix B)

Removing the bulk of the stool in a patient was believed to reduce the risk of complications; however, this remained unproven. Antibiotics were additionally used to further reduce the risk of wound infection and possibly other complications. In the initial phases, oral antibiotics were used and given over the days preceding surgery. More recently, there has been a major shift toward using parenteral antibiotics to do this job.

Neomycin and erythromycin were initially chosen as suitable oral antibiotics for prophylaxis of wound infection in colorectal cases. Such oral antibiotics are given at three time points the day before surgery (1 PM, 2 PM, and 11 PM the day before surgery for an 8 AM start time), in an effort to sterilize the bacteria within the bowel lumen. Antibiotics were shown to reduce bacterial counts by 1000-fold.[95] These agents were inexpensive, largely remained in the bowel lumen, and were therefore thought to be suitable for this technique. Erythromycin has now been replaced by metronidazole because of its improved activity against anaerobes, and less gastrointestinal side effects. Although these agents can be effective,[96] the results can be equaled or bettered by using parenteral medications.[97]

Over the last 20 years, many studies were performed to evaluate parenteral antibiotics for all forms of general surgery, and also for colorectal indications. Because of differences in trial design, antibiotics used, and definitions of wound infection and other outcome parameters, many of these studies are hard to compare with each other. Over this time, there was an evolution from using antibiotics for 5 days, down to the current situation in which they are generally given to cover the time of surgery itself, or used for 24 hours maximum, unless a therapeutic course is indicated for clinical reasons. This effort to minimize the number of doses of antibiotics that is given has been supported by microbiologists and infectious disease specialists, in the hope of reducing cases of nosocomial infection seen in association with prolonged antibiotic usage, particularly that with *Clostridium difficile*, which is being seen in epidemic proportions in some geographical areas and institutions. Furthermore, in the 17 trials comparing single-dose to multiple-dose (two or more doses) regimens, using the same antibiotic or combinations of antibiotics, no trial found a difference in wound infection rates, and a pooled analysis also showed no statistically significant difference.[96] This single-dose policy also reduces risk of toxicity, costs, and possibility of developing resistance to the antibiotic used.[98]

Further knowledge has also provided awareness that the essential time to have coverage (adequate systemic levels) with antibiotics is from the time of incision to the time of skin closure. Thus, prophylactic antibiotics are ideally given at the time of anesthetic induction, although the randomized, controlled trials permitted up to 1 hour after this time, and if necessary are repeated after 4–6 hours to keep adequate circulating levels, particularly if there has been significant blood loss.

Antibiotics need to cover Gram positive, negative, and anaerobic bacteria, and regimes such as ampicillin, gentamicin, and metronidazole used to be typical. Current choices usually include a second-generation cephalosporin with metronidazole, or an agent such as amoxicillin/clavulanic acid which avoids the need for metronidazole. In patients with penicillin allergy, ciprofloxacin may be used instead of the cephalosporin, or another alternative would be gentamicin, clindamycin, and metronidazole, although we prefer to avoid clindamycin because of concerns with nosocomial infection. These issues have been excellently reviewed elsewhere in a systematic review, documenting outcomes for each major antibiotic combination.[96]

A final issue relates to the combination of oral and parenteral agents. Some surgeons like this practice, thinking that this may further reduce infectious complications. One recent study has combined a randomized trial comparing oral neomycin and metronidazole with placebo in colonic surgery patients receiving parenteral amikacin and metronidazole. The combination of oral and intravenous antibiotics reduced wound infection rates, and this was supported by a meta-analysis of prior literature.[99]

Prophylaxis for Endocarditis and Prosthesis

Patients undergoing invasive colorectal procedures are at varying risk for endocarditis and infection of prosthesis. The American Society of Colon and Rectal surgeons has published Practice Parameters (Appendix B) to guide surgeons on selecting appropriate measures for at risk patients. For Additional discussion, see Chapter 9.

Communication with the Patient and Laying the Groundwork for Postoperative Recovery

No preoperative visit is complete without providing information on expected postoperative outcomes. This discussion helps the patient to build confidence and trust in the surgeon. Such discussion is likely to be an important component of any postoperative care pathway, and this may help lead to significant reduction in postoperative stay.[100–102]

Patients can be advised of the surgery they will undergo, their expected milestones in recovery, and possible complications, including issues such as readmission, which may occur in 10% or more of these patients undergoing major abdominal surgery.[103]

Conclusion

Assessment of the patient undergoing surgery is of extreme importance in providing patients with a safe recovery from their operation. This permits stratification of patients into groups that require intensive, moderate, or minimal investigation or treatment before anesthesia. Tests to investigate patients should be used selectively based on increasingly accepted guidelines. Patients who need such evaluation and treatment before surgery should also be seen by the relevant medical specialty when in the hospital, and receive any necessary instructions for appropriate medical follow-up after their surgery.

MBP continues to be used by the majority of colorectal surgeons, based on traditional practice patterns. Several randomized, controlled trials now suggest that this practice may be unnecessary. Patients undergoing bowel resection should be given antibiotic prophylaxis using one dose of parenteral broad-spectrum agents at the time of induction of anesthesia.

Appendix A: Practice Parameters for the Prevention of Venous Thromboembolism

Risk Classification

Low-risk Patients

The typical low-risk patient is one undergoing minor surgery who has one or no risk factors. No specific measures are recommended for patients at low risk other than early ambulation. Unprotected, these patients have a 2% chance of calf vein thrombosis and a negligible risk of pulmonary embolus.

Moderate-risk Patients

The typical moderate-risk patient is older than 40 years of age, undergoing major abdominal surgery, with no other major risk factors. Moderate-risk patients can be treated with either intermittent pneumatic compression (IPC) alone or low-dose unfractionated heparin (LDUH). Moderate-risk patients have two risk factors. Unprotected, these patients have a 10%–20% risk of calf vein thrombosis, and a 1%–2% chance of a pulmonary embolism.

High-risk Patients

High-risk patients have three or four risk factors. The typical high-risk patient is older than 40 years of age, is having major abdominal surgery, and harbors additional risk factors. High-risk patients can be treated with LDUH (bid or tid) or low-molecular-weight heparin (LMWH), although standard unfractionated heparin seems to be more cost effective. If heparin cannot or should not be used, IPC should be substituted. When heparin has not been started preoperatively, the patient should be reevaluated for postoperative heparin. Unprotected, these patients have a 20%–40% risk of calf vein thrombosis and a 2%–4% risk of pulmonary embolism.

Very High-risk Patients

A high-risk patient is upgraded to a highest-risk category when certain additional risk factors are present. These include a history of thromboembolic events, hypercoagulable states, and possibly malignancy. Assuming no contraindication, highest-risk patients ideally should receive pharmacologic treatment such as LDUH (bid or tid) or LMWH. Untreated,

TABLE 8-A.1. Recommendations for VTE prophylaxis by risk classification

	Thromboprophylaxis by risk classification*			
	Low	Moderate	High	Highest
Example	Ambulatory surgery, no risk factors	Major abdominal sx, age > 40 y, no other risk factors	Major abdominal sx, age > 60 y, additional risk factors	Major abdominal sx, prior VTE, malignancy, or hypercoagulable state
Calf vein thrombosis (without prophylaxis)	2	10–20	20–40	40–80
Clinical PE	0.2	1–2	2–4	4–10
Primary prophylaxis	None	IPC	LDUH (q 8–12 h) or LMWH	LDUH (q 8–12 h) or LMWH
Alternate prophylaxis	None	LDUH (q 12 h) or LMWH	IPC†	Heparin and IPC‡

Figures are percentages.

sx, symptoms; VTE, venous thromboembolism; PE, pulmonary embolism; q 8–12 h, every 8–12 hours.

*Modified with permission from Clagett GP, Anderson FA Jr, Geerts W, et al. Prevention of venous thromboembolism. Chest 1998;114:531S–560S.

†Intermittent pneumatic compression boots offer prophylaxis where the risk of bleeding is high. Heparin may be started postoperatively after the risk of bleeding has passed.

‡Some data suggest that IPC combined with heparin may offer increased protection. Where the risk of bleeding is high, IPC may be used intraoperatively and heparin may be added postoperatively after the risk of bleeding has passed.

these patients have a 40%–80% risk of calf vein thrombosis and a 4%–10% risk of pulmonary embolism.

Intuitively, there may be some advantage to a strategy of dual methods, i.e., combining intermittent pneumatic compression with heparin. Several investigators have suggested this. This has been shown to be efficacious for patients undergoing cardia and hip replacement surgery, but thus far there are no published data for colon and rectal surgery patients.

Appendix B: Practice Parameters for Antibiotic Prophylaxis to Prevent Infective Endocarditis or Infective Prosthesis During Colon and Rectal Endoscopy

These parameters are based in part on the recently updated recommendations made by the AHA and the previously published parameters developed by The American Society of Colon and Rectal Surgeons. According to the AHA, the risk for endocarditis is determined by the patient's preexisting cardiac condition and the surgical procedure in question. The major changes in the new AHA guidelines are the following: 1) it was emphasized that invasive procedures are not the cause of most cases of endocarditis; 2) cardiac conditions are stratified by the potential outcome if endocarditis develops; 3) procedures causing bacteremia are more clearly specified; 4) an algorithm for antibiotic prophylaxis for patients with mitral valve prolapse was developed; 5) prophylactic regimens for oral or dental procedures were modified; and 6) prophylactic regimens for genitourinary and gastrointestinal procedures were simplified. The AHA considers lower gastrointestinal endoscopy to be a low-risk procedure for initiating problematic bacteremia, and The Standards Task Force concurs. The Task Force considered other direct and indirect support for the use of antibiotic prophylaxis in patients with cardiac or other prostheses. It is the consensus of The Standards Task Force that prophylaxis be considered only for the high-risk groups listed in Table 8-B.1. The complex nature of individualized patient care does not allow standards to be spelled out for every clinical category.

TABLE 8-B.1. Conditions associated with endocarditis (high risk)

Prosthetic cardiac valves
History of endocarditis
Surgically constructed systemic pulmonary shunts
Complex cyanotic congenital heart disease
Vascular grafts (first 6 months after implantation)

Prepared by The Standards Task Force, The American Society of Colon and Rectal Surgeons.
Reprinted from Dis Colon Rectum 2000;43(9):1193–1200. Copyright 2003. All rights reserved. American Society of Colon and Rectal Surgeons.

References

1. Kiran RP, Delaney CP, Senagore AJ. Preoperative evaluation and risk assessment scoring. Clin Colorect Surg 2003;16: 75–84.
2. Bennett-Guerrero E, Hyam JA, Shaefi S, et al. Comparison of P-POSSUM risk-adjusted mortality rates after surgery between patients in the USA and UK. Br J Surg 2003;90:1593–1598.
3. Arvidsson S, Ouchterlony J, Sjostedt L, Svardsudd K. Predicting postoperative adverse events. Clinical efficiency of four general classification systems. The project perioperative risk. Acta Anaesthesiol Scand 1996;40(7):783–791.
4. Klotz HP, Candinas D, Platz A, et al. Preoperative risk assessment in elective general surgery. Br J Surg 1996;83:1788–1791.
5. Hartley MN, Sagar PM. The surgeon's 'gut feeling' as a predictor of post-operative outcome. Ann R Coll Surg Engl 1994;76(6 suppl):277–278.
6. Lawrence VA, Dhanda R, Hilsenbeck SG, et al. Risk of pulmonary complications after elective abdominal surgery. Chest 1996;110(3):744–750.
7. Mullen JL, Buzby GP, Waldman MT, et al. Prediction of operative morbidity and mortality by preoperative nutritional assessment. Surg Forum 1979;30:80–82.
8. Greenburg AG, Saik RP, Pridham D. Influence of age on mortality of colon surgery. Am J Surg 1985;150:65–70.
9. Buzby GP, Mullen JL, Matthews DC, et al. Prognostic nutritional index in gastrointestinal surgery. Am J Surg 1980;139(1):160–167.
10. Boyd JB, Bradford B Jr, Watne AL. Operative risk factors of colon resection in the elderly. Ann Surg 1980;192(6):743–746.
11. Cooperman M, Pflug B, Martin EW, et al. Cardiovascular risk factors in patients with peripheral vascular disease. Surgery 1978;84:505–509.
12. Detsky A, Abrams H, McLaughlin J, et al. Predicting cardiac complications in patients undergoing non-cardiac surgery. J Gen Intern Med 1986;1:211.
13. Goldman L, Caldera DL, Nussbaum SR, et al. Multifactorial index of cardiac risk in noncardiac surgical procedures. New Engl J Med 1977;297:845.
14. Anonymous. New classification of physical status. Anaesthesiology 1963;24:111.
15. Keats A. The ASA classification of physical status: a recapitulation. Anaesthesiology 1978;49:233–236.
16. Vacanti CJ, Van Houten RJ, Hill RC. A statistical analysis of the relationship of physical status to postoperative mortality in 63,388 cases. Anesth Analg 1970;49:564–566.
17. Menke H, Klein A, John KD, et al. Predictive value of ASA classification for the assessment of perioperative risk. Int Surg 1993;78:266–270.
18. Owens WD, Dykes MHM, Gilbert JP, et al. Development of two indices of postoperative morbidity. Surgery 1975;77: 586–592.
19. Wolters U, Wolf T, Stutzer H, et al. ASA classification and perioperative variables as predictors of postoperative outcome. Br J Anaesth 1996;77(2):217–222.
20. Klotz HP, Candinas D, Platz A, et al. Preoperative risk assessment in elective general surgery. Br J Surg 1996;83:1788–1791.
21. Mullen JL, Gertner MH, Buzby GP, et al. Implications of malnutrition in the surgical patient. Arch Surg 1979;114: 121–125.

22. Knaus WA, Zimmerman JE, Wagner DP, Draper EA, Lawrence DE. APACHE-acute physiology and chronic health evaluation: a physiologically based classification system. Crit Care Med 1981;9:591–597.

23. Knaus WA, Draper EA, Wagner DP, et al. APACHE II: a severity of disease classification system. Crit Care Med 1985;13: 818–829.

24. Goffi L, Saba V, Ghiselli R, et al. Preoperative APACHE II and ASA scores in patients having major general surgical operations: prognostic value and potential clinical applications. Eur J Surg 1999;165:730–735.

25. Koperna T, Semmler D, Marian F. Risk stratification in emergency surgical patients: is the APACHE II score a reliable marker of physiological impairment? Arch Surg 2001;136(1): 55–59.

26. Knaus WA, Wagner DP, Draper EA, et al. The APACHE III prognostic system. Risk prediction of hospital mortality for critically ill hospitalized adults. Chest 1991;100:1619–1636.

27. Le Gall JR, Loirat P, Alperovitch A, et al. A simplified acute physiology score for ICU patients. Crit Care Med 1984;12: 975–977.

28. Copeland GP, Jones D, Walters M. POSSUM: a scoring system for surgical audit. Br J Surg 1991;78:355–360.

29. Senagore AJ, Delaney CP, Duepree HJ, et al. An evaluation of POSSUM and p-POSSUM scoring systems in assessing outcomes with laparoscopic colectomy. Br J Surg 2003;90: 1280–1284.

30. Jones DR, Copeland GP, de Cossart L. Comparison of POSSUM with APACHE II for prediction of outcome from a surgical high-dependency unit. Br J Surg 1992;79:1293–1296.

31. Prytherch DR, Whiteley MS, Higgins B, Weaver PC, Prout WG, Powell SJ. POSSUM and Portsmouth POSSUM for predicting mortality. Physiological and Operative Severity Score for the enUmeration of Mortality and morbidity. Br J Surg 1998;85(9):1217–1220.

32. Wijesinghe LD, Mahmood T, Scott DJ, et al. Comparison of POSSUM and the Portsmouth predictor equation for predicting death following vascular surgery. Br J Surg 1998;85(2): 209–212.

33. Kuhan G, Abidia AF, Wijesinghe LD, et al. POSSUM and P-POSSUM overpredict mortality for carotid endarterectomy. Eur J Vasc Endovasc Surg 2002;23(3):209–211.

34. Midwinter MJ, Tytherleigh M, Ashley S. Estimation of mortality and morbidity risk in vascular surgery using POSSUM and the Portsmouth predictor equation. Br J Surg 1999;86(4): 471–474.

35. Tekkis PP, Kocher HM, Bentley AJ, et al. Operative mortality rates among surgeons: comparison of POSSUM and p-POSSUM scoring systems in gastrointestinal surgery. Dis Colon Rectum 2000;43(11):1528–1532; discussion 1532–1534.

36. Senagore AJ, Delaney CP, Duepree HJ, Brady K, Fazio VW. An evaluation of POSSUM and p-POSSUM scoring systems in assessing outcomes with laparoscopic colectomy. Br J Surg 2003;90:1280–1284.

37. Arvidsson S, Ouchterlony J, Nilsson S, et al. The Gothenburg study of perioperative risk. I. Preoperative findings, postoperative complications. Acta Anaesthesiol Scand 1994;38(7):679–690.

38. Cullen DJ, Civetta JM, Briggs BA, et al. Therapeutic intervention scoring system: a method for quantitative comparison of patient care. Crit Care Med 1974;2(2):57–60.

39. Keene AR, Cullen DJ. Therapeutic Intervention Scoring System: update 1983. Crit Care Med 1983;11(1):1–3.

40. Lemeshow S, Teres D, Pastides H, et al. A method for predicting survival and mortality of ICU patients using objectively derived weights. Crit Care Med 1985;13:519–525.

41. Matsusue S, Kashihara S, Koizumi S. Prediction of mortality from septic shock in gastrointestinal surgery by probit analysis. Jpn J Surg 1988;18(1):18–22.

42. Charlson ME, Pompei P, Ales KL, et al. A new method of classifying prognostic comorbidity in longitudinal studies: development and validation. J Chronic Dis 1987;40(5):373–383.

43. Champion HR, Sacco WJ, Carnazzo AJ, et al. Trauma score. Crit Care Med 1981;9(9):672–676.

44. Haga Y, Ikei S, Wada Y, et al. Estimation of Physiologic Ability and Surgical Stress (E-PASS) as a new prediction scoring system for postoperative morbidity and mortality following GI surgery. Surg Today 1999;29:219–225.

45. Haga Y, Wada Y, Takeuchi H, et al. Estimation of physiologic ability and surgical stress (E-PASS) for a surgical audit in elective digestive surgery. Surgery 2004;135:586–594.

46. Agarwal N, Leighton L, Mandile MA, et al. Outcomes of surgery for colorectal cancer in patients age 80 years and older. Am J Gastroenterol 1990;85:1096–1101.

47. Ondrula DP, Nelson RL, Prasad ML, et al. Multifactorial index of preoperative risk factors in colon resections. Dis Colon Rectum 1992;35:117–122.

48. Sagar PM, Hartley MN, Mancey-Jones B, et al. Comparative audit of colorectal resection with the POSSUM scoring system. Br J Surg 1994;81:1492–1494.

49. Sagar PM, Hartley MN, MacFie J, et al. Comparison of individual surgeon's performance. Risk-adjusted analysis with POSSUM scoring system. Dis Colon Rectum 1996;39:654–658.

50. Parker BM, Tetzlaff JE, Litaker DL, Maurer WG. Redefining the preoperative evaluation process and the role of the anesthesiologist. J Clin Anesth 2000;12:350–356.

51. Arvidsson S. Preparation of adult patients for anaesthesia and surgery. Acta Anaesthesiol Scand 1996;40:962–970.

52. Badner NH, Craen RA, Paul TL, Doyle JA. Anaesthesia preadmission assessment: a new approach through use of a screening questionnaire. Can J Anaesth 1998;45:87–92.

53. Mukherjee D, Eagle KA. Perioperative cardiac assessment for noncardiac surgery: eight steps to the best possible outcome. Circulation 2003;107:2771–2774.

54. King MS. Preoperative evaluation. Am Fam Physician 2000;62(2):387–396.

55. Mancuso CA. Impact of new guidelines on physicians' ordering of preoperative tests. J Gen Intern Med 1999;14(3):166–172.

56. Greer AE, Irwin MG. Implementation and evaluation of guidelines for preoperative testing in a tertiary hospital. Anaesth Intensive Care 2000;30:326–330.

57. Ricciardi G, Angelillo IF, Del Prete U, et al. Routine preoperative investigation. Results of a multicenter survey in Italy. Collaborator Group. Int J Technol Assess Health Care 1998; 14:526–534.

58. McKee RF, Scott EM. The value of routine preoperative investigations. Ann R Coll Surg 1987;69:160–162.

59. Muskett AD, McGreevy JM. Rational preoperative evaluation. Postgrad Med J 1986;62:925–928.

60. Pedersen T, Eliasen K, Henriksen E. A prospective study of mortality associated with anesthesia and surgery: risk indicators

of mortality in hospital. Acta Anaesthesiol Scand 1990;34(3): 176–182.

61. Roizen M. Preoperative evaluation. Can J Anaesth 1989;36: S13–19.

62. Macario A, Roizen MF, Thisted RA, Kim S, Orkin FK, Phelps C. Reassessment of preoperative laboratory testing has changed the test-ordering patterns of physicians. Surg Gynecol Obstet 1992;175:539–547.

63. Jakobsson A. Routine preoperative electrocardiograms. Lancet 1984;1:972.

64. Mantha S, Roizen MF, Barnard J, Thisted RA, Ellis JE, Foss J. Relative effectiveness of four preoperative tests for predicting adverse cardiac outcomes after vascular surgery: a meta-analysis. Anesth Analg 1994;79(3):422–433.

65. Eagle KA, Berger PB, Calkins H, et al. ACC/AHA guideline update for perioperative cardiovascular evaluation of noncardiac surgery—executive summary: a report of the ACC/AHA task force on practice guidelines (Committee to Update the 1996 Guidelines on Perioperative Cardiovascular Evaluation for Noncardiac Surgery). J Am Coll Cardiol 2002;39:542.

66. The Standards Task Force of the American Society of Colorectal Surgery. Practice parameters for the prevention of venous thromboembolism. Dis Colon Rectum 2000;43: 1037–1047.

67. Wille-Jorgensen P, Rasmussen MS, Andersen BR, Borly L. Heparin and mechanical methods for thromboprophylaxis in colorectal surgery. Cochrane Database Syst Rev 2003;(4): CD001217.

68. Brecher ME, Goodnough LT. The rise and fall of preoperative autologous blood donation. Transfusion 2001;41:1459–1462.

69. Waters JH, Lee SJ, Klein E, et al. Preoperative autologous donation versus cell salvage in the avoidance of allogeneic transfusion in patients undergoing radical retropubic prostatectomy. Anesth Analg 2004;98:537–542.

70. Charpak Y, Blery C, Chastang C, et al. Prospective assessment of a protocol for selective ordering of preoperative chest x-rays. Can J Anaesth 1988;35:259–264.

71. Archer C, Levy AR, McGregor M. Value of routine preoperative chest x-rays: a meta-analysis. Can J Anaesth 1993;40: 1022–1027.

72. Evans BA, Wijdicks EF. High-grade carotid stenosis detected before general surgery: is endarterectomy indicated? Neurology 2001;57:1328–1330.

73. American Diabetes Association. Clinical Practice Recommendations 1998. Screening for type 2 diabetes (position statement). Diabetes Care 1998;21(suppl 1):S20–22.

74. Campos AC, Meguid MM. A critical appraisal of the usefulness of perioperative nutritional support. Am J Clin Nutr 1992;55:117–130.

75. Solla JA, Rothenberger DA. Preoperative bowel preparation. A survey of colon and rectal surgeons. Dis Colon Rectum 1990;33:154–159.

76. Rosenberg IL, Graham NG, Dedombal FT, et al. Preparation of the intestine in patients undergoing major large bowel surgery, mainly for neoplasms of the colon and rectum. Br J Surg 1971;58:266–269.

77. Crapp AR, Tillotson P, Powis SJA, et al. Preparation of the bowel by whole-gut irrigation. Lancet 1975;ii:1239–1240.

78. Davis GR, Santa Ana CA, Morawski SG, et al. Development of a lavage solution associated with minimum water and electrolyte absorption or secretion. Gastroenterology 1980; 78:991–995.

79. Vanner SJ, MacDonald PH, Paterson WG, et al. A randomized prospective trial comparing oral sodium phosphate with standard polyethylene glycol-based lavage solution (golytely) in the preparation of patients for colonoscopy. Am J Gastroenterol 1990;85:422–427.

80. Oliveira L, Wexner SD, Daniel N, et al. Mechanical bowel preparation for elective colorectal surgery. A prospective randomized surgeon-blinded trial comparing sodium phosphate and polyethylene glycol-based oral lavage solutions. Dis Colon Rectum 1997;40:585–591.

81. Lee E, Roberts PL, Taranto R, et al. Inpatient vs. outpatient bowel preparation for elective colorectal surgery. Dis Colon Rectum 1996;39:369–373.

82. Aronchick CA, Lipshutz WH, Wright SH, et al. A novel tableted purgative for colonoscopic preparation: efficacy and safety comparisons with Colyte and Fleet Phosphosoda. Gastrointest Endosc 2000;52(3):346–352.

83. Kastenberg D, Chasen R, Choudhary C, et al. Efficacy and safety of sodium phosphate tablets compared with PEG solution in colon cleansing: two identically designed, randomized, controlled, parallel group, multicenter. Gastrointest Endosc 2001; 54(6):705–713.

84. Vukasin P, Weston L, Beart RW. Oral fleet phosphosoda laxative induced hyperphosphatemia and hypocalcemic tetany in an adult: report of a case. Dis Colon Rectum 1997;40:497–499.

85. Duthie GS, Foster ME, Price-Thomas JM, Leaper DJ. Bowel preparation or not for elective colorectal surgery. J R Coll Surg Edinb 1990;35:169–171.

86. van Geldere D, Fa-Si-Oen P, Noach LA, et al. Complications after colorectal surgery without mechanical bowel preparation. J Am Coll Surg 2002;194:40–47.

87. Demetriades D, Murray JA, Chan L, et al. Penetrating colon injuries requiring resection: diversion or primary anastomosis? An AAST prospective multicenter study. J Trauma 2001;50: 765–775.

88. Brownson P, Jenkins SA, Nott D, et al. Mechanical bowel preparation before colorectal surgery: results of a prospective randomized trial. Br J Surg 1992;79:461–462.

89. Burke P, Mealy K, Gillen P, et al. Requirement for bowel preparation in colorectal surgery. Br J Surg 1994;81:907–910.

90. Santos JC, Batista J, Sirimarco MT, et al. Prospective randomized trial of mechanical bowel preparation in patients undergoing elective colorectal surgery. Br J Surg 1994;81:1673–1676.

91. Miettinen R, Laitinen ST, Makela JT, Paakkonen ME. Bowel preparation with oral polyethylene glycol electrolyte solution vs. no preparation in elective open colorectal surgery: prospective randomized study. Dis Colon Rectum 2000;43:669–677.

92. Zmora O, Mahajna A, Bar-Zakai B, et al. Colon and rectal surgery without mechanical bowel preparation: a randomized, prospective trial. Ann Surg 2003;237:363–367.

93. Guenga KF, Matos D, Castro AA, Atallah AN, Wille-Jorgensen P. Mechanical bowel preparation for elective colorectal surgery. Cochrane Database Syst Rev 2003;2:CD001544.

94. Slim K, Vicaut E, Panis Y, et al. Meta-analysis of randomized clinical trials of colorectal surgery with or without mechanical bowel preparation. Br J Surg 2004;91:1125–1130.

95. Bartlett JG, Condon RE, Gorbach SL, et al. VA Cooperative Study on Bowel Preparation for Elective Colorectal

Operations: impact of oral antibiotic regimen on colonic flora, wound irrigation cultures and bacteriology of septic complications. Ann Surg 1978;188:249–254.

96. Song F, Glenny AM. Antibiotic prophylaxis in colorectal surgery: a systematic review of randomized controlled trials. Br J Surg 1998;85:1232–1241.

97. Schoetz DJ, Roberts PL, Murray JJ, Collier JA, Veidenheimer MC. Addition of parenteral cefoxitin to regimen of oral antibiotics for elective colorectal operations. A randomized prospective study. Ann Surg 1990;212:209–212.

98. Danielsen S, Midtvedt T, Giercksky KE. Preventive antibiotics in elective colorectal surgery. Nord Med 1989;104:247–249.

99. Lewis RT. Oral vs systemic antibiotic prophylaxis in elective colon surgery: a randomized study and meta-analysis send a message from the 1990s. Can J Surg 2002;45:173–180.

100. Delaney CP, Zutshi M, Senagore AJ, et al. Prospective randomized controlled trial between a pathway of Controlled Rehabilitation with Early Ambulation and Diet (CREAD) and traditional postoperative care after laparotomy and intestinal resection. Dis Colon Rectum 2003;46:851–859.

101. Delaney CP, Fazio VW, Senagore AJ, Robinson B, Halverson A, Remzi FH. "Fast track" post-operative management protocol for patients with high comorbidity undergoing complex abdominal and pelvic colorectal surgery. Br J Surg 2001;88:1533–1538.

102. Basse L, Jakobsen DH, Billesbolle P, Werner M, Kehlet H. A clinical pathway to accelerate recovery after colonic resection. Ann Surg 2000;232:51–57.

103. Kiran RP, Delaney CP, Senagore AJ, et al. Prediction and outcome of readmission after intestinal resection. J. Am Coll Surg 2004;198:877–883.

9
Postoperative Management: Pain and Anesthetic, Fluids and Diet

Tracey D. Arnell and Robert W. Beart, Jr.

Many of the major advancements and changes in the care and survival of the surgical patient have occurred in the postoperative period. This is frequently recognized in regard to critical care, but has been just as remarkable in the non–intensive care unit patient. Significant changes in reimbursement and patient population patterns have either driven, or allowed for, better survival, less morbidity, earlier discharge, and more ambulatory procedures. The major changes have been in the areas of postoperative feeding, activity, pain control, and ulcer and deep venous thrombosis (DVT) prophylaxis. In an attempt to incorporate this knowledge and in conjunction with physician extenders such as nurse practitioners and physician assistants, patient care pathways are being increasingly instituted and validated. The focus of this chapter will be on the non–intensive care unit inpatient.

Pain Control

The trends toward decreased length of hospital stay and more ambulatory procedures necessitate a good understanding of the mechanisms of pain and its relief. It has been clearly demonstrated that adequate pain control is necessary to maximize cardiac and respiratory function and decrease the risk of complications.[1–3] On a more practical note, the Joint Commission on Accreditation of Healthcare Organizations (JCAHO) now requires specific assessment and documentation of treatment of pain. Despite this, the management of acute pain is still less than ideal. In a survey of 250 patients who had undergone surgery (38% outpatient), 82% of respondents reported experiencing pain. Of these, 39% described severe to extreme pain and 47% moderate pain. One might think this is a result of the trend toward ambulatory procedures, but it was more common in the inpatient setting.[4] Although of course not all inclusive, what follows is a review of the components of pain and options for treatment.

Physiology

The subjective sensation of pain is made up of many components, both physical and psychological. One definition is that acute pain is "the initiation phase of an extensive, persistent nociceptive and behavioral cascade triggered by tissue injury." The cascade begins with tissue injury that causes nociceptive neurons to begin firing and the local release of inflammatory mediators in the periphery. Once nociceptors become sensitized, the threshold necessary for further activation is lowered and their discharge rate increases. Put simply, less painful stimuli ultimately result in more pain perception. This effect is amplified by the environment of inflammation and its mediators. The nociceptive signals are carried by A delta and C fibers to the spinal cord dorsal horn and the ascending pathways to the central nervous system. Integration of signals occurs at all levels in this pathway. Different analgesic choices will target different parts of this cascade. As a result, analgesic types can be combined to more effectively manage multiple components of pain.[5]

Techniques

In the inpatient setting of abdominopelvic surgery, the major modalities of postoperative pain control are patient-controlled anesthesia (PCA), opioids, nonsteroidal antiinflammatory drugs (NSAIDs), and epidural anesthesia. Preemptive analgesia is another tactic and includes preincisional infiltration of local anesthetics and administration of NSAIDs and intraoperative epidural anesthesia. Along less traditional lines, massage, acupuncture, and biofeedback therapy are being used in some institutions.

Opioids

Opioids are the most frequently used medication in perioperative pain management. Their mechanism is via specific opioid receptors as well as nonspecific antiinflammatory actions. They block transmission of nociceptive afferent signals in the spinal dorsal horn and involve efferent messaging by activating inhibitory pathways supraspinally. Additionally, they act locally in the areas of tissue injury to inhibit inflammation.[5]

Opioid side effects include respiratory depression, pruritus, nausea, vomiting, and constipation. Titration of morphine to pain is extremely important in avoiding respiratory depression because the respiratory center receives nociceptive input that counterbalances the depression. When pain is reduced by other means such as adjunct medications and nerve blocks, the amount of morphine must be reduced. Partial agonists have been developed (buprenorphine, tramadol) that may reduce these complications, but presently they are infrequently used and clinical experience is lacking.[6,7]

The most frequently used opioid is morphine, and it is against which all other choices are compared. The second most frequently used opioid is meperidine and it will be discussed specifically. Initially, it was developed as an anticholinergic agent but was found to have analgesic effects. The anticholinergic effect and the potential for less smooth muscle spasm in areas such as the colon, biliary tract, and renal system is one reason it continues to be used in acute pain management. In fact, when used in equianalgesic doses with morphine, meperidine has the same spasmodic effect on smooth muscle.[8] The analgesic effects of meperidine are inferior to those of morphine, and its duration of effectiveness is significantly less than 4 hours. Compounding this ineffectiveness is the use of the intramuscular (IM) route. The absorption is highly variable with variable blood levels resulting in poor pain control. In one series, only 30% of postoperative patients achieved 50% pain relief after injection of 100 mg of meperidine.[9,10] Meperidine causes central nervous system excitation, seizures, increased respiratory depression, has a propensity for addiction, and produces metabolites with little analgesic but significant neurotoxic potential.[8] All of these factors have led the JCAHO to discourage the use of meperidine in its pain guidelines. At best, meperidine, given its short duration of action and significant risk of serious side effects with repeated use, should have an extremely limited role in pain management of postoperative patients.

The route of administration of opioids is more important than the specific opioid used in terms of onset of action. For the intravenous (IV) route and the oral route, there is little difference among various opioids. The IV route is effective within minutes, whereas the oral route varies between 1 hour for standard release and 2–4 hours for sustained relief. The greatest variability occurs with IM administration based on the lipophilic nature of the drug. The more lipophilic, the quicker the onset of pain relief.[11]

For IV delivery, PCA has been used successfully for more than 30 years and is one of the recommended modes of pain control by the American Society of Anesthesiologists in their practice guidelines. Improved pain control, patients' satisfaction, and decreased pulmonary complications have been found in two large reviews comparing PCA with conventional opioid analgesia in postoperative patients.[12,13] Although more expensive, PCA opioid use is a safe and effective mode of delivery. Making the transition from IV pain control to oral pain control should be made with knowledge of the pain requirements based on the most current IV dosages. Table 9-1 lists equianalgesic doses of the IV and oral forms of several frequently used medications.

Nonopioid

Nonsteroidal Antiinflammatory Drugs

As previously described, the mechanism of pain production and perception is altered by the inflammatory cascade. By decreasing the production of mediators such as prostanoids, the perception of painful stimuli may also decrease. Nonsteroidal medications inhibit cyclooxygenase (COX) in the periphery and spinal cord and this may be the mechanism by which they are effective in diminishing hyperalgesia.[14] Their action is mediated by their effect on COX-2 receptors and result in analgesic and antiinflammatory effects. The side effects are largely a result of inhibition of COX-1 receptors which occur most frequently in the gastrointestinal (GI) tract, renal tissue, and platelets. The effectiveness of NSAIDs in the management of acute pain has been demonstrated in multiple disciplines of surgery including but not limited to orthopedic, oral, abdominal, and spinal surgery. There remain concerns regarding their safety in the surgical patient because of the risk of GI bleeding and, especially, surgical site bleeding. Overall, the use of these agents in postoperative surgical patients has been found to be safe, but there are risks of GI bleeding, renal injury, and surgical bleeding. In the largest review of the use of ketorolac in 1996, 10,272 patients receiving ketorolac were compared with 10,247 receiving opiates. The rate of complications for ketorolac compared with opiates was GI bleeding 2.1% versus 1.9%, serious operative site bleeding 1.5% versus 1.8%. In subanalysis, it was found that the major risk factors that significantly increased these

TABLE 9-1. Equianalgesic dosages of frequently prescribed IV and oral medications

| | Approximate equianalgesic | | Starting dosage, adults >50 kg | |
	IV/SC/IM	PO	IV/SC/IM	PO
Morphine	10 mg q 3–4 h	30 mg q 3–4 h	10 mg q 3–4 h	30 mg q 3–4 h
Codeine	75 mg q 3–4 h	130 mg q 3–4 h	60 mg q 2 h	60 mg q 3–4 h
Hydromorphone	1.5 mg q 3–4 h	7.5 mg q 3-4 h	1.5 mg q 3–4 h	6 mg q 3–4 h
Hydrocodone		30 mg q 3–4 h		10 mg q 3–4 h
Meperidine	100 mg q 3 h	300 mg q 2–3 h	100 mg q 3–4 h	
Oxycodone		30 mg q 3–4 h		10 mg q 3–4 h

Source: Tarascon Pocket Pharmacopeia, 2002 classic shirt pocket edition. Loma Linda, CA: Tarascon Publishing. PO, per os.

risks were patient age greater than 75, daily dosage exceeding 105 mg/day, and courses longer than 5 days.[15] Used within these parameters, NSAIDs are safe and effective as an adjunct or by themselves for the postoperative patient.

Antihistamines

Histamine is known to activate nociceptive fibers and may participate in mediating pain. For this reason, antihistamines have been proposed as adjuncts to pain management. The mechanism of antihistamines in analgesia is unclear but may involve opioid receptors or presynaptic inhibition of histamine receptors. Despite positive findings in animal models, clinical studies have been conflicting. The confounding factors of sedation and poor methodology do not allow for recommendations for their use as single agents. As adjuncts, they may have benefit although the same confounding factors exist in these data. As more selective antihistamines with less sedation become available, these questions may be answered.[16]

Epidural Anesthesia

Epidural anesthesia functions at the dorsal horn preventing afferent conduction of nociceptive stimuli. For patients undergoing laparotomy and lower abdominal and pelvic surgery, epidural anesthesia may have better pain control, patient satisfaction, and potentially return of bowel function with fewer side effects.[17,18] In a randomized study of colorectal patients undergoing thoracic epidural placement for colorectal resections, resolution of ileus and control of postoperative pain was significantly improved compared with those receiving a PCA.[19] These findings were supported in a series of patients undergoing proctocolectomy.[20] In a series of patients undergoing laparoscopic colon resection randomized to epidural versus PCA, the differences were not significant. The type of medication infused may also have a significant influence on the outcomes postoperatively as discussed in a Cochrane review in which those patients receiving local epidural anesthetics had reduced GI paralysis with comparable pain control.[21] The additional time and cost involved with an epidural has been the primary reason it has not been adopted in a more widespread manner.

Preemptive Analgesia

The debate over the effectiveness of preemptive analgesia continues. Initial animal studies demonstrated that the doses of analgesia necessary to prevent central hyperexcitability in rats was significantly less than that necessary to reverse it.[22] The concept is that by preventing the initial stimulation of central pain pathways, there will be decreased sensitization to noxious stimuli. When increased sensitization occurs, it is referred to as hyperalgesia and suggests that the same stimuli will produce different degrees of effects based on the state of the target. Hyperalgesia may result from upregulation of afferent pathways and the inflammatory mediators involved in the perception of pain.[23] This led to the evaluation of preemptive analgesia in human studies.

A review of the 80 randomized controlled trials regarding the comparison of preemptive and postoperative pain relief attempted to reach a consensus regarding preemptive analgesia trials in humans. The only end point examined was level of pain. The trials were divided into NSAIDs, IV opioids, epidural analgesia, caudal analgesia, and peripheral local anesthetics. Although there were a few studies that demonstrated improved pain control at various time points postoperatively, this was not consistent and not overall. The findings were that "timing of analgesia did not influence the quality of postoperative pain control, whatever the type of preemptive analgesia."[24] A comparison of preincisional versus postincisional epidural anesthesia with a combination of lidocaine and fentanyl including a control with a sham epidural showed very minimal difference between the former two groups in terms of postoperative morphine consumption. There was a 20% decrease in morphine use compared with the sham epidural as might be expected.[25] It has been suggested that the focus should shift from comparing preoperative and postoperative analgesia, to developing more comprehensive, multimodality paradigms of surgical pain control.

"Nontraditional" Adjuncts

Acupuncture and acupressure have been used for thousands of years and are now being increasingly used in Western medicine. There are many reports of their use in control of surgical pain, but few of these are randomized. The studies that have been randomized have been mixed in their findings as well as the type of acupuncture or acupressure. The methods include needles, pressure, and electrical stimulation and the number and location of sites is variable. The purported benefits are decreased need for opioids, decreased nausea, and lower plasma cortisol and epinephrine release.[26,27]

Modalities that address the psychological perception of pain, rather than only the physiologic, are being examined. It has been suggested that techniques such as massage may better address the psychological aspect. In the one randomized study of this in patients with acute surgical pain, there was no difference in the consumption of opioids in 202 patients.[28] For similar reasons, relaxation techniques and the use of music have been suggested.

Overall, the data are very limited for these therapies. Most have few risks associated with them (acupressure, psychological methods) and are becoming available in some hospitals. Their role in the management of acute postoperative pain remains to be seen in larger, randomized trials.

Perioperative Fluid Management

Basic fluid requirements under normal circumstances are approximately 2500 cc/day in a 70-kg adult. This allows for the 1500 cc of urine necessary to excrete waste products including urea, potassium, and sodium. A very simple formula for calculating basic fluid needs is 1500 cc for the first 20 kg with 20 cc/kg for the remaining weight. As a result of surgical stress, there is an increase in renin, aldosterone, and antidiuretic hormone release and activation of the sympathetic system resulting in sequestration of fluid (third spacing) and increased volume requirements. Additional losses may occur from blood loss, diarrhea, nasogastric tubes, and abdominal drains and these should be accounted for. Assuming a return to homeostasis, this fluid retention begins to resolve with a return to normal of the hormones and sympathetic nervous system. Table 9-2 lists the composition of the frequently administered colloids and should serve as a guide for replacement based on calculated fluid losses.

The management of perioperative fluid has not received much attention in terms of postoperative recovery and complications until recently. It may be that the routine administration of maintenance IV fluids is deleterious. In two randomized controlled trials of colorectal patients, a relatively restricted perioperative fluid administration schedule was used. The groups randomized to the restricted fluid had fewer complications in terms of cardiopulmonary events and tissue healing complications as well as quicker resolution of intestinal ileus.[29,30] The difference in cardiopulmonary complications was also found in a Cochrane review of patients undergoing orthopedic surgery.[31] There is still little information about perioperative fluid management of patients, but changes in standard regimens may be on the horizon.

Ulcer Prophylaxis

In many institutions, ulcer prophylaxis is a routine part of the postoperative orders. In patients without risk factors, or personal history, this is unnecessary. The incidence of clinically significant GI bleeding in hospitalized patients in this age of ulcer prophylaxis has been well characterized for the critically ill and is less than 0.2%.[32] In this population, mechanical ventilation, coagulopathy, prolonged hypotension, and organ failure have been the most consistently identified risk factors for the development of stress ulcer bleeding.[33,34] Despite this information, inappropriate use of these agents continues as demonstrated in a review of 226 patients admitted to the medical unit. In this population, prescribed ulcer prophylaxis was not indicated in 65% of patients yet a significant number of these patients were discharged on these medications.[35]

The choice of agents for prophylaxis has greatly increased. Table 9-3 lists the most common agents, mechanisms, and

TABLE 9-3. Mechanism of frequently used ulcer prophylaxis medications

	Mechanism
Antacids	• Neutralizes acid
Sucralfate	• Mucosal production
	• Stimulates mucous, HCO3, prostaglandin secretion (inhibits acid secretion)
	• Coat ulcer base
H2 Antagonists	• Blocks stimulation of histamine receptor and production of H+
Proton pump inhibitors	• Blocks H+/K+ ATPase pump (final step of acid production)

effectiveness. In a review of the studies comparing therapies for stress ulcer prophylaxis, Hiramoto et al.[36] concluded that H2 antagonists, sucralfate, and proton pump inhibitors are effective in decreasing the risk of clinically significant bleeding. Proton pump inhibitors, however, are the most potent gastric acid suppressant and, theoretically, may be more effective.

DVT Prophylaxis

Although the occurrence of a fatal pulmonary embolism (PE) is rare, venous thromboembolism (VTE), both symptomatic and asymptomatic, is relatively common in the surgical patient. In one study, 0.8% of patients admitted after surgical procedures developed symptomatic VTE. Of note, 66% of these occurred in the 3 months after discharge.[37] PE is the most preventable cause of death in hospitalized patients in the United States and was listed as the cause of death in 0.45% of deaths.[38] In light of the many available, low-risk forms of prophylaxis, this should be a part of the care of the postoperative patient.

Of the different therapies available, the costs and potential risks are variable. The potential risk factors are many, and are listed in Table 9-4.[39] Stratification of patients based on their risk for occurrence of VTE/PE should guide the choice of prophylaxis (Table 9-5). Each of the proposed therapies will be discussed in regard to institution, dosage, and effects.

Elastic Stockings

The literature available on the use of elastic stockings is based on the use of graduated compression stockings. They function by compressing the lower extremity in a gradual manner, with the greatest pressure at the ankle, encouraging venous return. If not fitted properly, they may actually be constrictive and increase the venous pressure below the knees, decreasing

TABLE 9-2. Composition of extracellular fluid and common crystalloid solutions

Type	Na+	Cl−	K+	Ca++	Mg++	HCO3−	Lactate
Extracellular fluid	142	103	4	5	3	27	
NaCl 0.9% (normal saline)	154	154					
Lactated Ringers	131	111	5	2			29
D5/0.45% saline	77	77					
Plasmalyte 148 + glucose (plasmalyte)	148	97	5		1	40	
Sodium bicarbonate 8.4%	1000					1000	

TABLE 9-4. Common causes of hypercoagulability

Risk factor
Age
Type of Surgery
  Orthopedic lower extremity
  Major surgery
Previous VTE
Malignancy
Pregnancy
Estrogen use
Obesity
Heart failure
Thrombophilic disorders
  Factor V Leiden
  Essential thrombocytosis
  Prothrombin G 20210 A mutation
Immobilization
Hospitalization

venous return.[40] In a Cochrane review, they did reduce the risk of VTE in moderate-risk patients.[41] As a solo prophylaxis, they should be reserved for the low-risk patient. Otherwise, they should be used in conjunction with other measures.

Sequential Compression Devices

These devices offer a very effective, low-risk prophylaxis for DVT. The mechanism is both direct and systemic. Locally, they compress the deep venous system decreasing stasis and encouraging venous return. On a systemic level, they increase the fibrinolytic activity by reducing plasminogen activator.[42] There are several types available including a foot pump, calf- and thigh-high devices. There are experimental and clinical data that suggest the devices may be equivalent, although the original studies were based on the thigh-high devices. Killewich et al.[43] studied the hemodynamics of the foot pump system and their conclusions were that there are measurable increases in the venous outflow with these devices. In patients undergoing hip replacement, the foot pump was equally effective as compared with low-molecular-weight heparin (LMWH).[44] No direct comparisons of the different devices are available.

An additional consideration is compliance. For maximal benefit in patients undergoing surgery, they should be placed before the induction of anesthesia and functioning throughout an operation. Postoperatively, their effectiveness can be compromised because of patient, physician, and nursing compliance. Cornwell et al.[45] observed the compliance of trauma patients with the use of sequential compression devices (SCDs). They defined full compliance as the SCDs being on the patient and functioning upon six observations. Based on this, 19% of patients were fully compliant and SCDs were on in 53% of observations.[45] When used properly, SCDs are a safe and effective prophylactic measure in the low- and moderate-risk patient.

Low-dose Unfractionated Heparin

Unfractionated heparin has been evaluated since the 1970s as a form of prophylaxis and has been shown to be safe in the majority of surgical patients. It consists of molecules that range in size from 3000 to 33,000 Da and binds to antithrombin (ATIII) and accelerates the inhibition of thrombin and other coagulation factors, particularly factor X. In a large randomized trial from 1970, low-dose unfractionated heparin (LDUH) decreased the risk of fatal PEs in the postoperative population from 0.7% to 0.1% in 4000 patients.[46] This was supported in a large metaanalysis of 70 randomized trials. The risk of DVT, PE, and fatal PE was decreased by more than 50%.[47] Although effective, one concern has been the risk of bleeding in the postoperative patient. There has been a small increase in postoperative bleeding in most studies, but the majority of these events are wound hematomas.

A more frequent side effect of heparin is heparin-induced thrombocytopenia (HIT). It is less common with prophylactic than therapeutic heparin, but may occur in 5%–15% of patients. HIT may cause a paradoxical hypercoagulable state with arterial and venous thrombosis. The platelet count should be followed in patients receiving routine heparin and discontinued immediately if diminishing.

It is recommended that subcutaneous (SC) heparin be started within 2 hours of an operation and continued until the patient is fully ambulatory. The dosage is generally 5000 U every (q) 12 hours. This may be increased in those patients in the high-risk category to 7500 U q 12 hours or 5000 U q 8 hours.

Low-Molecular-Weight Heparin

LMWH consists of heparin molecules in a smaller range and size than LDUH (3500–6000 Da). The mechanism is the same

TABLE 9-5. DVT prophylaxis guidelines

	Age (y)	Surgery	Risk factors	DVT	PE	Recommendation
Low	<40	Minor	None	0.4%	<0.5%	Early ambulation or Elastic stockings or IPC
Moderate				2%–4%	1%–2%	Early ambulation and Elastic stockings or IPC or LDUH or LMWH
A	Any	Minor	Present	4%		
B	<40	Major	None			
C	40–60	Minor	None			
High				4%–8%	2%–4%	Early ambulation and Elastic stockings and IPC or LDUH or LMWH
	>60	Minor	±Other			
	>40	Major	None			
	<40	Major	Present			

as LDUH regarding the acceleration of ATIII inactivation of Xa, but it does not inactivate thrombin. It also does not bind as strongly to plasma moieties so has greater bioavailability, longer half-life, and more predictable plasma levels. Because of this, partial thromboplastin time does not need to be monitored.[48] The incidence of HIT is also lower than LDUH (2.7% versus 0%).[49]

LMWH is at least as effective as LDUH in preventing DVT in postoperative general surgery and colorectal surgery patients without an increase in bleeding complications. A large European trial randomized 1351 patients undergoing abdominal surgery to LDUH or LMWH. The incidence of thromboembolic complications was equal (4.3% versus 4.7%), but patients in the LMWH group experienced fewer bleeding complications, primarily wound hematomas (8.3% versus 11.8%).[50] A metaanalysis of only prospective randomized trials of 5520 patients, including one trial with 1300 colorectal patients, confirmed these results.[51]

With this type of evidence, the question may be why LMWH is not the standard prophylaxis for surgical patients rather than LDUH. Primarily, it is the issue of cost-effectiveness. Based on their findings in a randomized prospective trial of 936 colorectal surgery patients, the authors of the Canadian Multicentre Colorectal Deep Vein Thrombosis Prophylaxis Trial attempted a cost analysis in both Canadian and US dollars for the use of LDUH and LMWH (enoxaparin). Based on their findings of equal effectiveness and a trend toward more bleeding in the LMWH group, they concluded that LDUH was more cost effective. Even with the assumption of greater effectiveness and equal bleeding, LMWH was twice as expensive as LDUH therapy. Their conclusion was: "Although heparin and enoxaparin are equally effective, low-dose heparin is a more economically attractive choice for thromboembolism prophylaxis after colorectal surgery."[52,53]

Duration

The risk of DVT and PE does not end with the discharge of the patient from the hospital. This is especially true given the decreasing lengths of stay and, therefore, the decreasing time available for prophylaxis while patients are hospitalized. In addition to the previous study cited by White et al. in which 66% of events occurred following discharge. Agnelli et al. found that 40% of DVT/PE events in patients operated on for cancer happened more than 21 days following surgery.[37,59a] It has been postulated that screening patients prior to discharge for DVT using ultrasound or venography and continuing anticoagulation in the population with positive findings would identify a population requiring continued anticoagulation. Pelligrini et al. reported in a prospective series of orthopedic patients that this was not successful in decreasing outpatient events, as 2.2% of patients with negative venograms developed a DVT requiring readmission with three deaths (0.15%).[60a] In a randomized prospective trial of 332 patients deemed high

risk having undergone curative pelvic or abdominal cancer resection, those patients who received 21 additional days of enoxaparin had a 4.8% rate of DVT versus 12.0% in the group receiving only in hospital prophylaxis.[61a] Given these findings, cosideration for extended prophylaxis in patients who are at moderate and high risk for thrombotic events must be given.

The American Society of Colon and Rectal Surgeons Practice Parameters for prevention of venous thromboembolism are presented in Appendix A, Chapter 8.

Anticoagulation

Although there are fairly well-defined recommendations available for the preoperative management of patients on chronic anticoagulation therapy, there is little regarding the postoperative resumption of therapy. The urgency and timing of postoperative anticoagulation can be inferred from the data regarding risk of adverse thromboembolism overall, tempered by an understanding of the risk of bleeding. Clearly, postoperative bleeding risks are influenced by the surgical procedure performed.

Overall, the risk of thrombotic and embolic events may be increased in the surgical patient and those in whom warfarin therapy has been abruptly stopped. In surgical patients not anticoagulated, changes in levels of fibrin D-dimer and other hemostatic markers associated with thrombosis have been found to be increased.[54,55] In those patients taking oral anticoagulation, there is biochemical evidence that there may be a rebound hypercoagulable state after the withdrawal of oral anticoagulation, perhaps increasing the risk even more.[56] Most studies have not borne this out in clinical practice, however.

An estimation of risk will help in guiding the need and timing for beginning anticoagulation postoperatively. A summary of the risk categories based on diagnosis and the general recommendation for anticoagulation is shown in Table 9-6.[57,58]

Diet

The resumption of a diet is critical to the recovery of the patient undergoing intestinal surgery. Before discharge, it is accepted that patients should tolerate oral analgesia, not require IV hydration, and demonstrate return of intestinal tract function. The order in which these occur varies by practitioner, however. The most traditional approach to these patients is postoperative nasogastric tube decompression, followed by advancement of oral intake based on demonstration of GI function by flatus and bowel movements. On the other extreme is the institution of a regular diet immediately after surgery with changes based on the clinical status. Much literature has accumulated in reference to the viability of these approaches.

Since the 1980s, many groups have evaluated the need for nasogastric tube decompression in the elective abdominal surgery patient.[58–61] The trials failed to show a benefit in

TABLE 9-6. Risk factors for adverse events based on diagnosis and anticoagulation recommendations

	Atrial fibrillation	Prosthetic valves	Thromboembolism
Adverse event risk	• 1%–8.5% strokes per year	• 8%/y without anticoagulation • 2%/y with anticoagulation	• 40%/y recurrence <1 mo • 10%–15%/y 1–3 mo • 5%/y >3 mo
Risk			
High	• Event <30 d • Mitral valve disease	• Event <30 d • Mural thrombus • Placement <90 d • Multiple valves • Caged-ball valve • Mitral position • Previous event • Atrial fibrillation • ↓LV function • Pregnancy	• Recent event <30 d
Intermediate	• Previous events • Age >75 y • ↓LV function • Left atrial enlargement • Ischemic disease • Hypertension • Diabetes	• Bi-leaflet or tilting-disc >90 d • Bioprosthetic valves 31–90 d	• Event 1–3 mo • Obesity • Malignancy • Familial prothrombotic state • Preoperative immobility
Low	• All others	• None	• Event >3 mo • No event

reduction of complications including anastomotic, hospital stay, or return to normal GI function. Combined with the patient discomfort and the loss of the lower esophageal sphincter as a protective mechanism, this has prompted most surgeons to abandon their routine use.

The advent of laparoscopic colon resection has facilitated a more aggressive approach to postoperative feeding regimens.[62,63] Several trials demonstrated that the majority of patients tolerated oral intake in the immediate postoperative period, regardless of the presence or absence of traditional markers of return of GI function. This approach has been used in the open colectomy patients as well. In a nonrandomized study of elderly patients (mean age, 77 years) undergoing open colon resection, 90% tolerated early feeding (clear liquids on day 2, regular diet day 3). There were no anastomotic leaks or abscesses in this group.[64] In a recent metaanalysis, 11 studies with 837 patients were identified which compared liberalized diet immediately postoperative to nothing by mouth until evidence of GI function. These included patients undergoing all types of GI surgery, not specifically colon surgery. Overall, there was a reduction in postoperative infections, both directly related to the surgical procedure and other infections such as pneumonia. There were actually fewer anastomotic complications and a shorter length of stay. The only negative finding was a small increase in the number of patients experiencing vomiting. This did not translate to more wound complications.[65]

In addition to having been shown to be safe and well tolerated, there are several theoretical advantages to early feeding. The potential benefits are related to maintenance of intestinal integrity from a biochemical and immunologic perspective. It has been clearly shown that malnutrition in the surgical patient is associated with increased morbidity and mortality.[66–68]

This has increased the interest in achieving adequate postoperative nutrition. In animal models, survival from peritonitis is significantly improved with enteral nutrition, and almost universally fatal with administration of TPN.[69] In one of the largest prospective, randomized clinical trials, Bozzetti et al.[70] randomized 159 malnourished postoperative cancer patients each to enteral versus parenteral nutrition. Seventy-nine of these patients underwent colon surgery, approximately equally divided between the two groups. Overall, there were fewer complications in the enterally fed group (34% versus 49%). Anastomotic leaks and intraabdominal abscesses were not significantly different between the groups. Of note, 21% of enterally fed patients required reduction in caloric intake or switch to parenteral nutrition (8%).[70]

In summation, early feeding after elective abdominal surgery and specifically colon surgery, has been shown to be safe and generally well tolerated. This may improve patients' comfort, and there is a growing body of evidence that early nutrition may improve outcome and reduce complications. These data are most convincing for the malnourished patient, and for the use of enteral nutrition.

Steroids

It is not infrequent that patients undergoing colorectal surgical procedures are taking exogenous steroids. Usually this is in the inflammatory bowel disease population, but there are many other clinical situations that may be encountered. Important considerations include identifying those patients at risk for adrenal insufficiency, equivalent oral and parenteral dosages, the effect of surgical stress on dosage requirements, and the timing of tapering to presurgical dosages or cessation of treatment. A brief review of the physiology of steroid homeostasis will help in understanding the recommendations.

Glucocorticoids are essential for protein, carbohydrate, and fat metabolism. Their overall effect is to increase gluconeogenesis by allowing for the production of amino acids by proteolysis and lipolysis. They also stimulate metabolism by their inotropic effects and enhancement of norepinephrine and epinephrine. Glucocorticoid production in the adrenal cortex is stimulated by the anterior pituitary gland via adrenocorticotropic hormone. The hypothalamus stimulates the pituitary by secreting corticotrophin-releasing hormone. Both of these regulatory hormones are inhibited by the end product cortisol by negative feedback. The usual production of cortisol in an unstressed individual is approximately 20 mg/day. During periods of maximal stress, this production may increase up to 150 mg/day.[71–74] The degree of stress is directly related to the magnitude of the procedure, and the anesthetic, with general anesthesia producing the greatest increases.[75]

It has been clearly demonstrated that adrenal atrophy and suppression occurs with exogenous steroid administration. This is a result of the negative feedback effect on adrenocorticotropic hormone by exogenous cortisol and the lack of stimulation of the adrenal cortex. This can take up to 1 year to recover and patients are frequently asymptomatic during this time if not exposed to stress. During this period, the potential for acute adrenal insufficiency exists.

In actuality, the occurrence of adrenal insufficiency in the surgical population is quite rare. The majority of reports are anecdotal. In fact, in one of the only randomized studies recently, those patients randomized to receiving only their usual daily dosage of steroid perioperatively did not experience symptoms of adrenal insufficiency. The numbers were too small (N = 18, N = 12 in the placebo group) to detect a small difference and the dosages of steroids in most patients were quite low, but this supports the rarity of the occurrence.[76] Salem et al.[77] reviewed the body of evidence regarding the perioperative use of steroid coverage. As they describe, the current usage is based on two anecdotal reports in 1952 which led to recommendations that became the standard of care. From their review, they conclude that the vast majority of patients are over-treated and recommendations should be tailored to identifiable populations at greatest risk. These populations are stratified based on the dosage and duration of treatment an individual patient has received. The risk of suppression can be predicted and this is shown in Table 9-7. As to the question of testing of the adrenal axis, it has not been clearly demonstrated that identified suppression leads to clinical insufficiency.[78,79]

The duration of the taper postoperatively is most impacted by the surgical procedure. For most outpatient procedures, the degree of postoperative stress is considered minor and patients can be returned to their preoperative dose immediately. For major surgery, stress dosages should be continued until signs of surgical stress have resolved. This varies from patient to patient as postoperative ileus, cardiac and pulmonary

TABLE 9-7. Risk of adrenal suppression from exogenous steroids and recommendations for replacement

	Dose	Duration	Recommendation
High risk*	>20 mg/d	>3 wk	• 100 mg at induction • 100 mg q 8 hrs throughout period of "stress"
Intermediate	>5 mg/d <20 mg/d	>3 wk	• Prophylaxis *or* • Testing of the axis
Low	Any dose <5 mg/d	>3 wk Any time	• No prophylaxis

*Patients with Cushing's syndrome are considered high risk regardless of dosage or duration of steroid administration.

complications and infections pose additional stress. For patients with an uncomplicated postoperative course, this generally begins on the third day. Once the taper begins, it can be carried out rapidly over a period of a few days to the preoperative dosage. Table 9-8 shows the equivalent steroid dosages for the parenteral and enteral steroids.[73,77,80]

It is important to recognize the signs of adrenal insufficiency because they may occur both in the immediate postoperative period and beyond in the event of a complication. These include bowel obstruction, anastomotic leak, surgical and nonsurgical infections. Symptoms may include hypoglycemia, cardiovascular collapse, fatigue, abdominal pain, nausea, and vomiting. In the postoperative patient presenting with a change in intestinal function, steroid withdrawal should be considered in the at-risk population. Stelzer et al.[81] reviewed their 60 steroid-dependent patients who underwent pouch surgery and developed signs and symptoms of a bowel obstruction. They found that 43 had no objective signs of mechanical obstruction and promptly resolved their symptoms within 4 hours of steroid administration. At the other extreme of intestinal function, Rai and Hemingway[82] reported on a patient presenting with high ileostomy output which was responsive to steroids.

Clinical Pathways

With an awareness of the benefits of practicing evidence-based medicine, the development of standardized postoperative protocols is a reasonable next step. Potential benefits include decreased length of stay with more efficient utilization of hospital beds and personnel, and potentially fewer mistakes because of standardization of care. Many groups have reported their successful application of such clinical pathways specifically in regard to colorectal surgery. The protocols are variable with respect to pain management and

TABLE 9-8. Equivalent steroid dosages

Glucocorticoid	Equivalent dose (mg)	Half-life (h)
Prednisone	5	18–36
Dexamethasone	0.5	36–54
Hydrocortisone	20	8–12
Methylprednisolone	4	18–36

the use of cathartics, but individually show a reduction in length of stay with acceptable outcomes. The major end points have been length of stay, readmission rate, complication rate, and patient satisfaction.

The trend toward earlier discharge began first with the laparoscopic colon resection patients. In 1995, Bardram et al.[83] prospectively followed eight patients over the age of 70 undergoing laparoscopic-assisted colectomy (extracorporeal anastomosis). The regimen involved thoracic epidural catheters intra- and postoperatively for pain control with the avoidance of opioids. A protein-enriched diet and ambulation were begun immediately according to a predetermined protocol. Patients were discharged after they had a normal bowel movement. Six of eight patients went home on the second day; two patients waited until day 3 because of "social" reasons. There were no readmissions and all patients were satisfied.[83] These results were reproduced in a group of 16 patients with a median age of 71 years undergoing open sigmoid colectomy. The protocol consisted of an epidural catheter during and after surgery for pain control. Immediately after surgery, a regimen of mobilization, cisapride and magnesium, and liberal diet including protein drinks was begun. The median length of stay was 2 days (range, 2–6 days) and readmissions were 3, not related to intestinal complications (headaches, social secondary to blindness) and there were no complications.[84]

Recently, a randomized trial compared patients undergoing open intestinal resection who followed a "fast-track" versus the "traditional" pathway. The traditional patients had a nasogastric tube placed that was removed when the drainage was low, and had sips of liquids until the occurrence of flatus and/or stool. The fast-tract patients began a regular diet if they tolerated liquids the evening of surgery and were encouraged to ambulate. No epidural catheters were used. The length of stay was significantly shorter (5.4 versus 7.1 days) and there was no difference in readmissions, complications, or patient satisfaction.[85] The same group has demonstrated that this approach is feasible and safe in the patient with significant comorbidity undergoing "complex" operations as well.[86]

Factors that are not necessarily emphasized in these studies, but are clearly present, include the involvement of ancillary staff and patient education. Preoperatively, patients should be educated regarding the expectations of the pathways in terms of their activity and diet. Additionally, an attempt to explain realistic expectations of what patients may expect in terms of pain and discomfort will help in compliance with the protocol. The caregivers, both family and hospital staff, must also be involved and aware of the pathway. Preoperative printed instructions and wall charts may help in achieving this understanding.

Conclusion

Clearly, the many facets to the postoperative care of the individual patient are complex and as varied as the population treated. The goal of this summary is to provide general recommendations and a framework on which to guide medical decision making. Consistency in postoperative care helps ancillary staff and patients in regard to expectations and understanding their course, but as the clinical situation evolves, changes may be necessary. A basic knowledge of the principles involved and the options available is crucial in delivering the appropriate care.

References

1. Gust R, Pecher S, Gust A, Hoffmann V, Bohrer H, Martin E. Effect of patient-controlled analgesia on pulmonary complications after coronary artery bypass grafting. Crit Care Med 1999;26:2218–2223.
2. Major CP, Greer MS, Russell WL, Roe SM. Postoperative pulmonary complications and morbidity after abdominal aneurysmectomy: a comparison of postoperative epidural versus parenteral opioid analgesia. Am Surg 1996;62:45–51.
3. Kouraklis G, Glinavou A, Raftopoulos L, Alevisou V, Lagos G, Karatzas G. Epidural analgesia attenuates the systemic stress response to upper abdominal surgery: a randomized trial. Int Surg 2000;85:353–357.
4. Apfelbaum JL, Chen C, Mehta SS, Gan TJ. Postoperative pain experience: results from a national survey suggest postoperative pain continues to be unmanaged. Anesth Analg 2003;97:534–540.
5. Carr DB, Goudas LC. Acute pain. Lancet 1999;353:2051–2058.
6. McQuay H. Opioids in pain management. Lancet 1999;353:2229–2232.
7. McQuay HJ. Potential problems of using both opioids and local anaesthetic. Br J Anaesth 1988;61:121.
8. Latta KS, Ginsberg B, Barkin RL. Meperidine: a critical review. Am J Ther 2002;9:53–68.
9. Austin KL, Stapleton JV, Mather LE. Multiple intramuscular injections: a major source of variability in analgesic response to meperidine. Pain 1980;8:47–62.
10. Erstad BL, Meeks ML, Chow H, et al. Site-specific pharmacokinetics and pharmacodynamics of intramuscular meperidine in elderly postoperative patients. Ann Pharmacother 1997;331:23–28.
11. Collins SL, Faura CC, Moore RA, Mcquay HJ. Peak plasma concentrations after oral morphine: a systematic review. J Pain Symptom Manage 1998;16:388–402.
12. Walder B, Schafer M, Henzi I, Tramer MR. Efficacy and safety of patient-controlled opioid analgesia for acute postoperative pain. A quantitative systematic review. Acta Anaesthesiol Scand 2001;45:795–804.
13. Ballantyne JC, Carr DB, Chalmers TC, Dear KB, Angelillo IF, Mosteller F. Postoperative patient-controlled analgesia: meta-analysis of initial randomized control trials. J Clin Anesth 1993;5:182–193.
14. McCormack K. Non-steroidal anti-inflammatory drugs and spinal nociceptive processing. Pain 1994;59:9–44.
15. Strom BL, Berlin J, Kinman JL, et al. Parenteral ketorolac and risk of gastrointestinal and operative site bleeding. A postmarketing surveillance study. JAMA 1996;275:376–382.
16. Raffa RB. Antihistamines as analgesics. J Clin Pharm Ther 2001; 26:81–85.
17. Mann C, Pouzeratte Y, Boccara G, et al. Comparison of intravenous or epidural patient-controlled analgesia in the elderly after major abdominal surgery. Anesthesiology 2000;92:433–441.
18. Eriksson-Mjoberg M, Svensson JO, Almkvist O, Olund A, Gustafsson LL. Extradural morphine gives better pain relief than

patient-controlled i.v. morphine after hysterectomy. Br J Anaesth 1997;78:10–16.

19. Carli F, Trudel JL, Belliveau P. The effect of intraoperative thoracic epidural anesthesia and postoperative analgesia on bowel function after colorectal surgery: a prospective randomized trial. Dis Colon Rectum 2001;44:1083–1089.

20. Scott AM, Starling JR, Ruscher AE, DeLessio ST, Harms BA. Thoracic versus lumbar epidural anesthesia's effect of pain control and ileus resolution after restorative proctocolectomy. Surgery 1996;120:688–695.

21. Jorgensen H, Wetterslev J, Moiniche S, Dahl JB. Epidural local anaesthetics versus opioid based analgesic regimens on postoperative gastrointestinal paralysis, PONV, and pain after abdominal surgery. Cochrane Database Syst Rev 2000;4:CD001893.

22. Woolf CJ. Evidence for a central component of postinjury pain hypersensitivity. Nature 1983;308:386–388.

23. Coderre TJ, Katz J, Vaccarino AL, Melzack R. Contribution of central neuroplasticity to pathological pain. Review of clinical and experimental evidence. Pain 1993;52:259–285.

24. Moiniche S, Kehlet H, Dahl JB. A qualitative and quantitative systematic review of preemptive analgesia for postoperative pain relief. Anesthesiology 2002;96:725–741.

25. Katz J, Cohen L, Schmid R, Chan VWS, Wowk A. Postoperative morphine use and hyperalgesia are reduced by preoperative but not intraoperative epidural analgesia. Implications for preemptive analgesia and the prevention of central sensitization. Anesthesiology 2003;98:1449–1460.

26. Sakurai M, Suleman MI, Morioka N, Akca O, Sessler DI. Minute sphere acupressure does not reduce postoperative pain or morphine consumption. Anesth Analg 2003;96:493–497.

27. Kotani N, Hashimoto H, Sata Y, et al. Preoperative intradermal acupuncture reduces postoperative pain, nausea and vomiting, analgesic requirement and sympathoadrenal responses. Anesthesiology 2001;95:349–356.

28. Piotrowski MM, Paterson C, Mitchinson A, Kim HM, Kirsh M, Hinshaw DB. Massage as adjuvant therapy in the management of acute postoperative pain: a preliminary study in men. J Am Coll Surg 2003;197:1037–1046.

29. Lobo DN, Bostock KA, Neal KR, et al. Effect of salt and water balance on recovery of gastrointestinal function after elective colonic resection: a randomised controlled trial. Lancet 2002; 359:1812–1818.

30. Brandstrup B, Tonnesen H, Beier-Holgersen R, et al. Effects of intravenous fluid restriction on postoperative complications: comparison of two perioperative fluid regimens. Ann Surg 2003;238:641–648.

31. Price J, Sear J, Venn R. Perioperative fluid volume optimization following proximal femoral fracture. Cochrane Database Syst Rev 2002;(1):CD003004.

32. Pimental M, Roberts DE, Bernstein CN, Hoppensack M, Duerksen DR. Clinically significant gastrointestinal bleeding in critically ill patients. Am J Gastroenterol 2000;95:2801–2806.

33. Terdiman JP, Ostroff JW. Gastrointestinal bleeding in the hospitalized patient: a case-control study to assess risk factors, causes, and outcome. Am J Med 1998;104:349–354.

34. Cook DJ, Fuller HD, Guyatt GH, et al. Risk factors for gastrointestinal bleeding in critically ill patients. N Engl J Med 1994; 330:377–381.

35. Nardino RJ, Vender RJ, Herbert PN. Overuse of acid-suppressive therapy in hospitalized patients. Am J Gastroenterol 2000;95: 3118–3122.

36. Hiramoto JS, Terdiman JP, Norton JA. Evidence based analysis: postoperative gastric bleeding: etiology and prevention. Surg Oncol 2003;12:9–19.

37. White RH, Romano PS, Zhou H. A population-based comparison of the 3 month incidence of thromboembolism after major elective/urgent surgery. Thromb Haemost 2001;86:2255.

38. Horlander KT, Mannino DM, Leeper KV. Pulmonary embolism mortality in the United States, 1979–1998: an analysis using multiple-cause mortality data. Arch Intern Med 2003;163: 1711–1717.

39. Kaboli P, Henderson MC, White RH. DVT prophylaxis and anticoagulation in the surgical patient. Med Clin North Am 2004;87: 77–110.

40. Best AJ, Williams S, Crozier A, Bhatt R, Gregg PJ, Hui AC. Graded compression stockings in elective orthopedic surgery. An assessment of the in vivo performance of commercially available stockings in patients having hip and knee arthroplasty. J Bone Joint Surg Br 200;82:116–118.

41. Amarigiri SV, Lees TA. Elastic compression stockings for prevention of deep vein thrombosis. Cochrane Database Syst Rev 2000:CD001484.

42. Camerota AJ, Chouhan V, Harada RN, et al. The fibrinolytic effects of intermittent pneumatic compression: mechanism of enhanced fibrinolysis. Ann Surg 1997;226:306–313.

43. Killewich LA, Sandager GP, Nguyen AH, Lilly MP, Flinn WR. Venous hemodynamics during impulse foot pumping. J Vasc Surg 1995;22:598–605.

44. Warwick D, Harrison J, Glew D, Mitchelmore A, Peters TJ, Donovan J. Comparison of the use of a foot-pump with the use of low molecular weight heparin for the prevention of deep-vein thrombosis after total hip replacement. J Bone Joint Surg Am 1998;80:1158–1166.

45. Cornwell EE, Chang D, VelmahosG, et al. Compliance with sequential compression device prophylaxis in at-risk trauma patients: a prospective analysis. Am Surg 2002;68:470–473.

46. Prevention of fatal postoperative pulmonary embolism by low doses of heparin. An international multicentre trial. Lancet 1975;2:45–51.

47. Collins R, Scrimgeour A, Yusuf S, Peto R. Reduction in fatal pulmonary embolism and venous thrombosis by perioperative administration of subcutaneous heparin. Overview of results of randomized trials in general, orthopedic, and urologic surgery. N Engl J Med 1988;318:1162–1173.

48. Simmons ED. In: Bongard FS, Sue DY, eds. Antithrombotic Therapy. In Current Critical Care Diagnosis and Treatment. 2nd ed. New York: McGraw Hill; 2002;905–924.

49. Warkentin TE, Levine MN, Hirsh J, et al. Heparin-induced thrombocytopenia in patients treated with low-molecular weight heparin or unfractionated heparin. N Engl J Med 1995;332:1330–1335.

50. Kakkar VV, Boeckl O, Boneu B, et al. Efficacy and safety of a low-molecular-weight heparin and standard unfractionated heparin for prophylaxis of postoperative venous thromboembolism. European multicenter trial. World J Surg 1997;2:2–8.

51. Mismetti P, Laporte S, Darmon JY, Buchmuller A, Decousus H. Meta-analysis of low molecular weight heparin in the prevention of venous thromboembolism in general surgery. Br J Surg 2001; 88:913–930.

52. Etchells E, McCleod RS, Geerts W, Barton P, Detsky AS. Economic analysis of low-dose heparin vs the low-molecular weight heparin enoxaparin for prevention of venous thromboembolism after colorectal surgery. Arch Intern Med 1999;159:1221–1228.

53. McLeod RS, Geerts WH, Sniderman KW, et al. Subcutaneous heparin versus low-molecular-weight heparin as thromboprophylaxis

in patients undergoing colorectal surgery: results of the Canadian colorectal DVT prophylaxis trial: a randomized, double-blind trial. Ann Surg 2001;233:438–444.

54. Palareti G, Legnani C, Guazzaloca G, et al. Activation of blood coagulation after abrupt or stepwise withdrawal of oral anticoagulants: a prospective study. Thromb Haemost 1994;72:222.

55. Genewein U, Haeberli A, Straub PW, Beer JH. Rebound after cessation of oral anticoagulant therapy: the biochemical evidence. Br J Haematol 1996;92:479.

56. Watts SA, Gibbs NM. Outpatient management of the chronically anticoagulated patient for elective surgery. Anaesth Intensive Care 2003;31:145–154.

57. Kearon C, Hirsh J. Current concepts: management of anticoagulation before and after elective surgery. N Engl J Med 1997;336:1506–1511.

58. Bauer JJ, Gelernt IM, Salky BA, Kreel I. Is routine postoperative nasogastric decompression really necessary? Ann Surg 1985;201:233–236.

59. Argov S, Goldstein I, Barzilai A. Is routine use of the nasogastric tube justified in upper abdominal surgery? Am J Surg 1980;130:849–850.

59a. Agnelli G, Boli G, Capussotti L. et al. A clinical outcome based prospective study on venous thromboembolism after cancer surgery. Ann Surg 2006;243:89–95.

60. Meltvedt R, Knecht B, Gibbons G, et al. Is nasogastric suction necessary after elective colon resection? Am J Surg 1985;149:620–622.

60a. Pelligrini VD, Donaldson CT, Farber DC, Lehman EB, Evarts CM. Prevention of readmission for venous thromboembolic disease after total hip arthroplasty. Clin Ortho and Related Research 2005;441:56–62.

61. Wolff BG, Pemberton JH, Van Heerden JA, et al. Elective colon and rectal surgery without nasogastric decompression. Ann Surg 1987;154:640–642.

61a. Bergqvist D, Agnelli G, Cohen AT, et al. ENOXACAN II Investigators. Duration of prophylaxis against venous thromboembolism with enoxaparin after surgery for cancer. N Engl J Med 2002;346:971–980.

62. Wexner SD, Cohen SM, Johansen OB, et al. Laparoscopic colorectal surgery: a prospective assessment and current perspective. Br J Surg 1993;80:1602–1605.

63. Jacobs M, Verdeja JC, Goldstein HS. Minimally invasive colon resection (laparoscopic colectomy). Surg Laparosc Endosc 1992;1:144–150.

64. DiFronzo LA, Yamin N, Patel K, O'Connell TX. Benefits of early feeding and early hospital discharge in elderly patients undergoing open colon resection. J Am Coll Surg 2003;197:747–752.

65. Lewis SJ, Egger M, Sylvester PA, Thomas S. Early enteral feeding versus "nil by mouth" after gastrointestinal surgery: systemic review and meta-analysis of controlled trials. BMJ 2001;323:773–776.

66. Apelgren KN, Rombeau JL, Twomey PL, Miller RA. Comparison of nutritional indices and outcomes in critically ill patients. Crit Care Med 1982;10:305–307.

67. Klonoff-Cohen H, Barrett-Connor EL, Edelstein SL. Albumin levels as a predictor of mortality in the healthy elderly. J Clin Epidemiol 1992;45:207–212.

68. Dervenis C, Augerinos C, Lytres D, Dells S. Benefits and limitations of enterol nutrition in the early postoperative period. Arch Surg 2003;387:441–449.

69. Petersen SR, Kudsk KA, Carpenter G, Sheldon G. Malnutrition and immunocompetence: increased mortality following an infectious challenge during hyperalimentation. J Trauma 1981;21:528–533.

70. Bozzetti F, Braga M, Gianotti L, Gavazzi, Mariani L. Postoperative enteral versus parenteral nutrition in malnourished patients with gastrointestinal cancer: a randomized mulitcentre trial. Lancet 2001;358:1487–1492.

71. Chernow B, Alexander HR, Smallridge RC, et al. Hormonal responses to graded surgical stress. Arch Intern Med 1987;145:1273–1278.

72. Kehlet H. A rational approach to dosage and preparation of parenteral glucocorticoid substitution therapy during surgical procedure. Acta Anaesthesiol Scand 1975;19:260–264.

73. Orth DN, Kovacs WJ. The adrenal cortex. In: Wilson JD, Foster DW, Kronenberg HM, et al., eds. Williams Textbook of Endocrinology. 9th ed. Philadelphia: WB Saunders; 1988:517–664.

74. White PC, Pescovitz OH, Cutler GB. Synthesis and metabolism of corticosteroids. In: Becker KL, ed. Principles and Practice of Endocrinology and Metabolism. 2nd ed. Philadelphia: Lippincott; 1995:647–662.

75. Udelsman R, Norton JA, Jelenich SE, et al. Responses of the hypothalamic-pituitary adrenal and rennin-angiotensin axis and the sympathetic system during controlled surgical and anesthetic stress. J Clin Endocrinol Metab 1987;64:986–994.

76. Glowniak JV, Loriaux DL. A double-blind study of perioperative steroid requirements in secondary adrenal insufficiency. Surgery 1997;121:123–129.

77. Salem M, Tainsh RE, Brombert J, Loriaux DL, Chernow B. Perioperative glucocorticoid coverage. A reassessment 42 years after emergence of a problem. Ann Surg 1994;219:416–425.

78. Bromberg JS, Baliga P, Cofer JB, et al. Stress steroids are not required for patients receiving a renal allograft and undergoing operation. J Am Coll Surg 1995;180:532–536.

79. Boots JMM, van den Ham ECH, Christiaans MHL, van Hooff JP. Risk of adrenal insufficiency with steroid maintenance therapy in renal transplantation. Transplant Proc 2002;34:1696–1697.

80. Rolih C, Ober K. The endocrine response to critical illness. Med Clin North Am 1995;79:211–224.

81. Stelzer M, Phillips JD, Fonkalsrud EW. Acute ileus from steroid withdrawal simulating intestinal obstruction after surgery for ulcerative colitis. Arch Surg 1990;125:914–917.

82. Rai S, Hemingway D. Acute adrenal insufficiency presenting as high output ileostomy. Ann R Coll Surg 2003;85:105–106.

83. Bardram L, Funch-Jensen P, Jensen P, Crawford ME, Kehlet H. Recovery after laparoscopic colonic surgery with epidural analgesia, and early oral nutrition and mobilization. Lancet 1995;345:763–764.

84. Kehlet H, Mogensen T. Hospital stay of 2 days after open sigmoidectomy with a multimodal rehabilitation programme. Br J Surg 1999;86:227–230.

85. Delaney CP, Fazio VW, Senagore AJ, Robinson B, Halverson AL, Remzi FH. "Fast track" post-operative management protocol for patients with high co-morbidity undergoing complex abdominal and pelvic colorectal surgery. Br J Surg 2001;88:1533–1538.

86. Delaney CP, Zutshi M, Senagore AJ, Remzi FH, Hammel J, Fazio VW. Prospective, randomized, controlled trial between a pathway of controlled rehabilitation with early ambulation and diet and traditional postoperative care after laparotomy and intestinal resection. Dis Colon Rectum 2003;46:851–859.

10
Postoperative Complications

David W. Dietz and H. Randolph Bailey

The ability to minimize, recognize, and treat postoperative complications is one of the most important aspects of surgery. This chapter will focus on those surgical complications most often encountered by colorectal surgeons: injuries to the bowel and genitourinary structures, pelvic hemorrhage, small bowel obstruction, wound infections, abscesses, and anastomotic leaks, strictures, and bleeding.

Unrecognized Enterotomies and Enterocutaneous Fistulae

Patients undergoing extensive adhesiolysis are at highest risk for enterotomies. An enterotomy in and of itself is not a complication, rather it is the failure to recognize and adequately repair an enterotomy that leads to trouble. In cases in which any significant degree of adhesiolysis is performed, the entire bowel should be carefully inspected at the end of the procedure. Although the natural history of serosal tears is unknown, they should be repaired when recognized with imbricating seromuscular sutures. Full-thickness enterotomies can be repaired using a number of different and equally effective techniques; one common method is a two-layer closure using an inner layer of absorbable seromuscular stitches (i.e., 3-0 Vicryl) and an outer layer of permanent Lembert stitches (i.e., 4-0 Ethibond). In cases in which multiple enterotomies have occurred within a short segment of bowel, resection of the involved segment with primary anastomosis is performed. If the mesentery has also been injured during the course of adhesiolysis, the viability of the bowel ends should be confirmed before anastomosis.

Failure to recognize an enterotomy at the time of surgery will lead to one of several postoperative complications. The patient may develop peritonitis within the first 24 to 48 hours after surgery. This may be difficult to detect in the background of narcotic analgesia and the surgeon and patient's expectation of postoperative incisional pain. The diagnosis is purely based on patient appearance and examination. The usual markers of bowel perforation (leukocytosis, fever, and pneumoperitoneum) are not reliable, because they are normal findings in the early postoperative patient. A high index of suspicion should be maintained with a low threshold for reexploration. Reoperation within the first several days is usually not difficult because significant adhesions have not yet formed. Most enterotomies found in this situation can be repaired primarily, provided that the bowel edges are viable. Should the repair fail, if the repair can be placed directly under the midline fascial closure, this may result in the development of a direct enterocutaneous fistula rather than recurrent peritonitis. If conditions are not favorable for primary repair, a stoma should be created. An especially difficult situation is that in which bilious fluid is encountered at reexploration but no enterotomy can be found. After running both the small and large bowel at least twice and excluding a duodenal, gastric, or gallbladder injury, the only remaining option may be to place drains in both paracolic gutters and the pelvis in hopes of creating a controlled enterocutaneous fistula. Insufflation of the small bowel with carbon dioxide gas through a nasogastric tube has also been described as a method for localizing small enterotomies. Gas bubbles may be seen emanating from the site of injury after the abdomen has been filled with saline.

An unrecognized enterotomy may also present as an enterocutaneous fistula, with enteric drainage emanating from the incision or wound later in the postoperative course. If there are no signs of sepsis, a nonoperative approach may be considered, especially if the patient is more than 1 week removed from surgery. The patient is placed on complete bowel rest, a nasogastric tube is placed, broad-spectrum antibiotic coverage is initiated, and a computed tomography (CT) scan is obtained to assess for an associated abscess or fluid collection. If a fluid collection greater than 4 cm in diameter is present, percutaneous, radiologically guided drainage should be used. If available, an enterostomal therapist should be involved to assist with pouching the fistula in order to protect the skin from irritating enteric contents. In most cases, parenteral nutrition will be started to meet the patient's caloric and protein requirements in anticipation of a prolonged period of fasting. H2 antagonists should be added to decrease gastric secretions. Somatostatin analogs may also be used to decrease the volume of fistula output, although they do not seem to increase the rate of spontaneous fistula closure.[1] The rate of spontaneous small bowel fistula closure varies but is typically less than 50%. Chances of spontaneous closure are thought to be reduced by high output because of proximal location, distal obstruction, local sepsis, radiation exposure, a short or epithelialized tract, malignancy, a foreign body in the tract (e.g., mesh, sutures), Crohn's disease, and malnutrition.[2]

Most enterocutaneous fistulae that close spontaneously will do so within the first month. If the fistula persists, fibrin glue injection can be attempted. Several reports have been published describing this technique and successful closure has been achieved in some cases.[3–5] Although no large series exists to define the success rate, little is lost in making the attempt. Surgical intervention should be delayed until all sepsis has resolved, adequate nutrition has been restored, and intraabdominal adhesions have softened to the point of allowing safe reoperation. Most authors recommend a delay of at least 6 weeks since the last laparotomy, but 3–6 months may be more appropriate.[6,7] The ultimate healing rate after definitive surgical repair is approximately 80%.[7]

Anastomotic Complications

Anastomotic complications are among the most feared in colorectal surgery. They can lead to emergent reoperation and/or a prolonged, complicated, and costly postoperative hospitalization. If the patient recovers from the acute event, chronic sequelae may develop because of stricture or pelvic fibrosis leading to poor bowel function and the possibility of further revisionary surgery or permanent fecal diversion.

Anastomotic complications are usually related to technical factors (ischemia, tension, poor technique, stapler malfunction) or preexisting conditions in the patient such as local sepsis, poor nutrition, immunosuppression, morbid obesity, and radiation exposure. The contribution of the former may be minimized by a careful, methodical approach to construction of the anastomosis (Table 10-1). For colorectal anastomoses, a tension-free anastomosis may be achieved by full division of the lateral attachments of the descending colon, complete mobilization of the splenic flexure, high ligation of the

TABLE 10-1. Steps to minimize risk of leak from colorectal or coloanal anastomoses

1. Ensure good blood supply (pulsatile bleeding from marginal artery at level of anastomosis)
2. Ensure tension-free anastomosis by complete mobilization of splenic flexure (includes high ligation of IMA and ligation of inferior mesenteric vein at lower border of pancreas)
3. Avoid use of sigmoid colon in creation of anastomoses
4. Inspection of anastomotic donuts for completeness after circular stapled anastomoses
5. Air or fluid insufflation test to rule out anastomotic leak immediately after construction in the operating room

inferior mesenteric artery (IMA), separation of the omentum from the distal transverse colon and mesocolon, and division of the inferior mesenteric vein at the lower edge of the pancreas. Adequate blood supply should be confirmed by cutting across the marginal artery or bowel wall with anything less than pulsatile bleeding considered unacceptable. Further colon resection should be performed until adequate bleeding is encountered. If necessary, anastomoses between the hepatic flexure or distal ascending colon and rectum are easily achieved by passing the colon through a window in the mesentery of the terminal ileum.

Nutritional status, degree of immunosuppression, and general medical condition should be considered when deciding whether or not to perform a primary anastomosis. If severe malnutrition (albumin <2.0 or weight loss >15%) or significant immunosuppression (chemotherapy, high-dose steroids) are present, an end colostomy and Hartmann stump will minimize the risk of complications. Colostomy takedown can then be performed if and when these factors have been corrected. Preoperative weight loss, if able to be accomplished by the morbidly obese patient, will make the construction of deep pelvic anastomoses easier. When operating in the radiated pelvis, one end of the bowel used to construct the anastomosis should come from outside the field of radiation.

Bleeding

Anastomotic bleeding is common and varies greatly in severity. In most cases, bleeding is minor and is manifested by the passage of dark blood with the patient's first bowel movements after surgery. In rare instances, bleeding can be massive and require transfusion and active intervention.

Bleeding can occur after either stapled or hand-sewn anastomoses, but is probably more common with the former. This complication can be reduced by careful inspection of the staple line, particularly in the case of side-to-side/functional end-to-end anastomoses. Before closing the enterotomy through which the stapler was introduced, the linear staple line can be everted and inspected. Bleeding points should be controlled with sutures rather than cautery to prevent a deep burn injury which may lead to delayed leak. The incidence of bleeding from the linear staple line can be minimized by using the antimesenteric borders of each limb to construct the anastomosis, thus avoiding inclusion of the mesentery in the staple line.

Bleeding from circular stapled anastomoses or from the staple lines of ileal or colonic J pouches is usually not diagnosed until after the patient has left the operating room. After performing proctoscopy to evacuate clot from the rectum or neorectum, a rectal tube is inserted and a 1:100,000 solution of saline and epinephrine is instilled. The tube is then clamped for 15 minutes. If bleeding persists after the solution is allowed to drain, the procedure may be repeated. If bleeding continues or hypotension develops, the patient should be returned to the operating room for transanal examination of the anastomosis or pouch under anesthesia. Bleeding from anastomoses that are not accessible using these techniques (i.e., ileocolic or small bowel to small bowel) may be managed with supportive care and correction of any underlying coagulopathy. If bleeding is severe, angiography may be required to localize the site and allow selective infusion of vasopressin. Alternatively, colonoscopy may be used. If the anastomosis can be visualized, the bleeding site can be treated with either cautery or injection of epinephrine. In rare cases, reoperation with resection of the bleeding anastomosis is required.

Leaks

The incidence of anastomotic leak varies widely and is related to the factors listed above as well as the type of anastomosis. The lowest leak rates are seen after small bowel or ileocolic anastomosis (1%–3%) whereas the highest occur after coloanal anastomosis (10%–20%). Vignali et al. reported on 1014 colorectal anastomoses. The overall clinical leak rate was 2.9%. The incidence of leak was strongly associated with the distance of the anastomosis from the anal verge. Eight percent of low anastomoses (<7 cm from anal verge) leaked compared with only 1% of high anastomoses (>7 cm from anal verge). Although diabetes mellitus, use of a pelvic drain, and duration of surgery were each related to anastomotic leak in the univariate analysis, only low anastomosis was predictive in the multivariate model.

Another high-risk anastomosis is the ileal pouch-anal anastomosis. Leak rates of 5%–10% have been reported.[8–10] Data from series of ileal pouch-anal anastomosis in patients with ulcerative colitis identify prednisone dosage >40 mg/day as a significant risk factor.

Role of Fecal Diversion

The creation of a proximal diverting stoma minimizes the severe consequences of an anastomotic leak but it does not reduce the incidence of leak itself.[11–13] A diverting stoma should be considered for any high-risk anastomosis [coloanal, low colorectal (<6 cm from anal verge)]. In addition, patient factors such as severe malnutrition, significant immunosuppression, and purulent peritonitis or pelvic sepsis should be considered as indications for diversion. Consideration should also be given to the patient's comorbidities and general condition; in cases in which the "physiologic reserve" necessary to tolerate an anastomotic leak does not exist, the use of a proximal stoma should be strongly entertained. Neoadjuvant radiation therapy does not seem to increase the incidence of anastomotic leak in patients undergoing restorative proctectomy for rectal cancer[14,15] but this may be because of the tendency for surgeons to cover these anastomoses with a proximal stoma, thus reducing the clinical manifestations of a leak. In fact, recent data from a large randomized trial assessing the efficacy of short-course neoadjuvant radiation therapy in rectal cancer found that a protecting stoma reduces the need for surgical intervention should an anastomotic leak occur.[16]

Role of Pelvic Drains

The use of pelvic drains is controversial. Whereas surgeons have long believed that preventing the collection of fluid or hematoma in the pelvis minimizes risk of anastomotic leak, the use of drains has not been shown to be of benefit or harm in a recent, large randomized study[17] and in a metaanalysis.[18] However, examination of the data from the Dutch TME trial showed that the use of pelvic drains reduced the incidence of clinical anastomotic leak after short-course neoadjuvant radiation therapy from 23% to 9%. In the absence of data suggesting harm, the authors routinely drain low colorectal or coloanal anastomoses, especially after neoadjuvant therapy.

Management of Anastomotic Leak

Anastomotic leaks can be divided into "free" and "contained" varieties. Free leaks are those in which fecal contents leak from the anastomosis and spread throughout the abdominal cavity. Patients usually present with fever, tachycardia, leukocytosis, and diffuse peritonitis. Feculent fluid may present itself through the surgical incision or via the pelvic drains. Hypotension and other signs of systemic sepsis may ensue. If the patient is stable, radiologic investigation is helpful to localize the leak and to determine its size and severity.

Patients with "free" leaks should be taken to the operating room after fluid resuscitation and administration of broad-spectrum intravenous antibiotics. Surgical treatment will be dictated by the findings at operation. Most leaking colorectal anastomoses will require abdominal washout and takedown of the anastomosis with creation of an end-colostomy and Hartmann stump. If the stump cannot be stapled or sutured closed because of the friability of the tissues, transabdominal pelvic and peranal drains should be placed. However, leaking ileocolic or small bowel to small bowel anastomoses can occasionally be repaired primarily in carefully selected circumstances, i.e., small defect with viable edges. However, resection of the anastomosis with either reconstruction or creation of a stoma is the wisest and most conservative option. Placing the repaired anastomosis directly under the midline incision will usually result in an enterocutaneous fistula rather than a second bout of peritonitis should the repair fail. If the viability of the bowel ends is questionable, takedown of the anastomosis and creation of a stoma is mandatory. Small defects in colorectal anastomoses may also, under ideal circumstances, be repaired primarily and covered with a proximal ileostomy. This is contraindicated, however, if there is a significant fecal load present between the ileostomy and the site of repair.

"Contained" leaks are those in which the extravasation of contrast material is limited to the pelvis and usually result in the development of a pelvic abscess (Figure 10-1). If the abscess cavity is small and contrast flows freely back into the bowel, the patient may be treated with intravenous antibiotics, bowel rest, and observation. If the abscess is larger or somewhat removed from the site of the anastomosis, then

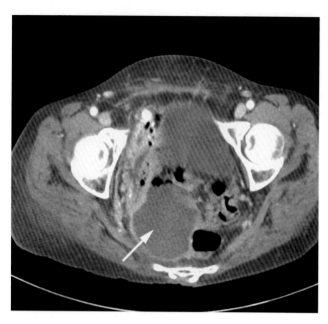

FIGURE 10-1. Pelvic abscess resulting from ileocolic anastomotic leak (white arrow). Extravasated enteric contrast can be seen in the right pelvis tracking down toward the abscess.

percutaneous abscess drainage using CT or ultrasound guidance may avoid laparotomy. Such leaks rarely require subsequent fecal diversion.

Fistulae

Anastomotic leaks may also result in fistulae to the skin, vagina, male genitourinary system, or chronic presacral abscess (presacral sinus). Colocutaneous fistulae will frequently close with conservative management consisting of either bowel rest with total parenteral nutrition or a low residue diet and pouching of the fistula to protect the surrounding skin. If drainage persists, reoperation for fistula takedown and reconstruction of the anastomosis can be performed after a delay of 3–6 months. Patients can usually eat a normal diet during this time period to maintain nutritional status. Fibrin glue injection has been reported as a successful alternative to surgery (see above).

Colovaginal fistulae are usually the consequence of either an anastomotic leak necessitating through the vaginal cuff in a patient who has undergone a prior hysterectomy or the inclusion of the vagina during creation of a stapled anastomosis. In either case, spontaneous closure is rare. If the vaginal drainage is copious and intolerable to the patient, proximal fecal diversion may be necessary. An alternative measure to avoid a stoma during the period of fistula maturation is to use a large-volume daily enema to evacuate the colonic contents at a predictable time each day. After a waiting period of 6–12 weeks, reoperation may be performed. Options include attempts at local repair using mucosal flaps (colonic or vaginal)/sleeve advancements or laparotomy with redo coloanal

anastomosis, either primary or delayed ("Turnbull-Cutait pullthrough").

Chronic presacral abscess or sinus may result from a posterior leak in a coloanal or ileal pouch-anal anastomosis. Patients may have an occult presentation consisting of vague pelvic pain, fevers, frequency of stool, urgency, and bleeding. A pelvic CT scan will usually show presacral inflammatory changes and a contrast enema will confirm the presence of a sinus tract originating from the posterior midline of the anastomosis and extending cephalad into the presacral space. Examination under anesthesia can then be performed with careful inspection of the anastomosis. A probe or clamp is placed through the anastomotic defect and the chronic presacral cavity is simply lain open using cautery and gently curetted of granulation tissue. This will allow free drainage of the presacral abscess and healing by secondary intention. This may result in a chronic posterior sinus or "pseudo-diverticulum."

Stricture

Anastomotic stricture may be the end result of anastomotic leak or ischemia. It typically presents 2–12 months after surgery with increasing constipation and difficulty evacuating. If the initial resection was done for malignancy, recurrence as a cause of the stricture must be excluded with a combination of CT scan and fluorodeoxyglucose–positron emission tomography (PET) scan. Biopsy is mandated if a mass or abnormality is identified. Low colorectal, coloanal, or ileal pouch-anal anastomotic strictures may be successfully treated with repeated dilatations using an examining finger or rubber dilators. Dilation is more successful if initiated within the first few weeks after surgery. In fact, almost all coloanal or ileoanal anastomoses will stricture to some degree during the early postoperative period, especially if a diverting stoma is present. All such anastomoses should undergo digital examination at 4–6 weeks after surgery and just before stoma closure (usually at 2–3 months). Strictures are usually soft and easily dilated during these examinations. Higher colorectal, colocolic, or ileocolic strictures may be approached using endoscopic balloon dilatation (Figure 10-2). If these measures fail, or if the stricture is extremely tight or long, revisionary surgery may be required. These are difficult operations, however, because of the pelvic fibrosis that develops after anastomotic leak and complications are common. In some cases, permanent fecal diversion is the only option.[19,20]

Genitourinary Complications

Ureteral Injuries

Injury to the ureters typically occurs at one of four specific points in the procedure. The first is during high ligation of the IMA where the junction between the upper and middle thirds of the left ureter lies in close proximity to the vessels. Failure

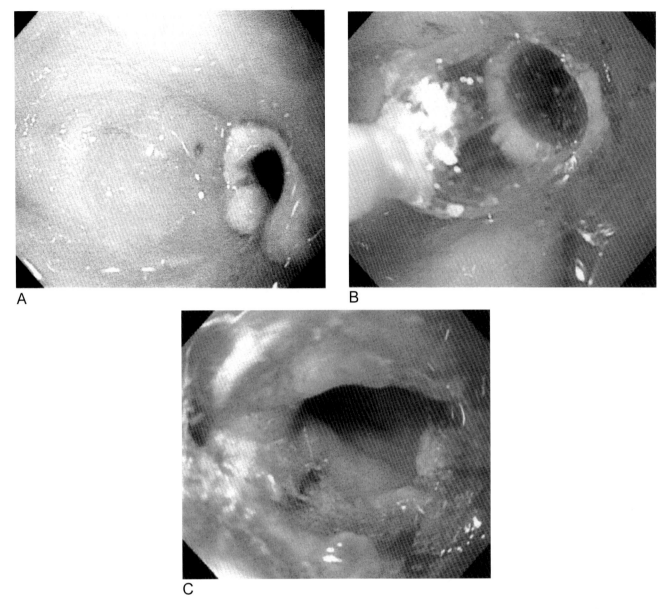

FIGURE 10-2. Endoscopic balloon dilatation of a colorectal anastomotic stricture. **A** Five-millimeter colorectal anastomotic stricture. **B** Balloon dilator inflated. **C** Result.

to mobilize the ureter laterally before ligation of the IMA may result in its inclusion with the vascular pedicle when clamped and subsequent division. It is good practice to always confirm the position of the left ureter before and after applying clamps to the IMA and before division of the vessel. Injury at this level is usually limited to transection and can be repaired primarily using an end-to-end, spatulated anastomosis performed over a stent. The second point of danger is during mobilization of the upper mesorectum near the level of the sacral promontory. It is at this point that the ureters cross over the bifurcation of the iliac artery and course medially as they enter the pelvis. The left ureter may be closely associated with the sigmoid colon and can even be adherent secondary to prior inflammatory processes. The injury may be tangential

and not readily recognized in the setting of a phlegmon or abscess. Ureteral stents in this setting are most beneficial in identifying the injury rather than preventing it. Injury at this level is usually managed by either primary repair or ligation of the distal stump and creation of a ureteroneocystostomy with a Boari flap or psoas hitch repair.

The third point of risk is during the deepest portion of the abdominal phase of the operation. Anterolateral dissection in the plane between the lower rectum, pelvic sidewall, and bladder base can result in ureter injury at the ureterovesical junction. The ureter may also be injured at this level during division of the lateral stalks. The final area of risk is during the most cephalad portion of the perineal phase of the operation. If exposure is limited (obese patient, android pelvis), the ureter may be unknowingly divided near the ureterovesical junction. In either of these circumstances, the injury can be managed by creating a ureteroneocystostomy. The ureter is reimplanted into the bladder by tunneling the ureter through the bladder wall and creating a mucosa to mucosa anastomosis.

Should ureteral injury occur, the key to minimizing its consequence is immediate (intraoperative) recognition and repair of the injury. In cases in which a difficult pelvic dissection is anticipated, because of prior pelvic surgery, inflammation, or a locally advanced tumor, the preoperative placement of ureteral stents can be invaluable. Although the literature does not demonstrate that stents prevent ureteral injuries, palpation of the stents can aid in localization of the ureters and can also facilitate identification and repair should injury occur. In cases in which the surgeon is suspicious of occult injury, indigo carmine can be administered intravenously. After several minutes, the urine will turn blue-green and the operative field can then be inspected for staining. Unfortunately, the literature suggests that less than 50% of ureteral injuries are identified intraoperatively, usually because the injury is not suspected. Ureteral stents should be used selectively, however, because their use can lead to complications such as obstruction secondary to hematoma, perforation, or acute renal failure.

Urethral Injuries

Iatrogenic injury to the urethra may be the result of abdominoperineal resection (APR). The injury typically occurs during the perineal portion of the procedure and usually involves the membranous or prostatic portion. Intraoperatively, urethral injury may be recognized by visualization of the Foley catheter through the defect. These injuries may be difficult to avoid in the presence of a large, deeply penetrating anterior tumor in which involvement of the prostate gland can occur. Desmoplastic reaction to the tumor or edema from neoadjuvant radiation therapy may also obscure anatomic planes. Small injuries can be repaired at the time of surgery using 5-0 chromic sutures with the Foley catheter left in place to stent the repair for 2–4 weeks. Larger injuries or those not presenting until the postoperative period (urine draining from the perineal wound) require proximal urinary diversion via suprapubic catheter and delayed repair. This should be performed by a skilled urologist with experience in urethral reconstruction and typically utilizes a gracilis muscle flap.

Bladder Injury

Bladder injuries are relatively frequent and are, in most cases, related to resection of an adherent rectosigmoid tumor or diverticular phlegmon. When created purposefully or recognized immediately, defects in the bladder dome are easily repaired in two layers with a Foley catheter then left in place for 7–10 days postoperatively. Before removal, a cystogram

may be obtained to confirm healing. Injuries to the base of the bladder are more problematic. The major risk of repair in this situation is occlusion of the ureteral orifice at the trigone. Most urologists advocate opening of the bladder dome to gain access to the bladder lumen with subsequent repair of the trigone injury under direct vision from the interior. Ureteral patency is confirmed at the conclusion of the repair before closing the cystotomy. Injuries not recognized at the time of surgery will present in the postoperative period with urine in the abdominal cavity, pneumaturia, or fecaluria. Initially, fecal and urinary diversion may be necessary to temporize the situation until reoperation can be safely performed. At that time, takedown of the colovesical fistula is performed with primary repair of the bladder. If available, omentum should be interposed between the bladder repair and any bowel anastomosis. Catheter drainage of the bladder is maintained for 1–2 weeks.

Urinary Dysfunction

Urinary dysfunction is one of the most common urinary complications of APR.[21] Some degree of voiding difficulty occurs in up to 70% of patients after APR, but it is usually confined to the early postoperative period. In most instances, urinary retention is the result of denervation of the detrusor muscle causing partial paralysis. Bladder contractility is under parasympathetic control via pelvic nerve branches originating from the inferior hypogastric plexus. These nerves can be injured if the endopelvic fascia is breached, especially during blunt dissection of the rectum. Temporary dysfunction of these nerves is nearly universal after APR, even when a meticulous sharp dissection is used. Most patients, however, will only require maintenance of a Foley catheter for 5–7 days postoperatively. In a small percentage of patients, the problem persists beyond several months and urologic consultation is required. A small percentage of these patients may require prostatectomy or even intermittent self-catheterization on a long-term basis.

Sexual Dysfunction

Recent series report an incidence of sexual dysfunction of 15%–50% in male patients undergoing APR for rectal cancer.[22–24] This wide range is likely attributable to several factors such as patient age, preoperative libido, use of adjuvant radiation therapy, varying definitions of dysfunction, time point of follow-up, and social barriers preventing a frank discussion of the problem. The type of dysfunction is dependent on the pattern of nerve injury. Damage to the superior hypogastric (sympathetic) plexus during high ligation of the IMA or to the hypogastric nerves at the sacral promontory during mobilization of the upper mesorectum, results in ejaculatory problems such as retrograde ejaculation. This is the most common type of sexual dysfunction seen in male patients after APR and is also the type most likely to resolve with time (6–12 months). Damage to the pelvic plexus during the lateral dissection or to the nervi erigentes or cavernous nerves while dissecting the anterior plane (abdominal or perineal phase) may result in erectile dysfunction. The cavernous nerves arise from branches of the pelvic plexus and course anterior to Denonvillier's fascia at the lateral border of the seminal vesicles. Parasympathetic innervation from these routes controls the inflow to and retention of blood within the corpora cavernosa. The important anatomic relations of the pelvic nerves are illustrated in Figure 10-3.

Risk of injury to these nerves may be reduced by tailoring the anterior dissection based on the location of the tumor. The highest risk of parasympathetic nerve injury occurs when dissection is performed in the plane anterior to Denonvillier's fascia and flush with the posterior aspect of the seminal vesicles and prostate. Whereas some believe that this plane is a vital part of total mesorectal excision for any low rectal cancer, others will only include Denonvillier's fascia in the resection specimen for an anterior tumor where it may help obtain a clear radial margin.[25] For posterior tumors, Denonvillier's fascia is preserved by dissecting between it and the fascia propria of the rectum in order to protect the small cavernous nerves. Using a "nerve sparing" approach to total mesorectal excision, several authors have reported an incidence of erectile dysfunction of 5%–15% after proctectomy for rectal cancer. Factors shown to increase risk are older age, poor preoperative libido, and low rectal tumor requiring APR (two- to threefold increase compared with low anterior resection).

Although harder to quantify, sexual dysfunction also occurs in women after proctectomy. It is characterized by dyspareunia and inability to produce vaginal lubricant and achieve orgasm. The incidence is lower than that seen in males and varies between 10% and 20%.[26]

Female Infertility

Several recent studies have documented decreased fertility in women who have undergone restorative proctocolectomy for ulcerative colitis or familial adenomatous polyposis.[27,28] The postoperative infertility rate exceeds 50% in this group when defined as "one year of unprotected intercourse without conception." This has important implications in both preoperative patient counseling and in the modification of operative technique to minimize the effect of pelvic adhesions on fertility. Women of childbearing age should be informed of this potential complication before elective restorative proctocolectomy because it may influence the timing of surgery. In addition, because pelvic adhesions are thought to interfere with egg transit from the ovary to the fallopian tube, measures to minimize their occurrence may be of benefit. Tacking the ovaries to the anterior abdominal wall outside of the pelvis and wrapping the adnexa with an anti-adhesion barrier sheet are frequently used techniques but there are no data to support their efficacy.

Trapped Ovary Syndrome

Trapped ovary syndrome is a fairly common complication after restorative proctocolectomy in young women. The adhesions that form after ileal pouch-anal anastomosis trap the ovaries in the pelvis and cover the fallopian tubes. With each ovulatory cycle, there is release of fluid into the pelvic cavity defined by these adhesions. As fluid accumulates and the cavity expands, patients will complain of pelvic or lower abdominal pain relevant to the side of the trapped ovary. A CT scan or ultrasound will reveal a cystic lesion in the pelvis containing no air and with no surrounding inflammatory reaction. Operative findings are a cyst containing clear or tan fluid, surrounded by adhesions and with the ovary attached. Treatment consists of unroofing and evacuation of the cyst, pelvic adhesiolysis, and suspension of the ovary to the pelvic brim or iliac fossa with sutures. Trapped ovary syndrome may be prevented by suspending the ovaries at the time of restorative proctocolectomy and by placement of an adhesion barrier film in the pelvis.

Small Bowel Obstruction

Perhaps the most critical components in the management of patients with bowel obstruction are the recognition and prevention of the disastrous effects of bowel ischemia. Timely

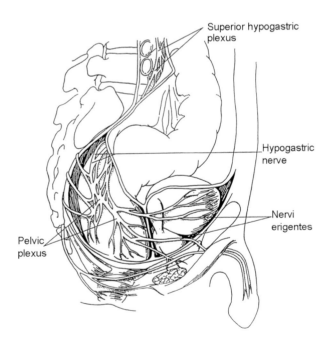

FIGURE 10-3. Anatomic relations of the pelvic nerves. Damage to the superior hypogastric plexus during high ligation of the IMA or to the hypogastric nerves at the sacral promontory during mobilization of the upper mesorectum results in retrograde ejaculation. Damage to the pelvic plexus during the lateral dissection or to the nervi erigentes or cavernous nerves while dissecting the anterior plane may result in erectile dysfunction.

surgical intervention, before the development of transmural necrosis, will limit complications and improve outcome. In one recently published series of more than 1000 patients undergoing surgery for small bowel obstruction, nonviable strangulated bowel was present at laparotomy in only 16% of cases but the risk of death in this group was increased four-fold.[29] It is also important to distinguish between early (<30 days) and late postoperative small bowel obstruction.

Presentation and Diagnosis

Nausea and vomiting, colicky pain, abdominal bloating, and obstipation are the hallmark signs of small bowel obstruction. The degree to which each of these contributes to the clinical picture will depend on the location, degree, and duration of the obstruction.

The commonly regarded hallmarks of strangulated bowel are fever, tachycardia, leukocytosis, sepsis, peritoneal signs, and the presence of continuous as opposed to intermittent pain. If any of these are found, the suspicion of ischemia should be high. These signs may also be found in patients without strangulation and are, therefore, nonpathognomonic. In many cases, however, this determination is not made until laparotomy, and timely surgical intervention in symptomatic patients may be the best means of avoiding the progression to bowel ischemia. This fact is underscored by a report from Sarr and colleagues[30] who found that the traditional clinical parameters frequently used to predict strangulation were neither sensitive nor specific. Nearly one-third of patients with strangulation were not diagnosed until the time of surgery.

Radiographic Studies

Plain Radiographs

An acute abdominal series is the initial imaging study performed in most patients suspected of having small bowel obstruction and consists of both upright and supine abdominal films and an upright chest X-ray. Typical findings include dilated, air-filled loops of small bowel, air-fluid levels, and an absence or paucity of colonic air. These findings may be absent, however, when the obstruction is proximal or the dilated bowel loops are mostly fluid filled. The sensitivity of plain radiographs in detecting small bowel obstruction is approximately 60%. The findings of pneumatosis intestinalis or portal vein gas is worrisome for advanced bowel ischemia.

CT Scan

Abdominopelvic CT scanning is increasingly used as a primary imaging modality in patients suspected of having small bowel obstruction. In addition to establishing the diagnosis, CT may also be able to precisely define a transition point and reveal secondary causes of obstruction such as tumor, hernia, intussusception, volvulus, or inflammatory conditions such as Crohn's disease and radiation enteritis. CT may also reveal closed loop obstructions or signs of progressing ischemia such as bowel wall thickening, pneumatosis, or portal vein gas. Several studies have shown that the sensitivity of CT in diagnosing small bowel obstruction approaches 90%–100%.

Contrast Studies

Contrast studies using water-soluble agents are frequently used in patients with acute small bowel obstruction. In patients with distal small bowel obstruction, a contrast enema is an efficient means by which colonic obstruction can be excluded. Antegrade studies of the small bowel can help to differentiate partial from complete obstruction, and may therefore predict the need for surgical intervention. In fact, some authors have used small bowel contrast studies as a "screening test" for patients presenting with adhesive obstructions. Failure of contrast material to reach the colon by 24 hours is used as an indication for prompt surgical exploration. Several studies have also shown that the antegrade administration of contrast agents may speed the resolution of partial small bowel obstruction, presumably through an osmotic effect. However, conflicting data also exist and the therapeutic effects of the small bowel contrast study remain to be defined.

Initial Therapy and Nonoperative Management

Once the diagnosis of small bowel obstruction is made, the patient is admitted to the hospital. Those with peritonitis, perforation, or signs of ischemic bowel are immediately prepared for laparotomy with expeditious correction of fluid and electrolyte deficits. A urinary catheter is inserted to guide resuscitation with the end points being resolution of tachycardia and hypotension and/or achieving a urine output of at least 0.5 cc/kg/h. Broad-spectrum antibiotic coverage is initiated. A nasogastric tube is inserted preoperatively to decompress the stomach, because these patients are at risk for aspiration on induction of general anesthesia.

If signs of perforation or ischemia are not present, a trial of expectant management may be undertaken. Patients with partial small bowel obstructions secondary to adhesions will resolve with a nonoperative approach in 80% of cases.[31–33] The success rate for patients initially presenting with complete obstruction is significantly lower. The nonoperative management of small bowel obstruction consists of fluid and electrolyte replacement, bowel rest, and tube decompression. The debate between standard nasogastric tube versus long nasoenteric tube decompression has mostly settled in favor of the nasogastric tube. This is in part attributable to the fact that long tubes with mercury-weighted tips (Miller-Abbott) are no longer available for use (because of concern about the elemental Mercury) and have been replaced with a balloon-tipped tube (Gowen tube) that requires endoscopic placement. Long tubes are more difficult to place, requiring special expertise, serial radiographic studies, or endoscopy to guide insertion. There has been some recent resurgence in interest in the use of nasoenteric tubes, mostly among radiologists. Indications for long tube management of small bowel obstruction include early postoperative obstruction and recurrent partial obstruction where the transition point is difficult to identify on contrast studies.

Narcotic analgesics may be administered to comfort the patient, but not to the point of diminishing mental status. The practice of withholding pain medication to avoid masking the signs of perforation or ischemia is probably unnecessary. Serial abdominal examinations (ideally just before the next dose of analgesics) should be performed to assess for increasing tenderness or the presence of peritoneal signs. Any change in the patient's condition that suggests developing bowel ischemia mandates exploratory laparotomy. In general, a nonoperative course may be followed for 24–48 hours. If the obstruction has not resolved within that time period, it is unlikely to do so and laparotomy is advised.

Decision to Operate

Several studies have attempted to define certain criteria that would reliably predict the presence or absence of strangulated bowel. Unfortunately, none have been shown to be particularly accurate and the best tool remains sound clinical judgment. Certainly, patients with fever, peritonitis, pneumoperitoneum, or overt sepsis should undergo emergent laparotomy because these are hard signs of transmural bowel necrosis. The presence of early ischemia, however, is much more difficult to discern. It is not uncommon for patients with small bowel obstruction to present with tachycardia, relative hypotension, mild acidosis, and leukocytosis, all of which may be secondary to dehydration. These patients should be aggressively rehydrated with isotonic intravenous fluids and the above parameters should be reassessed. Persistence of any of these signs after fluid resuscitation should prompt immediate laparotomy. Adherence to this simple algorithm should minimize the progression to strangulation while limiting the number of unnecessary laparotomies.

Distinguishing between partial and complete obstruction is also a key element in deciding which patients should be taken for early operation. As stated above, the likelihood of resolution of a complete obstruction with expectant management is low (20%). Delaying operative therapy until after a nonviable strangulation or perforation has occurred will substantially increase the mortality rate. Although this distinction may be difficult to make clinically, there are some useful caveats. The passage of stool or flatus cannot be relied on as an accurate predictor because patients with complete obstruction may continue to pass stool and flatus until the bowel distal to the site of obstruction is evacuated. However, if this continues for more than 12 hours after the onset of obstructive symptoms, the likelihood of complete obstruction is diminished. The passage of large volumes of nonbloody, watery stool along with

vomiting and distension is pathognomonic for partial small bowel obstruction. The onset of flatus, however, usually signals the beginning of resolution of the obstruction because flatus is produced from swallowed air.

Surgical Technique

After the adequacy of resuscitation is confirmed and broad-spectrum antibiotics active against enteric pathogens are administered, the peritoneal cavity is entered through a midline incision. This is a point in the operation where the risk of inadvertent enterotomy is very high because bowel loops are distended and often adherent to the undersurface of the abdominal wall. Once the fascia is encountered, the application of gentle pressure with the bevel of the scalpel blade, rather than a cutting stroke, is used to breach the peritoneal cavity. Using this technique, it is usually possible to recognize an adherent bowel loop before enterotomy occurs.

In the most favorable scenario, a single constricting band will be encountered that can be sharply divided to relieve the obstruction. In the worst cases, the peritoneal cavity will be totally obliterated by scar tissue. An orderly and systematic approach to adhesiolysis is advised in these instances. First, the underside of the midline scar is cleared so that the entire length of the incision can be opened if necessary. Next, adhesions to the abdominal wall are dissected laterally until both paracolic gutters are reached. This will allow the placement of a self-retaining retractor to facilitate exposure. In cases in which bowel distension is severe, needle decompression may be used to gain additional working space. Particularly severe adhesions that defy identification of the bowel and peritoneal surfaces ("frozen abdomen") may be injected with saline through a fine-gauge needle to separate the surfaces and thus facilitate adhesiolysis. Attention is then turned to the pelvis where the most difficult adhesions are often encountered. Rather than separating individual bowel loops at this stage, the small bowel residing in the pelvis should be mobilized "en-masse" by lysing adhesions to the pelvic structures in an anterior to posterior manner in order to roll the mass of intestine up and out of the pelvis. The final portion of this stage of the operation involves mobilizing the plane between the small bowel mesentery and the retroperitoneum until the duodenum is encountered. Only at this point are all adhesions between individual bowel loops lysed in order to free the entire length of the small intestine. The bowel is then inspected for any coexisting pathology and for enterotomies or serosal tears created in the course of mobilization.

Assessment of bowel viability is usually possible by using the triad of color, peristalsis, and mesenteric pulsations. In cases in which these signs are questionable, the ischemic segment should be wrapped in warm, wet packs and viability reassessed after 15 minutes. If viability is still in doubt, use of the Doppler probe or systemic injection of fluorescein dye followed by inspection of the bowel under a Wood's lamp may aid in decision making. If the area in question is a short segment, it may be best to proceed with resection. If an extensive segment of questionable viability is present, then a second-look operation 24 hours later should be planned before committing the patient to a massive small bowel resection.

There is some debate as to the need for complete adhesiolysis when the point of obstruction is encountered early in the operation. It is our policy to divide the majority of adhesions if this can be done safely. This will facilitate inspection of the entire length of the small bowel and allows for the placement of anti-adhesion barriers if desired (see below).

Special Situations

Early Postoperative Bowel Obstruction

Early postoperative bowel obstruction is generally defined as mechanical obstruction occurring within 1 month of abdominal or pelvic surgery. This condition is special in that attempts at relaparotomy in the early postoperative period frequently result in disastrous complications. The mantra of "never let the sun rise or set on a patient with bowel obstruction" should not be broadly applied in this group. An intense inflammatory response usually begins within the abdomen at 7–10 days postoperatively and persists for at least 6 weeks. If forced to operate during this period of time, the surgeon is likely to encounter dense hypervascular adhesions that may obliterate the peritoneal cavity. The risk of enterotomy and subsequent fistulization is extremely high. In addition, vascular or extensive serosal injury of the bowel may lead to massive resections. Therefore, immediate reoperation for early postoperative bowel obstruction is not advised, especially considering the fact that the development of strangulation in this setting is extremely rare. These patients should be managed conservatively with nasogastric or long tube suction and intravenous fluids. If resolution does not occur within the first 5–7 days, a percutaneous gastrostomy tube may be placed for longer-term decompression, and the patient is started on hyperalimentation. Patients may be discharged from the hospital on this regimen and laparotomy performed in 6 weeks if the obstruction has not resolved. However, if peritonitis or signs of sepsis are present initially or develop during the course of nonoperative therapy, a CT scan should be performed immediately. Any abscess or fluid collection caused by an enteric leak can be percutaneously drained and a controlled enterocutaneous fistula established. Exploration is usually only required in cases of ischemic or necrotic bowel. There is a place for very early exploration within the first 10 days postoperatively if obstruction is recognized promptly. The adhesions encountered during this time period have not usually become severe and can be dealt with safely.

Anastomotic "Overhealing"

Anastomotic overhealing is a rare cause of postoperative small bowel obstruction. It is most often attributable to early adhesion and healing of the staple lines of the linear cutter between the limbs of a functional end-to-end/side-to-side anastomosis. This is best prevented by maximally distracting the two staple lines as the transverse staple line is placed to close the enterotomy made to introduce the side-to-side stapler. When this occurs in the early postoperative period, it will be easily diagnosed with a water-soluble contrast study, especially if administered via a long tube near the point of obstruction. The treatment should be conservative initially and may include long tube decompression. In some cases, the balloon-tipped catheter itself has broken through the healing web and relieved the obstruction. In the case of an obstructed ileocolic anastomosis, colonoscopic balloon dilatation may be carefully used. Operative intervention should be a last resort and usually requires resection and reanastomosis.

Prevention of Adhesions

More than 90% of patients undergoing abdominal surgery will develop some degree of intraabdominal adhesions. Adhesion formation can occur wherever the visceral or parietal peritoneum has been disturbed. Once an area of injury is established, fibrin is deposited and then organizes to form a matrix for collagen deposition. Bowel motility and endogenous lubricants attempt to counteract this process, but in most cases, adhesions will eventually result as the deposited collagen matures. As discussed earlier, the progression from early to mature adhesions usually takes approximately 6 weeks.

Several strategies have been developed to minimize, prevent, or influence adhesion formation. Gentle handling of tissues, avoiding the deposition of talc by wearing powder-free gloves, and copious lavage of the peritoneal cavity at the conclusion of the operative procedure are simple means that should be used in all cases. In instances in which particularly severe adhesion formation can be anticipated, for instance patients with multiple recurrences of small bowel obstruction, the use of long intestinal tubes placed at the conclusion of surgery to "splint" the bowel open during adhesion formation has been advocated. This is usually accomplished by inserting a Baker tube via a proximal jejunostomy.

Recently, several chemoprophylactic agents have been developed in an attempt to reduce or eliminate adhesions through a barrier mechanism. The best studied of these is a bioresorbable membrane of modified sodium hyaluronate and carboxymethylcellulose. A large multicenter study by Becker et al.[34] has shown that this material substantially reduces the extent, incidence, and severity of adhesion formation. Its efficacy in reducing the incidence of adhesive bowel obstruction has recently been reported.[35] However, the decrease in incidence of bowel obstruction from 3.4% in the control group to 1.8% in the treatment group is of uncertain clinical significance. The use of adhesion barriers in patients at high risk for subsequent reoperation because of disease or previous adhesions may be justified by the likely improvement in the ease and safety of the subsequent abdominal reentry and explorations. One of the problems with the barrier material is that it only prevents adhesions between the surfaces where it is applied.

Pelvic Bleeding

Serious pelvic bleeding may be encountered during proctectomy and is usually caused by injury to the presacral venous plexus or the internal iliac vessels or their branches. Although rare, pelvic bleeding can be a devastating event and is a significant cause of operative mortality. Presacral venous hemorrhage is especially challenging because the anatomy and fragility of the presacral venous plexus make control of bleeding difficult. Attempts at electrocoagulation or suture ligation of these vessels usually results in an increase in bleeding and is not advised. Direct finger pressure should be used to gain temporary control of bleeding while allowing the anesthesia team to "catch up" with the resuscitation. Once the patient is stabilized, several methods exist for permanent hemostasis. The most common of these is the use of sterile thumbtacks or specially designed "occluder pins" that are driven into the sacrum at right angles and directly over the site of bleeding.[36,37] If this is unsuccessful, a rectus abdominus muscle flap may be rotated down into the pelvis based on the inferior epigastric pedicle. Heavy sutures are then placed on either side of the sacrum and tied down to compress the rectus flap against the sacrum to tamponade the bleeding.[38] Other methods to control presacral bleeding have also been described[39–42] such as removing a 2×2 cm square of rectus muscle and tacking this to the sacrum with absorbable sutures placed on either side of the bleeding site and tied tightly to secure the muscle patch. Application of electrocautery to the muscle then produces a secure coagulum on the surface of the bleeding venous plexus. If these measures fail, pelvic bleeding may be controlled by packing several laparotomy sponges tightly into the pelvis with the ends being brought out through the lower portion of the abdominal wound. The abdomen is then closed and the patient is taken to the intensive care unit for blood transfusion, fluid resuscitation, correction of coagulopathy, and general support. After 24–48 hours, the patient is returned to the operating room for removal of the packs.[43]

Wound Infection and Intraabdominal Abscess

Wound Infection

Because of the large bacterial content of the colon (10^{10} anaerobes and 10^8 aerobes/gram of stool), wound infection rates are high after colorectal surgical procedures.[44,45] The introduction of an oral antibiotic preparation before surgery by Nichols and Condon reduced wound infection rates from 40% historically to the present day level of 5%–10%. In many centers, a single parenteral dose of antibiotics at induction has replaced the more complicated "Nichol's prep." Several

single-agent or combination choices exist, each with adequate gram-negative and anaerobic coverage. Risk factors for wound infection have been identified and include malnutrition, diabetes mellitus, immunosuppression, age >60 years, American Society of Anesthesia score >2, fecal contamination, length of hospitalization before surgery, and extensive surgery.[46] Recently, there is a growing body of literature that shows that mechanical bowel preparation does not decrease the incidence of wound infection. Several metaanalyses have examined this question and are in agreement.[47–49] The largest and most recent also found that the risk of anastomotic leak was actually increased in patients receiving a bowel preparation (odds ratio 1.75).[50]

Wound infections typically present on or around the fifth postoperative day and are characterized by erythema, warmth, tenderness, fever, and purulent drainage. Initial treatment consists of opening a portion of the skin incision over the area of maximal change to allow drainage. Antibiotics are not prescribed unless there is cellulitis present. If a significant amount of necrotic tissue is present, it should be débrided. Once the wound is adequately drained, a packing regimen is begun and the wound is allowed to heal by secondary intention. Large wounds may be treated with application of a vacuum-assisted wound closure device. After the wound has been débrided by several days of wet to dry dressing changes, the vacuum-assisted closure device is applied (V.A.C.; KCI Therapeutic Services, San Antonio, TX). The advantages of this system are simplification of wound care and quicker closure. The dressing only needs to be changed every 4–5 days and wounds typically close within several weeks.

Several situations require more aggressive treatment. Deep infection involving the rectus muscle and fascia may occur and result in dehiscence. These patients should be taken back to the operating room for debridement of the necrotic fascial edges and repair of the dehiscence. Invasive wound infections with either clostridium perfringens or beta-hemolytic streptococcus is a potentially life-threatening complication. These infections may have an atypical presentation in that they can occur within the first 1–2 days after surgery and may be associated with minimal skin changes. The combination of fever and unusually severe wound pain early in the postoperative course should prompt opening of the skin incision. A necrotizing infection is suggested by the drainage of thin gray fluid. The key to timely diagnosis and treatment of these severe infections is a high level of suspicion. The patient should be taken to the operating room for a thorough wound exploration. All devitalized tissue should be removed and the fascia excised back to healthy, bleeding edges. Broad-spectrum antibiotic coverage should include high-dose penicillin.

Intraabdominal Abscess

Intraabdominal abscesses can result from anastomotic leaks, enterotomies, or spillage of bowel contents at the time of surgery. Patients will usually present with fever, leukocytosis, and abdominal or pelvic pain 5–7 days after surgery. The diagnostic modality of choice is a CT scan of the abdomen and pelvis performed with intravenous and oral contrast (and rectal contrast in the patient with a colorectal anastomosis). The finding of a fluid collection with a thickened, enhancing rim and surrounding inflammatory stranding is diagnostic. Air bubbles may also be present in the collection. Proximity to a staple line and the presence of contrast material in the abscess suggest an anastomotic leak as its cause.

Most intraabdominal or pelvic abscesses can be successfully treated with percutaneous catheter drainage performed under ultrasound or CT guidance. Intravenous antibiotics should also be administered. The CT scan is repeated 48 hours after drainage to assess its efficacy. Further follow-up is usually performed by contrast studies obtained by injecting the drainage catheter. Once the abscess cavity has collapsed and no fistula to the bowel is identified, the catheter can be

safely removed. Some abscesses cannot be drained percutaneously because of their location and lack of a safe "radiographic window" for drainage. Reported success rates for percutaneous drainage of intraabdominal abscesses range from 65% to 90% and depend on size, complexity, etiology, and microbial flora.[51–54]

Perineal Wound Infection

Perineal wound infection and delayed healing are major causes of morbidity after APR with the incidence ranging from 11% to 50%.[55–58] The rigidity of the lower pelvis combined with wide resection of the perineal soft tissues and levator muscles is mostly to blame, because this results in dead space cephalad to the skin closure which is easily infected.[59] Technical modifications that may help reduce the incidence of perineal wound problems include reapproximation of the

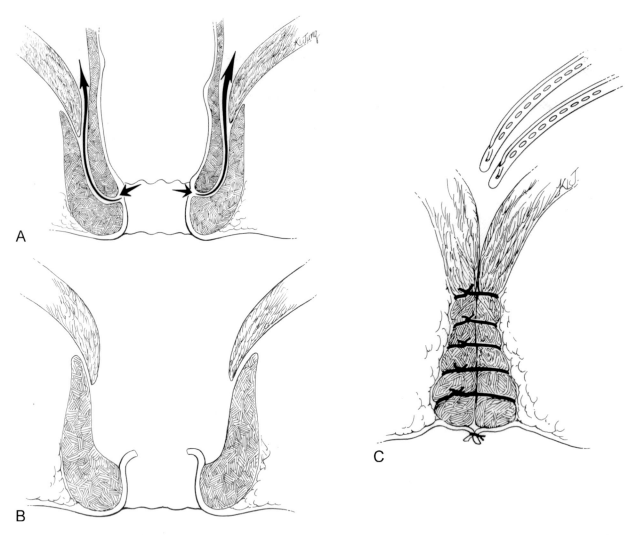

FIGURE 10-4. Technique of intersphincteric proctectomy. **A** The mucosa overlying the intersphincteric groove is incised near the dentate line and the dissection is carried cephalad between the internal and external sphincters. **B** This results in retention of the external sphincters and levators which are then able to be closed in the midline **C**.

subcutaneous tissues, suction drainage of the pelvis (with or without irrigation) to prevent hematoma formation and resultant fibrosis,[60] and filling of the dead space with an omental pedicle graft.[61–65] The area of raw surface deep in the pelvis also frequently fills with small bowel and may lead to small bowel obstruction. The bowel can be excluded from the pelvis by closing the pelvic peritoneum when possible, pulling the uterus posteriorly to close the defect, or by rotating the cecum into the pelvis. The use of absorbable mesh has also been described, but this has been associated with multiple reports of obstruction and fistulization. If possible, based on oncologic factors, a cuff of levator muscle can be left by incising the pelvic floor just outside of the external sphincter muscle. This should always be possible for small rectal cancers. This allows closure of the levator muscles in the midline and prevents dead space formation and perineal hernia. Several risk factors for perineal wound complications have been identified. Foremost among these is the use of neoadjuvant radiation therapy. In one study, the incidence of perineal wound infection increased from 13% to 34% with the addition of preoperative radiation whereas the rate of nonhealing at 30 days increased from 19% to 51%. Rates of perineal wound complications were even higher if intraoperative radiation was used.[66] Other factors are long operative time (>300 minutes), intraoperative hypothermia, and fecal contamination during the perineal dissection.[67,68] Patients with anorectal Crohn's disease are also at increased risk when undergoing APR for rectal cancer. However, an intersphincteric dissection in patients with inflammatory bowel disease allows closure of the external sphincter and may improve wound healing (Figure 10-4).

If infection does occur, the skin should be opened to allow drainage and a program of wet to dry packing begun. A vacuum-assisted closure device can then be placed, as described above. In cases in which a chronic perineal sinus develops, closure of the defect will require wound debridement and myocutaneous flap reconstruction with gracilis, inferior gluteus, or rectus abdominus muscle.

References

1. Sancho JJ, di Costanzo J, Nubiola P, et al. Randomized double-blind placebo-controlled trial of early octreotide in patients with postoperative enterocutaneous fistula. Br J Surg 1995;82(5):638–641.
2. Berry SM, Fischer JE. Enterocutaneous fistulas. Curr Probl Surg 1994;31(6):469–566.
3. Huang CS, Hess DT, Lichtenstein DR. Successful endoscopic management of postoperative GI fistula with fibrin glue injection: report of two cases. Gastrointest Endosc 2004;60(3):460–463.
4. Okamoto K, Watanabe Y, Nakachi T, et al. The use of autologous fibrin glue for the treatment of postoperative fecal fistula following an appendectomy: report of a case. Surg Today 2003;33(7):550–552.
5. Lamont JP, Hooker G, Espenschied JR, Lichliter WE, Franko E. Closure of proximal colorectal fistulas using fibrin sealant. Am Surg 2002;68(7):615–618.
6. Fazio VW, Coutsoftides T, Steiger E. Factors influencing the outcome of treatment of small bowel cutaneous fistula. World J Surg 1983;7(4):481–488.
7. Hollington P, Mawdsley J, Lim W, Gabe SM, Forbes A, Windsor AJ. An 11-year experience of enterocutaneous fistula. Br J Surg 2004;91(12):1646–1651.
8. Fazio VW, Ziv Y, Church JM, et al. Ileal pouch-anal anastomoses complications and function in 1005 patients. Ann Surg 1995;222(2):120–127.
9. Dayton MT, Larsen KR, Christiansen DD. Similar functional results and complications after ileal pouch-anal anastomosis in patients with indeterminate vs ulcerative colitis. Arch Surg 2002;137(6):690–694.
10. Sugerman HJ, Sugerman EL, Meador JG, Newsome HH Jr, Kellum JM Jr, DeMaria EJ. Ileal pouch anal anastomosis without ileal diversion. Ann Surg 2000;232(4):530–541.
11. Marusch F, Koch A, Schmidt U, et al. Value of a protective stoma in low anterior resections for rectal cancer. Dis Colon Rectum 2002;45(9):1164–1171.
12. Pakkastie TE, Ovaska JT, Pekkala ES, Luukkonen PE, Jarvinen HJ. A randomised study of colostomies in low colorectal anastomoses. Eur J Surg 1997;163(12):929–933.
13. Dehni N, Schlegel RD, Cunningham C, Guiguet M, Tiret E, Parc R. Influence of a defunctioning stoma on leakage rates after low colorectal anastomosis and colonic J pouch-anal anastomosis. Br J Surg 1998;85(8):1114–1117.
14. Enker WE, Merchant N, Cohen AM, et al. Safety and efficacy of low anterior resection for rectal cancer: 681 consecutive cases from a specialty service. Ann Surg 1999;230(4):544–552.
15. Kapiteijn E, Marijnen CA, Nagtegaal ID, et al. Preoperative radiotherapy combined with total mesorectal excision for resectable rectal cancer. N Engl J Med 2001;345(9):638–646.
16. Peeters KC, Tollenaar RA, Marijnen CA, et al. Risk factors for anastomotic failure after total mesorectal excision of rectal cancer. Br J Surg 2004;92(2):211–216.
17. Merad F, Hay JM, Fingerhut A, et al. Is prophylactic pelvic drainage useful after elective rectal or anal anastomosis? A multicenter controlled randomized trial. French Association for Surgical Research. Surgery 1999;125(5):529–535.
18. Urbach DR, Kennedy ED, Cohen MM. Colon and rectal anastomoses do not require routine drainage: a systematic review and meta-analysis. Ann Surg 1999;229(2):174–180.
19. Di Giorgio P, De Luca L, Rivellini G, Sorrentino E, D'amore E, De Luca B. Endoscopic dilation of benign colorectal anastomotic stricture after low anterior resection: a prospective comparison study of two balloon types. Gastrointest Endosc 2004;60(3):347–350.
20. Suchan KL, Muldner A, Manegold BC. Endoscopic treatment of postoperative colorectal anastomotic strictures. Surg Endosc 2003;17(7):1110–1113.
21. Hollabaugh RS Jr, Steiner MS, Sellers KD, Samm BJ, Dmochowski RR. Neuroanatomy of the pelvis: implications for colonic and rectal resection. Dis Colon Rectum 2000;43(10):1390–1397.
22. Walsh PC, Schlegel PN. Radical pelvic surgery with preservation of sexual function. Ann Surg 1988;208(4):391–400.
23. Havenga K, Enker WE, McDermott K, Cohen AM, Minsky BD, Guillem J. Male and female sexual and urinary function after total mesorectal excision with autonomic nerve preservation for carcinoma of the rectum. J Am Coll Surg 1996;182(6):495–502.

24. Masui H, Ike H, Yamaguchi S, Oki S, Shimada H. Male sexual function after autonomic nerve-preserving operation for rectal cancer. Dis Colon Rectum 1996;39(10):1140–1145.

25. Lindsey I, Mortensen NJ. Iatrogenic impotence and rectal dissection. Br J Surg 2002;89(12):1493–1494.

26. Havenga K, Enker WE, McDermott K, Cohen AM, Minsky BD, Guillem J. Male and female sexual and urinary function after total mesorectal excision with autonomic nerve preservation for carcinoma of the rectum. J Am Coll Surg 1996;182(6):495–502.

27. Gorgun E, Remzi FH, Goldberg JM, et al. Fertility is reduced after restorative proctocolectomy with ileal pouch anal anastomosis: a study of 300 patients. Surgery 2004;136(4):795–803.

28. Olsen KO, Joelsson M, Laurberg S, Oresland T. Fertility after ileal pouch-anal anastomosis in women with ulcerative colitis. Br J Surg 1999;86(4):493–495.

29. Fevang BT, Fevang J, Stangeland L, Soreide O, Svanes K, Viste A. Complications and death after surgical treatment of small bowel obstruction: a 35-year institutional experience. Ann Surg 2000;231(4):529–537.

30. Sarr MG, Bulkley GB, Zuidema GD. Preoperative recognition of intestinal strangulation obstruction. Prospective evaluation of diagnostic capability. Am J Surg 1983;145(1):176–182.

31. Biondo S, Pares D, Mora L, Marti RJ, Kreisler E, Jaurrieta E. Randomized clinical study of gastrografin administration in patients with adhesive small bowel obstruction. Br J Surg 2003;90(5):542–546.

32. Choi HK, Chu KW, Law WL. Therapeutic value of gastrografin in adhesive small bowel obstruction after unsuccessful conservative treatment: a prospective randomized trial. Ann Surg 2002; 236(1):1–6.

33. Chen SC, Lin FY, Lee PH, Yu SC, Wang SM, Chang KJ. Water-soluble contrast study predicts the need for early surgery in adhesive small bowel obstruction. Br J Surg 1998;85(12):1692–1694.

34. Becker JM, Dayton MT, Fazio VW, et al. Prevention of postoperative abdominal adhesions by a sodium hyaluronate-based bioresorbable membrane: a prospective, randomized, double-blind multicenter study. J Am Coll Surg 1996;183(4):297–306.

35. Fazio VW, Cohen Z, Fleshman JW, et al. Adhesion Study Group. Reduction in adhesive small bowel obstruction by Seprafilm® adhesion barrier after intestinal resection. Dis Colon Rectum 2006;48:1–9.

36. Nivatvongs S, Fang DT. The use of thumbtacks to stop massive presacral hemorrhage. Dis Colon Rectum 1986;29(9):589–590.

37. Stolfi VM, Milsom JW, Lavery IC, Oakley JR, Church JM, Fazio VW. Newly designed occluder pin for presacral hemorrhage. Dis Colon Rectum 1992;35(2):166–169.

38. Remzi FH, Oncel M, Fazio VW. Muscle tamponade to control presacral venous bleeding: report of two cases. Dis Colon Rectum 2002;45(8):1109–1111.

39. Cosman BC, Lackides GA, Fisher DP, Eskenazi LB. Use of tissue expander for tamponade of presacral hemorrhage. Report of a case. Dis Colon Rectum 1994;37(7):723–726.

40. Losanoff JE, Richman BW, Jones JW. Cyanoacrylate adhesive in management of severe presacral bleeding. Dis Colon Rectum 2002;45(8):1118–1119.

41. Remzi FH, Oncel M, Fazio VW. Muscle tamponade to control presacral venous bleeding: report of two cases. Dis Colon Rectum 2002;45(8):1109–1111.

42. Xu J, Lin J. Control of presacral hemorrhage with electrocautery through a muscle fragment pressed on the bleeding vein. J Am Coll Surg 1994;179(3):351–352.

43. Metzger PP. Modified packing technique for control of presacral pelvic bleeding. Dis Colon Rectum 1988;31(12):981–982.

44. Rau HG, Mittelkotter U, Zimmermann A, Lachmann A, Kohler L, Kullmann KH. Perioperative infection prophylaxis and risk factor impact in colon surgery. Chemotherapy 2000;46(5):353–363.

45. Platell C, Hall JC. The prevention of wound infection in patients undergoing colorectal surgery. J Hosp Infect 2001;49(4):233–238.

46. Platell C, Hall JC. The prevention of wound infection in patients undergoing colorectal surgery. J Hosp Infect 2001;49(4):233–238.

47. Slim K, Vicaut E, Panis Y, Chipponi J. Meta-analysis of randomized clinical trials of colorectal surgery with or without mechanical bowel preparation. Br J Surg 2004;91(9):1125–1130.

48. Platell C, Hall J. What is the role of mechanical bowel preparation in patients undergoing colorectal surgery? Dis Colon Rectum 1998;41(7):875–882.

49. Guenaga KF, Matos D, Castro AA, Atallah AN, Wille-Jorgensen P. Mechanical bowel preparation for elective colorectal surgery. Cochrane Database Syst Rev 2003;(2):CD001544.

50. Slim K, Vicaut E, Panis Y, Chipponi J. Meta-analysis of randomized clinical trials of colorectal surgery with or without mechanical bowel preparation. Br J Surg 2004;91(9):1125–1130.

51. Khurrum BM, Hua ZR, Batista O, et al. Percutaneous postoperative intra-abdominal abscess drainage after elective colorectal surgery. Tech Coloproctol 2002;6(3):159–164.

52. Schechter S, Eisenstat TE, Oliver GC, Rubin RJ, Salvati EP. Computerized tomographic scan-guided drainage of intra-abdominal abscesses. Preoperative and postoperative modalities in colon and rectal surgery. Dis Colon Rectum 1994;37(10):984–988.

53. Benoist S, Panis Y, Pannegeon V, et al. Can failure of percutaneous drainage of postoperative abdominal abscesses be predicted? Am J Surg 2002;184(2):148–153.

54. Cinat ME, Wilson SE, Din AM. Determinants for successful percutaneous image-guided drainage of intra-abdominal abscess. Arch Surg 2002;137(7):845–849.

55. Pollard CW, Nivatvongs S, Rojanasakul A, Ilstrup DM. Carcinoma of the rectum. Profiles of intraoperative and early postoperative complications. Dis Colon Rectum 1994;37(9): 866–874.

56. Rosen L, Veidenheimer MC, Coller JA, Corman ML. Mortality, morbidity, and patterns of recurrence after abdominoperineal resection for cancer of the rectum. Dis Colon Rectum 1982; 25(3):202–208.

57. Rothenberger DA, Wong WD. Abdominoperineal resection for adenocarcinoma of the low rectum. World J Surg 1992;16(3):478–485.

58. Nissan A, Guillem JG, Paty PB, et al. Abdominoperineal resection for rectal cancer at a specialty center. Dis Colon Rectum 2001;44(1):27–35.

59. Silen W, Glotzer DJ. The prevention and treatment of the persistent perineal sinus. Surgery 1974;75(4):535–542.

60. Wang JY, Huang CJ, Hsieh JS, Huang YS, Juang YF, Huang TJ. Management of the perineal wounds following excision of the rectum for malignancy. Gaoxiong Yi Xue Ke Xue Za Zhi 1994;10(4):177–181.

61. Hay JM, Fingerhut A, Paquet JC, Flamant Y. Management of the pelvic space with or without omentoplasty after abdominoperineal resection for carcinoma of the rectum: a prospective multicenter study. The French Association for Surgical Research. Eur J Surg 1997;163(3):199–206.

62. Rice ML, Hay AM, Hurlow RH. Omentoplasty in abdominoperineal resection of the rectum. Aust N Z J Surg 1992;62(2):147–149.

63. Ferguson CM. Use of omental pedicle grafts in abdominoperineal resection. Am Surg 1990;56(5):310–312.

64. Smith SR, Swift I, Gompertz H, Baker WN. Abdominoperineal and anterior resection of the rectum with retrocolic omentoplasty and no drainage. Br J Surg 1988;75(10):1012–1015.

65. Moreaux J, Horiot A, Barrat F, Mabille J. Obliteration of the pelvic space with pedicled omentum after excision of the rectum for cancer. Am J Surg 1984;148(5):640–644.

66. Nissan A, Guillem JG, Paty PB, et al. Abdominoperineal resection for rectal cancer at a specialty center. Dis Colon Rectum 2001; 44(1):27–35.

67. Baudot P, Keighley MR, Alexander-Williams J. Perineal wound healing after proctectomy for carcinoma and inflammatory disease. Br J Surg 1980;67(4):275–276.

68. Irvin TT, Goligher JC. A controlled clinical trial of three different methods of perineal wound management following excision of the rectum. Br J Surg 1975;62(4):287–291.

11
Benign Anorectal: Hemorrhoids

José R. Cintron and Herand Abcarian

Anatomy

Hemorrhoids are cushions of specialized, highly vascular tissue found within the anal canal in the submucosal space. The term "hemorrhoidal disease" should be reserved for those vascular cushions that are abnormal and cause symptoms in patients. These cushions of thickened submucosa contain blood vessels, elastic tissue, connective tissue, and smooth muscle.[1] The anal submucosal smooth muscle (Treitz's muscle) originates from the conjoined longitudinal muscle (see Figure 11-1). These smooth muscle fibers then pass through the internal sphincter and anchor themselves into the submucosa, thereby contributing to the bulk of the hemorrhoids and suspending the vascular cushions at the same time.[2] Some of the vascular structures within the cushion when examined microscopically lack a muscular wall. The lack of a muscular wall characterizes these vascular structures more as sinusoids and not veins. Studies have shown that hemorrhoidal bleeding is arterial and not venous because hemorrhage from disrupted hemorrhoids occurs from presinusoidal arterioles that communicate with the sinusoids in this region.[1] This is supported by the bright red appearance and the arterial pH of the blood.[3] The venous plexus and sinusoids below the dentate line which constitute the external hemorrhoidal plexus drain primarily via the inferior rectal veins into the pudendal veins which are branches of the internal iliac veins. Venous drainage also occurs to a lesser extent via the middle rectal veins to the internal iliac veins. This overlying tissue is somatically innervated and is therefore sensitive to touch, pain, stretch, and temperature. The subepithelial vessels and sinuses above the dentate line which constitute the internal hemorrhoid plexus are drained by way of the middle rectal veins to the internal iliacs.

The vascular cushions within the anal canal contribute to anal continence and function as a compressible lining that protects the underlying anal sphincters. Additionally, the cushions are critical in providing complete closure of the anus, further aiding in continence. As an individual coughs, strains, or sneezes, these fibrovascular cushions engorge and maintain closure of the anal canal to prevent leakage of stool in the presence of increased intrarectal pressure. These cushions account for approximately 15%–20% of the anal resting pressure.[4] Additionally, this tissue likely supplies important sensory information that enables individuals to discriminate between liquid, solid, and gas, further aiding in continence. It is essential to consider that while undertaking any treatment for hemorrhoidal disease the fibrovascular cushions are a part of normal anorectal anatomy and are important in the continence mechanism. Therefore, surgical removal may result in varying degrees of incontinence particularly in individuals with marginal preoperative control. There are three main vascular cushions that are found anatomically in health as well as in disease. The cushions are located in the left lateral, right anterior, and right posterior positions of the anus. This specific configuration has been shown in cadaver studies to be present only 19% of the time.[1] Most individuals have additional smaller accessory cushions present in between the main cushions. This anatomic configuration apparently bears no relationship to the terminal branching of the superior rectal artery. The position of hemorrhoids within the anal canal, however, remains remarkably consistent. The configuration of these cushions is quite constant and borne out by the fact that the same configuration can be found in children, the fetus, and even in the embryo.[1] The topographic location of pathology around the anus should be described in anatomic terms (anterior, posterior, right lateral, left lateral, etc.) and not by the numbers on the face of a clock. In this way, regardless of whether the patient is in a prone, supine, or lateral position, the pathology can always be accurately located.

Etiology

Etiologic factors thought to be contributory to the pathologic changes in the vascular cushions include constipation, prolonged straining, irregular bowel habits, diarrhea, pregnancy, heredity, erect posture, absence of valves within the hemorrhoidal sinusoids, increased intraabdominal pressure with

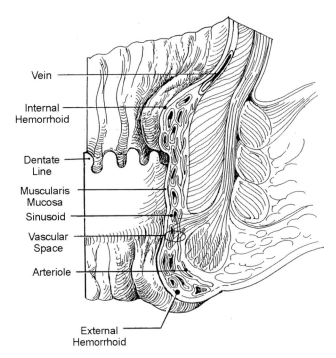

Vein

Internal
Hemorrhoid

Dentate
Line

Muscularis
Mucosa

Sinusoid

Vascular
Space

Arteriole

External
Hemorrhoid

FIGURE 11-1. Anal cushion showing Treitz's muscle derived from the conjoined longitudinal muscle of the anal canal.

obstruction of venous return, aging (deterioration of anal supporting tissues), and internal sphincter abnormalities. Patients with hemorrhoid disease have been shown to have increased anal resting pressures when compared with controls.[5,6] This increased resting pressure returns to normal after hemorrhoidectomy, but it is unclear whether the hemorrhoids are the cause of this increase.[7] Manometry also shows the presence of increased ultra slow waves in patients with hemorrhoid disease but the exact significance of this is unclear.[8] In pregnant women, approximately 0.2% require an urgent hemorrhoidectomy for incarcerated and prolapsed hemorrhoids.[9] Rigorous proof of the theories mentioned, however, is lacking. One of the most important etiologic theories is the "sliding anal cushion theory."[1] Thompson concluded that a sliding downward of the anal lining is responsible for the development of hemorrhoids. Repeated stretching of the anal supporting tissues (submucosal Treitz's muscle and elastic connective tissue framework) which normally functions to anchor and suspend the anal canal lining causes fragmentation of the supporting tissues and subsequent prolapse of the vascular cushions. Furthermore, straining and irregular bowel habits may be associated with engorgement of the vascular cushions making their displacement more likely. This theory is further supported by histologic studies that have shown deterioration of the anal supporting tissues by the third decade of life.[10] Additionally, vascular changes that seem to be associated with the development of hemorrhoids include increased arteriovenous communications, vascular hyperplasia, and increased neovascularization with increased CD105 immunoactivity.[3,5,11]

Epidemiology

The reported prevalence of hemorrhoids in the United States is 4.4%, peaking between the ages of 45 and 65. Increased prevalence rates are seen in Caucasians and in individuals with higher socioeconomic status.[12] Whether this is secondary to differences in health-seeking behavior rather than true prevalence remains to be proven. The prevalence of hemorrhoids is reported to have decreased during the later half of the 20th century; however, this is based on population-based surveys and needs to be interpreted with caution because it reflects self-reporting of symptoms without corroboration via physical examination.[13]

Classification

Hemorrhoids are divided into two types, external and internal. External hemorrhoids are located in the distal one-third of the anal canal, distal to the dentate line, and are covered by anoderm (modified squamous epithelium lacking any skin appendages) or by skin. Internal hemorrhoids are located proximal to the dentate line and are covered by columnar or transitional epithelium. Because this overlying tissue is viscerally innervated, it is not sensitive to touch, pain, or temperature, making it easily amenable to office procedures. Internal hemorrhoids are further subclassified into degrees based on size and clinical symptoms as initially reported by Banov et al.[14] (see Table 11-1). Mixed or combined hemorrhoids are defined as the presence of both internal and external hemorrhoids.

Symptoms

Patients with anal complaints from whatever etiology frequently present at the office complaining of "hemorrhoids or piles." Many patients referred or coming into the office complaining of "hemorrhoids" frequently are found to have other anal problems such as pruritus ani, anal fissures, fistulas, and skin tags. A careful history and physical examination including anoscopy by an experienced individual is mandatory and will frequently lead to the correct diagnosis. The presence, quantity, frequency, and timing of bleeding and prolapse should be noted. Patients with hemorrhoid disease may complain of bleeding, mucosal protrusion, pain, mucus, discharge, difficulties with perianal hygiene, a sensation of incomplete evacuation, and cosmetic deformity.[5,15] A thorough dietary and medication history should also be done because certain medications, diets, and or dietary indiscretions cause or exacerbate constipation or diarrhea.

Symptoms from external hemorrhoids are usually secondary to thrombosis and physical examination shows a tender, bluish-colored lump at the anus distal to the dentate line associated with acute pain. Thrombosed external hemorrhoids can bleed secondary to pressure necrosis and subsequent

Table 11-1. Classification of internal hemorrhoids

	First degree	Second degree	Third degree	Fourth degree
Finding	Bulge into the lumen of the anal canal ± painless bleeding	Protrude at the time of a bowel movement and reduce spontaneously	Protrude spontaneously or with bowel movement, require manual replacement	Permanently prolapsed and irreducible
Symptoms	Painless bleeding	• Painless bleeding • Anal mass with defecation • Anal burning or pruritus	• Painless bleeding • Anal mass with defecation • Feeling of incomplete evacuation • Mucous leakage • Fecal leakage • Perianal burning or pruritus ani • Difficulty with perianal hygiene	• Painless or painful bleeding • Irreducible anal mass • Feeling of incomplete evacuation • Mucous leakage • Fecal leakage • Perianal burning or pruritus ani • Difficulty with perianal hygiene
Signs	• Bright red bleeding • Bleeding at end of defecation • Blood drips or squirts into toilet • Bleeding may be occult	• Bright red bleeding • Prolapse with defecation	• Bright red bleeding • Blood drips or squirts into toilet • Prolapsed hemorrhoids reduce manually • Perianal stool or mucous • Anemia extremely rare	• Bright red bleeding • Blood drips or squirts into toilet • Prolapsed hemorrhoids always out • Perianal stool or mucous • Anemia extremely rare

ulceration of the overlying skin. External skin tags are folds of skin that arise from the anal verge. These tags may be the end result of prior episodes of thrombosed external hemorrhoids. Enlarged skin tags or external hemorrhoids may interfere with anal hygiene leading to perianal burning or pruritus.

Internal hemorrhoids are painless unless thrombosis, strangulation, gangrene, or prolapse with edema occurs. Despite what is written, patients will frequently come to the office complaining of "painful hemorrhoids" even when none of these conditions exist. Once other sources of pain are ruled out, careful inquiry regarding the description of their pain further elucidates that patients frequently describe their anal pain as "burning" in nature. This may be secondary to perianal irritation from mucous or fecal leakage leading to secondary pruritus ani. Bleeding from internal hemorrhoids is bright red and associated with bowel movements. The bleeding usually occurs at the end of defecation. The patient may complain of blood dripping or squirting into the toilet or blood on the toilet tissue. Bleeding may also be occult leading to guaiac-positive stools or rarely to anemia. Prolapse of the hemorrhoid cushions may manifest itself as an anal mass, mucous discharge, or a sensation of incomplete evacuation. The examiner should ascertain whether the hemorrhoids reduce spontaneously or require manual reduction.

Differential Diagnosis

Because most patients that come into the office or emergency room with anal symptomatology complain of "hemorrhoids," it is important to rule out other causes (see Table 11-2). If the patient's main complaint is anal pain, then other diagnoses should routinely be sought unless thrombosis or prolapse of hemorrhoids is obvious. The causes of pain are almost invariably found in pathology distal to the dentate line, i.e., fissure, abscess, fistula, external hemorrhoid thrombosis, or prolapsed thrombosed internal hemorrhoids.

Examination

After a general patient assessment, the patient is ideally examined in the prone jackknife position on a proctologic table. Patients with a history suggestive of hemorrhoid disease with an unremarkable examination in the prone jackknife position should be examined in a sitting position on the commode while asking the patient to strain. Oftentimes, pathology is uncovered when gravity assists in the examination. In patients who are unable to tolerate the jackknife position (morbidly obese, pregnant, elderly, patient with knee or hip

Table 11-2. Differential diagnoses

	Acute pain	Chronic pain	Bleeding	Pruritus or discharge	Lump or mass
Possible diagnoses	• Fissure • Abscess • Fistula • Thrombosed hemorrhoid	• Fissure • Abscess • Fistula • Anal stenosis • Anal Crohn's • Thrombosed hemorrhoid	• Fissure • Polyps • Colorectal cancer • Inflammatory bowel disease • Proctitis • Internal hemorrhoids • Ruptured thrombosed external hemorrhoid	• Fistula • Anal warts • Anal incontinence • Rectal prolapse • Pruritus ani • Hypertrophied anal papilla • Prolapsed hemorrhoid	• Abscess • Skin tags • Anal tumor • Rectal tumor • Rectal polyps • Rectal prolapse • Anal Crohn's • Prolapsed anal papilla • Thrombosed or prolapsed hemorrhoid

joint pathology, pulmonary disease) or when a proctologic table is not available, examination should be performed in the modified left lateral (Sims) position. The location of all anal pathology is described anatomically (anterior, posterior, left lateral, right lateral, etc.) and not by the numbers on the face of a clock. In this way, the pathology can easily be located regardless of what position the patient is in. Calmly reassure your patients at the start of the examination and routinely discuss what you are about to do before actually carrying out anal inspection, palpation, digital rectal examination, anoscopy, and proctoscopy, which should be performed on all patients if feasible.

Gentle spreading of the buttocks allows careful inspection of the squamous portion of the anal canal as well as the perianal, genital, perineal, and sacrococcygeal regions. Skin tags, external hemorrhoids, fissures, fistulas, infection, hemorrhoid prolapse, mucosal prolapse, rectal prolapse, tumors, skin lesions, thrombosis, and rashes all can be diagnosed on careful visual inspection if present. Palpation of the perianal region can localize pain, tenderness, induration, or masses. Digital examination gently performed localizes pain, masses, abscesses, and assesses sphincter tone. Anoscopy permits visualization of the anoderm and internal hemorrhoidal cushions. Anoscopy is best performed with a side-viewing anoscope especially when hemorrhoid ligation is being considered. A multi-slotted anoscope is also available and was developed to facilitate the synchronous exposure and placement of multiple hemorrhoid bands without the need to reposition the anoscope. This may offer less postligation pain and decreased need for repeat ligation in comparison to the conventional anoscope for banding.[16] Although the degree of prolapse may be ascertained if the patient is asked to strain, a more accurate assessment of prolapse can be made if inspection takes place while the patient is sitting and straining on a commode. Proctoscopy or flexible sigmoidoscopy must be performed when possible to assess the rectum and lower colon for neoplasms and inflammatory bowel disease.

At a minimum, all patients with anorectal complaints must undergo anoscopy, rigid proctosigmoidoscopy, and/or flexible sigmoidoscopy and further work-up depends on findings at physical examination, patient age, and history. Although patients may be too uncomfortable to undergo these procedures at the initial visit, it is important that they are performed before discharging the patient from your care. Sole reliance on a patient's description of hematochezia to make a diagnosis is inaccurate and further workup is warranted.[17] Practice guidelines from the American Society for Gastrointestinal Endoscopy and the Society for Surgery of the Alimentary Tract suggest, at a minimum, anoscopy and flexible sigmoidoscopy for bright-red rectal bleeding.[18] Total colon examination via colonoscopy or air-contrast barium enema is indicated when no source is evident on anorectal examination, the bleeding is atypical for hemorrhoids, anemia or Hemoccult-positive stool is present, or significant risk factors for colonic neoplasia exist (age, family history, or personal history of polyps).[18–20] Because hemorrhoids are rarely the cause of anemia (0.5 patients/100,000 population), total colon examination is indicated even in the very young patient.[21,22] Patients less than 40 years of age with hemorrhoid disease compatible with their symptomatology probably require no further work-up. Patients older than 40 years of age with minimal hemorrhoid disease, additional symptoms, or positive family history for colorectal cancer should undergo a total colon examination with either a colonoscopy or double contrast barium enema to identify other etiologies for bleeding that are not obvious on initial examination.

Treatment

Treatment for symptomatic internal hemorrhoids varies from simple reassurance to operative hemorrhoidectomy. Treatments are classified into three categories: 1) dietary and lifestyle modification; 2) nonoperative/office procedures; and 3) operative hemorrhoidectomy. In general, less symptomatic hemorrhoids, such as those that cause only minor bleeding, can be treated with simple measures such as dietary modification, change in defecatory habits, or office procedures. More symptomatic hemorrhoids such as third or fourth degree are more likely to require operative intervention.

Dietary and Lifestyle Modification

Because prolonged attempts at defecation, either secondary to constipation or diarrhea, have been implicated in the development of hemorrhoids, the main goal of this treatment is to minimize straining at stool. This is usually achieved by increasing fluid and fiber in the diet, recommending exercise, and adding supplemental fiber agents (psyllium) to the diet in patients unable to consume sufficient amounts of fiber in their diets. Despite common teaching, little good evidence exists regarding the benefit of fiber in preventing or managing hemorrhoid disease. Reduced hemorrhoidal bleeding has been shown with the use of psyllium in a double-blind, placebo controlled trial; however, other studies are less favorable.[23–26] Psyllium works in conjunction with water to add moisture to the stool and subsequently decrease constipation. Psyllium may also be therapeutic in treating diarrhea. It may add bulk to liquid stools therefore increasing the consistency and decreasing the volume. Dietary modification with fiber supplementation (psyllium, methylcellulose, calcium polycarbophil) is one of the mainstays of therapy for patients with hemorrhoidal disease. In the majority of cases, symptoms of bleeding and pain improve over a 6-week period. A diet high in fiber (20–35 g/day) including the consumption of plenty of fruits and vegetables is recommended especially if the patient has a history of constipation or straining. A common problem with fiber supplementation is noncompliance because of either poor palatability or symptoms of bloating, increased flatus, and abdominal cramps. Compliance is improved by

TABLE 11-3. Fiber supplements

Type of fiber	Trade name	Available fiber
Psyllium	Metamucil™	3.4 g/teaspoon
	Metamucil capsules™	0.52 g/capsule
	Konsyl™	6.0 g/teaspoon
Methylcellulose	Citrucel™	2.0 g/dose
Calcium polycarbophil	FiberCon™	0.5 g/capsule
	Konsyl fiber tablets™	0.5 g/tablet

starting at lower doses and slowly increasing the quantity of fiber ingested until the desired stool consistency is achieved. Some common fiber products currently available are listed in Table 11-3. If dietary modification fails to relieve symptoms, then further therapy is indicated (see Table 11-4).

Frequently, a change in defecatory habits will resolve symptoms. Oftentimes, simply asking an individual to curtail reading on the commode resolves the hemorrhoidal symptoms. Lifestyle and dietary modifications along with ruling out proximal sources of bleeding are all that is required for the majority of patients complaining of hemorrhoidal disease.

Medical Therapy

Rigorous levels of evidence do not exist to support the use of topical therapies, whether physical or pharmacologic (sitz baths, anesthetics, phlebotonics, corticosteroids, or ice). Most studies have used poor methods with lack of controls, multiple associated components, and heterogeneous preparations. Therefore, firm recommendations cannot be made at the time of the writing of this chapter. Cochrane reviews on related registered Cochrane titles are listed in Table 11-5.[27–29]

Despite the lack of any rigorous evidence, probably the most effective topical treatment for the relief of symptoms comes in the way of warm (40°C) sitz baths. Soaking time should be limited (15 minutes) to prevent edema of the perianal and perineal skin. The application of ice packs to the anal region also may relieve symptoms and is acceptable provided that contact time is not prolonged. Pharmaceutical preparations such as creams, ointments, foams, and suppositories have little pharmacologic rationale in the management of hemorrhoidal disease. Suppositories never remain within the anal canal and usually end up in the lower rectum where they may provide an emollient effect or lubrication to the stool. Popular topical soothing agents are frequently combined with corticosteroids and or anesthetics. Although individuals may report empirical symptomatic benefit with their use, patients must be advised against prolonged use because of possible local allergic effects or sensitization of the skin.

There have been several phlebotonics that have been evaluated in the literature. Citrus bioflavonoids and related substances are widely used in Europe to treat diseases of the blood vessels and lymph system, including hemorrhoids, chronic venous insufficiency, leg ulcers, easy bruising, nosebleeds, and lymphedema after breast cancer surgery. These compounds are thought to work by strengthening the walls of blood vessels, increasing venous tone, lymphatic drainage, and normalizing capillary permeability. The major bioflavonoids found in citrus fruits are diosmin, hesperidin, rutin, naringin, tangeretin, diosmetin, narirutin, neohesperidin, nobiletin, and quercetin. Flavonoids are reported to have numerous health benefits. They are the natural pigments in fruits and vegetables. Our body cannot produce bioflavonoids. Diosmin (Daflon) is

TABLE 11-4. Management of internal hemorrhoids by classification

Treatments	First degree	Second degree	Third degree	Fourth degree	Acute prolapse with thrombosis
Dietary	X	X	X	X	X
Banding	X	X	X		
Sclerotherapy	X	X	X		
Infrared coagulation	X	X	X		
Excisional hemorrhoidectomy			X	X	Emergent
Stapled hemorrhoidopexy		X	X	X (?)	
Multiple thrombectomies and multiple bandings					X

TABLE 11-5. Registered Cochrane review titles on hemorrhoid management

Cochrane review title	Author	Primary aim
Laxatives and topical treatments for hemorrhoids[27]	Alonso-Coello and Lopez-Yarto[27]	To determine the efficacy of laxatives and topical treatments in improving the symptoms derived from symptomatic hemorrhoids
Nonoperative treatment for hemorrhoidal disease[28]	Thaha, Campbell, and Steele[28]	To determine the long-term therapeutic efficacy of various nonoperative treatment methods in controlling hemorrhoidal symptoms
Phlebotonics for hemorrhoids[29]	Alonso, Johanson, Lopez-Yarto,[29] and Martinez	To determine the efficacy of phlebotonics in improving the symptoms derived from symptomatic hemorrhoids
Circular stapled anopexy versus excisional hemorrhoidectomy for the treatment of hemorrhoidal disease	Thaha, Campbell, Staines, Nyström, Steele[180–182]	To assess stapled anopexy with excisional methods

probably the best studied but has not been approved for use in the United States.[30–32] Other phlebotonics include:

Natural products: flavonoids;[33,34] rutosides[35–37] (troxerutin, buckwheat herb extract, *Ruscus aculeatus*), diosmine, hidrosmin, gingko biloba, saponosides; escin (horse chestnut seed extract).

Synthetic products: calcium dobesilate, naftazone, aminaftone, chromocarbe, and others: iquinosa, flunarizine, sulfomucopolysaccharide.

Calcium dobesilate (calcium 2,5-dihydroxybenzenesulfonate) is a drug with previously demonstrated efficacy in the treatment of diabetic retinopathy and chronic venous insufficiency. These beneficial effects of the drug are related to its ability to decrease capillary permeability, platelet aggregation, and blood viscosity and to increase lymphatic transport. A randomized, double-blind, controlled study was conducted to investigate the efficacy of oral calcium dobesilate therapy in treating acute attacks of internal hemorrhoids. Twenty-nine well-documented adult patients with first- or second-degree internal hemorrhoids were treated with calcium dobesilate for 2 weeks, whereas 16 patients received only a high-fiber diet to serve as control. The symptom and anoscopic inflammation scores obtained with calcium dobesilate treatment were significantly better than those with diet only ($P = .0017$ and $P = .0013$, respectively). Together with recommendations about diet and bowel discipline, oral calcium dobesilate treatment provided efficient, fast, and safe symptomatic relief from acute symptoms of hemorrhoidal disease. This symptomatic healing is associated with a significant improvement in the anoscopically observed inflammation.[38] Symptomatic improvement has been shown in other studies but results are not always consistent, especially when fiber is included.[30–32,39]

Office Treatments

Rubber Band Ligation

Rubber band ligation is a method of tissue fixation and one of the most widely used techniques in the United States. It can be used to treat first-, second-, and third-degree internal hemorrhoids. The most common method currently in use for the outpatient treatment for hemorrhoids was originally described by Barron[40] in 1963. He reported satisfactory results in 150 patients, the majority of which were treated in the outpatient setting. The rubber band is placed on the redundant mucosa a minimum of 2 cm above the dentate line which causes strangulation of the blood supply to the banded tissue, which sloughs off in 5–7 days leaving a small ulcer that heals and fixes the tissue to the underlying sphincter. Rubber band ligation is frequently recommended for individuals with first- or second-degree hemorrhoids and, in some circumstances, third-degree hemorrhoids.

Several commercially available types of hemorrhoid ligators are available including a suction ligator (McGown™,

Pembroke Pines, FL) (see Figure 11-2A) that draws the hemorrhoid tissue into the ligating barrel via suction, and closing the handle inserts a band around the hemorrhoid.[41] The advantage of this ligator is that only one hand is required for placement of the band, making an assistant unnecessary for the procedure. The disadvantage of the suction ligator is that the ligating barrel is smaller than other ligators, hence less tissue is banded. With the conventional ligators, an atraumatic clamp is used to draw hemorrhoid tissue into the barrel of the ligator and a small rubber band is placed (see Figure 11-2B). A disadvantage compared with the suction ligator is that two hands are required for placement of a band necessitating an additional assistant for the procedure. An advantage is that a greater amount of excess hemorrhoid tissue can be eliminated with these ligators. Ligation of internal hemorrhoids using an endoscopic variceal ligator has been shown to be safe and reportedly controls bleeding and prolapse in approximately 95% and 90% of patients, respectively, with a major complication rate of less than 4%.[42–44] Malposition of bands utilizing the endoscopic ligator approach requiring their removal has been reported as high as 5% in patients.[43] Cost effectiveness of this endoscopic ligation procedure has not been compared with hemorrhoid banding with traditional instruments. An alternative device developed for hemorrhoid banding consists of a disposable syringe-like hemorrhoid ligator, invented to

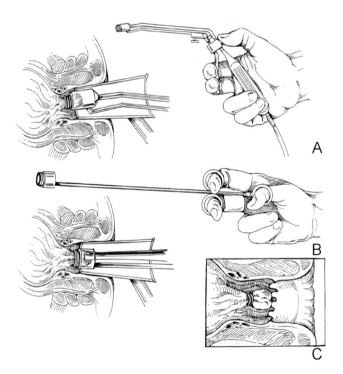

FIGURE 11-2. Banding an internal hemorrhoid. **A** The internal hemorrhoid is teased into the barrel of the ligating gun with a McGown suction ligator, or **B** a McGivney type ligator. **C** The apex of the banded hemorrhoid is well above the dentate line in order to minimize pain. (Reprinted from Beck D, Wexner S. Fundamentals of Anorectal Surgery. 2nd ed. Copyright 1998, with permission from Elsevier.)

simplify the banding procedure for both patient and surgeon[45] (see Figure 11-3). This single-operator ligator, with its own suction mechanism, was designed for use without the need of an assistant or an anoscope. By pointing the ligator directly toward the appropriate site and by measuring the distance from the anal margin using reference markings on the ligator, the bands can be placed accurately in a blind manner inside the rectum for the treatment of symptomatic internal hemorrhoids. Before the band is discharged, rotating the ligator 180 degrees while applying suction will alert the operator if the application site is not appropriate. O'Regan[45] reported a 97% success rate with two major complications (one episode of bleeding and one of perianal sepsis) in 480 patients.

Rubber band ligation can be performed safely with the patient in various positions; however, the prone jackknife position provides the best exposure. Anesthesia is not required for this procedure. Rectal preparation with enemas is not required but may be used if desired. A standard

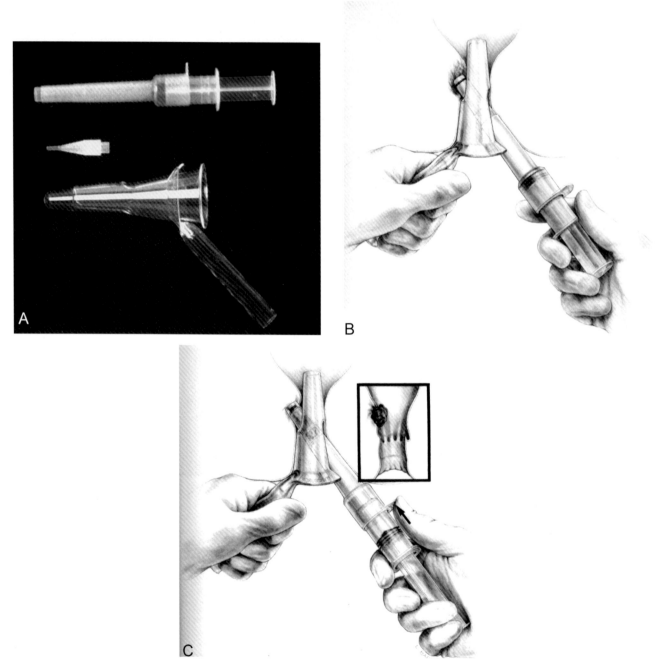

FIGURE 11-3. **A** O'Regan disposable banding system (Medsurge Medical Products Corp., Vancouver, Canada). **B, C** Technique of internal hemorrhoid ligation using the O'Regan ligating system.

commercially available ligator, good lighting, and a slotted anoscope are all that is required. The largest hemorrhoid bundle is routinely banded first. A single or double band is placed on one hemorrhoid bundle. Care is taken to place the band at least 2–3 cm above the dentate line approximately at the level of the anorectal ring or apex of the hemorrhoid. It is imperative to avoid banding too close to the dentate line or incorporating internal sphincter into the ligator because this can potentially lead to severe pain or pelvic sepsis. It has been shown that multiple hemorrhoid groups can be banded at a single session with no significant increase in morbidity when compared with single ligation.[16,46–50] Some surgeons prefer banding one group initially to monitor patient response and then perform multiple bandings at a subsequent session if the initial banding was well tolerated.

Patients are instructed that normal activities may be resumed immediately after banding and they may experience a feeling of incomplete evacuation or anal pressure. Approximately 5–7 days after the procedure, the banded tissue sloughs off at which time the patient may notice a small amount of bleeding. Patients should be advised to avoid aspirin or platelet-altering drugs after banding for a period of 7–10 days to minimize delayed hemorrhage; however, there is no level I evidence to support this recommendation. It is an absolute contraindication to band patients on sodium warfarin or heparin therapy because subsequent sloughing of tissue may lead to massive hemorrhage.

Complications of hemorrhoid banding include pain, thrombosis, bleeding, and life-threatening perineal or pelvic sepsis. The most common complication of rubber band ligation is pain, which is reported in 5%–60% of patients.[21,48,51–53] Pain is usually minor and relieved with sitz baths and analgesics. A dull, persistent ache is common for the first 1–2 days after banding. Significant anal pain is rare but is often secondary to a malpositioned rubber band placed too close to the dentate line. If the pain is experienced immediately after the banding, then the rubber band can be removed with a hooked cutting probe or hooked scissors. The subsequent development of aching pain is generally treated with sitz baths and analgesics. Constipation should be avoided during this period because it has been shown to worsen the outcome of rubber band ligation.[54] Rarely, hemorrhoid banding can result in thrombosis of internal and external hemorrhoids resulting in significant pain. Bleeding when it occurs is generally minor and occurs immediately after banding or 7–10 days later when the band falls off. Massive bleeding is a rare occurrence but may require operative intervention to control persistent hemorrhage. This may be minimized by having patients withhold aspirin or other nonsteroidals during the postbanding period. Other complications such as abscess, thrombosis, band slippage, priapism, and urinary dysfunction occur in less than 5% of patients.[55] There have been several reported cases of life-threatening perineal and/or pelvic sepsis after hemorrhoid banding.[56–58] This necrotizing perineal or pelvic sepsis is rare but mandates emergent attention. The triad of increasing pain, fever, and urinary dysfunction or retention either alone or together suggests the diagnosis.[59] These patients require intensive care unit admission, intravenous antibiotics, emergent examination under anesthesia, and debridement of all necrotic tissue. The risk of necrotizing infection seems to be increased in individuals with immune compromised states, including patients with uncontrolled acquired immunodeficiency syndrome, neutropenia, and severe diabetes mellitus.[60] Although the evidence is anecdotal in nature, caution is recommended in selecting these patients for rubber band ligation treatment.

Success rates with rubber band ligation will vary depending on length of follow-up, degree treated, and criteria for success.[21,49,53,61] Approximately two-thirds to three-quarters of all individuals with first- and second-degree hemorrhoids respond to banding although this may need to be repeated at a later date.[54,62,63] More than one banding session is usually required. The majority of patients experience relief of symptoms without further treatment. As previously mentioned, hemorrhoids can be banded at a single session or at multiple sessions. A retrospective study comparing single versus multiple banding identified greater discomfort (29% versus 4.5%) and more vasovagal symptoms (12.3% versus 0%) with multiple hemorrhoids being banded at a single session.[49] Bat et al.[55] prospectively studied complications in 512 patients undergoing hemorrhoid banding. Minor complications developed in 4.6% of patients including pain, band slippage, mucosal ulcer, and priapism. Hospitalization for major complications was necessary in 2.5%, and included massive hemorrhage, severe pain, urinary retention, and perianal sepsis. Savioz et al.[62] investigated relapse rates after banding in 92 individuals. They found 23% of patients required repeat banding over 5 years and 32% at 10 years, and believed hemorrhoid banding to be a durable procedure. Bayer et al.[64] followed 2934 patients banded over a 12-year period. Seventy-nine percent required no further therapy, whereas 18% required repeat banding because of recurrence. Hemorrhoidectomy was necessary in 2.1% related to persistent symptoms.

Infrared Photocoagulation, Bipolar Diathermy, and Direct-Current Electrotherapy

These techniques rely on coagulation, obliteration, and scarring which eventually produce fixation of the hemorrhoid tissue. Infrared photocoagulation utilizes infrared radiation generated by a tungsten-halogen lamp applied onto the hemorrhoid tissue through a solid quartz light guide[65] (Redfield Corporation, Montvale, NJ) (see Figure 11-4). The infrared coagulator light is converted to heat which coagulates tissue protein and evaporates water from cells leading to inflammation, eschar formation, and eventual scarring which assists in fixation of the hemorrhoid group.

The amount of destruction depends on the intensity and the duration of application. The procedure is performed by applying the tip of the infrared coagulator near the apex of the

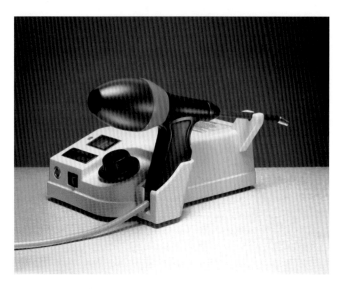

Figure 11-4. Infrared coagulator IRC2100™ (Redfield Corporation, Rochelle Park, NJ).

hemorrhoid for a 1.0- to 1.5-second pulse of energy. Approximately three to four applications per hemorrhoid are performed and one to three hemorrhoids undergo treatment per session.[53] The application of the tip to the hemorrhoid produces a 3- to 4-mm^2-diameter area of coagulation with a depth of penetration of approximately 2.5 mm that ulcerates and scars in 2 weeks providing fixation of the hemorrhoid and cessation of bleeding[66] (see Figure 11-5). Complications are very infrequent and may include pain or fissure secondary to inappropriate placement of the tip too close to the dentate line

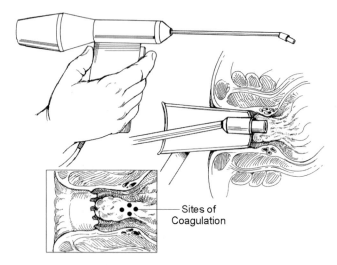

Sites of Coagulation

Figure 11-5. Infrared photocoagulation. The infrared photocoagulator creates a small thermal injury. Thus, several applications are required for each hemorrhoidal column. [Reprinted from Beck D. Hemorrhoids. Handbook of Colorectal Surgery. 2nd ed. Copyright 2003 by Taylor & Francis Group LLC (B). Reproduced with permission of Taylor & Francis Group LLC (B) in the format Textbook via Copyright Clearance Center.]

or bleeding caused by excessive application of the probe tip. The infrared coagulator works best with small, bleeding, first- and second-degree hemorrhoids. It has been described to be slightly less painful than rubber banding.[67] In three randomized trials, hemorrhoid bleeding was successfully controlled in the majority of patients with first- and second-degree hemorrhoids.[53,66,67]

Bipolar diathermy or coagulation (BICAP; Circon ACMI, Stamford, CT) is essentially electrocautery in which the heat does not penetrate as deeply as in monopolar coagulation.[68,69] The diathermy is applied in 1-second pulses at approximately 20 watts until the underlying tissue coagulates. The depth of injury is 2.2 mm and, unlike infrared photocoagulation, the depth does not increase with multiple applications at the same site which frequently is necessary.[66,69] First-, second-, and third-degree hemorrhoids have been treated with success rates varying from 88% to 100% whereas up to 20% of patients may need excisional hemorrhoidectomy for prolapsing tissue.[21,51,66,68–70]

Direct-current electrotherapy is applied through a probe placed via an anoscope onto the mucosa at the apex of the hemorrhoid. Application of the 110-volt direct current is set to the maximal tolerable level (approximately 16 mA) and then left in place for approximately 10 minutes.[51,69–73] Multiple treatments are required to the same site in up to 30% of patients with second- and third-degree hemorrhoids.[71] Adequate control of bleeding in up to 88% of patients is obtained when adequate current levels and contact time are used.[51,69] This technique, however, has not been widely accepted primarily because of the lengthy treatment times and limited effect in higher-degree hemorrhoids.[73] Reported complications include pain, ulcer formation, and bleeding.

Sclerotherapy

This office method relies on the injection of chemical agents into hemorrhoids that create fibrosis, scarring, shrinkage, and fixation of the hemorrhoid by obliterating the vascularity with a sclerosant solution. This procedure takes minutes to perform in the office and does not require anesthesia. Frequently used agents include 5% phenol in oil, 5% quinine and urea, or hypertonic salt solution. Approximately 2–3 mL of the sclerosant is injected into the submucosa of each hemorrhoid bundle at least 1 cm proximal to the dentate line with a 25-guage spinal needle or specialized hemorrhoid needle (Gabriel). Care should be taken to avoid intramucosal or intramuscular injection in order to prevent mucosal sloughing with ulceration or excessive pain, respectively. Sclerotherapy should not be performed in the face of anorectal infection or with prolapsed thrombosed hemorrhoids. Sclerotherapy can be used in patients on long- or short-term anticoagulation. Repetitive sclerotherapy should be used with caution because of the potential of scarring and stricture formation. Complications are infrequent and usually related to incorrect placement of the sclerosant.[53,74] Rarely, a patient may develop impotence, urinary symptoms, or an abscess secondary to a misplaced injection or granulomatous reaction to the oil-based sclerosant.[75] Sclerotherapy works best for first- and second-degree hemorrhoids. Walker et al.[53] reported a 30% recurrence rate of symptoms 4 years after initial successful injection. Khoury et al.[76] performed a prospective, randomized study in 120 consecutive patients looking at single versus multiple phenol injections for the treatment of hemorrhoids in patients who have had prior medical therapy. Results from that study showed that injection sclerotherapy, whether single or multiple, is an effective form of therapy for patients with first- or second-degree hemorrhoids with improvement or cure in almost 90% of patients.[76] Another randomized, prospective study, however, showed no difference in bleeding rates at 6 months follow-up when comparing sclerotherapy plus bulk laxative to bulk laxative alone.[77]

Anal Dilatation or Stretch

This method of treating hemorrhoids by manual dilatation of the anus was reported and popularized by Lord in 1968.[78] Although it has had its proponents, primarily in European countries, subsequent reports have shown endosonographic evidence of sphincter injury as well as high rates of associated incontinence especially with long-term follow-up.[79–81] In addition to its higher failure rate in comparison to surgical hemorrhoidectomy, and because of the risk of incontinence, most authorities advocate abandoning this approach for the treatment of hemorrhoids.[81,82]

Cryotherapy

Cryotherapy is based on the concept that freezing the internal hemorrhoid at low temperatures can lead to tissue destruction. A special probe is required through which nitrous oxide at $-60°$ to $-80°C$ or liquid nitrogen at $-196°C$ is circulated. Initial enthusiasm with cryotherapy essentially has disappeared because of very disappointing results. The procedure is time consuming and associated with a foul-smelling profuse discharge, irritation, and pain.[83–85] Furthermore, improper application can lead to anal stenosis and or incontinence from sphincter destruction. The procedure should no longer be recommended for the treatment of internal hemorrhoids.

External Hemorrhoids

Acute Thrombosis

Patients with a thrombosed external hemorrhoid typically present with complaints of a painful mass in the perianal region. The pain is frequently described as burning in nature. The pain associated with the abrupt onset of an anal mass usually peaks at around 48 hours and subsides significantly after the fourth day (see Figure 11-6). The skin overlying the thrombosed hemorrhoid may necrose and ulcerate, resulting in bleeding, discharge, or infection.

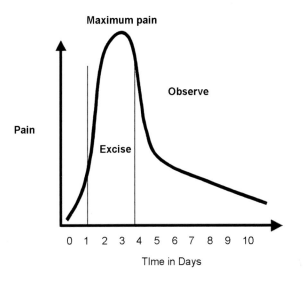

FIGURE 11-6. Timing of excision of a thrombosed external hemorrhoid.

Treatment should be aimed at relief of pain. The management will depend, therefore, on the patient's symptoms at the time seen. If the pain is intense, then excision of the thrombosed external hemorrhoid should be offered. If the pain is subsiding, then conservative nonoperative management is warranted. Nonoperative treatment consists of warm sitz baths, nonconstipating analgesics, and bulk-producing fiber supplements. Anoscopy and proctoscopy to rule out associated anorectal disease are postponed to a later date when the patient is not in acute pain.

The operative treatment of a thrombosed external hemorrhoid demands excision of the entire thrombus. This can be done in the clinic, office, or emergency room under local anesthesia (0.5% lidocaine mixed with equal amounts of 0.25% bupivacaine containing 1:200,000 epinephrine). The overlying skin and surrounding area are prepped with Betadine swabs or alcohol and then anesthetized. A small radial elliptical incision is performed directly over the thrombosed hemorrhoid and the thrombus is excised in total with the aid of a fine scissors and forceps. Hemostasis is obtained with either Monsel's solution (ferric subsulfate) on cotton-tipped applicator or with silver nitrate. Although the skin edges can be reapproximated loosely with absorbable sutures, leaving the wounds open to heal by secondary intention gives greater assurance that rethrombosis will not occur in the same location. Postoperatively the patients are given a prescription for analgesics, instructed to take warm sitz baths two to three times daily, and to take bulk-producing fiber supplements.

Operative Hemorrhoidectomy

Hemorrhoidectomy is indicated for patients with symptomatic combined internal and external hemorrhoids who have failed or are not candidates for nonoperative treatments. This would include patients with extensive disease, patients with

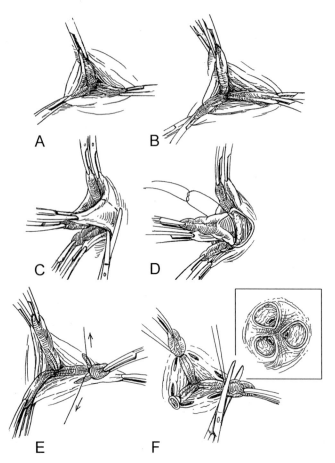

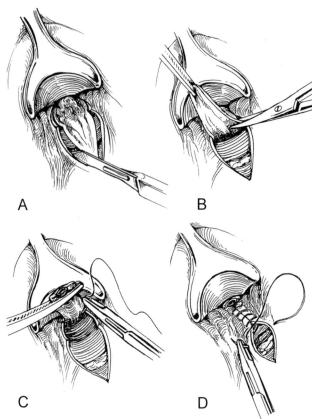

FIGURE 11-7. Open (Milligan-Morgan) hemorrhoidectomy. **A** External hemorrhoids grasped with forceps and retracted outward. **B** Internal hemorrhoids grasped with forceps and retracted outward with external hemorrhoids. **C** External skin and hemorrhoid excised with scissors. **D** Suture placed through proximal internal hemorrhoid and vascular bundle. **E** Ligature tied. **F** Tissue distal to ligature is excised. Insert depicts completed three bundle hemorrhoidectomy.

FIGURE 11-8. Modified Ferguson excisional hemorrhoidectomy. **A** Double elliptical incision made in mucosa and anoderm around hemorrhoidal bundle with a scalpel. **B** The hemorrhoid dissection is carefully continued cephalad by dissecting the sphincter away from the hemorrhoid. **C** After dissection of the hemorrhoid to its pedicle, it is either clamped, secured, or excised. The pedicle is suture ligated. **D** The wound is closed with a running stitch. Excessive traction on the suture is avoided to prevent forming dog ears or displacing the anoderm caudally.

concomitant conditions such as fissure or fistula, and patients with a preference for operative therapy. Only about 5%–10% of patients need surgical hemorrhoidectomy.[15,86] Recurrence with operative hemorrhoidectomy is uncommon and hemorrhoidectomy is the most effective treatment for hemorrhoids, especially those that are third degree.[87,88] Hemorrhoidectomy can be performed using a variety of techniques or instruments; however, most are variants of either a closed or open technique.[89,90] The Milligan-Morgan technique (open) is widely used in the United Kingdom (Figure 11-7). It involves excision of the external and internal hemorrhoid components leaving the skin defects open to heal by secondary intention over a 4- to 8-week period.[90] The Ferguson hemorrhoidectomy (closed) involves excision of the external and internal hemorrhoid components with closure of the skin defects primarily (Figure 11-8).[89]

Circular excision of the internal hemorrhoids and prolapsing rectal mucosa proximal to the dentate line has also been described for the surgical management of hemorrhoids (Whitehead procedure, Figure 11-9).[91–94] This technique involves circumferential excision of hemorrhoidal veins and mucosa beginning at the dentate line and proceeding proximally. It was used often in Great Britain but has fallen out of favor. It is rarely used in the United States because of technical difficulties and the potential for ectropion but has attracted the attention of some surgeons using a modification of the original technique.[93,95]

Table 11-6 lists four randomized prospective studies comparing open versus closed hemorrhoidectomy.[96–99] The majority of trials showed no difference in pain, analgesic use, hospital stay, and complications, whereas complete wound healing shows mixed results. There essentially seems to be no difference in both techniques and, therefore, recommendations for either should be based on surgeon experience and patient preference.

One of the most significant obstacles to patients seeking surgical management of their hemorrhoids is postoperative pain. Narcotics are often required to control pain and patients are frequently not back to their usual activities including work for 2–4 weeks.[100–103] A number of trials have looked at results with a variety of different excision techniques including scissors, diathermy, laser, bipolar diathermy (LigaSure™; Valleylab, Boulder, CO), and the ultrasonically activated scalpel.[104–117] Although some of these newer instruments have come into vogue for performing operative hemorrhoidectomy such as the Harmonic Scalpel® or LigaSure™ device, no long-term results have been published utilizing these modalities[104,105,113] (see Tables 11-7 and 11-8). Furthermore, the additional costs accrued through the use of this equipment and the lack of documented superior results with these techniques precludes recommendation for routine use. The majority of randomized trials have shown no difference between diathermy or scissor excision hemorrhoidectomy[106,116,117] (see Table 11-7). Laser hemorrhoidectomy was initially suggested to be associated with decreased postoperative pain; however, a randomized trial comparing Nd:YAG laser versus cold scalpel did not detect any difference.[107–109] Furthermore, the trial reported increased costs and decreased wound healing with use of the laser.[109]

Other strategies or procedures developed in an attempt to reduce postoperative pain include use of limited incisions, suturing the vascular pedicle without any incisions, performing a concomitant lateral internal sphincterotomy, use of metronidazole, using anal sphincter relaxants, injecting local anesthetics, using anxiolytics, and parasympathomimetics. All these strategies, however, have had mixed results and therefore cannot be recommended for routine use.[118–127]

Complications associated with hemorrhoidectomy include urinary retention (2%–36%), bleeding (0.03%–6%), anal stenosis (0%–6%), infection (0.5%–5.5%), and incontinence (2%–12%).[86,107,109,128–134]

Another method recently developed to reduce pain and treat hemorrhoidal disease has recently come into favor. Over the past 6–7 years, stapled "hemorrhoidectomy" has been developed as an alternative to standard Ferguson or Milligan-Morgan hemorrhoidectomy mainly because of the pain associated with traditional hemorrhoid surgery. It was first alluded to by Pescatori et al.[135] for mucosal prolapse but refined by Longo[136] using a specially developed circular stapling device (see Figure 11-10). The procedure involves the use of a specially designed circular stapler (Ethicon Endo-Surgery), which performs a circumferential resection of mucosa and submucosa above the hemorrhoids and then staples closed the

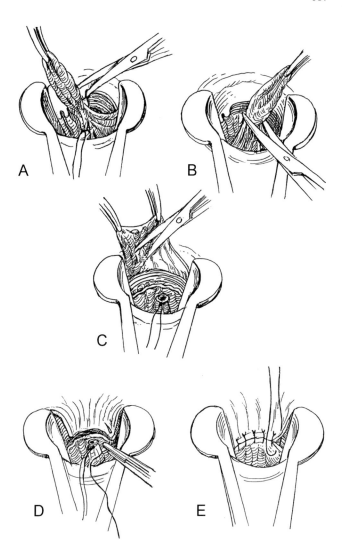

FIGURE 11-9. Whitehead hemorrhoidectomy. **A** Suture placed through proximal internal hemorrhoid for orientation. Excision started at dentate line and continued to proximal bundle. **B** Internal hemorrhoidal tissue excised above ligated bundle. **C** Vascular tissue excised from underside of elevated anoderm. **D** End of anoderm reapproximated with sutures to original location of dentate line. **E** Completed procedure.

defect (see Figure 11-11). This procedure is more of a hemorrhoidopexy than a hemorrhoidectomy and is also known by other names (stapled anopexy, stapled prolapsectomy, stapled circumferential mucosectomy). None of the hemorrhoids are necessarily removed by this procedure, rather they are simply returned to their physiologic position. The preservation of the

TABLE 11-6. Randomized, prospective studies of open versus closed hemorrhoidectomy

Author	N	Pain	Complete wound healing	Analgesics	Hospital stay	Complications
Ho	67	n.s.	O > C	n.s.	n.s.	n.s.
Carapeti	36	n.s.	n.s.	n.s.	n.s.	n.s.
Arbman	77	n.s	C > O	n.s.	n.s.	n.s.
Gencosmanoglu	80	C > O	C > O	C > O	n.s.	C > O

C, close; O, open; n.s., not significant.

TABLE 11-7. Randomized, prospective studies of LigaSure™ versus diathermy hemorrhoidectomy

Author	N	Operative time	Blood loss	Hospital Stay	Postoperative pain	Complications
Jayne	40	L < D	L < D	L < D	n.s.	n.s.
Palazzo	34	L < D	?	n.s.	n.s.	n.s.
Franklin	34	L < D	?	n.s.	L < D	?

L, LigaSure™; D, diathermy; n.s., not significant; ?, not reported; N, number.

TABLE 11-8. Randomized, prospective studies of ultrasonic scalpel (Harmonic) versus diathermy hemorrhoidectomy

Author	N	OR time	Postoperative pain	QOL	Complications
Khan	30	n.s.	Day 1 = n.s. Day 7 HS > D	n.s.	n.s.
Tan	50	n.s.	n.s.	?	n.s.
Armstrong	50	?	H < D	?	n.s.
Chung*	86	NS	H < BS H < S	n.s.	n.s.

H, Harmonic Scalpel; D, diathermy; n.s., not significant; BS, bipolar scissors; S, scissors; QOL, quality of life.
*This study compared results between the ultrasonic scalpel and either bipolar scissors or regular scissors.

anal cushions within the anal canal may in fact contribute to the low rate of incontinence after this operation. This procedure can be used for patients with all degrees of hemorrhoids, however is best reserved for patients with second- and third-degree hemorrhoids that do not respond to banding and fourth-degree hemorrhoids that are reducible under anesthesia.[137] The cost and anesthetic risks do not make stapling a practical option for grade 1 and 2 disease, which should continue to be treated with traditional methods. The stapling

device cuts and staples well above the dentate line, therefore postoperative pain is minimal, and usually absent. The stapling procedure does not create any external wounds.

A number of randomized, controlled trials comparing stapled hemorrhoidopexy with conventional hemorrhoidectomy have been published as well as reviewed and are listed in Table 11-9.[100–103,138–149] Cochrane review on a registered Cochrane title comparing stapled anopexy with excisional methods is pending. The majority of studies show that stapled

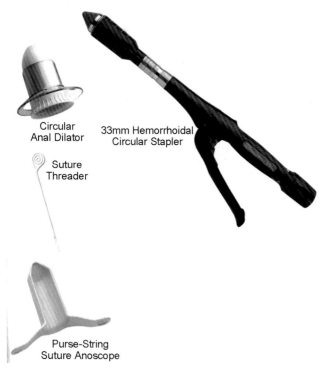

FIGURE 11-10. Second generation PPH-03 hemorrhoid stapler. Shown are 33-mm hemorrhoidal circular stapler, suture threader, circular anal dilator, and pursestring suture anoscope. (Reprinted with permission from Ethicon Endo-Surgery.)

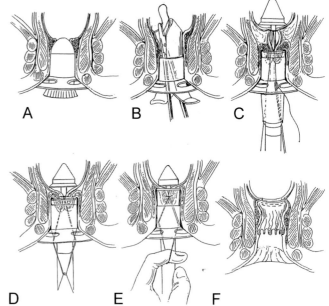

FIGURE 11-11. Stapled anoplasty (procedure for prolapse and hemorrhoids). **A** Retracting anoscope and dilator inserted. **B** Monofilament pursestring suture (eight bites) placed using operating anoscope approximately 3–4 cm above anal verge. **C** Stapler inserted through pursestring. Pursestring suture tied and ends of suture manipulated through stapler. **D** Retracting on suture pulls anorectal mucosa into stapler. **E** Stapler closed and fired. **F** Completed procedure.

TABLE 11-9. Prospective, randomized trials comparing stapled hemorrhoidopexy with excisional hemorrhoidectomy

Author	Year	Location	No. PPH patients	No. excisional patients	Follow-up	Conclusions regarding stapled hemorrhoidopexy
Ho[138]	2000	Singapore	57	62 MM	3 mo	Similar LOS, less pain at bowel movement, less analgesics, earlier return to work, similar complications, similar manometry and U/S data
Mehigan[103]	2000	United Kingdom	20	20 MM	4 mo	Less pain, same LOS, similar complications, earlier return to activity
Rowsell[139]	2000	United Kingdom	11	11 MM	6 wk	Shorter LOS, less pain, earlier return to activity
Boccasanta[100]	2001	Italy	40	40 MM	20 mo	Less OR time, less pain, similar complications, earlier return to work, same recurrence
Brown[140]	2001	Singapore	15	15 MM	6 wk	For thrombosed internal hemorrhoids: less pain, more complications, earlier return to work
Shalaby[102]	2001	Egypt	100	100 MM	1 y	Less OR time and LOS, less pain, earlier return to work, less anal discharge, fewer complications
Correa-Rovelo[141]	2002	Mexico	42	42 Ferg	6 mo	Less OR time, less pain, fewer complications, shorter time to BM, earlier return to activity
Hetzer[101]	2002	Switzerland	20	20 Ferg	1 y	Less OR time, less pain, similar complications, earlier return to work, same recurrence
Ortiz[142]	2002	Spain	27	28 MM	1 y	Less OR time, less pain, similar return to work, similar complications, more recurrent prolapse
Pavlidis[143]	2002	Greece	40	40 MM	1 y	Less OR time, shorter LOS, less pain, less analgesics, greater satisfaction, similar symptom control
Wilson[144]	2002	United Kingdom	32	30 MM	8 wk	Less OR time, shorter LOS, shorter postoperative time with anal pad, more postoperative bleeding, reduced anal discharge, shorter time to work
Cheetham[145]	2003	United Kingdom	15	16 MM	18 mo	Less pain, earlier time to work, two PPH patients with persistent pain/fecal urgency, same satisfaction, similar symptom control
Kairaluoma[146]	2003	Finland	30	30 MM	1 y	Less pain, earlier return to work, similar complications, more treatment failures
Maw[147]	2003	Singapore	101	98 MM	Perioperative	No difference in rate of bacteremia
Palimento[148]	2003	Italy	37	37 MM	6 mo	Less OR time, less pain, less pain with BM, similar return to activity, similar symptom control
Senagore[149]	2003	United States	77	79 Ferg	1 y	Less pain, less pain at BM, less analgesics, fewer re-treatments, similar symptom control

Los = length of stay   OR = operating room   PPH = procedure for prolapse and hemorrhoids
uls = ultrasound   BM = bowel movement   wk = week
MM = Milligam-Morgan   Ferg = Ferguson   mo = month   y = years

hemorrhoidopexy is less painful, and allows earlier return to work compared with conventional hemorrhoidectomy. A systematic review of stapled hemorrhoidopexy concluded that the procedure was as safe as conventional hemorrhoidectomy and was associated with shorter operative time, convalescence, and postoperative disability.[150] Senagore et al.[149] reported results from a U.S. multicenter, randomized, prospective study on stapled anopexy versus Ferguson hemorrhoidectomy at the American Society of Colon and Rectal Surgeons annual meeting in 2003. The results showed less pain, less pain at bowel movement, less analgesic use, and fewer re-treatments, with similar symptom control in comparison to Ferguson hemorrhoidectomy. Despite these early encouraging results and safety profile, several serious complications have been reported including rectal perforation,

retroperitoneal sepsis, and pelvic sepsis.[151,152] Other studies have indicated the presence of smooth muscle fibers in the excised specimens as well as a 14% incidence of internal sphincter fragmentation in those procedures in which the standard 37-mm anal dilator is used.[153,154] What long-term sequelae this may have remains to be seen.

The main complication of the procedure is bleeding from the staple line, which can be easily controlled by oversewing the bleeding point on the staple line.[155] With the second generation 33-mm hemorrhoidal circular stapler (Ethicon Endo-Surgery; PPH03) and a closed staple height of 0.75 mm, bleeding has been markedly decreased. One other disadvantage of the stapling procedure is that it does not address fibrotic external hemorrhoids or additional anorectal pathology such as fissures or skin tags.

Stapling Technique

The stapling procedure can be done with the patient in the prone jackknife, lithotomy, or left lateral position while under local, spinal, or general anesthesia. A circular anal dilator is introduced into the anal canal, which reduces the prolapsed tissues. The obturator is removed, and the prolapsed tissue falls into the lumen of the dilator. A circumferential pursestring suture is placed 4–6 cm above the dentate line into the submucosa. The circular stapler is opened and the head is introduced proximal to the pursestring. The pursestring sutured is tied and the suture threader is used to pull the free ends of the pursestring suture through a pair of holes on the lateral sides of the stapler. Traction is applied to the pursestring while the stapler is being closed, which causes the prolapsed mucosa and some hemorrhoidal tissue to be drawn into the casing. The stapler is fully tightened and then fired. The instrument should be left closed for 20 seconds after firing to enhance hemostasis. The staple line should be carefully examined for hemostasis and any bleeding areas should be oversewn. Anoscopic examination will reveal persistent internal hemorrhoids. It is important to remember that this technique does not completely excise the hemorrhoids; rather, it returns the tissues to their physiologic location. The circular specimen will contain the excised tissue and the pursestring suture.

Strangulated Hemorrhoids

Strangulated hemorrhoids arise from prolapsed third- or fourth-degree hemorrhoids that become incarcerated and irreducible because of prolonged swelling. Patients usually have a long-standing history of prolapse and may present with complaints of severe pain and urinary retention. Examination shows a rosette of thrombosed external hemorrhoids and prolapsed incarcerated internal hemorrhoids with marked edema. This can progress to subsequent ulceration and necrosis if left untreated.

Treatment usually consists of urgent or emergent hemorrhoidectomy in an operating room. An open or closed technique can be performed unless tissues are necrotic in which case the open technique should be performed. Emergency hemorrhoidectomy in the presence of strangulation and necrosis is safe provided all necrosis is excised.[134]

An alternative treatment that can be performed in the office or emergency department setting consists of locally anesthetizing the area, collapsing the tissues via massage, reducing the internal hemorrhoids and performing multiple external thrombectomies, and multiple rubber band ligations. This can provide immediate relief and future hemorrhoidectomy is seldom needed.[156] A randomized trial comparing open hemorrhoidectomy versus incision and ligation for acute hemorrhoidal disease showed both techniques to be safe and with a trend toward earlier recovery from the incision ligation technique.[156]

Hemorrhoids, Varices, and Portal Hypertension

The etiology of "hemorrhoids" in patients with portal hypertension must be distinguished from anorectal varices especially when bleeding is present. The upper anal canal (internal hemorrhoids) is drained by the middle rectal vein which drains into the iliac veins and subsequently into the systemic circulation. The inferior rectal veins drain the lower part of the anal canal (external hemorrhoids) into the internal iliac veins. Anorectal varices essentially provide a collateral pathway to decompress the portal system into the systemic circulation. Despite this communication between the portal and systemic systems, the incidence of hemorrhoidal disease in patients with portal hypertension is no greater than in the general population.[157–159]

Chawla and Dilawari[160] observed anorectal varices endoscopically in approximately 78% of their patients. Hosking et al.[157] observed varices in 59% of cirrhotic patients with portal hypertension. Hence, anorectal varices are actually quite common in patients with portal hypertension. However, unlike esophageal varices, anorectal varices rarely bleed and are implicated in less than 1% of massive bleeding episodes in patients with portal hypertension.[161] Nevertheless, bleeding from anorectal varices has been reported and may be continuous or intermittent and massive. Treatment of bleeding from anorectal varices has include a conservative medical management, direct suture ligation,[162] stapled anopexy,[163] transjugular intrahepatic portosystemic shunt,[164–166] ligation of the inferior mesenteric vein,[167] inferior mesocaval shunt,[168] inferior mesorenal vein shunt,[169] sigmoid venous to ovarian vein shunt.[170]

Hemorrhoids in Pregnancy

Although hemorrhoidal symptoms often occur and are exacerbated during pregnancy, the majority that intensify during delivery usually resolve. Hemorrhoidectomy during pregnancy should only be offered for acutely thrombosed and prolapsed hemorrhoidal disease. If required, the procedure should be performed under local anesthesia with the patient in the left anterolateral position to rotate the uterus off the inferior vena cava.[9,171]

Hemorrhoids and Crohn's Disease

Crohn's disease of the intestine in and of itself is not an absolute contraindication to hemorrhoidectomy. However, extreme caution and careful patient selection are warranted. In a study published from St. Mark's hospital, the rate of severe complications was high.[172] Approximately 30% of their Crohn's patients treated for hemorrhoids required a proctectomy for complications possibly related to the treatment. In contrast, Wolkomir and Luchtefeld[173] reported a 2-month healing rate of almost 90% in Crohn's patients with quiescent ileal or colonic disease undergoing hemorrhoidectomy. Nevertheless, hemorrhoidectomy in patients with anorectal Crohn's disease or Crohn's proctitis should not be performed because of a substantially increased risk of local complications and subsequent need for proctectomy.[172]

Hemorrhoids and the Immunocompromised

Management of hemorrhoidal disease in the immunocompromised patient is challenging and fraught with difficulties secondary to poor wound healing and infectious complications. Although it does not appear that surgery increases the mortality in patients with hematologic malignancies (leukemia, lymphoma), hemorrhoidectomy should be performed as a last resort to relieve pain and sepsis.[174] Stapled hemorrhoidopexy may offer an alternative to excisional hemorrhoidectomy, avoiding external wounds and hence problems with wound healing; however, data in this group of patients are anecdotal at best. Although infection with the human immunodeficiency virus is not a contraindication to hemorrhoidectomy, it cannot be recommended for patients with the acquired immunodeficiency syndrome because of increased complications.[175]

Posthemorrhoidectomy Hemorrhage

Severe hemorrhage after hemorrhoidectomy is a rare complication occurring in approximately 2% (0.6%–5.4%) of patients.[176,177] Traditionally, sepsis of the ligated pedicle has been considered an important etiological factor, although this has been challenged by a recent study by Chen et al.[178] who found male patients and operating surgeon as risk factors. The majority of patients will respond to packing or tamponade with a Foley catheter balloon. Approximately 15%–20% of patients may need suture ligation to control the postoperative bleed. Initial rectal irrigation has been suggested as a technique to separate patients that have stopped bleeding from those that need to go to the operating room.[179] Another helpful technique is to irrigate the rectum free of clots and blood at the initial hemorrhoid operation, to prevent postoperative passage of old clots that could cause clinical confusion.

Appendix: Practice Parameters for Ambulatory Anorectal Surgery

Prepared by The Standards Task Force, The American Society of Colon and Rectal Surgeons

Drs. Ronald Place and Neal Hyman, Project Coordinators; Clifford Simmang, Committee Chairman; Peter Cataldo; James Church; Jeff Cohen; Frederick Denstman; John Kilkenny; Juan Nogueras; Charles Orsay; Daniel Otchy; Jan Rakinic; Joe Tjandra

Ambulatory Facilities

Anorectal Surgery May Be Safely and Cost-Effectively Performed in an Ambulatory Surgery Center.

Level of Evidence—Class III (*Appendix A*). It has been estimated that 90% of anorectal cases may be suitable for ambulatory surgery. A wide variety of anorectal conditions including condylomata, fissures, abscesses, fistulas, tumors, hemorrhoids, pilonidal disease, and various miscellaneous conditions have been shown to be amenable to surgery on an outpatient basis. An admission rate of 2% has been reported. A reduction in hospital charges of 25%–50% has also been noted.

Patients with American Society of Anesthesiology (ASA) Classifications I and II Are Generally Considered Suitable Candidates for Outpatient Anorectal Surgery (Appendix B). Selected ASA Category III Patients May Also Be Appropriate Candidates.

Level of Evidence—Class III. Multiple factors must be considered in determining the appropriateness of performing anorectal surgery in the ambulatory setting. The ASA physical status classification is useful to determine the risk of anesthesia. The magnitude of the proposed surgery, type of anesthesia, availability of appropriate instrumentation, ability of the patient to follow instructions, distance of the patient's home from the surgical center, and home support structure all need to be considered.

Preoperative Evaluation

Preoperative Investigations (e.g., Laboratory Studies and Electrocardiograms) Should Be Dictated by History and Physical Examination.

Level of Evidence—Class III. Multiple studies have documented that patient history and physical examination are the key elements of an appropriate preoperative evaluation. Routine preoperative investigations that are not warranted on the basis of history and physical seem to provide little further information. There is clear evidence that nonselective preoperative screening yields few abnormal results.

One study of 1200 patients undergoing ambulatory surgery revealed that the vast majority of abnormalities could have been predicted by history and physical examination. These abnormalities did not predict perioperative complications or the need for hospital admission. A separate study of 1109 patients undergoing elective surgery revealed that 47% of laboratory investigations duplicated tests performed within the previous year. Meaningful changes in the repeat laboratory values were very rare. Such abnormalities were predictable by the patient's history. A further study of 5003 preoperative screening tests revealed 225 abnormal results. Only 104 were of potential importance and the abnormality caused action in only 17 cases. It was believed that only four patients could have had a conceivable benefit from their preoperative screening test.

Similar studies have been performed to investigate the value of specific tests. A study of 12,338 patients undergoing invasive procedures was performed to examine the value of determining activated partial thromboplastin time as a routine. Ninety-two percent of the patients were believed to be at low risk (there were no clinical factors to suggest the bleeding tendency). In these patients, it was shown that no information was gained from activated partial thromboplastin time, and therefore, clotting studies had no role as a screening test in asymptomatic patients. Similarly, routine cardiac workup seems unjustified. The risk of a perioperative myocardial infarction in patients without clinical evidence of heart disease is 0.15%. This risk increases significantly in patients who had a previous myocardial infarction. History and physical examination are the cornerstones of appropriate preoperative evaluation.

Intraoperative Considerations

Most Anorectal Surgery May Be Safely and Cost-Effectively Performed Under Local Anesthesia; Regional or General Anesthesia May Be Used Depending on Patient or Physician Preference.

Level of Evidence—III. The use of local anesthetics such as monitored anesthetic care for anorectal surgery is safer and has fewer complications than other anesthetic techniques. Perianal infiltration of local anesthetics is a simple procedure that is easily learned. Injection of the local anesthetics can be accomplished in less than 5 minutes and the operation begun immediately. However, the anesthetic technique used for any procedure should be the one that provides for maximal safety and efficacy.

Postoperative Considerations

Anorectal Surgery Patients May Safely Be Discharged from the Postanesthesia Care Unit.

Level of Evidence—II. The time course for recovery from anesthesia includes early recovery, intermediate recovery, and late recovery. Early recovery is the time interval for anesthesia emergence and recovery of protective reflexes and motor activity. The Aldrete score has been used for 30 years to determine release from phase 1 (early) recovery to a hospital bed or phase 2 (intermediate) recovery. Intermediate recovery is the period during which coordination and physiology normalize to an extent that the patient can be discharged from phase 2 recovery in a state of "home readiness" and be able to return home in the care of a responsible adult. The Post-Anesthetic Discharge Scoring System has been shown to be efficacious for discharge.

Multiple Modalities May Be Used to Achieve Adequate Postoperative Pain Control.

Level of Evidence—II. If local anesthetics are not used as the primary anesthetic technique, their use will provide prolonged postoperative analgesia. Oral narcotics may be used as primary postoperative analgesia. The use of nonsteroidal antiinflammatory drugs, particularly intramuscular or intravenous Toradol® (Roche Pharmaceuticals, Nutley, NJ) or sulindac suppositories has also shown improved analgesia, lower narcotic usage, and lower rates of urinary retention. Although the effect is unknown, oral metronidazole shows improved postoperative pain control.

Postoperative Urinary Retention Can Be Reduced by Limiting Perioperative Fluid Intake.

Level of Evidence—III. Multiple studies have shown that limiting perioperative fluid lowers the incidence of postoperative urinary retention. These same studies show conflicting evidence over the relationship between gender, age, and the quantity of narcotic medication and urinary retention. Hemorrhoidectomy and the performance of multiple anorectal procedures have higher rates of urinary retention.

Postoperative Education Should Include Recommendations for Sitz Baths, Fluid Intake, and Activity Limitations.

Level of Evidence—III. Textbooks of anorectal surgery advocate consistent instructions before discharge from ambulatory surgery. Although derived from common sense, scientific justification does not exist. With appropriate communication, ambulatory anorectal surgery may be performed with a high degree of patient satisfaction.

TABLE 11-A1. Levels of evidence

Level I: Evidence from properly conducted randomized, controlled trials.
Level II: Evidence from controlled trials without randomization, or cohort or case-control studies, or multiple times series, dramatic uncontrolled experiments.
Level III: Descriptive case series or opinions of expert panels.

TABLE 11-A2. ASA physical status classification

Class I: Patient has no systemic disturbance (e.g., healthy, no medical problems).
Class II: Patient has mild to moderate systemic disturbance (e.g., hypertension, diabetes).
Class III: Patient has severe systemic disturbance (e.g., heart disease that limits activity).
Class IV: Patient has severe systemic disturbance that is life-threatening (e.g., unstable angina, active congestive heart failure).
Class V: Patient is moribund and has little chance of survival (e.g., ruptured abdominal aortic aneurysm).

References

1. Thomson WH. The nature of haemorrhoids. Br J Surg 1975;62(7):542–552.
2. Hansen HH. The importance of the musculus canalis ani for continence and anorectal diseases (author's transl). Langenbecks Arch Chir 1976;341(1):23–37.

3. Thulesius O, Gjores JE. Arterio-venous anastomoses in the anal region with reference to the pathogenesis and treatment of haemorrhoids. Acta Chir Scand 1973;139(5):476–478.

4. Lestar B, Penninckx F, Kerremans R. The composition of anal basal pressure. An in vivo and in vitro study in man. Int J Colorectal Dis 1989;4(2):118–122.

5. Loder PB, Kamm MA, Nicholls RJ, Phillips RK. Haemorrhoids: pathology, pathophysiology and aetiology. Br J Surg 1994;81(7):946–954.

6. Galizia G, Lieto E, Castellano P, Pelosio L, Imperatore V, Pigantelli C. Lateral internal sphincterotomy together with haemorrhoidectomy for treatment of haemorrhoids: a randomised prospective study [comment]. Eur J Surg 2000;166(3):223–228.

7. Read MG, Read NW, Haynes WG, Donnelly TC, Johnson AG. A prospective study of the effect of haemorrhoidectomy on sphincter function and faecal continence. Br J Surg 1982;69(7):396–398.

8. Sun WM, Read NW, Shorthouse AJ. Hypertensive anal cushions as a cause of the high anal canal pressures in patients with haemorrhoids. Br J Surg 1990;77(4):458–462.

9. Saleeby RG Jr, Rosen L, Stasik JJ, Riether RD, Sheets J, Khubchandani IT. Hemorrhoidectomy during pregnancy: risk or relief? Dis Colon Rectum 1991;34(3):260–261.

10. Haas PA, Fox TA Jr, Haas GP. The pathogenesis of hemorrhoids. Dis Colon Rectum 1984;27(7):442–450.

11. Chung YC, Hou YC, Pan AC. Endoglin (CD105) expression in the development of haemorrhoids. Eur J Clin Invest 2004;34(2):107–112.

12. Johanson JF, Sonnenberg A. The prevalence of hemorrhoids and chronic constipation. An epidemiologic study. Gastroenterology 1990;98(2):380–386.

13. Johanson JF, Sonnenberg A. Temporal changes in the occurrence of hemorrhoids in the United States and England. Dis Colon Rectum 1991;34(7):585–591; discussion 591–593.

14. Banov L Jr, Knoepp LF Jr, Erdman LH, Alia RT. Management of hemorrhoidal disease. J S C Med Assoc 1985;81(7):398–401.

15. Dennison AR, Whiston RJ, Rooney S, Morris DL. The management of hemorrhoids. Am J Gastroenterol 1989;84(5):475–481.

16. Armstrong DN. Multiple hemorrhoidal ligation: a prospective, randomized trial evaluating a new technique. Dis Colon Rectum 2003;46(2):179–186.

17. Segal WN, Greenberg PD, Rockey DC, Cello JP, McQuaid KR. The outpatient evaluation of hematochezia. Am J Gastroenterol 1998;93(2):179–182.

18. Clinical Practice Committee, American Gastroenterological Association. American Gastroenterological Association medical position statement: diagnosis and treatment of hemorrhoids. Gastroenterology 2004;126(5):1461–1462.

19. Nakama H, Kamijo N, Fujimori K, Horiuchi A, Abdul Fattah S, Zhang B. Immunochemical fecal occult blood test is not suitable for diagnosis of hemorrhoids. Am J Med 1997;102(6):551–554.

20. Korkis AM, McDougall CJ. Rectal bleeding in patients less than 50 years of age. Dig Dis Sci 1995;40(7):1520–1523.

21. Madoff RD, Fleshman JW. American Gastroenterological Association technical review on the diagnosis and treatment of hemorrhoids. Gastroenterology 2004;126(5):1463–1473.

22. Kluiber RM, Wolff BG. Evaluation of anemia caused by hemorrhoidal bleeding. Dis Colon Rectum 1994;37(10):1006–1007.

23. Moesgaard F, Nielsen ML, Hansen JB, Knudsen JT. High-fiber diet reduces bleeding and pain in patients with hemorrhoids: a double-blind trial of Vi-Siblin. Dis Colon Rectum 1982;25(5):454–456.

24. Perez-Miranda M, Gomez-Cedenilla A, Leon-Colombo T, Pajares J, Mate-Jimenez J. Effect of fiber supplements on internal bleeding hemorrhoids. Hepatogastroenterology 1996;43(12):1504–1507.

25. Broader JH, Gunn IF, Alexander-Williams J. Evaluation of a bulk-forming evacuant in the management of haemorrhoids. Br J Surg 1974;61(2):142–144.

26. Webster DJ, Gough DC, Craven JL. The use of bulk evacuant in patients with haemorrhoids. Br J Surg 1978;65(4):291–292.

27. Alonso-Coello P, Lopez-Yarto M. Laxatives and topical treatments for hemorrhoids. Cochrane Database Syst Rev 2005;2.

28. Thaha MA, Campbell KL, Steele RJC. Non-operative treatment for haemorrhoidal disease. Cochrane Database Syst Rev 2004;2.

29. Alonso P, Johanson J, Lopez-Yarto M, Martinez MJ. Phlebotonics for haemorrhoids. Cochrane Database Syst Rev 2003;2.

30. Thanapongsathorn W, Vajrabukka T. Clinical trial of oral diosmin (Daflon) in the treatment of hemorrhoids. Dis Colon Rectum 1992;35(11):1085–1088.

31. Godeberge P. Daflon 500 mg in the treatment of hemorrhoidal disease: a demonstrated efficacy in comparison with placebo. Angiology 1994;45(6 pt 2):574–578.

32. Cospite M. Double-blind, placebo-controlled evaluation of clinical activity and safety of Daflon 500 mg in the treatment of acute hemorrhoids. Angiology 1994;45(6 pt 2):566–573.

33. Ho YH, Foo CL, Seow-Choen F, Goh HS. Prospective randomized controlled trial of a micronized flavonidic fraction to reduce bleeding after haemorrhoidectomy. Br J Surg 1995;82(8):1034–1035.

34. Misra MC, Parshad R. Randomized clinical trial of micronized flavonoids in the early control of bleeding from acute internal haemorrhoids [comment]. Br J Surg 2000;87(7):868–872.

35. Wijayanegara H, Mose JC, Achmad L, Sobarna R, Permadi W. A clinical trial of hydroxyethylrutosides in the treatment of haemorrhoids of pregnancy. J Int Med Res 1992;20(1):54–60.

36. Squadrito F, Altavilla D, Oliaro Bosso S. Double-blind, randomized clinical trial of troxerutin-carbazochrome in patients with hemorrhoids. Eur Rev Med Pharmacol Sci 2000;4(1–2):21–24.

37. Basile M, Gidaro S, Pacella M, Biffignandi PM, Gidaro GS. Parenteral troxerutin and carbazochrome combination in the treatment of post-hemorrhoidectomy status: a randomized, double-blind, placebo-controlled, phase IV study. Curr Med Res Opin 2001;17(4):256–261.

38. Mentes BB, Gorgul A, Tatlicioglu E, Ayoglu F, Unal S. Efficacy of calcium dobesilate in treating acute attacks of hemorrhoidal disease. Dis Colon Rectum 2001;44(10):1489–1495.

39. Ho YH, Tan M, Seow-Choen F. Micronized purified flavonidic fraction compared favorably with rubber band ligation and fiber alone in the management of bleeding hemorrhoids: randomized controlled trial [comment]. Dis Colon Rectum 2000;43(1):66–69.

40. Barron J. Office ligation treatment of hemorrhoids. Dis Colon Rectum 1963;6:109–113.

41. Budding J. Solo operated haemorrhoid ligator rectoscope. A report on 200 consecutive bandings. Int J Colorectal Dis 1997; 12(1):42–44.

42. Su MY, Chiu CT, Wu CS, et al. Endoscopic hemorrhoidal ligation of symptomatic internal hemorrhoids. Gastrointest Endosc 2003;58(6):871–874.

43. Berkelhammer C, Moosvi SB. Retroflexed endoscopic band ligation of bleeding internal hemorrhoids. Gastrointest Endosc 2002;55(4):532–537.

44. Trowers EA, Ganga U, Rizk R, Ojo E, Hodges D. Endoscopic hemorrhoidal ligation: preliminary clinical experience. Gastrointest Endosc 1998;48(1):49–52.

45. O'Regan PJ. Disposable device and a minimally invasive technique for rubber band ligation of hemorrhoids. Dis Colon Rectum 1999;42(5):683–685.

46. Law WL, Chu KW. Triple rubber band ligation for hemorrhoids: prospective, randomized trial of use of local anesthetic injection. Dis Colon Rectum 1999;42(3):363–366.

47. Poon GP, Chu KW, Lau WY. Conventional vs. triple rubber band ligand for hemorrhoids. A prospective, randomized trial. Dis Colon Rectum 1986;29(12):836–838.

48. Khubchandani IT. A randomized comparison of single and multiple rubber band ligations. Dis Colon Rectum 1983;26(11): 705–708.

49. Lee HH, Spencer RJ, Beart RW Jr. Multiple hemorrhoidal bandings in a single session. Dis Colon Rectum 1994;37(1):37–41.

50. Lau WY, Chow HP, Poon GP, Wong SH. Rubber band ligation of three primary hemorrhoids in a single session. A safe and effective procedure. Dis Colon Rectum 1982;25(4):336–339.

51. Templeton JL, Spence RA, Kennedy TL, Parks TG, Mackenzie G, Hanna WA. Comparison of infrared coagulation and rubber band ligation for first and second degree haemorrhoids: a randomised prospective clinical trial. Br Med J Clin Res Ed 1983;286(6375):1387–1389.

52. Ambrose NS, Hares MM, Alexander-Williams J, Keighley MR. Prospective randomised comparison of photocoagulation and rubber band ligation in treatment of haemorrhoids. Br Med J Clin Res Ed 1983;286(6375):1389–1391.

53. Walker AJ, Leicester RJ, Nicholls RJ, Mann CV. A prospective study of infrared coagulation, injection and rubber band ligation in the treatment of haemorrhoids. Int J Colorectal Dis 1990;5(2):113–116.

54. Mattana C, Maria G, Pescatori M. Rubber band ligation of hemorrhoids and rectal mucosal prolapse in constipated patients. Dis Colon Rectum 1989;32(5):372–375.

55. Bat L, Melzer E, Koler M, Dreznick Z, Shemesh E. Complications of rubber band ligation of symptomatic internal hemorrhoids. Dis Colon Rectum 1993;36(3):287–290.

56. O'Hara VS. Fatal clostridial infection following hemorrhoidal banding. Dis Colon Rectum 1980;23(8):570–571.

57. Russell TR, Donohue JH. Hemorrhoidal banding. A warning. Dis Colon Rectum 1985;28(5):291–293.

58. Scarpa FJ, Hillis W, Sabetta JR. Pelvic cellulitis: a life-threatening complication of hemorrhoidal banding. Surgery 1988;103(3):383–385.

59. Quevedo-Bonilla G, Farkas AM, Abcarian H, Hambrick E, Orsay CP. Septic complications of hemorrhoidal banding. Arch Surg 1988;123(5):650–651.

60. Shemesh EI, Kodner IJ, Fry RD, Neufeld DM. Severe complication of rubber band ligation of internal hemorrhoids. Dis Colon Rectum 1987;30(3):199–200.

61. Marshman D, Huber PJ Jr, Timmerman W, Simonton CT, Odom FC, Kaplan ER. Hemorrhoidal ligation. A review of efficacy. Dis Colon Rectum 1989;32(5):369–371.

62. Savioz D, Roche B, Glauser T, Dobrinov A, Ludwig C, Marti MC. Rubber band ligation of hemorrhoids: relapse as a function of time. Int J Colorectal Dis 1998;13(4):154–156.

63. Wrobleski DE, Corman ML, Veidenheimer MC, Coller JA. Long-term evaluation of rubber ring ligation in hemorrhoidal disease. Dis Colon Rectum 1980;23(7):478–482.

64. Bayer I, Myslovaty B, Picovsky BM. Rubber band ligation of hemorrhoids. Convenient and economic treatment. J Clin Gastroenterol 1996;23(1):50–52.

65. Leicester RJ, Nicholls RJ, Mann CV. Infrared coagulation: a new treatment for hemorrhoids. Dis Colon Rectum 1981;24(8):602–605.

66. Dennison A, Whiston RJ, Rooney S, Chadderton RD, Wherry DC, Morris DL. A randomized comparison of infrared photocoagulation with bipolar diathermy for the outpatient treatment of hemorrhoids. Dis Colon Rectum 1990;33(1):32–34.

67. Poen AC, Felt-Bersma RJ, Cuesta MA, Deville W, Meuwissen SG. A randomized controlled trial of rubber band ligation versus infra-red coagulation in the treatment of internal haemorrhoids. Eur J Gastroenterol Hepatol 2000;12(5):535–539.

68. Jensen DM, Jutabha R, Machicado GA, et al. Prospective randomized comparative study of bipolar electrocoagulation versus heater probe for treatment of chronically bleeding internal hemorrhoids. Gastrointest Endosc 1997;46(5):435–443.

69. Randall GM, Jensen DM, Machicado GA, et al. Prospective randomized comparative study of bipolar versus direct current electrocoagulation for treatment of bleeding internal hemorrhoids. Gastrointest Endosc 1994;40(4):403–410.

70. Hinton CP, Morris DL. A randomized trial comparing direct current therapy and bipolar diathermy in the outpatient treatment of third-degree hemorrhoids. Dis Colon Rectum 1990;33(11):931–932.

71. Norman DA, Newton R, Nicholas GV. Direct current electrotherapy of internal hemorrhoids: an effective, safe, and painless outpatient approach. Am J Gastroenterol 1989;84(5):482–487.

72. Zinberg SS, Stern DH, Furman DS, Wittles JM. A personal experience in comparing three nonoperative techniques for treating internal hemorrhoids. Am J Gastroenterol 1989;84(5): 488–492.

73. Varma JS, Chung SC, Li AK. Prospective randomised comparison of current coagulation and injection sclerotherapy for the outpatient treatment of haemorrhoids. Int J Colorectal Dis 1991;6(1):42–45.

74. Sim AJ, Murie JA, Mackenzie I. Three year follow-up study on the treatment of first and second degree hemorrhoids by sclerosant injection or rubber band ligation. Surg Gynecol Obstet 1983;157(6):534–536.

75. Bullock N. Impotence after sclerotherapy of haemorrhoids: case reports. BMJ 1997;314(7078):419.

76. Khoury GA, Lake SP, Lewis MC, Lewis AA. A randomized trial to compare single with multiple phenol injection treatment for haemorrhoids. Br J Surg 1985;72(9):741–742.

77. Senapati A, Nicholls RJ. A randomised trial to compare the results of injection sclerotherapy with a bulk laxative alone in the treatment of bleeding haemorrhoids. Int J Colorectal Dis 1988;3(2):124–126.

78. Lord PH. A new regime for the treatment of haemorrhoids. Proc R Soc Med 1968;61(9):935–936.

79. Speakman CT, Burnett SJ, Kamm MA, Bartram CI. Sphincter injury after anal dilatation demonstrated by anal endosonography. Br J Surg 1991;78(12):1429–1430.

80. MacDonald A, Smith A, McNeill AD, Finlay IG. Manual dilatation of the anus. Br J Surg 1992;79(12):1381–1382.

81. Konsten J, Baeten CG. Hemorrhoidectomy vs. Lord's method: 17-year follow-up of a prospective, randomized trial. Dis Colon Rectum 2000;43(4):503–506.

82. Hiltunen KM, Matikainen M. Anal dilatation, lateral subcutaneous sphincterotomy and haemorrhoidectomy for the treatment of second and third degree haemorrhoids. A prospective randomized study. Int Surg 1992;77(4):261–263.

83. O'Callaghan JD, Matheson TS, Hall R. Inpatient treatment of prolapsing piles: cryosurgery versus Milligan-Morgan haemorrhoidectomy. Br J Surg 1982;69(3):157–159.

84. Goligher JC. Cryosurgery for hemorrhoids. Dis Colon Rectum 1976;19(3):213–218.

85. Smith LE, Goodreau JJ, Fouty WJ. Operative hemorrhoidectomy versus cryodestruction. Dis Colon Rectum 1979;22(1):10–16.

86. Bleday R, Pena JP, Rothenberger DA, Goldberg SM, Buls JG. Symptomatic hemorrhoids: current incidence and complications of operative therapy. Dis Colon Rectum 1992;35(5):477–481.

87. Granet E. Hemorrhoidectomy failures: causes, prevention and management. Dis Colon Rectum 1968;11(1):45–48.

88. MacRae HM, Temple LK, McLeod RS. A meta-analysis of hemorrhoidal treatments. Semin C R Surg 2002;13:77–83.

89. Ferguson JA, Mazier WP, Ganchrow MI, Friend WG. The closed technique of hemorrhoidectomy. Surgery 1971;70(3):480–484.

90. Milligan ET, Morgan CN, Jones LE. Surgical anatomy of the anal canal and the operative treatment of hemorrhoids. Lancet 1937;2:119–1124.

91. Devien CV, Pujol JP. Total circular hemorrhoidectomy. Int Surg 1989;74(3):154–157.

92. Boccasanta P, Venturi M, Orio A, et al. Circular hemorrhoidectomy in advanced hemorrhoidal disease. Hepatogastroenterology 1998;45(22):969–972.

93. Wolff BG, Culp CE. The Whitehead hemorrhoidectomy. An unjustly maligned procedure. Dis Colon Rectum 1988;31(8):587–590.

94. Whitehead W. The surgical treatment of hemorrhoids. Br Med J 1882;1:148–150.

95. Bonello JC. Who's afraid of the dentate line? The Whitehead hemorrhoidectomy. Am J Surg 1988;156(3 pt 1):182–186.

96. Ho YH, Seow-Choen F, Tan M, Leong AF. Randomized controlled trial of open and closed haemorrhoidectomy. Br J Surg 1997;84(12):1729–1730.

97. Carapeti EA, Kamm MA, McDonald PJ, Chadwick SJ, Phillips RK. Randomized trial of open versus closed day-case haemorrhoidectomy. Br J Surg 1999;86(5):612–613.

98. Arbman G, Krook H, Haapaniemi S. Closed vs. open hemorrhoidectomy—is there any difference? Dis Colon Rectum 2000;43(1):31–34.

99. Gencosmanoglu R, Sad O, Koc D, Inceoglu R. Hemorrhoidectomy: open or closed technique? A prospective, randomized clinical trial. Dis Colon Rectum 2002;45(1):70–75.

100. Boccasanta P, Capretti PG, Venturi M, et al. Randomised controlled trial between stapled circumferential mucosectomy and conventional circular hemorrhoidectomy in advanced hemorrhoids with external mucosal prolapse. Am J Surg 2001;182(1):64–68.

101. Hetzer FH, Demartines N, Handschin AE, Clavien PA. Stapled vs excision hemorrhoidectomy: long-term results of a prospective randomized trial. Arch Surg 2002;137(3):337–340.

102. Shalaby R, Desoky A. Randomized clinical trial of stapled versus Milligan-Morgan haemorrhoidectomy. Br J Surg 2001;88(8):1049–1053.

103. Mehigan BJ, Monson JR, Hartley JE. Stapling procedure for haemorrhoids versus Milligan-Morgan haemorrhoidectomy: randomised controlled trial. Lancet 2000;355(9206):782–785.

104. Chung YC, Wu HJ. Clinical experience of sutureless closed hemorrhoidectomy with LigaSure. Dis Colon Rectum 2003;46(1):87–92.

105. Franklin EJ, Seetharam S, Lowney J, Horgan PG. Randomized, clinical trial of Ligasure vs conventional diathermy in hemorrhoidectomy. Dis Colon Rectum 2003;46(10):1380–1383.

106. Seow-Choen F, Ho YH, Ang HG, Goh HS. Prospective, randomized trial comparing pain and clinical function after conventional scissors excision/ligation vs. diathermy excision without ligation for symptomatic prolapsed hemorrhoids. Dis Colon Rectum 1992;35(12):1165–1169.

107. Wang JY, Chang-Chien CR, Chen JS, Lai CR, Tang RP. The role of lasers in hemorrhoidectomy. Dis Colon Rectum 1991;34(1):78–82.

108. Iwagaki H, Higuchi Y, Fuchimoto S, Orita K. The laser treatment of hemorrhoids: results of a study on 1816 patients. Jpn J Surg 1989;19(6):658–661.

109. Senagore A, Mazier WP, Luchtefeld MA, MacKeigan JM, Wengert T. Treatment of advanced hemorrhoidal disease: a prospective, randomized comparison of cold scalpel vs. contact Nd:YAG laser. Dis Colon Rectum 1993;36(11):1042–1049.

110. Khan S, Pawlak SE, Eggenberger JC, et al. Surgical treatment of hemorrhoids: prospective, randomized trial comparing closed excisional hemorrhoidectomy and the Harmonic Scalpel technique of excisional hemorrhoidectomy. Dis Colon Rectum 2001;44(6):845–849.

111. Tan JJ, Seow-Choen F. Prospective, randomized trial comparing diathermy and Harmonic Scalpel hemorrhoidectomy. Dis Colon Rectum 2001;44(5):677–679.

112. Armstrong DN, Ambroze WL, Schertzer ME, Orangio GR. Harmonic Scalpel vs. electrocautery hemorrhoidectomy: a prospective evaluation. Dis Colon Rectum 2001;44(4):558–564.

113. Chung CC, Ha JP, Tai YP, Tsang WW, Li MK. Double-blind, randomized trial comparing Harmonic Scalpel hemorrhoidectomy, bipolar scissors hemorrhoidectomy, and scissors excision: ligation technique. Dis Colon Rectum 2002;45(6):789–794.

114. Palazzo FF, Francis DL, Clifton MA. Randomized clinical trial of Ligasure versus open haemorrhoidectomy. Br J Surg 2002;89(2):154–157.

115. Jayne DG, Botterill I, Ambrose NS, Brennan TG, Guillou PJ, O'Riordain DS. Randomized clinical trial of Ligasure versus conventional diathermy for day-case haemorrhoidectomy. Br J Surg 2002;89(4):428–432.

116. Ibrahim S, Tsang C, Lee YL, Eu KW, Seow-Choen F. Prospective, randomized trial comparing pain and complications between diathermy and scissors for closed hemorrhoidectomy. Dis Colon Rectum 1998;41(11):1418–1420.

117. Andrews BT, Layer GT, Jackson BT, Nicholls RJ. Randomized trial comparing diathermy hemorrhoidectomy with the scissor dissection Milligan-Morgan operation. Dis Colon Rectum 1993;36(6):580–583.

118. Ui Y. Anoderm-preserving, completely closed hemorrhoidectomy with no mucosal incision. Dis Colon Rectum 1997;40(10 suppl):S99–101.

119. Patel N, O'Connor T. Suture haemorrhoidectomy: a day-only alternative. Aust N Z J Surg 1996;66(12):830–831.

120. Mathai V, Ong BC, Ho YH. Randomized controlled trial of lateral internal sphincterotomy with haemorrhoidectomy. Br J Surg 1996;83(3):380–382.

121. Carapeti EA, Kamm MA, McDonald PJ, Phillips RK. Double-blind randomised controlled trial of effect of metronidazole on pain after day-case haemorrhoidectomy. Lancet 1998; 351(9097):169–172.

122. Hussein MK, Taha AM, Haddad FF, Bassim YR. Bupivacaine local injection in anorectal surgery. Int Surg 1998;83(1):56–57.

123. Pryn SJ, Crosse MM, Murison MS, McGinn FP. Postoperative analgesia for haemorrhoidectomy. A comparison between caudal and local infiltration. Anaesthesia 1989;44(12):964–966.

124. Chester JF, Stanford BJ, Gazet JC. Analgesic benefit of locally injected bupivacaine after hemorrhoidectomy. Dis Colon Rectum 1990;33(6):487–489.

125. Ho YH, Seow-Choen F, Low JY, Tan M, Leong AP. Randomized controlled trial of trimebutine (anal sphincter relaxant) for pain after haemorrhoidectomy. Br J Surg 1997;84(3):377–379.

126. Gottesman L, Milsom JW, Mazier WP. The use of anxiolytic and parasympathomimetic agents in the treatment of postoperative urinary retention following anorectal surgery. A prospective, randomized, double-blind study. Dis Colon Rectum 1989;32(10):867–870.

127. Wasvary HJ, Hain J, Mosed-Vogel M, Bendick P, Barkel DC, Klein SN. Randomized, prospective, double-blind, placebo-controlled trial of effect of nitroglycerin ointment on pain after hemorrhoidectomy. Dis Colon Rectum 2001;44(8):1069–1073.

128. Denis J, Dubois N, Ganansia R, du Puy-Montbrun T, Lemarchand N. Hemorrhoidectomy: Hospital Leopold Bellan procedure. Int Surg 1989;74(3):152–153.

129. Reis Neto JA, Quilici FA, Cordeiro F, Reis Junior JA. Open versus semi-open hemorrhoidectomy: a random trial. Int Surg 1992;77(2):84–90.

130. Tajana A. Hemorrhoidectomy according to Milligan-Morgan: ligature and excision technique. Int Surg 1989;74(3):158–161.

131. Lacerda-Filho A, Cunha-Melo JR. Outpatient haemorrhoidectomy under local anaesthesia. Eur J Surg 1997;163(12):935–940.

132. Johnstone CS, Isbister WH. Inpatient management of piles: a surgical audit. Aust N Z J Surg 1992;62(9):720–724.

133. Leff EI. Hemorrhoidectomy—laser vs. nonlaser: outpatient surgical experience. Dis Colon Rectum 1992;35(8):743–746.

134. Eu KW, Seow-Choen F, Goh HS. Comparison of emergency and elective haemorrhoidectomy. Br J Surg 1994;81(2):308–310.

135. Pescatori M, Favetta U, Dedola S, Orsini S. Transanal stapled excision of rectal mucosal prolapse. Tech Coloproctol 1997;1:96–98.

136. Longo A. Treatment of hemorrhoidal disease by reduction of mucosa and haemorrhoidal prolapse with a circular stapling device: a new procedure—6th World Congress of Endoscopic Surgery. Mundozzi Editore 1998:777–784.

137. Corman ML, Gravie JF, Hager T, et al. Stapled haemorrhoidopexy: a consensus position paper by an international working party—indications, contra-indications and technique. Colorectal Dis 2003;5(4):304–310.

138. Ho YH, Cheong WK, Tsang C, et al. Stapled hemorrhoidectomy—cost and effectiveness. Randomized, controlled trial including incontinence scoring, anorectal manometry, and endoanal ultrasound assessments at up to three months. Dis Colon Rectum 2000;43(12):1666–1675.

139. Rowsell M, Bello M, Hemingway DM. Circumferential mucosectomy (stapled haemorrhoidectomy) versus conventional haemorrhoidectomy: randomised controlled trial. Lancet 2000;355(9206):779–781.

140. Brown SR, Ballan K, Ho E, Ho Fams YH, Seow-Choen F. Stapled mucosectomy for acute thrombosed circumferentially prolapsed piles: a prospective randomized comparison with conventional haemorrhoidectomy. Colorectal Dis 2001; 3(3):175–178.

141. Correa-Rovelo JM, Tellez O, Obregon L, Miranda-Gomez A, Moran S. Stapled rectal mucosectomy vs. closed hemorrhoidectomy: a randomized, clinical trial. Dis Colon Rectum 2002;45(10):1367–1374.

142. Ortiz H, Marzo J, Armendariz P. Randomized clinical trial of stapled haemorrhoidopexy versus conventional diathermy haemorrhoidectomy. Br J Surg 2002;89(11):1376–1381.

143. Pavlidis T, Papaziogas B, Souparis A, Patsas A, Koutelidakis I, Papaziogas T. Modern stapled Longo procedure vs. conventional Milligan-Morgan hemorrhoidectomy: a randomized controlled trial [comment]. Int J Colorectal Dis 2002;17(1):50–53.

144. Wilson MS, Pope V, Doran HE, Fearn SJ, Brough WA. Objective comparison of stapled anopexy and open hemorrhoidectomy: a randomized, controlled trial. Dis Colon Rectum 2002;45(11):1437–1444.

145. Cheetham MJ, Cohen CR, Kamm MA, Phillips RK. A randomized, controlled trial of diathermy hemorrhoidectomy vs. stapled hemorrhoidectomy in an intended day-care setting with longer-term follow-up. Dis Colon Rectum 2003;46(4):491–497.

146. Kairaluoma M, Nuorva K, Kellokumpu I. Day-case stapled (circular) vs. diathermy hemorrhoidectomy: a randomized, controlled trial evaluating surgical and functional outcome. Dis Colon Rectum 2003;46(1):93–99.

147. Maw A, Concepcion R, Eu KW, et al. Prospective randomized study of bacteraemia in diathermy and stapled haemorrhoidectomy. Br J Surg 2003;90(2):222–226.

148. Palimento D, Picchio M, Attanasio U, Lombardi A, Bambini C, Renda A. Stapled and open hemorrhoidectomy: randomized controlled trial of early results. World J Surg 2003;27(2): 203–207.

149. Senagore AJ, Singer M, Abcarian H, et al. A prospective, randomized, controlled, multicenter trial comparing stapled hemorrhoidopexy and Ferguson hemorrhoidectomy: perioperative and one year results. American Society of Colon and Rectal Surgeons Annual Meeting, New Orleans, LA, June 21–26, 2003.

150. Sutherland LM, Burchard AK, Matsuda K, et al. A systematic review of stapled hemorrhoidectomy. Arch Surg 2002;137(12): 1395–1406; discussion 1407.

151. Ripetti V, Caricato M, Arullani A. Rectal perforation, retropneumoperitoneum, and pneumomediastinum after stapling procedure for prolapsed hemorrhoids: report of a case and subsequent considerations. Dis Colon Rectum 2002;45(2):268–270.

152. Maw A, Eu KW, Seow-Choen F. Retroperitoneal sepsis complicating stapled hemorrhoidectomy: report of a case and review of the literature. Dis Colon Rectum 2002;45(6): 826–828.

153. George BD, Shetty D, Lindsey I, Mortensen NJ, Warren BF. Histopathology of stapled haemorrhoidectomy specimens: a cautionary note. Colorectal Dis 2002;4(6):473–476.

154. Ho YH, Seow-Choen F, Tsang C, Eu KW. Randomized trial assessing anal sphincter injuries after stapled haemorrhoidectomy. Br J Surg 2001;88(11):1449–1455.

155. Singer M, Cintron J, Fleshman J, et al. Early experience with stapled hemorrhoidectomy in the United States. Dis Colon Rectum 2002;45:360–367.

156. Rasmussen OO, Larsen KG, Naver L, Christiansen J. Emergency haemorrhoidectomy compared with incision and banding for the treatment of acute strangulated haemorrhoids. A prospective randomised study. Eur J Surg 1991;157(10):613–614.

157. Hosking SW, Smart HL, Johnson AG, Triger DR. Anorectal varices, haemorrhoids, and portal hypertension. Lancet 1989;1(8634):349–352.

158. Goenka MK, Kochhar R, Nagi B, Mehta SK. Rectosigmoid varices and other mucosal changes in patients with portal hypertension. Am J Gastroenterol 1991;86(9):1185–1189.

159. Bernstein WC. What are hemorrhoids and what is their relationship to the portal venous system? Dis Colon Rectum 1983;26(12):829–834.

160. Chawla Y, Dilawari JB. Anorectal varices—their frequency in cirrhotic and non-cirrhotic portal hypertension. Gut 1991; 32(3):309–311.

161. Johansen K, Bardin J, Orloff MJ. Massive bleeding from hemorrhoidal varices in portal hypertension. JAMA 1980; 244(18):2084–2085.

162. Hosking SW, Johnson AG. Bleeding anorectal varices—a misunderstood condition. Surgery 1988;104(1):70–73.

163. Biswas S, George ML, Leather AJ. Stapled anopexy in the treatment of anal varices: report of a case. Dis Colon Rectum 2003;46(9):1284–1285.

164. Shibata D, Brophy DP, Gordon FD, Anastopoulos HT, Sentovich SM, Bleday R. Transjugular intrahepatic portosystemic shunt for treatment of bleeding ectopic varices with portal hypertension. Dis Colon Rectum 1999;42(12):1581–1585.

165. Godil A, McCracken JD. Rectal variceal bleeding treated by transjugular intrahepatic portosystemic shunt. Potentials and pitfalls. J Clin Gastroenterol 1997;25(2):460–462.

166. Fantin AC, Zala G, Risti B, Debatin JF, Schopke W, Meyenberger C. Bleeding anorectal varices: successful treatment with transjugular intrahepatic portosystemic shunting (TIPS). Gut 1996;38(6):932–935.

167. Yeh T Jr, McGuire HH Jr. Intractable bleeding from anorectal varices relieved by inferior mesenteric vein ligation. Gastroenterology 1994;107(4):1165–1167.

168. Montemurro S, Polignano FM, Caliandro C, Rucci A, Ruggieri E, Sciscio V. Inferior mesocaval shunt for bleeding anorectal varices and portal vein thrombosis. Hepatogastroenterology 2001;48(40):980–983.

169. Rahmani O, Wolpert LM, Drezner AD. Distal inferior mesenteric veins to renal vein shunt for treatment of bleeding anorectal varices: case report and review of literature. J Vasc Surg 2002;36(6):1264–1266.

170. Sato Y, Yokoyama N, Suzuki S, Tani T, Nomoto M, Hatakeyama K. Double selective shunting for esophagogastric and rectal varices in portal hypertension due to congenital hepatic polycystic disease. Hepatogastroenterology 2002; 49(48):1528–1530.

171. Nivatvongs S. Alternative positioning of patients for hemorrhoidectomy. Dis Colon Rectum 1980;23(5):308–309.

172. Jeffery PJ, Parks AG, Ritchie JK. Treatment of haemorrhoids in patients with inflammatory bowel disease. Lancet 1977; 1(8021):1084–1085.

173. Wolkomir AF, Luchtefeld MA. Surgery for symptomatic hemorrhoids and anal fissures in Crohn's disease. Dis Colon Rectum 1993;36(6):545–547.

174. Grewal H, Guillem JG, Quan SH, Enker WE, Cohen AM. Anorectal disease in neutropenic leukemic patients. Operative vs. nonoperative management. Dis Colon Rectum 1994; 37(11):1095–1099.

175. Morandi E, Merlini D, Salvaggio A, Foschi D, Trabucchi E. Prospective study of healing time after hemorrhoidectomy: influence of HIV infection, acquired immunodeficiency syndrome, and anal wound infection. Dis Colon Rectum 1999; 42(9):1140–1144.

176. Rosen L, Sipe P, Stasik JJ, et al. Outcome of delayed hemorrhage following surgical hemorrhoidectomy. Dis Colon Rectum 1993;36:743.

177. Basso L, Pescatori M. Outcome of delayed hemorrhage following surgical hemorrhoidectomy [letter]. Dis Colon Rectum 1994;37:288–289.

178. Chen HH, Wang JY, Changchien RC, et al. Risk factors associated with posthemorrhoidectomy secondary hemorrhage. A single institution prospective study of 4880 consecutive hemorrhoidectomies. Dis Colon Rectum 2003;45:1096–1099.

179. Chen HH, Wang J, Changchien CR, Yeh CY, Tsai WS, Tang R. Effective management of posthemorrhoidectomy secondary hemorrhage using rectal irrigation. Dis Colon Rectum 2002; 45:234–238.

180. Jayaraman S, Colquhoun PHD, Malthaner RA. Circular stapled anopexy versus excisional hemorrhoidectomy for hemorrhoidal disease. (Protocol) *The Cochrane Database of Systematic Reviews* 2005;3: CD005393. DOI: 10.1002/ 14651858.CD005393.

181. Shanmugam V, Thaha MA, Rabindranath KS, Campbell KL, Steele RJC, Loudon MA, Rubber band ligation versus excisional hemorrhoidectomy for hemorrhoids. *The Cochrane Database of Systematic Reviews* 2005;1: Art.No.: CD005034. DOI: 10.1002/14651858.CD005034.

182. Quijano CE, Abalos E. Conservative management of symptomatic and/or complicated haemorrhoids in pregnancy and the puerperium. *The Cochrane Database of Systematic Reviews* 2005;3: Art.No.: CD004077. DOI: 10.1002/14651858. CD004077.pub2.

12
Benign Anorectal: Anal Fissure

Sharon L. Dykes and Robert D. Madoff

Epidemiology

An anal fissure, or fissure-in-ano, is an oval, ulcer-like, longitudinal tear in the anal canal, distal to the dentate line. Although the exact incidence is unknown, it is a common disorder, with equal gender distribution. Fissures can occur at any age, but are usually seen in younger and middle-aged adults. In almost 90% of cases, fissures are identified in the posterior midline, but can be seen in the anterior midline in up to 25% of affected women and 8% of affected men. An additional 3% of patients have both anterior and posterior fissures. Fissures occurring in lateral positions should raise suspicions for other disease processes, such as Crohn's disease, tuberculosis, syphilis, human immunodeficiency virus (HIV)/ acquired immunodeficiency syndrome (AIDS), or anal carcinoma (Figure 12-1).

Early, or acute, fissures have the appearance of a simple tear in the anoderm, whereas chronic fissures, defined by symptoms lasting more than 8–12 weeks, are further characterized by edema and fibrosis. Typical inflammatory manifestations of chronic fissures include a sentinel pile, or skin tag, at the distal fissure margin and a hypertrophied anal papilla proximal to the fissure in the anal canal. In addition, fibers of the internal anal sphincter (IAS) are often visible at the fissure base.

Etiology

The cause of anal fissure has been long debated. Trauma to the anal canal secondary to the passage of a hard stool is believed to be a common initiating factor. A history of constipation is not universally obtained, however, and some patients report an episode of diarrhea before the onset of symptoms.

The persistence of a fissure after any initiating event is associated with increased resting anal pressure—an observation first reported in the mid-1970s.[1,2] Physiologic studies using ambulatory manometry have confirmed the presence of sustained resting hypertonia in fissure patients.[3] Further observations have delineated an inverse relationship between anal canal pressure and perfusion of the anoderm. Ischemia was initially proposed as an instigator of fissure persistence by Gibbons and Read[4] in 1986. Later support was provided by angiographic studies of the inferior rectal artery in cadavers, which demonstrated a paucity of blood vessels in the posterior midline of the anal canal in 85% of those examined.[5] Schouten et al.[6] measured anodermal blood flow in healthy individuals using Doppler laser flowmetry, and found that the posterior midline had the lowest perfusion when compared with the other three quadrants. In addition, there was a significant inverse correlation between posterior midline anodermal blood flow and maximum resting anal pressure in a large cohort of patients that included normal controls and fissure patients. Those with fissures demonstrated the highest resting anal pressures and the lowest posterior blood flow of any group. Improvement in posterior midline blood flow was noted to occur after reduction of anal pressure with anesthesia. These same authors were able to demonstrate normalization of sphincter hypertonia and anodermal blood flow after lateral internal sphincterotomy (LIS) in anal fissure patients.

Symptoms

The clinical hallmark of an anal fissure is pain during, and particularly after, defecation. In acute fissures, pain may be short-lived, but it can last several hours or even all day in the presence of a chronic fissure. The pain is frequently described as passing razor blades or glass shards. Understandably, patients with anal fissures may often fear bowel movements. Rectal bleeding, although not uncommon, is usually limited to minimal bright red blood seen on the toilet tissue.

Diagnosis

Diagnosis is suggested by patient history and confirmed by physical examination. Most fissures are readily visible by simply spreading the buttocks with opposing traction of the

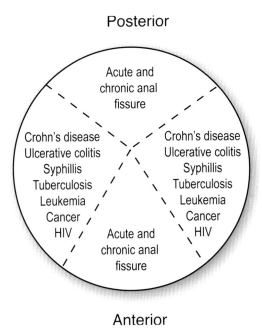

FIGURE 12-1. The location of anal fissure suggests their cause.

thumbs (Figure 12-2). Once the presence of a fissure is verified, further attempt to examine the anal canal with insertion of a finger or endoscopic instrumentation (anoscopy or proctoscopy) is not appropriate. Most patients are far too tender to justify such invasive evaluation, which should be delayed or deferred until symptoms have resolved.

Fissures may be frequently misdiagnosed as hemorrhoids by primary care providers. The differential diagnosis includes perianal abscess, anal fistula, inflammatory bowel disease, sexually transmitted disease, tuberculosis, leukemia, and anal carcinoma. Atypical fissures, such as those occurring off the midline, multiple, painless, and nonhealing fissures, warrant

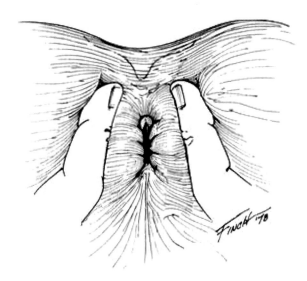

FIGURE 12-2. Examination revealing an anal fissure.

further evaluation, via examination under anesthesia and possible biopsy and cultures.

Management

Conservative

Almost half of all patients diagnosed with an acute fissure will heal with conservative measures, i.e., sitz baths and psyllium fiber supplementation, with or without the addition of topical anesthetics or anti-inflammatory ointments. In a retrospective review, Shub et al.[7] were able to demonstrate healing in 44% of fissure patients using psyllium fiber, sitz baths, and emollient suppositories. During a 5-year follow-up period, there were treatment failures in 27% of patients initially reported as healed. A second retrospective review almost 20 years later demonstrated similar findings. Hananel and Gordon[8] reported initial healing in 44% and recurrence in 18.6% of their fissure patients. Therapy consisted of bulking agents and sitz baths.

Jensen[9] has conducted two randomized, controlled trials examining the effects of unprocessed bran in both initial treatment and maintenance therapy of acute fissures. In the first, 103 patients with acute posterior anal fissures were randomized to receive lignocaine ointment (33), hydrocortisone ointment (35), or sitz baths and unprocessed bran (35) for 3 weeks, with symptomatic relief and fissure healing as endpoints. After weeks 1 and 2, patients treated with sitz baths and bran were found to have significant improvement in symptomatic relief as compared with the other two groups. By the 3-week endpoint, there was no symptomatic difference between the three groups; however, healed fissures occurred most frequently in the bran/sitz bath group (87%), when compared with patients receiving hydrocortisone (82.4%) or lignocaine (60%). In a double-blind, placebo-controlled trial, fissure recurrence was measured after 1 year in three groups. Significantly fewer recurrences (16%) were seen in patients receiving 15 g of unprocessed bran daily, when compared with 60% of patients receiving 7.5 g daily or 68% of patients on placebo.[10]

Operative Treatment

The primary goal in the treatment of a nonhealing anal fissure is to decrease abnormally elevated resting anal tone. Operative procedures, such as manual anal dilatation or internal sphincterotomy, have been advocated as initial modes of treatment because they produce permanent reductions in maximum resting anal pressures.

Anal Dilatation

Manual dilatation of the anus for anal fissure was first reported in 1964.[11] Ensuing endorsements have described a variety of means to enlarge the anal canal, such as the "four-finger method" and an assortment of instrumentation, including rectal dilators and retractors. Inconsistencies with regard to technique, specifically extent and duration of sphincter stretch, have cast some doubt about true success rates of this procedure. Reports as recent as 1995, however, support the use of gentle anal dilatation as a "first management choice in the treatment of anal fissure."[12–15] In 1992, Sohn et al.[16] standardized the extent of anal dilatation using either a Parks' retractor opened to 4.8 cm or a pneumatic balloon inflated to 40 mm. These authors reported up to 93%–94% healing of anal fissures after these procedures, which were associated with relatively few complications.

Long-term outcomes of anal dilatation are sparse. Additional widespread criticism of the technique stems from reported complications of incontinence, secondary to diffuse sphincter damage. In a retrospective analysis by MacDonald et al.,[14] patient outcomes after manual anal dilatation were reviewed. Not only was dilatation unsuccessful in 56% of patients diagnosed with fissures, incontinence occurred in 27% of patients overall. Speakman et al.[17] performed endoanal ultrasound and anorectal physiology studies on 12 men with fecal incontinence after anal dilatation. Internal and external anal sphincter defects were identified in 11 and 3 patients, respectively. Sphincter defects after anal dilatation were also recognized by Nielsen et al.,[18] who reported minor incontinence in 12.5% of patients overall. Ultrasound was ultimately performed in 20 patients, 13 of whom had IAS defects. Deficits were identified in 61% (11/18) of the continent and 100% (2/2) of the incontinent patients.

One retrospective review comparing treatment outcomes of anal dilatation and lateral subcutaneous sphincterotomy was reported by Collopy and Ryan.[19] Questionnaires were sent to 160 patients who underwent either of the two procedures. Fissure recurrence and incontinence were reported less often in the sphincterotomy group. Early prospective, randomized trials did not support these findings.[20–22] In one study, recurrence and incontinence rates were equal between both groups[20]; in another, significantly worse after lateral sphincterotomy.[21] Four months after randomization in the trial by Marby et al., symptomatic improvement was reported in 93% after dilatation versus 78% after sphincterotomy ($P < .05$). During the same time period, recurrence rates were 10% after dilatation and 29% after sphincterotomy ($P < .02$). Later randomized trials demonstrated better functional results, in terms of incontinence, after lateral sphincterotomy.[23] Whereas recurrence rates were 3.5%–10% up to 1 year after lateral sphincterotomy, higher rates of 26%–30% were observed after anal dilatation.[22,24]

Lateral Internal Sphincterotomy

The use of internal sphincterotomy in the treatment of anal fissure was introduced by Eisenhammer[25] in the early 1950s. His initial approach through the bed of the fissure in the posterior midline often resulted in a scarred groove, or "keyhole deformity," as often referred today. The functional impairment that ensued resulted in incontinence to gas and/or stool for many patients. Lateral subcutaneous sphincterotomy was popularized by Notaras[26] in 1969, and was believed to be associated with less functional impairment. In a retrospective review of 300 patients, comparing LIS to fissurectomy and midline sphincterotomy, Abcarian[27] reported a low recurrence rate of 1.3% and no incontinence after LIS—his procedure of choice for uncomplicated anal fissures. Several retrospective studies support the use of LIS as the preferred operative method for the treatment of anal fissures.[28–30] Exceptional healing and low recurrence rates have invariably been reported, and LIS has emerged as the "gold standard" for the treatment of anal fissure[31] (Table 12-1).

Persistent incontinence to gas and stool has emerged as a major concern after sphincterotomy. Incontinence rates of up to 36% have been reported, but these vary widely among studies.[32–36] Much of this variation can be attributed to differences in definition and assiduousness of follow-up. Reasons for incontinence after LIS have been related to the type and extent of sphincter muscle divided. Sultan et al.[37] prospectively performed endoanal ultrasonography before and 2 months after sphincterotomy in 15 patients. IAS defects were identified in 14 patients. In 90% of the women examined, the defect comprised the full length of the sphincter. Incontinence to flatus was reported in 3 of 10 women, in whom *external* sphincter defects were found in 2. The authors concluded that the complete sphincter deficits observed in women were the consequences of lack of appreciation for shorter anal canals in this population and suggested that postsphincterotomy incontinence may be further lessened if external anal sphincter deficits are recognized preoperatively.

Littlejohn and Newstead[38] reported a retrospective review of 287 patients who underwent tailored sphincterotomy, i.e., division of the IAS for the length of the fissure, rather than to the dentate line. There were no reports of incontinence to liquid or solid stool. The incidence of urgency was 0.7%; gas incontinence, 1.4%; and minor staining, 35%. Pescatori et al.[39] reported the results of a prospective, randomized study of tailored LIS on the basis of preoperative manometry. When increased resting anal tone was not demonstrated preoperatively, fissurectomy with anoplasty was performed. For elevated anal pressures (70–90 mm Hg), the extent of sphincterotomy was 0.5–1.5 cm and up to 2.5 cm for higher pressures. Continence worsened in only 11% of patients, and recurrences were limited to 4% of patients after sphincterotomy.

Inadvertent division of the external sphincter during sphincterotomy affects overall healing rates as well. In a study by Farouk et al.,[40] ultrasound evaluations performed in patients with persistent fissures after sphincterotomy demonstrated a lack of internal sphincter defects in almost 70% of patients. External sphincter defects were identified, however.

Other technical variations that have influenced patient outcomes after LIS have been described (Figures 12-3 and 12-4).

TABLE 12-1. Results of LIS

Year	Author	n	Success (%)	Recurrence (%)	Incontinence (%)[*]	Follow-up (type)	Follow-up (mo)
1980	Abcarian[27]	150	100	1.3	0	C	NS
1981	Keighley et al.[107]	71	100	25	2	I, E	12
1982	Ravikumar et al.[108]	60	97	0	5	C	24
1984	Hsu and MacKeigan[28]	89	100	5.6	0	C	NS
1984	Jensen et al.[24]	30	100	3	0	Q, E	18
1985	Walker et al.[43]	306	100	0	15	I	52
1987	Gingold[109]	86	100	3.5	0	C	24
1987	Weaver et al.[20]	39	93	5.1	2.5	I, E	17
1988	Lewis et al.[41]	350	94	6	6	I	37
1988	Zinkin[110]	151	94.7	NS	NS	None	0
1989	Khubchandani and Reed[33]	717	97.7	NS	35.1	Q	52.9
1992	Kortbeek et al.[42]	112	95.5	NS	NS	I	1.5
1994	Pernikoff et al.[34]	500	99	2	16	Q	78
1994	Romano et al.[35]	44	100	0	9	E	8
1995	Leong and Seow-Choen[46]	20	100	NS	0	I, E	6.5
1995	Prohm and Bonner[111]	177	96	3.3	1.6	E	1.5
1995	Usatoff and Polglase[29]	98	90	20	18	Q	41
1996	Garcia-Aguilar et al.[32]	864	96	11	37.8	Q	63.5
1997	Hananel and Gordon[30]	312	98.6	1.4†	—	C	NS
1997	Littlejohn and Newstead[38]	352	99.7	1.4	1.4	C	9
1999	Nyam and Pemberton[36]	585	96	8	15	Q	72
2004	Wiley et al.[112]	76	96	NS	6.8	Q	12
2004	Parellada[113]	27	100	NS	15	E	2.5

C, chart review; E, examination; I, interview; Q, questionnaire; NS, not stated.

[*]Includes seepage and incontinence to flatus and stool.

†Recurrence and persistence combined.

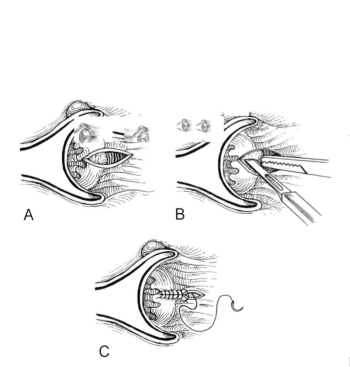

FIGURE 12-3. Open lateral internal anal sphincterotomy. **A** Radial skin incision distal to the dentate line exposing the intersphincteric groove. **B** Elevation and division of the internal sphincter. **C** Primary wound closure.

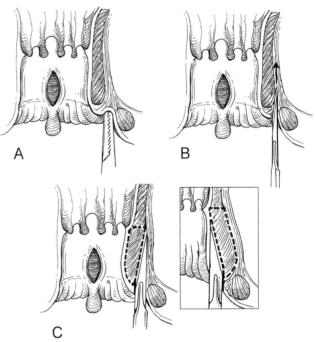

FIGURE 12-4. Closed lateral internal anal sphincterotomy. **A** Location of the intersphincteric groove. **B** Insertion of knife blade in the intersphincteric plane in performing a "blind" lateral subcutaneous internal anal sphincterotomy. **C** Lateral to medial division of the IAS (insert: medial to lateral division of the muscle).

With regard to open or closed sphincterotomy, several retrospective analyses[41] and at least one randomized trial[42] report similar rates of initial healing and fissure recurrence. In these studies, incontinence to flatus or stool occurred in 15%–17% of patients overall. Although there was no significant difference in *acute* complications in another randomized study, long-term persistent complications were more frequent in the open (55%) than the closed (20%) sphincterotomy group in retrospective review.[43] In a separate study, in which the degree of continence after open versus closed sphincterotomy was assessed by questionnaire, closed internal sphincterotomy was again favored. A significant difference was reported with regard to postoperative incontinence to gas (27.6% versus 30.6%), stool (3.1% versus 11.3%), and seepage (16.1% versus 26.7%).[32]

Excision of hypertrophied anal papillae and fibrous anal polyps has been advocated by Gupta and Kalaskar.[44] In a randomized trial, patient satisfaction was rated as excellent or good after removal of these structures in 84% of patients, compared with 58% of patients whose polyps and papillae were left intact. In a separate prospective study, earlier wound healing rates were achieved with primary closure after LIS, as compared with healing by secondary intention.[45]

Advancement Flaps

One prospective trial of the use of advancement flaps for chronic anal fissures has been conducted to date.[46] When patients were randomized to receive LIS or advancement flap, there was no significant difference between healing rates (100% in the sphincterotomy group versus 85% in the flap group, $P = .12$). Incontinence was not observed in either group.

Medical Management

Sphincter Relaxants

Increasing concerns with long-term complications associated with the operative management of anal fissures has led to the development of "chemical sphincterotomy," aimed at reducing mean maximum resting anal pressures, without permanent sphincter injury. Preparations have included: 1) various nitrate formulations, including nitroglycerin (NTG) ointment, glyceryl trinitrate (GTN), and isosorbide dinitrate (ISDN); 2) oral and topical calcium channel blockers, including nifedipine and diltiazem (DTZ); 3) adrenergic antagonists; 4) topical muscarinic agonists, i.e., bethanechol; 5) phosphodiesterase inhibitors; and 6) botulinum toxin (BT). However, there is increasing controversy in this area. Whereas one recent review concluded "first-line use of medical therapy cures most chronic fissures cheaply and conveniently,"[47] a systematic review of the literature published at the same time concluded "medical therapy for chronic anal fissure . . . may be applied with a chance of cure that is only marginally better than placebo . . . [and] far less effective than surgery."[48]

Topical Nitrates

The IAS is a smooth muscle whose tone is affected by both intrinsic myogenic properties and extrinsic neural influences. Nitric oxide is the predominant nonadrenergic, noncholinergic neurotransmitter in the IAS. Release of nitric oxide results in IAS relaxation. Exogenous nitrates release nitric oxide in vivo and have been used as nitric oxide donors.

Studies by Loder et al.[49] and Guillemot et al.[50] demonstrated decreased resting anal pressure with 0.2% GTN. This led to a series of retrospective and prospective reports, as well as randomized trials, supporting the use of various nitrate preparations in the treatment of anal fissures (Table 12-2). An early clinical trial in 1997 by Bacher et al.[51] randomized 35 patients with acute and chronic anal fissures to receive either 0.2% NTG ointment or 2% lidocaine gel for 4 weeks. After 1 month, the healing rate was 80% for patients receiving NTG (11 of 12 acute and 5 of 8 chronic fissures), which was significantly higher than the 40% healing rate reported for patients receiving topical lidocaine (5 of 10 acute and 1 of 5 chronic fissures). Manometry was performed on the 28th day of treatment. Overall maximum resting anal pressures were found to decrease from a mean of 110 to 87 cm H_2O, although this difference was not observed for patients with chronic fissures or patients receiving lidocaine ointment. The authors postulated that the persistence and recurrence of chronic anal fissures was secondary to lack of sphincter tone reduction.

Subsequent randomized, placebo-controlled trials have attempted to determine whether higher doses of NTG ointment promote healing and lessen recurrence in chronic anal fissures. Carapeti et al.[52] found no difference in chronic fissure healing between patients randomized to receive an 8-week treatment of either 0.2% GTN 3 times daily or 0.2% GTN titrated in 0.1% increments (to maximum of 0.6%). Higher dosing did not result in accelerated healing. Patients treated actively with either GTN preparation demonstrated 67% healing rate, compared with 32% in those receiving placebo. Bailey et al.[53] and Scholefield et al.[54] reported similar findings when patients with chronic anal fissures were randomized to receive placebo, 0.1%, 0.2%, or 0.4% GTN ointment 2–3 times daily. In the study by Bailey et al., there were no significant differences in fissure healing among treatment groups. In fact, healing rates were approximately 50% for all groups, including placebo.[53] Scholefield et al. also demonstrated similar healing rates among all groups (37.5% for placebo, 46.9% for 0.1% GTN, 40.4% for 0.2% GTN, and 54.1% for 0.4% GTN) with no significant improvement over the placebo response.[54]

Additional randomized, placebo-controlled trials have demonstrated comparable healing rates of 46%–70% in patients with chronic anal fissures after application of 0.2% GTN ointment 2–3 times daily for 4–8 weeks. Supportive data have included statistically significant decreases in pain scores and maximal anal resting pressures in patients treated with GTN as compared with placebo. In a study by Altomare et al.,[55] 132 patients with chronic fissures were randomized to receive

TABLE 12-2. Randomized trials of NTG therapy

Year	Author	n	Treatment	Follow-up	Success (%)
1997	Lund et al.[114]	80	0.2% GTN bid placebo	8 wk	68 39
1997	Oettle[56]	24	0.2% GTN tid LIS	4 wk	83.3 100
1997	Bacher et al.[51]	35	0.2% GTN 2% lidocaine	4 wk	80 40
1999	Kennedy et al.[115]	43	0.2% GTN placebo	4 wk	46 16
1999	Carapeti et al.[52]	70	0.2% GTN tid 0.2% GTN tid (titrated to 0.6%) placebo	8 wk	67 32
2000	Altomare et al.[55]	132	0.2% GTN bid placebo	4 wk	49.2 51.7
2000	Zuberi et al.[60]	42	0.2% GTN 10mg NTG patch LIS	8 wk	66.7 63.2 91.7
2000	Richard et al.[58]	82	0.2% GTN LIS	6 mo	27.2 92.1
2001	Evans et al.[57]	65	0.2% GTN tid LIS	8 wk	60.6 97
2001	Chaudhuri et al.[116]	19	0.2% GTN bid placebo	6 wk	70 22.2
2002	Libertiny et al.[59]	70	0.2% GTN LIS	2 y	45.7 97.1
2002	Bailey et al.[53]	304	0.1%, 0.2%, and 0.4% GTN bid/tid placebo	8 wk	50% across board
2003	Scholefield et al.[54]	200	0.1%, 0.2%, and 0.4% GTN bid/tid placebo	8 wk	46.9, 40.4, 54.1, 37.5

GTN, glyceryl trinitrate; NTG, nitroglycerin; LIS, lateral internal sphincterotomy; bid, twice daily; tid, three times daily.

0.2% GTN or placebo bid for 4 weeks. These authors confirmed the effects of GTN on anodermal blood flow and sphincter pressure, but unlike similarly designed trials, they demonstrated no significant difference in healing rates between GTN and placebo (49.2% versus 51.7%). They concluded that the use of GTN as a substitute for surgery should be discouraged.

Several simultaneous randomized trials whose treatment arms consisted of 0.2% GTN and LIS support the findings of Altomare et al. Although initial healing rates during 4- to 8-week evaluation periods were similar to those in placebo-based trials (and up to 83.3% in a study by Oettle[56]), healing rates were far superior for LIS (91.7%–100%). Evans et al.[57] demonstrated healing in 20 (60.6%) of 33 patients treated with GTN, in comparison to 26 (97%) of 27 patients treated with sphincterotomy. Of the patients initially treated with GTN, 12 eventually underwent sphincterotomy for persistent fissures. Of the 20 patients whose fissures healed with GTN treatment, nine developed recurrences. The authors acknowledge that GTN will heal the majority of fissures, but concluded "a significant minority have little improvement and require conventional surgical treatment."[57] Richard et al.[58] also found LIS "superior to topical NTG . . . in the treatment of chronic anal fissure, with a high rate of healing, few side effects, and low risk of early incontinence." After 6-week follow-up in a multi-center, randomized, controlled trial, 89.5% of patients in the LIS group compared with 29.5% in the NTG group had complete healing of fissures. At 6 months, fissure healing had occurred in 92.1% versus 27.2% in the LIS and NTG groups, respectively. Side effects were observed more frequently in patients treated with NTG (28.9%), compared with LIS (84%).

Although findings were similar in other randomized, controlled trials, conclusions still favor the use of GTN. Libertiny et al.[59] randomized 70 patients with chronic anal fissure to receive 0.2% GTN or LIS. Only 16 of 35 patients initially treated with GTN healed without recurrence during 24-month follow-up, in contrast to operative cure in 34 of 35 patients treated with LIS. The authors concluded that chemical sphincterotomy with GTN should be the initial treatment in patients with chronic anal fissure, and despite its effectiveness, LIS should be reserved for treatment failures. Zuberi et al.[60] similarly concluded that GTN ointment and NTG patch were effective treatment options in patients with anal fissures. In their study of 42 patients, healing rates were 66.7% in patients receiving 0.2% GTN, 63.2% for those receiving a 10-mg NTG patch applied at a distance from the fissure, and 91.7% in patients who underwent LIS. Their findings support the use of GTN as a first line agent in chronic anal fissures, as the difference in healing rates was not statistically significant between groups.

Other nitrate preparations have been used in the treatment of anal fissures. A prospective, uncontrolled study by Schouten et al.[61] demonstrated reduction in anal pressure and improvement in anodermal blood flow in patients with chronic anal fissure treated with ISDN. The authors demonstrated an 88% fissure healing rate after 12 weeks. Two randomized, placebo-controlled trials confirmed these findings. Werre et al.[62] were able to achieve healing in 17 of 20 patients (85%) with chronic anal fissure treated with ISDN for 5 weeks, as compared with 6 of 17 patients (35.3%) who received placebo. Tankova et al.[63] subsequently reported fissure healing in 80% of patients actively treated with mononitrate for 3 weeks, compared with 22% of the control group. In a dose finding study, Lysy et al.[64] found that 2.5 mg of topically applied ISDN 3 times daily resulted in a greater reduction in maximum anal resting pressure than 1.25 mg. By 1 month, 34 patients (83%) were able to achieve complete healing of their fissures. During the mean follow-up period of 11 months, six healed patients had fissure recurrence, which responded to additional treatment with ISDN.

Endogenous nitric oxide donors, such as L-arginine, have also been shown to be effective in relaxation of the anal sphincter. Preliminary in vivo studies in rats have demonstrated a decline in sphincter pressure with administration of 10 mg L-arginine rectally. This effect was reversed with the use of L-arginine antagonists. In a placebo-controlled trial, 46% reduction in resting anal pressure was observed 5 minutes after topical application of L-arginine, and maintained for 2 hours. The decrease in pressure observed in the placebo group was not significant.[65]

Despite these encouraging results regarding initial healing rates with topical nitrates, concerns about long-term outcomes and adverse reactions have limited their use. In studies summarizing long-term follow-up, recurrence rates up to 35% have been documented. For example, in a retrospective study by Dorfman et al.,[66] of 31 patients treated with 0.2% GTN bid, only 67% were compliant with treatment. Although there was an overall healing rate of 56%, recurrence occurred in 27% of patients initially healed. More than 75% of patients had side effects, including headache in 63% and lightheadedness in 52% of patients. In a nonrandomized, prospective trial, Graziano et al.[67] demonstrated a 67% recurrence rate for chronic fissures during a 9-month follow-up period. Patients were treated with a 2-week course of 0.25% NTG, which produced headache in 77% of patients actively treated.

Side effects have invariably been reported in randomized, controlled trials as well. Mild headaches were described by Bacher et al.[51] in 20% of patients receiving 0.2% GTN. Altomare et al.[55] reported that 34% of chronic fissure patients treated with GTN had headaches and nearly 6% of patients had orthostatic hypotension. Carapeti et al. reported headaches in 72% of patients receiving GTN versus 27% of controls receiving placebo.[52] In the L-arginine study, no side effects were noted during the study period.[65]

Calcium Channel Blockers

The effect of nifedipine on the anal sphincter was first evaluated by Chrysos et al.[68] in a prospective, controlled trial in 1996. Anorectal manometry was performed on 10 patients with hemorrhoids and/or anal fissure and 10 controls before and 30 minutes after receiving 20 mg of sublingual nifedipine. Anal resting pressure was reduced by almost 30% in both groups. This study set the stage for further prospective, clinical trials examining the efficacy of nifedipine and other calcium channel blockers in treating anal fissures. Carapeti et al.[69] investigated the use of topical DTZ in the treatment of anal fissure, after a prior randomized trial demonstrated that the majority of fissure patients treated with GTN developed headaches. After application of 2% DTZ gel 3 times daily in 10 patients, 67% obtained healed fissures after 8 weeks of treatment. No headaches or side effects were reported.

Further prospective trials substantiated these findings. Knight et al.[70] also evaluated the effects of 2% DTZ gel in 71 patients and were able to achieve healing in 75%, after 9 weeks of treatment. An additional 8 weeks of treatment was administered to incompletely healed fissures in 17 patients, 8 of whom healed. Side effects were reported in five patients overall: four with perianal dermatitis and one with headache. Agaoglu et al.[71] demonstrated 60% healing in patients treated with 20 mg of oral nifedipine twice daily. Headache was reported in only one patient. Ansaloni et al.[72] reported even more encouraging results regarding efficacy of 6 mg of oral lacidipine and warm sitz baths. At 2 months' follow-up, 90.4% of patients treated healed without evidence of fissure recurrence; however, 33% of patients had side effects.

Randomized, controlled trials comparing topical nifedipine gel with a combination of topical lidocaine and hydrocortisone gels have also demonstrated superiority of nifedipine in the treatment of anal fissures. Antropoli et al.[73] randomized 283 patients to either receive 0.2% nifedipine gel every 12 hours or 1% lidocaine/1% hydrocortisone gels. Complete healing occurred in 95% of patients receiving nifedipine, as compared with 50% of controls. Perrotti et al.[74] similarly randomized 110 patients with anal fissure to receive 0.3% nifedipine gel with 1.5% lidocaine or 1.5% lidocaine with 1% hydrocortisone twice daily. Of the 52 patients treated with nifedipine, 94.5% healed completely versus 16.4% of controls. During 1-year follow-up, three of the 52 patients healed with nifedipine had recurrent fissures; two healed after additional treatment. No side effects were observed in either study.

Jonas et al.[75] performed a randomized, controlled trial to ascertain whether different routes of administration had similar healing rates. The authors randomized 50 patients to receive 60 mg of oral DTZ or 2% topical DTZ gel twice daily. Complete healing occurred in 38% of patients taking oral treatment versus 65% of patients using topical therapy. Side effects were reported in 33% of patients treated orally.

Although long-term follow-up studies are lacking, several randomized, controlled trials comparing calcium channel

12. Benign Anorectal: Anal Fissure

blockers and nitrates have been performed. Kocher et al.[76] randomized 61 patients with chronic anal fissures to receive 0.2% GTN or 2% DTZ. After 6–8 weeks of treatment, 21 of 29 patients in the GTN group and 13 of 31 in the DTZ group experienced side effects. Therapeutic efficacy was similar between both groups. In the GTN group, 25 of 29 patients (86.2%) were healed or improved, compared with 24 of 31 patients (77.4%) in the DTZ group ($P = .21$). Bielecki et al.[77] also found equal healing rates between topical 0.2% GTN and 2% DTZ, as well as fewer headaches with 2% DTZ (0% versus 33% with 0.2% GTN). In a prospective, double-blind trial by Ezri and Susmallian,[78] 52 patients were randomized to receive topical GTN or nifedipine. The healing rate was higher ($P < .04$) with nifedipine (89%) as compared with GTN (58%). Side effects occurred more frequently ($P < .01$) with GTN (40%) than nifedipine (5%), a finding that was similar to the other trials. Recurrences within a 6-month period were common in both groups: 31% for GTN and 42% for nifedipine. Based on these study results, topical calcium channel blockers appear to be as effective as topical nitrates, with fewer side effects. Initial data suggest that long-term recurrences may be similar between both treatment groups, but further studies are warranted. Currently, topical calcium channel blocker preparations are not commercially available in the United States.

Adrenergic Antagonists

The effect of alpha-1 adrenergic blockade on anal sphincter pressure has been studied in two prospective trials. Pitt et al.[79,80] administered 20 mg of indoramin, an alpha-1 blocker, to seven patients with chronic anal fissure and six healthy controls. Reduction in anal pressure was observed in both groups: 35.8% in patients with fissure and 39.9% in those without. In a placebo-controlled trial, 23 patients with chronic anal fissure were randomized to receive 20 mg of indoramin or placebo twice daily.[79] Although a 29.8% reduction in maximum anal resting pressure was observed 1 hour after active treatment, healing occurred in only 1 patient (7%), despite 6 weeks of therapy. That patient developed a recurrence within 3 months. In the placebo group, 22% of patients achieved healing, although no significant change in anal pressure was observed. The trial was not completed because of lack of efficacy.

Cholinergic Agonists

Carapeti et al.[81] documented reduced anal sphincter pressure using bethanechol in a dose-finding study. Using increasing concentrations of bethanechol gel in healthy volunteers, they demonstrated a 24% reduction in maximal anal resting pressure using 0.1% dose. In a subsequent study, they reported fissure healing in 9 of 15 patients treated with 0.1% bethanechol gel 3 times daily for 8 weeks.[69] Maximum resting sphincter pressure was significantly lower after treatment ($P = .02$) compared with pretreatment values. No side effects were reported.

Phosphodiesterase Inhibitors

Early work by Jones et al.[82] has demonstrated an in vitro effect of increasing concentrations of various phosphodiesterase inhibitors on internal sphincter tone. This may spark future clinical trials in the treatment of anal fissure.

Botulinum Toxin

Botulinum Toxin (BT) is an exotoxin produced by the bacterium *Clostridium botulinum*. When injected locally, BT binds to the presynaptic nerve terminal at the neuromuscular junction, thereby preventing release of acetylcholine and resulting in temporary paralysis of skeletal muscle. Its mechanism of action on smooth muscle, such as the internal sphincter, has been evaluated in recent animal studies. In a series of experiments, Jones et al.[83] injected BT into porcine anal sphincters, which responded with decreased mean anal resting pressure in subsequent manometric studies. Strips of sphincter muscle were then isolated and examined in vitro. Application of electrical field stimulation and nicotinic agonists resulted in increased myogenic tone, which was blocked by guanethidine and attenuated by BT injection. These findings suggested that the predominant effect of BT on the IAS is sympathetic blockade.

BT injections can be given easily, on an outpatient basis, and are well tolerated. The commercial availability of BT has prompted several prospective trials examining its efficacy in the treatment of anal fissure (Table 12-3). An early placebo-controlled trial randomized 30 patients to receive either two injections of 20 U BT-A or saline.[84] After 2 months, complete healing occurred in 11 of 15 patients (73.3%) receiving BT and 2 of 15 patients (13.3%) receiving placebo. Subsequent BT injections were offered and given to 10 patients in the control group; there were seven healed fissures. Repeat BT injections (25 U) were given to four treatment failures, all of which healed after 2 months. No recurrences were observed during 16 months' follow-up. In a randomized trial comparing BT and lidocaine pomade in the treatment of anal fissure, Colak et al.[85] demonstrated superiority ($P = .006$) of BT in 62 patients, with complete epithelialization in 70.58% of patients in the BT group versus 21.42% in the lidocaine group.

The dose of BT injected is critical to successful healing in anal fissures. Siproudhis et al.[86] reported that a single 20-U injection of BT was not superior to that of placebo in a randomized, double-blind trial of 44 patients with chronic anal fissure. In a dose-finding study, Brisinda et al.[87] randomized 150 patients to two treatment arms. Initial treatment with 20 U of BT, followed by 30 U of BT for fissure persistence, was given to the first group, and 30 U of BT, followed by 50 U of BT, was given to the second group. One month after BT injections, there were no significant differences in resting anal pressures between the two groups; however, complete healing was more frequent in the second group (87%) than the first (73%). Fissures remained unhealed in two patients in the first, and three patients in the second group, despite additional BT

TABLE 12-3. Prospective BT trials

Year	Author	n	Treatment	Follow-up	Success (%)	Side effects
1998	Maria et al.[84]	30	BT 20 U (2 doses)		73.3	
			Saline	2 mo	13.3 (P = .003)	
1999	Brisinda et al.[90]	50	BT 20 U (2 doses)		96	
			0.2% NTG	2 mo	60 (P = .005)	20% headaches
2002	Colak et al.[85]	62	BT		70.6	
			Lidocaine	2 mo	21.4 (P = .006)	
2002	Brisinda et al.[87]	150	BT 20 U, 30 U		89	
			BT 30 U, 50 U	2 mo	96	
2003	Siproudhis et al.[86]	44	BT 20 U (1 dose)		22.7	
			Saline	4 wk	22.7	
2003	Mentes et al.[91]	101	BT 0.3 U/kg		75.4	
			LIS	12 mo	94 (P = .008)	16% incontinence

BT, botulinum toxin; U, units; LIS, lateral internal sphincterotomy.

injections. Temporary incontinence to flatus was reported in 6.6% of the second group only.

Optimal dosing of BT therapy was evaluated in a separate study by Madalinski et al.[88] Fourteen patients with chronic anal fissures resistant to topical nitrates and a subsequent 25-U BT injection were offered a second application of topical nitrates, which resulted in healing in only one patient. A higher dose of BT (50 U) was given to the 13 remaining patients and healing achieved in seven. The use of BT injections for GTN treatment failures was further supported in a prospective trial conducted by Lindsey et al.[89] Forty patients with chronic anal fissures despite GTN therapy were treated with 20 U of BT. Initial success, which included patients with symptomatic relief in the presence of an unhealed fissure, was observed in 29 patients (73%). Less than one-third of patients eventually underwent a surgical procedure. Transient incontinence was noted in 18% of patients. The authors concluded that BT should be considered as a second-line, and perhaps a first-line, agent in the treatment of chronic anal fissures before pursuing surgical options.

In a prospective, randomized trial, Brisinda et al.[90] directly compared BT injection and topical NTG as first-line agents in the treatment of chronic anal fissures. BT injections (20 U) were given on each side of the IAS and 0.2% NTG ointment was applied twice daily for 6 weeks. Fissures healed in 96% of the patients in the BT group and 60% of the patients in the NTG group. Moderate to severe headaches were reported in 20% of the NTG group, whereas no side effects were observed after BT injections. Regarding nonsurgical treatment of chronic anal fissure, the authors concluded that BT was more effective than NTG therapy.

There has been only one prospective, randomized trial to date comparing BT to LIS in the treatment of chronic anal fissures. Mentes et al.[91] reported the results of 61 patients receiving a total of 0.3 U/kg BT in two divided doses and 50 patients who underwent sphincterotomy. Fissure healing was evaluated at 1 and 4 weeks postprocedure, as well as at 2-, 6-, and 12-month intervals. Patients in the BT group had a second injection if healing was incomplete after 2 months. After 1 month, fissures were completely healed in 62.3% of patients in the BT group versus 82% of patients in the LIS group (P = .023). By 2 months, healing rates were 73.8% in the BT group and 98% in the LIS group (P < .0001). Six months after treatment, 86.9% of patients in the BT group had healed fissures. In the LIS group, two patients developed recurrences, decreasing the healing rate to 94%, not significantly different from the BT group. By 12 months, however, fissure recurrence in seven patients in the BT group resulted in a decrease in the overall healing rate to 75.4%, significantly lower than 94% rate still observed in the LIS group (P = .008). Anal incontinence, predominantly to flatus, was reported in 16% of patients in the LIS group. No side effects were observed with BT injections. Although initial success and fewer complications were found with BT therapy, long-term results were not as encouraging when compared with LIS.

Late recurrence rates 42 months after BT treatment of chronic anal fissures have been reported in a prospective trial by Minguez et al.[92] Only patients with complete healing 6 months after BT injections were included for reassessment in 6-month intervals. Fissure recurrence was demonstrated in 41.5% of patients. Stratification by various clinical parameters revealed that higher risks of recurrence were associated with anterior location, chronicity of disease (longer than 12 months), multiple injections, and dosage greater than 21 U. They comment that lack of recurrence cited in earlier reports by Maria et al. and Brisinda et al. may have been influenced by their use of strict exclusion criteria, such as patients with anterior fissures. Furthermore, standard doses of BT were not used in all trials. Optimal dosing and appropriate patient selection remain uncertain.

Complications reported after BT injections of anal fissures have included perianal hematomas in 2 of 10 patients treated by Tilney et al.[93] and perianal thrombosis in early reports by Jost et al.,[94] although this has not been reproduced in his recent experience.[95]

Special Situations

Low Pressure Fissures

Unlike the classic anal fissures described previously, low pressure fissures are not appropriate candidates for operative sphincterotomy. Patients within this category include those with impaired continence and fissure recurrence after sphincterotomy. Anal fissures sustained after childbirth are also associated with reduced anal canal pressures. Corby et al.[96] prospectively studied 209 primigravid women with anal manometry 6 weeks before and after childbirth. Of those women, 9% developed postpartum fissures. Manometric evaluations demonstrated similar antepartum resting and squeeze pressures in women who developed fissure and those who did not. In addition, postpartum resting and squeeze pressures were decreased in both groups. For this group of patients, "surgical interference with the anal sphincter mechanism should be avoided."[96]

Optimal treatment of low-pressure fissures is unclear. Nyam et al.[97] reported the results of an island flap in 21 patients with preoperative median resting anal pressures and squeeze pressures significantly lower than controls or patients with high-pressure fissures. Sphincter defects were recognized ultrasonographically in 15 of 21 patients (71%). During an 18-month follow-up, all fissures healed and incontinence was not observed. The authors concluded that the island advancement flap "provides a useful alternative" for recurrent anal fissures, or low-pressure anal fissures, in which sphincterotomy "might jeopardize continence."[97]

Crohn's

The incidence of perianal Crohn's fissures varies widely among reports. In one retrospective review by Platell et al.,[98] symptomatic anal disease was documented in 42.4% of patients with Crohn's disease. More than one-quarter of those patients (27.6%) had anal fissures. In a separate analysis in which 3.8% of patients with Crohn's disease required surgery for perianal symptoms, Sangwan et al.[99] found that 31.8% had anal fissures. Fleshner et al.[100] specifically examined fissures in Crohn's disease and found 84% were symptomatic. Multiple fissures were noted in one-third of patients and only 66% were located in the posterior midline. Sweeney et al.[101]

reviewed the natural history of Crohn's fissures in 61 patients, in whom anal fissure was the only anal pathology. Fissure healing occurred in 42 of 69 patients (60.8%) during medical treatment for Crohn's disease. Ten patients developed additional anal lesions. Six patients (9.8%) eventually underwent anorectal surgery.

Traditionally, anorectal surgery in patients with Crohn's disease has been approached with caution. Complications resulting in proctectomy and fears regarding postoperative incontinence, exacerbated by preexisting diarrhea, have precluded perianal operations in these patients (although impairment of continence after such operations has not been studied in this population). As a result, most authorities argue that initial treatment of Crohn's fissures should be focused on controlling diarrhea. If fissure persists despite conservative measures, examination under anesthesia and limited sphincterotomy should be performed. Currently, there are no data to support the use of topical sphincter relaxants or BT in the treatment of fissures in Crohn's disease.

Outcomes after surgery in patients with Crohn's fissures have been reported, albeit in small retrospective series. Wolkomir and Luchtefeld[102] reported uncomplicated wound healing in 22 of 25 patients. In the series by Fleshner et al.,[100] 88% of patients healed after anorectal surgery, compared with 49% of patients after medical treatment and 29% after abdominal surgery. Of treatment failures, perianal abscess or fistula was observed in 26% of patients.

Anal dilatation for Crohn's fissures has also been reported with some success. Isbister and Prasad[12] reported that "three patients with anal fissures and Crohn's disease were successfully managed by anal dilatation." Allan and Keighley[103] described improvement in 4 of 7 patients, in whom 1 became incontinent.

Human Immunodeficiency Virus

Distinction between HIV-associated fissures and HIV-associated ulcers is necessary for optimization of fissure management in this patient population. Fissures in HIV-positive patients have a typical appearance, whereas HIV ulcers are deep and broad based and can occur anywhere within the anal canal.[104,105] Early pessimistic reports of poor wound healing and high rates of incontinence after sphincterotomy for HIV-associated fissures may have been skewed by inclusion of HIV ulcers in the fissure group.[105] In addition, these data preceded the era of highly effective antiviral therapy. In fact, there is a paucity of current information on HIV-associated fissures, and no available data about risk of postoperative incontinence or use of topical sphincter relaxants or BT as treatment options.

Barrett et al.[106] reported fissure prevalence in 32% of HIV-positive patients. Although sphincterotomies were performed in 18 patients, specific outcomes were not reported. Viamonte et al.[104] compared alternative treatments for anal fissures in 33 HIV-positive patients. Ten patients were lost to follow-up.

Improvement was noted in 10 patients treated nonoperatively and in 12 of 13 patients who underwent LIS. Actual healing rates were not provided, but no cases of incontinence were observed.

Conclusions

Anal fissure is a common, symptomatic disorder. Diagnosis is often established by history alone, but is easily confirmed by physical examination without the need for additional instrumentation. After instigation by anal trauma, anal fissure is sustained by elevated resting anal pressure. Treatment of anal fissure has consequently been aimed at reducing anal tone.

Surgery has been highly effective, although alterations in continence have been documented. Although proponents of anal dilatation exist, LIS has been advocated as the operation of choice. Regarding nonoperative treatment options, the early GTN literature has been promising, but varies significantly with regard to rates of healing, relapse, and side effects. Topical calcium channel blockers have shown similar efficacy to GTN, but fewer side effects have been reported. In at least one randomized trial, BT demonstrated superiority to GTN, but long-term outcomes of BT have uncovered high fissure recurrence rates. In general, the success of medical therapies has been controversial, with lack of consensus demonstrably evident after dichotomous analyses in the recent literature: a review by Lindsey et al.[47] that determines that most chronic anal fissures are successfully treated by inexpensive medical therapies and a systematic evaluation by Nelson[48] that concludes that medical therapy offers only a slight advantage when compared with placebo, but is significantly inferior to surgery.

References

1. Hancock BD. The internal sphincter and anal fissure. Br J Surg 1977;64(2):92–95.
2. Nothmann BJ, Schuster MM. Internal anal sphincter derangement with anal fissures. Gastroenterology 1974;67(2):216–220.
3. Farouk R, Duthie GS, MacGregor AB, Bartolo DC. Sustained internal sphincter hypertonia in patients with chronic anal fissure. Dis Colon Rectum 1994;37(5):424–429.
4. Gibbons CP, Read NW. Anal hypertonia in fissures: cause or effect? Br J Surg 1986;73:443–445.
5. Klosterhalfen B, Vogel P, Rixen H, Mittermayer C. Topography of the inferior rectal artery: a possible cause of chronic, primary anal fissure. Dis Colon Rectum 1989;32(1):43–52.
6. Schouten WR, Briel JW, Auwerda JJ, De Graaf EJ. Ischaemic nature of anal fissure. Br J Surg 1996;83(1):63–65.
7. Shub HA, Salvati EP, Rubin RJ. Conservative treatment of anal fissure: an unselected, retrospective and continuous study. Dis Colon Rectum 1978;21:582–583.
8. Hananel N, Gordon PH. Re-examination of clinical manifestations and response to therapy of fissure-in-ano. Dis Colon Rectum 1997;40:229–233.
9. Jensen SL. Treatment of first episodes of acute anal fissure: prospective randomised study of lignocaine ointment versus hydrocortisone ointment or warm sitz baths plus bran. Br Med J (Clin Res Ed) 1986;292(6529):1167–1169.
10. Jensen SL. Maintenance therapy with unprocessed bran in the prevention of acute anal fissure recurrence. J R Soc Med 1987;80(5):296–298.
11. Watts JM, Bennett RC, Goligher JC. Stretching of anal sphincters in treatment of fissure-in-ano. Br Med J 1964;342–343.
12. Isbister WH, Prasad J. Fissure in ano. Aust N Z J Surg 1995; 65(2):107–108.
13. O'Connor JJ. Lord procedure for treatment of postpartum hemorrhoids and fissures. Obstet Gynecol 1980;55(6):747–748.
14. MacDonald A, Smoth A, McNeill AD, Finlay IG. Manual dilatation of the anus. Br J Surg 1992;79:1381–1382.
15. Giebel GD, Horch R. Treatment of anal fissure: a comparison of three different forms of therapy. Nippon Geka Hokan 1989;58:126–133.
16. Sohn N, Eisenberg MM, Weinstein MA, Lugo RN, Ader J. Precise anorectal sphincter dilatation: its role in the therapy of anal fissures. Dis Colon Rectum 1992;35:322–327.
17. Speakman CT, Burnett SJ, Kamm MA, Bartram CI. Sphincter injury after anal dilatation demonstrated by anal endosonography. Br J Surg 1991;78:1429–1430.
18. Nielsen MB, Rasmussen OO, Pedersen JF, Christiansen J. Risk of sphincter damage and anal incontinence after anal dilatation for fissure-in-ano. An endosonographic study. Dis Colon Rectum 1993;36(7):677–680.
19. Collopy B, Ryan P. Comparison of lateral subcutaneous sphincterotomy with anal dilatation in the treatment of fissure in ano. Med J Aust 1979;2:461–462, 487.
20. Weaver RM, Ambrose NS, Alexander-Williams J, Keighley MR. Manual dilatation of the anus vs. lateral subcutaneous sphincterotomy in the treatment of chronic fissure-in-ano. Results of a prospective, randomized, clinical trial. Dis Colon Rectum 1987;30(6):420–423.
21. Marby M, Alexander-Williams J, Buchmann P, et al. A randomized controlled trial to compare anal dilatation with lateral subcutaneous sphincterotomy for anal fissure. Dis Colon Rectum 1979;22(5):308–311.
22. Olsen J, Mortensen PE, Krogh Petersen I, Christiansen J. Anal sphincter function after treatment of fissure-in-ano by lateral subcutaneous sphincterotomy versus anal dilatation. A randomized study. Int J Colorectal Dis 1987;2(3):155–157.
23. Saad AM, Omer A. Surgical treatment of chronic fissure-in-ano: a prospective randomised study. East Afr Med J 1992;69:613–615.
24. Jensen SL, Lund F, Nielsen OV, Tange G. Lateral subcutaneous sphincterotomy versus anal dilatation in the treatment of fissure in ano in outpatients: a prospective randomised study. Br Med J (Clin Res Ed) 1984;289(6444):528–530.
25. Eisenhammer S. The evaluation of the internal anal sphincterotomy operation with special reference to anal fissure. Surg Gynecol Obstet 1959;109:583–590.
26. Notaras MJ. Lateral subcutaneous sphincterotomy for anal fissure: a new technique. Proc R Soc Med 1969;62:713.
27. Abcarian H. Surgical correction of chronic anal fissure: results of lateral internal sphincterotomy vs. fissurectomy: midline sphincterotomy. Dis Colon Rectum 1980;23(1):31–36.
28. Hsu TC, MacKeigan JM. Surgical treatment of chronic anal fissure. A retrospective study of 1753 cases. Dis Colon Rectum 1984;27(7):475–478.

29. Usatoff V, Polglase AL. The longer term results of internal anal sphincterotomy for anal fissure. Aust N Z J Surg 1995;65(8): 576–578.

30. Hananel N, Gordon PH. Lateral internal sphincterotomy for fissure-in-ano: revisited. Dis Colon Rectum 1997;40(5):597–602.

31. Hyman N. Incontinence after lateral internal sphincterotomy: a prospective study and quality of life assessment. Dis Colon Rectum 2004;47:35–38.

32. Garcia-Aguilar J, Belmonte C, Wong WD, Lowry AC, Madoff RD. Open vs. closed sphincterotomy for chronic anal fissure: long-term results. Dis Colon Rectum 1996;39(4):440–443.

33. Khubchandani IT, Reed JF. Sequelae of internal sphincterotomy for chronic fissure in ano. Br J Surg 1989;76(5):431–434.

34. Pernikoff BJ, Eisenstat TE, Rubin RJ, Oliver GC, Salvati EP. Reappraisal of partial lateral internal sphincterotomy. Dis Colon Rectum 1994;37(12):1291–1295.

35. Romano G, Rotondano G, Santangelo M, Esercizio L. A critical appraisal of pathogenesis and morbidity of surgical treatment of chronic anal fissure. J Am Coll Surg 1994;178(6):600–604.

36. Nyam DC, Pemberton JH. Long-term results of lateral internal sphincterotomy for chronic anal fissure with particular reference to incidence of fecal incontinence. Dis Colon Rectum 1999;42:1306–1310.

37. Sultan AH, Kamm MA, Nicholls RJ, Bartram CI. Prospective study of the extent of internal anal sphincter division during lateral sphincterotomy. Dis Colon Rectum 1994;37(10):1031–1033.

38. Littlejohn DR, Newstead GL. Tailored lateral sphincterotomy for anal fissure. Dis Colon Rectum 1997;40(12):1439–1442.

39. Pescatori M, Ayabaca SM, Cafaro D. Tailored sphincterotomy or fissurectomy and anoplasty? Dis Colon Rectum 2002; 45(11):1563–1564; author reply 1564.

40. Farouk R, Monson JR, Duthie GS. Technical failure of lateral sphincterotomy for the treatment of chronic anal fissure: a study using endoanal ultrasonography. Br J Surg 1997;84:84–85.

41. Lewis TH, Corman ML, Prager ED, Robertson WG. Long-term results of open and closed sphincterotomy for anal fissure. Dis Colon Rectum 1988;31(5):368–371.

42. Kortbeek JB, Langevin JM, Khoo RE, Heine JA. Chronic fissure-in-ano: a randomized study comparing open and subcutaneous lateral internal sphincterotomy. Dis Colon Rectum 1992;35(9):835–837.

43. Walker WA, Rothenberger DA, Goldberg SM. Morbidity of internal sphincterotomy for anal fissure and stenosis. Dis Colon Rectum 1985;28(11):832–835.

44. Gupta PJ, Kalaskar S. Removal of hypertrophied anal papillae and fibrous anal polyps increases patient satisfaction after anal fissure surgery. Tech Coloproctol 2003;7:155–158.

45. Aysan E, Aren A, Ayar E. A prospective, randomized, controlled trial of primary wound closure after lateral internal sphincterotomy. Am J Surg 2004;187:291–294.

46. Leong AF, Seow-Choen F. Lateral sphincterotomy compared with anal advancement flap for chronic anal fissure. Dis Colon Rectum 1995;38(1):69–71.

47. Lindsey I, Jones OM, Cunningham C, Mortensen NJ. Chronic anal fissure. Br J Surg 2004;91(3):270–279.

48. Nelson R. A systematic review of medical therapy for anal fissure. Dis Colon Rectum 2004;47(4):422–431.

49. Loder PB, Kamm MA, Nicholls RJ, Phillips RK. 'Reversible chemical sphincterotomy' by local application of glyceryl trinitrate. Br J Surg 1994;81:1386–1389.

50. Guillemot F, Leroi H, Lone YC, Rousseau CG, Lamblin MD, Cortot A. Action of in situ nitroglycerin on upper anal canal pressure of patients with terminal constipation. A pilot study. Dis Colon Rectum 1993;36:372–376.

51. Bacher H, Mischinger HJ, Werkgartner G, et al. Local nitroglycerin for treatment of anal fissures: an alternative to lateral sphincterotomy? Dis Colon Rectum 1997;40(7):840–845.

52. Carapeti EA, Kamm MA, McDonald PJ, Chadwick SJ, Melville D, Phillips RK. Randomised controlled trial shows that glyceryl trinitrate heals anal fissures, higher doses are not more effective, and there is a high recurrence rate. Gut 1999;44(5):727–730.

53. Bailey HR, Beck DE, Billingham RP, et al. A study to determine the nitroglycerin ointment dose and dosing interval that best promote the healing of chronic anal fissures. Dis Colon Rectum 2002;45:1192–1199.

54. Scholefield JH, Bock JU, Marla B, et al. A dose finding study with 0.1%, 0.2%, and 0.4% glyceryl trinitrate ointment in patients with chronic anal fissures. Gut 2003;52:264–269.

55. Altomare DF, Rinaldi M, Milito G, et al. Glyceryl trinitrate for chronic anal fissure: healing or headache? Results of a multicenter, randomized, placebo-controlled, double-blind trial. Dis Colon Rectum 2000;43(2):174–179.

56. Oettle GJ. Glyceryl trinitrate vs. sphincterotomy for treatment of chronic fissure-in-ano: a randomized, controlled trial. Dis Colon Rectum 1997;40:1318–1320.

57. Evans J, Luck A, Hewett P. Glyceryl trinitrate vs. lateral sphincterotomy for chronic anal fissure: prospective, randomized trial. Dis Colon Rectum 2001;44:93–97.

58. Richard CS, Gregoire R, Plewes EA, et al. Internal sphincterotomy is superior to topical nitroglycerin in the treatment of chronic anal fissure: results of a randomized, controlled trial by the Canadian Colorectal Surgical Trials Group. Dis Colon Rectum 2000;43(8):1048–1057; discussion 1057–1048.

59. Libertiny G, Knight JS, Farouk R. Randomised trial of topical 0.2% glyceryl trinitrate and lateral internal sphincterotomy for the treatment of patients with chronic anal fissure: long-term follow-up. Eur J Surg 2002;168:418–421.

60. Zuberi BF, Rajput MR, Abro H, Shaikh SA. A randomized trial of glyceryl trinitrate ointment and nitroglycerin patch in healing of anal fissures. Int J Colorectal Dis 2000;15:243–245.

61. Schouten WR, Briel JW, Boerma MO, Auwerda JJ, Wilms EB, Graatsma BH. Pathophysiological aspects and clinical outcome of intra-anal application of isosorbide dinitrate in patients with chronic anal fissure. Gut 1996;39:465–469.

62. Werre AJ, Palamba HW, Bilgen EJ, Eggink WF. Isosorbide dinitrate in the treatment of anal fissure: a randomised, prospective, double blind, placebo-controlled trial. Eur J Surg 2001;167:382–385.

63. Tankova L, Yoncheva K, Muhtarov M, Kadyan H, Draganov V. Topical mononitrate treatment in patients with anal fissure. Aliment Pharmacol Ther 2002;16:101–103.

64. Lysy J, Israelit-Yatzkan Y, Sestiere-Ittah M, Keret D, Goldin E. Treatment of chronic anal fissure with isosorbide dinitrate: long-term results and dose determination. Dis Colon Rectum 1998;41:1406–1410.

65. Griffin N, Zimmerman DD, Briel JW, et al. Topical L-arginine gel lowers resting anal pressure: possible treatment for anal fissure. Dis Colon Rectum 2002;45:1332–1336.

66. Dorfman G, Levitt M, Platell C. Treatment of chronic anal fissure with topical glyceryl trinitrate. Dis Colon Rectum 1999;42:1007–1010.

67. Graziano A, Svidler Lopez L, Lencinas S, Masciangioli G, Gualdrini U, Bisisio O. Long-term results of topical nitroglycerin in the treatment of chronic anal fissures are disappointing. Tech Coloproctol 2001;5:143–147.

68. Chrysos E, Xynos E, Tzovaras G, Zoras OJ, Tsiaoussis J, Vassilakis SJ. Effect of nifedipine on rectoanal motility. Dis Colon Rectum 1996;39:212–216.

69. Carapeti EA, Kamm MA, Phillips RK. Topical diltiazem and bethanechol decrease anal sphincter pressure and heal anal fissures without side effects. Dis Colon Rectum 2000;43: 1359–1362.

70. Knight JS, Birks M, Farouk R. Topical diltiazem ointment in the treatment of chronic anal fissure. Br J Surg 2001;88: 553–556.

71. Agaoglu N, Cengiz S, Arslan MK, Turkyilmaz S. Oral nifedipine in the treatment of chronic anal fissure. Dig Surg 2003;20: 452–456.

72. Ansaloni L, Bernabe A, Ghetti R, Riccardi R, Tranchino RM, Gardini G. Oral lacidipine in the treatment of anal fissure. Tech Coloproctol 2002;6:79–82.

73. Antropoli C, Perrotti P, Rubino M, et al. Nifedipine for local use in conservative treatment of anal fissures: preliminary results of a multicenter study. Dis Colon Rectum 1999;42(8): 1011–1015.

74. Perrotti P, Bove A, Antropoli C, et al. Topical nifedipine with lidocaine ointment vs. active control for treatment of chronic anal fissure: results of a prospective, randomized, double-blind study. Dis Colon Rectum 2002;45:1468–1475.

75. Jonas M, Neal KR, Abercrombie JF, Scholefield JH. A randomized trial of oral vs. topical diltiazem for chronic anal fissures. Dis Colon Rectum 2001;44:1074–1078.

76. Kocher HM, Steward M, Leather AJ, Cullen PT. Randomized clinical trial assessing the side-effects of glyceryl trinitrate and diltiazem hydrochloride in the treatment of chronic anal fissure. Br J Surg 2002;89:413–417.

77. Bielecki K, Kolodziejczak M. A prospective randomized trial of diltiazem and glyceryltrinitrate ointment in the treatment of chronic anal fissure. Colorectal Dis 2003;5:256–257.

78. Ezri T, Susmallian S. Topical nifedipine vs. topical glyceryl trinitrate for treatment of chronic anal fissure. Dis Colon Rectum 2003;46:805–808.

79. Pitt J, Dawson PM, Hallan RI, Boulos PB. A double-blind randomized placebo-controlled trial of oral indoramin to treat chronic anal fissure. Colorectal Dis 2001;3:165–168.

80. Pitt J, Craggs MM, Henry MM, Boulos PB. Alpha-1 adrenoceptor blockade: potential new treatment for anal fissures. Dis Colon Rectum 2000;43:800–803.

81. Carapeti EA, Kamm MA, Evans BK, Phillips RK. Topical diltiazem and bethanechol decrease anal sphincter pressure without side effects. Gut 1999;45(5):719–722.

82. Jones OM, Brading AF, McC Mortnensen NJ. Phosphodiesterase inhibitors cause relaxation of the internal anal sphincter in vitro. Dis Colon Rectum 2002;45:530–536.

83. Jones OM, Moore JA, Brading AF, Mortensen NJ. Botulinum toxin injection inhibits myogenic tone and sympathetic nerve function in the porcine internal anal sphincter. Colorectal Dis 2003;5:552–557.

84. Maria G, Cassetta E, Gui D, Brisinda G, Bentivoglio AR, Albanese A. A comparison of botulinum toxin and saline for the treatment of chronic anal fissure [see comments]. N Engl J Med 1998;338(4):217–220.

85. Colak T, Ipek T, Kanik A, Aydin S. A randomized trial of botulinum toxin vs lidocain pomade for chronic anal fissure. Acta Gastroenterol Belg 2002;65:187–190.

86. Siproudhis L, Sebille V, Pigot F, Hemery P, Juguet F, Bellissant E. Lack of efficacy of botulinum toxin in chronic anal fissure. Aliment Pharmacol Ther 2003;18:515–524.

87. Brisinda G, Maria G, Sganga G, Bentivoglio AR, Albanese A, Castagneto M. Effectiveness of higher doses of botulinum toxin to induce healing in patients with chronic anal fissures. Surgery 2002;131:179–184.

88. Madalinski MH, Slawek J, Zbytek B, et al. Topical nitrates and the higher doses of botulinum toxin for chronic anal fissure. Hepatogastroenterology 2001;48:977–979.

89. Lindsey I, Jones OM, Cunningham C, George BD, Mortensen NJ. Botulinum toxin as second-line therapy for chronic anal fissure failing 0.2 percent glyceryl trinitrate. Dis Colon Rectum 2003;46:361–366.

90. Brisinda G, Maria G, Bentivoglio AR, Cassetta E, Gui D, Albanese A. A comparison of injections of botulinum toxin and topical nitroglycerin ointment for the treatment of chronic anal fissure [see comments]. N Engl J Med 1999;341(2): 65–69 [published erratum appears in N Engl J Med 1999; 341(8):624].

91. Mentes BB, Irkorucu O, Akin M, Leventoglu S, Tatlicioglu E. Comparison of botulinum toxin injection and lateral internal sphincterotomy for the treatment of chronic anal fissure. Dis Colon Rectum 2003;46:232–237.

92. Minguez M, Herreros B, Espi A, et al. Long-term follow-up (42 months) of chronic anal fissure after healing with botulinum toxin. Gastroenterology 2002;123:112–117.

93. Tilney HS, Heriot AG, Cripps NP. Complication of botulinum toxin injections for anal fissure. Dis Colon Rectum 2001; 44:1721–1724.

94. Jost WH, Schanne S, Mlitz H, Schimrigk K. Perianal thrombosis following injection therapy into the external anal sphincter using botulin toxin. Dis Colon Rectum 1995;38:781.

95. Jost WH. Ten years' experience with botulin toxin in anal fissure. Int J Colorectal Dis 2002;17:298–302.

96. Corby H, Donnelly VS, O'Herlihy C, O'Connell PR. Anal canal pressures are low in women with postpartum anal fissure. Br J Surg 1997;84(1):86–88.

97. Nyam DC, Wilson RG, Stewart KJ, Farouk R, Bartolo DC. Island advancement flaps in the management of anal fissures. Br J Surg 1995;82:326–328.

98. Platell C, Mackay J, Collopy B, Fink R, Ryan P, Woods R. Anal pathology in patients with Crohn's disease. Aust N Z J Surg 1996;66(1):5–9.

99. Sangwan YP, Schoetz DJ Jr, Murray JJ, Roberts PL, Coller JA. Perianal Crohn's disease. Results of local surgical treatment. Dis Colon Rectum 1996;39(5):529–535.

100. Fleshner PR, Schoetz DJ Jr, Roberts PL, Murray JJ, Coller JA, Veidenheimer MC. Anal fissure in Crohn's disease: a plea for aggressive management. Dis Colon Rectum 1995;38(11): 1137–1143.

101. Sweeney JL, Ritchie JK, Nicholls RJ. Anal fissure in Crohn's disease. Br J Surg 1988;75(1):56–57.

102. Wolkomir AF, Luchtefeld MA. Surgery for symptomatic hemorrhoids and anal fissures in Crohn's disease. Dis Colon Rectum 1993;36(6):545–547.

103. Allan A, Keighley MR. Management of perianal Crohn's disease. World J Surg 1988;12(2):198–202.

104. Viamonte M, Dailey TH, Gottesman L. Ulcerative disease of the anorectum in the HIV+ patient. Dis Colon Rectum 1993; 36(9):801–805.

105. Weiss EG, Wexner SD. Surgery for anal lesions in HIV-infected patients. Ann Med 1995;27(4):467–475.

106. Barrett WL, Callahan TD, Orkin BA. Perianal manifestations of human immunodeficiency virus infection: experience with 260 patients. Dis Colon Rectum 1998;41(5):606–611; discussion 611–602.

107. Keighley MR, Greca F, Nevah E, Hares M, Alexander-Williams J. Treatment of anal fissure by lateral subcutaneous sphincterotomy should be under general anaesthesia. Br J Surg 1981;68(6):400–401.

108. Ravikumar TS, Sridhar S, Rao RN. Subcutaneous lateral internal sphincterotomy for chronic fissure-in-ano. Dis Colon Rectum 1982;25(8):798–801.

109. Gingold BS. Simple in-office sphincterotomy with partial fissurectomy for chronic anal fissure. Surg Gynecol Obstet 1987;165(1):46–48.

110. Zinkin L. Left lateral internal sphincterotomy for anal fissure: as an office procedure. N J Med 1988;85(1):43–45.

111. Prohm P, Bonner C. Is manometry essential for surgery of chronic fissure-in-ano? Dis Colon Rectum 1995;38(7): 735–738.

112. Wiley M, Day P, Rieger N, Stephens J, Moore J. Open vs. closed lateral internal sphincterotomy for idiopathic fissure-in-ano: a prospective, randomized, controlled trial. Dis Colon Rectum 2004;47(6):847–852.

113. Parellada C. Randomized, prospective trial comparing 0.2 percent isosorbide dinitrate ointment with sphincterotomy in treatment of chronic anal fissure: a two-year follow-up. Dis Colon Rectum 2004;47(4):437–443.

114. Lund JN, Scholefield JH. A randomised, prospective, double-blind, placebo-controlled trial of glyceryl trinitrate ointment in treatment of anal fissure [see comments]. Lancet 1997; 349(9044):11–14 [published erratum appears in Lancet 1997; 349(9052):656].

115. Kennedy ML, Sowter S, Nguyen H, Lubowski DZ. Glyceryl trinitrate ointment for the treatment of chronic anal fissure: results of a placebo-controlled trial and long-term follow-up. Dis Colon Rectum 1999;42(8):1000–1006.

116. Chaudhuri S, Pal AK, Acharya A, et al. Treatment of chronic anal fissure with topical glyceryl trinitrate: a double-blind, placebo-controlled trial. Indian J Gastroenterol 2001;20(3):101–102.

13
Benign Anorectal: Abscess and Fistula

Carol-Ann Vasilevsky and Philip H. Gordon

Anorectal abscesses and fistula-in-ano represent different stages along the continuum of a common pathogenic spectrum. The abscess represents the acute inflammatory event whereas the fistula is representative of the chronic process.

Abscess

Anatomy

Successful eradication of anorectal suppuration and fistula-in-ano requires an in-depth understanding of anorectal anatomy. Essential is an understanding of the existence of potential anorectal spaces[1] (Figure 13-1A). The perianal space is located in the area of the anal verge. It becomes continuous with the ischioanal fat laterally while it extends into the lower portion of the anal canal medially. It is continuous with the intersphincteric space. The ischioanal space extends from the levator ani to the perineum. Anteriorly it is bounded by the transverse perineal muscles; the lower border of the gluteus maximus and the sacrotuberous ligament form its posterior border. The medial border is formed by the levator ani and external sphincter muscles; the obturator internus muscle forms the lateral border. The intersphincteric space lies between the internal and external sphincters and is continuous inferiorly with the perianal space and superiorly with the rectal wall. The supralevator space is bounded superiorly by peritoneum, laterally by the pelvic wall, medially by the rectal wall, and inferiorly by the levator ani muscle. The deep postanal space is located between the tip of the coccyx posteriorly and lies below the levator ani and above the anococcygeal ligament (Figure 13-1B).

At the level of the dentate line, the ducts of the anal glands empty into the anal crypts. Some 80% of the anal glands are submucosal in extent, 8% extend to the internal sphincter, 8% to the conjoined longitudinal muscle, 2% to the intersphincteric space, and 1% penetrate the internal sphincter.[2]

Pathophysiology

Etiology

Ninety percent of all anorectal abscesses result from nonspecific cryptoglandular infection whereas the remainder result from the causes as listed in Table 13-1. According to the cryptoglandular theory championed by Parks,[3] abscesses result from obstruction of the anal glands and ducts. Obstruction of a duct may result in stasis, infection, and formation of an abscess. Persistence of anal gland epithelium in part of the tract between the crypt and the blocked part of the duct results in the formation of a fistula. Predisposing factors include diarrhea and trauma in the form of a hard stool. Associated factors may be anal fissures, infection of a hematoma, or Crohn's disease.

Classification

Abscesses are classified according to their location in the aforementioned potential anorectal spaces: perianal, ischioanal, intersphincteric, and supralevator (Figure 13-2). Perianal abscesses are the most common type whereas supralevator abscesses are the rarest. Pus can also spread circumferentially through the intersphincteric, supralevator, or ischioanal spaces, the latter via the deep postanal space, resulting in a horseshoe abscess.

Evaluation and Treatment

Symptoms

Pain, swelling, and fever are the hallmarks associated with an abscess. The patient with a supralevator abscess may complain of gluteal pain.[4] Rectal bleeding has been reported. Severe rectal pain accompanied by urinary symptoms such as dysuria, retention, or inability to void may be suggestive of an intersphincteric or supralevator abscess.

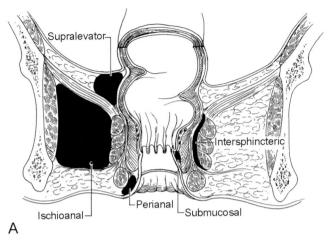

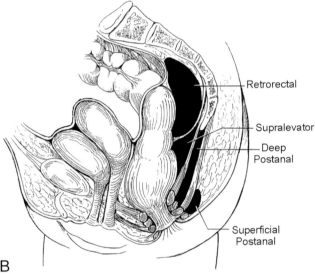

FIGURE 13-1. Anorectal spaces. **A** Coronal section. **B** Sagittal section. (From Vasilevsky CA. Anorectal abscess and fistula-in-ano. In: Beck D, ed. Handbook of Colorectal Surgery. 2nd ed. Copyright 2003 by Taylor & Francis Group LLC (B). Reproduced with permission of Taylor & Francis Group LLC (B) in the format Textbook via Copyright Clearance Center.)

TABLE 13-1. Etiology of anorectal abscess

Nonspecific
  Cryptoglandular
Specific
  Inflammatory bowel disease
    Crohn's disease
    Ulcerative colitis
    Infection
    Tuberculosis
    Actinomycosis
    Lymphogranuloma venereum
  Trauma
    Impalement
    Foreign body
    Surgery
      Episiotomy
      Hemorrhoidectomy
      Prostatectomy
  Malignancy
    Carcinoma
    Leukemia
    Lymphoma
    Radiation

Treatment

General Principles

Essentially, the treatment of an anorectal abscess involves incision and drainage. Watchful waiting under the cover of antibiotics is ineffective and may allow the suppurative process to progress resulting in the creation of a more complicated abscess and thus possible injury to the sphincter mechanism. Rarely, delay in diagnosis and management of anorectal abscesses may result in life-threatening necrotizing infection and death.[5]

Physical Examination

Inspection will reveal erythema, swelling, and possible fluctuation. It is crucial to recognize that no visible external manifestations will be present with the intersphincteric or supralevator abscesses despite the patient's complaint of excruciating pain.[1] Although digital examination may not be possible because of extreme tenderness, palpation, if possible, will demonstrate tenderness and a mass. With a supralevator abscess, a tender mass may be palpated on rectal or vaginal examination.[4] Anoscopy and sigmoidoscopy are inappropriate in the acute setting.

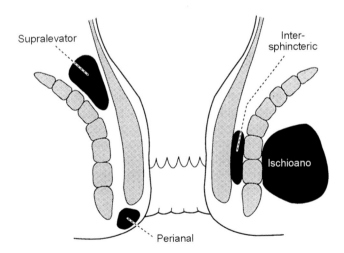

FIGURE 13-2. Classification of anorectal abscess. (Reprinted from Vasilevsky CA. Fistula-in-ano and abscess. In: Beck DE, Wexner SD, eds. Fundamentals of Anorectal Surgery. London: WB Saunders, copyright 1998, with permission from Elsevier.)

Operative Management

Incision and Drainage

Perianal abscesses can be effectively drained under local anesthesia.[4,6] After the most tender point has been determined, the area is infiltrated with 0.5% lidocaine with 1:200,000 epinephrine. A cruciate or elliptical incision is made and the edges are trimmed to prevent coaptation which may result in poor drainage or recurrence (Figure 13-3). No packing is required.

Most ischioanal abscesses can be incised and drained in a similar manner with the site of incision shifted close to the anal side of the abscess, minimizing the complexity of a subsequent fistula. Large ischioanal or horseshoe abscesses often require drainage with the patient under a regional or general anesthetic and in the prone jackknife or left lateral (Sim's) position. The location of infection is often in the deep postanal space. Access to this space may be achieved by a midline incision between the coccyx and anus, spreading the superficial external sphincter to enter the space. An opening is made in the posterior midline and the lower half of the internal sphincter is divided to drain the anal gland in which the infection originated.[4] Counter-incisions are made over each ischioanal fossa to allow drainage of the anterior extensions of the abscess (Hanley procedure)[5,7] (Figure 13-4).

Because the diagnosis of an intersphincteric abscess is entertained when the patient presents with pain out of proportion to the physical findings, an examination under anesthesia is mandatory to completely assess the cause of the pain. Once the diagnosis is established, either by palpation of a protrusion into the anal canal or by needle aspiration in the intersphincteric plane, treatment consists of dividing the internal sphincter along the length of the abscess cavity. The wound is then marsupialized to allow adequate drainage and quicker healing.

Before the treatment of a supralevator abscess, it is essential to determine its origin because it may arise from an upward extension of an intersphincteric or an ischioanal abscess, or downward extension of a pelvic abscess.[1,4] The treatment in each case will be different. If the origin is an intersphincteric abscess, it should be drained through the rectum by dividing the internal sphincter and not through the ischioanal fossa, because this will result in the creation of a suprasphincteric fistula. However, if it arises from an ischioanal abscess, it should be drained through the perineal skin and not through the rectum; otherwise, an extrasphincteric fistula will occur (Figure 13-5). If the abscess is of pelvic origin, it may be drained through the rectum, ischioanal fossa, or abdominal wall via percutaneous drainage depending on the direction to which it is pointing.

Catheter Drainage

An alternative method of treatment for selected patients is catheter drainage. Patients suitable for this technique should not have severe sepsis or any serious systemic illness.[8] The patient is placed in the prone jackknife position or left lateral

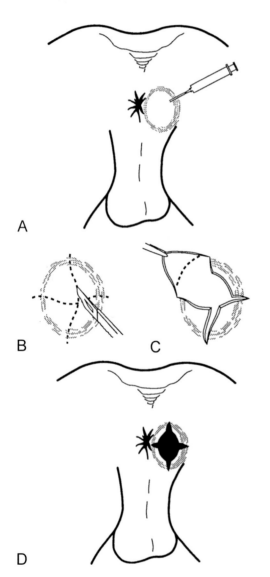

FIGURE 13-3. Drainage of abscess. **A** Injection of local anesthesia. **B** Cruciate incision. **C** Excision of skin. **D** Drainage cavity.

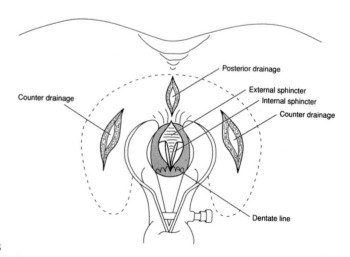

FIGURE 13-4. Drainage of horseshoe abscess.

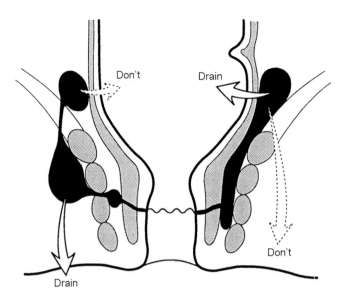

FIGURE 13-5. Drainage of a supralevator abscess.

(Sim's) position. The skin is prepared with a proviodine-iodine solution and the fluctuant point of the abscess is selected. Local anesthesia consisting of 0.5% lidocaine with 1:200,000 epinephrine is injected in a 1-cm area of skin and a stab incision is made to drain the pus. The lidocaine should be injected into the skin around, rather than immediately over, the point of maximal fluctuation because the acid environment may otherwise preclude adequate anesthesia (Figure 13-6A). A 10- to 16-French soft latex mushroom catheter is inserted over a probe into the abscess cavity. When released, the shape of the catheter tip will hold the catheter in place, obviating the need for sutures. The external portion of the catheter is shortened to leave 2–3 cm outside the skin with the tip in the depth of the abscess cavity (Figure 13-6B). This reduces the chances of the catheter falling out of or into the abscess cavity. A small bandage is placed over the catheter.

Several portions of this technique deserve further comment. First, the stab incision should be placed as close as possible to the anus, minimizing the amount of tissue that must be opened if a fistula is found after resolution of inflammation (Figure 13-6A). Second, the size and length of the catheter should correspond to the size of the abscess cavity (Figure 13-7A). A catheter that is too small or too short may fall into the wound (Figure 13-7B). Third, the length of time that the catheter should be left in place requires clinical judgment. Factors involved in this decision should include the size of the original abscess cavity, the amount of granulation tissue around the catheter, and the character and amount of drainage. If there is doubt, it is better to leave the catheter in place for a longer period of time.

Primary Fistulotomy

A point of controversy is whether primary fistulotomy should be performed at the time of initial abscess drainage. Proponents[5,9–11] believe that in the acute phase one can better

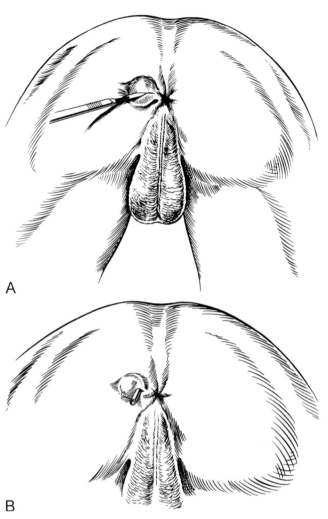

FIGURE 13-6. Catheter drainage of an abscess. **A** Stab incision. **B** Catheter in abscess cavity.

trace the suppurative process because of the presence of pus. Primary fistulotomy eliminates the source of infection and decreases the rate of recurrence, obviating the need for subsequent surgery with the potential to decrease disability and morbidity. Fucini[11] reported no recurrences in 51 of 58 primary

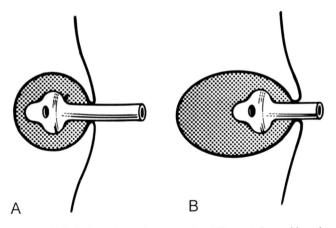

FIGURE 13-7. Catheter in an abscess cavity. **A** Correct size and length of catheter. **B** Catheter too short.

fistulotomies when internal openings could be identified. No major incontinence was reported, but impaired control of flatus was seen in 17%. In eight patients in whom only incision and drainage were performed because of failure to identify an internal opening, recurrences were reported in 87%.[11]

Opponents[6,12] are reluctant to perform primary fistulotomy in the presence of acute inflammation because the search for an internal opening may lead to creation of false passages resulting in neglect of the main source of infection. Failure to identify an internal opening has been reported to occur in as high as 66% of patients.[10] In addition, 34%–50% of patients who present with an abscess for the first time will not develop a fistula.[6,12] Thus, primary fistulotomy in these patients would be unnecessary and may result in needless disturbances of continence. Of those patients whose abscesses are drained, 11% may develop a fistula whereas 37% may develop a recurrent abscess.[6] This is most often observed in conjunction with ischioanal abscesses.[6] The search for an internal opening converts the operative procedure from one that can be performed under local anesthesia to one that requires regional or general anesthesia. A prospective, randomized trial of drainage alone versus drainage and fistulotomy for acute perianal abscesses with proven internal openings revealed that incision and drainage alone demonstrated no statistical significance in recurrence compared with concurrent fistulotomy although there was a tendency to recurrence in the former group.[13] Another prospective study advocated a conservative approach in the treatment of anorectal abscess, reserving fistulotomy as a second-stage procedure if necessary.[14]

If the internal opening of a low transsphincteric fistula is readily apparent at the time of abscess drainage, primary fistulotomy is feasible with the following exceptions: 1) patients with Crohn's disease, 2) patients with acquired immunodeficiency syndrome (AIDS), 3) elderly patients, 4) patients with high transsphincteric fistulas, and 5) women with anterior fistulas and episiotomy scars.

The decision to perform a primary fistulotomy should be individualized but should only be attempted by a surgeon with a sound knowledge of the regional anatomy. Insistence upon finding a fistula may encourage creation of a false passage and unnecessary division of sphincter muscle.[11]

As will be seen in the discussions of the use of fibrin glue ranal plug in the treatment of fistula-in-ano further on in this chapter, many of the former proponents of primary fistulotomy have abandoned this approach and have instead elected to await the appearance of a fistula after drainage only to treat it with fibrin glue ranal plug so as to avoid cutting any sphincter muscle.

Antibiotics

There is little if any role for antibiotics in the primary management of anorectal abscesses except as an adjunct in patients with valvular heart disease or prosthetic valves, extensive soft tissue cellulitis, prosthetic devices, diabetes, immunosuppression, or systemic sepsis.

Postoperative care

Patients are instructed to continue with a regular diet and to take a bulk-forming agent, non-codeine-containing analgesic, and sitz baths. Patients are generally seen in follow-up in 2–4 weeks or for intersphincteric or supralevator abscesses, 2 weeks postoperatively. Those patients in whom catheter drainage has been performed are seen within 7–10 days after the procedure. If the cavity has closed around the catheter and drainage has ceased, the catheter is removed. If the cavity has not healed, the catheter is left in place or replaced with a smaller one. In all cases, patients are observed until complete healing has occurred.

Complications

Recurrence

After incision and drainage, ischioanal and intersphincteric abscesses are associated with the development of recurrent abscesses or fistulas in as many as 89% of patients.[6,14,15] Recurrence is more likely to occur in patients with a history of abscess drainage[6,14,15] perhaps because the natural barriers to infection have been destroyed.

Reasons for recurrence of anorectal infections include missed infection in adjacent anatomic spaces, the presence of an undiagnosed fistula or abscess at initial abscess drainage, and failure to completely drain the abscess.[5]

If a patient waits too long for follow-up after catheter drainage, the skin may seal and a second incision may be required to retrieve the catheter or redrain a recurrent abscess.

Failure to detect a primary opening at the time of primary fistulotomy and abscess drainage may result in persistence of the infection.

Extra-anal Causes

Extra-anal disease should be considered once the usual causes of recurrence have been ruled out. Hidradenitis suppurativa and downward extension of a pilonidal abscess should be considered.[1] A prospective review of recurrent anorectal abscesses by Chrabot et al.[16] reported hidradenitis in one-third of patients with recurrent abscesses. In addition, the possibility of Crohn's disease should be suspected.

Incontinence

Incontinence may result after incision and drainage of an abscess either from iatrogenic damage to the sphincter or inappropriate wound care. Continence may be compromised if the superficial external sphincter is inadvertently divided during drainage of a perianal or deep postanal abscess in a patient with preoperative borderline continence. Drainage of a supralevator abscess may lead to incontinence if the puborectalis is inappropriately divided.[17] Prolonged packing of a drained abscess may impair continence by preventing the development of granulation tissue and promoting the formation of excess scar tissue.[18]

Although advocated to decrease recurrence rates, primary fistulotomy may result in unnecessary division of sphincter muscle in acutely inflamed tissue. Schouten and van Vroonhoven[14] reported a 39% rate of continence disturbances in a prospective, randomized trial.

Special Considerations

Necrotizing Anorectal Infection

Rarely, anorectal abscesses may result in necrotizing infection and death. Factors thought to be responsible include delay in diagnosis and management, virulence of the organism involved, bacteremia and metastatic infections, or underlying disorders such as diabetes, blood dyscrasias, heart disease, chronic renal failure, hemorrhoids, and previous abscess or fistula.[5]

Symptoms and Signs

Spreading soft tissue infection of the perineum can be classified into two groups.[19] The first group includes anorectal sepsis in which the infection extends superficially around the perineum resulting in necrosis of skin, subcutaneous tissue, fascia, or muscle. Perianal crepitation, erythematous, indurated skin, blistering, or gangrene may be present (Figure 13-8). A black spot may appear early and indicates a widespread necrotizing infection.[20] The second group includes sepsis in which the preperitoneal or retroperitoneal spaces have become involved.[19] Subtle signs may be present which include abdominal wall induration, tenderness, or a vague mass. It is important to realize that systemic symptoms such as fever, tachycardia, and vascular volume depletion may precede the appearance of overt signs of infection.[21]

Treatment

Treatment consists of vigorous intravenous fluid hydration, restoration of electrolyte balance, and insertion of a Foley catheter. Accompanying coagulopathy, respiratory insufficiency, and renal failure must be aggressively treated. Invasive monitoring and ventilatory support may be necessary.[22] Pus or necrotic tissue from the infected region must be cultured for aerobes and anaerobes. A Gram stain can be used to distinguish between the presence of clostridial and nonclostridial organisms.[23] Empiric broad-spectrum antibiotic therapy should be instituted regardless of Gram stain and culture results. The chosen antibiotic regimen should be effective against staphylococci and streptococci, Gram-negative coliforms, *Pseudomonas*, *Bacteroides*, and *Clostridium*. For Gram-positive rods seen on Gram stain, antibiotics administered should include sodium penicillin G in doses of 24–30 million units per day and an aminoglycoside. Tetanus toxoid should also be administered.[22]

Surgical treatment consists of wide radical debridement until healthy tissue is encountered. The goals of surgical debridement are to remove all nonviable tissue, halt the progression of infection, and alleviate the systemic toxicity.[21] It is crucial to realize that the preoperative skin changes may be minimal compared with the operative findings which may include edema, liquefactive necrosis of subcutaneous tissues, watery pus formation, and extensive necrosis of underlying fascia.[22] Reexamination under anesthesia is usually necessary because this is the only manner by which adequate wound examination can be conducted.[22] The need for colostomy is a debatable issue and has been recommended if the sphincter muscle is grossly infected, if there is colonic or rectal perforation, if the rectal wound is large, if the patient is immunocompromised, or if incontinence is present.[19,21] Whereas some authors[23] believe that colostomy is seldom necessary, fecal diversion may also be accomplished with the use of a "medical colostomy" consisting of enteral or parenteral nutrition. Controversy also exists with regard to the need for urinary diversion by suprapubic catheterization. It has been suggested that this may be indicated in the presence of known stricture and urinary extravasation with phlegmon.[24]

Although antibiotics and adequate surgical drainage are thought to be sufficient, the use of hyperbaric oxygen (HBO) has been advocated as an adjunct to treatment, particularly in patients with diffuse spreading infections who do not have chronic obstructive pulmonary disease.[25] It is postulated that HBO has a direct antibacterial effect on anaerobic bacteria by diminishing the effect of endotoxins and optimizing leukocyte phagocytic function.[20] HBO may also promote wound healing by facilitating fibroblast proliferation.[25] HBO is delivered as 100% oxygen through an oronasal mask or endotracheal tube at 3 atm for one or two cycles each lasting 2 hours. If HBO is to be used as an adjunctive therapy, appropriate surgical intervention with wide debridement cannot be compromised because ischemic tissue cannot be salvaged by HBO.[21]

Despite aggressive surgical and multidisciplinary management of anorectal sepsis, mortality rates ranging from 8% to 67% have been reported.[19,21] This high mortality rate is attributable in part to the aggressive nature of the infection and to the underlying comorbid diseases that are present in these

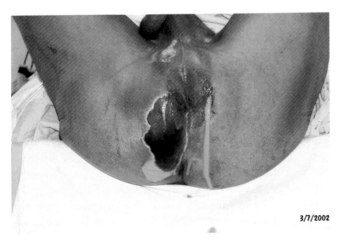

3/7/2002

FIGURE 13-8. Necrotizing anorectal infection.

patients.[21] Mortality rates are 2–3 times higher in diabetics, in elderly patients, and in patients in whom treatment is delayed.[21]

Anal Infection and Hematologic Diseases

Acute anorectal suppuration poses an interesting and often life-threatening problem in patients with acute hematologic diseases. In patients with acute leukemia, mortality rates of 45%–78% have been reported.[26] There is a definite relationship between the number of circulating granulocytes and the incidence of perianal infection in patients with hematologic diseases. In one study, patients with neutrophil counts below 500 per cubic millimeter had an incidence of anorectal infections of 11% whereas those with counts greater than 500 per cubic millimeter had an incidence of 0.4%.[27] Glenn et al.[28] reported that 63% of anorectal infectious episodes occurred when fewer than 500 neutrophils were present per cubic millimeter. The risk of developing anorectal infection in this patient population has been found to be related to the severity and duration of the neutropenia.[26] The most important prognostic indicator was the number of days of neutropenia during the infectious episode.[28]

The most common presenting symptoms include fever which precedes pain, and urinary retention. Point tenderness and poorly demarcated induration constitute the earliest signs,[26] whereas external swelling and fluctuation often appear late in the course of infection.[28]

Controversy surrounds the treatment of acute anorectal infections in patients with hematologic malignancies. Surgery has generally been avoided because what may seem to be simple incision and drainage may produce scant or no pus and may instead cause hemorrhage, poor wound healing, or expanding soft tissue infection.[28]

Any patient with perianal pain is assumed to have a perianal complication and is started on precautionary measures which consist of no digital rectal examinations, suppositories, or enemas.[29] Sitz baths, stool softeners, bulk agents, and analgesia are advised. On aspiration of most abscesses in this group, the most common organisms have been found to be *Escherichia coli* and group D streptococcus.[28] Consequently, infections are successfully controlled with a third-generation cephalosporin combined with anaerobic coverage or an extended spectrum penicillin in combination with an aminoglycoside and an anti-anaerobic antibiotic. This combination has been associated with an 88% success rate.[28]

Barnes et al.[26] recommend an aggressive surgical approach. Through this approach, 13 of 15 patients who were severely neutropenic with neutrophil counts of fewer than 100 per cubic millimeter recovered with incision and drainage. It must be noted that these patients were found to have extensive soft tissue infection. Because appropriate antibiotic coverage has been found to control infection successfully, surgery has generally been recommended only if there is obvious fluctuation, progression of soft tissue infection, or persistent sepsis after a trial of antibiotic therapy.[28]

With severe neutropenia of fewer than 500 neutrophils per cubic millimeter, low-dose radiation therapy of 300–400 rads for a period of 1–3 days has been suggested. Spontaneous drainage or subsidence of induration has been found to occur in 3–5 days.[29] A randomized, controlled study, however, has failed to confirm the utility of this approach.[30]

Anorectal Sepsis in the Patient Positive for the Human Immunodeficiency Virus

Patients who are human immunodeficiency virus (HIV) positive and present with abscesses require drainage either by incision and drainage or use of catheter drainage. Because these patients are immunosuppressed, adjunctive antibiotics should be used. Efforts should be directed at keeping wounds small because these patients are at risk of poor wound healing.[31] An increased incidence of perianal sepsis[32] may be observed in HIV-positive patients. Serious septic complications or uncommon presentations of anorectal sepsis were found in 13% of patients who initially presented with anorectal suppuration in one study.[31] In another study, perianal sepsis was associated with in situ neoplasia.[33]

Fistula-in-ano

Familiarity of the surgeon with the anatomy of the anorectal area and with the pathogenesis and classification of fistulas is essential for their adequate management.

Pathophysiology

Etiology

A fistula is defined as an abnormal communication between any two epithelium-lined surfaces. A fistula-in-ano is an abnormal tract or cavity communicating with the rectum or anal canal by an identifiable internal opening. Most fistulas are thought to arise as a result of cryptoglandular infection.

Classification

The most helpful yet complicated classification of fistula-in-ano is that described by Parks et al. (Table 13-2). It has been suggested that its use is particularly applicable to the treatment of recurrent fistulas.[10]

Intersphincteric Fistula-in-ano

This fistula is the result of a perianal abscess. The tract passes within the intersphincteric space (Figure 13-9A). This is the most common type of fistula and accounts for approximately 70% of fistulas.[34] A high blind tract passing from the fistula tract to the rectal wall may occur; in addition, the tract may also pass into the lower rectum. The infectious process may pass into the intersphincteric plane and terminate as a blind tract. There is no downward extension to the anal margin, and

TABLE 13-2. Classification of fistula-in-ano

Intersphincteric
  Simple low tract
  High blind tract
  High tract with rectal opening
  Rectal opening without perineal opening
  Extrarectal extension
  Secondary to pelvic disease
Transsphincteric
  Uncomplicated
  High blind tract
Suprasphincteric
  Uncomplicated
  High blind tract
Extrasphincteric
  Secondary to anal fistula
  Secondary to trauma
  Secondary to anorectal disease
  Secondary to pelvic inflammation

thus no external opening is present. Infection may also spread in the intersphincteric plane to reach the pelvic cavity to lie above the levator ani muscles. Lastly, an intersphincteric fistula may originate in the pelvis as a pelvic abscess but manifest itself in the perianal area.

Transsphincteric Fistula-in-ano

In its usual variety, this fistula results from an ischioanal abscess and constitutes approximately 23% of fistulas seen.[34] The tract passes from the internal opening through the internal and external sphincters to the ischioanal fossa (Figure 13-9B). A high blind tract may also occur in this situation in which the upper arm of the tract may pass toward the apex of the ischioanal fossa or may extend through the levator ani muscles and thereby into the pelvis. One form of transsphincteric

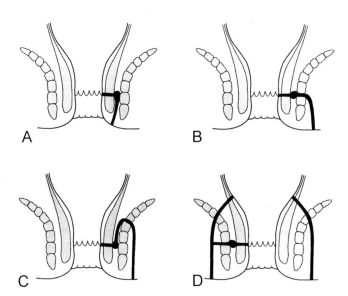

FIGURE 13-9. Classification of fistula-in-ano. **A** Intersphincteric. **B** Transsphincteric. **C** Suprasphincteric. **D** Extrasphincteric.

fistula is the rectovaginal fistula. This is discussed further in Chapter 14.

Suprasphincteric Fistula-in-ano

This fistula results from a supralevator abscess and accounts for approximately 5% of fistulas in some series.[34] The tract passes above the puborectalis after arising as an intersphincteric abscess. The tract curves downward lateral to the external sphincter in the ischioanal space to the perianal skin (Figure 13-9C). A high blind tract may also occur in this variety and result in a horseshoe extension.

Extrasphincteric Fistula-in-ano

This constitutes the rarest type of fistula and accounts for 2% of fistulas.[34] The tract passes from the rectum above the levators and through them to the perianal skin via the ischioanal space (Figure 13-9D). This fistula may result from foreign body penetration of the rectum with drainage through the levators, from penetrating injury to the perineum, or from Crohn's disease or carcinoma or its treatment. However, the most common cause may be iatrogenic secondary to vigorous probing during fistula surgery.[4]

Evaluation and Treatment

Symptoms

A patient with a fistula-in-ano will often recount a history of an abscess that has been drained either surgically or spontaneously. Patients may complain of drainage, pain with defecation, bleeding caused by the presence of granulation tissue at the internal opening, swelling, or decrease in pain with drainage. Additional bowel symptoms may be present when the fistula is secondary to proctocolitis, Crohn's disease, actinomycosis, or anorectal carcinoma.[35] Systemic diseases such as HIV, carcinoma, and lymphoma should be entertained.[35]

Physical Examination

The external or secondary opening may be seen as an elevation of granulation tissue discharging pus. This may be elicited on digital rectal examination. In most cases, the internal or primary opening is not apparent. The number of external openings and their location may be helpful in identifying the primary opening. According to Goodsall's rule (Figure 13-10), an opening seen posterior to a line drawn transversely across the perineum will originate from an internal opening in the posterior midline. An anterior external opening will originate in the nearest crypt. Generally, the greater the distance from the anal margin, the greater the probability of a complicated upward extension. Cirocco and Reilly[36] found that Goodsall's rule was accurate in describing the course of anal fistulas with a posterior external opening. It was inaccurate in patients with anterior external openings because 71% of these fistulas tracked to a midline anterior primary opening. This

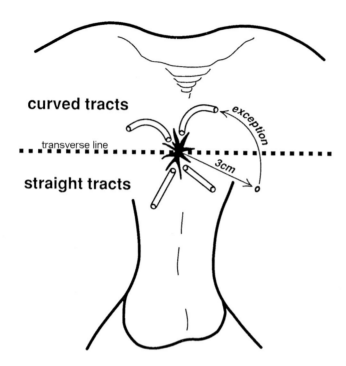

FIGURE 13-10. Goodsall's rule.

was especially true in women in whom fistulas with anterior external openings tracked in a radial manner in only 31%.[36]

Digital rectal examination may reveal an indurated cord-like structure beneath the skin in the direction of the internal opening with asymmetry between right and left sides. Internal openings may be felt as indurated nodules or pits leading to an indurated tract.[36] Posterior or lateral induration may be palpable indicating fistulas deep in the postanal space or horseshoe fistulas.[35,36] Bidigital rectal examination will define the relationship of the tract to the sphincter muscles and provides information as to preoperative sphincter tone, bulk, and voluntary squeeze pressure which need to be assessed preoperatively because of a possible risk of incontinence.[17,35]

Investigations

Anoscopy should be done before operation in an attempt to identify the primary opening. Sigmoidoscopy should be performed to locate a proximal internal opening and to exclude underlying pathology such as proctitis or neoplasia. Colonoscopy or barium enema and a small bowel series are indicated in patients who have symptoms suggestive of inflammatory bowel disease and in patients with multiple or recurrent fistulas. Although anal manometry is not generally required, it may be useful as an adjunct to planning the operative approach in women with previous obstetric trauma, in an elderly patient, a patient with Crohn's disease or AIDS, or in a patient with a recurrent fistula.[37]

The role of preoperative imaging is to demonstrate clinically undetected sepsis, to serve as a guide at the time of the initial surgery, to determine the relationship of the fistula tract to the sphincter mechanism, and to reveal the site of sepsis in a recurrent fistula, all serving to decrease recurrence rates associated with fistula surgery. Imaging may take the form of fistulography, computed tomography (CT) scan, endoanal ultrasound, and magnetic resonance imaging (MRI).

Fistulography

Fistulography, which involves cannulation of the external opening with a small feeding tube and injection of water-soluble contrast may be useful in the evaluation of recurrent fistulas or in Crohn's disease where previous surgical forays or disease may have altered anorectal anatomy[38] (Figure 13-11). Contrast is introduced at low pressures for fear of tissue disruption. This may not allow secondary tracts to fill with contrast. It is difficult to distinguish between an abscess located high in the ischioanal fossa and one located in the supralevator space. In addition, the level of the internal opening may be difficult to see because of the absence of precise landmarks. Contrast may reflux into the rectum wrongly suggesting an extrasphincteric tract with a rectal opening thus resulting in injudicious probing. Accuracy rates in identifying the internal openings and extensions in one study were found to be 16%, whereas a subsequent study found fistulography to be useful in 96%.[38,39] Its use resulted in altered surgical management or revealed other surgical pathology in 48%.[38] It was found, for reasons outlined previously, to have a false-positive rate of 12%.[39] Fistulography is invasive and potentially may result in the dissemination of sepsis.

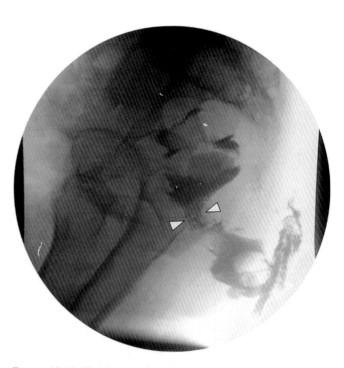

FIGURE 13-11. Fistulogram. Arrowheads indicate fistula tract.

CT Scan

CT scanning performed with intravenous and rectal contrast is a noninvasive method used to assess the perirectal spaces. Its use may be to distinguish an abscess requiring drainage from perirectal cellulitis. It does not permit visualization of tracts in relation to the levators.

Endoanal Ultrasound

The role of endoanal ultrasound is to establish the relation of the primary tract to the anal sphincters, to determine if the fistula is simple or complex with extensions, and to determine the location of the primary opening. It may aid in the identification of complex fistulas and may serve as an adjunct in the evaluation of complex suppuration to assess the adequacy of drainage[40] (Figure 13-12a). A prospective study that compared this modality to digital examination found that although endosonography was able to detect a large portion of intersphincteric and transsphincteric tracts, it was unable to detect primary superficial, extrasphincteric and suprasphincteric tracts or secondary supralevator or infralevator tracts.[41] A study conducted 10 years later[42] using a 10-mHz probe along with injection of hydrogen peroxide into the tract, was able to identify the internal opening in 93%. Although this investigative modality is rapid and well tolerated, it is operator dependent and scars or defects caused by previous sepsis, surgery, or trauma will confuse ultrasonographic interpretation and make delineation of fistula tracts difficult.[41] The concomitant use of hydrogen peroxide (Figure 13-12b) or Levovist™[43] at the time of ultrasound examination has been found to improve its accuracy.

Magnetic Resonance Imaging

MRI in the form of endoanal coil, body coil, and phase array coil (Figure 13-13) may be of value in the assessment of patients with complex fistulas and in those with anatomic distortion resulting from previous surgery. Because MRI can provide multiplanar visualization of the sphincter muscles, differentiation of supralevator from infralevator lesions is easier.[44] MRI has been found to accurately delineate the presence and course of a primary fistulous tract but also demonstrates the site and presence of any secondary extensions.[45] It also provides the most accurate imaging technique of localizing the site of the internal opening because its location can be inferred from the proximity of the tract in the intersphincteric space.[45] A prospective study that compared the accuracy of MRI in the preoperative assessment of anal fistulas to operative findings found concordance rates of 88% for the presence and course of the primary tract, 91% for the presence and site of secondary extensions or abscesses and 97% for the presence of horseshoeing, and 80% for the position of the internal openings.[45] In the same study, failure of healing in 9% was found to be related to pathology missed at the time of surgery which had been documented on preoperative MRI.[45] Difficulties in interpretation, however, may occur because neural and vascular structures could be mistaken for fistulas and chemical shift artifacts may simulate a fistula filled with fluid.[46] The use of the endoanal coil has been found to be superior to external MRI for the identification of complex sphincter anatomy especially in the demonstration of the morphology of the internal and external sphincters[47]; however, definition may fall off outside the sphincter and may fail to show the tracts that lie beyond its range. It is also painful. A prospective study comparing hydrogen peroxide endoanal ultrasound to endoanal MRI found good agreement for the classification of the primary fistula tract and the location of the internal opening. These results also demonstrated good agreement with the surgical findings enabling both to be reliable for the preoperative evaluation of fistulas.[48]

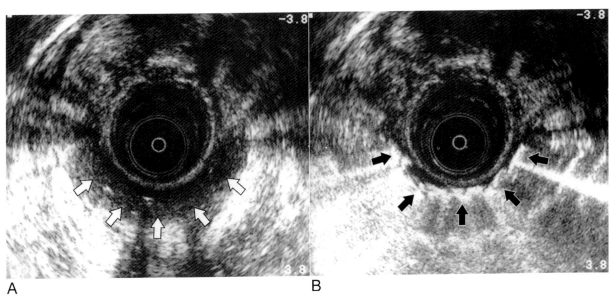

A   B

FIGURE 13-12. **A** Anal endosonogram; arrows indicate fistula tract; **B** with hydrogen peroxide; arrows indicate better delineation of fistula tract. (Courtesy Dr. Julio Faria.)

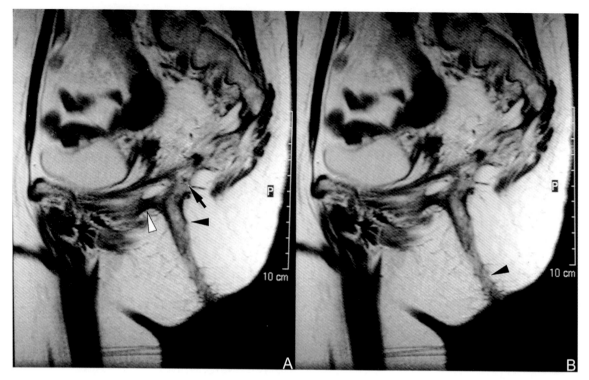

FIGURE 13-13. Phase array MRI. **A** White arrowhead indicates levators; black arrowhead indicates fistula tract to rectum; black arrow shows tract crossing levator. **B** Arrowhead indicates tract going to skin.

A prospective trial comparing the use of the endoanal coil to the body coil found that surgical concordance for the endoanal coil was 68% versus 96% for the body coil, presumably because of field of view limitations.[49] This can be overcome with the use of the phase array coil which has a larger field of view and may be useful in Crohn's disease and recurrent fistulas.[50]

Buchanan et al.,[51] in a prospective study to determine the impact of MRI with primary fistulas, found that MRI changed the surgical approach in 10%. In another study with respect to recurrent fistulas, recurrence rates were found to be higher for those surgeons who never used MRI.[52] They concluded that MRI-guided surgery can decrease recurrence rates by 75% in surgery for recurrent fistulas.

Treatment

General Principles

The principles of fistula surgery are to eliminate the fistula, prevent recurrence, and preserve sphincter function. Success is usually determined by identification of the primary opening and dividing the least amount of muscle possible.

Several methods have been proposed to identify the primary opening in the operating room[1,4]:

1. Passage of a probe or probes from the external opening to the internal opening or vice versa.
2. Injection of a dye such as dilute solution of methylene blue, milk, or hydrogen peroxide, and noting their appearance at the dentate line. Although methylene blue may stain surrounding tissues, diluting it with saline or hydrogen peroxide will obviate this problem.
3. Following the granulation tissue present in the fistula tract.
4. Noting puckering of an anal crypt when traction is placed on the tract. This may be useful with simple fistulas but is less successful in the more complicated varieties.

Operative Management

Lay-open Technique

For the treatment of simple intersphincteric and low transsphincteric fistulas, the patient is placed in the prone jack-knife position after induction of a regional anesthetic. Local anesthesia consisting of 0.5% lidocaine or 0.25% bupivacaine hydrochloride with 1:200,000 epinephrine is injected along the fistula tract for hemostasis after insertion of an anal speculum. Use of bupivacaine provides analgesia of longer duration than most regional anesthetics. A probe is inserted from the external opening along the tract to the internal opening at the dentate line. The tissue overlying the probe is incised and the granulation tissue curetted and sent for pathologic evaluation. A gentle probe is used to identify any high blind tracts or extensions, which are unroofed, if found. If desired, the wound may be marsupialized on either edge by sewing the edges of the incision to the tract with a running locked absorbable suture. There is no need to insert packing if an adequate unroofing has been accomplished (Figure 13-14A–C).

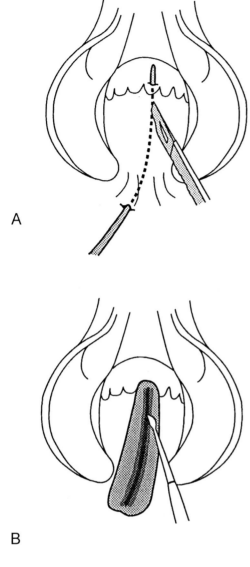

A

B

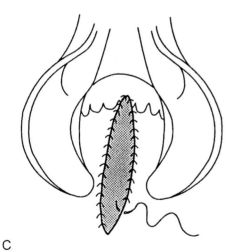

C

FIGURE 13-14. Technique of laying open. **A** Insertion of probe and incision of tissue overlying probe. **B** Curettage of granulation tissue. **C** Marsupialization of wound edges.

Seton

The problem of preserving anal continence and treating the fistula is more complicated when managing high transsphincteric fistulas. If the tract is seen to cross the sphincter muscle at a high level, the use of the lay-open technique in combination with insertion of a seton is safer. A seton may be any foreign substance that can be inserted into the fistula tract to encircle the sphincter muscles. Materials frequently used include silk or other nonabsorbable suture material, Penrose drains, rubber bands, vessel loops, and silastic catheters.[17] The lower portion of the internal sphincter is divided along with the skin to reach the external opening and a nonabsorbable suture or elastic suture is inserted into the fistulous tract. The ends of the suture or elastic are tied with multiple knots to create a handle for manipulation (Figure 13-15). This form of seton, known as a cutting seton, is tightened at regular intervals to slowly cut through the sphincter. This allows the tract to become more superficial, converting a high fistula into a low one. The proximal fistulotomy subsequently heals by stimulating fibrosis behind it reestablishing continuity of the anorectal ring to prevent separation of the sphincter muscle at a second-stage repair 8 weeks later when the remaining external sphincter is divided. The seton also allows delineation of the amount of remaining muscle thus enabling improved postoperative assessment by outlining the tract. A seton may also be used as a drain which is left loosely in place to facilitate prolonged drainage. Specific indications for seton use include the following:[53] 1) to identify and promote fibrosis around a complex anal fistula that encircles most or all of the sphincter mechanism; 2) to mark the site of a transsphincteric fistula in cases of massive anorectal sepsis where the normal anatomic landmarks have been distorted; 3) anterior, high transsphincteric fistulas in women. Because the

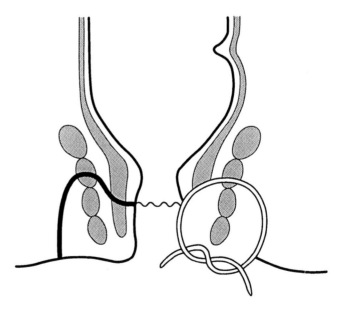

FIGURE 13-15. Seton.

puborectalis is absent in this area and the external sphincter is quite tenuous, primary fistulotomy may result in incontinence; 4) the presence of a high transsphincteric fistula in a patient with AIDS in whom healing is known to be poor; 5) to avoid premature skin closure and formation of recurrent abscesses and promote long-term drainage in patients with Crohn's disease. In these patients, a silastic catheter can be left in place for a prolonged period of time to promote epithelialization of the fistula tract or tracts; 6) when there is suspicion that primary fistulotomy will result in incontinence such as in those patients with multiple simultaneous fistulas, patients who have undergone multiple prior sphincter operations such as fistulotomy or internal sphincterotomy, and in elderly patients with weakened sphincter muscles.

Another option available to treat transsphincteric fistulas without division of muscle involves the use of a dermal island flap.[54] Division of muscle was able to be avoided in 90%; however, a 23% failure rate was reported. This was found to be more likely in males, patients who had previous treatment of their fistulas, patients with large fistulas requiring combined flaps, and patients who underwent simultaneous fibrin glue injection.

Treatment of suprasphincteric fistulas requires an appreciation that the tract involves the entire external sphincter complex as well as the puborectalis muscle. Laying open the entire tract would render the patient incontinent. Thus, several methods have been proposed to manage this fistula without the ensuing devastating consequences. The use of a seton has been advocated in combination with division of the internal sphincter and the superficial portion of the external sphincter to the external opening. The seton is placed around the remaining external sphincter as was previously described.[55]

A modification of this approach has been proposed by Kennedy and Zegarra[56] in which an internal sphincterotomy is performed, followed by opening of the tracts outside the external sphincter without division of any portion of the external sphincter which is encircled by a seton to promote fibrosis and assure adequate drainage. Complete healing using the latter approach has been reported in 66% with posterior fistulas and in 88% with anterior fistulas.[56] Parks and Stitz[55] obtained healing in 63%. Another method that has been proposed to treat this type of fistula is the anorectal advancement flap which will be described.

The horseshoe variety of the suprasphincteric fistula also presents the problem of complete sphincter involvement combined with the presence of multiple external openings a great distance from the cryptoglandular source. Treatment consists of identification of the internal opening and proper drainage of the postanal space as was previously described. The horseshoe extensions are enlarged for counter-drainage and the granulation tissue is curetted.

The treatment of an extrasphincteric fistula depends on its etiology. If the fistula arises secondary to an anal fistula, a secondary opening above the puborectalis is thought to be iatrogenic because of extensive probing of a transsphincteric fistula. The lower portion of the internal sphincter is divided and the rectal opening is closed with a nonabsorbable suture. A temporary colostomy may be necessary but a medical colostomy consisting of preoperative mechanical and antibiotic bowel preparation followed by enteral feeding may suffice. If the fistula is the result of entrance of a foreign body, it must be removed, drainage must be established, the internal opening closed, and a temporary colostomy constructed to decrease rectal pressure. This type of fistula may also be a manifestation of Crohn's disease. Treatment will depend on the nature of the anorectal mucosa and drainage may be assisted by placement of a seton. Finally, the fistula may be the result of downward tracking of a pelvic abscess which must be drained so that the fistula can heal.

Anorectal Advancement Flap

When the traditional laying-open technique may be inappropriate, for example, in anterior fistulas in women, in patients with inflammatory bowel disease, in patients with high transsphincteric and suprasphincteric fistulas, as well as in those with previous multiple sphincter operations, multiple and complex fistulas, the use of an anorectal advancement flap has been advocated[57] (Figure 13-16A–D). Advantages of this technique include a reduction in the duration of healing, reduced associated discomfort, lack of deformity to the anal canal, as well as little potential additional damage to the sphincter muscles because no muscle is divided.[17]

After full mechanical and antibiotic bowel preparation, the patient is placed in the prone jackknife or left lateral position. Under a regional or general anesthetic, after insertion of a Foley catheter, the fistula tract is identified with a probe and either cored out or curetted. The internal opening is identified and excised. The external opening is enlarged to allow for drainage. A full-thickness flap of rectal mucosa, submucosa, and part of the internal sphincter is raised. The residual internal opening is closed with absorbable suture. The flap is then advanced 1 cm below the internal opening. The tip of the flap containing the fistulous opening is excised and the flap is sewn into place with absorbable sutures ensuring that the mucosal and muscular suture lines do not overlap. The base of the flap should be twice the width of the apex to maintain good blood supply. Successful results have reported in more than 90% of patients.[58] Factors associated with poor outcomes include Crohn's disease and steroids.[59] Cigarette smoking was found to be another significant variable in another study.[60]

Fistulectomy

Although excision of the fistula or fistulectomy was thought to be a satisfactory method of treatment of fistula-in-ano, its use is no longer recommended. Larger wounds are created significantly prolonging wound healing time.[61] A greater separation of muscle ends occurs[1] and there is greater risk of injuring or excising underlying muscle[57] thereby increasing the risk of incontinence. Schouten and van Vroonhoven[14]

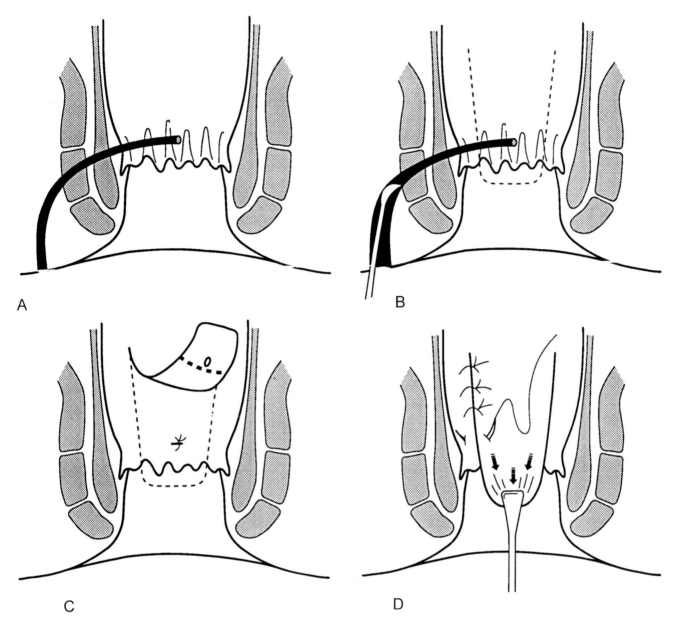

FIGURE 13-16. Anorectal advancement flap. **A** Transsphincteric fistula-in-ano. **B** Enlargement of external opening and curettage of granulation tissue. **C** Mobilization of flap and closure of internal opening. **D** Suturing of flap in place covering internal opening.

have found that fistulectomy, whether primary or secondary, was associated with a clinically significant disturbance in anal function.

Fibrin Glue

The use of fibrin glue as a primary treatment alone or in combination with an advancement flap has come into vogue. This treatment modality is appealing because it is a noninvasive approach that avoids the risk of incontinence associated with fistulotomy. In the case of failure, it may be repeated several times without jeopardizing continence. The technique involved is simple. As with fistulotomy, the fistula tract along with its internal and external openings is identified and curetted (with curettes or flexible brushes). Fibrin glue is injected into the fistula tract through a Y connector so that the entire tract is filled and the glue can be seen emerging from the internal opening. The injecting catheter is slowly withdrawn so that the entire tract is filled. Petrolatum jelly gauze may be placed over the external opening.

Enthusiasm generated because of short-term success rates of 70%–74%[62,63] has been tempered because of delayed fistula recurrence despite initial apparent healing.[64] With longer follow-up, 60% of fistulas were found to have healed in a recent study[65] although patients underwent a two-stage approach consisting of seton placement followed by glue injection at a second stage. Patients who failed underwent repeat injection which allowed 69% to heal. The 29% who failed to heal underwent either fistulotomy or advancement flap. Late recurrences (6%) occurred more than 6 months postoperatively and were treated with reinjection. Buchanan et al.[66] found fibrin glue injection to be useful in 14% with complex anal fistulas without extensions.

Although the exact mechanisms responsible for failure have not been entirely appreciated, it has been suggested that curettage may not adequately remove all granulation or epithelialized tissue thus failing to provide the correct environment for the glue to work.[66] Other adverse factors shown to influence healing include the presence of a short tract which may make it easier for the fibrin glue plug to become dislodged as well as the presence of a cavity on endoanal ultrasound.[67] The latter was associated with a complication of perianal abscess because the tract may not have been entirely filled with glue.[68] It has been suggested that fibrin glue be considered as first-line treatment for complex anal fistulas in appropriately selected patients.

Bioprosthetic Fistula Plug

Recently, the use of a bioprosthetic plug made from lyophilized porcine intestinal submucosal has been described for complex anal fistulas.[117] This porcine fistula plug (Surgisis anal fistula plug) is commercially available from Cook Surgical Inc, Bloomington, IN. Following rehydration of the plug, the following technique is used. The fistula tract is identified but not debrided. A solution of peroxide may be used to gently clean the tract. A fistula probe is placed through the tract and a 2–0 suture is placed through the tapered end of the plug and the ends of this suture are attached to the fistula probe at the primary opening. The suture is pulled from the primary opening, through the fistula tract to exit at the secondary opening. For patients with a "horseshoe" fistula, an incision is made over the fistula tract distal to the anal verge to create a secondary opening that the ends of the suture are brought through. With gentle traction on the suture, the porcine plug is pulled into the primary opening of the fistula until "wrinkling" of the superficial layer of the plug is first seen. The plug is not forced tightly. Excess plug is removed by transecting the plug at the level of the primary opening. The plug is secured in the primary opening using a 2–0 absorbable suture placed in a figure of 8 fashion with the suture crossing through the center of the plug and incorporating a generous portion of the sphincter mechanism on both sides. Any plug protruding through the secondary opening is also excised. The distal end of the plug is not sutured to the fistula tract and the distal opening is left open for drainage. Patients are advised to avoid vigorous physical activity for two weeks after plug placement to minimize the chance of plug dislodgement.

The prospective study by Johnson, et al., compared the procine plug to fibrin glue in twenty-five patients with high transsphincteric or deeper fistuals.[117] Patients with Crohn's dis-

ease or superficial fistulas were excluded. Ten patients underwent fibrin glue closure, and 15 used a fistula plug. Patient's age, gender, fistula tract characteristics, and number of previous closure attempts was similar in both groups. In the fibrin glue group, six patients (60 percent) had persistence of one or more fistulas at three months, compared with two patients (13 percent) in the plug group (p < 0.05, Fisher exact test). The authors concluded that closure of the primary opening of a fistula tract using a suturable biologic anal fistula plug is an effective method of treating anorectal fistulas.

The technique has appeal for its simplicity and avoidance of sphincter injury. The technique seems to work best with long tracts without active sepsis. It is not suitable for short rectovaginal fistulas. An additional limitation has been the relatively high cost of the plug and the lack of large scale controlled multi-center trials. Although the early has been positive, further prospective, long-term studies are warranted.

Postoperative Care

After the lay-open technique, patients are placed on regular diets, bulk agents, and non-codeine-containing analgesia. Patients are instructed to take frequent sitz baths to ensure perianal hygiene. Patients are evaluated at 2-week intervals to ensure that healing has occurred from the depths of the tract. Granulation tissue can be cauterized using silver nitrate sticks and cotton-tipped swabs are often used to probe the depths of the incision to ensure that adequate healing is occurring.

After the advancement flap technique, the Foley catheter is removed on the following day. The authors prefer to maintain patients on intravenous therapy and no oral nutrition for 5 days to allow adequate healing of the flap. After elapse of this time, the diet is progressed and routine management is instituted. The editor (D.E.B.) prefers to feed patients as soon as they can tolerate a diet.

Complications

Incontinence

Minor disorders of continence after fistulotomy have been reported to range from 18% to 52% whereas soiling and insufficiency have been reported in as many as 35% to 45%[69] (Table 13-3). The occurrence of continence disorders has been found to be related to the complexity of the fistula and to the level and location of the internal opening.[69]

Patients with complicated fistulas, high openings, posterior openings, and fistula extensions have been found to be at higher risk.[69] In the treatment of complicated fistulas and those with high openings, more muscle is divided, thus decreasing anal pressures whereas posterior fistula wounds have been associated with higher rates of incontinence because of their more circuitous routes.[69] Drainage of extensions may accidentally damage small nerves and create more scar tissue around the anorectum.[69] If the edges of the

TABLE 13-3. Results of Fistula Surgery

Author	Year	No. of patients	Recurrence (%)	Incontinence (%)
Marks and Ritchie[70]	1977	793	—	3, 17, 25*
Vasilevsky and Gordon[71]	1985	160	6.3	0.7, 2.0, 3.3†
Fucini[11]	1991	99	3.0	0, 0.2, 0.5‡
Van Tets[69]	1994	19	—	33.0
Sangwan[72]	1994	461	6.5	2.8
Garcia-Aguilar et al.[73]	1996	293	7.0	42.0
Mylonakis et al.[74]	2001	100	3.0	0, 6.0, 3.0§
Malouf et al.[75]	2002	98	4.0	10
Westerterp et al.[76]	2003	60	0	50

*3% solid stool, 17% liquid stool, 25% flatus.
†0.7% solid stool, 2.0% liquid stool, 3.3% flatus.
‡0% solid stool, 0.2% liquid stool, 0.5% flatus.
§0% solid stool, 6.0% soiling, 3.0% gas.

fistulotomy wound do not approximate precisely, the anus may be unable to properly close, resulting in intermittent leakage of gas and stool.[53] In addition to these factors, impaired continence was associated with increasing age[70] and female gender.[69,70] The latter is probably the result of partial anal sphincter disruption and/or traction injury to the pudendal nerves sustained during vaginal delivery.[70]

Although excellent results using a seton have been reported,[77] its use does not protect against the development of impaired continence.[69] Minor continence disorders were reported in 73%[69] whereas Williams et al.[78] reported minor disturbances in 54%. Parks and Stitz[55] found that minor incontinence occurred in 39% with the two-stage approach versus 17% when only the first stage was performed and the seton was removed rather than dividing the muscle. Major fecal incontinence was reported in 6.7%[53] after a review of several series (Table 13-4). The degree of incontinence is thought to be influenced by the patient's preoperative state of control as well as to how the anal wound heals.[53] Excellent results with respect to continence have been reported with the use of the advancement flap[59] although recent reports have observed disturbances in continence in 9%–35%.[82,83]

Recurrence

Recurrence rates after fistulotomy range from 0% to 18%.[72] Results from selected references are cited in Table 13-3. Causes include failure to identify a primary opening or recognize lateral or upward extensions of a fistula.[71,72]

TABLE 13-4. Results of staged fistulotomy using a seton

Author	Year	Recurrence (%)	Incontinence (%)
Ramanujam et al.[77]	1983	1/45 (2)	1/45 (2)
Fasth et al.[79]	1990	0/7 (0)	0/7 (0)
Williams et al.[78]	1991	2/28 (8)	1/24 (4)
Pearl et al.[53]	1993	3/116 (3)	5/116 (5)
Van Tets[69]	1994	—	15/29 (54)
Graf et al.[80]	1995	2/25 (8)	11/25 (44)
Garcia-Aguilar et al.[73]	1996	6/63 (9)	39/61 (64)
Hasegawa et al.[81]	2000	8/32 (25)	15/32 (4.8)

Inability to locate the primary opening may imply a circuitous tract,[72] spontaneous closure of the primary opening,[71] or a microscopic opening.[72] The presence of secondary tracts[71] which can be easily missed accounted for early recurrence in 20%.[72] Premature closure of the fistulotomy wound can be obviated by producing an external wound twice the size of the anal wound resulting in proper healing of the internal wound before the external wound.[72] Diligent postoperative care can also reduce recurrence rates by avoiding bridging and pocketing of the wound.[84] Epithelialization of the fistula tract from internal or external openings rather than chronic infection of an anal gland has also been suggested as the cause of a persistent anal fistula.[85]

Recurrence rates after staged repairs using a seton range from 0% to 29%.[53] Results from selected references are cited in Table 13-4.

Although recurrence rates after anorectal advancement flaps were initially reported to be low, with long-term follow-up, recurrence rates of 40% have been reported.[83] Recurrence can be minimized provided that care has been taken to avoid necrosis or retraction of the flap. The use of full-thickness rectal wall has been advocated to prevent ischemic necrosis of the flap.[86]

Early postoperative complications that have been reported after fistula surgery include urinary retention, hemorrhage, fecal impaction, and thrombosed external hemorrhoids, which were found to occur in less than 6% of cases.[18] Later complications such as pain, bleeding, pruritus, and poor wound healing have been reported in 9% of patients.[57] Anal stenosis may occur and is usually the result of loose stools allowing healing of the anal canal by scar contracture.[35] Mucosal prolapse caused by extensive division of sphincter muscle may also occur and can be treated by band ligation, sclerosis, or excision.[57] With attention to both operative detail and postoperative follow-up, these complications can be reduced to a minimum.

Special Considerations

Crohn's Disease

Anal fistulas are the most difficult and challenging complication of Crohn's disease to manage. They constitute the most common perianal manifestations, occurring in 6%–34% of patients.[87] The location of Crohn's disease in the bowel has an impact on the frequency of fistulas. Patients with colonic Crohn's have a higher incidence with the rate approaching 100% in those with rectal Crohn's.[88]

As discussed previously, patients with Crohn's disease should undergo sigmoidoscopy, colonoscopy, and small bowel follow through to determine the extent of disease. Delineation of the fistulous tract is especially important in Crohn's disease because many fistulas may be complex in nature. In this context, endoanal ultrasound has been found to be as useful as MRI. MRI has been found to detect abscesses that were clinically unsuspected on clinical examination[89] and has been helpful in determining the relationship of the fistulous tract to the sphincter muscles.

Therapeutic goals in managing anorectal fistulas in Crohn's disease remain the alleviation of symptoms and preservation of continence. Surgical treatment of fistulas is associated with poor and delayed wound healing and with the risk of sphincter injury. Alexander-Williams stated that "incontinence is likely to be the result of aggressive surgeons, not of aggressive disease." A conservative approach has therefore been advocated, especially because 38% of such fistulas have been reported to heal spontaneously without any surgical intervention.[90] Medications used in the treatment of fistulas include antibiotics such as metronidazole and ciprofloxacin and immunomodulators such as corticosteroids, 6MP, azathioprine, and infliximab. Although several studies have reported spontaneous closure of fistulas in 34%–50% of patients treated with metronidazole,[88] improvement is usually seen after 6–8 weeks of treatment with relapses common once the medication is discontinued. A recent study that looked at the long-term effects of 6MP and azathioprine found that these medications were efficacious in only one-third of patients with fistulizing perianal disease.[91] These effects seemed unrelated to their effects on intestinal disease. The authors concluded that their results did not support the use of these medications solely for the improvement of perianal disease. The use of infliximab has been associated with a 62% reduction in draining fistulas.[92] The combination of infliximab and 6MP may prolong the effect of initial infliximab treatment on fistula closure.[93] Selective seton placement combined with infusion of infliximab and maintenance therapy with azathioprine or methotrexate resulted in complete healing in 67% with Crohn's fistulas in a recently reported retrospective study.[94] Maintenance therapy with infliximab has been reported to result in absence of draining fistulas in 36% of patients compared with 19% in placebo patients at 54-week follow-up.[95]

Although fistulas may occur in as many as 73% of patients after previous abscess drainage,[87] it is imperative that primary fistulotomy not be performed because of the high risk of creating false passages and injuring the sphincter mechanism. Asymptomatic fistulas require no treatment. Low fistulas with simple tracts can be managed with the standard lay-open method in the absence of active proctitis. Successful outcome as gauged by healing has been reported to occur in 42%–100%, mostly in the 70%–80% range of procedures.[96]

The advent of fibrin glue has certainly offered another option in the armamentarium of treating fistulous Crohn's disease. A closure rate of 60% has been reported in one study.[97] This may also be combined with an endorectal advancement flap in the absence of rectal involvement.

Fistulotomy has been associated with prolonged healing.[98] Factors associated with delayed healing are rectal involvement,[10,73] anorectal complications (especially strictures),[98] and the presence or absence of an internal opening.[99] Successful healing has occurred in patients with a classic internal opening at the dentate line and in those without rectal involvement[99] although Halme and Sainio[98] found that delayed healing occurred in 80% of patients despite the presence of a normal rectum; Van Dongen and Lubbers[100] found no difference in healing even in the presence of rectal involvement. Nonetheless, initial therapy should be directed at resolving inflammation in the rectum. This can be accomplished with the use of topical steroid or 5-acetylsalicylic enemas or suppositories. In addition, oral medication may be necessary.

Incontinence has been reported in patients with proctitis who have not undergone anal surgery.[100] A patient with severe rectal involvement and even a simple low fistula is not a candidate for fistulotomy. Division of any sphincter muscle in this situation may result in frank incontinence because the noncompliant rectum acts as a conduit rather than as a reservoir. Continence problems have been reported in 25% of patients after simple incision and drainage of abscesses during which the sphincter mechanism has not been touched.[100] Allan and Keighley[101] reported a 50% frequency of major fecal incontinence and minor incontinence has been described in 33% of patients who have undergone only simple drainage or local surgery.[98] It is thought that diarrhea from either associated intestinal involvement or multiple previous small bowel resections is important in control disorders in these patients.[87,98,100] Appropriate medical therapy should be used to control the diarrhea.

Complex fistulas with high rectal openings might best be managed conservatively, because impaired continence may certainly result if the sphincter muscle is divided. Eradication of the fistula in this situation may not be possible because of the complexity of the tracts. Seton placement has been advocated to promote drainage, limit recurrent suppuration, and preserve sphincter function.[102] Rectal advancement flaps have been used in the absence of severe rectal disease.[103] These have been found to succeed in patients without concomitant small bowel Crohn's.[104]

The importance of quiescent intestinal disease for successful outcome of local fistula surgery has been suggested[105] but not generally accepted and practical. Proximal fecal diversion has also been suggested as an option to ameliorate severe perianal disease because diversion of the fecal stream may reduce perianal inflammation. However, improvement is temporary because fistulas will reactivate after restoration of intestinal continuity.[106]

Complicated fistulas are more likely to recur because of the reluctance of the surgeon to divide sphincter muscle. The use of a long-term in-dwelling seton as a drain is therefore recommended.[102] Fistula recurrence may be as high a 39% after removal of the seton and may necessitate the use of concomitant medical therapy.[87] The use of a rectal advancement flap has been successful; however, breakdown is possible because of sepsis.[103] In patients with mild proctitis, a 20% success rate has been reported.[103] The presence of a protective stoma in this situation does not guarantee success, with failure reported in 55% of patients.[103] A covering stoma may be beneficial in the patient who has undergone multiple unsuccessful repairs.[103] Many fistulas may require repeat fistulotomy to achieve complete healing[98] or repeat injections of fibrin glue. For severe intractable disease, an intersphincteric proctectomy may ultimately become necessary. The intersphincteric technique reduces the size of the resulting wound and reduces the incidence of unhealed sinuses.

Fistula-in-ano in the HIV-positive Patient

Anal fistulas are prevalent in the anoreceptive HIV-positive individual.[107] Disturbed locoregional defenses may allow infection to occur.[107] Although anal fistulas in HIV-positive patients arise from the dentate line similar to those in HIV-negative patients, they are more likely to have incomplete anal fistulas leading to blind sinus tracts.[108] Concern for wound healing has tempered enthusiasm for operative intervention. However, selective operative management will result in a high rate of complete or partial wound healing with symptomatic relief without excessive morbidity or mortality.[107] Severity of illness must be assessed before operative intervention because patients with more advanced disease are less likely to heal their wounds. Data are conflicting as to whether preoperative CD4+ lymphocyte counts can be related to poor wound healing[107]; however, Consten et al.[31] found that low CD4+ lymphocyte counts in patients with perianal sepsis were a risk factor for disturbed wound healing. Use of Highly Active Antiviral therapy (HAART) may reduce the incidence of opportunistic infections and anorectal disease and aid healing.[109]

Asymptomatic fistulas require no treatment. Perioperative antibiotic therapy over a 5-day course has been recommended because of the high risk of infectious complications.[107] Care should be exercised to avoid creation of large wounds and to preserve as much sphincter muscle as possible because these patients may be prone to diarrhea which may overwhelm a partially divided sphincter.[107] In patients who are good operative risks, fistulotomy is appropriate in patients with intersphincteric or low transsphincteric fistulas. For high or complex fistulas as well as for those patients who are poor operative risks, liberal use of draining setons is recommended.[35,107] It is important to realize that cellulitis may be seen with a fistula without

concomitant underlying exudate.[107] Metastatic abscesses to other organs including brain, liver, and mediastinum have been reported with asymptomatic perianal fistulas.[31] Healing has been reported in 55%–80% of patients.[31,107]

Rectourethral Fistulas

Pathophysiology

Rectourethral fistulas are rare but devastating complications that may occur after radical prostatectomy, radiation treatment for prostate cancer, trauma, recurrent perineal abscess, or after treatment with radiofrequency hyperthermia for benign prostatic hypertrophy. It may occur after trauma, as a result of Crohn's disease.

The prostatic urethra is the most common site for fistulization to occur because this portion of the urethra is adjacent to the rectal wall.

Evaluation and Treatment

Symptoms

The most common symptoms include leakage of urine through the rectum during voiding, pneumaturia, and fecaluria. These symptoms will tend to occur during the early postoperative period after prostatectomy. In addition, recurrent urinary tract infections resistant to antibiotic treatment after one of the aforementioned causes should suggest this diagnosis.

Investigations

Prostate-specific antigen determination should be done to rule out recurrence of carcinoma. Digital rectal examination should always be performed to determine if there is any anorectal pathology that could be the cause. Sigmoidoscopy will show the fistula opening which is located on the anterior rectal wall and in addition rule out rectal pathology as a source. Cystoscopy and retrograde urethral cystography should be performed to determine the presence of a urethral stricture. Assessment of urinary continence should be done before any attempt at surgical repair.

Operative Treatment

Operative repair of rectourethral fistulas is challenging because of technical difficulties that are often encountered as a result of difficult exposure. Multiple repairs have been developed but there is no consensus as to which is best. Traditionally, it has been suggested that the first attempt at repair is the best and that subsequent repairs become more difficult.[110]

Treatment consisting of fecal diversion with either colostomy or ileostomy and urinary diversion with suprapubic catheterization under cover of antibiotics has been described in the management of rectourethral fistulas secondary to radiation when the urethral defect has been found to be too large to repair. This has been associated with bouts of recurrent sepsis and persistent symptoms.[111]

Transabdominal Approach

The transabdominal approach combines the use of abdominoanal pullthrough in combination with omental interposition. Difficulties with this procedure include limited exposure deep in the male pelvis making closure of the urethral defect very difficult. A fenestrated splinting catheter apposed to the omentum has been used when leaving the prostatic defect open. Complications associated with this approach include impotence and urethral stricture.[110]

Perineal Approach

Perineal approaches using the gracilis muscle, dartos, or Martius flap have been described. Access through scarred tissue limits exposure and may result in limited space available for the muscle to be placed. Important repair principles include excision of the fistula, development of layers on the urinary and rectal sides if the fistula and closure of nonoverlapping suture lines with interposition of the levators when possible. Zmora et al.[112] retrospectively reported on the effectiveness of the gracilis transposition in healing all rectourethral fistulas with minimal morbidity. Complications with this procedure include urinary incontinence and stricture as well as complications associated with the muscle harvest.

Anterior Trans-anorectal Approach

In this approach, a midline perineal incision is deepened by incising all structures superficial to the prostatic capsule which include the superficial perineal fascia, the central tendon of the perineum, and the internal and external sphincters.[110] This approach allows better access in the repair of complicated membranoprostatic fistulas with preservation of continence and erectile function.

Per-anal Approach

This approach has the theoretical advantages of minimal scarring and fewer wound infections although it suffers from limited exposure. Initially described by Parks and Motson,[113] it involves the use of a full-thickness advancement of anterior rectal wall protected by diverting colostomy. Success rates of 83% have recently been reported when combined with fecal diversion, urinary diversion, both, or none at all.[114] Success rates have been found to be higher when the flap was done for fistulas secondary to iatrogenic causes or trauma as opposed to Crohn's disease.[114] Advancement flap repair can be achieved with minimal morbidity and good postoperative quality of life without compromise to future interventions if needed.

Kraske Laterosacral Approach

This approach provides excellent exposure without division of the sphincter mechanism. The need to excise two to three sacral segments as well as the nerves, muscles, and ligaments around them pose a disadvantage.[110]

York Mason (Trans-sphincteric) Approach

This approach affords a rapid, bloodless exposure through fresh territory and allows for complete separation of the urinary and fecal streams. It avoids the neurovascular bundles and pelvic floor structures essential in maintaining continence and sexual function. It may be performed in combination with a diverting colostomy or a so-called medical colostomy consisting of mechanical preparation and postoperative elemental diet.

It has been associated with longer operative times and more postoperative pain than the other procedures mentioned but has a reported 100% success rate.[115]

Transanal Endoscopic Microsurgery

This highly specialized technique allows for a meticulous two-layer closure of the rectal wall and may be combined with transurethral fulguration of the opposite urethral opening of the fistula.[116] There has been no reported morbidity associated with this procedure although experience is very limited.

Cystectomy and Ileal Conduit

Cystectomy and ileal conduit may be considered for those patients with a low probability of success in resolving the fistula or in maintenance of urinary continence.[110]

Appendix: Practice Parameters for Treatment of Fistula-in-ano

Prepared by The Standards Task Force, American Society of Colon and Rectal Surgeons

Acute Suppuration (Abscess)

Presentation and Management

An abscess should be drained in a timely manner; lack of fluctuance is not a reason for delay in treatment. If the abscess is superficial, it may be drained in the office setting using a local anesthetic. If the patient is too tender to permit examination and drainage, then these measures should be undertaken in the operating room. Antibiotics may have a role as adjunctive therapy in special circumstances, including valvular heart disease, immunosuppression, extensive cellulitis, or diabetes. Location of the abscess should be documented. If possible, anoscopy should be performed to reveal the primary site of infection. Patients should notify the physician if pain recurs after abscess drainage.

Chronic Suppuration (Fistula)

Physical Examination

Inspection and palpation form the basis of the initial evaluation. Specifically, external (secondary) openings are sought, because their relationship to the anal canal provides a clue to the origin of the abscess-fistula. Anoscopy may be useful to identify an internal opening. If clinically indicated, proctosigmoidoscopy or colonoscopy may be suggested to exclude more proximally located inflammatory disorders with which fistulas can be associated.

Radiographic Evaluation

Ultrasound, fistulography, computed tomography, and magnetic resonance imaging are not routinely indicated in the initial evaluation of fistulas but may be helpful in identifying an occult cause of recurrent fistula.

Treatment

Simple Fistulas May Be Treated by Fistulotomy. Fistulotomy is preferred to fistulectomy, because the former technique does not involve excision of the sphincter. Primary fistulotomy is appropriate in cases of intersphincteric and low transsphincteric fistulas. Exceptions may include an anteriorly based transsphincteric fistula in a female, a diabetic patient, or a patient with a weakened sphincter. Patients with irritable bowel syndrome or increased stool frequency may require staged fistulotomy with a seton.

Recurrent Abscess-Fistula/Incontinence. Repeat fistulotomy can be used in treatment of recurrent fistula. If the patient with a recurrent fistula has symptomatic incontinence, then a physiologic investigation may be warranted.

Selective Complex Fistulas May Require Treatment Other Than Fistulotomy. These indications include: 1) high transsphincteric fistula, 2) extrasphincteric fistula, 3) anterior fistulas in females, 4) patients with coexisting inflammatory disease, 5) patients with immunosuppressive disease such as human immunodeficiency virus, 6) elderly patients with poor sphincter function, 7) uncertainty by the surgeon of level of fistula in relation to sphincter, 8) multiple simultaneous fistulas, and 9) patients with multiple prior sphincter surgeries or injuries. Either seton placement or advancement flap closure should be considered. The seton may be used in either a cutting or draining manner, depending on the clinical situation and the patient's underlying condition.

Special Considerations

Rectovaginal Fistulas

For a traumatic (postobstetric) fistula, a 3- to 6-month waiting period after injury is generally useful to promote fibrosis of the injured muscle. A fistulotomy is not generally used if it results in undue amounts of sphincter division. Treatment alternatives include transanal or transvaginal advancement flap closure, closure of the rectovaginal septum, conversion to a complete perineal laceration with layered closure, sphincteroplasty, and muscle interposition.

Radiation-associated Fistulas

Interposition flap or transabdominal approaches have the highest success rates, depending on the level of the fistula.

High Fistulas

For some surgeons, the transabdominal approach is more familiar and involves division of the fistula with layered closure and interposition of omentum. Alternatively, an anterior resection or coloanal anastomosis may be considered.

Suprasphincteric Fistulas

Treatment requires an appreciation that the tract involves the entire external sphincter complex and the puborectalis muscle. Useful treatment options include division of the internal sphincter with concomitant seton placement, excision and drainage of the tract with closure of the internal opening, and advancement flap closure.

Horseshoe Fistula

The internal opening and postanal (or deep anterior anal) space should be drained with or without a seton. The horseshoe portion of the fistula should be curetted and counterdrained rather than unroofed.

Human Immunodeficiency Virus Infection

Large open wounds and sphincter division should be avoided. In general, minimally immunocompromised patients can undergo standard fistulotomy, whereas patients with higher degrees of immunosuppression should undergo placement of a noncutting (draining) seton.

Crohn's Disease

Initial management should be directed at resolving rectal inflammation. Such medical management may include antidiarrheals, topical enemas, antibiotics, suppositories, or systemic steroids and/or immunosuppressive agents. Fistulotomy is a reasonable alternative in most cases of intersphincteric or low transsphincteric fistulas. More complex fistulas can be treated with drainage, seton placement, or flap closure based on the patient's level of continence or extent of concomitant intestinal disease. Ultimately, a temporary or permanent stoma may be indicated.

Reprinted from Dis Colon Rectum 1996;39(12):1361–1372. Copyright © 1996. All rights reserved. American Society of Colon and Rectal Surgeons.

References

1. Gordon PH. Anorectal abscess and fistula-in-ano. In: Gordon PH, Nivatvongs S, eds. Principles and Practice of Surgery for the Colon, Rectum and Anus. St. Louis: Quality Medical Publishing; 1999:241–286.

2. Seow-Choen F, Ho JMS. Histoanatomy of anal glands. Dis Colon Rectum 1994;37:1215–1218.

3. Parks AG. Pathogenesis and treatment of fistula-in-ano. Br Med J 1961;1:463–469.

4. Goldberg SM, Gordon PH, Nivatvongs S. Essentials of Anorectal Surgery. Philadelphia: JB Lippincott; 1980:100–127.

5. Abcarian H. Surgical management of recurrent anorectal abscess. Contemp Surg 1982;21:85–91.

6. Vasilevsky CA, Gordon PH. The incidence of recurrent abscesses or fistula-in-ano following anorectal suppuration. Dis Colon Rectum 1984;27:126–130.

7. Hanley PH, Ray JE, Pennington EE, Grablowsky OM. A ten year follow up study of horseshoe-abscess fistula-in-ano. Dis Colon Rectum 1976;19:507–515.

8. Beck DE, Fazio VW, Lavery IC, et al. Catheter drainage of ischiorectal abscesses. South Med J 1988;81:444–446.

9. Hanley PH. Anorectal abscess fistula. Surg Clin North Am 1978;58:487–503.

10. Read DR, Abcarian H. A prospective survey of 474 patients with anorectal abscess. Dis Colon Rectum 1979;22:566–569.

11. Fucini C. One stage treatment of anal abscesses and fistulas. A clinical appraisal on the basis of two different classifications. Int J Colorectal Dis 1991;6:12–16.

12. Scoma JA, Salvati EP, Rubin RJ. Incidence of fistulas subsequent to anal abscesses. Dis Colon Rectum 1974;17:357–359.

13. Tang C-L, Chew S-P, Soew-Choen F. Prospective randomized trial of drainage alone vs drainage and fistulotomy for acute perianal abscesses with proven internal opening. Dis Colon Rectum 1996;39:1415–1417.

14. Schouten WR, van Vroonhoven TMJV. Treatment of anorectal abscesses with or without primary fistulectomy: results of a prospective randomized trial. Dis Colon Rectum 1991;34:60–63.

15. Buchan R, Grace RH. Anorectal suppuration: the results of treatment and factors influencing the recurrence rate. Br J Surg 1973;60:537–540.

16. Chrabot CM, Prasad ML, Abcarian H. Recurrent anorectal abscesses. Dis Colon Rectum 1984;27:126–130.

17. Seow-Choen F, Nicholls RJ. Anal fistula. Br J Surg 1992;79:197–205.

18. Mazier WP. The treatment and care of anal fistulas: a study of 1000 patients. Dis Colon Rectum 1971;14:134–144.

19. Huber P Jr, Kissack AS, Simonton ST. Necrotizing soft tissue infection from rectal abscess. Dis Colon Rectum 1983;26:507–511.

20. Bubrick MP, Hitchcock CR. Necrotizing anorectal and perineal infections. Surgery 1979;86:655–662.

21. Laucks SS. Fournier's gangrene in anorectal surgery. Surg Clin North Am 1994;74:1339–1352.

22. Kovalcik P, Jones J. Necrotizing perineal infections. Am Surg 1983;49:163–166.

23. Abcarian H, Eftaiha M. Floating free-standing anus. A complication of massive anorectal infection. Dis Colon Rectum 1983;26:516–521.

24. Bode WE, Ramos R, Page CP. Invasive necrotizing infection secondary to anorectal abscess. Dis Colon Rectum 1982;25:416–419.

25. Lucca M, Unger H, Devenny A. Treatment of Fournier's gangrene with adjunctive hyperbaric oxygen therapy. Am J Emerg Med 1990;8:385–387.

26. Barnes SG, Sattler FR, Ballard JO. Perirectal infections in acute leukemia. Improved survival after incision and debridement. Ann Intern Med 1984;100:515–516.

27. Vanheuverzwyn R, Delannoy A, Michaux JL, Dive C. Anal lesions in hematologic diseases. Dis Colon Rectum 1980;23:310–312.

28. Glenn J, Cotton D, Wesley R, Pizzo P. Anorectal infections in patients with malignant diseases. Rev Infect Dis 1988;10:42–52.

29. Sehdev MK, Daviing MD, Seal SH, Stearns MW. Perianal and anorectal complications in leukemia. Cancer 1973;31:149–152.

30. Levi JA, Schimpff SC, Slawson RC, Wiernik PH. Evaluation of radiotherapy for localized inflammatory skin and perianal lesion in adult leukemia: a prospectively randomized double-blind study. Cancer Treat Rep 1977;61:1301–1305.

31. Consten CJ, Siors FJM, Noten HJ, et al. Anorectal surgery in human immunodeficiency virus-infected patients. Dis Colon Rectum 1995;38:1169–1175.

32. Sim A. Anorectal infection in HIV infection and AIDS: diagnosis and management. Baillieres Clin Gastroenterol 1992;6:95–103.

33. Miles AJG, Mellor CH, Gazzard B, et al. Surgical management of anorectal disease in HIV-positive homosexuals. Br J Surg 1990;77:869–871.

34. Parks AG, Gordon PH, Hardcastle JD. A classification of fistula-in-ano. Br J Surg 1976;63:1–12.

35. Wexner SD, Rosen L, Roberts PL, et al. Practice parameters for treatment of fistula-in-ano: supporting documentation. Dis Colon Rectum 1996;39:1363–1372.

36. Cirocco WC, Reilly JC. Challenging the predictive accuracy of Goodsall's rule for anal fistulas. Dis Colon Rectum 1992;35:537–542.

37. Sainio P, Husa A. A prospective manometric study of the effect of anal fistula surgery on anorectal function. Acta Chir Scand 1985;151:279–288.

38. Weisman RI, Orsay CP, Pearl RK, Abcarian H. The role of fistulography in fistula-in-ano. Report of five cases. Dis Colon Rectum 1991;34:181–184.

39. Kuijpers HC, Schulpen T. Fistulography for fistula-in-ano: is it useful? Dis Colon Rectum 1985;28:103–104.

40. Cataldo P, Senagore J, Luchtefeld MA, et al. Intrarectal ultrasound in the evaluation of perirectal abscesses. Dis Colon Rectum 1993;36:554–558.

41. Soew-Choen F, Burnett S, Bartram CI, Nicholls RJ. Comparison between anal endosonography and digital examination in the evaluation of anal fistulas. Br J Surg 1991;78:445–447.

42. Lengyel AJ, Hurst NG, William JG. Preoperative assessment of anal fistulas using endoanal ultrasound. Colorectal Dis 2002;4:436–440.

43. Chew SSB, Yang JL, Newstead GL, et al. Anal fistula: Levovist™-enhanced endoanal ultrasound. A pilot study. Dis Colon Rectum 2003;46:377–384.

44. Rafal RB, Nicholls JN, Cennerazzo WJ, et al. MRI for evaluation of perianal inflammation. Abdom Imaging 1995;20:248–252.

45. Barker PG, Lunniss PJ, Armstrong P, et al. Magnetic resonance imaging of fistula-in-ano: technique, interpretation and accuracy. Clin Radiol 1994;49:7–13.

46. Myhr GE, Myrvold HE, Nilsen G, et al. Perianal fistulas: use of MR imaging for diagnosis. Radiology 1994;191:545–549.

47. Stoker J, Hussain SM, van Kempen D, et al. Endoanal coil in MR imaging of anal fistulas. AJR Am J Roentgenol 1996;166: 360–362.

48. West RL, Zimmerman DE, Dwarkasing S, et al. Prospective comparison of hydrogen peroxide 3-dimensional endoanal ultrasonography and endoanal magnetic resonance imaging of perianal fistulas. Dis Colon Rectum 2003;46:1407–1415.

49. Halligan S, Bartram CI. MR imaging of fistula-in-ano: are endoanal coils the gold standard? AJR Am J Roentgenol 1998; 171:407–412.

50. Beets-Tan RGH, Beets GL, van de Hoop AG, et al. Preoperative MR imaging of anal fistulas: does it really help the surgeon? Radiology 2001;218:75–84.

51. Buchanan GN, Halligan S, Williams AB, et al. Magnetic resonance imaging for primary fistula in ano. Br J Surg 2003;90: 877–881.

52. Buchanan G, Halligan A, Cohen CRG, et al. Effect of MRI on clinical outcome of recurrent fistula-in-ano. Lancet 2002;360: 1661–1662.

53. Pearl RK, Andrews JR, Orsay CP, et al. Role of the seton in the management of anorectal fistulas. Dis Colon Rectum 1993;36:573–579.

54. Nelson RL, Cintron J, Abcarian H. Dermal-island flap anoplasty for transsphincteric fistula-in-ano: assessment of treatment failures. Dis Colon Rectum 2000;43:681–684.

55. Parks AG, Stitz RW. The treatment of high fistula-in-ano. Dis Colon Rectum 1976;19:487–499.

56. Kennedy HL, Zegarra JP. Fistulotomy without external sphincter division for high anal fistulae. Br J Surg 1990;77: 898–901.

57. Fazio VW. Complex anal fistulae. Gastroenterol Clin North Am 1987;16:93–114.

58. Kodner IJ, Mazor A, Shemesh GI, et al. Endorectal advancement flap repair of rectovaginal and other complicated anorectal fistulas. Surgery 1993;114:682–690.

59. Sonoda T, Hull T, Piedmonte MR, Fazio VW. Outcomes of primary repair of anorectal and rectovaginal fistulas using the endorectal advancement flap. Dis Colon Rectum 2002;45: 1622–1628.

60. Zimmerman DD, Delemarre JB, Gosselink MP, et al. Smoking affects the outcome of transanal mucosal advancement flap repair of transsphincteric fistulas. Br J Surg 2003;90:351–354.

61. Kronberg O. To lay open or excise a fistula-in-ano. Br J Surg 1985;72:970.

62. Cintron JR, Park JJ, Orsay CP, et al. Repair of fistula-in-ano using autologous fibrin tissue adhesive. Dis Colon Rectum 1999;42:607–613.

63. Patrij L, Kooman B, Mortina CM, et al. Fibrin glue-antibiotic mixture in the treatment of anal fistulae: experience with 69 cases. Dig Surg 2000;17:77–80.

64. Cintron JR, Park JJ, Orsay CP, et al. Repair of fistulas-in-ano using fibrin adhesive. Long term follow up. Dis Colon Rectum 2000;43:944–950.

65. Sentovitch SM. Fibrin glue for anal fistulas: long-term results. Dis Colon Rectum 2003;46:498–502.

66. Buchanan GN, Bartram CI, Phillips RKS, et al. Efficacy of fibrin sealant in the management of complex anal fistulas. A prospective trial. Dis Colon Rectum 2003;46:1167–1174.

67. You SY, Mizrahi N, Zmora O, et al. The role of endoanal ultrasound as a predictive factor in endoanal advancement flap surgery [abstract]. Colorectal Dis 2001;3(suppl)76.

68. Lindsey I, Smilgen-Humphreys MM, Cunningham C, et al. Randomized controlled trial of fibrin glue vs conventional treatment for anal fistula. Dis Colon Rectum 2002;45: 1608–1615.

69. Van Tets WF, Kuijpers HC. Continence disorders after anal fistulotomy. Dis Colon Rectum 1994;37:1194–1197.

70. Marks CG, Ritchie JK. Anal fistulas at St. Mark's Hospital. Br J Surg 1977;64:84–91.

71. Vasilevsky CA, Gordon PH. Results of treatment of fistula-in-ano. Dis Colon Rectum 1985;28:225–231.

72. Sangwan YP, Rosen L, Riether RD, et al. Is simple fistula-in-ano simple? Dis Colon Rectum 1994;37:885–889.

73. Garcia-Aguilar JC, Belmonte C, Wong WD, et al. Surgical treatment of fistula-in-ano. Factors associated with recurrence and incontinence. Dis Colon Rectum 1996;39:723–729.

74. Mylonakis E, Katsios C, Godevenos D, et al. Quality of life of patients after surgical treatment of anal fistula; the role of anal manometry. Colorectal Dis 2001;3:417–421.

75. Malouf AJ, Buchanan GN, Carapeti A, et al. A prospective audit of fistula-in-ano at St. Mark's Hospital. Colorectal Dis 2002;4:13–19.

76. Westerterp M, Volkers NA, Poolman RW, van Tets WF. Anal fistulotomy between Skylla and Charybdis. Colorectal Dis 2003;5:549–555.

77. Ramanujam PS, Prasad ML, Abcarian H. The role of seton in fistulotomy of the anus. Surg Gynecol Obstet 1983;157: 419–422.

78. Williams JG, Macleod CAH, Goldberg SM. Seton treatment of high anal fistula. Br J Surg 1991;78:1159–1161.

79. Fasth SB, Nordgren S, Hulten L. Clinical course and management of suprasphincteric and extrasphincteric fistula-in-ano. Acta Chir Scand 1990;156:397–402.

80. Graf W, Pahlman L, Egerbald S. Functional results after seton treatment of high transsphincteric anal fistulas. Eur J Surg 1995;161:289–291.

81. Hasegawa H, Radley S, Keighley MR. Long term results of cutting seton fistulotomy. Acta Chir Iugosl 2000;47(4 suppl 1): 19–21.

82. Schouten WR, Zimmerman DD, Briel JW, Briel JW. Transanal advancement flap repair of transsphincteric fistulas. Dis Colon Rectum 1999;42:1419–1423.

83. Mizrahi N, Wexner SD, Zmora O, et al. Endorectal advancement flap: are there predictors of failure? Dis Colon Rectum 2002;45:1616–1621.

84. Soew-Choen F, Phillips RKS. Insights gained from the management of problematical anal fistulae at St. Mark's Hospital, 1984–88. Br J Surg 1991;78:539–541.

85. Lunniss PJ, Sheffield JP, Talbot IC, et al. Persistence of idiopathic anal fistula may be related to epithelialization. Br J Surg 1995;82:32–33.

86. Lewis P, Bartolo DCC. Treatment of trans-sphincteric fistulae by full thickness anorectal advancement flaps. Br J Surg 1990; 77:1187–1189.

87. Williams JG, Rothenberger DA, Nemer FD, Goldberg SM. Fistula-in-ano in Crohn's disease. Results of aggressive surgical treatment. Dis Colon Rectum 1991;34:378–384.

88. Schwartz DA, Pemberton JH, Sandborn WJ. Diagnosis and treatment of perianal fistulas in Crohn's disease. Ann Intern Med 2001;135:906–918.

89. Jenss H, Starlinger M, Skaleij M. Magnetic resonance imaging in perianal Crohn's disease. Lancet 1992;340:1286.

90. Buchmann P, Keighley MRB, Allan RN, et al. Natural history of perianal Crohn's disease: ten-year follow-up. A plea for conservatism. Am J Surg 1980;140:642–644.

91. Lecomte T, Contou JF, Beaugerie L, et al. Predictive factors of response of perianal Crohn's disease to azathioprine or 6-mercaptopurine. Dis Colon Rectum 2003;46:1469–1475.

92. Present DH, Rutgeerts P, Targan S, et al. Infliximab for the treatment of fistulas in patients with Crohn's disease. N Engl J Med 1999;340:1398–1405.

93. Ochsonkuhn T, Goke B, Sackman M. Combining infliximab with 6MP for fistula therapy in Crohn's disease. Am J Gastroenterol 2002;97:2022–2025.

94. Topstad D, Panaccione R, Heine JA, et al. Combined seton placement, infliximab infusion and maintenance immunosuppressives improve healing rate in fistulizing anorectal Crohn's disease. A single center experience. Dis Colon Rectum 2003; 46:577–583.

95. Sands BE, Anderson FH, Bernstein CN, et al. Infliximab maintenance therapy for fistulizing Crohn's disease. N Engl J Med 2004;350:876–885.

96. Nivatvongs S, Gordon PH. Crohn's disease. In: Gordon PH, Nivatvongs S, eds. Principles and Practice of Surgery for the Colon, Rectum and Anus. St. Louis: Quality Medical Publishing; 1999:952–954.

97. Beck DE. Management of anorectal Crohn's fistulas. Clin Colon Rectal Surg 2001;14:117–128.

98. Halme L, Sainio P. Factors related to frequency, type and outcome of anal fistulas in Crohn's disease. Dis Colon Rectum 1995;38:55–59.

99. Levien DH, Surrell J, Mazier WP. Surgical treatment of anorectal fistula in patients with Crohn's disease. Surg Gynecol Obstet 1989;169:133–136.

100. Van Dongen LM, Lubbers GJC. Perianal fistulas in Crohn's disease. Arch Surg 1986;121:1187–1190.

101. Allan A, Keighley MRB. Management of perianal Crohn's disease. World J Surg 1988;12:198–202.

102. White RA, Eisenstat TE, Rubin RJ, Salvati EP. Seton management of complex anorectal fistulas in patients with Crohn's disease. Dis Colon Rectum 1990;33:587–589.

103. Jones OJ, Fazio VW, Jagelman DG. The use of transanal rectal advancement flaps in the management of fistulas involving the anorectum. Dis Colon Rectum 1987;30:919–923.

104. Joo JS, Weiss EG, Nogueras JJ, Wexner SD. Endorectal advancement flap in perianal Crohn's disease. Am Surg 1998;64:147–150.

105. Wolff BE, Culp CE, Beart RW, et al. Anorectal Crohn's disease: a long term prospective. Dis Colon Rectum 1985;28:709–711.

106. McLeod RS. Management of fistula-in-ano: 1990 Roussel Lecture. Can J Surg 1991;34:581–585.

107. Savafi A, Gottesman L, Dailey TH. Anorectal surgery in the HIV+ patient: update. Dis Colon Rectum 1991;34:299–304.

108. Manookian CM, Sokol TP, Hendrick C. Does HIV status influence the anatomy of anal fistulas. Dis Colon Rectum 1998;41:1529–1533.

109. Aleali M, Gottesman L. Anorectal disease in HIV-positive patients. Clin Colon Rectal Surg 2001;14:265–273.

110. Bukowski TP, Chakrabarty A, Powell IJ, et al. Acquired rectourethral fistula: methods of repair. J Urol 1995;153:730–733.

111. Thompson IM, Marx AC. Conservative therapy of rectourethral fistula: five-year follow up. Urology 1990;6: 533–536.

112. Zmora O, Potenti FM, Wexner SD, et al. Gracilis muscle transposition for iatrogenic rectourethral fistula. Ann Surg 2003;237:483–487.

113. Parks AG, Motson RW. Peranal repair of rectoprostatic fistula. Br J Surg 1983;70:725–726.

114. Garofalo TE, Delaney CP, Jones SM, et al. Rectal advancement flap repair of rectourethral fistula. A 20-year experience. Dis Colon Rectum 2003;46:762–769.

115. Prasad ML, Nelson R, Hambrick E, Abcarian H. York Mason procedure for repair of postoperative rectoprostatic urethral fistula. Dis Colon Rectum 1983;26:716–720.

116. Wilbert DM, Buess G, Bichler K-H. Combined endoscopic closure of rectourethral fistula. J Urol 1996;155:256–258.

117. Johnson EK, Gaw JU, Armstrong DN. Efficacy of anal fistula plug vs fibrin glue in closure of anorectal fistulas. Dis Colon Rectum 2006;49:371–376.

14
Benign Anorectal: Rectovaginal Fistulas

Ann C. Lowry and Barton Hoexter

Although typically small in size and seemingly simple, rectovaginal fistulas are an aggravation to the patients and surgeons. Passing flatus or stool through the vagina is understandably distressing to patients; the lack of a uniformly successful repair is frustrating to surgeons.

Etiology

Obstetric injury is the most frequent cause of acquired rectovaginal fistulas but infection and other forms of trauma may also result in these fistulas. After an obstetric injury, the fistula may be manifest immediately but more frequently appears 7–10 days after delivery. Fistulas occur most often after a third- or fourth-degree laceration. Inadequate repair, breakdown of the repair, or infection may result in fistula formation. In developed nations, rectovaginal fistulas occur after 0.06%–0.1% of vaginal deliveries.[1–3] In developing countries, however, the incidence of rectovaginal and vesicovaginal fistula after childbirth is almost 3 times higher, with more than half of these fistulas being larger than 4 cm in diameter.[4,5] In these countries, prolonged labor, causing necrosis of the rectovaginal septum, leads to the formation of a fistula.

Disease processes may also cause rectovaginal fistulas. Cryptoglandular infection may result in an abscess spontaneously draining into the vagina resulting in a fistula. Rectal and gynecologic malignancies may result in fistulas as a result of local extension of the tumor or secondary to treatment with radiotherapy. Women with inflammatory bowel disease, Crohn's disease more frequently than ulcerative colitis, may develop rectovaginal fistulas. In a 23-year population-based study of patients with Crohn's disease in Olmsted County, MN, 88 fistulas developed in 59 patients.[6] Eight (9%) of the fistulas were rectovaginal fistulas. Over a period of approximately 30 years, 90 of the 886 women seen at St. Mark's Hospital with Crohn's disease and an intact rectum developed a rectovaginal fistula.[7]

Operative trauma may also result in a rectovaginal fistula. Complications of rectal or vaginal surgery usually result in fistulas opening low in the rectum. High fistulas are most frequently complications of low stapled colorectal or ileoanal anastomoses. In one series of 140 patients undergoing low anterior resection for rectal carcinoma, four (2.9%) developed a rectovaginal fistula.[8] The mechanism is usually that a portion of the posterior vaginal wall is included in the anastomosis or that an abscess secondary to an anastomotic leak drains into the vagina. Pouch vaginal fistulas are reported in 3%–12% of patients.[9–12] Rectovaginal fistulas are also a complication of neovaginal construction for congenital abnormalities or as sex-change procedures.[13]

Fistulas have also been reported after vaginal dilatation of a radiated vaginal cuff, fecal impaction, viral and bacterial infection in human immunodeficiency virus patients and sexual assault.[14–17] Congenital rectovaginal fistulas occur but are outside the scope of this chapter.

Evaluation

There are two primary goals in the evaluation of women with possible rectovaginal fistulas: identification of the fistula site and assessment of the surrounding tissue. The type of investigation required varies with the underlying etiology of the fistula.

Identification of Fistula Site

In most women with complaints consistent with a rectovaginal fistula, the site can be readily identified on examination. Visual examination may show the dark red rectal mucosa contrasting with the pale mucosa of the vagina. A dimple may be palpable in the anterior midline on rectal examination. The rectal opening is frequently visible on anoscopy. In some women, the diagnosis may be elusive. A methylene blue test may confirm the presence of a communication and aid in locating the site. During this test, a vaginal tampon is inserted and then the patient is given an enema colored with methylene blue. If the patient retains the enema, staining on the tampon is highly suggestive of a rectovaginal fistula. Alternatively, saline can be instilled in the vagina with the patient in the lithotomy position. The rectum is then insufflated with air and the vagina observed for bubbles.

Radiographic tests may help identify an elusive fistula. One option is vaginography. The examination is performed by instilling contrast into the vagina through a Foley catheter with the balloon inflated to occlude the vaginal opening. The technique has a sensitivity of 79%–100% for the detection of the fistula tract. Vaginography is most helpful for colovaginal and enterovaginal fistulas; it is less useful for low rectovaginal fistulas.[18,19] Computed tomography scans may identify the fistula tract and characterize the surrounding tissue. Contrast material in the vagina after oral or rectal administration is diagnostic of a fistula. Suggestive evidence includes air or fluid in the vagina if there is no history of recent instrumentation.

Both magnetic resonance imaging (MRI) and ultrasound are used to identify fistulas. Small studies of endoanal ultrasound with and without contrast, MRI with and without endoluminal coils, and transperineal and transvaginal ultrasounds are available. One study comparing MRI with a coil to endoanal ultrasound found the same positive predictive value for identification of the fistula site for both tests.[20] Accuracy could not be determined in this retrospective study. In an earlier study of endoanal ultrasound, positive predictive value was good but ultrasound only identified 28% of rectovaginal fistulas.[21] Fistulas above the dentate line were more frequently identified than ones at or below the dentate line. Contrast enhanced ultrasound using hydrogen peroxide seems to be more accurate than nonenhanced studies.[22] Contrast enhanced ultrasound has not been directly compared with MRI. Another group reported the use of transperineal and transvaginal ultrasound in the assessment of fistulas. The examinations successfully identified fistulas.[23] The accuracy of the technique could not be determined because only 56% of patients underwent surgery. At present it is not clear which radiologic examination is optimal to detect elusive fistulas.

Assessment of Local Tissue

The second goal of evaluation is to determine the etiology and to assess the surrounding tissue. The necessary tests are determined by the suspected etiology of the fistula. Symptoms of incontinence should be elicited during the history. If the mechanism of injury is childbirth, the patient with a fistula is at significant risk of a sphincter defect. In a review by the University of Minnesota, 48% of women with rectovaginal fistulas complained of incontinence preoperatively.[24] Ultrasound or MRI should be done to assess the anal sphincter. One study found that 100% of women presenting with a rectovaginal fistula after a delivery had a sphincter defect.[21] In another study, only 3 of 34 women with rectovaginal fistulas had an isolated rectovaginal fistula without abnormality in the perineal body or sphincter muscles.[25] Symptoms of the fistula

frequently mask anal incontinence; failure to study the sphincter may lead to a poor choice of repair and persistent incontinence postoperatively.[24,26] Endoanal ultrasound and MRI are reported to be essentially equivalent in detection of a sphincter defect.[20]

Multiple perianal fistulas suggest Crohn's disease as the etiology. Evaluation of the intestinal tract by colonoscopy and contrast studies is indicated in patients with known or suspected inflammatory bowel disease. One must be careful to consider the patient's obstetric history even if she carries the diagnosis of Crohn's disease.

Biopsy of a detectable mass should be done for suspected malignancy. The presence of a known malignancy may dictate a workup for metastatic disease. It is critical that recurrent carcinoma be distinguished from irradiation injury. In patients with a history of malignancy treated by radiation, examination under anesthesia with biopsies is often necessary. Two series report an approximately 50% incidence of recurrent cancer on biopsies of these fistulas.[27,28]

Classification

A variety of classification systems exist for rectovaginal fistulas. Most systems classify by size, location, and etiology. Daniels[29] classified fistulas by their location along the rectovaginal septum as low, middle, or high. The rectal opening is at the dentate line and the vaginal opening just inside the vaginal fourchette in low fistulas. The vaginal opening is at or near the cervix in high fistulas. Middle fistulas are located between high and low fistulas. This system is useful in that high fistulas are more likely to require laparotomy; perineal approaches are appropriate for most low and middle fistulas. However, beyond that, these categories are not very useful in guiding treatment decisions. In addition, this terminology is not applied consistently because some authors would term the low fistulas anovaginal fistulas. Others state that the rectal opening is below the dentate line in anovaginal fistulas.

Another system classifies fistulas into simple and complex categories.[30] Simple fistulas are small (<2.5 cm), low, and secondary to trauma or infection. Complex fistulas are large, high, caused by inflammatory bowel disease, radiation, or malignancy, or persistent despite multiple failed repairs. This system separates fistulas amenable to local repairs and ones likely to require resection or the interposition of well-vascularized tissue. Simple fistulas tend to have healthy surrounding tissue and complex fistulas occur in diseased tissue which dictates the type of repair necessary.

Saclarides[31] argues that a classification system based on etiology is the most useful for the treating physician. A system determined by etiology would take into consideration the state of the surrounding tissue both anatomically and functionally as well as the health of the patient.

None of these systems have been tested to see whether they are predictive of outcome but a strong case can be made that etiology is the best guide to patient management. Research in this area would benefit from standardized terminology and a valid classification system.

Conservative Management

For women with small fistulas and minimal symptoms, medical management is appropriate. Optimizing the patient's bowel function, particularly controlling diarrhea, is beneficial. Unfortunately, for the majority of women with rectovaginal fistulas, the symptoms are intolerable.

Surgical Techniques

Local Repairs

General Considerations

A local repair is appropriate for the first or second repair in women with rectovaginal fistulas and intact sphincter muscles. The type of repair is determined by surgeon expertise and size of the fistula. Colorectal surgeons typically prefer an endorectal or perineal approach whereas gynecologists favor a transvaginal approach.

Patients undergo mechanical and antibiotic preparation preoperatively. General anesthesia is used in most cases although the repairs may be performed under regional anesthesia. A urinary catheter is inserted. Prone jackknife position provides the best exposure for transanal and perineal approaches whereas lithotomy position is better for transvaginal repairs. Exposure is optimized by the use of a headlight, taping of the buttocks, and a Lone Star retractor. A Pratt bivalve anoscope will be helpful in repair of low fistulas; Wylie renal vein retractors, narrow Deaver, or malleable retractors are preferable for higher fistulas.

Simple fistulotomy is reported as an option but should be avoided because of the risk of incontinence. It is not acceptable to divide a significant portion of intact sphincter muscle and leave it to heal by secondary intention.

Fibrin Sealant

Fibrin glue instillation has been used for fistula-in-ano with some success. The technique does not differ when fibrin glue is applied to rectovaginal fistulas. Most studies that include rectovaginal fistulas report discouraging results of 0%–33% success in very small numbers of patients.[32–34] The one exception is a study by Venkatesh and Ramanujam[35] who report that six of eight patients with rectovaginal fistulas were cured with fibrin glue.

Advancement Flaps

Advancement flaps may be approached transrectally, vaginally, or through the perineum. An advantage of the transanal approach is direct access to the rectal side of the fistula which is the high pressure side. Several variations of the technique for endorectal advancement flaps have been reported but the general principles are the same. With the patient in the prone jackknife position and adequate exposure, a U-shaped flap is outlined with the distal end below the fistula opening. The flap should have a base 2–3 times wider than the apex. A flap of mucosa, submucosa, and circular muscle is raised for a distance sufficient to allow a tension-free repair, usually 4–5 cm. The fistula tract is debrided but not excised. Anoderm is elevated off the internal sphincter and circular muscle laterally. The muscles are approximated over the fistula opening with long-acting absorbable suture in one to two layers. The distal end of the flap including the fistula site is excised and the flap sutured in place with absorbable suture. The vaginal side is left open for drainage (Figure 14-1). Patients are typically observed overnight. They resume a normal diet with fiber supplements to prevent constipation. Diarrhea must also be controlled because it will affect healing as much as constipation. There is usually minimal discomfort and a brief recovery period. Patients are cautioned to avoid intercourse and the use of tampons for 6 weeks.

The literature contains many case series of endorectal advancement flaps[24,26,36–50] (Table 14-1). The reported outcome measure is usually successful repair of the fistula; continence is rarely included. The explanation of the wide range of results is not clear. Perhaps it is the surgeon's technique or patient selection that explains the reports with high success rates. Other considerations are that some studies include patients with concomitant sphincter repairs. One would expect that group to have a higher closure rate than patients undergoing an endorectal advancement flap alone. Some series include fistulas of multiple etiologies which may influence outcome. Even within a group of patients whose etiology is all obstetric injury, early series mix patients with and without sphincter defects. The presence of scar rather than healthy muscle under the flap intuitively would decrease the success of the repair. A recent series of endorectal advancement flaps in women with intact sphincter muscles supports that view. Eleven of 12 fistulas healed.[38] In addition, some series report ultimate closure rates combining patients with one attempt at repair and those with repeated attempts. Watson and Phillips[50] reported a primary success rate in 7 of 12 patients and an ultimate success in 10 of 12 patients illustrating the difference that would occur depending on the reporting method. Not all authors include both data. The number of previous repairs has been reported to affect the success rate and is not always reported.[51] Lowry and colleagues[40] reported a success rate of more than 80% in first and second repairs but only 55% in patients with two prior repairs. Follow-up techniques vary and may influence the accuracy of the data.

Recent investigations sought explanations for the failure rate. One group presented a retrospective study of 116 consecutive endorectal advancement flaps done for both fistulas-in-ano and rectovaginal fistulas. Recurrence was not associated with prior attempts at repair, type of fistula,

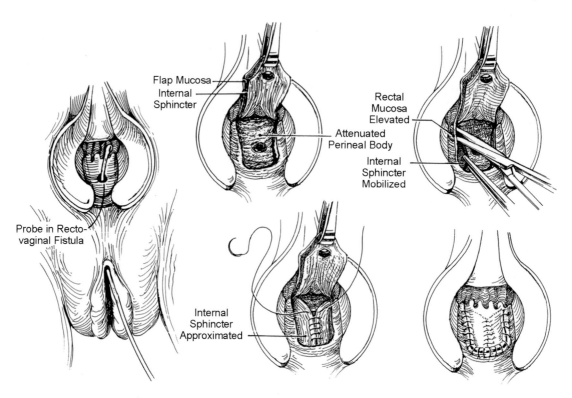

FIGURE 14-1. Endorectal advancement flap.

origin, steroid use, antibiotic usage, bowel confinement, or presence of a diverting stoma.[41] There was a higher rate of recurrence in patients with Crohn's disease. Sonoda and colleagues[43] also found that a diagnosis of Crohn's disease was associated with a higher failure rate in their study of 105 endorectal advancement flaps. In distinction to the first study, however, patients with rectovaginal fistulas secondary to obstetric injury also had a lower success rate. Smoking was linked to failure of endorectal advancement flap in another study.[52] In an attempt to improve the results, that group added labial fat transposition to endorectal advancement flap.[45]

Unfortunately, the results were no different from an advancement flap alone.

Sliding flaps may also be performed on the vaginal side. An incision is made in the posterior vaginal wall near the introitus and a flap of vaginal wall is raised. Dissection is extended laterally to the ischial tuberosities to provide adequate mobility. The vaginal and rectal defects are closed with absorbable sutures. The levator ani muscles are approximated in the midline; this portion of the repair is believed to be critical to its success. The vaginal flap is then sutured in place. Success rates of 84%–100% are reported with vaginal flaps.[50,53–57]

TABLE 14-1. Results of endorectal advancement flaps

Author	Year	No. of patients	Success (%)	Comments
Greenwald & Hoexter[36]	1978	20	100	Tract excised, layered closure under flap
Hoexter et al.[37]	1985	15	100	Repair as above
Wise et al.[44]	1991	40	85	15 concomitant sphincteroplasty
Lowry[68]	1991	85	78	25 concomitant sphincteroplasty
Kodner et al.[47]	1993	71	93	Unknown no. sphincteroplasty
Khanduja et al.[26]	1994	16	100	Patients without incontinence
MacRae et al.[48]	1995	28	29	50% obstetric, previous failed repairs
Mazier et al.[49]	1995	19	95	67% simple
Watson & Phillips[50]	1995	12	58%	Ultimate success 83%, 25% stomas
Tsang et al.[24]	1998	27	41	All obstetric
Hyman[38]	1999	12	91	Etiology not reported
Joo et al.[39]	1998	20	75	Ultimate success, all Crohn's
Baig et al.[46]	2000	19	74	7 concomitant sphincteroplasty
Mizrahi et al.[41]	2002	32	56	Mixture of etiologies
Sonoda et al.[43]	2002	37	43	Mixture of etiologies
Zimmerman et al.[45]	2002	21	48	6 concomitant sphincteroplasty 12 labial flap transposition

Anocutaneous flaps are an option for distal rectovaginal or anovaginal fistulas. A flap of anoderm and perineal skin is raised and advanced into the anal canal. After the fistula track is debrided, the flap is sutured into place.[58] A diamond-shaped cutaneous flap has also been used on the vaginal side in conjunction with an endoanal advancement flap.[59] Only a few cases have been reported with either technique.

Rectal Sleeve Advancement

An alternative transrectal approach is a rectal sleeve advancement involving mobilization of the distal rectum and advancement to cover the fistula. A circumferential incision is made at the dentate line and deepened through the submucosa. This plane is continued in a cephalad direction exposing internal sphincter muscle. Above the anorectal ring the dissection becomes full thickness. The mobilization continues until healthy, nonscarred tissue is reached and that tissue can be pulled down to the dentate line without tension. The rectum is pulled through the anal canal, the diseased portion excised, and healthy tissue sutured to anoderm below the dentate line. This technique is reported in patients with a rectovaginal fistula and inflamed anal canal and distal rectum from Crohn's disease. In a series of five patients with rectovaginal fistulas and Crohn's disease reported by the Cleveland Clinic, three of the patients with fecal diversion healed.[60] One patient required two rectal sleeve advancements before healing occurred. Of the two patients without fecal diversion, one healed. Simmang et al.[61] emphasized that this technique is useful for someone with a rectovaginal fistula and a stricture because both problems will be corrected with the procedure.

A variation is the modified Noble-Mengert-Fish technique.[25] With this procedure, the full thickness of the anterior rectal wall is mobilized. A curvilinear incision is made at the mucocutaneous junction over the anterior 180 degrees of the anal canal. The dissection continues until the rectovaginal septum is entered. The superior limit is the vault of the vagina; the lateral margin is the full width of the rectovaginal space. There needs to be adequate dissection to ensure that the flap will reach the area of the external sphincter without tension. The flap is then anchored to the external anal sphincter and the perineal skin, forming a new mucocutaneous junction. Older reports of this technique documented successful repair of rectovaginal fistulas in 86%–100%. Minor incontinence troubled 25% of patients.[42,62,63] The only recent report combined this repair with sphincter reconstruction or perineal body repair in the majority of patients.[25] The overall anatomic success was 94%; the results for the anterior rectal wall advancement alone were not reported separately.

Excision of Fistula with Layered Closure

Another option is excision of the fistula tract and layered closure. Layered closure may actually be performed through the rectum, vagina, or perineum. If done through the rectum or vagina, an elliptical incision is made around the fistula and

mucosal flaps are raised for 2–3 cm. The fistula tract is excised. Vaginal mucosa, rectovaginal septum, rectal muscle, and rectal mucosa are closed in succession. Plication of the levator muscles is added by some surgeons. If done through the perineum, a transverse incision is made and extended down to the fistula tract. The fistula is then cored out of the rectal and vaginal walls and a layered closure performed.

Using layered closure, successful repair is reported in 88%–100% of patients in the small series published.[53–56]

Perineo-proctotomy

Perineo-proctotomy or conversion to a fourth-degree laceration is usually performed with the patient in the lithotomy position; this approach begins with the identification of the fistula and division of the bridge of skin, subcutaneous tissue, sphincter muscle, rectal and vaginal walls overlying the fistula. The tract is excised and both the rectal and vaginal walls are dissected away from the muscle. After repair of both the rectal and vaginal defects, the external sphincter muscle is reapproximated. The muscle must be adequately mobilized to avoid tension on the repair. The perineal body is reconstructed and the skin closed (Figure 14-2).

The use of perineo-proctotomy or conversion to a fourth-degree laceration for rectovaginal fistulas is reported in women with intact sphincter muscles as well as ones with a sphincter disruption. Success rates for fistula closure range from 87% to 100% in small series.[35,49,56,64] In most series, postoperative continence is not documented. Mazier and colleagues[49] did report that none of 38 women undergoing this repair were incontinent postoperatively.

Inversion of Fistula

Inversion of the fistula is a simple technique usually performed through the vagina. The vaginal mucosa is mobilized circumferentially around the fistula. The tract is excised and a pursestring suture used to invert the fistula into the rectum. The vaginal wall is then closed over the inversion.[65] One small series reports success in 8 of 11 patients[66]; a more recent series reports a 100% success rate in 47 women.[67]

Complex Repairs

The complex repairs involve the interposition of well-vascularized tissue between the rectum and the vagina; that tissue may be muscle, omentum, or healthy bowel. With the exception of transposition of the rectus muscle, the initial dissection for muscle interposition is typically through the perineum. The interposition of omentum or healthy bowel requires an abdominal procedure.

Tissue Interposition: Muscle

The most common tissue interposition technique is a sphincteroplasty utilized when a defect in the external sphincter is

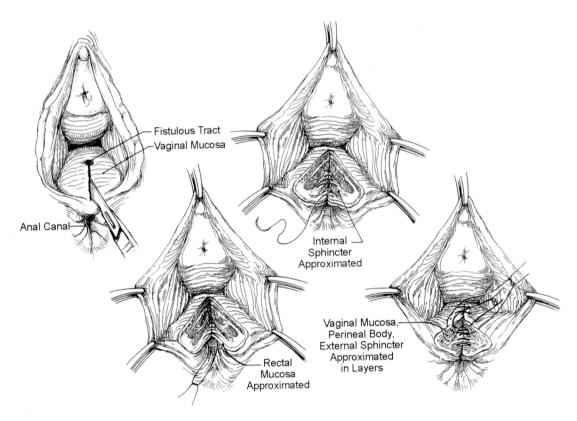

Figure 14-2. Perineo-proctotomy.

present with the rectovaginal fistula. In that situation, an over-lapping sphincteroplasty will correct the fistula and the incontinence. The technical details are described and illustrated in Chapter 46 on incontinence. Successful closure of rectovaginal fistulas with this operation is reported in 65%–100% of patients (Table 14-2).[21,26,42,44,48,68,69]

When the sphincter muscle is intact or the fistula is above the sphincter muscles, rectus, bulbocavernous, gracilis, gluteus, and sartorius muscles have been used to repair rectovaginal fistulas.[4,70–82] The perineal dissection is similar regardless of the muscle used. Preoperatively, the patients undergo a full mechanical bowel preparation and receive preoperative antibiotics. For these dissections, a Lone Star retractor and a headlight are very useful for exposure. With the patient in the prone jackknife position, a transverse perineal incision close to the vaginal introitus is made. The posterior

TABLE 14-2. Results of sphincteroplasty for rectovaginal fistula

Author	Year	No. of patients	Success (%)
Russell & Gallagher[42]	1977	9	96
Lowry[68]	1991	29	93
Wise et al.[44]	1991	15	100
Khanduja et al.[26]	1994	11	100
MacRae et al.[48]	1995	7	86
Tsang et al.[24]	1998	35	80
Yee et al.[21]	1999	22	91
Halverson et al.[69]	2001	14	65

vaginal wall is separated from the anal sphincter and anterior rectal wall until soft, pliable tissue is reached. This dissection is often difficult because of dense scarring. Care must be taken to avoid entering the rectum; a finger or anoscope in the rectum is helpful to identify the appropriate plane. The rectal and vaginal walls are closed with absorbable sutures. It is generally not necessary to trim the vaginal or rectal wall and doing so often only makes a significantly larger defect. The mobilized muscle is then inserted between the rectum and the vagina and tacked to the posterior vaginal wall. The incision is loosely closed often with a drain in place. For transposition of the rectus muscle, a midline abdominal incision is also made to allow dissection between the rectum and vagina from above as well as from the perineal side.

If the labial fat pad is chosen for transposition, the patient is placed in modified lithotomy position. Once the perineal dissection is completed, a longitudinal incision is made over the labial majora. Skin flaps are raised laterally and medially. There is often a plane similar to Scarpa's fascia for this portion of the dissection. The dissection is continued to the periosteum of the pubis posteriorly. Superiorly the tissue is mobilized to the pubic symphysis. Once the entire fat pad with the bulbocavernous muscle is mobilized, the superior end is divided. The posterior pedicle is left intact to preserve the perineal branch of the pudendal artery. A subcutaneous, subvaginal tunnel is created from the base of the pedicle to the perineal incision. The flap is pulled through this tunnel and sutured to the posterior vaginal wall above the vaginal and rectal closures. The labial incision is closed in two layers over a suction drain. The perineal incision is closed loosely often over a drain (Figure 14-3). When vaginal stenosis is a concern, inclusion of an island of skin from the inner thigh with the pedicle is an alternative.[4] The use of the Martius graft is reported primarily in fistulas secondary to radiation. Aartsen and Sindram[83] reported 100% success in 14 patients initially; they do caution, however, that after a 10-year follow-up, 8 of the 14 patients required diversion for progressive radiation damage. Others report success in 78%–84%.[74,75,84]

The details of mobilization of the rectus, gracilis, and sartorius muscles are beyond the scope of this chapter.

Tissue Interposition: Bowel

Healthy bowel may be interposed in one of two ways. An extended low anterior resection may be done with excision of the rectum containing the fistula and an anastomosis below. The vaginal defect is closed and if possible separated from the new anastomosis with omentum. Parks and associates[85] described a sleeve coloanal technique when the fistula is very low. The rectum is mobilized to a level below the fistula and divided. From a perineal approach, a distal rectal mucosectomy is performed. The proximal healthy colon is pulled through the muscular sleeve covering the fistula. A handsewn coloanal anastomosis is then completed. Technical success is reported in 78%–100% of patients.[85–87] In a review of functional results after stoma closure, 64% of patients were completely continent at 6 months and 75% at 1 year.[87]

An alternative is a procedure described by Bricker and Johnston.[88] Through an abdominal incision the fistula is divided. The sigmoid colon is mobilized and divided. The proximal end is used for a temporary colostomy; the distal end is rotated upon itself and sutured in an end to side manner to the debrided edges of the defect in the rectal wall. When healing is confirmed with a contrast study, the proximal sigmoid colon is sutured to the loop of colon used in the repair (Figure 14-4). Bricker and colleagues[89] reported excellent or satisfactory results in 19 of 26 patients.

Choice of Treatment

For any patient with a rectovaginal fistula, conservative management is an option if the symptoms are tolerable. In addition, fibrin glue instillation may reasonably be attempted particularly in low, small fistulas. The success rate is unproven but the procedure is very well tolerated and carries minimal risk. For fistulas resulting in significant symptoms, the choice of treatment largely depends on the etiology of the fistula.

Rectovaginal Fistulas Secondary to Obstetric Injury

Rectovaginal fistulas may close spontaneously in the early postpartum period[67,90]; all others require surgery to close. It is important that the surrounding tissue be free of infection and induration before proceeding with surgery. For most patients, treatment of infection and time will allow the surrounding tissue to soften. Once the surrounding tissue is amenable to repair, timing of the repair may be chosen by the patient. Patients with significant symptoms need not wait until their childbearing is complete, although depending on the choice of repair, subsequent babies should be delivered by Cesarean section.

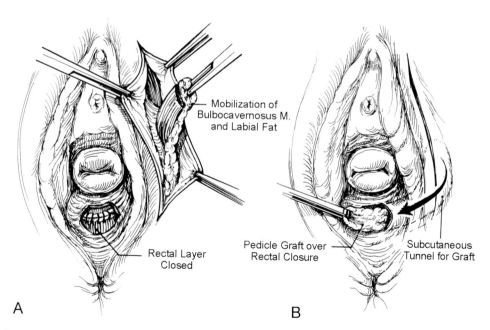

FIGURE 14-3. Martius graft. **A** Perineal dissection and mobilization of graft. **B** Interposition of labial graft.

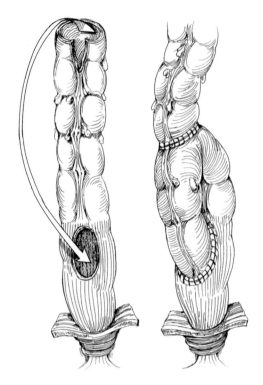

FIGURE 14-4. Onlay patch (Bricker procedure).

As mentioned above, an important part of the evaluation of women with rectovaginal fistulas caused by obstetric injury is assessment of anal sphincter anatomy and function. In multiple studies, the incidence of associated sphincter defect is close to 100% in this subset of patients.[21,24,26] Therefore, both closure of the fistula and continence should be considered important outcome measures.

For women with intact sphincters and a rectovaginal fistula after childbirth, a simple local repair is recommended. Because data comparing the various repairs do not exist, the choice of the repair should be based on the surgeon's experience. In most practices, these women represent only a small portion of the patients with rectovaginal fistulas because the majority will have a concomitant sphincter defect.

For women with sphincter defects, sphincteroplasty closes the fistula and repairs the sphincter defect. A perineoproctotomy is also appropriate. The advantage of this technique is the excellent exposure it provides; the disadvantage is the risk of incontinence if intact sphincter muscle is divided. No direct comparison of this approach and sphincteroplasty exists but sphincteroplasty is more widely accepted.

Rectovaginal Fistulas Secondary to Cryptoglandular Disease

When rectovaginal fistulas secondary to cryptoglandular disease are reported, they represent only a small portion of most series. Evaluation must include a search and treatment of associated local sepsis with the possible use of a seton.

Endoanal ultrasound should be performed to exclude an occult sphincter defect. If none is found, an endorectal advancement flap is the most frequently used procedure. Fistula closure rate is rarely documented separately for cryptoglandular fistulas so the success rate is not well established. In some series, it seems that these fistulas heal less well than other types. Insertion of fibrin glue, a vaginal advancement flap, and an anocutaneous flap would be reasonable alternatives but no data exist regarding their efficacy in this specific situation. In addition, there are no data comparing any two procedures.

Rectovaginal Fistulas Secondary to Crohn's Disease

The treatment of patients with rectovaginal fistulas secondary to Crohn's disease differs from other patients with rectovaginal fistulas in several ways. Given the nature of Crohn's disease, control of symptoms becomes the primary goal as opposed to elimination of the fistula in this subset of patients. In addition, the treatment is in more flux than any other subset of patients.

Medical management with antibiotics and immunosuppressive medication was able to control symptoms but rarely close fistulas. Surgical therapy often required proctectomy because of associated proctitis and was not uniformly successful even in the absence of inflammation.[7,91] Over a period of approximately 30 years, Radcliffe and colleagues at St. Mark's Hospital identified 90 women with Crohn's disease and a rectovaginal fistula.[7] Eight were diverted, 34 underwent early proctectomy, and another 12 required proctectomy later. The indications for proctectomy were severe colitis or proctitis or an associated anal lesion in the majority of patients. Twelve were managed conservatively and 24 underwent a local repair. Heyen and colleagues[91] traced the course of 28 women with Crohn's disease and a vaginal fistula. Five required early proctectomy and seven underwent proctectomy later. Of the 16 fistulas managed conservatively, none healed. Malignancy developed in the fistula tract of two patients.

The introduction of infliximab is a recent addition to the treatment options for Crohn's perianal fistulas. A randomized, controlled trial found that infliximab was significantly better than placebo in healing fistulas in Crohn's disease.[92] Subsequent studies have confirmed a 24%–55% healing rate by assessment of clinical symptoms.[93,94] Most of these studies reported healing rates after a course of three infusions. Data are accumulating that some patients will require a longer course, perhaps maintenance therapy, to control symptoms. In addition, several studies using follow-up ultrasound or MRI revealed that the radiologic healing rate is lower than the clinical healing rate.[95] One recent study showed that there was continued radiologic healing with a longer course of therapy.[96] It also seems that a combination of surgery and infliximab is necessary in a substantial portion of patients. Results are better when drainage of local sepsis and placement of a seton are done before initiating infliximab.[93] If the goal is complete healing, the seton must be removed before the completion of the course of infliximab. Another unresolved detail is whether the addition of immunosuppressive medication improves the response rate or maintenance of a response. Although this therapy is promising for perianal fistulas, it is not clear that rectovaginal fistulas respond as well. One study reported that only one of eight patients with a rectovaginal fistula had a complete response[93] whereas another study reported no difference between simple and complex fistulas.[96]

At the present time, the following treatment program seems reasonable. Each patient should be assessed to determine the presence of associated proctitis and undrained local sepsis. Patients with associated proctitis require appropriate medical or surgical management for that condition. In either case, any local sepsis should be drained, all tracts identified, and setons placed if appropriate. Until more definitive data are available, a trial of infliximab should be considered. Setons should be removed before the last infusion. If symptoms resolve or are minimal, then conservative therapy is appropriate. No clear recommendation regarding maintenance infliximab or immunosuppressive medication is possible at this time.

If a persistent fistula results in significant symptoms and any associated proctitis resolves, then surgical intervention is appropriate. A multitude of repairs is reported. Vaginal flaps succeeded in 13 of 14 patients in one series.[97] All patients had diverting stomas at the time of the repair. Eradication of the fistula with an endorectal advancement flap is reported in 30%–70% of patients.[43] Kodner reported an initial healing rate of 71% which increased to 92% with additional procedures.[47] The Cleveland Clinic surgeons tailor the advancement flap according to the height and length of the fistula and the presence of rectal ulceration or inflammation. They report an initial healing rate of 54% and an overall success rate of 68% including repeat repairs. The necessity of diversion is controversial but it is often performed in this subset of patients. All of these results predate the introduction of infliximab. Whether the use of infliximab or other new medications will result in improved outcomes remains to be seen.

Rectovaginal Fistulas Secondary to Malignancy

The treatment of these fistulas is dictated by the type of underlying malignancy. For rectal cancer invading the vagina, resection with or without reconstruction is required. If preoperative adjuvant therapy is given, diversion before initiation of treatment may be necessary for the patient's comfort. If reconstruction is possible, interposition of tissue between the colorectal anastomosis and closure of the vagina may prevent a postoperative fistula if a pelvic abscess or anastomotic leak occurs. For squamous cell carcinoma of the anus, a preexisting fistula or one that develops during chemoradiation often requires diversion for symptom control. If there is complete resolution of the tumor after chemoradiation, repair of the fistula with interposition of the bulbocavernous or gracilis

muscle is indicated after a waiting period to allow for resolution of any acute radiation changes. It is unlikely that a local repair would be successful. If tumor persists after chemoradiation, an abdominal perineal resection is necessary. Low rates of perineal wound healing in this situation have led to the use of primary muscle flaps for wound closure. Presumably those muscles flaps would be particularly indicated if a rectovaginal fistula exists. The same principles apply when invasion of the rectum by gynecologic malignancy occurs.

Rectovaginal Fistulas Secondary to Radiation Therapy

The evaluation of patients with fistulas secondary to radiation must be more intensive than most other patients with rectovaginal fistulas. Because of their usual age, they are more likely to have significant medical conditions. In addition, it is paramount that the fistula site be biopsied to exclude recurrent cancer. Diversion for a minimum of 6 months is recommended to allow inflammation in the surrounding tissue to resolve. Decisions about surgical intervention center on the patient's overall medical condition, the degree of symptoms caused by the fistula and any associated abnormalities, and the risk of a proposed corrective procedure. Not uncommonly, the combination of those factors makes a colostomy alone the most reasonable choice. This is particularly appropriate if the patient is experiencing significant fecal incontinence. If, however, the patient's condition allows, a variety of surgical options exist. If the fistula is low and the rectum is relatively normal, muscle interposition through the perineum is a reasonable choice. If the fistula is high, tissue interposition through the abdomen is preferable. If a stricture or severe radiation damage exists in the rectum, rectal resection with reconstruction would eliminate that problem and the fistula. However, the morbidity can be high, e.g., 24% in one series.[99] A Bricker procedure is less morbid and can relieve a stricture but does not avoid the potential bleeding, pain, or malignant transformation associated with leaving the rectum in place. Patient selection and operative choice must be made based on clinical experience because comparative studies do not exist.

Iatrogenic Rectovaginal Fistulas

The choice of treatment for an iatrogenic fistula is based on the causative operation. Fistulas developing after rectal resection almost always arise at the anastomosis. They have been reported after both hand-sewn and stapled anastomoses.[100,101] Radiation and prior or concomitant hysterectomy increase the risk of fistula formation. Incorporation of the vaginal wall in the stapler is probably the most common explanation but necessitation of pelvic infection into the vagina may also occur. Obviously, prevention with adequate dissection of the rectum from the vagina before inserting the stapler and careful attention to the separation of the rectum and vagina as the stapler is fired is optimal. Once a fistula occurs, temporary diversion is often necessary to control pelvic sepsis. Some fistulas will close spontaneously although this is less likely if the patient has received pelvic radiation.[102] Repair is determined by the level of the fistula. High fistulas usually require repeat resection with anastomosis or interposition of omentum or muscle. Low fistulas may be amenable to rectal or vaginal advancement flaps. Large fistulas or one failing initial attempts at repair will require tissue interposition.

Persistent Rectovaginal Fistulas

There are few data regarding fistulas that persist after an attempted repair. Repeat repairs after one attempt seem to have a reasonable success rate.[40,50,51] However, several studies report a higher failure rate after two or more procedures so subsequent options should be chosen carefully.[40,51] Two reports specifically address the issue of persistent fistulas. MacRae and colleagues[48] retrospectively reviewed 28 patients who had at least one previous attempt at repair. The etiology was obstetric injury in 14, Crohn's disease in 5, and miscellaneous in 9. Five of the last group had fistulas considered simple; one fistula was caused by radiation. In the 14 patients with a history of obstetric injury, advancement flaps, sphincteroplasty, or coloanal anastomoses were performed. Eleven flaps were performed in nine patients with four resulting in healed fistulas. All five of the patients undergoing sphincteroplasty had successful outcomes as did the two patients undergoing coloanal anastomoses. Overall, 5 of 23 advancement flaps (29%) in 17 patients were successful. Sphincteroplasty succeeded in six of seven patients (86%); four of six coloanal anastomoses (67%) and both of two gracilis muscle interpositions succeeded.

In a report from the Cleveland Clinic, Halverson et al.[69] retrospectively reviewed 35 patients with recurrent rectovaginal fistulas. Causes of the fistulas included obstetric injury in 15, Crohn's disease in 12, pouch vaginal fistulas in 5, cryptoglandular disease in 2, and iatrogenic after low anterior resection in 1. Advancement flap, sphincteroplasty, rectal sleeve advancement, insertion of fibrin glue, and ileal pouch revision were used. The results are presented by etiology and by type of repair but not stratified by both. All 15 obstetric patients were ultimately healed after 23 repairs. Two of the four cryptoglandular fistulas were eradicated. Nine of the 30 mucosal advancement flaps (30%) and 9 of 14 sphincteroplasty procedures (65%) successfully closed the fistulas. Rectal sleeve advancement resulted in healing in two of three fistulas. Crohn's disease, the presence of a diverting stoma, and decreased time interval from a prior repair were associated with a poor outcome regardless of the technique used. The authors commented that the presence of a stoma likely was a marker for more complex disease.

From the data available, it seems that a reasonable approach to recurrent rectovaginal fistulas would begin with a planned waiting period of a minimum of 3 months. In the interval, the status of the sphincter muscle and surrounding tissue should be evaluated. Any areas of sepsis must be drained. For low fistulas, the treatment choice depends on the status of the sphincter and the number of prior repairs. If the sphincter muscle is intact and the patients had undergone only one or perhaps two previous repairs, a repeat advancement flap or rectal sleeve advancement would be appropriate. Insertion of fibrin glue is a safe alternative but there are few data regarding the expected success rate. If there is a defect in the sphincter muscle, sphincteroplasty is the appropriate choice. Conversion to a fourth-degree laceration followed by a layered repair may be chosen by some surgeons. If the muscle is intact and two or more repairs have failed, a tissue interposition technique should be considered. Tissue interposition may also be required for recurrent fistulas with anatomically intact sphincter wraps. The insertion of bulbocavernous muscle is the least morbid transposition method but there are no comparative data regarding outcomes of the various interposition methods. The role of diversion is not established but seems to be primarily control of symptoms except perhaps in patients with Crohn's disease.

Recurrent fistulas involving the middle of the vagina almost always require tissue interposition. The choice depends on the level of the fistula and the body habitus of the patient. The bulbocavernous muscle may not reach if the patient is obese or the fistula is in the upper middle third of the vagina. Gracilis muscle would be a good alternative in those situations. High fistulas require resection or tissue interposition through an abdominal approach.

Conclusion

The literature on rectovaginal fistulas documents a wealth of clinical experience. However, there is a definite lack of uniform terminology, standardized evaluation, and comparative studies. Given the multitude of etiologies and the varying nature of the anatomy and condition of surrounding tissue, improving the quality of research will be challenging. However, continued work is necessary to determine appropriate patient selection and optimal surgical repair.

References

1. Homsi R, Daikoku NH, Littlejohn J, Wheeless CR Jr. Episiotomy: risks of dehiscence and rectovaginal fistula. Obstet Gynecol Surv 1994;49:803–808.
2. Venkatesh KS, Ramanujam PS, Larson DM, Haywood MA. Anorectal complications of vaginal delivery. Dis Colon Rectum 1989;32:1039–1041.
3. Beynon CL. Midline episiotomy as a routine procedure. J Obstet Gynaecol Br Commonw 1974;81:126–130.
4. Margolis T, Elkins TE, Seffah J, Oparo-Addo HS, Fort D. Full-thickness Martius grafts to preserve vaginal depth as an adjunct in the repair of large obstetric fistulas. Obstet Gynecol 1994; 84:148–152.

5. Hamlin C, Turnbull GB. The treatment of rectovaginal and vesicovaginal fistulas in women with childbirth injuries in Ethiopia. J Wound Ostomy Continence Nurs 1997;24:187–189.

6. Schwartz DA, Loftus EV Jr, Tremaine WJ, et al. The natural history of fistulizing Crohn's disease in Olmsted County, Minnesota. Gastroenterology 2002;122:875–880.

7. Radcliffe AG, Ritchie JK, Hawley PR, Lennard-Jones JE, Northover JM. Anovaginal and rectovaginal fistulas in Crohn's disease. Dis Colon Rectum 1988;31:94–99.

8. Nakagoe T, Sawai T, Tuji T, et al. Avoidance of rectovaginal fistula as a complication after low anterior resection for rectal cancer using a double-stapling technique. J Surg Oncol 1999; 71:196–197.

9. Groom JS, Nicholls RJ, Hawley PR, Phillips RK. Pouch-vaginal fistula. Br J Surg 1993;80:936–940.

10. O'Kelly TJ, Merrett M, Mortensen NJ, Dehn TC, Kettlewell M. Pouch-vaginal fistula after restorative proctocolectomy: aetiology and management. Br J Surg 1994;81:1374–1375.

11. Paye F, Penna C, Chiche L, Tiret E, Frileux P, Parc R. Pouch-related fistula following restorative proctocolectomy. Br J Surg 1996;83:1574–1577.

12. Wexner SD, Rothenberger DA, Jensen L, et al. Ileal pouch vaginal fistulas: incidence, etiology, and management. Dis Colon Rectum 1989;32:460–465.

13. Schult M, Wolters HH, Lelle RJ, Winde G, Senninger N. Outcome of surgical intervention for rectoneovaginal fistulas in Mayer-Rokitansky-Kuester-Hauser syndrome. World J Surg 2001;25:438–440.

14. Schwartz J, Rabinowitz H, Rozenfeld V, Leibovitz A, Stelian J, Habot B. Rectovaginal fistula associated with fecal impaction. J Am Geriatr Soc 1992;40:641.

15. Hoffman MS, Wakeley KE, Cardosi RJ. Risks of rigid dilation for a radiated vaginal cuff: two related rectovaginal fistulas. Obstet Gynecol 2003;101:1125–1126.

16. Sharland M, Peake J, Davies EG. Pseudomonal rectovaginal abscesses in HIV infection. Arch Dis Child 1995;72:275.

17. Parra JM, Kellogg ND. Repair of a recto-vaginal fistula as a result of sexual assault. Semin Perioper Nurs 1995;4:140–145.

18. Bird D, Taylor D, Lee P. Vaginography: the investigation of choice for vaginal fistulae? Aust N Z J Surg 1993;63:894–896.

19. Giordano P, Drew PJ, Taylor D, Duthie G, Lee PW, Monson JR. Vaginography: investigation of choice for clinically suspected vaginal fistulas. Dis Colon Rectum 1996;39:568–572.

20. Stoker J, Rociu E, Schouten WR, Lameris JS. Anovaginal and rectovaginal fistulas: endoluminal sonography versus endoluminal MR imaging. AJR Am J Roentgenol 2002;178:737–741.

21. Yee LF, Birnbaum EH, Read TE, Kodner IJ, Fleshman JW. Use of endoanal ultrasound in patients with rectovaginal fistulas. Dis Colon Rectum 1999;42:1057–1064.

22. Sudol-Szopinska I, Jakubowski W, Szczepkowski M. Contrast-enhanced endosonography for the diagnosis of anal and anovaginal fistulas. J Clin Ultrasound 2002;30:145–150.

23. Stewart LK, McGee J, Wilson SR. Transperineal and trans-vaginal sonography of perianal inflammatory disease. AJR Am J Roentgenol 2001;177:627–632.

24. Tsang CB, Madoff RD, Wong WD, et al. Anal sphincter integrity and function influences outcome in rectovaginal fistula repair. Dis Colon Rectum 1998;41:1141–1146.

25. Veronikis DK, Nichols DH, Spino C. The Noble-Mengert-Fish operation-revisited: a composite approach for persistent rectovaginal fistulas and complex perineal defects. Am J Obstet Gynecol 1998;179:1411–1416; discussion 1416–1417.

26. Khanduja KS, Yamashita HJ, Wise WE Jr, Aguilar PS, Hartmann RF. Delayed repair of obstetric injuries of the anorectum and vagina. A stratified surgical approach. Dis Colon Rectum 1994;37:344–349.

27. Allen-Mersh TG, Wilson EJ, Hope-Stone HF, Mann CV. The management of late radiation-induced rectal injury after treatment of carcinoma of the uterus. Surg Gynecol Obstet 1987;164:521–524.

28. van Nagell JR Jr, Parker JC Jr, Maruyama Y, Utley J, Luckett P. Bladder or rectal injury following radiation therapy for cervical cancer. Am J Obstet Gynecol 1974;119:727–732.

29. Daniels B. Rectovaginal Fistula: A Clinical and Pathological Study. Pathology. Minneapolis: University of Minnesota; 1949.

30. Rothenberger DA, Goldberg SM. The management of rectovaginal fistulae. Surg Clin North Am 1983;63:61–79.

31. Saclarides TJ. Rectovaginal fistula. Surg Clin North Am 2002;82:1261–1272.

32. Abel ME, Chiu YS, Russell TR, Volpe PA. Autologous fibrin glue in the treatment of rectovaginal and complex fistulas. Dis Colon Rectum 1993;36:447–449.

33. Buchanan GN, Bartram CI, Phillips RK, et al. Efficacy of fibrin sealant in the management of complex anal fistula: a prospective trial. Dis Colon Rectum 2003;46:1167–1174.

34. Loungnarath R, Dietz DW, Mutch MG, Birnbaum EH, Kodner IJ, Fleshman JW. Fibrin glue treatment of complex anal fistulas has low success rate. Dis Colon Rectum 2004;47:432–436.

35. Venkatesh KS, Ramanujam P. Fibrin glue application in the treatment of recurrent anorectal fistulas. Dis Colon Rectum 1999;42:1136–1139.

36. Greenwald JC, Hoexter B. Repair of rectovaginal fistulas. Surg Gynecol Obstet 1978;146:443–445.

37. Hoexter B, Labow SB, Moseson MD. Transanal rectovaginal fistula repair. Dis Colon Rectum 1985;28:572–575.

38. Hyman N. Endoanal advancement flap repair for complex anorectal fistulas. Am J Surg 1999;178:337–340.

39. Joo JS, Weiss EG, Nogueras JJ, Wexner SD. Endorectal advancement flap in perianal Crohn's disease. Am Surg 1998;64:147–150.

40. Lowry AC, Thorson AG, Rothenberger DA, Goldberg SM. Repair of simple rectovaginal fistulas. Influence of previous repairs. Dis Colon Rectum 1988;31:676–678.

41. Mizrahi N, Wexner SD, Zmora O, et al. Endorectal advancement flap: are there predictors of failure? Dis Colon Rectum 2002;45:1616–1621.

42. Russell TR, Gallagher DM. Low rectovaginal fistulas. Approach and treatment. Am J Surg 1977;134:13–18.

43. Sonoda T, Hull T, Piedmonte MR, Fazio VW. Outcomes of primary repair of anorectal and rectovaginal fistulas using the endorectal advancement flap. Dis Colon Rectum 2002;45: 1622–1628.

44. Wise WE Jr, Aguilar PS, Padmanabhan A, Meesig DM, Arnold MW, Stewart WR. Surgical treatment of low rectovaginal fistulas. Dis Colon Rectum 1991;34:271–274.

45. Zimmerman DD, Gosselink MP, Briel JW, Schouten WR. The outcome of transanal advancement flap repair of rectovaginal fistulas is not improved by an additional labial fat flap transposition. Tech Coloproctol 2002;6:37–42.

46. Baig MK, Zhao RH, Yuen CH, et al. Simple rectovaginal fistulas. Int J Colorectal Dis 2000;15:323–327.

47. Kodner IJ, Mazor A, Shemesh EI, Fry RD, Fleshman JW, Birnbaum EH. Endorectal advancement flap repair of rectovaginal and other complicated anorectal fistulas. Surgery 1993;114:682–689; discussion 689–690.

48. MacRae HM, McLeod RS, Cohen Z, Stern H, Reznick R. Treatment of rectovaginal fistulas that has failed previous repair attempts. Dis Colon Rectum 1995;38:921–925.

49. Mazier WP, Senagore AJ, Schiesel EC. Operative repair of anovaginal and rectovaginal fistulas. Dis Colon Rectum 1995; 38:4–6.

50. Watson SJ, Phillips RK. Non-inflammatory rectovaginal fistula. Br J Surg 1995;82:1641–1643.

51. Ozuner G, Hull TL, Cartmill J, Fazio VW. Long-term analysis of the use of transanal rectal advancement flaps for complicated anorectal/vaginal fistulas. Dis Colon Rectum 1996; 39:10–14.

52. Zimmerman DD, Delemarre JB, Gosselink MP, Hop WC, Briel JW, Schouten WR. Smoking affects the outcome of transanal mucosal advancement flap repair of trans-sphincteric fistulas. Br J Surg 2003;90:351–354.

53. Hibbard LT. Surgical management of rectovaginal fistulas and complete perineal tears. Am J Obstet Gynecol 1978;130:139–141.

54. Lawson J. Rectovaginal fistulae following difficult labour. Proc R Soc Med 1972;65:283–286.

55. Lescher TC, Pratt JH. Vaginal repair of the simple rectovaginal fistula. Surg Gynecol Obstet 1967;124:1317–1321.

56. Tancer ML, Lasser D, Rosenblum N. Rectovaginal fistula or perineal and anal sphincter disruption, or both, after vaginal delivery. Surg Gynecol Obstet 1990;171:43–46.

57. Wiskind AK, Thompson JD. Transverse transperineal repair of rectovaginal fistulas in the lower vagina. Am J Obstet Gynecol 1992;167:694–699.

58. Hesterberg R, Schmidt WU, Muller F, Roher HD. Treatment of anovaginal fistulas with an anocutaneous flap in patients with Crohn's disease. Int J Colorectal Dis 1993;8:51–54.

59. Haray PN, Stiff G, Foster ME. New option for recurrent rectovaginal fistulas. Dis Colon Rectum 1996;39:463–464.

60. Hull TL, Fazio VW. Surgical approaches to low anovaginal fistula in Crohn's disease. Am J Surg 1997;173:95–98.

61. Simmang CL, Lacey SW, Huber PJ Jr. Rectal sleeve advancement: repair of rectovaginal fistula associated with anorectal stricture in Crohn's disease. Dis Colon Rectum 1998; 41:787–789.

62. Mengert WF, Fish SA. Anterior rectal wall advancement: technique for repair of complete perineal laceration and recto-vaginal fistula. Obstet Gynecol 1955;5:262–267.

63. Hilsabeck JR. Transanal advancement of the anterior rectal wall for vaginal fistulas involving the lower rectum. Dis Colon Rectum 1980;23:236–241.

64. Pepe F, Panella M, Arikian S, Panella P, Pepe G. Low rectovaginal fistulas. Aust N Z J Obstet Gynaecol 1987;27:61–63.

65. Hudson CN. Acquired fistulae between the intestine and the vagina. Ann R Coll Surg Engl 1970;46:20–40.

66. Given FT Jr. Rectovaginal fistula. A review of 20 years' experience in a community hospital. Am J Obstet Gynecol 1970;108:41–46.

67. Rahman MS, Al-Suleiman SA, El-Yahia AR, Rahman J. Surgical treatment of rectovaginal fistula of obstetric origin: a review of 15 years' experience in a teaching hospital. J Obstet Gynaecol 2003;23:607–610.

68. Lowry AC, Goldberg SM. Simple rectovaginal fistula. In: Cameron J, ed. Current Surgical Therapy. 4th edition. St. Louis: Mosby; 1991.

69. Halverson AL, Hull TL, Fazio VW, Church J, Hammel J, Floruta C. Repair of recurrent rectovaginal fistulas. Surgery 2001;130:753–757; discussion 757–758.

70. Pinedo G, Phillips R. Labial fat pad grafts (modified Martius graft) in complex perianal fistulas. Ann R Coll Surg Engl 1998;80:410–412.

71. Rius J, Nessim A, Nogueras JJ, Wexner SD. Gracilis transposition in complicated perianal fistula and unhealed perineal wounds in Crohn's disease. Eur J Surg 2000;166:218–222.

72. Shah NS, Remzi F, Massmann A, Baixauli J, Fazio VW. Management and treatment outcome of pouch-vaginal fistulas following restorative proctocolectomy. Dis Colon Rectum 2003;46:911–917.

73. Tran KT, Kuijpers HC, van Nieuwenhoven EJ, van Goor H, Spauwen PH. Transposition of the rectus abdominis muscle for complicated pouch and rectal fistulas. Dis Colon Rectum 1999;42:486–489.

74. White AJ, Buchsbaum HJ, Blythe JG, Lifshitz S. Use of the bulbocavernosus muscle (Martius procedure) for repair of radiation-induced rectovaginal fistulas. Obstet Gynecol 1982; 60:114–118.

75. Zacharin RF. Grafting as a principle in the surgical management of vesicovaginal and rectovaginal fistulae. Aust N Z J Obstet Gynaecol 1980;20:10–17.

76. Byron RL Jr, Ostergard DR. Sartorius muscle interposition for the treatment of the radiation-induced vaginal fistula. Am J Obstet Gynecol 1969;104:104–107.

77. Chitrathara K, Namratha D, Francis V, Gangadharan VP. Spontaneous rectovaginal fistula and repair using bulbocavernosus muscle flap. Tech Coloproctol 2001;5:47–49.

78. Elkins TE, DeLancey JO, McGuire EJ. The use of modified Martius graft as an adjunctive technique in vesicovaginal and rectovaginal fistula repair. Obstet Gynecol 1990;75:727–733.

79. Gorenstein L, Boyd JB, Ross TM. Gracilis muscle repair of rectovaginal fistula after restorative proctocolectomy. Report of two cases. Dis Colon Rectum 1988;31:730–734.

80. Horch RE, Gitsch G, Schultze-Seemann W. Bilateral pedicled myocutaneous vertical rectus abdominus muscle flaps to close vesicovaginal and pouch-vaginal fistulas with simultaneous vaginal and perineal reconstruction in irradiated pelvic wounds. Urology 2002;60:502–507.

81. Kaman L, Singh R, Kaplish B, Virk SS, Patel F. Gracilis repair for a case of radiation induced rectovaginal fistulae. Trop Gastroenterol 1999;20:92–93.

82. Onodera H, Nagayama S, Kohmoto I, Maetani S, Imamura M. Novel surgical repair with bilateral gluteus muscle patching for intractable rectovaginal fistula. Tech Coloproctol 2003;7: 198–202.

83. Aartsen EJ, Sindram IS. Repair of the radiation induced rectovaginal fistulas without or with interposition of the bulbocavernosus muscle (Martius procedure). Eur J Surg Oncol 1988;14:171–177.

84. Boronow RC. Repair of the radiation-induced vaginal fistula utilizing the Martius technique. World J Surg 1986;10:237–248.

85. Parks AG, Allen CL, Frank JD, McPartlin JF. A method of treating post-irradiation rectovaginal fistulas. Br J Surg 1978;65:417–421.

86. Nowacki MP, Szawlowski AW, Borkowski A. Parks' coloanal sleeve anastomosis for treatment of postirradiation rectovaginal fistula. Dis Colon Rectum 1986;29:817–820.

87. Cooke SA, de Moor NG. The surgical treatment of the radiation-damaged rectum. Br J Surg 1981;68:488–492.

88. Bricker EM, Johnston WD. Repair of postirradiation rectovaginal fistula and stricture. Surg Gynecol Obstet 1979;148:499–506.

89. Bricker EM, Kraybill WG, Lopez MJ. Functional results after postirradiation rectal reconstruction. World J Surg 1986;10:249–258.

90. Mattingly R. Anal incontinence and rectovaginal fistulas. In: Mattingly R, ed. TeLindefs Operative Gynecology. Philadelphia: Lippincott; 1977:618–626.

91. Heyen F, Winslet MC, Andrews H, Alexander-Williams J, Keighley MR. Vaginal fistulas in Crohn's disease. Dis Colon Rectum 1989;32:379–383.

92. Present DH, Rutgeerts P, Targan S, et al. Infliximab for the treatment of fistulas in patients with Crohn's disease. N Engl J Med 1999;340:1398–1405.

93. Topstad DR, Panaccione R, Heine JA, Johnson DR, MacLean AR, Buie WD. Combined seton placement, infliximab infusion, and maintenance immunosuppressives improve healing rate in fistulizing anorectal Crohn's disease: a single center experience. Dis Colon Rectum 2003;46:577–583.

94. Ricart E, Sandborn WJ. Infliximab for the treatment of fistulas in patients with Crohn's disease. Gastroenterology 1999;117:1247–1248.

95. Van Assche G, Vanbeckevoort D, Bielen D, et al. Magnetic resonance imaging of the effects of infliximab on perianal fistulizing Crohn's disease. Am J Gastroenterol 2003;98:332–339.

96. Rasul I, Wilson SR, MacRae H, Irwin S, Greenberg GR. Clinical and radiological responses after infliximab treatment for perianal fistulizing Crohn's disease. Am J Gastroenterol 2004;99:82–88.

97. Sher ME, Bauer JJ, Gelernt I. Surgical repair of rectovaginal fistulas in patients with Crohn's disease: transvaginal approach. Dis Colon Rectum 1991;34:641–648.

98. Morrison JG, Gathright JB Jr, Ray JE, Ferrari BT, Hicks TC, Timmcke AE. Results of operation for rectovaginal fistula in Crohn's disease. Dis Colon Rectum 1989;32:497–499.

99. Nowacki MP. Ten years of experience with Parks' coloanal sleeve anastomosis for the treatment of post-irradiation rectovaginal fistula. Eur J Surg Oncol 1991;17:563–566.

100. Rex JC Jr, Khubchandani IT. Rectovaginal fistula: complication of low anterior resection. Dis Colon Rectum 1992;35:354–356.

101. Sugarbaker PH. Rectovaginal fistula following low circular stapled anastomosis in women with rectal cancer. J Surg Oncol 1996;61:155–158.

102. Civelli EM, Gallino G, Valvo F, et al. Correlation between radiotherapy and suture fistulas following colo-anal anastomosis for carcinoma of the rectum evaluation of 152 consecutive patients. Tumori 2002;88:321–324.

15
Pilonidal Disease and Hidradenitis Suppurativa[*]

Jeffery M. Nelson and Richard P. Billingham

Pilonidal Disease

Background and Incidence

"Pilonidal disease" refers to a subcutaneous infection occurring in the upper half of the gluteal cleft. It may present as an acute "pilonidal abscess," or as an indolent wound, resistant to spontaneous healing, and causing drainage and discomfort. It typically presents in the second decade of life, but also occurs in teenagers and in patients in their thirties.[1] It afflicts men more often than women at a ratio of three or four to one, and is more common in individuals with more body hair.[1] It is not known to be more common in any one racial group. During World War II, soldiers filled up whole hospital wards to convalesce from the large excisional operations used at the time to treat pilonidal disease.[2] It became such a problem that the Surgeon General forbade wide local excision as primary therapy, because this treatment had hospitalized 79,000 soldiers for an average hospital stay of 55 days.[3] Akinci et al.[4] reported an 8.8% incidence of pilonidal disease in Turkish Army recruits and found associations with family history, obesity, being a vehicle driver, and having a history of a furuncle at another site on the body. Sondenaa et al.[5] studied 322 patients with pilonidal disease prospectively and calculated the incidence of the disease at 26 per 100,000 persons. It occurred 2.2 times more often in men than in women. He also found the following significant associations: family history in 38%; obesity in 37%; preceding local irritation or trauma in 34%; and a sedentary occupation in 44%. Since World War II, a paradigm shift has occurred in favor of conservative measures, mainly in the form of shaving and hygiene.

Patients typically present initially with pain, redness, and swelling in the midline gluteal cleft region overlying the sacrum and coccyx. Many patients will spontaneously drain their abscesses, which will temporarily relieve the symptoms. This may set up a chronic cycle of drainage and recrudescence of the abscess before the patient eventually seeks medical attention. Thus, some patients may already have a chronic condition at the time of their initial presentation. Patients may also present with a history of having had many different surgical procedures performed in the past for their disease. They may have a persistent wound from a midline excision or a failed flap procedure. Those patients with long-standing disease typically have multiple sinuses that usually extend cephalad from where the midline pits lie. Uncommonly, this process can be quite destructive with large sinus cavities extending out into the lateral gluteal regions.

Pilonidal disease first appeared in the medical literature in 1833 when William Mayo published his first descriptions of this problem.[6] The term "pilonidal," which means "hair nest," however, was first used by Hodges in 1880.[7,8] The term pilonidal "cyst" is a misnomer, because no epithelialized wall exists in the cavities this disease creates. Pilonidal "sinus" or "disease" are the more accurate terms. Pilonidal disease itself, and the surgical and medical treatment related to it, can be a source of disability. This disease disables patients primarily because of pain and its inconvenient location in the gluteal cleft.

Pathogenesis

Empiric data currently support the theory that pilonidal disease is an acquired condition. Pilonidal disease has been observed in the hands of barbers and sheep shearers, implying that shed hairs may initiate the condition.[6] In addition, pilonidal lesions appear to have the pathologic characteristics of a foreign body reaction, presumably from burrowed hair and debris.[1] Pilonidal disease likely results from problems that attack epidermis in the gluteal cleft, rather than from a problem in the deep tissues, or problems with midline skin itself.[3] John Bascom believes that the skin in the natal cleft is perfectly normal, but that conditions that exist there may predispose a patient to pilonidal disease.[3,9] Treatment, therefore, should be directed at changing those conditions. Bascom sur-

---

[*]The opinions or assertions contained herein are the private views of the authors and are not to be construed as official or as reflecting the views of the Department of the Army or the Department of Defense.

mises that the natal cleft is probably a hypoxic environment, and cites as empiric evidence the fact that anaerobic bacteria can be cultured from pilonidal wounds and abscesses.[3,10] However, no experiments have directly shown that the natal cleft is hypoxic at all, or even to what degree it may be hypoxic. In addition, Bascom theorizes that vacuum forces and negative suction in the natal cleft draws hair and debris into the midline pits, which are stretched and ruptured hair follicles, resulting in obstruction.[6] These stretched follicles, he believes, stretch and eventually rupture into the subcutaneous tissue, causing the classic pilonidal abscess.[10] The midline "pits" communicate with chronic abscesses containing trapped hair and debris via sinus tracts. If these sinus tracts become epithelialized, excision is the only option for cure. Presently, the ideas of Bascom and others about the pathogenesis of pilonidal disease are based on empiric evidence. No published experiments exist that directly prove or refute the current theories about how pilonidal disease occurs.

Initial Presentations: Pilonidal Abscess

The presenting symptoms for many patients include pain, swelling, and erythema near the top of the natal cleft, with or without spontaneous drainage. A few definitions at this point are in order. An *acute pilonidal abscess* is no different from an acute abscess in any other location on the body. It requires incision and drainage before considering any other definitive therapy. A *chronic abscess* is really an established pilonidal sinus cavity, which chronically drains and fails to heal because of retained hair and foreign material. A *recurrent abscess* is an acute abscess, which occurs after apparent complete healing of pilonidal disease in the past. Excision in a patient in the presence of acute inflammation and swelling is ill advised. Many times the midline pits will not be visible until after the inflammation subsides. Abscesses should be drained with an incision parallel to the midline and at least 1 cm lateral to it (if possible) to facilitate healing of the wound (Figure 15-1). It is prudent to remove a small ellipse of skin from the wound to prevent the skin edges from sealing and reforming the abscess. Packing of such wounds serves no good purpose, is painful, and potentially interferes with drainage and healing. Antibiotics are only necessary in the patient with significant cellulitis. Simply cover the wound with a dressing and have the patient do sitz baths or use a hand-held shower 2–3 times a day. The patient should return to the office every week or two until the wound heals. Any hair that has grown back within 2 inches of the entire gluteal cleft is shaved at each visit (Figure 15-2).

Initial Presentation: Draining Pilonidal Chronic Abscess

Pilonidal disease has been treated in many different ways, but no treatment has proved completely satisfactory. The ideal treatment would at least meet the following criteria: ease of

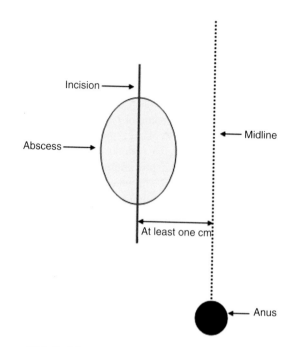

FIGURE 15-1. Incision placement for acute pilonidal abscess.

performance; short or no hospitalization; low recurrence rate; minimal pain and wound care; fast return to normal activity; and cost effectiveness. No current treatment meets all these criteria.

Nonsurgical Approach

Shaving

For the initial treatment of chronic disease (which can be a chronic sinus that has never been treated or any persistent disease that has failed to heal despite treatment), shaving alone has been advocated as the sole alternative treatment for pilonidal disease. In 1994, Armstrong and Barcia[9] tested the hypothesis that wide, meticulous shaving was equal or superior to surgical therapy of any kind. They performed a pilot

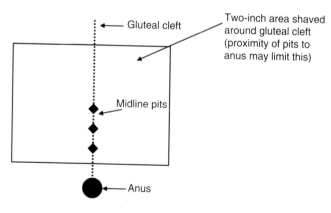

FIGURE 15-2. Shaving technique.

nonrandomized cohort study, which also included a follow-up retrospective study, which remains one of the largest studies to date looking at any aspect of pilonidal disease. One group of patients was treated with weekly strip shaving (5 cm circumferentially around the entire gluteal cleft) until healing occurred and the other with surgery (midline excision with or without marsupialization, closure or partial closure, and open packing; rotational flaps; Z-plasty; and skin grafting). The article does not clarify if the patients treated with surgery received one or more of these procedures. They then followed the patients for 3 years, comparing the groups as to the number of occupied bed days and number of operations needed. They found a highly statistically significant difference in favor of the group that received only shaving. This study received criticism for several reasons. First, they did not control for the type of surgery the nonconservative group received, or for the severity of disease. They also did not look at healing or recurrence rates. One might surmise that even though the conservatively treated patients were not occupying hospital beds, they still could have been suffering for long periods from their disease. They may have also sought treatment elsewhere. Despite these limitations, this study provides evidence that conservative nonsurgical treatment, when applied with a dedicated effort, can work. Physicians should consider shaving as the initial therapy in all patients without an acute or chronic abscess and localized disease. However, no one knows how long one should continue shaving in order to prevent recurrence. Currently, we recommend shaving until complete healing has occurred. Recently, several authors have described laser hair removal as an alternative to shaving.[11–13]

Surgical Approaches

Midline Excision

The most frequently performed operation for pilonidal disease is midline excision, with or without primary closure of the wound, because most chronic or recurrent disease presents while localized to the midline. In this procedure, only the clearly abnormal tissue in the midline is excised. It is not necessary to always excise down to presacral fascia. Surprisingly, the literature contains only four randomized, prospective studies comparing open excision to excision and primary closure. In 1985, Kronborg et al.[14] randomized 88 patients to one of three treatment groups: excision, leaving the wound open; excision and wound closure; and excision and closure with postoperative clindamycin coverage. This article is important because it was the first to look at the utility of using antibiotics after pilonidal excision. The authors then looked at recurrence and healing rates. They followed each patient for 3 years. Healing rates among each of the primary closure groups were not statistically significant, and there was no benefit shown from the addition of clindamycin (14 versus 11 days, $P > .10$). Healing took a substantially longer amount of time in the open group compared with the primary closure

groups (64 versus 15 days, $P > .001$). Recurrence rates were not significant in any of the groups ($P > .40$); however, there was a tendency toward more recurrences in the primary closure group (7 versus 0 at 3 months and 7 versus 4 at 3 years).

Fuzun et al.[15] randomized 91 patients to either excision without closure or excision with primary closure. The authors then followed the patients for a minimum of 4 months. They primarily looked at infection and recurrence rates. In the two patients who experienced infection in the closed group, this was treated with simple suture removal and healing by secondary intent without the need for further hospitalization. They used no antibiotics. Patients whose wounds were left open had a lower infection rate (1.8% versus 3.6%, $P < .01$) and no instances of recurrence, whereas the recurrence rate for those undergoing wound closure was 4.4% ($P < .01$). They did not specify the duration of healing for either group. The only patients that had delayed healing were those few patients who developed a wound infection. Despite the statistically significant differences in favor of open excision, the authors concluded that either method is acceptable.

Sondenaa et al.[16] randomized 153 patients to midline excision and primary closure with or without cefoxitin prophylaxis. After following the patients for 4 weeks, they found no differences in healing or recurrence. Based on these data, the authors did not recommend cefoxitin prophylaxis. In a follow-up article a year later, the same authors published the results of a study that randomized 120 patients to either open excision or excision with primary closure.[17] They followed the patients for a median of 4.2 years. The authors detected no significant difference between the groups, and concluded that either method was acceptable.

Based on the results of these studies, no clear benefit exists for the use of primary closure after midline excision. Proponents of primary closure cite the accelerated healing rate in patients in whom this approach is successful. However, this comes with the price of a significantly increased chance of more wound infections.

Unroofing and Secondary Healing

Midline excision without primary closure leaves a large wound, which is associated with long healing times. If wound closure is not indicated (i.e., with an associated abscess), a smaller wound with much shorter healing times can be achieved with unroofing or laying open of the pilonidal sinus (Figure 15-3A). Open wounds require dressing changes and wound care, but unroofing is associated with half the healing time of wide and deep excision.[18,19] The recurrence rate is less than 13% with this technique.

Bascom's Chronic Abscess Curettage and Midline Pit Excision (Bascom I)

Bascom bases this procedure on the premise that efforts to help patients with pilonidal disease should be directed at changing the gluteal cleft conditions rather than excising a

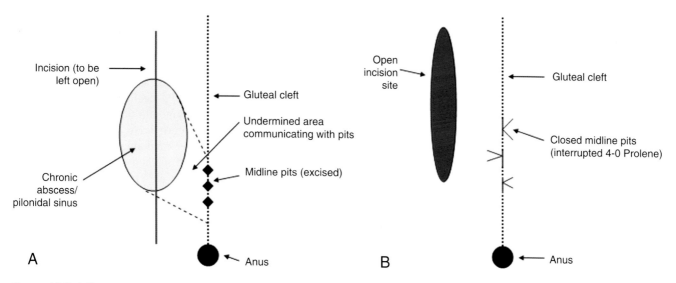

FIGURE 15-3. **A** Bascom procedure. Lateral incision and debridement of cavity. **B** Bascom procedure. Removal of a midline pits with small incisions after lateral debridement, and closure of midline wounds without closure of the lateral incision.

large amount of normal tissue associated with the diseased areas. In patients who present initially with a chronic abscess, this procedure has given excellent results. He does this by making a generous, vertically oriented incision through the site of the abscess cavity more than 1 cm off the midline (in some cases more than one chronic abscess is present) and then curetting it out, without excising the fibrous abscess wall. The connecting tracts to the midline pits are also identified and the overlying skin undermined so that they drain to the site of the incision. The midline pits are then excised using a small diamond-shaped incision to circumferentially remove each of them.[3,10] According to Bascom,[10] the excised pit should be about the size of a grain of rice. The undermined flap of skin, between the incision and drainage site and the excised midline pits, is then tacked down, and the pit excision sites are closed with either subcuticular or vertical mattress, nonabsorbable suture (4-0 or 3-0) (Figure 15-3B). Once this has been accomplished, meticulous shaving of the gluteal cleft should continue at least once a week until the wound has healed. Shaving can be done in the physician's office, or at home by a family member or friend who has been given the proper instruction.

Senapati et al.[20] published a prospective series of 218 patients treated with Bascom's operation described above. The patients had a mean age of 27 years, and a mean duration of symptoms of 2.4 years. The mean duration of follow-up was 12.1 months (range, 1–60). Follow-up consisted of phone calls, office visits, and mailed questionnaires. All but one patient healed his or her pit excision sites. The lateral wound in one patient failed to heal and required further excision. All the other wounds healed after a mean of 4 weeks (range, 1–15 weeks). Four percent of patients experienced bleeding that required either external pressure or cautery to stop. Eight percent of patients reformed their abscesses when the lateral skin

wound healed before the underlying cavity completely healed. This required reopening the lateral wound. Ninety percent of patients healed completely with only 21 patients (10%) ultimately requiring further surgery for recurrent pilonidal disease. Given the overall good results and the fact that patients who failed to heal or recurred were not any worse off than when they initially presented, they recommended the use of this technique. To date, no trials compare Bascom's procedure with another approach to chronic abscess.

Treatment: Recurrent Disease and Severe Disease

Controversy exists over how to treat and follow patients who heal, but continue to present with multiply recurrent disease despite attempts at limited surgery and the other conservative measures discussed above. In addition to midline excision, the surgical options often used today, after initial shaving and hygiene methods have failed, include rhomboid flaps, Z-plasty (Figure 15-5), the Karydakis procedure, Bascom's cleft lift procedure, V-Y plasty, gluteus maximus myocutaneous flaps, and skin grafting (Table 15-1). Some level-one evidence exists regarding flap-based or asymmetric closures off the midline

TABLE 15-1. Complex Pilonidol Procedure Results

Procedure	% Healing (mean)	% Complications (mean)	% Recurrence (mean)
Rhomboid flap[21,22]	100	13.5	4.9
Karydakis[24]	—	8.5	1
Bascom cleft lift[3]	100	—	0
V-Y plasty[25]	100	8	0
Z-plasty[26]	100	—	0
Myocutaneous flap[287]	100	100	0
Skin graft[29]	96.6	—	1.7

for pilonidal disease, but most data come from patient series reports. The major disadvantages with flaps are longer operative times, greater blood loss, potential flap loss, and infection. However, these flaps do offer a quicker time to healing than midline excision, with no increase in infection rate.

Rhomboid Flap

The rhomboid, or Limberg flap, is a cutaneous rotational flap used to fill soft tissue defects and is ideally suited for this purpose with regard to pilonidal disease (Figure 15-4A–D). One large recent prospective series used the rhomboid flap on 102 patients regardless of the severity of their disease.[21] All of the patients healed eventually, but they did not specify a time frame. They reported a 6% complication rate consisting of three seromas, two partial wound dehiscences, and one wound infection. The recurrence rate was 4.9%. The authors also used the rhomboid flap to treat recurrences. Patients returned to normal activity by 7 days, on average. Although this study is not level-one evidence, it does show us that the majority of patients treated with this method generally do

well in the short term. Abu Galala et al.[22] randomized 46 patients with chronic sinuses to either the rhomboid flap, or to midline excision with primary closure, and followed them for healing and recurrence. Patients with acute abscesses or recurrent sinuses were excluded. All of the rhomboid flap patients healed versus only 77% healing in the midline closure group ($P > .02$). After 18 months of follow-up, 9% of the midline suture group had recurred. No one in the rhomboid flap group recurred. Another randomized, prospective trial regarding the rhomboid flap method evaluated the use of drains after surgery. Erdem et al.[23] randomized 40 patients and used a drain in half of them. The study found no difference in wound healing or recurrence ($P > .05$). The drain group, however, had a longer hospital stay ($P < .001$).

Despite the overall good results with use of the rhomboid flap for recalcitrant pilonidal disease, this technique necessitates excision of a large amount of normal tissue and subsequently creates a large scar at the flap site (Figure 15-4D). Also, many patients with chronic abscesses have their abscesses located so lateral and cephalad to the midline area containing the pits, that it makes the use of this technique

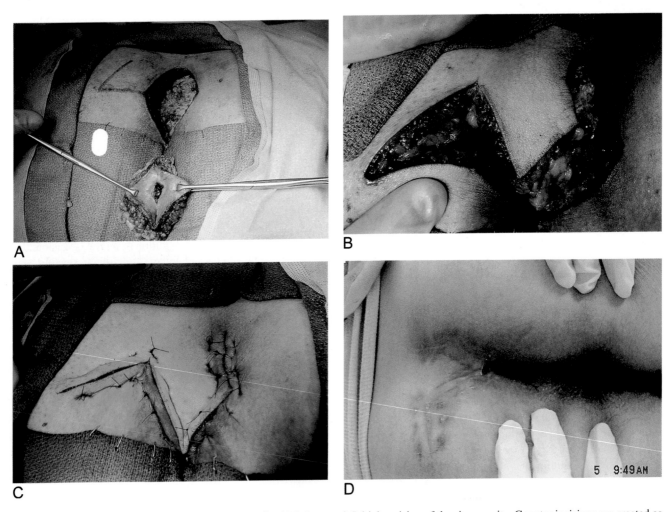

FIGURE 15-4. Rhomboid flap technique for recurrent pilonidal disease. **A** Initial excision of the sinus cavity. Counter incisions are created as shown. **B** Flaps are raised and maneuvered as shown to close defect. **C** Final surgical result. **D** Result at 1 month postoperatively.

more morbid because of the size of the flap required to cover the excised area. With disease localized more or less to the midline, however, any abscess cavities and all the pits are easily excised. In addition, this technique works particularly well for flap coverage of chronic wounds (as a result of midline excisions) in the gluteal cleft that have failed to heal over a prolonged period of time.

Karydakis Flap

The Karydakis operation has been used by Dr. Karydakis in Athens, Greece since 1965. The two goals of this procedure are: 1) to eccentrically excise "vulnerable" tissue in the midline, or laterally displace it; and 2) to laterally displace the surgical wound out of the midline gluteal cleft. An elliptical incision is made parallel to the midline at a distance at least 1 cm from the midline. Skin and gluteal fat are then excised down to the sacral fascia eccentrically (Figure 15-5). By necessity, some normal tissue needs to be excised to create a flap. This flap is then sutured down to the sacral fascia. The closed incision should be entirely lateral to the cleft.

In 1992 Karydakis reported the results of this approach in 7471 patients over a period of 24 years from 1966 to 1990, which is one of the largest series in the surgical literature.[24] Follow-up ranged from 2 to 20 years, and was possible in 95% of cases. He reported a recurrence rate of 1% in the first 6545 cases, finding that new disease occurred from new midline pits. The overall complication rate was 8.5%, mainly from infections and fluid collections. Antibiotics were not routinely used, but a drain was always placed at the upper end of the wound for 2–3 days.

The large numbers of patients that have received this operation along with the good reported results make this an attractive option to consider. However, no one else has ever studied this or reported their results, nor are there any comparative trials.

Bascom Cleft Lift (Bascom II)

Bascom developed this procedure, which may be the most technically challenging of all the techniques dealing with multiply recurrent and severe pilonidal disease. It also may prove to be the most revolutionary technique to come along since the Karydakis procedure. The key difference between the cleft lift procedure and other flap-based procedures is that the cleft lift procedure excises no normal subcutaneous tissue. As described above, the Karydakis procedure does excise normal fat to create the flap. The only tissue excised during the cleft lift is a portion of skin. The goal of the cleft lift procedure is to undermine and completely obliterate the gluteal cleft in the diseased area. This procedure detaches the skin of the gluteal cleft from the underlying subcutaneous tissue as a flap. A portion of this flap containing the diseased skin is then excised from the side of the buttocks to which the flap will be sutured (Figure 15-6A). When the flap is pulled across the midline, the gluteal subcutaneous tissue is approximated underneath the flap, thus obliterating the gluteal cleft. Any open chronic wounds or sinus cavities are simply curetted out, but not excised. The raised skin flaps cover these prior wound sites in addition to coapting the normal gluteal fat. The final suture line lies parallel to, but well away from, the midline, and is free from tension (Figure 15-6B). Bascom[3] studied 28 consecutive patients with recurrent, festering wounds who

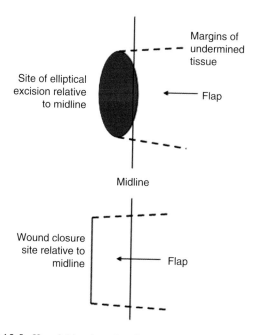

FIGURE 15-5. Karydakis advancing flap operation.

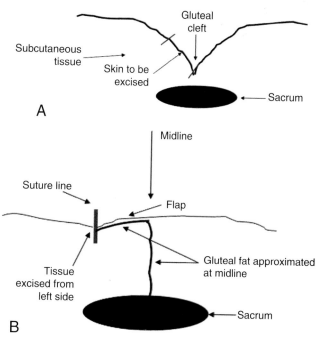

FIGURE 15-6. **A** Cleft-lift technique as described by Bascom for non-healing midline wounds. **B** Final result after flaps are raised and underlying gluteal fat is approximated.

received this treatment. Twenty-two patients healed their wounds immediately and had their sutures removed at 1 week. Six patients took longer to heal because of small wound separations. Three patients required operative revision to achieve healing. Finally, one obese patient took 13 months to heal. The median follow-up was 20 months (range, 1 month to 15 years) and all patients remained healed. This procedure has enjoyed spectacular results in Dr. Bascom's hands, but it awaits duplication elsewhere.

V-Y Plasty

Schoeller et al.[25] retrospectively investigated the use of the V-Y advancement flap in 24 patients with a mean follow-up of 4.5 years. They reported two wound dehiscences, but achieved healing in all cases. They noted no recurrences. Overall, they found the method to be satisfactory, but demanding, and recommended a simpler approach. However, it may have applicability in some situations in which other flaps have failed, such as the rhomboid flap.

Z-plasty

Hodgson and Greenstein[26] published the only other randomized, prospective study on flap closure for pilonidal disease in 1981. This study looked at Z-plasty versus midline excision with or without marsupialization. The Z-plasty group required no further surgery, but 40% of the open excision group did go on to have repeat operations. This study gives us the best available evidence that even open excision, although not prone to wound breakdown, does not completely rectify a patient's wound issues, at least in the short term.

Petersen et al.[27] reviewed these asymmetric closure techniques, which utilize cutaneous flaps, examining the results of 74 articles published in the last 35 years. Wound infections occurred in up to 38.5% of all patients undergoing any surgery for pilonidal disease. However, they found no consistent trend that all flap procedures had significantly lower infection rates than midline excision. Similarly, wound failure occurred in up to 52.4% of all patients. No individual technique showed consistently better results in this regard, compared with all flap procedures as a group. Pilonidal recurrence proved to be the only area in which the flap techniques showed a consistent advantage. Recurrence occurred in up to 26.8% of all the patients. The midline pits recurred less often in the asymmetric closure/flap group compared with midline excision. Overall, they concluded that asymmetric closures and flap techniques were superior to midline excision despite the limitations of the study. Also, they recommended that an asymmetric closure, such as the Karydakis, be considered initially before using the rotational flap procedures, because these may be unnecessarily complex.[27]

Myocutaneous Flaps

Larger areas of disease with large, deep wounds may require myocutaneous flaps. Rosen and Davidson[28] treated five patients with severe disease with gluteus myocutaneous flaps.

They were all young males and had received an average of six previous procedures. All patients healed with an average follow-up of 40 months and 13 hospital days. Most surgeons reserve this technique for the most severe cases, usually after failure of simpler techniques.

Skin Grafting

No study looking at skin grafting for pilonidal disease has been published since 1983 when Guyuron et al.[29] published their retrospective study of 58 patients so treated. Seventy-two percent of these patients initially presented to the authors' institution with recurrent disease. The patients all underwent excision of their pilonidal disease with split-thickness skin grafting. They noted a 1.7% recurrence rate and a 3.4% graft failure rate. The authors recommended use of this method for recurrent or extensive pilonidal disease.

Summary

The algorithm in Figure 15-7 delineates an approach to pilonidal disease based on the evidence presented in this section. Conservative treatment ought to form the cornerstone of therapy—specifically, wide, meticulous shaving and hygiene. The best evidence available suggests that shaving should be done until healing is complete, either in patients treated primarily this way, or those treated with surgery. When patients present initially with simple midline pits, sinuses, and various symptoms, such as pain and occasional drainage, but no acute abscess, shaving can again be offered as the initial treatment. A patient who presents with an acute pilonidal abscess should have incision and drainage, ideally making the incision lateral to the midline whenever possible. At the same time, one should do a 2-inch strip shave circumferentially around the affected area. Anyone familiar with the procedure (doctor, medical assistant, significant other, etc.) repeats the shaving

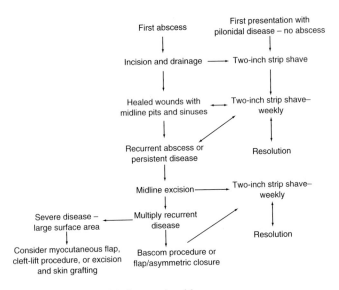

FIGURE 15-7. Pilonidal disease algorithm.

weekly. Continue dressing changes and sitz baths without packing until the wound has healed. If this is the initial presentation of the patient's pilonidal disease, then simply continue shaving. This shaving must be meticulous and ritualistic to be successful. One single hair protruding from a midline pit will keep it open. The majority of patients do not recur after conservative treatment consisting of incision and drainage and shaving. For these reasons, we do not recommend continued shaving once healing is complete.

Patients who present with multiply recurrent pilonidal disease, meaning disease occurring sometime after healing of prior episodes (i.e., abscesses, new pits) are more challenging. The usual case is the patient with a chronic abscess that persists despite shaving and other conservative measures. Continued shaving in this situation is unlikely to succeed, because the abscess cavity and the epithelialized tracts connecting it to the midline pits will contain a great deal of burrowed hair. In this case, we prefer to move on to the Bascom chronic abscess curettage and midline pit excision, or a cutaneous flap procedure. For the initial management of the chronic abscess, virtually all cases can be done as an outpatient in the operating room under local anesthesia with conscious sedation. Sungurtekin et al.[30] found no benefit to the use of spinal anesthesia over local anesthesia in the outpatient surgical treatment of pilonidal disease. They randomized 60 patients receiving the rhomboid flap operation to either spinal anesthesia or local anesthesia. The local group also received intravenous midazolam for sedation. They found no differences regarding patient satisfaction, side effects, or pain scores. However, two spinal patients suffered urinary retention. In addition, both the amount of time spent recovering before discharge, and the total cost of the spinal anesthetic patients' care were significantly higher ($P < .05$).

Neither antibiotics nor drains have been shown to be helpful on a routine basis. However, when taking on complex flap procedures or skin grafts, antibiotics may be used perioperatively based on evidence from other arenas of surgery proving their benefit. The evidence presented here also shows that more complications and recurrences occur with midline excision and primary closure than with open excision alone. However, time to healing is greater with open excision. Despite the good results reported with the flaps and asymmetric closures for pilonidal disease, midline excision or unroofing does seem to work most of the time, and has the advantage of simplicity. Cutaneous rotational flaps and asymmetric closures may best be reserved for the patient with a laterally located chronic abscess, multiply recurrent disease, a large area of involvement, or a nonhealing wound.

In response to the question, "Which procedure should be tried first for the new pilonidal patient?" the answer is, "It depends." If the patient presents with a draining sinus, alternately known as a chronic abscess, the surgeon first needs to note the location of the sinus relative to the midline. In the case in which all the disease, sinuses, and pits are located near and in the midline, then a conservative midline excision is a reasonable first-line treatment. A Bascom procedure for a chronic abscess/sinus is also reasonable. Many times, however, multiple draining sinuses exist and can be located far enough away from the midline that a simple midline excision becomes impractical because of the larger wound created. In this case, we typically make a choice between a Bascom I and a rhomboid flap. For patients who have failed midline excisions, a rhomboid flap or a Bascom I are our procedures of choice for the patient whose disease is easily encompassed within the rhomboid excision specimen. If this is not the case, then another Bascom I is again a good option for this type of presentation, primarily because it is nonexcisional in nature (except for the midline pits). As always, shaving should continue with the proper vigilance until healing is complete. For a small, chronic nonhealing wound from a prior operation for pilonidal disease, a rotational flap is ideal. We prefer the rhomboid flap for this purpose. For extensive recurrence in the midline with abscesses and multiple nonhealing wounds, the Bascom II procedure has shown great promise.

Hidradenitis Suppurativa

Background

Hidradenitis suppurativa is a cutaneous condition that involves skin containing apocrine sweat glands. Areas of the body where this often occurs include the perineum, the axilla, and the groin. It presents initially as an abscess, but is typically multiply recurrent in the affected area and ultimately can lead to severe scarring and disability for the patient. This section will focus on disease that presents perianally. Velpeau first described this entity in 1839 as an inflammatory process causing superficial skin abscesses affecting the axillary, mammary, and perineal regions. It was not until 1854, however, that Verneuil ascribed this process specifically to sweat glands. Verneuil also named the disease "hidradenitis suppurativa," although it has also been called Verneuil's disease, as well as "the follicular occlusion triad," "acne inverse," and "acne vulgaris." Schieffendecker classified sweat glands as eccrine or apocrine in 1922. He then localized hidradenitis suppurativa to the apocrine glands of the perineal, mammary, axillary, inguinal, and umbilical areas.[31] Finally, Lane in 1933 and Brunsting in 1939, defined the histology of this disorder and implicated luminal obstruction of the apocrine sweat glands as the inciting event.[32,33]

Incidence and Etiology

The exact incidence of hidradenitis suppurativa in general is unknown. However, one in every 300 individuals may be affected in some way.[32] African-Americans seem to be affected more often than Caucasians, and perianal disease seems to be more common in males.[31,32] Almost all patients present after puberty and before the age of 40, implicating hormones and the development of secondary sexual characteristics as causative.[32] Other endocrine associations include diabetes mellitus, hypercholesterolemia, and Cushing's disease. It can theoretically occur in any skin that contains apocrine glands, but the most common locations are axillary and inguinal-perineal. Obesity has been implicated as a predisposing factor presumably from shearing forces in the affected areas.[32] In a series from the Lahey clinic, 70% of affected patients were smokers, but no causal relationship could be shown.[32] Perianal hidradenitis affects males twice as often as females, but hidradenitis in all locations may be more common in females and African-American persons.[32] Fortunately for sufferers of perianal hidradenitis, it seems to recur less often after surgical treatment (<0.5%) than does inguinal-perineal disease (37%–74%).[31,33]

Bacteriology

Wound cultures from hidradenitis patients have grown *Staphylococcus epidermidis*, *Escherichia coli*, *Klebsiella*, *Proteus*, alpha *Streptococcus*, anaerobic bacteria, and diptheroids, although negative cultures are common. Lapins et al.[34] showed that *S. epidermidis* was the most frequently cultured bacteria from deep portions of hidradenitis suppurativa lesions in 25 patients. *Chlamydia trachomatis*, often associated with lymphogranuloma venereum, and *Bilophila wadsworthia* infection have also been implicated, but the clinical significance is not known.[31,32]

Pathogenesis

Most authors agree that hidradenitis suppurativa originates from obstruction of apocrine sweat glands by keratin. However, it is unknown why this occurs in some people and not in others (females, African-Americans, etc). Attanoos et al.[35] examined 118 pathologic hidradenitis specimens and found some degree of keratin plugging in all cases along with an active deep folliculitis. They concluded that plugging of the hair follicle itself led to apocrine inflammation making the actual apocrine gland destruction of hidradenitis suppurativa a secondary process. These glands secrete a milky, odorless fluid that only becomes malodorous after it interacts with bacteria on the skin. The apocrine glands secrete into the hair follicle as opposed to directly onto the skin like eccrine sweat glands. The function of apocrine secretion is unknown. Nevertheless, obstruction leads to secondary bacterial infection and rupture of the gland into the dermis and subcutaneous tissue, thus causing cellulitis, abscess, and draining sinuses. This process then leads to the characteristic "pit-like" scars from chronic fibrosis of the destroyed glandular unit. With time, this disease can become not only disfiguring, but debilitating. Microscopically, the pathognomonic serpentine epithelialized sinus tracks with giant cells and granulomas are typically seen.[31,32,36,37]

Differential Diagnosis

Differentiating hidradenitis suppurativa from other inflammatory conditions of the perianal region can be difficult, and many of them may coexist. Cutaneous infections such as furuncles, carbuncles, lymphogranuloma venereum, erysipelas, epidermoid or dermoid cysts, and tuberculosis can be particularly troublesome. In particular, it must be distinguished from other fistulizing or sinus-forming processes of the perineum. Crohn's disease typically affects the anus and rectum with fistulas arising from the dentate line or higher in the rectum. Ordinary perianal abscesses and fistulas of cryptoglandular origin will arise from the dentate line and traverse the sphincter mechanism. In contrast, hidradenitis does not affect the rectum, because apocrine glands only exist in the lower two-thirds of the anal canal and do not penetrate into the sphincter complex. Thus, patients will not have sinus or fistula tracks to or from the rectum.[31,32] If fistulas are present, then the surgeon should perform anoscopy to rule out the possibility of fistula-in-ano from a cryptoglandular source. Fistulas from hidradenitis should only connect areas of involved skin, and not penetrate the anal sphincters. If they do, then another, or concomitant, diagnosis should be entertained. Several case reports have been published describing the association of Crohn's disease and hidradenitis, but no definitive link between the two conditions has ever been proven.[38–42] Nonspecific granulomas (required for a pathologic diagnosis of Crohn's disease) are seen in pathologic specimens in both diseases and may be confused with one another.

Several cases of squamous cell carcinoma in chronic hidradenitis wounds have also been published.[43–46] A retrospective review of a Swedish database of hospital discharge diagnoses from 1965 to 1997 revealed a 50% increased risk of developing *any* cancer in patients with hidradenitis suppurativa over the general population. Specifically, the authors observed significant increases for nonmelanoma skin cancers, buccal cancer, and primary liver cancer.[47] The association seems to be rare with affected patients, who usually have had untreated disease for longer than 20 years. One report found a 3.2% incidence in 125 patients with perianal hidradenitis lasting 20–30 years.[46] One should at least keep a high index of suspicion for this entity in patients with long-standing disease and extensive scarring in the affected areas.

Treatment: Initial

Hidradenitis suppurativa typically presents with pain, erythema, and swelling in the affected area. Patients with cellulitis and no definable clinical abscess may be successfully treated with antibiotics that cover skin flora, such as staphylococcus species, over 1–2 weeks. The safest course of action with any patient who presents with an obvious abscess is incision and drainage. No evidence exists supporting the use of prophylactic antibiotics beyond the initial treatment course. Jemec and Wendelboe[48] conducted the only double-blinded randomized, prospective study looking at antibiotic use for hidradenitis suppurativa (or any other aspect of this disease). They evaluated 46 patients with mild hidradenitis (not more than 10 lesions; no extensive sinus tracts) after 3 months of therapy with either systemic tetracycline or topical clindamycin. The patients also received a placebo of the other agent. Patients selected for the study did not undergo incision and drainage. The authors found no benefit of topical clindamycin versus systemic tetracycline for treatment of acute disease. The study did not include a control arm, which received no antibiotics, so we cannot conclude that these topical antibiotics provide no benefit or some benefit versus no topical antibiotic treatment at all.

Sadly, 83% of patients will have recurrent localized sepsis of some sort after initial incision and drainage or limited excision. Our preference is to leave the wounds open to heal by secondary intent, after excising the involved area. Pathologic examination may show apocrine involvement providing histologic confirmation of hidradenitis.[31]

Treatment: Chronic

Chronic disease is simply any hidradenitis disease persisting or recurring after initial treatment. This could present as recurrent abscesses, nodules, sinuses, fistulas, cellulitis, or any combination of these problems. Unroofing of all sinus tracts is a simple method that may control the hidradenitis, but disease remains, by definition, and recurrence is highly likely for this reason. More specifically, unroofing of abscesses does not control the underlying problem in patients who get hidradenitis. It is a problem with the apocrine glands located in susceptible perianal skin. Unless the surgeon excises all this skin, the patient will technically be at risk for recurrence, although not every patient eventually goes on to radical excision.

Excision with healing by secondary intention is probably the most widely used surgical treatment. The literature reports various recurrence rates after removal of a portion, or all, of the apocrine gland bearing skin. Only the grossly involved apocrine bearing skin (but all of it) in the perianal area should be excised full thickness into the uninvolved gluteal fat. No evidence exists supporting any need for a wide excisional margin, however. This method is simple and almost never requires fecal diversion. It also allows completion of the procedure as an outpatient. Perioperative antibiotics are unnecessary. Patients with large areas of involvement may undergo staged excision. The extent of excision should remain outside the anal verge as long as there is no obvious involvement or history of involvement in the anal canal. If excision is necessary near the anal canal, because of extensive involvement at the anal verge, it should be limited, or staged, in order to prevent a stricture. The major disadvantage of this method is that the wounds take 1 month or much longer to heal, and they require daily wound care. The disability associated with this treatment, however, is minimal. With either of the methods mentioned above, the patient should do sitz baths, or use a

handheld shower, at least twice daily along with dressing changes.

Recently, reports on the use of negative pressure dressings have appeared as a way to promote healing and shorten the time to wound closure.[49] The purported benefits of these dressings, which have never been validated, include increased wound oxygen tension, decreased bacterial counts, better control of fluid produced by the wound, increased granulation tissue formation, and decreased shear forces. Negative pressure dressings have been used successfully on open wounds and on skin grafts.[49,50] However, the expense and mechanical difficulties inherent with all dressings placed in the perianal area are rarely justified. These dressings require an air-tight seal at all times, which is difficult to achieve near the anal verge.

Patients with chronic disease, extensive scarring, and sinus tracts rarely respond to conservative measures. The gold standard of care remains wide excision of all skin bearing involved apocrine glands. Reconstruction then can follow a number of paths—unroofing of sinus tracts with or without marsupialization, cutaneous flap closure, myocutaneous flap closure, or excision and simple healing by secondary intent. Cutaneous or myocutaneous flaps are typically taken from the posterior thigh, gluteus muscle, or lumbosacral region. They are analogous to those used for pilonidal disease. Flaps are almost never necessary, however. Which of these options to choose, however, depends on the extent of involvement around the anus and the severity of disease. Patients who might benefit from diversion are those who cannot take care of their wounds long term and those who have both hidradenitis and Crohn's disease, although this is rarely needed.[32,51]

Summary

The algorithm in Figure 15-8 depicts our suggested approach to treating patients with perianal hidradenitis suppurativa. Patients who present initially with an acute abscess, and a

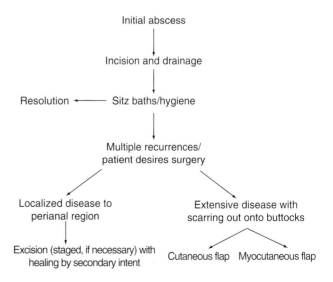

FIGURE 15-8. Perianal hidradenitis suppurativa algorithm.

history and examination consistent with hidradenitis, should have incision and drainage, ideally in an office setting.[52] Physicians should reserve antibiotics for those patients with a component of cellulitis as discussed above, or those who are immunocompromised. This process can be repeated as many times as is necessary. It is important to rule out other causes of perianal sepsis in the early stages of the disease, such as Crohn's disease or perirectal abscesses from a cryptoglandular source. For those patients with chronic and/or recurring disease, we proceed to definitive excision, as long as the diagnosis is not in doubt and we have exhausted the simpler alternatives. Flap procedures are reserved for patients with extensive scarring and tissue damage out onto skin distant from the anus, such as the buttocks. By the time a patient reaches the point at which they desire surgery, they have usually suffered for many years with recurrent abscesses in the affected area.

Even relatively large open wounds around the anus heal remarkably well in the absence of Crohn's disease and other inflammatory, malignant, or infectious processes, compared with how similar wounds typically heal in other areas of the body. Because of this, it is usually not necessary to use flaps after skin excisions for hidradenitis around the anus, especially when using a staged approach. If circumferential disease is present and requires excision, we excise half of the involved perianal skin down to subcutaneous fat and allow the wound to heal by secondary intent, which may take up to 3 months. We excise the other half after complete healing of the first wound. If circumferential excision of perianal skin is considered in a single procedure, we take care not to excise the skin at or inside the anal verge. This diminishes the risk of anal stricture. For patients whose disease does not extend out more than 5 or 6 cm from the anal verge, this approach works very well. We consider a flap-based procedure for those patients with much wider involvement extending out onto the buttocks. Negative pressure dressings are only rarely of potential help.

References

1. da Silva JH. Pilonidal cyst: cause and treatment. Dis Colon Rectum 2000;43(8):1146–1156.
2. Casberg MA. Infected pilonidal cysts and sinuses. Bull US Army Med Dept 1949;9:493–496.
3. Bascom J, Bascom T. Failed pilonidal surgery: new paradigm and new operation leading to cures. Arch Surg 2002;137:1146–1150.
4. Akinci OF, Bozer M, Uzunkoy A, Duzgun SA, Coskun A. Incidence and aetiological factors in pilonidal sinus among Turkish soldiers. Eur J Surg 1999;165(4):339–342.
5. Sondenaa K, Andersen E, Nesvik I, Soreide JA. Patient characteristics and symptoms in chronic pilonidal sinus disease. Int J Colorectal Dis 1995;10(1):39–42.
6. Hull TL, Wu J. Pilonidal disease. Surg Clin North Am 2002;82:1169–1185.
7. Mayo OH. Observations on Injuries and Diseases of the Rectum. London: Burgess and Hill; 1833:45–46.
8. Hodges RM. Pilonidal sinus. Boston Med Surg J 1880;103:485–486.
9. Armstrong JH, Barcia PJ. Pilonidal sinus disease. The conservative approach. Arch Surg 1994;129(9):914–917; discussion 917–919.
10. Bascom JU. Pilonidal sinus. Curr Pract Surg 1994;6:175–180.
11. Lavelle M, Jafri Z, Town G. Recurrent pilonidal sinus treated with epilation using a ruby laser. J Cosmet Laser Ther 2002;4(2):45–47.
12. Downs AM, Palmer J. Laser hair removal for recurrent pilonidal sinus disease. J Cosmet Laser Ther 2002;4(3–4):91.
13. Odili J, Gault D. Laser depilation of the natal cleft: an aid to healing the pilonidal sinus. Ann R Coll Surg Engl 2002;84(1):29–32.
14. Kronborg O, Christensen K, Zimmermann-Nielsen C. Chronic pilonidal disease: a randomized trial with a complete 3-year follow-up. Br J Surg 1985;72(4):303–304.
15. Fuzun M, Bakir H, Soylu M, et al. Which technique for treatment of pilonidal sinus: open or closed? Dis Colon Rectum 1994;37(11):1148–1150.
16. Sondenaa K, Nesvik I, Gullaksen FP, et al. The role of cefoxitin prophylaxis in chronic pilonidal sinus treated with excision and primary suture. J Am Coll Surg 1995;180(2):157–160.
17. Sondenaa K, Nesvik I, Anderson E, Soreide JA. Recurrent pilonidal sinus after excision with closed or open treatment: final result of a randomised trial. Eur J Surg 1996;162(4):351.
18. Beck DE. Pilonidal disease. In: Bland KI, ed. The Practice of General Surgery. Philadelphia: WB Saunders; 2002:509–514.
19. Beck DE, Karulf RE. Pilonidal disease. In: Beck DE, ed. Handbook of Colorectal Surgery. 2nd ed. New York: Marcel Dekker; 2003:391–404.
20. Senapati A, Cripps NP, Thompson MR. Bascom's operation in the day-surgical management of symptomatic pilonidal sinus. Br J Surg 2000;87(8):155–156.
21. Urhan MK, Kukukel F, Topgul K, Ozer I, Sari S. Rhomboid excision and Limberg flap for managing pilonidal sinus. Dis Colon Rectum 2002;45(5):656–659.
22. Abu Galala KH, Salam IMA, Samaan KRA, et al. Treatment of pilonidal sinus by primary closure with a transposed rhomboid flap compared with deep suturing: a prospective randomised clinical trial. Eur J Surg 1999;165(5):468–472.
23. Erdem E, Sungurtekin U, Nessar M. Are postoperative drains necessary with the Limberg flap for treatment of pilonidal sinus? Dis Colon Rectum 1998;41(11):1427–1431.
24. Karydakis GE. Easy and successful treatment of pilonidal sinus disease after explanation of its causative process. Aust N Z J Surg 1992;62(5):385–389.
25. Schoeller T, Wechselberger G, Otto A, Papp C. Definite surgical treatment of complicated recurrent pilonidal disease with a modified fasciocutaneous V-Y advancement flap. Surgery 1997;121(3):258–263.
26. Hodgson WJ, Greenstein RJ. A comparative study between Z-plasty and incision and drainage or excision with marsupialization for pilonidal sinus. Surg Gynecol Obstet 1981;153(6):842–844.
27. Petersen S, Koch R, Stelzner S, Wendlandt TP, Ludwig K. Primary closure techniques in chronic pilonidal sinus: a survey of the results of different surgical approaches. Dis Colon Rectum 2002;45(11):1458–1467.
28. Rosen W, Davidson JS. Gluteus maximus musculocutaneous flap for the treatment of recalcitrant pilonidal disease. Ann Plast Surg 1996;37(3):293–297.

29. Guyuron B, Dinner MI, Dowden RV. Excision and grafting in treatment of recurrent pilonidal sinus disease. Surg Gynecol Obstet 1983;156(2):201–204.

30. Sungurtekin H, Sungurtekin U, Erdem E. Local anesthesia and midazolam versus spinal anesthesia in ambulatory pilonidal surgery. J Clin Anesth 2003;15(3):201–205.

31. Rubin RJ, Chinn BT. Perianal hidradenitis suppurativa. Surg Clin North Am 1994;74(6):1317–1325.

32. Mitchell KM, Beck DE. Hidradenitis suppurativa. Surg Clin North Am 2002;82:1187–1197.

33. Banerjee AK. Surgical treatment of hidradenitis suppurativa. Br J Surg 1992;79:863–866.

34. Lapins J, Jarstrand C, Emtestam L. Coagulase-negative staphylococci are the most common bacteria found in cultures from the deep portions of hidradenitis suppurativa lesions, as obtained by carbon dioxide laser surgery. Br J Dermatol 1999;140:90–95.

35. Attanoos RL, Appleton MAC, Douglas-Jones AG. The pathogenesis of hidradenitis suppurativa: a closer look at apocrine and apoeccrine glands. Br J Dermatol 1995;133:254–258.

36. Jemec GBE, Hansen U. Histology of hidradenitis suppurativa. J Am Acad Dermatol 1996;34:994–999.

37. Gilliland R, Wexner SD. Complicated anorectal sepsis. Surg Clin North Am 1997;77(1):115–148.

38. Burrows NP, Jones RR. Crohn's disease in association with hidradenitis suppurativa [letter to the editor]. Br J Dermatol 1992;126:523–529.

39. Katsanos KH, Christodoulou DK, Tsianos EV. Axillary hidradenitis suppurativa successfully treated with infliximab in a Crohn's disease patient [letter to the editor]. Am J Gastroenterol 2002;97(8):2155–2156.

40. Tsianos EV, Dalekos GN, Tzermias C, Merkouropoulos, Hatzis J. Hidradenitis suppurativa in Crohn's disease: a further support to this association. J Clin Gastroenterol 1995;20(2):151–153.

41. Roy MK, Appleton MAC, Delicata RJ, Sharma AK, Williams GT, Carey PD. Probable association between hidradenitis suppurativa and Crohn's disease: significance of epithelioid granuloma. Br J Surg 1997;84:375–376.

42. Ostlere LS, Langtry JAA, Mortimer PS, Staughton RCD. Hidradenitis suppurativa in Crohn's disease. Br J Dermatol 1991; 125:384–386.

43. Anstey AV, Wilkinson JD, Lord P. Squamous cell carcinoma complicating hidradenitis suppurativa. Br J Dermatol 1990;123: 527–531.

44. Gur E, Neligan PC, Shafir R, Reznick R, Cohen M, Shpitzer T. Squamous cell carcinoma in perineal inflammatory disease. Ann Plast Surg 1997;38(6):653–657.

45. Dufresne RG, Ratz JL, Bergfeld WF, Roenigk RK. Squamous cell carcinoma arising from the follicular occlusion triad. J Am Acad Dermatol 1996;35:475–477.

46. Malaguanera M, Pontillo T, Pistone G, Succi L. Squamous-cell cancer in Verneuil's disease (hidradenitis suppurativa). Lancet 1996;348:1449.

47. Lapins J, Weimin Y, Nyren O, Emtestam L. Incidence of cancer among patients with hidradenitis suppurativa. Arch Dermatol 2001;137:730–734.

48. Jemec GBE, Wendelboe P. Topical clindamycin versus systemic tetracycline in the treatment of hidradenitis suppurativa. J Am Acad Dermatol 1998;39:971–974.

49. Elwood ET, Bolitho DG. Negative-pressure dressings in the treatment of hidradenitis suppurativa. Ann Plast Surg 2001;46: 49–51.

50. Blackburn JH, Boemi L, Hall WW, et al. Negative-pressure dressings as a bolster for skin grafts. Ann Plast Surg 1998;40:453–457.

51. Ger R. Fecal diversion in management of large infected perianal lesions. Dis Colon Rectum 1996;39:1327–1329.

52. Beck DE. Miscellaneous disorders of the colon, rectum and anus: stricture, pruritus ani, proctalgia, colitis cystica profunda, solitary rectal ulcer, hidradenitis. In: Pemberton SH (ed). Shackleford's Surgery of the Alimentary Tract. Vol 4, 5th ed. Philadelphia: WB Saunders; 2002:501–518.

16
Perianal Dermatology and Pruritus Ani

Charles O. Finne

Perianal skin is subject to virtually all of the diseases that affect skin in other areas of the body. The differential diagnosis of perianal skin is presented in Table 16-1. This list includes a variety of diagnoses, which almost never present as isolated perianal disease, but there are common diseases such as psoriasis that may present in isolation without obvious ties to other areas of the body unless a careful search is made. Successful treatment of perianal disease requires accurate diagnosis to eliminate diseases that have specific cause and treatment (e.g., psoriasis, candida, Bowen's disease). Recognition of important treatable causes requires a disciplined, organized approach to diagnosis with frequent use of biopsy. This chapter's objective is to lay out a strategy to facilitate accurate diagnosis and successful treatment of perianal and anal skin conditions. Implicit in this strategy is the ability to properly examine the anus with appropriate instruments and bright light and to understand diseases peculiar to the anal area, hence, the importance of the colorectal surgeon who has the skills to accomplish this task. The importance of complete, accurate evaluation is emphasized by a St. Louis University series in which a study of 209 patients with the presenting symptom of pruritus over a 2-year period revealed that 75% of patients had coexisting anal or colorectal pathology. The diagnoses included 11% with rectal cancer, 6% with anal canal cancer, and 2% with colon cancer, although the majority of patients had hemorrhoids or fissure.[1]

Definitions

Pruritus ani is a term of Latin derivation, which means itchy anus. Not only is it a symptom, but the term is a Medline MeSH searchable diagnosis and is also used to designate a specific condition of disputed etiology recognized since antiquity.[2,3] Pruritus used alone simply means itchy: there is no distinction between it and itch, an unpleasant sensation that provokes the desire to scratch.[4] To avoid confusion in this chapter, the syndrome will always be referred to as pruritus ani. Pruritus ani has been classified into primary and second-

ary. The primary form is the classic syndrome of idiopathic pruritus ani, whereas the secondary form implies an identifiable cause or a specific diagnosis.

Accurate description of the morphology of skin lesions can aid in the diagnosis and follow-up of patients with pruritic complaints. Macules are flat spots. Papules are elevated circumscribed solid lesions, raised spots. Vesicles are separations of the epidermis and dermis filled with serum. Bulla are larger vesicles or blisters. Pustules contain pus. Ulcers are surface lesions with loss of continuity of the skin and may result from rupture of vesicular lesions, infection, or trauma. Intertrigo is inflammation seen between two opposing skin surfaces, often the result of mixed bacterial, fungal infection associated with moisture, obesity, and poor hygiene.

Physiologic Considerations

Itch is a surface phenomenon mediated by pain fibers in the epidermis that may have a lower threshold for stimulation than pain. Itch receptors may be located more superficially than those dedicated to pain. Because receptors are superficial, innocuous, nondamaging stimuli such as wearing wool, or other minor mechanical stimuli may induce itching. In addition to histamine, kallikrein, bradykinin, papain, and trypsin experimentally produce itching, but these substances do not respond to blockade with histamine antagonists such as diphenhydramine, hence topical antihistamines are not always effective against itching.[5] The phenomenon of hyperesthesia with chronic pain may have a parallel with itching, whereas minimal stimulation of the skin may induce itching; scratching with subsequent injury may produce an enlarging patch of itchy skin. Scratching produces inadequate feedback to inhibit itching; more scratching occurs with cutaneous injury, which provides an additional stimulus to scratch in a self-defeating loop. Substituting heat, cold, painful or stinging stimulus for the itch by applying alcohol or pepper extract may provoke an inhibitory feedback not supplied by scratching alone and lead to inhibition of the urge to scratch.[5] Itching

TABLE 16-1. Differential diagnosis of anal dermatoses

Inflammatory disease	Nonsexual infectious disease
Pruritus ani	Pilonidal disease
Psoriasis	Hidradenitis suppurativa
Lichen planus	Fistula-in-ano
Lichen sclerosis et atrophicus	Crohn's disease
Atrophoderma	Tuberculosis
Contact (allergic) dermatitis	Actinomycosis
Seborrheic dermatitis	Herpes zoster
Atopic dermatitis	Vaccinia
Radiation dermatitis	Fournier's gangrene
Behçet's syndrome	Tinea cruris
Lupus erythematosus	Candidiasis
Dermatomyositis	"deep" mycoses
Scleroderma	Amebiasis cutis
Erythema multiforme	Trichomoniasis
Familial chronic pemphigus	Schistosomiasis cutis
(Hailey-Hailey)	Bilharziasis
Pemphigus vulgaris	*Oxyuris* (pinworm)
Cicatricial pemphigoid	Creeping eruption (larva migrans)
	Larva currens
	Cimicosis (bed bugs)
	Pediculosis (lice)
	Scabies
Sexually transmitted disease	**Premalignant and malignant disease**
Gonorrhea	Acanthosis nigricans
Syphilis	Leukoplakia
Chancroid	Mycosis fungoides
Granuloma inguinale	Leukemia cutis
Lymphogranuloma venereum	Basal cell carcinoma
Molluscum contagiosum	Squamous cell carcinoma
Herpes simplex	Melanoma
Condyloma acuminata	Bowen's disease (AIN)
	Extramammary Paget's disease

Source: Modified from Corman.[2]

attending the healing of surgical wounds and scars probably results from the combination of histamine release, release of other kinins and prostaglandins involved in the inflammatory phase of healing, and regeneration of nerves that may be thinly myelinated in immature scars. Antihistamines, topical anti-inflammatory agents (steroids), topical anesthetics, and aloe preparations (prostaglandin inhibitors) all have beneficial effects on the itching of healing wounds.[5]

Etiology of Pruritus

Because pruritus is a symptom that may have protean causes, it is useful to consider diagnoses that have been associated with pruritus ani. Table 16-2 is a list of diagnoses and conditions modified from Stamos and Hicks.[6] Specific causes are considered below.

Localized Itch Syndromes

Notalgia paresthetica is a defined syndrome with itching or pain of the upper mid back to either side of the scapular region. This has been attributed to spinal nerve damage or entrapment, but an inherited form with eight affected family members has been described. Skin biopsies have shown increases in sensory innervation in the area, and other changes that could be attributed to repeated rubbing and scratching. Treatment by application of pepper cream (capsaicin 0.025%) has been effective. Such treatment may exacerbate the symptoms during the first week of application, but thereafter both the symptoms and the side effects of the treatment subside. Topical application of EMLA® (2.5% lignocaine + 2.5% prilocaine), a topical anesthetic cream, has also been effective.[5] Dermographism has been reported as a cause of anogenital pruritus.[7,8] It is not unreasonable to propose that the idiopathic form of pruritus ani may be a related disorder, and that the skin changes are the sole result of skin trauma. The effectiveness of the anal tattooing procedures, discussed later, lends some support to this hypothesis.

TABLE 16-2. Proposed etiologies of idiopathic pruritus ani

Anatomic factors	Obesity, deep clefts, hirsutism, tight clothing
Anorectal disease	Fissure, fistula, tags, prolapsing papilla, hemorrhoids, mucosal prolapse, sphincter insufficiency, deforming scars
Antibiotics	
Contact dermatitis	Chemicals in topical preparations, toilet paper, wet wipes, alcohol, witch hazel, "caine" anesthetics, fecal soiling
Dermatoses	Psoriasis, seborrheic dermatitis, atopic dermatitis, lichen planus, lichen simplex, LS, dermographism
Diet	Coffee (caffeinated and decaffeinated), chocolate, spicy foods, citrus fruits, tomatoes, beer, dairy products, vitamin A and D deficiencies, fat substitutes, consumption of large volumes of liquids
Diarrhea	Infectious diarrhea, irritable bowel syndrome, Crohn's disease, ulcerative colitis
Drugs	Quinidine, colchicine, intravenous steroids
Gynecologic conditions	Pruritus vulvae, vaginal discharge of infection
Idiopathic	
Infection	Viruses: herpes simplex, cytomegalovirus, papillomavirus; bacteria: *S. aureus*, beta hemolytic strep, mixed infections; fungi: dermatophytes, *Candida* species; parasites: pinworms, scabies, pediculosis; spirochetes: syphilis
Neoplasms	Bowen's disease (AIN), extramammary Paget's disease, squamous cell carcinoma variants, secreting villous tumors
Personal hygiene	Poor cleansing habits, over-meticulous cleansing producing mechanical trauma, use of soaps
Psychogenic/neurogenic	Anxiety, neurosis, psychosis, neurodermatitis, neuropathy, "itch syndromes"
Radiation	Radiation dermatitis, sphincter compromise or leakage caused by radiation proctitis
Systemic disease	Jaundice, diabetes mellitus, chronic renal failure, iron deficiency, thyroid disorders, lymphoma, polycythemia vera

Source: Modified from Stamos and Hicks, 1998.[6]

Fecal Contamination

Systematic, rigorous studies of anal pruritus are rare, but good evidence supports fecal contamination as one cause of symptoms. Caplan[9] performed a study in 27 Caucasian men in which fresh autologous feces was applied as a patch test both perianally and on the inner arm, and perianal skin was also cultured for fungi. There were 10 control subjects where feces samples were collected; the skin was spatulated but feces not applied to the skin. The patch-tested subjects had several pH-adjusted samples applied to the skin in addition to the unadulterated samples. Twelve of the 27 had a history of pruritus ani. pH of the perianal skin varied from 5.0 to 7.0 and was not different between the two groups. Five of 12 pruritus subjects (42%) grew yeast (non–*Candida albicans*) but no dermatophytes, whereas 4 of 15 nonpruritus subjects (27%) grew *C. albicans* (3) or *Geotrichum*. Twelve of 27 (44%) with feces applied to the skin developed symptoms from the feces. Four of 12 (33%) of the pruritus group developed symptoms, 8 of 15 (53%) of the nonpruritus group developed symptoms, whereas none of the control group developed symptoms. Symptoms occurred within 1–6 hours in all but one subject and were relieved by washing the skin. Only one of the 27 subjects reacted to feces on the arms patch test, suggesting that the skin in different locations reacts differently. The prompt appearance of symptoms and relief with cleansing was believed to indicate an irritant effect rather than an allergic effect.

Smith and colleagues[10] in a rigorous study of 75 patients with pruritus found that half of their patients had poorly formed stools and 41% of their patients complained of soiling from daily to several times a week. Seepage of liquid and mucous was believed to be an important factor in the etiology of the symptoms. Coffee was demonstrated to lower anal resting pressure in 8 of 11 patients.

Allan et al.[11] showed that leakage during a saline infusion test occurred sooner in patients with pruritus ani than in nonpruritic controls (median leak point 600 mL versus 1300 mL in controls). This is consistent with findings by Farouk et al.[12] and Eyers and Thomson[13] who both found that the anal inhibitory reflex was more pronounced in patients with pruritus ani. Rectal distension, because the decrease in anal pressure from baseline is greater in patients with pruritus ani, makes these patients more prone to leak and soil.

Viral Infection

Condylomata acuminata are a common cause of itching, but the diagnosis is easily recognizable and should not be confused with idiopathic pruritus ani. Condylomata, papilloma virus infection, and anal intraepithelial neoplasia (AIN) will be discussed extensively elsewhere. Herpes syndromes are usually accompanied by pain rather than itching and the clinical course is accompanied by a characteristic eruption consisting of red macules, which progress to vesicles that rupture, ulcerate, and may become secondarily infected. Culture or biopsy shows specific diagnostic findings. Likewise, molluscum contagiosum produces characteristic lesions, papular, 2- to 5-mm diameter, with central umbilication, usually clustered. Human immunodeficiency virus–associated lesions are rarely associated with chronic itching except for secondary fungal infections. No credible evidence exists for a viral etiology in idiopathic pruritus ani.

Fungal Infection

Smith et al.[10] found no instances of fungal infection in their investigation of pruritus in which each of 75 patients had scrapings and fungus cultures. In contrast, Dodi et al.[14] found *C. albicans* had no relationship to pruritus (culture positive in 23% of control subjects, 26% of those with pruritus, and 28% of those without pruritus), but 10 patients who cultured dermatophytes all had itching. None of these patients had exposure to steroids or antibiotics. Their conclusion was that *C. albicans* was saprophytic in the absence of steroids, but that dermatophytes were always pathogenic. Prolonged courses of steroids are said to enhance pathogenicity of *C. albicans* and to mask *Candida* infection.[15]

Verbov[3] found 7 of 47 patients (15%) with pruritus ani whose itching was attributed to *Candida* out of a review of his dermatologic practice (3000 patients surveyed on the basis of their primary complaint). Pirone et al.[16] claim that surgical treatment of anal disorders (hemorrhoids, fissure, spasm, mucosal prolapse) eliminated *Candida* and dermatophyte infections in all but 3 of 23 patients who were culture positive and symptomatic with itching before surgery. Two of these three failures responded to antifungal treatment, but the final patient continued to itch.

In another study of 200 patients evaluated by colorectal surgeons and dermatologists, thrush was found in 28 (14%), only one of whom was diabetic. Fourteen patients had local steroid therapy, and 6 occurred after a course of systemic antibiotics. Only one case of dermatophyte infection was found.[17]

Perianal dermatophyte infection, all *Trichophyton rubrum*, was reported to be infrequent by Alexander[15] (4 of nearly 300 cases). Topical steroids may render direct scrapings negative for hyphae.

Bacterial Infection

Several non–sexually transmitted bacterial infections are reported to cause longstanding pruritus. Weismann et al.[17A] reported that 19 patients (16 males and 3 females) with pruritus of duration 1–20 years had beta hemolytic streptococci cultured (four also had *Staphylococcus aureus*) from the perianal area but not from nasal or throat swabs. Treatment with various regimens resulted in cure of 42% and amelioration of symptoms in the others.

Erythrasma was reported to cause pruritus in 15 of 81 patients (18%) who had failed to respond to routine treatment.[18] Wood's light fluorescence (coral pink) was the most reliable diagnostic maneuver, being positive in every case, but cultures of *Corynebacterium minutissimum* were positive in only four cases. Groin, thighs, and toes were also involved in every case and cure was achieved in all patients with erythromycin. Smith et al.[10] found erythrasma in only 1 of their 75 patients, each of whom had Wood's light examination. *C. minutissimum* is probably present in normal skin flora, but the moisture, diabetes, and obesity predispose to infection which is usually found in the body folds (axilla, groin, intergluteal, inframammary) and toe webs.[19] The St. Mark's series found erythrasma in 16% of their 200 cases, but 27% of the group were symptomatic for more than 5 years.[17] Their patients had disease in more than one site, in common with other quoted series.

S. aureus has been anecdotally implicated as a cause of treatable pruritus.[20] Intertrigo was reported in 27% of the St. Mark's series and was highly treatable with topical agents.[17]

Contact Dermatitis

Contact dermatitis has been reported from a wide variety of preparations including topical anesthetics, topical antibiotics, topical antiseptics, topical antihistamines, and nickel.[17,21] Common sensitizing agents identified in the dermatologic literature are listed in Table 16-3. The role of feces and seepage as a contact agent has been emphasized in almost every article devoted to pruritus ani. Contact dermatitis may have an irritant or allergic basis, but is recognized by being an eczematous inflammation characterized by erythema, scale, and vesicles.[22] Avoidance of contact with the inciting agent is the obvious treatment, and topical steroids may be useful unless secondary infection is present. It is preferable to avoid soaps. Bath oils and emollient creams may be useful for cleansing. The cause of contact dermatitis may be obscure. Dasan et al.[21] reported one patient who had pruritus associated with bathing in a tub of water in which his wife shampooed her hair with para phenyl diamine, a dye. When the patient's wife stopped shampooing her hair in the tub, his symptoms resolved.

A large study of patch testing in 80 patients with pruritus ani in Sheffield, England, emphasized the importance of

TABLE 16-3. Common sensitizing agents

Ethylenediaminetetraacetic acid
Formalin
Lanolin (wood wax alcohol)
Mercury
   [$Hg(NH_2)Cl$, thimerosal]
Neomycin
Nickel
Paraben mixtures
Paraphenylenediamine
Potassium dichromate
Rubber ingredients
Topical anesthetics
   (benzocaine, dibucaine)
Turpentine oil

contact dermatitis as an aggravating factor. Fifty-five patients tested positive. Thirty-eight of the positives were to medicaments or their constituents including neomycin, fragrance mix, Peru balsam, and cinchocaine. After counseling, two-thirds of these 55 patients experienced improvement or resolution of their symptoms.[23] These authors disputed the recommendation to use "wet wipes" for cleansing because of possible sensitization. Bruynzeel[24] corroborates the potential sensitization from use of moist wipes containing methyldibromoglutaronitrile. Rohde believes that excessive exposure to water and the act of excessive cleansing itself may incite symptoms, and recommends the use of oils for cleaning.

Alexander[15] found lanolin, neomycin, procaine, and parabens to be offending agents and emphasized the difficulty of identifying these types of products when incorporated with a local anesthetic or steroid because the anesthetic suppresses the itching and the steroid suppresses the inflammation giving paradoxical temporary relief. Temporary relief leads to increasing application of the offending agent over a wider area, escalating the process.[15]

Psoriasis

Psoriasis has been an important underlying cause of pruritus in every series on this subject. In a combined colorectal dermatologic clinic established to prospectively evaluate patients with pruritus, 22 of 40 patients were found to have psoriasis.[21] Alexander[15] confirms that psoriasis may present as an isolated lesion in the perianal area, and emphasizes that lesions in this location do not appear as typical because of maceration. Smith et al.[10] found 6 cases (8%) of psoriasis in his series, 5 of which had not been previously diagnosed. The St. Marks-Guy's hospital series found 5.5% of their 200 patients had psoriasis.[17] They also emphasized the nontypical appearance of the perianal lesions. Lochridge[25] claimed the diagnosis of perianal psoriasis in 81 patients, all of whom responded to fluocinolone acetonide 0.025% (Synalar®) with normalization of the skin. He recommended a search for lesions elsewhere including elbows, knees, ankles, extensor surfaces of the forearm, base of the scalp, ear canals, eyelids, nipples, penis, vulva, or navel. Biopsy was rarely diagnostic because of secondary changes as a result of drugs or trauma and limited experience of pathologists with diagnosis of perianal skin.

Lichen Sclerosis

Lichen sclerosis (formerly lichen sclerosus et atrophicus) (LS) is a chronic disease of unknown cause, almost always occurring in women (female/male 10:1, usually seen on the penis in the male) which in females has a predilection for the vulva and perianal area. The skin has a characteristic appearance that is white, atrophic, and wrinkled.[22,26–29] Involvement of the labia gives this condition a characteristic distribution that makes recognition easy once the diagnosis is considered. Biopsy is characteristic and may be especially indicated in a lesion not responding to treatment because of rare occurrence of squamous cell carcinoma.[30–32] Treatment of LS with a potent topical steroid (clobetasol propionate 0.05%, Temovate®) for 6–8 weeks is highly successful, often resulting in normalization of the skin.[5,27,29] Other recent reports suggest that tacrolimus ointment may avoid the skin atrophy that may accompany potent steroid use.[33,34] Patients with LS in the vulva probably have a 4%–5% incidence of squamous cell carcinoma arising in or adjacent to the LS.[31] These patients should be followed periodically for raised lesions or ulcers that fail to heal. The exact role LS has in the development of cancer is not certain, but is thought to be independent of human papilloma virus.[30]

Food Factors

No controlled trials have been done to examine food stuffs or diet as a cause for itching, but strong opinions have garnered a revered place in the literature. Friend[35] states that virtually all patients with idiopathic pruritus ani consume enormous quantities of liquids, are almost never constipated, and usually have loose stools. Because it helps their symptoms, patients with severe pruritus usually maintain good anal hygiene. Friend states that there are six common foods that unequivocally cause idiopathic pruritus: coffee, tea, cola, beer, chocolate, and tomato (ketchup) and that total elimination will result in remission of itching in 2 weeks. After a 2-week elimination period, the food may be reintroduced to determine the threshold above which consumption causes symptoms. Thresholds are typically between 2–3 cups of coffee, 4 cups of tea, and less than 2 cans of beer.

Smith et al.[10] demonstrated that coffee lowered anal resting pressure in 8 of 11 patients tested. An elimination diet gave partial or complete relief in 27 of 56 (48%) of their patients. Specific dietary items identified by elimination as a cause were coffee (8), alcohol (5), peanuts (3), chocolate (2), milk products (3), cola (1), and citrus (1). Alcohol was an equivocal factor in this study because 41% did not consume alcohol and only a third of patients drank more than 1 ounce per day. Smith et al. confirm the importance of poorly formed stool and coffee which may contribute to seepage and recommend a bulk agent taken at the same time of day to promote regular, complete emptying of stool.

Daniel et al.[1] reported that average coffee intake in patients with primary pruritus ani averaged 6 cups per day, compared with those with secondary pruritus who averaged about 3.5 cups per day.

Akl[36] reported an 8-year-old boy with asthma, intolerant of milk with abdominal pain, whose pruritus ani disappeared after elimination of yogurt.

Coexisting Anal Disease

Coexisting surgical anal conditions (hemorrhoids, fissure, fistulas) may of themselves produce itching or aggravate any

tendency to itch. Most authors agree that correcting these disorders in selected patients is indicated. Smith et al. reported that 8 of his 75 patients required treatment of hemorrhoids (four operations, four Barron ligations) which by virtue of prolapse may induce soiling.[10] These authors note, however, that correction of the hemorrhoids eliminated itching in only one patient. Another with scars from previous fissure surgery also had soiling not amenable to surgical correction. Murie et al.,[37] in a study of 82 hemorrhoidal patients with and without pruritus, believe that pruritus is more common in patients with hemorrhoids than in age- and sex-matched controls without hemorrhoids and that correction of the hemorrhoids usually eliminates itching along with the other symptoms of bleeding, pain, soiling, and protrusion. Bowyer and McColl[17] reported that hemorrhoids were the sole cause of itching in 16 of their 200 patients, contributory in 27 others, and that correction of fissure was required in five patients before symptoms were relieved. Five others had skin tags which when removed eliminated symptoms. These patients could point to the skin tag as the source of the itching. Dasan et al.[21] in a study of 40 patients with pruritus found two that required surgery, one to remove complex skin tags and the other to correct a fistula. The St. Louis University group found that 52% of 109 patients with the sole presenting complaint of itching had anorectal disease as the cause.[1] The diagnoses included hemorrhoids, fissure, idiopathic proctitis, condyloma, ulcerative proctitis, abscess, and fistula.

Pirone et al.,[16] as mentioned above, believe that correction of hemorrhoids, fissure, mucosal prolapse, and spasm can resolve fungal infection and the consequent pruritus.

Psychologic Factors

Smith et al.[10] studied 25 of their patients who completed an MMPI (Minnesota Multiphasic Personality Inventory). They found no deviations on the clinical scales but a trend toward inhibition of aggression, and denial of feeling of social and emotional alienation. Anxiety, stress, and fatigue added to personality, coping skills, and obsessive compulsive disorders probably have a role in the exacerbation of pruritus ani.[38] Because of this, psychiatric drugs may have a role in its management in isolated cases, but the preponderance of evidence suggests, in my opinion, that idiopathic pruritus ani does not have a psychiatric basis except as a form of neurodermatitis. The fact that it responds to simple topical treatment with resolution of physical findings in most cases and is so common argues against an obscure etiology.

Steroid-induced Itching

Anogenital itching has been reported after bolus administration of intravenous dexamethasone.[39] More often, itching occurs as a rebound phenomenon after withdrawal of steroids leading to their reinstitution and chronic use because symptoms always exacerbate after withdrawal. This syndrome has been characterized as steroid addiction[40] and can lead to permanent deformity and dependence.[41] Experimental application of potent steroids under occlusion for as little as 3 weeks has been shown to produce an acute dermatitis resembling that seen with a blister that has been unroofed and exposed to air.[40] In my view, steroids should always be viewed as potentially dangerous and should be used to achieve specific effects. Potency and dosing should be tapered in a planned manner with the goal of eliminating steroids altogether from a maintenance regimen. If elimination is not possible, alternate day therapy or intermittent therapy once or twice a week is to be preferred.

Skin Trauma

Trauma can arise from physiologic processes such as diarrhea or frequent stools which may be associated with frequent wiping and maceration. Scratching either consciously or nocturnally while asleep may result in the classic lesion of lichen simplex chronicus. Alexander-Williams[42] puts it nicely: "Perianal dermatitis is a cross between a nappy rash, athlete's foot, and a self inflicted injury. In most patients the problem is due either to inadequate cleansing of the anus or to over vigorous attempts to polish it clean." There is controversy about the best way to clean the anus. Rohde[43] takes issue with the standard method using water or wet wipes and advocates a smooth, dry article with olive oil if necessary, believing that water breaks down the barrier function of the skin. Most authors agree that contact dermatitis is a contributing cause of perianal irritation and that attempts to discontinue over-the-counter preparations (OTCs), perfumed, or scented products including toilet paper, should be made because of potential sensitizing agents (Table 16-3). Bland emollients, Acid Mantle®-based creams, and waterless cleansing agents are reasonable substitutes that may be used with tissue paper or cotton balls for cleansing and left on the skin. My own experience suggests that dilute white vinegar (1 tablespoon in 8 ounces of water) and Burow's solution (Domeboro®) are effective cleansing agents associated with little adverse reaction. Burow's solution and acetic acid have been found to be an effective antibacterial in chronic otitis with little toxicity.[44–47]

Neoplasms

Perianal Paget's disease is rare and large series do not exist, but more than half of patients in most series have itching, often for longer than 3 months.[48–50] Perianal Bowen's disease (intraepithelial squamous cell carcinoma in situ) is also rare, but in a series of 47 patients reviewed at the Cleveland Clinic, 28 (60%) had perianal itching as a presenting complaint.[51] AIN is the sequel to human papillomavirus infection (associated with itching) and refers to premalignant change in the area of the dentate line and anal transitional zone. Although pruritus has not been described in large series looking at AIN[52,53] (because of their study design), it

would seem prudent to be alert for neoplastic change in any patient with a history of warts who presents with pruritus. Higher-grade tumors such as melanoma or squamous cell cancer usually present with bleeding or pain, not with pruritus.[54–56] Further discussion of anal neoplastic disease is found in Chapter 35.

Diagnosis of Perianal Disease

Given the variety of possible diagnoses as cataloged so far, it is important to identify the specific diagnoses that are treatable for cure, and to engage a strategy that will avoid mistakes. It is often helpful in the differential diagnosis of anal and perianal disease processes to divide them into the general classifications of mass (inflammatory or neoplastic), rash, or fissure (primary or secondary). The morphology of a lesion is a starting point for diagnosis, but may not be specific, and the same disease may have several different appearances (Table 16-4). As an example, candidiasis may be present as an erythematous lesion, a papular lesion, or as an ulcerative lesion. Specific techniques are necessary, therefore, to establish or eliminate a diagnosis. Bacterial culture is a time-honored technique for identification of organisms, but proper media and collection techniques must be used to avoid killing certain species.[57]

TABLE 16-4. Morphology of perianal skin lesions

Ulcers	Papules
Herpes genitalis	Venereal warts
Syphilis	Scabies
Trauma	Molluscum contagiosum
Chancroid	Candidiasis
Fixed drug eruption	Syphilis
Lymphogranuloma venereum	
Tularemia	
Behçet's syndrome	
Malignancy	
Donovanosis (granuloma inguinale)	
Candidiasis	
Histoplasmosis	
Mycobacterioses	
Amebiasis	
Gonorrhea	
Trichomoniasis	

Diffuse erythema	Crusts
Candidiasis	Herpes genitalis
Trauma	Scabies
Contact dermatitis	
Fixed drug eruption	

Miscellaneous findings
  Linear tracks: scabies
  Reddish flecks: crab louse excreta
  Maculae ceruleae (sky-blue spots): crab lice
  Nits: crab lice
  Hypertrophic: donovanosis

History and Physical Examination

History and physical examination, often overlooked in our technologic arrogance, is still the most basic maneuver for diagnosis of any disease (see Table 16-5). Inquiry about other skin diseases, allergic conditions such as asthma or urticaria, or sites of involvement may be the first clue to diagnosis of unrecognized psoriasis or atopic dermatitis. Patients may not relate the itch on their elbow to the itch around their anus. Erythrasma usually involves the groin and toes, usually is chronic, and is often associated with hyperpigmentation. Patients frequently do not consider OTC or nonprescription preparations as medicines, but these may modify the appearance of a condition or even cause it. Specific questions about the use of these products are necessary to uncover their use and exposure to unsuspected ingredients. Knowledge of a patient's allergies is important not only for avoidance, but may aid in uncovering an unsuspected exposure to an occult ingredient. Patients sometimes have had patch testing and allergy consultation, and will not volunteer that information unless specifically asked. Patch testing, dermatologic consultation, and withdrawal of medication may be in order. Specific questions about infections, colds, or diarrheal illnesses treated with pills may be necessary to uncover antibiotic use. Patients sometimes will not list prednisone in their list of medications until asked a question pertinent to an illness such as arthritis or asthma or myalgias. A condition that has come and gone for years or that has seasonal exacerbation may be a clue to anal fissure, but could reflect dietary changes, type of clothes worn, or laundry practices.

Physical examination should specifically look for other sites of involvement. The groin is a classic intertriginous area that is easily accessible in the prone jackknife or the lateral position and should be the first place one looks to confirm a suspected yeast or fungus diagnosis. Hyperpigmentation in the buttock cleft or other intertriginous area is a clue to a chronic inflammatory condition or the presence of chronically

infected drainage or secretion. Effective treatment of a patient with changes in the groin as well as the cleft requires attention to each area of involvement. If a condition is infectious, steps to eliminate the infection will be more successful if the environment of the host is made inhospitable to the organism in each area of involvement. A sharply defined border usually points to a definable diagnosis such as tinea, especially when accompanied by scale (Figure 16-1). Psoriasis usually has a sharply defined border, but in the cleft may lack the classic scale seen in skin that is exposed to air. In the confined, occluded area of the cleft, there usually is no scale (Figure 16-2). Neoplastic changes may appear sharply marginated, but margins may be microscopically involved, especially around the dentate line, even if grossly normal (Figure 16-3, Bowen's disease). Infiltrative processes may be less well defined as in Paget's disease of the anus with the same caveat about margins (Figure 16-4). Inflammatory changes of idiopathic nature often have borders that are indistinct and nondescript (Figures 16-5 and 16-6). Bright red erythema often is seen with perianal yeast (Figure 16-6). Erythema may be seen with chronic steroid use (Figure 16-7). Patient A had used hydrocortisone daily for 20 years or more and came in with recurrent warts and carcinoma in situ when the cortisone failed to control his symptoms. Treatment of his warts, carcinoma in situ, and withdrawal of his steroids resulted in resolution of his symptoms and normalization of his skin. Patient B had used Mycolog® cream daily for several years, having had radiation therapy for prostate cancer. He was also treated with withdrawal of steroids. Acute severe injury from prolonged diarrhea with frequent wiping produced the picture of lichen simplex chronicus (Figure 16-8), which was treated by specific treatment of the patient's diarrhea, cleansing with Burow's solution, and topical silver sulfadiazine to which

TABLE 16-5. Historical and physical factors aiding diagnosis of anal and perianal disease

Historical
    Other skin conditions, asthma, urticaria
    Prior treatments/OTC topicals
    Allergies
    Chemicals/clothes/laundry
    Antibiotic use
    Systemic disease
    Chronicity
Physical findings
    Multiple sites (elbows, groins, intertriginous areas, labia, toe webs)
    Mass or woody induration
    Hyperpigmentation
    Scale
    Lichenification
    Ulceration
    Groin adenopathy
    Defined edge or margin

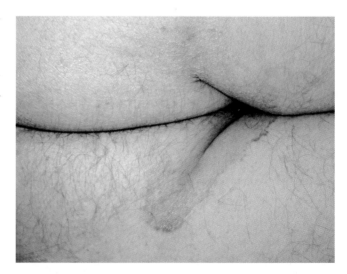

FIGURE 16-1. Dermatophyte infection. Note the sharp border, the scale at the edges, and its involvement of the groin crease. As this type of infection moves into the anal cleft, the characteristic edge at the border of the cleft and involvement of the groin may be the only clues.

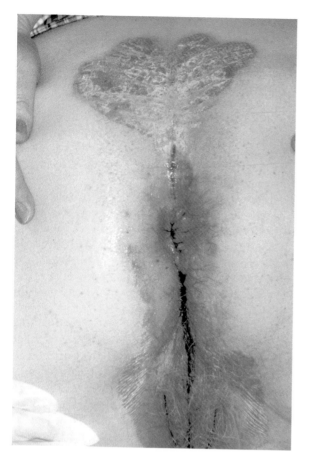

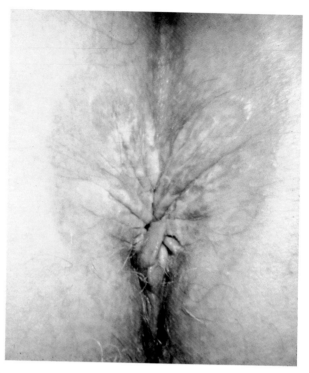

FIGURE 16-4. Perianal Paget's disease may present as a nondescript rash that itches. This clinical appearance is not specific and requires biopsy to confirm the diagnosis. Unlike Paget's of the breast, there is rarely an underlying invasive adenocarcinoma, and local excision with clear margins is the treatment of choice. Margins of excision require frozen section confirmation because clinically normal skin may be involved.

FIGURE 16-2. Psoriasis often appears atypical in the cleft and around the labia, lacking the silvery scale that is so characteristic. Isolated areas of involvement in the cleft occur and require biopsy confirmation by a competent skin pathologist.

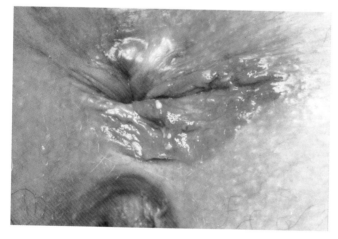

FIGURE 16-3. Anal Bowen's disease or squamous cell carcinoma in situ may have a varied appearance and be indistinguishable from Paget's Disease (Figure 5) by clinical examination. The white pearls on the red background are often present and are a clue to the diagnosis. Despite sharp-appearing edges, the process often involves normal-looking skin and requires frozen section to confirm negative margins.

cortisone was added. Chronic infected discharge may lead to hyperpigmentation in the cleft (Figure 16-9) in this case caused by chronic pilonidal disease, but may also occur with fistulas, chronic yeast or fungus infection, or hidradenitis. Treatment complications can result in a rash in this patient with a contact dermatitis from clotrimazole (Figure 16-10). Severe symptoms, especially paresthesias, coupled with scattered lesions may be a clue to herpes virus infection (Figure 16-11). LS characteristically involves the perineum and labia in the female and has a distinctive appearance with wrinkling of the skin (Figure 16-12). Biopsy is characteristic.

Groin adenopathy, and whether or not the nodes are tender, can have specific relevance to diagnosis of perianal and anal disease (Table 16-6), especially sexually transmitted disease.

Laboratory Examination

Ideally, infected material should be aspirated with a syringe and expelled into a sterile container. Next best is a swab of exudate collected from a deep portion of the lesion. Bacterial and fungal cultures should be placed into a bacterial transport medium and refrigerated if any delay in transport to the laboratory occurs. Anaerobic specimens require transport in a special anaerobic medium, and should not be refrigerated. Viral

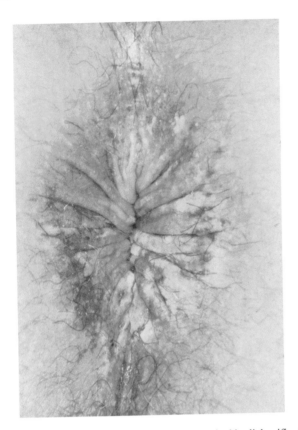

FIGURE 16-5. Classic severe pruritus ani is marked by lichenification (leathery thickening of the skin), accentuation of folds, fissuring of the skin, and erosions and an indistinct border. Changes this severe require short-term aggressive therapy with high-potency steroids for 4–8 weeks which then are rapidly tapered to a maintenance program, if possible without steroids. It is important to rule out secondary infection, which requires specific treatment.

cultures require a viral transport medium and should be kept on ice. Vesicular lesions should be unroofed and cultures taken from the base of the vesicle. Microscope slides can be pressed against the base of the lesion for Tzanck smears, but inoculation of the fluid or exudate from the lesion base onto cell culture is more sensitive (viral culture).[57]

The office should have arrangements with a laboratory, which will supply culture swabs with transport media appropriate for aerobic, anaerobic, fungal, and viral culture. These become outdated and can result in rejection of specimens for processing. The practitioner should check the appropriateness of the media and its date before using it. Because staph and strep have been documented as causal agents, it is prudent to culture for pathogens in almost all cases in which treatment is not obvious. Conventional water-soluble lubricant is bactericidal for some organisms (*Neisseria gonorrhoeae*). Swabs should be lubricated with saline if lubricated at all. Ulcerated lesions should have the base vigorously swabbed. Biopsy should be accomplished early with a representative lesion and should include an area of adjacent normal skin. Specific query should be made to the pathologist about suspected diagnoses, and if possible a pathologist with skin expertise should be consulted. Highly reliable histologic criteria exist for viral lesions, pyoderma, syphilis, and neoplastic lesions. EMLA® cream, applied as a lubricant at the time of examination, may facilitate injection of local anesthetic, and biopsy may conveniently be done with either an 11 blade or skin punch blades that come in numerous sizes in separate sterile packages (Figure 16-13). Bleeding from punch biopsy holes is readily controlled with sliver nitrate sticks or GELFOAM® packing.

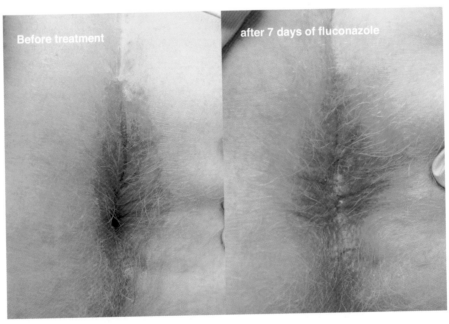

FIGURE 16-6. Perianal yeast may present as a bright red rash without the cheesy exudate sometimes seen elsewhere and may follow treatment with antibiotics for some other condition. This infection is easy to treat but has a tendency to recur. Rendering the cleft environment inhospitable by drying with a hair dryer after bathing and using athletes foot powder to coat the skin and absorb moisture can help maintain remission.

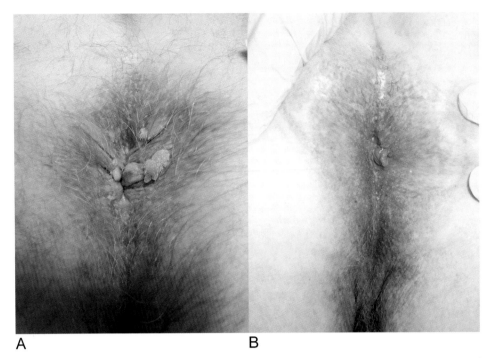

A   B

FIGURE 16-7. Chronic steroid use may cause itching or mask other processes. **A** An elderly man who had used 1% cortisone daily for more than 20 years, but had worsening of his symptoms despite increasing use. Treatment of his warts and carcinoma in situ along with withdrawal of steroids resolved his symptoms. The erythema has disappeared and he had remained free of symptoms for over a year. **B** A similar erythema superimposed on radiation dermatitis from treatment of prostate cancer. Withdrawal of Mycolog®, which had been used for years without interruption and substitution of a barrier cream with menthol relieved his symptoms.

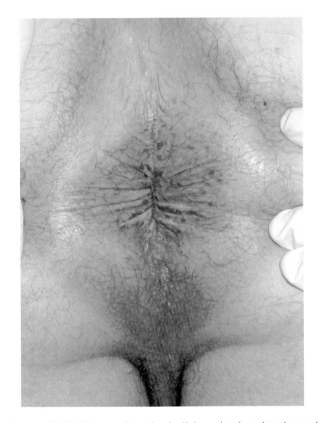

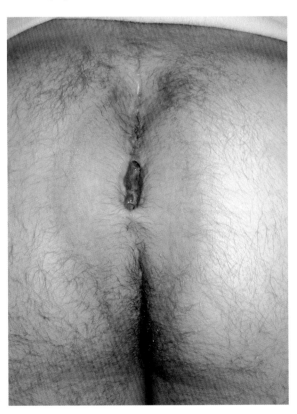

FIGURE 16-8. This man has classic lichen simplex chronicus with inflammation and erosion resulting from unremitting diarrhea of 3 weeks' duration with wiping five times a day. Treatment of the patient's diarrhea and topical silver sulfadiazine with 2% cortisone achieved rapid healing and relief of symptoms.

FIGURE 16-9. Hyperpigmentation may result from chronic inflammatory changes in the skin for whatever reason. In this particular case, infected drainage from a chronic pilonidal sinus was the cause, but fistula disease, chronic dermatophyte infection, erythrasma may produce the same picture. This finding should emphasize the need to modify environmental conditions within the cleft and surrounding area as an adjunct to healing.

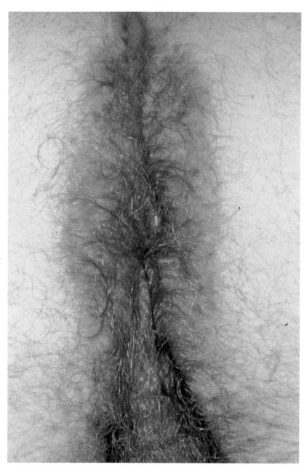

FIGURE 16-10. This patient had a reaction to topical clotrimazole in use for 1 week.

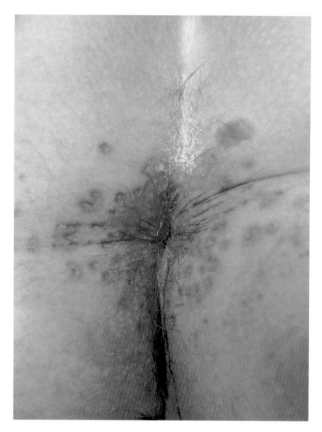

FIGURE 16-11. Scattered lesions, especially when accompanied by severe symptoms suggest herpes virus infection. Herpes simplex type 1 was cultured from the base of these ulcerations that were 9 days old at the time of this picture. Treatment caused prompt resolution of symptoms.

Skin scrapings may be submitted for fungus culture, and if available examined by KOH prep for hyphae. Most colorectal offices are not set up for KOH prep and rarely are we trained in this technique, therefore culture is probably more reliable.

Treatment of Pruritus Ani

A general strategy is presented in Table 16-7. Directed treatment for a specific, curable diagnosis is the ideal, and diagnostic efforts should be directed to avoid overlooking curable disease.

Many investigators have alluded to the importance of controlling seepage and fecal contamination of the skin. Diet may directly contribute to itching and it is prudent to give patients a list of potential foods implicated in itching for an elimination trial. Patients with loose stools may benefit from the addition of fiber to absorb moisture and add bulk and improve emptying with defecation. Many patients who have tried fiber without benefit may benefit from judicious use of Imodium® or Lomotil® to lessen frequency and firm up stools. Questran®, in varied doses, has been helpful in my practice to firm loose stools.

Environmental factors should be altered as much as possible with removal of irritants such as soaps, perfumes, dyes in clothes or wiping tissues, alcohol- or witch hazel-containing agents, and moisture. Dove® is free of conventional soap and is the preferred bathing agent. Bidets are not common in the United States, but detachable shower heads are common and inexpensive and when equipped with long tubing and handle may be a useful item for cleansing the perianal skin and anal canal and eliminating soap residues by flushing with water in the squatting position. Subsequent drying with a hair dryer can eliminate moisture, and application of an athlete's foot powder or barrier cream will lubricate and prevent maceration of the skin in the cleft and anal canal. Zeasorb® is an alternate lubricating, drying agent in powder form. Cornstarch is to be avoided because it is culture medium for yeast. Cornmeal agar is used to identify different species of yeast in the laboratory.[57] Dilute white vinegar (1 tablespoon in an 8-ounce glass of water) on a cotton ball is a cheap effective nonsoapy cleanser that can be kept at the toilet when bathing is not handy. Burow's solution, 1:40 (Domeboro® tablet one in 12 ounces of water, or one in 6 ounces for 1:20) is another nonirritating cleanser that can be kept refrigerated in a plastic squeeze bottle and used in lieu of soap or plain water. Burow's

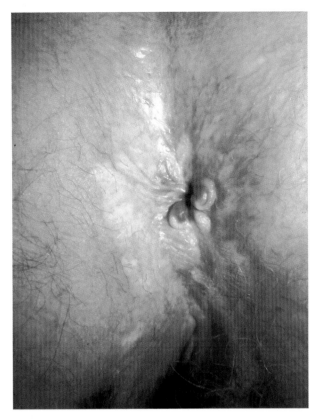

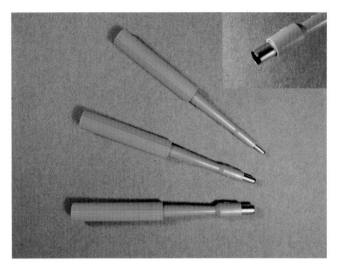

FIGURE 16-13. Skin punch biopsy tools come in various sizes up to 1 cm in diameter (2, 3, and 5 mm pictured). They may be purchased as autoclavable sets which may be sterilized and reused, or for the occasional user, disposable punches are supplied in individually wrapped sterile packages. One advantage of the disposable instruments is that they are always sharp.

FIGURE 16-12. LS has a distinctive appearance with cigarette paper thinning and wrinkling of the skin. It almost always involves the labial skin and perineum, making it easy to recognize. Biopsy is characteristic and is especially indicated for any areas that are raised, ulcerated, or unresponsive to treatment because of a 5% risk of squamous cell carcinoma developing within its distribution.

orally) is available topically as an effective antihistamine (Zonalon®), but orally is 1000 times more potent than diphenhydramine (Benadryl®) for elimination of itching and may a useful adjunct at bedtime to avoid nocturnal scratching. Nocturnal scratching, of which the patient may be unaware, is probably a significant contributing factor in most cases of idiopathic pruritus ani. Patients who are awakened by the urge to scratch should be instructed to gently cleanse the area to eliminate any fecal seepage and reapply their steroid or barrier cream (whichever is in effect at the time) but not to scratch. Pepper creams may be useful in breaking the overwhelming urge to scratch by substituting a more powerful temporary burning stimulus.

No data exist on the influence of clothes or other fomites on pruritus, but from a practical standpoint, loose underwear that

may be used as an antibacterial soak for 5–15 minutes and then dried. Balneol® is a commercially available mineral oil–based preparation that can be kept in a pocket and squeezed onto toilet paper to make a soothing cleansing agent when using public facilities. Breaks in the skin caused by scratching or over-vigorous cleansing efforts must be avoided, so an attempt to control symptoms with application of topical anesthetics, menthol, phenol, camphor, or a combination of ingredients may be appropriate. These agents may be used in combination with topical steroids, topical antifungal agents, and topical antibacterials. Doxepin (Sinequan®

TABLE 16-6. Differential diagnosis of groin adenopathy

Benign reactive (shoeless walking)
Lymphoma
Carcinoma (penis,vulva, anal canal)
Sarcoidosis
Syphilis (nontender)
Leishmaniasis
Chancroid (tender)
Herpes genitalis (tender)
Lymphogranuloma venereum

TABLE 16-7. Treatment of pruritus ani

1. Specific directed treatment for a diagnosis
2. Eliminate offending agent [contact irritant (perfume, soap, toilet paper), organism]
3. Eliminate scratching (especially nocturnal)
4. Control symptoms
5. Hygienic measures (Dove® soap, detachable shower head, hair dryer to dry)
6. Withdraw inappropriate steroids
7. Treat infection (silver sulfadiazine cream, gentamicin or clindamycin topically, nystatin, clotrimazole)
8. Protect skin [barrier creams, powders (especially athlete's foot powder)]
9. Correct anal disease (fissure, hemorrhoids)
10. Judicious use of appropriate steroids
11. Emphasize control as a chronic condition
12. Reassess diagnosis if response to treatment is not appropriate
13. Anal tattooing in extreme cases

allows air circulation and promotes dryness makes sense. Fresh clothes should be used daily that have been laundered without perfume, perhaps with the addition of a small amount of chlorine bleach to secure lowered bacterial counts.

Patients who come to the office with acute moderate to severe changes of the skin are treated by application of Berwick's dye (combination of gentian violet and brilliant green) which has alcohol content and stings, often relieving the itch. The dye is dried with compressed air or a hair dryer. Benzoin tincture is applied over top of this as a barrier and dried similarly. This preparation will stay in place for several days if only water is used to cleanse and gives excellent temporary relief of symptoms and allows reepithelialization of broken skin. Berwick's is suitable as an office applied remedy but is generally not for home application.

Patients who have mild to moderate symptoms with minimal skin changes will often respond to topical 1% hydrocortisone cream which can be combined with menthol, 0.5%–1.0%, and topical antibiotics (gentamicin, clindamycin, or bacitracin) or antifungals (clotrimazole, nystatin). This preparation is applied at night and in the morning after bathing, being used daily until symptoms subside. Thereupon a tapering regimen is instituted, ending with substitution of a barrier cream such as Calmoseptine® to keep the skin covered. Elimination of the steroids and substitution of an innocuous agent to maintain attention to the hygiene is an important goal. Patients with thickened skin and chronic moderate or severe changes should be approached with higher intensity therapy, with a medium or high potency steroid for a limited, defined period of time (Table 16-8; nonsteroidal topical therapies are listed in Table 16-9). My preference is to prescribe brand names when dealing with topical steroids because of the vehicle in which it is delivered, and the particular salt matter as to potency (Table 16-8). For instance, betamethasone as Diprolene® is more than 1000 times more potent than Valisone® cream, with Valisone® ointment

TABLE 16-8. Relative potency of topical steroids (descending order)

Group 1 (most potent)	Group 4
Betamethasone dipropionate 0.05% (Diprolene®)	Desoximetasone 0.05% (Topicort LP®)
Clobetasol propionate 0.05% (Temovate®)	Flurandrenolide 0.05% (Cordran®)
Group 2	**Group 5**
Desoximetasone 0.25% (Topicort®)	Betamethasone valerate cream 0.1% (Valisone®)
Fluocinonide 0.05% (Lidex®)	Hydrocortisone butyrate 0.1% (Locoid®)
	Triamcinolone acetonide 0.1% (Kenalog®)
Group 3	**Group 6 (least potent)**
Betamethasone valerate ointment 0.1% (Valisone®)	Alclometasone dipropionate 0.05% (Aclovate®)
Triamcinolone acetonide 0.5% (Aristocort®)	Hydrocortisone 1%

TABLE 16-9. Nonsteroidal topical therapy for itching

Berwick's dye (crystal violet 1% + brilliant green 1% + 95% ethanol 50% + distilled H_2O q.s.ad. 100%) with benzoin barrier
Burow's solution 1:40
Calmoseptine®
Camphor® (0.1%–3%)
Capsaicin (Zostrix® 0.025%, Dolorac® 0.25%)
Cold compress (ice cube)
Doxepin 5% (Zonalon®)
EMLA (eutectic mixture of local anesthetics)
Hot compress (120°F)
Macrolide topical agents (Tacrolimus and Pimecrolimus)
Menthol (0.125%–1%)
Phenol (0.125%–2%)
Pramoxine
Shake lotions (calamine + additives)
Topical "caines"

somewhere in between. These differences can lead to a great deal of confusion when prescribing by generic name without spelling out every tiny detail. Emphasize to patients that a high-potency steroid should be used for a limited period of time, generally 4–8 weeks. When normalization of the skin has been achieved, switch them to a mild steroid such as hydrocortisone 1% or Locoid® 0.1% with tapering frequency of application down to once or twice a week or to total elimination. Patients who have frankly eroded or denuded skin may benefit from topical antibiotics. Silver sulfadiazine cream to which hydrocortisone or triamcinolone and menthol have been added may be soothing and promote regrowth of epidermis over ulcerated areas while suppressing the inflammation that can cause fissuring in the skin.

Skin atrophy is a serious problem with prolonged use of potent steroids, but each of the steroid preparations differs in its tendency to cause trouble. Creams cause comparatively greater atrophy than ointment preparations containing identical ingredients.[58] Newer, double-ester, nonfluorinated steroids may prove to be less atrophogenic than the older preparations,[58,59] but the package stuffers for prednicarbate and mometasone furoate still quote 8% and 6% incidence of mild skin atrophy for these compounds. Macrolide topical immune modulators (tacrolimus and pimecrolimus) seem to be free of the problem of skin atrophy, a fact that enhances their appeal for use on the apposed skin of the cleft.[60] These compounds may have some intrinsic antifungal activity as well.[61] I have had a very limited, good anecdotal experience with these compounds, but there are currently no published data on topical macrolide use in pruritus ani. Table 16-10 lists the

TABLE 16-10. Adverse reactions to topical steroids

Skin atrophy with telangiectasia, pseudoscars, purpura, striae, spontaneous bleeding
Tinea, impetigo, scabies incognito
Allergic contact dermatitis
Systemic absorption with adrenal suppression
Burning, itching, dryness from vehicle
Rebound worsening after withdrawal

potential complications of topical steroids, which are not to be taken lightly, and are all the more important because they are preventable complications of treatment excess.

Anal Tattooing

Every practice has a small number of patients who respond poorly to treatment and whose symptoms are severe enough to alter life and happiness. These refractory patients may benefit from a technique originally described by a Russian surgeon, but espoused in the United States by Wolloch and Dintsman[62] who described nine patients, eight of whom got relief after one treatment, one requiring a second injection to obtain a good result. Eusebio et al.[63] reported 23 patients: 13 with complete relief, 8 with incomplete relief but much improved, and 2 who were not improved, but who had presented with burning, not itching. Three cases of skin necrosis resulted in modification of their technique, and treatment of 11 subsequent patients was without complication with good result.[64] The modified technique consists of the intradermal and subcutaneous injection of the following solution with the patient under intravenous sedation in the prone jackknife position: 10 mL 1% methylene blue + 5 mL normal saline + 7.5 mL 0.25% bupivacaine with epinephrine (1/200,000) + 7.5 mL 0.5% lidocaine. Farouk and Lee[65] reported six patients treated with a similar volume to the modified technique of Eusebio et al. Five patients got substantial relief of symptoms with follow-up of 2–5 years. Three of the six required a repeat injection at 1, 3, and 5 years after the initial treatment.

I have personally used this technique on four patients, infiltrating the skin with the same solution as Eusebio et al. using a modified technique. I use a 30- or 27-gauge needle and infiltrate the skin as I would for cutaneous anesthesia with multiple injection sites sufficient to cover the perianal-involved skin up to the dentate line (Figure 16-14). All four of my patients have gotten results lasting at least 1 year, during which time all have had relative cutaneous hypoesthesia. They describe the sensation as having the side of one's face numb after a dental block. Certain individuals have found this sensation very disagreeable, so I am careful to warn them in detail before treatment. The skin changes of severe pruritus in all cases rapidly and dramatically regressed and resolved. In one case with return of skin sensation at about a year, the pruritus returned and required topical therapy to be reinstituted, but was milder and did not require repeat injection. The response of these patients during the time of hypalgesia lends some credence to the idea of skin trauma from nocturnal scratching of which patients are not aware.

Conclusion

Skin conditions around the anus are common and often poorly diagnosed and treated. The appearance of a lesion is rarely pathognomonic, but may place it into a diagnostic category

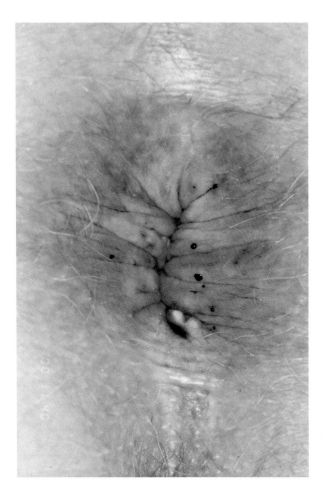

FIGURE 16-14. Tattooing with methylene blue is a simple technique to treat intractable itching that does not respond to traditional vigorous therapy. Patients experience hypalgesia and numbness of the perianal skin that can be bothersome, but rapid resolution of itching occurs and the chronic skin changes normalize quickly.

that can be either treated or investigated in a systematic way to arrive at a logical successful outcome. Follow-up of treatment plans, reevaluation of patients with chronic conditions, and reconsideration of ongoing prescriptions should be standard practice and help to avoid the pitfall of misdiagnosis.

References

1. Daniel GL, Longo WE, Vernava AM 3rd. Pruritus ani. Causes and concerns. Dis Colon Rectum 1994;37(7):670–674.
2. Corman ML. Colon and Rectal Surgery. 2nd ed. Philadelphia: Lippincott; 1989:287.
3. Verbov J. Pruritus ani and its management: a study and reappraisal. Clin Exp Dermatol 1984;9(1):46–52.
4. Quine WV. Quiddities: An Intermittently Philosophical Dictionary. Cambridge: Harvard University Press; 1987.
5. Bernhard JD. Itch: mechanisms and management of pruritus. New York: McGraw-Hill; 1994.
6. Stamos MJ, Hicks TC, eds. Pruritus Ani: Diagnosis and Treatment. New York: Thieme Medical Publishers; 1998.

7. Sherertz EF. Clinical pearl: symptomatic dermatographism as a cause of genital pruritus. J Am Acad Dermatol 1994;31(6): 1040–1041.

8. Bernhard JD, Kligman AM, Shelley WB. Dermographic pruritus: invisible dermographism. J Am Acad Dermatol 1995;33(2 pt 1): 322.

9. Caplan RM. The irritant role of feces in the genesis of perianal itch. Gastroenterology 1966;50(1):19–23.

10. Smith LE, Henrichs D, McCullah RD. Prospective studies on the etiology and treatment of pruritus ani. Dis Colon Rectum 1982;25(4):358–363.

11. Allan A, Ambrose NS, Silverman S, Keighley MR. Physiological study of pruritus ani. Br J Surg 1987;74(7):576–579.

12. Farouk R, Duthie GS, Pryde A, Bartolo DC. Abnormal transient internal sphincter relaxation in idiopathic pruritus ani: physiological evidence from ambulatory monitoring. Br J Surg 1994;81(4):603–606.

13. Eyers AA, Thomson JP. Pruritus ani: is anal sphincter dysfunction important in aetiology? Br Med J 1979;2(6204):1549–1551.

14. Dodi G, Pirone E, Bettin A, et al. The mycotic flora in proctological patients with and without pruritus ani. Br J Surg 1985; 72(12):967–969.

15. Alexander S. Dermatological aspects of anorectal disease. Clin Gastroenterol 1975;4(3):651–657.

16. Pirone E, Infantino A, Masin A, et al. Can proctological procedures resolve perianal pruritus and mycosis? A prospective study of 23 cases. Int J Colorectal Dis 1992;7(1):18–20.

17. Bowyer A, McColl I. A study of 200 patients with pruritus ani. Proc R Soc Med 1970;63(suppl):96–98.

17A. Weismann K, Sand Petersen C, Roder B. Pruritus ani caused by heto-hoemolytic streptocacel Acta Derm Venereal 1996;76:415.

18. Bowyer A, McColl I. Erythrasma and pruritus ani. Acta Derm Venereol 1971;51(6):444–447.

19. Sindhuphak W, MacDonald E, Smith EB. Erythrasma. Overlooked or misdiagnosed? Int J Dermatol 1985;24(2):95–96.

20. Baral J. Pruritus ani and *Staphylococcus aureus*. J Am Acad Dermatol 1983;9(6):962.

21. Dasan S, Neill SM, Donaldson DR, Scott HJ. Treatment of persistent pruritus ani in a combined colorectal and dermatological clinic. Br J Surg 1999;86(10):1337–1340.

22. Habif TP. Clinical Dermatology: A Color Guide to Diagnosis and Therapy. 3rd ed. St. Louis: Mosby; 1996.

23. Harrington CI, Lewis FM, McDonagh AJ, Gawkrodger DJ. Dermatological causes of pruritus ani. BMJ 1992;305(6859):955.

24. Bruynzeel DP. Dermatological causes of pruritus ani. BMJ 1992;305(6859):955.

25. Lochridge E Jr. Pruritis ani: perianal psoriasis. South Med J 1969;62(4):450–452.

26. Meffert JJ, Davis BM, Grimwood RE. Lichen sclerosus. J Am Acad Dermatol 1995;32(3):393–416; quiz 7–8.

27. Neill SM, Tatnall FM, Cox NH. Guidelines for the management of lichen sclerosus. Br J Dermatol 2002;147(4):640–649.

28. Wong YW, Powell J, Oxon MA. Lichen sclerosus. A review. Minerva Med 2002;93(2):95–99.

29. Powell JJ, Wojnarowska F. Lichen sclerosus. Lancet 1999;353 (9166):1777–1783.

30. Carli P, De Magnis A, Mannone F, Botti E, Taddei G, Cattaneo A. Vulvar carcinoma associated with lichen sclerosus. Experience at the Florence, Italy, Vulvar Clinic. J Reprod Med 2003;48(5): 313–318.

31. Carli P, Cattaneo A, De Magnis A, Biggeri A, Taddei G, Giannotti B. Squamous cell carcinoma arising in vulval lichen sclerosus: a longitudinal cohort study. Eur J Cancer Prev 1995; 4(6):491–495.

32. Byren I, Venning V, Edwards A. Carcinoma of the vulva and asymptomatic lichen sclerosus. Genitourin Med 1993;69(4): 323–324.

33. Assmann T, Becker-Wegerich P, Grewe M, Megahed M, Ruzicka T. Tacrolimus ointment for the treatment of vulvar lichen sclerosus. J Am Acad Dermatol 2003;48(6):935–937.

34. Bohm M, Frieling U, Luger TA, Bonsmann G. Successful treatment of anogenital lichen sclerosus with topical tacrolimus. Arch Dermatol 2003;139(7):922–924.

35. Friend WG. The cause and treatment of idiopathic pruritus ani. Dis Colon Rectum 1977;20(1):40–42.

36. Akl K. Yogurt-induced pruritus ani in a child. Eur J Pediatr 1992;151(11):867.

37. Murie JA, Sim AJ, Mackenzie I. The importance of pain, pruritus and soiling as symptoms of haemorrhoids and their response to haemorrhoidectomy or rubber band ligation. Br J Surg 1981;68(4):247–249.

38. Koblenzer CS. Psychologic and psychiatric aspects of itching. In: Bernhard JD, ed. Itch: Mechanisms and Management of Pruritus. New York: McGraw-Hill; 1994:347–365.

39. Andrews D, Grunau VJ. An uncommon adverse effect following bolus administration of intravenous dexamethasone. J Can Dent Assoc 1986;52(4):309–311.

40. Kligman AM, Frosch PJ. Steroid addiction. Int J Dermatol 1979;18(1):23–31.

41. Goldman L, Kitzmiller KW. Perianal atrophoderma from topical corticosteroids. Arch Dermatol 1973;107(4):611–612.

42. Alexander-Williams J. Pruritus ani. Br Med J (Clin Res Ed) 1983;287(6386):159–160.

43. Rohde H. Routine anal cleansing, so-called hemorrhoids, and perianal dermatitis: cause and effect? Dis Colon Rectum 2000; 43(4):561–563.

44. Thorp MA, Oliver SP, Kruger J, Prescott CA. Determination of the lowest dilution of aluminium acetate solution able to inhibit in vitro growth of organisms commonly found in chronic suppurative otitis media. J Laryngol Otol 2000;114(11):830–831.

45. Thorp MA, Kruger J, Oliver S, Nilssen EL, Prescott CA. The antibacterial activity of acetic acid and Burow's solution as topical otological preparations. J Laryngol Otol 1998;112(10): 925–928.

46. Thorp MA, Gardiner IB, Prescott CA. Burow's solution in the treatment of active mucosal chronic suppurative otitis media: determining an effective dilution. J Laryngol Otol 2000;114(6): 432–436.

47. Dibb WL. In vitro efficacy of Otic Domeboro against *Pseudomonas aeruginosa*. Undersea Biomed Res 1985;12(3): 307–313.

48. Sarmiento JM, Wolff BG, Burgart LJ, Frizelle FA, Ilstrup DM. Paget's disease of the perianal region: an aggressive disease? Dis Colon Rectum 1997;40(10):1187–1194.

49. Jensen SL, Sjolin KE, Shokouh-Amiri MH, Hagen K, Harling H. Paget's disease of the anal margin. Br J Surg 1988;75(11):1089–1092.

50. Helwig EB, Graham JH. Anogenital (extramammary) Paget's disease. A clinicopathological study. Cancer 1963;16:387–403.

51. Marchesa P, Fazio VW, Oliart S, Goldblum JR, Lavery IC. Perianal Bowen's disease: a clinicopathologic study of 47 patients. Dis Colon Rectum 1997;40(11):1286–1293.

52. Chang GJ, Berry JM, Jay N, Palefsky JM, Welton ML. Surgical treatment of high-grade anal squamous intraepithelial lesions: a prospective study. Dis Colon Rectum 2002;45(4):453–458.

53. Goldstone SE, Winkler B, Ufford LJ, Alt E, Palefsky JM. High prevalence of anal squamous intraepithelial lesions and squamous-cell carcinoma in men who have sex with men as seen in a surgical practice. Dis Colon Rectum 2001;44(5):690–698.

54. Goldman S, Glimelius B, Pahlman L. Anorectal malignant melanoma in Sweden. Report of 49 patients. Dis Colon Rectum 1990;33(10):874–877.

55. Brady MS, Kavolius JP, Quan SH. Anorectal melanoma. A 64-year experience at Memorial Sloan-Kettering Cancer Center. Dis Colon Rectum 1995;38(2):146–151.

56. Enker WE, Heilwell M, Janov AJ, et al. Improved survival in epidermoid carcinoma of the anus in association with preoperative multidisciplinary therapy. Arch Surg 1986;121(12):1386–1390.

57. McClatchey KD. Clinical Laboratory Medicine. 2nd ed. Philadelphia: Lippincott Williams & Wilkins; 2002.

58. Kerscher MJ, Korting HC. Comparative atrophogenicity potential of medium and highly potent topical glucocorticoids in cream and ointment according to ultrasound analysis. Skin Pharmacol 1992;5(2):77–80.

59. Kerscher MJ, Hart H, Korting HC, Stalleicken D. In vivo assessment of the atrophogenic potency of mometasone furoate, a newly developed chlorinated potent topical glucocorticoid as compared to other topical glucocorticoids old and new. Int J Clin Pharmacol Ther 1995;33(4):187–189.

60. Robinson N, Singri P, Gordon KB. Safety of the new macrolide immunomodulators. Semin Cutan Med Surg 2001;20(4):242–249.

61. Ling MR. Topical tacrolimus and pimecrolimus: future directions. Semin Cutan Med Surg 2001;20(4):268–274.

62. Wolloch Y, Dintsman M. A simple and effective method of treatment for intractable pruritus ani. Am J Proctol Gastroenterol Colon Rectal Surg 1979;30(1):34–36.

63. Eusebio EB, Graham J, Mody N. Treatment of intractable pruritus ani. Dis Colon Rectum 1990;33(9):770–772.

64. Eusebio EB. New treatment of intractable pruritus ani. Dis Colon Rectum 1991;34(3):289.

65. Farouk R, Lee PW. Intradermal methylene blue injection for the treatment of intractable idiopathic pruritus ani. Br J Surg 1997;84(5):670.

17
Sexually Transmitted Diseases

Charles B. Whitlow and Lester Gottesman

There are more than 25 diseases spread primarily by sexual means with an annual incidence of approximately 15 million cases in the United States.[1] In 1994, the overall cost related to major sexually transmitted diseases (STDs) was estimated to be 17 billion dollars. In the United Kingdom, the incidence of STDs has increased substantially over the past 6 years and has led to a new government strategy to counteract these increases.[2,3]

Site and route of infection determine the symptoms caused by STDs. Infections of the distal anal canal, anoderm, and perianal skin are similar to lesions in other parts of the genitalia and perineum caused by the same organisms. These are typically the result of anal receptive intercourse but in some instances represent contiguous spread from genital infections. Proctitis from sexually transmitted organisms is almost always from anal intercourse. Direct or indirect fecal–oral contact produces infection with organisms that cause proctocolitis or enteritis but are generally thought of as food or waterborne diseases instead of STDs. Included in this group are *Entamoeba histolytica*, *Campylobacter*, *Shigella*, *Giardia lamblia*, and hepatitis A. Although it seems that male homosexual activity and the use of the anorectum for sexual gratification is increasing, data regarding the frequency of these behaviors both past and present are limited. Current estimates are that less than 2% of adult males regularly practice anal receptive intercourse and between 2% to 10% participate in homosexual activity at any point in their life.[4] Between 5% and 10% of females engage in anal receptive intercourse "with some degree of regularity" and females seem to be more likely than men to have unprotected anal intercourse.[4]

Difficulty in correct diagnosis and appropriate treatment of STDs of the anorectum is caused by several factors. 1) The signs and symptoms of infection are more organ related than organism related so that no symptom or symptom complex or physical finding is diagnostic for many STDs. 2) The presence of more than one organism is not uncommon, especially with anogenital ulcerations. 3) Determining true pathogen from colonizing organisms may be difficult. 4) Lastly, there is a lack of rapid sensitive diagnostic tests for many STDs so that empiric treatment is frequently required.

This chapter discusses the STDs that are most often seen by colorectal surgeons. Entire texts are devoted to the STDs; however, we will confine most of our comments to the diagnosis, treatment, and prevention of the anorectal component of these infections. Infections, which manifest as one of the colitides, are covered in Chapter 43.

Overview of Anorectal Immunology

The optimal state of health of the anus requires the integrity of the skin which acts as the primary protection against invasive pathogens. The mucosa shed from the rectum contains immunoglobulin A which traps foreign antigens and expels them with stool, preventing them from reaching the anorectal crypt cells.[5] Cellular immunity is controlled by the Langerhans, or dendritic cells which communicate with the T cells through a complicated mechanism and essentially prime the T cells to identify foreign cells.[6] This then allows the entire complement of cell-mediated immunity to destroy that which is alien. Although study of anal immunology is still in its infancy, it seems that certain pathogens may alter the balance of cellular elements. It is known that whereas human papilloma virus (HPV) increases Langerhans cells, human immunodeficiency virus (HIV) may damage their effectiveness. In addition, pathogens such as HPV and herpes simplex virus (HSV) invade into the host cell, combining with cellular elements or the genome, thus evading surveillance mechanisms. In addition, in the case of HPV, the identifying foreign antigens are placed onto the frame of the new virus near the epidermis, where the virus normally sheds and where an attack by the host has little value.[7]

HIV is known to deplete cell-mediated immunity by depletion of T cells and destruction of Langerhans cells. This allows, through unknown mechanisms, propagation of oncogenic processes such as HPV to become dysplastic. The exact switches are not understood but seem to be related to the coexistence of perhaps HSV and the highly active antiretroviral therapy (HAART) drugs.

Breakdown of the mucous complex protecting the rectum is seen in various diseases contracted through anal intercourse. The physical act of intercourse abrades the mucous lining and delivers pathogens directly to the crypt and columnar cells allowing for easy entry. Depending on their mechanism of action, they may burrow into the cells (ameba) or proliferate on the cells without damaging them (*G. neisseria*). Invasive pathogens (*LGV*) unleash nefarious cytokines that can destroy the cell. The immune response is usually too late to contain an acute attack. In the case of recurrent viral attacks (HPV, HSV), it seems that the level of functioning T cells may have an impact on recurrence of warts or herpes outbreaks. The mechanics of anoreceptive intercourse, as compared with vaginal intercourse, almost always results in denuding of the protecting cellular and mucous layer of the anus and rectum.

Latex allergies, with condom use, may also be seen causing severe invasive and erosive proctitis and should be in the differential of a caustic burn to the rectum after sexual anoreceptive intercourse.

Diagnosis and Management of Bacterial Pathogens

Gonorrhea

Neisseria gonorrhoeae, the Gram-negative diplococcus (Figure 17-1) responsible for gonorrhea, was first described by Albert Neisser in 1879 from exudates from urethritis and cervicitis.[8] It is probably the most common bacterial STD affecting the anorectum. Whereas gonorrhea rates decreased over the last several decades, in the mid-1990s the incidence slowly increased to the current rate of about 650,000 cases per year. Similar recent increases have been noted in Canada and the United Kingdom.[9] Peak incidence for all forms of gonorrhea is in the late teens for females and early 20s for males. African-Americans have a 30-fold higher rate of infection than white Americans.

Infection from *N. gonorrhoeae* occurs in columnar, cuboidal, or noncornified epithelial lined cells of the urethra, endocervix, rectum, and pharynx and is frequently asymptomatic. The incubation period ranges from 3 days to 2 weeks. Untreated infection may lead to disseminated gonococcal infection with transient bacteremia, arthritis, and dermatitis. Rare but severe sequelae include endocarditis and meningitis.

Anorectal transmission in homosexual males and some females is by anoreceptive intercourse with an infected partner. Thirty-five to fifty percent of women with gonococcal cervicitis have concomitant rectal infection which is believed to be from contiguous spread from the genital infection.[10] Oral-anal sex has been suggested as another mode of anorectal gonococcal infection.[11] A large percentage of patients who culture positive for rectal gonorrhea are asymptomatic—up to 50% of males and 95% of females. Asymptomatic rectal infection constitutes the main reservoir of gonococcal disease in homosexual men.

Symptomatic anorectal gonococcal infection results in pruritus, tenesmus, bloody discharge, mucopurulent discharge, and/or severe pain. External inspection of the anus is generally unremarkable; however, nonspecific erythema and superficial ulceration may occur (Figure 17-2). Anoscopy reveals a thick purulent discharge, which classically is expressed from the anal crypts as pressure is applied externally on the anus. Nonspecific proctitis may be present with erythema, edema, friability, and pus. Diagnosis is confirmed by culture on selective media (Thayer-Martin or Modified New York City) incubated in a CO_2-rich environment and Gram's stain of directly visualized discharge.[12] The use of lubricants other than water may introduce antibacterial agents during anoscopy and decrease diagnostic yield. Nonculture detection of gonorrhea is being used more frequently especially in urethral and cervical infections. Nucleic acid amplification tests (NAATs) such as polymerase chain reaction

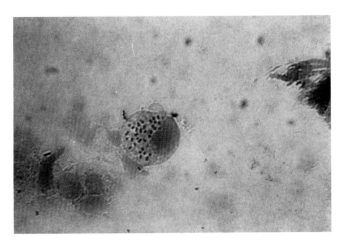

FIGURE 17-1. Gram-negative intracellular diplococcus.

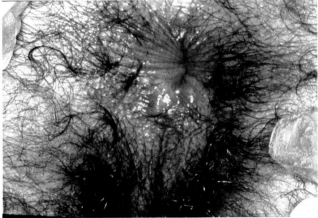

FIGURE 17-2. Anorectal gonorrhea.

(PCR) and ligase chain reaction (LCR) and nonamplified DNA probes provide sensitivities of greater than 95% but do not provide antibiotic susceptibility data. There are no NAATs currently licensed for detection of rectal gonorrhea.[13]

Because of the prevalence of penicillinase-producing *N. gonorrhoeae* starting in the 1970s, penicillin G is no longer the drug of choice for gonorrhea. The most current recommended treatment regimens from the Centers for Disease Control (CDC) were published in 2002 and are listed in Table 17-1. Since publication of these guidelines, cefixime has become unavailable in the United States. Alternative regimens include spectinomycin (2 g as a single intramuscular injection), other cephalosporins (ceftizoxime, cefoxitin, and cefotaxime), and other quinolones. Only a few isolates reported by the Gonococcal Isolate Surveillance Report in the past 10 years showed decreased susceptibility to the cephalosporins listed in Table 17-1.[15] Quinolone-resistant *N. gonorrhoeae* (QRNG) have been detected in the past decade with increasing frequency in Asia and the Pacific. In the United States, this is particularly important in Hawaii (where QRNG may account for as much as 14% of gonorrhea isolates) and California. In the United Kingdom, the overall rate of QRNG was reported at 9.8% for 2002.[16] Concurrent HIV infection does not alter treatment for anorectal gonorrhea. Because of the high rate of concomitant infection with chlamydia, patients treated for gonococcal infections should be given appropriate treatment for chlamydia at the same visit or measures to rule out chlamydial infection should be taken.

Routine follow-up at 3 months is no longer necessary because current treatment provides near 100% efficacy. Patients with persistent symptoms after treatment should be followed and cultured as should those treated with nonstandard antibiotics. Sexual partners from the past 60 days should be treated and patient should abstain from intercourse until treatment is completed and symptoms resolved.

Chlamydia/Lymphogranuloma Venereum

Chlamydia trachomatis is an obligate intracellular bacterium that is sexually transmitted and results in clinical infections that are similar to those caused by *N. gonorrhoeae*. Simultaneous infection with both organisms is common. Chlamydia is the most frequently reported STD in the United States with an annual incidence of about 3 million cases per year.[17] Aggressive screening programs are credited with the decline of the chlamydia infection rate from its peak of more than 4 million per year in the early 1970s.

Anorectal transmission of chlamydia is through anoreceptive intercourse although secondary involvement can occur as a late manifestation of genital infection. Different serovars of *C. trachomatis* produce differing clinical illness. Serovars D through K [non–lymphogranuloma venereum (LGV)] are responsible for proctitis and common genital infections. Lymphogranuloma venereum is caused by LGV serovars L1–L3. The incubation period for chlamydia is 5 days to 2 weeks. Non-LGV serovars are less invasive and cause mild proctitis (manifested by tenesmus, pain, and discharge) but asymptomatic infection is common. LGV serovars produce a much more aggressive infection with perianal, anal, and rectal ulceration. The proctitis produced can be difficult to distinguish from Crohn's disease (including microscopic findings of granulomas) with resulting rectal pain and discharge. Anoscopy and sigmoidoscopy demonstrate friable rectal mucosa, which is more severe in appearance (and extends above the rectum in some cases) in LGV strains.[18–20] Perianal abscesses, fistulas, and stricturing may also occur. Lymphadenopathy develops in draining nodal basins—iliac, perirectal, inguinal, and femoral—several weeks after initial infection. Large indurated matted nodes (Figure 17-3) and overlying erythema may produce a clinical picture similar to syphilis.

Diagnosis of chlamydia as the causative agent in proctitis can be difficult. Proper specimen collection increases diagnostic yield and consists of a cotton or Dacron swab with an inert shaft (plastic or metal). Specimen for tissue culture should be transported on specific medium and kept refrigerated or on ice until inoculated onto culture plates. Specimens that are to be tested by a nonculture technique are transported and stored in accordance with the test manufacturer's guidelines. In patients with a clinical presentation consistent with chlamydia proctitis, rectal Gram's stain showing polymorphonuclear leukocytes without visible gonococci is presumptive for a diagnosis of chlamydia.[20] Tissue culture for chlamydia is relatively insensitive and is not widely available because of cost and technical requirements.[21]

TABLE 17-1. Treatment of anorectal gonococcal infection[14]

One of the following as a single dose:	
Ceftriaxone	125 mg intramuscularly
Ciprofloxacin	500 mg orally
Ofloxacin	400 mg orally
Levofloxacin	250 mg orally
Cefixime	400 mg orally

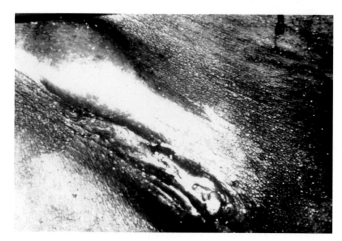

FIGURE 17-3. Inguinal adenopathy of LGV.

Antigen detection by direct fluorescent antibody (DFA) or enzyme immunoassay DFA is highly specific, widely available, and does not require rapid transportation or refrigeration. A trained microscopist is needed for interpretation. As with gonorrhea, newer NAATs are available. Their use is increasing in genital infection but unproven for anorectal chlamydia. A pilot study using both PCR and LCR techniques showed that these techniques can be effective for making this diagnosis but there are few additional data on the use of NAATs in anorectal chlamydia.[22]

The two recommended treatment regimens for rectal chlamydia (non-LGV) are azithromycin, 1 g orally as a single dose or doxycycline, 100 mg orally, twice a day for 7 days.[14] Alternative regimens include erythromycin (less effective, more gastrointestinal side effects), ofloxacin (7-day course, more expensive), or levofloxacin (7-day course, no data on efficacy). Treatment of LGV is with doxycycline or erythromycin for 21 days. In patients with HIV and LGV, prolonged therapy may be required. Management of sexual contacts is the same as for gonorrhea. Abstinence from sexual intercourse should last until 7 days after treatment with azithromycin or completion of 7 days of doxycycline.

Syphilis

Syphilis is an STD caused by the spirochete *Treponema pallidum* that can present in one of several progressive stages—primary (chancre or proctitis), secondary (condyloma lata), or tertiary. The incidence of syphilis had its recent peak of 107 cases per 100,000 people in the United States in 1991, but decreased to 2.2 per 100,000 in 2001, meaning that only 6103 cases were reported. A slight increase in primary and secondary syphilis cases reported occurred in 2002.[23] These low rates have led to a national plan for eliminating syphilis.[24]

The primary stage of anorectal syphilis appears within 2–10 weeks of exposure via anal intercourse. The chancre begins as a small papule that eventually ulcerates. Anal ulcers are frequently painful (in contrast to genital ulcers) and without exudates. They may be single or multiple (Figures 17-4 and 17-5) and located on the perianal skin, in the anal canal, or distal rectum. Differentiation from idiopathic anal fissures may be difficult. Painless but prominent lymphadenopathy is common. Proctitis from syphilis may occur with or without chancres.[18] Untreated lesions in this stage will usually heal in several weeks.

Hematogenous dissemination of untreated syphilis leads to a secondary stage that occurs 4–10 weeks after primary lesions appear. Nonspecific systemic symptoms from this infection include fever, malaise, arthralgias, weight loss, sore throat, and headache. A maculopapular rash is seen on the trunk and extremities. Condyloma lata, another secondary manifestation, are gray or whitish, wart-like lesions that appear adjacent to the primary chancre and are laden with spirochetes. Untreated, the symptoms of syphilis usually resolve after 3–12 weeks—of these patients, approximately one-fourth will have a relapse of symptoms in the first year. This is called early latent syphilis.

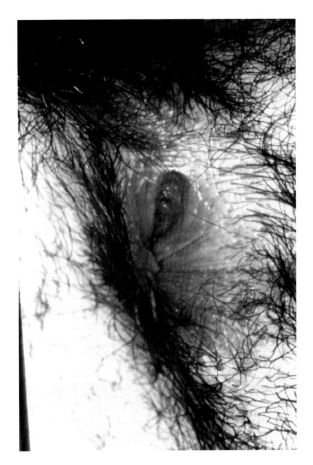

FIGURE 17-4. Solitary anal chancre.

Diagnosis in the primary or secondary stage is made by visualization of spirochetes on dark-field microscopic examination of scrapings from chancres (Figure 17-6). Alternatively, spirochetes may be demonstrated on Warthin-Starry silver stain of biopsy specimens. A direct fluorescent antibody test for *T. pallidum* (DFA-TP) is performed by some laboratories.[18,25] Serologic tests, rapid plasma reagin (RPR) and Venereal Disease Research Laboratory (VDRL), have a false-negative rate of up to 25% in primary syphilis and are

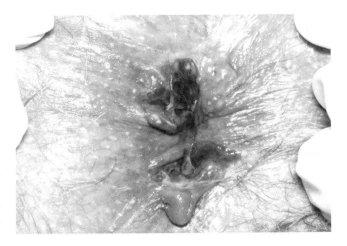

FIGURE 17-5. Multiple anal chancres.

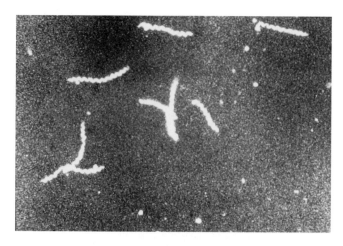

FIGURE 17-6. Spirochetes demonstrated on dark-field microscopy.

called nontreponemal tests because they are not specific for *T. pallidum* infection. Positive nontreponemal tests should be confirmed by a treponemal test such as the fluorescent treponemal antibody absorption test (FTA-ABS), which remains positive for life.

A single intramuscular injection of 2.4 million units of benzathine penicillin G is the treatment for primary and secondary syphilis. Penicillin-allergic patients are treated with doxycycline (100 mg orally, twice daily for 14 days) or tetracycline (500 mg orally, four times a day for 14 days). Follow-up serology (VDRL or RPR) should be checked at 6 months after therapy for HIV-negative patients and every 3 months for HIV-positive patients.[14] Treatment failures are re-treated with the same dose of penicillin but at weekly intervals for a total of 3 weeks. Partner notification, testing, and treatment depends on stage at diagnosis of the index case. At-risk partners include sexual contacts a) within the prior 3 months plus duration of symptoms for patients with primary syphilis; b) within the prior 6 months plus duration of symptoms for patients with secondary syphilis; and c) within the prior year for those with early latent syphilis.[26]

Chancroid

Chancroid is an ulcerating STD caused by the Gram-negative, facultative anaerobic bacillus *Haemophilus ducreyi*. Whereas there were approximately 5000 cases reported per year in the late 1980s and early 1990s in the United States, there were fewer that 200 cases reported in 1999.[1] It is much more common in developing countries with a global incidence estimated at 6 million.[27]

Transmission of *H. ducreyi* is strictly via sexual contacts through breaks in the skin during intercourse and results in genital ulcers. The initial manifestation (hour to days after exposure) is as infected tender papules with erythema that subsequently develop into pustules and then (days to weeks) become ulcerated and eroded. Multiple ulcers are common and are generally painful, especially in males. Although chancroid ulcers are most frequently located on the genitalia,

perianal abscesses and ulceration may occur. Anal ulcerations in females may be the result of drainage from adjacent genital infections. Differentiation of other ulcerating STDs cannot be made on gross appearance in most cases.[28] Painful inguinal adenopathy accompanies half of cases in males and is usually unilateral. Females are less likely to develop adenopathy from *H. ducreyi* infection.[29] Abscess formation may result, necessitating drainage. Besides causing genital ulcers, *H. ducreyi* facilitates transmission of HIV and vice versa.

Diagnosis of chancroid is made by Gram stain and culture of *H. ducreyi* (on selective medium agar) from the base of ulcers. Gram stain is only 40%–60% sensitive relative to culture and demonstrates nonmotile Gram-negative rods in small groups. *H. ducreyi* is difficult to culture and many laboratories in the United States are not equipped to perform this test. PCR is more sensitive than culture for detecting *H. ducreyi* but is not commercially available at this time.[30] Treatment for *H. ducreyi* is single-dose treatment with azithromycin (1 g, orally) or ceftriaxone (250 mg, intramuscularly). Alternatively, regimens include ciprofloxacin, 500 mg orally twice a day for 3 days or erythromycin 500 mg three times a day for 1 week.[14]

Granuloma Inguinale (Donovanosis)

Donovanosis is an ulcerating infection of the genitalia and anus caused by *Calymmatobacterium granulomatis* (also called *Donovania granulomatis*). Transmission is believed to occur from both sexual and nonsexual contact. It is rarely seen in the United States but is common in parts of Africa, South America, and Australia. Morphologic manifestations include an ulcerogranulomatous form (nontender, fleshy, beefy red ulcers), hypertrophic or verrucous lesions, necrotic ulcers, or cicatricial. Genital involvement is most common but contiguous involvement of the anorectum occurs. Development of sclerotic lesions causes anal stenosis.[31]

C. granulomatis cannot be cultured by routine techniques. Diagnosis can be made by tissue smear or biopsy that reveals Donovan bodies (small inclusions) within macrophages. Several antibiotic regimens have been recommended. The most recent CDC guidelines are doxycycline (100 mg orally, twice daily for 1 week) or trimethoprim-sulfamethoxazole (one 800 mg/160 mg tablet orally, twice a day for at least 3 weeks).[14] Alternative treatments include at least 3 weeks of ciprofloxacin, azithromycin, or erythromycin. Some authors believe azithromycin to be the preferred treatment.[31]

Diagnosis and Management of Viral Pathogens

Herpes Simplex Virus

HSV is a DNA virus of the family *Herpesviridae* that includes varicella-zoster virus, Epstein-Barr virus, and Cytomegalovirus. Herpes is the most prevalent STD in the United States with the current seroprevalence rate for HSV-2 estimated to be 20% for the general population.[32] Black females are the subgroup with the highest seroprevalence at 55%. Two serotypes of HSV are described. HSV-2 has been most associated with anogenital herpes infections. HSV-1 infection most often presents as labial, oral, or ocular lesions but accounts for about 30% of genital infections. Several recent reports have shown an increasing percentage of genital infections caused by HSV-1.[33,34] Asymptomatic infection with HSV is common.

Transmission is via close contact with an individual who is shedding the virus and infection results from penetration of mucosal surfaces or breaks in the skin. Productive infection causes viral replication within cells and cell death. Clinical infection presents first with systemic symptoms (fever, headache, myalgias), followed by local symptoms (pain, pruritus). Vesicles appear over the anogenital area, increase in number and size, and eventually ulcerate and coalesce (Figures 17-7 and 17-8). Vesicles and ulcerations heal over a mean time of 3 weeks.

Anorectal involvement by HSV-2 is acquired by anorectal intercourse and is second only to gonorrhea as a cause of proctitis in homosexual men. Herpetic infection of the anorectum results in severe anal pain, tenesmus, hematochezia, and rectal discharge. The proctitis seen is typically limited to the distal 10 cm of the rectum with diffuse friability. Simultaneous with infection, HSV moves through peripheral sensory nerves to sensory or autonomic nerve root ganglia. Sacral radiculopathy of the lower sacral roots from this infection causes sacral paresthesias and neuralgias, urinary retention, constipation, and impotence. Tender inguinal adenopathy occurs in half of patients with HSV proctitis.[35]

Herpes has the ability to persist in their host because of latency—the viral genome maintained in a stable condition in host cell nuclei. For HSV, the site of latent infection is the sensory ganglia of nerves innervating the site of infection. Reactivation of latent virus results in recurrent infection but the stimuli for this process are poorly understood.[36]

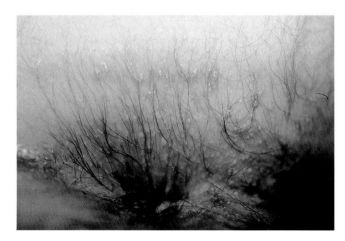

FIGURE 17-7. Perianal herpes.

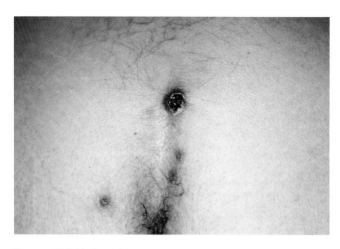

FIGURE 17-8. Perianal herpes.

Recurrent attacks are generally milder, shorter in duration, and without the constitutional symptoms that occur with initial infection.

Diagnosis is frequently made on clinical grounds alone. Cultures taken from ulcerations, rectal swabs, or biopsies confirm the diagnosis. Multinucleated giant cells with intranuclear inclusion bodies (ground-glass appearance) on Pap smear or Tzank prep are less sensitive than viral culture. Direct immunofluorescence has also been used for diagnosing HSV.[18] For cases in which cultures are not available, paired type-specific serology demonstrating seroconversion is diagnostic. In the past 5 years, the Food and Drug Administration (FDA) has approved several commercially available HSV serology tests. These tests have specificities and sensitivities of greater than 90% and are sure to become more frequently used in the diagnosis of HSV.[37,38] It should be noted that seroconversion may take several weeks after initial infection and repeat testing intervals are dependent on the particular serology kit used.[39]

Treatment of patients with anorectal herpes includes comfort measures such as warm soaks and oral analgesics. The only prospective, randomized trial of antiviral treatment for herpes proctitis demonstrated a shortened duration of symptoms and period of viral shedding with oral acyclovir 400 mg, five times a day for 10 days.[40] A three times per day dosing has been shown to be effective for genital herpes but has not been evaluated for herpes proctitis.[41] Other antiviral agents (valacyclovir and famciclovir) used for genital herpes are most likely effective for HSV proctitis at the same doses used for genitourinary infection but also lack clinical studies for this indication. Severe mucocutaneous HSV infection in which the patient cannot tolerate oral medication warrants intravenous acyclovir. Topical acyclovir has limited efficacy and is not recommended. Treatment of initial episodes of HSV do not prevent latency, asymptomatic viral shedding, or the course of subsequent episodes. Recurrent episodes may be treated with oral antiviral agents. Valacyclovir (500 mg twice a day) and acyclovir (200 mg five times a day) have demonstrated equal efficacy in treating genitourinary HSV recurrences.[42] Prompt initiation of treatment at onset of symptoms of HSV recurrence reduces duration of symptoms and healing times. Patients who experience more than five recurrences per year are considered for suppressive treatment. Valacyclovir, acyclovir, and famciclovir have all demonstrated 70% or greater reduction compared with placebo.

As with all STDs, counseling of patients with HSV is an important part of treatment and prevention.[41,42] Specific items that should be addressed are: 1) infectivity is not isolated to symptomatic outbreaks; most sexual HSV transmission occurs during asymptomatic periods; 2) latent infection and the risk of recurrence; suppressive therapy does not eliminate latent infection or viral shedding; 3) abstinence is recommended while lesions are present. Condoms are advised for all other times although they likely provide incomplete protection. Most recently, once-daily administration of valacyclovir has been shown to reduce the risk of HSV-2 transmission between HSV-2-seropositive patients and their seronegative sexual partners.[43]

Human Papilloma Virus

HPV is a DNA papovirus. Although HPV is not a reportable STD, it is probably the most common STD in the United States with an estimated incidence of more than 5 million cases per year (in contrast to chlamydia, being the most common of the reportable STDs).[1] There are more than 80 subtypes of HPV, almost one-third of which cause anogenital warts. Subtypes 6 and 11 are the most common of the low-risk HPV subtypes, whereas subtypes 16 and 18 have the greatest associated risk of anal dysplasia and anal cancer. Transmission is via sexual contact with infected individuals with or without gross lesions, and asymptomatic infection is common. Perianal involvement can occur in the absence of receptive anal intercourse.

Presenting complaints of perianal or anal condyloma acuminata include presence of a growth, pruritus, bleeding, chronic drainage, pain, and difficulty with hygiene. Physical examination is generally all that is required for diagnosis and shows the characteristic gray or pink fleshy, cauliflower-like growths of variable size in the perianal region (Figure 17-9). Anoscopy is an integral part of the evaluation. In the anal canal, the lesions tend to be small papules and involvement above the dentate line is rare. Examination should include the genitalia (including vaginal speculum examination and Pap smear), perineum, and groin folds.

The goal of treatment of condyloma acuminata is destruction or removal of all gross disease while minimizing morbidity, although this does not ensure eradication of infection. Tangential excision, cryotherapy, or fulguration of small lesions can be performed as an office procedure with a local anesthetic with little discomfort or inconvenience to the patient. Larger lesions are treated by electrodesiccation. The patient is placed in the lateral or prone jackknife position.

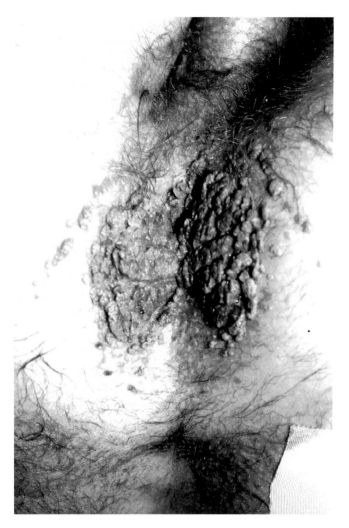

FIGURE 17-9. Perianal condyloma.

Depending on the size and number of lesions, local, spinal, or general anesthesia is used. The superficial-most layer of the condyloma is fulgurated with the electrosurgery tip until the lesion takes on a gray-white appearance. This is followed by curettage or simply abrading the fulgurated tissue with gauze. The process is repeated until the condyloma is completely removed without burning into the deep dermis or subcutaneous fat. Pedunculated warts are simply transected at their base. Tissue from HIV+ patients, recurrent lesions, flat lesions, or those that are suspicious (ulcerated, friable, hypervascular) should be sent for histopathologic evaluation. Topical 5% lidocaine is helpful in decreasing postoperative pain. Oral analgesics and daily cleansing with mild soap and water are all that is required for postoperative care in most patients. Silver sulfadiazine or mupirocin are applied in cases in which postoperative bacterial infection is suspected. Overall condyloma clearance rates for surgical techniques range from 60% to 90% with recurrence rates of 20% to 30%.[44]

The patient can apply topical agents such as podofilox and imiquimod but neither is approved for use in the anal canal.

Podofilox is the purified active component of the antimitotic plant resin podophyllin and is available as a 0.5% gel or solution. A treatment cycle consists of twice-daily application for 3 days followed by no treatment for 4 days. This is repeated for up to 1 month. Toxicity concerns are less than those with podophyllin and clearance rates for condyloma of 35%–80% have been reported. Recurrence rates in patients treated with podofilox are 10%–20%.[44–48] Imiquimod is an immune response modifier that increases local production of interferon. Complete response can be expected in 50% of patients treated with imiquimod with 11% of patients experiencing a recurrence.[44,49–51] It is applied at bedtime three times a week, left in place for 6–8 hours, and then removed by washing. Treatment may take up to 16 weeks. One study demonstrated no benefit to increased dosing frequency (from once to two or three times daily).[52] Side effects of imiquimod include pain, burning, itching, and ulceration which may require cessation of therapy. Imiquimod is used 1) as initial treatment with electrodesiccation reserved for those who have incomplete response, or 2) after destructive treatment and epithelial healing to treat remaining disease or decrease recurrence. Although there are no published randomized data to support this use, one of the authors (L.G.) has noted substantial diminution of wart recurrence (unpublished data). Currently, imiquimod is not approved for anal canal use but this application is being investigated.[53] Trichloracetic acid is applied topically and is useful for treating small lesions in the anal canal. Topical and intralesional interferon have been used to treat condyloma acuminata with mixed results. Other agents that have been used to treat anogenital condyloma but are not in widespread use include 5-FU cream, cidofovir, and autologous vaccine.

Bushke and Loewenstein first described giant condyloma acuminata (GCA) in 1925. They are most associated with HPV types 6 and 11 but histologically demonstrate some differences from ordinary condyloma—marked papillomatosis, acanthosis, thickened rete ridges, and increased mitotic activity. The substantial percentage of cases with in situ or invasive squamous cell cancers have led to speculation that GCA represents part of a continuum from condyloma to invasive squamous cell cancer.

Wide local excision with a 1-cm margin is the treatment of choice for these lesions. Local tissue flaps or grafted skin may be required to repair surgical defects. Abdominal-perineal resection has been used for GCA involving the anal sphincters. Chemoradiation is also an option in the treatment of GCA, especially in those patients who are poor surgical candidates or in whom clear surgical margin are not attainable.[54] Complete regression of GCA with chemoradiation has been reported.[55]

HPV, Anal Intraepithelial Dysplasia, and Anal Cancer

Although it is clear that HPV has a significant role in the development of cervical cancer, its significance in the development of anal cancer and its presumed precursor (anal

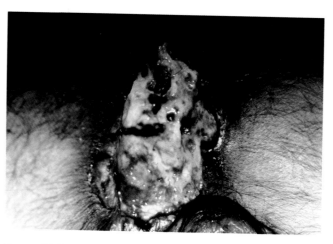

FIGURE 17-10. Anal cancer in an HIV-positive patient.

intraepithelial dysplasia) are not as well defined (Figure 17-10). Histologic and epidemiologic similarities between the two exist. Histologically, the anal canal resembles the cervix in that they are both transition zones from columnar epithelium to squamous epithelium. Epidemiologic studies before the HIV infection epidemic showed the incidence of anal cancer in homosexual males to be 12.5–37 per 100,000 in the United States.[56] This is similar to the incidence of cervical cancer prior to routine Pap testing. The risk of anal cancer developing in an HIV+ homosexual male is estimated to be 38 times that of the general population and twice the risk of an HIV− homosexual male.[56,57] HPV infection has been reported in 93% of HIV+ homosexual males compared with 60% of HIV− homosexual males.[54]

Anal cytology has been suggested as a screening tool for detecting patients with anal dysplasia. Applying the current cervical cytology terminology, specimens are designated normal, atypical squamous cells of indeterminate significance (ASCUS), low-grade squamous intraepithelial lesions (LSIL), or high-grade squamous intraepithelial lesions (HSIL). The benefit and best timing of this screening are undetermined. Evaluation and treatment algorithms as well as recommended testing schedules have been reported.[58,59] One such evaluation and treatment algorithm recommends high-resolution (with acetowhitening and staining with Lugol's solutions) anoscopy with biopsy.[59] Subsequent treatment is based on histologic findings which are typically reported as normal or AIN (anal epithelial neoplasia) I, II, or III. Options for treatment include local destruction (with topical agents, cryotherapy, or fulguration), excision, or observation. However, there are limitations of our understanding of the relationship among HPV, AIN, and anal cancer that prevent the dogmatic recommendation and widespread acceptance of such an approach. First, the incidence and predictability of the progression of AIN to invasive cancer is unclear.[60,61] The lack of inter- and intraobserver agreement in the interpretation of AIN no doubt contributes to this lack of understanding.[62] Second, data demonstrating efficacy (defined as long-term removal of AIN, prevention of anal cancer) of treatment is lacking. There is no evidence that destroying AIN III has any impact on survival. Chang et al.[63] reported 37 patients with HSIL who underwent incisional biopsy and fulguration. Staged procedures were performed in patients with circumferential disease. Morbidity was mostly uncontrolled pain that lasted a mean of 2.9 weeks. Recurrence of HSIL at 12 months was 79% in HIV+ patients. The absence of established benefit combined with the morbidity of treatment lead us and others to the recommendation that AIN (regardless of grade) be observed unless there are gross or ulcerated lesions present. Clinical trials are needed to establish and justify the benefit of more aggressive treatment. It is our belief that because the acquisition of anal cytology specimens require no particular expertise, this procedure should remain the domain of the patients' primary managing physicians who are most likely to have frequent contact with these patients (internist, general practitioner, infectious disease specialist). Patients with abnormal cytology should be referred to the colon and rectal surgeon who should evaluate patients with staining and magnification if possible to determine if biopsy or excision is required (Table 17-2).

TABLE 17-2. Algorithm for management of patients with abnormal anal cytology

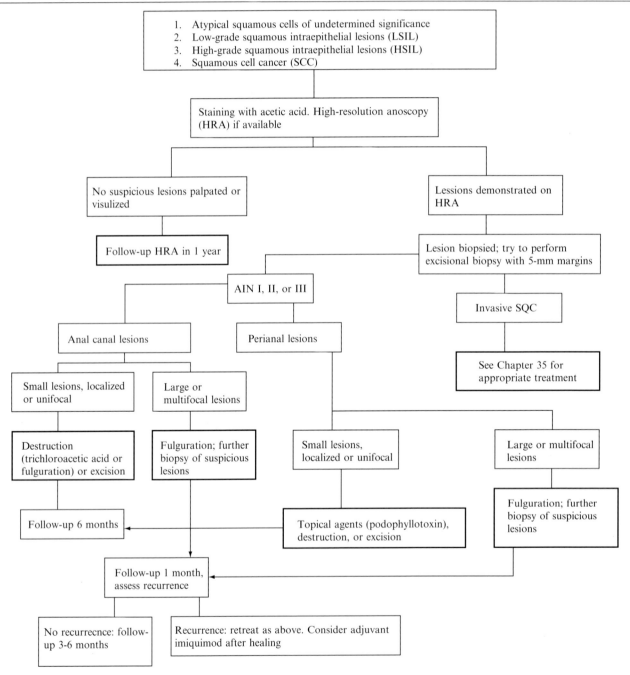

Two additional comments with regard to the association of HPV, HIV, and AIN should be made. First, the use of HAART (discussed in more detail later in the section on HIV) does not reduce the incidence of AIN.[64] The clinical implications of this fact are: a) anal cytology screening should not be stopped just because a patient is treated with HAART; and b) with HIV patients living longer secondary to HAART, the incidence of anal cancers may increase. Second, the prevalence of HPV and AIN is high in HIV-positive males with CD4+ counts less than 500×10^6 cells/L even in the absence of a history of anal intercourse.[65] These patients should also be considered for cytologic screening.

Molluscum Contagiosum

The molluscum contagiosum virus is a member of the poxvirus family and causes a benign papular condition of the skin. Transmission is by sexual and nonsexual contact. The incubation period is 1–6 months, followed by development of 2- to 6-mm flesh-colored, umbilicated papules.[66] Symptoms are uncommon although pruritus or tenderness may occur. Immunocompromised hosts such as those with HIV are more prone to infection with molluscum contagiosum (compared with HIV negative) and may have a more severe form of the disease with hundreds of lesions. Diagnosis is usually made on clinical grounds but excisional biopsy demonstrates enlarged epithelial cell with intracytoplasmic molluscum bodies. Treatment is generally through eradication with curettage, electrodesiccation, or cryotherapy. Podophyllotoxin (0.5%) and imiquimod (5%) have both been used as self-applied topical preparations with success.[67,68] Neither is FDA approved for this use.

HIV and the Acquired Immunodeficiency Syndrome

Infection from the HIV (at that time called human t-lymphotropic virus) related to acquired immunodeficiency syndrome (AIDS) was first described in 1983.[69] The most current data available show that in 2001 there were approximately 344,000 people in the United States with AIDS and another 162,000 with HIV infection not meeting the criteria for AIDS.[70] Cumulative totals showed 807,075 cases of AIDS in the United States through 2001 and a death rate of 57% in this group. Whereas the incidence of HIV infection has apparently leveled, the numbers of new AIDS cases and deaths from AIDS have decreased. This is in large part attributable to HAART—combinations of potent anti-HIV drugs that are nucleoside analogs, non-nucleoside reverse transcriptase inhibitors, or protease inhibitors. Table 17-3 shows the current classification system for patients who are HIV positive.

Surgery for anorectal diseases is the most common indication for surgery in HIV-infected patients and in 5% of patients whose anorectal complaints are the presenting symptom of their HIV infection.[72] Most of the indications for surgery are common to the population at large but some are unique to

TABLE 17-3. Revised classification system for HIV and AIDS[71]

CD4+ T lymphocyte categories
Category 1: ≥500 cells/μL
Category 2: 200–499 cells/μL
Category 3: <200 cells/μL

Clinical categories
Category A: HIV positive; asymptomatic; persistent generalized lymphadenopathy
Category B: Symptomatic conditions not listed in clinical category C; are conditions that are attributed to HIV infection; or conditions that have a clinical course or require management that is complicated by HIV infection. Examples include: bacillary angiomatosis, oropharyngeal or vulvovaginal candidiasis, cervical dysplasia, diarrhea (more than 1 month in duration), more than one episode of herpes zoster, pelvic inflammatory disease, peripheral neuropathy
Category C: Diagnoses included in the AIDS surveillance case definition—candidiasis (pulmonary or esophageal), invasive cervical cancer, Coccidiomycosis, extrapulmonary cryptococcosis, chronic intestinal cryptosporidiosis, Cytomegalovirus disease (other than liver, spleen, nodes) or retinitis, HIV-encephalopathy, HSV (chronic ulcers, pulmonary, or esophageal), histoplasmosis (disseminated or extrapulmonary), isosporiasis (chronic intestinal), Kaposi's sarcoma, Burkitt's lymphoma, immunoblastic lymphoma, primary brain lymphoma, *Mycobacterium avium* complex or any mycobacterium species other than *M. tuberculosis* (extrapulmonary or disseminated), *M. tuberculosis*, *Pneumocystis carinii* pneumonia, progressive focal leukoencephalopathy, recurrent *Salmonella septicemia*, toxoplasmosis of the brain, HIV wasting syndrome.

	Clinical categories		
CD4+ categories	A1	B1	**C1**
	A2	B2	**C2**
	A3	**B3**	**C3**

Bolded groups are defined as AIDS.

AIDS patients. Several studies demonstrate poor wound healing and increased morbidity in the surgical treatment of anorectal disease in AIDS patients.[72–74] Delayed or failed wound healing has been associated with presence of AIDS, decreased absolute leukocyte count, and decreased CD4 count. Morandi et al.[73] found that at 32 weeks after hemorrhoidectomy, 50% of AIDS patients had incompletely healed wounds. The overall complication rate was significantly higher in the AIDS group than in HIV+ patients without AIDS. Lord[75] reported decreased wound healing in HIV+ patients with T lymphocyte count of less than 50. Others have shown longer interval and decreased complete wound healing in HIV+ patients with CD4+ T lymphocyte counts of less than 200.[74] The studies reviewed above describe patients who were not treated with HAART. There is a lack of data describing wound healing in anorectal surgery since the widespread use of HAART; however, the observation of the authors is that compensated HIV+ patients are at no significant risk of increased complications from anorectal surgery. Other factors to be considered in selecting appropriate treatment include any untreatable diarrheal conditions, degree of existing fecal incontinence, and the effect of the proposed surgical procedure on incontinence.

Anal fissures that occur in HIV+ patients must be distinguished from idiopathic AIDS-related anal ulcers (Figure 17-11) and ulcerating STDs such as HSV or syphilis. Anal

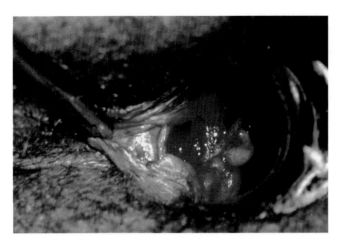

FIGURE 17-11. AIDS anal ulcer.

fissures in this patient population are indistinguishable from those in the general population and their treatment is similar—initial conservative management with surgery for treatment failures.[76,77] Treatment of fissures in HIV+ patients is modified by the factors described above and include controlling diarrhea when possible and encouraging abstinence from anoreceptive intercourse.

Although data on the incidence of AIDS-related anal ulcers are lacking, it seems that they are less common with HAART because the lesions are most frequently associated with clinical AIDS and lower CD4+ counts. These ulcers can be distinguished from typical anal fissures because they are more proximal in the anal canal (frequently above the dentate line or anorectal ring), broader based, deeply ulcerating with destruction of sphincter planes, and may demonstrate mucosal bridging. Debilitating pain is a common presenting symptom of these ulcers. Surgical debridement allows for adequate drainage of feculent or purulent material trapped in the ulcer and removal of necrotic debris. Biopsy and culture identify potentially treatable causes for ulceration—malignancy, acid-fast bacilli, HSV, *H. ducreyi*, *T. pallidum*. Cytomegalovirus has been cultured from these ulcers by some authors but is apparently not causal and therefore does not require treatment. Intralesional injection with steroids (methylprednisolone 80–160 mg, in 1 cc 0.25% bupivacaine) provides relief in the majority of patients but not healing.[78] Those who have persistent pain are reinjected.

Perianal suppurative diseases are common conditions in AIDS patients. Abscesses should be drained using small incisions, and placement of a mushroom catheter will lessen recurrent sepsis. Broad-spectrum antibiotics should be given in immune-compromised patients especially if cellulitis is present. Culture (to include mycobacterium) and histopathologic evaluation will help identify infection from atypical organisms and malignancy.

Nadal et al.[74] reported on fistulotomies performed in 31 HIV+ patients. Seven patients had failure of wound healing and all had clinical AIDS, CD4+ counts of less than 200, and

absolute leukocyte counts of less than 3000/mm³. Based on this, the authors treat anal fistulas in AIDS patients with high viral loads and low CD4+ counts similar to Crohn's patients. Draining setons are placed liberally with selective use of fistulotomy for low uncomplicated fistulas. Fistulotomy in HIV+ patients with AIDS and normal CD4+ counts is based on criteria similar to HIV− patients.

Thrombosed external hemorrhoids in patients with AIDS are treated the same as for HIV− patients. Acute thrombosis (24–48 hours after onset of symptoms) is treated with excision. Subacute thrombosis (longer than 48 hours from symptom onset) is treated conservatively with sitz baths and oral analgesics.

Internal hemorrhoids present with symptoms of bleeding or prolapse. Initial treatment in patients with AIDS is with a high fiber diet and bulking agents. Proximal colonic sources of bleeding should be excluded via colonoscopy. Patients who fail initial conservative measures are treated with rubber band ligation or infrared coagulation. Other nonoperative techniques such as bipolar coagulation, cryotherapy, or injection sclerotherapy are acceptable. There are conflicting recommendations for operative treatment of hemorrhoids published within the last decade. In a retrospective study, Hewitt et al.[79] found no difference in wound healing between HIV+ and HIV− patients. The mean CD4+ count was 301 but they classified 81% of patients as having AIDS based on symptoms or CD4 count less than 200. In the discussion, the authors comment that the majority of their patients were well nourished and otherwise healthy. They conclude that HIV status should not alter the indications for surgery in patients with symptomatic hemorrhoids. In contrast, as mentioned above, Morandi et al.[73] prospectively evaluated healing time after hemorrhoidectomy. Functional status and presence of AIDS were the two factors that correlated with poor wound healing. AIDS patients with nonhealing had a mean CD4+ count of 79. Unfortunately, they do not comment on relief of hemorrhoid symptoms. It seems that asymptomatic HIV+ patients who do not meet the clinical or CD4+ count diagnostic criteria for AIDS (see Table 17-2) can be treated with hemorrhoidectomy with the expectation that they will have good symptomatic relief and normal wound healing. AIDS patients with more advanced disease (clinical category C) or low CD4+ counts (especially less than 100) are at increased risk for wound healing problems. The benefit of symptomatic relief may still warrant performing surgical treatment in this group.[76]

References

1. Centers for Disease Control and Prevention. Tracking the hidden epidemics. Trends in STDs in the United States. April 2001:1–26.
2. British Medical Association. Sexually transmitted infections. February 2002:1–25.
3. Kinghorn G. A sexual health and HIV strategy for England. Br Med J 2001;323:243–244.

4. Halperin DT. Heterosexual anal intercourse: prevalence, cultural factors, and HIV infection and other health risks. Part 1. AIDS Patient Care STDS 1999;13:717–730.

5. Kozlowski PA, Neutra MR. The role of mucosal immunity in prevention of HIV transmissions. Curr Mol Med 2003;3: 217–228.

6. Sobhani I, Walker F, Aparicio T, et al. Effect of anal epidermoid cancer-related viruses on the dendritic (Langerhans') cells of the human anal mucosa. Clin Cancer Res 2002;8:2862–2869.

7. Middleton K, Peh W, Southern S, et al. Organization of human papillomavirus productive cycle during neoplastic progression provide a basis for selection of diagnostic markers. J Virol 2003;77:10186–10201.

8. Kampmeier RH. Identification of the gonococcus by Albert Neisser. Sex Transm Dis 1978;5:71–72.

9. Hansen L, Wong T, Perrin M. Gonorrhoea resurgence in Canada. Int J STD AIDS 2003;14:727–731.

10. Hook EW III, Handsfield HH. Gonococcal infection in the adult. In: Holmes KK, Sparling PR, Mardh PA, et al., eds. Sexually Transmitted Diseases. New York: McGraw-Hill; 1999:451–466.

11. McMillan A, Young H, Moyes A. Rectal gonorrhoea in homosexual men: source of infection. Int J STD AIDS 2000;11:284–287.

12. Ison C, Martin D. Gonorrhea. In: Morse SA, Ballard RC, Holmes KK, Moreland AA, eds. Atlas of Sexually Transmitted Diseases and AIDS. Edinburgh: Mosby; 2003:109–125.

13. Young H, Manavi K, McMillan A. Evaluation of ligase chain reaction for the non-cultural detection of rectal and pharyngeal gonorrhea in men who have sex with men. Sex Transm Infect 2003;79:484–486.

14. Centers for Disease Control and Prevention. Sexually transmitted diseases treatment guidelines 2002. MMWR 2002;51 (RR-6):1–77.

15. Centers for Disease Control and Prevention. Sexually transmitted disease surveillance 2002 supplement. Gonococcal isolate surveillance project annual report. Atlanta, Georgia: U.S. Department of Health and Human Services; October, 2003.

16. Fenton KA, Ison C, Johnson AP, et al. Ciprofloxacin resistance in Neisseria gonorrhoeae in England and Wales in 2002. Lancet 2003;361:1867–1868.

17. Cates W. Estimates of the incidence and prevalence of sexually transmitted diseases in the United States. Sex Transm Dis 1999;26(supplement):S2–7.

18. Rampalo AM. Diagnosis and treatment of sexually acquired proctitis and proctocolitis: an update. Clin Infect Dis 1999;28 (suppl 1):S84–90.

19. Gregory A, Gottesman L. Sexually transmitted and infectious diseases. In: Beck DE, Wexner SD, eds. Fundamentals of Anorectal Surgery. London: WB Saunders; 1998:414–431.

20. Stamm W. Chlamydia trachomatis infections of the adult. In: Holmes KK, Sparling PR, Mardh PA, et al., eds. Sexually Transmitted Diseases. New York: McGraw-Hill; 1999:407–422.

21. Schacter J, Stephens R. Infections caused by Chlamydia trachomatis. In: Morse SA, Ballard RC, Holmes KK, Moreland AA, eds. Atlas of Sexually Transmitted Diseases and AIDS. Edinburgh: Mosby; 2003:73–96.

22. Golden MR, Astete SG, Galvan R, et al. Pilot study of COBAS PCR and ligase chain reaction for detection of rectal infections due to Chlamydia trachomatis. J Clin Microbiol 2003;41:2174–2175.

23. Centers for Disease Control and Prevention. Primary and secondary syphilis—United States 2002. MMWR 2003;52: 1117–1120.

24. Centers for Disease Control and Prevention. The national plan to eliminate syphilis from the United States. Atlanta: U.S. Department of Health and Human Services; 1999:1–84. Available at: http://www.cdc.gov/stopsyphilis/plan.pdf.

25. Cox D, Liu H, Moreland A, Levine W. Syphilis. In: Morse SA, Ballard RC, Holmes KK, Moreland AA, eds. Atlas of Sexually Transmitted Diseases and AIDS. Edinburgh: Mosby; 2003:23–51.

26. Kohl KS, Farley T, Ewell J, Scioneaux J. Usefulness of partner notification for syphilis control. Sex Transm Dis 1999;26:201–207.

27. Spinola SM, Bauer ME, Munson RS. Immunopathogenesis of Haemophilus ducreyi infection (chancroid). Infect Immun 2002;70:1667–1676.

28. DiCarlo RP, Martin DH. The clinical diagnosis of genital ulcer disease in men. Clin Infect Dis 1997;25:292–298.

29. Ballard R, Morse S. Chancroid. In: Morse SA, Ballard RC, Holmes KK, Moreland AA, eds. Atlas of Sexually Transmitted Diseases and AIDS. Edinburgh: Mosby; 2003:53–71.

30. Orle KA, Gates CA, Martin DH, et al. Simultaneous PCR detection of Haemophilus ducreyi, Treponema pallidum, and herpes simplex virus types 1 and 2 from genital ulcers. J Clin Microbiol 1996;34:49–54.

31. O'Farrell N. Donovanosis. Sex Transm Dis 2002;78:452–457.

32. Fleming DT, McQuillan GM, Johnson RE, et al. Herpes simplex virus type 2 in the United States, 1976 to 1994. N Engl J Med 1997;337:1105–1111.

33. Roberts CM, Pfister JR, Spear SJ. Increasing proportion of herpes simplex virus type 1 as a cause of genital herpes infection in college students. Sex Transm Dis 2003;30:797–800.

34. Lafferty WE. The changing epidemiology of HSV-1 and HSV-2 and implications for serological testing. Herpes 2002;9:51–55.

35. Goodell SE, Quinn TC, Mkrtichian E, et al. Herpes simplex virus proctitis in homosexual men. Clinical, sigmoidoscopic, and histopathological features. N Engl J Med 1983;308:868–871.

36. Pertel PR, Spear PG. Biology of herpesviruses. In: Holmes KK, Sparling PR, Mardh PA, et al., eds. Sexually Transmitted Diseases. New York: McGraw-Hill; 1999:269–283.

37. Wald A, Ashley-Morrow R. Serological testing for herpes simplex virus (HSV)-1 and HSV-2 infection. Clin Infect Dis 2002;35 (suppl 2):S173–182.

38. Slomka MJ. Current diagnostic techniques in genital herpes: their role in controlling the epidemic. Clin Lab 2000;46:591–607.

39. Ashley RL. Performance and use of HSV type-specific serology test kits. Herpes 2002;9:38–45.

40. Rompalo AM, Mertz GJ, Davis LG, et al. A double-blind study of oral acyclovir for the treatment of first episode herpes simplex virus proctitis in homosexual men. JAMA 1988;259:2879–2881.

41. Wald A. New therapies and prevention strategies for genital herpes. Clin Infect Dis 1999;28(suppl):S4–13.

42. Patel R. Progress in meeting today's demands in genital herpes: an overview of current management. J Infect Dis 2002:186(suppl 1):S47–56.

43. Corey L, Wald A, Patel R, et al. Once-daily valacyclovir to reduce the risk of transmission of genital herpes. N Engl J Med 2004;350:11–20.

44. Wiley DJ, Douglas J, Beutner K, et al. External genital warts: diagnosis, treatment, and prevention. Clin Infect Dis 2002; 35(suppl 2):S210–224.

45. von Krogh G, Longstaff E. Podophyllin office therapy against condyloma should be abandoned. Sex Transm Infect 2001;77: 409–412.

46. von Krogh G, Lacey CJN, Gross G, et al. European course on HPV associated pathology: guidelines for primary care physicians for the diagnosis and management of anogenital warts. Sex Transm Infect 2000;76:162–168.

47. Greenberg MD, Rutledge LH, Reid R, et al. A double-blind, randomized trial of 0.5% podofilox and placebo for the treatment of genital warts in women. Obstet Gynecol 1991;77:735–739.

48. Edwards L, Ferenczy A, Eron L, et al. Self-administered topical 5% imiquimod cream for external anogenital warts. Arch Dermatol 1998;134:25–30.

49. Tyring S, Edwards L, Cherry LK, et al. Safety and efficacy of 0.5% podofilox gel in the treatment of anogenital warts. Arch Dermatol 1998;134:33–38.

50. Maitland JE, Maw R. An audit of patients who have received imiquimod cream 5% for the treatment of anogenital warts. Int J STD AIDS 2000;11:268–270.

51. Beutner K, Tyring SK, Trofatter KF Jr, et al. Imiquimod, a patient-applied immune-response modifier for treatment of external genital warts. Antimicrob Agents Chemother 1998;42:789–794.

52. Fife KH, Ferenczy A, Douglas JM, et al. Treatment of external warts in men using 5% imiquimod cream applied three times a week, once daily, twice daily, or three times a day. Sex Transm Dis 2001;28:226–231.

53. Kaspari M, Gutzmer, Kaspari T, et al. Application of imiquimod by suppositories (anal tampons) efficiently prevents recurrences after ablation of anal canal condyloma. Br J Dermatol 2002;147:757–759.

54. Trombetta LJ, Place RJ. Giant condyloma acuminatum of the anorectum: trends in epidemiology and management. Report of a case and review of the literature. Dis Colon Rectum 2001;44:1878–1886.

55. Butler TW, Gefter J, Kleto D, et al. Squamous-cell carcinoma of the anus in condyloma acuminatum: successful treatment with pre-operative chemotherapy and radiation. Dis Colon Rectum 1987;30:293–295.

56. Frisch M, Biggar RJ, Goedert JJ. Human papillomavirus-associated cancers in patients with immunodeficiency virus infection and acquired immunodeficiency syndrome. J Natl Cancer Inst 2000;92:1500–1510.

57. Goedert JJ, Cote TR, Virgo P, et al. Spectrum of AIDS-associated cancers in patients with human immunodeficiency virus infection and acquired immunodeficiency syndrome. Lancet 1998;351:1833–1839.

58. Chin-Hong PV, Palefsky JM. Natural history and clinical management of anal human papillomavirus disease in men and women infected with human immunodeficiency virus. Clin Infect Dis 2002;35:1127–1134.

59. Palefsky JM. Anal human papillomavirus infection and anal cancer in HIV-positive individuals: an emerging problem. AIDS 1994;8:293–295.

60. Cleary RK, Shaldenbrand JD, Fowler JJ, et al. Perianal Bowen's disease and anal intraepithelial neoplasia. Dis Colon Rectum 1999;42(7):945–951.

61. Caruso ML, Valentini AM. Different human papillomavirus genotypes in anogenital lesions. Anticancer Res 1999;19:3049–3053.

62. Colquhoun P, Nogeras JJ, Dipasquale B, et al. Interobserver and intraobserver bias exists in the interpretation of anal dysplasia. Dis Colon Rectum 2003;46:1338.

63. Chang GJ, Berry JM, Jay N, Palefsky JM, Welton ML. Surgical treatment of high-grade anal squamous intraepithelial lesions. A prospective study. Dis Colon Rectum 2002;45:453–458.

64. Piketty C, Darragh TM, Heard I, et al. High prevalence of anal squamous intraepithelial lesions in HIV-positive men despite the use of highly active antiretroviral therapy. Sex Transm Dis 2004; 31:96–99.

65. Piketty C, Darragh TM, Da Costa M, et al. High prevalence of anal human papillomavirus infection and anal cancer precursors among HIV-infected persons in the absence of anal intercourse. Ann Intern Med 2003;183:453–459.

66. Douglas JM Jr. Molluscum contagiosum. In: Holmes KK, Sparling PR, Mardh PA, et al., eds. Sexually Transmitted Diseases. New York: McGraw-Hill; 1999:385–389.

67. Skinner RB. Treatment of molluscum contagiosum with imiquimod 5% cream. J Am Acad Dermatol 2002;47:S221–224.

68. Syed TA, Lundin S, Ahmad M. Topical 0.3% and 0.5% podophyllotoxin cream for self-treatment of molluscum contagiosum in males. A placebo-controlled, double-blind study. Dermatology 1994;189:65–68.

69. Barre-Sinoussi F, Chermann JC, Rey F, et al. Isolation of a T-lymphotropic retrovirus from a patient at risk for acquired immune deficiency syndrome (AIDS). Science 1983;220:868–871.

70. Centers for Disease Control and Prevention. HIV/AIDS surveillance report. 2001;13:5–6.

71. Centers for Disease Control and Prevention. MMWR 1992; 41CRR-13:1–19.

72. Barrett WL, Callahan TD, Orkin BA. Perianal manifestations of human immunodeficiency virus infection. Experience with 260 patients. Dis Colon Rectum 1998;41:606–612.

73. Morandi E, Merlini D, Salvaggio A, et al. Prospective study of healing time after hemorrhoidectomy. Influence of HIV infection, acquired immunodeficiency syndrome, and anal wound infection. Dis Colon Rectum 1999;42:1140–1144.

74. Nadal SR, Manzione CR, Galvao VM, et al. Healing after fistulotomy. Comparative study between HIV+ and HIV− patients. Dis Colon Rectum 1998;41:177–179.

75. Lord RVN. Anorectal surgery in patients infected with human immunodeficiency virus. Factors associated with delayed wound healing. Ann Surg 1997;226:92–99.

76. Brar HS, Gottesman L, Surawicz C. Anorectal pathology in AIDS. Gastrointest Endosc Clin North Am 1998;8:913–931.

77. Bernstein M. Anal fissure and the human immunodeficiency virus. Semin Colon Rectal Surg 1997;8:40–45.

78. Modesto VL, Gottesman L. Surgical debridement and intralesional steroid injection in the treatment of idiopathic AIDS-related anal ulcerations. Am J Surg 1997;174:439–441.

79. Hewitt WR, Sokol TP, Fleshner RP. Should HIV status alter indications for hemorrhoidectomy? Dis Colon Rectum 1996;39:615–618.

18
Benign Colon: Diverticular Disease

Alan G. Thorson and Stanley M. Goldberg

The term "diverticular disease" of the colon represents a continuum of anatomic and pathophysiologic change within the colon related to the presence of diverticula. These changes most often occur in the sigmoid colon. The continuum can range from the presence of a single diverticulum (a sac or pouch in the wall of an organ) to many diverticula (which may be too numerous to count). It can refer to an asymptomatic state (diverticulosis) or any one of a number of diverse combinations of inflammatory symptoms, changes, and complications (diverticulitis).

Symptoms may variably result from simple physiologic changes in colonic motility related to altered neuromuscular activity in the sigmoid colon, varying degrees of localized inflammatory response, or complex inflammatory interactions leading to diffuse peritonitis and septic shock. These more complex symptoms and resulting complications arise from breaches in the integrity of the wall of one or more diverticula. Diverticula may be true, containing all layers of the bowel wall (congenital), or false, lacking the muscular layer (acquired or pulsion diverticula).

This chapter will deal with inflammatory diverticular disease and its associated complications. Bleeding from diverticular disease is discussed in Chapter 20 (Lower Gastrointestinal Hemorrhage).

Incidence

Diverticulosis was first described in the mid-19th century as more of a curiosity than a significant disease entity. However, since the early 20th century, an increasing prevalence of the disease has been recognized in industrialized countries. The incidence increases with age and the adoption of a diet high in red meat, refined sugars, and milled flour but low in whole grain breads, cereals, and fruits and vegetables. Although the exact incidence is not well established, numerous autopsy, radiographic, and endoscopic series have shown that the incidence has increased dramatically over the past 75 years,[1–4]

from around 5% near the turn of the century to 50% or more by 1975.[2,3]

It is now estimated that the risk of developing diverticular disease in the United States approximates 5% by age 40 and may increase to more than 80% by age 80.[5]

This increase in observed incidence was originally attributed to new imaging techniques [the introduction of the barium enema (BE) in the early 20th century] and bias inherent to estimates based on a population presenting with symptoms requiring an investigation.[6] It is now clear that not only diverticulosis but the incidence of related complications are increasing. This is exemplified by increasing costs in the treatment of diverticular disease which accounts for nearly 450,000 hospital admissions, 2 million office visits, 112,000 disability cases, and 3000 fatalities each year in the United States.[7] It is estimated that costs will continue to increase as the population continues to age in the next several decades.

Proportionately few people become symptomatic from the presence of diverticula. An estimated 10%–20% of people with diverticula develop symptoms of diverticulitis, and only 10%–20% of these will require hospitalization. Of those that require hospitalization, 20%–50% will require operative intervention. The percentage of hospitalized patients requiring operation has been increasing as outpatient management becomes more common and those admitted as inpatients are more seriously ill.[8] Overall, less than 1% of patients with diverticula will ultimately require surgical management.[9]

There is some evidence that males are more frequently affected at a younger age and females at an older age; however, significant bias may influence this impression. Young females may frequently be underdiagnosed because of confusion with gynecologic diseases in the young. Older females may be overdiagnosed because of confusion with irritable bowel syndrome (IBS). There also seems to be a dichotomy in age and sex with regard to complications of diverticular disease, particularly perforation. The incidence of perforation is higher in males younger than age 50 but in females older than 50.[10]

Pathophysiology

Diverticulosis is associated with high intraluminal pressures. Pressures in patients with diverticular disease have been found as high as 90 mm Hg during peak contraction. This represents a value nearly 9 times higher than seen in patients with normal colons.[11] It is theorized that such pressures lead to segmentation. Segmentation refers to a process whereby the colon effectively functions as a series of separate compartments rather than a continuous tube.

The high pressures that each compartment is capable of producing are directed toward the colonic wall rather than as propulsive waves. These pressures predispose to herniation of mucosa through the muscular defects that exist where blood vessels penetrate to reach the submucosa and mucosa (vasa recta brevia). Most of these penetrations occur between the mesenteric and anti-mesenteric tinea where, not coincidentally, most diverticula occur. As the mucosa herniates, it does so without dragging the muscular layer along, leaving the diverticula denuded of muscle and consistent with the definition of an acquired process. Thus, the most common diverticula are acquired or pulsion diverticula.

These high pressures are consistent with the sigmoid colon being the most common site of involvement. This can be explained by the law of Laplace which states that the tension in the wall of a hollow cylinder is proportional to its radius times the pressure within the cylinder. Because of segmentation, the sigmoid generates pressures so high that the effect of a smaller radius is overcome resulting in total tension in the wall of the sigmoid colon being higher than the rest of the colon and thus the sigmoid has the highest risk of diverticulum formation. It is hypothesized that at least a part of fiber's protective effect is a result of stool bulking which maintains a larger lumen, prevents segmenting contractions, and decreases high pressures.

Complementary to these theories of pathogenesis is the consistent colonic wall muscle abnormality associated with sigmoid diverticular disease. Both the circular and longitudinal muscle wall is typically thickened resulting in a reduction in the size of the lumen and a shortening of the sigmoid. The reduced lumen size may be further enhanced by secondary pericolic fibrosis.

The source of this muscular thickening is not clear. It has been observed that in the normal process of left colon peristalsis, smooth muscle in the rectosigmoid will relax in response to a stimulus, causing contraction of the colon above and the rectum below. A combination of poor diet, aging, and constipation could lead to malfunction of this relaxation response leading to a functional obstruction and the hypertrophy seen in the muscle.[12] Cellular hypertrophy, cellular hyperplasia, and elastosis have all been described. Elastosis seems to precede the development of diverticulosis. It is not found in any other inflammatory conditions of the colon.

Several alternative concepts have been advanced to explain the differences in presentation of diverticular disease. Although the most common finding in diverticular disease is the muscular changes already discussed, some patients fail to demonstrate this characteristic. These patients are more likely to have diffuse diverticula throughout the colon, and are noted to have a higher incidence of bleeding. They may have an underlying connective tissue abnormality. This would explain the development of diverticula in the absence of high intraluminal pressures. The high incidence of bleeding in these patients could be related to associated inadequate vascular support in the diverticular wall.

Pain associated with diverticular disease may be related to muscle spasm as well as inflammation. Perforation can occur in the absence of inflammation and may be secondary to the extremely high intraluminal pressure.[13]

Etiology

The etiology of diverticulitis remains complex and relatively poorly understood. Pathophysiologic studies reveal that complications do not occur until there is microperforation through the wall of a diverticulum into the pericolic tissue. A single diverticulum experiences a change in the permeability of its isolated mucosa from physical, biochemical, or physiologic means. It is postulated that a free perforation then occurs leading to a characteristic response and progressing to varying degrees of inflammation. The perforation might be small and cause a microabscess, develop into a phlegmon, or form into a large abscess. Free perforation occurs rarely, but fistulization does frequently occur, most often to the bladder.[14]

The original communication with the lumen of the bowel is usually rapidly obliterated by the inflammatory process. Occasional failure of the diverticular neck to obliterate may lead to a free communication between the bowel and the peritoneal cavity with resultant fecal peritonitis. Rupture of a noncommunicating abscess may lead to purulent peritonitis.[15]

Low-grade inflammation of colonic mucosa, induced by changes in bacterial microflora, can affect the enteric nervous system and alter gut function, leading to symptom development. This explanation has been postulated as a source of symptoms in IBS. The same explanation can be easily extrapolated to symptoms in diverticular disease because some patients with diverticular disease demonstrate bacterial overgrowth.[16] This common source of symptoms reinforces the difficulty in sorting through the differential in patients with symptoms of bowel disease.

Recent clinical investigations have shown that disturbances in cholinergic activity may contribute to diverticular disease. Cholinergic stimulation in patients with diverticular disease leads to unsynchronized slow waves of relatively low frequency as opposed to bursts of action potentials normally associated with peristalsis.[17,18] This suggests a possible role for cholinergic denervation hypersensitivity in colonic smooth muscle with upregulation of smooth muscle muscarinic receptors.[19]

The colon with diverticular disease has more cholinergic innervation than normal colon. In addition, there is less noncholinergic, nonadrenergic inhibitory nerve activity. This increased cholinergic activity and the relative paucity of inhibitory activity may contribute to the high intraluminal pressures and segmentation seen in the diverticular colon.[20]

Epidemiology

Diet

Large cohort and case-control studies in the United States and Greece have shown that diets high in red meat and low in fruit and vegetable fiber increase diverticular symptoms by as much as threefold.[21,22] Vegetables and brown bread have been shown to be protective.[22] Fiber may be protective by increasing stool weight and water content which decrease colonic segmentation pressures and transit times.[23] Fiber, through the process of fermentation, also provides short-chain fatty acids to the colonic epithelial cells, an important source of fuel and mucosal health.[24–26] Red meat has been associated with heterocyclic amines, a factor in colon mucosal apoptosis.[27] Dietary heme has been shown to be highly cytotoxic to rat colons.[28]

Age and Sex

Population-based studies have reported differences in disease presentation according to age and sex. However, it is not clear that all of these associations would remain valid in the global population of diverticular disease. McConnell et al.[29] reported that female patients present with complications requiring surgery an average of 5 years later than males. Men have a higher incidence of bleeding and women a higher incidence of fistula. Younger men present with fistula and older men bleeding. Young females present with perforation whereas older females with chronic disease and stricture. Overall, patients younger than age 50 present more often with chronic or recurrent diverticulitis.[29] Finally, more patients at younger and younger ages are being diagnosed with diverticular disease.

Nonsteroidal Inflammatory Drugs

Nonsteroidal inflammatory drugs (NSAIDs) have been linked to increased rates of complications related to diverticular disease. The plausible mechanism of action is indirect through known inhibition of cyclooxygenase and resultant decreased prostaglandin synthesis in the gut. Prostaglandins are important in the maintenance of mucosal blood flow and an effective colonic mucosal barrier. A direct mechanism also exists through mucosal damage caused by NSAIDs which leads to increased translocation of toxins and bacteria.[30–32]

Immunocompromise

The use of corticosteroids is associated with a higher risk of perforation and more severe inflammatory complications. The postulated mechanism is immunosuppressive and antiinflammatory effects hinder confinement of perforation in its early stages. The use of other immunosuppressive drugs has also been associated with such increased risks. The main risk seems to be more virulent complications once complications occur.[33]

Opiates

The use of opiate pain medications has been shown to increase intracolonic pressure and slow intestinal transit, both risks for complications of diverticular disease. Case series have shown high percentages of patients with perforation taking opiate analgesics.[30,34]

Smoking

A recent large case-control study showed that smokers had 3 times the risk of developing complications from diverticular disease than did nonsmokers.[35] However, a large cohort study involving more than 46,000 men in the United States did not find this same association.[36]

Alcohol

A Danish cohort study showed the risk of diverticulitis was 3 times higher in female alcoholics than the general population and 2 times higher in male alcoholics. However, the data may be biased because of dietary and smoking habits associated with alcoholics.[37]

Clinical Manifestations

Clinical Patterns

Diverticular disease may be classified into diverticulosis (asymptomatic) and diverticulitis (symptomatic) (Table 18-1). Diverticulosis refers to the presence of diverticula with no related symptoms. This applies to the vast majority (80%–90%) of patients with diverticular disease. Diverticulitis can be subclassified into noninflammatory, acute (simple or

TABLE 18-1. The classification of diverticular disease

Diverticulosis	Asymptomatic
Diverticulitis	
Noninflammatory	Symptoms without inflammation
Acute	Symptoms with inflammation
Simple	Localized
Complicated	With perforation
Chronic	Persistent, low grade
Atypical	Symptoms without systemic signs
Recurring, persistent	Symptoms with systemic signs (may be intermittent)
Complex	With fistula, stricture, obstruction
Malignant	Severe, fibrosing

complicated), chronic (atypical or recurring/persistent), and complex disease. The term "malignant diverticulitis" has been used to describe a particularly severe form of fibrosing disease with phlegmonous inflammation extending below the peritoneal reflection, frequent fistula formation, obstruction, and high postoperative morbidity and mortality.[38] Many consider this form to be misdiagnosed Crohn's disease.

Noninflammatory Diverticular Disease

Noninflammatory diverticular disease describes those patients with symptoms of diverticulitis but without associated inflammation.[39] The diagnosis is made at the time of elective operation when no inflammatory changes are found in the specimen. This has been reported in 15%–35% of resections.[39] Some would consider this a missed diagnosis (IBS). However, if that were always the case, then one would expect a very low resolution of symptoms after resection. In fact, although a lack of inflammatory changes in the resected specimen has been associated with lesser degrees of symptom relief, the success rate is not zero.[40–42] One could conclude that resections are being performed for the right indication but the wrong pathology, delays in surgery may lead to complete resolution of previous inflammation, or noninflammatory diverticular disease is a real entity that sometimes requires surgical intervention. Careful follow-up on the long-term outcomes in these patients could go a long way in answering this question.

The term atypical has been applied to patients with chronic symptoms who never develop the necessary clinical and laboratory criteria to be judged as having acute diverticulitis. Up to 24% of these patients are found to lack inflammatory changes in the resected specimen thus fulfilling the criteria for noninflammatory diverticular disease. The remaining members of this group could be considered as having had acute diverticulitis based on histologic findings of inflammation. A high percentage of atypical patients (88%) become pain free at least on short-term (12 months) follow-up.[42]

Acute Diverticulitis

Acute diverticulitis is heralded by signs and symptoms of acute inflammation and may be simple (limited to the colonic wall and adjacent tissues) or complicated (with perforation). Simple acute disease is usually accompanied by systemic signs of fever and leukocytosis whereas complicated acute disease may have the added signs of tachycardia and hypotension.

Complicated acute diverticulitis can be classified according to the extent of spread of the inflammatory process. A common classification for diverticulitis with perforation was first described by Hughes et al.[43] in 1963 and slightly revised and popularized by Hinchey et al.[44] in 1978. Stage I diverticulitis is a localized pericolic or mesenteric abscess, stage II is a confined pelvic abscess, stage III is generalized purulent peritonitis, and stage IV is generalized fecal peritonitis (Figure 18-1).

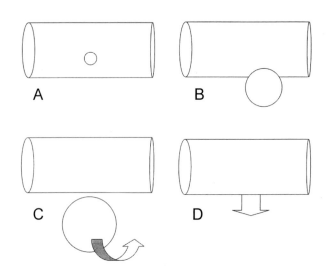

FIGURE 18-1. Diagrammatic representation of classification system for diverticular abscesses in which the cylinders represent the colon, the circles an abscess, and the arrows perforation. **A** Hinchey stage I: localized pericolic or mesenteric abscess. **B** Hinchey stage II: confined pelvic abscess. **C** Hinchey stage III: generalized purulent peritonitis resulting from perforation of an abscess. **D** Hinchey stage IV: generalized fecal peritonitis secondary to free colonic perforation.

Chronic Diverticulitis

Patients with chronic diverticulitis remain symptomatic (left lower quadrant pain) despite standard treatment. It is considered atypical if systemic signs never develop. With systemic signs, chronic disease may manifest as recurring, intermittent episodes of acute disease or as persistent, symptomatic low-grade disease. This is frequently associated with the presence of a phlegmon. If resection is performed, there will be evidence of inflammatory changes within the specimen.

Complex Diverticular Disease

Complex diverticulitis refers to disease in those patients who manifest sequelae of chronic inflammation including fistula, stricture, and obstruction. Each of these complications will be addressed later in this chapter.

Natural History

The natural history of diverticular disease is one of increasing risk with increasing age and a diet low in fiber and high in red meat. The number and size of diverticula may increase with age; however, progression from one segment of bowel to another does not typically occur. The most common location for complications is in the sigmoid colon. It is unusual for complications to develop in the proximal colon after resection of the diseased sigmoid colon.

Most patients who develop a first episode of symptomatic diverticulitis have been asymptomatic until 1 month before presentation. Most will respond to bowel rest and antibiotics as an outpatient. It is difficult to reliably estimate how many outpatients will have recurrent episodes because outpatient data are generally not reflective of a primary care population. However, it has been reported that up to 10% of patients with a first episode who have responded to outpatient management will develop recurrent or persistent symptoms which will require hospitalization.[45]

Data are more readily available on recurrence for patients who were initially treated as inpatients. But our understanding of the natural history continues to evolve as antibiotics become more effective and inpatient status means increasingly severe disease. These changes make historical data regarding these issues of less value. In today's world, inpatients might be expected to be at a greater risk of recurrence. In fact, 10%–20% or more of these patients will develop a recurrence.[45] Some, but not all of these patients, will require a second hospitalization. The interval between acute events may be prolonged (median 5 years).[46] After a second hospital admission, up to 70% will continue with symptoms and more than half of those that require a third admission will do so within 1 year. The more complicated the attack, the higher the risk of recurrence.[4,14,47–50]

It has been estimated that up to 1% of all patients with diverticulosis will eventually require operative intervention.[9] However, with an increasing overall number of individuals affected with diverticulosis and better antibiotics for managing infections, this estimate may now be too high.

Presenting Symptoms

Patients with acute diverticulitis typically complain of left lower quadrant abdominal pain. However, in a patient with a redundant sigmoid colon, an inflamed segment might present with pain in the right lower quadrant, thus complicating the differential diagnosis with appendicitis. The pain is generally constant in nature, not colicky. Radiation may occur to the back, ipsilateral flank, groin, and even down the leg. The pain may be preceded or accompanied by episodes of constipation or diarrhea. It often is progressive in nature if appropriate treatment is not instituted.

Historically, age was used as a primary determinant in distinguishing the most likely etiology of such pain. However, as increasing numbers of young people are found to have diverticular disease, the overlap between age groups has broadened and the need for diagnostic acumen has significantly sharpened. Classically, there is no prodromal epigastric pain with diverticulitis as one might expect to see with appendicitis.

Nausea and vomiting are unusual in the absence of obstruction, although secondary ileus with abdominal distention is common in more severe cases. Bleeding is not a typical associated finding, and, if present, suggests an alternative diagnosis (e.g., cancer). Symptoms of dysuria or urgency suggest possible bladder involvement because of an adjacent inflammatory mass or a colovesical fistula. Pneumaturia, fecaluria, or passage of gas and stool through the vagina suggest a colovesical or colovaginal fistula, respectively. Fever is common and proportional to the amount of inflammatory response present. A high fever suggests a perforation with abscess or peritonitis.

Occasionally, diverticular disease will present in unusual ways. These include lower extremity (hip) joint infections of a chronic nature that culture positive for enteric bacteria. Other unusual presentations include female adnexal masses on the left; inflammation/necrosis of the perineum and genitalia including complex anal fistula and Fournier's gangrene; subcutaneous emphysema of the lower extremities, neck, and abdominal wall; isolated hepatic abscess caused by enteric organisms; brain abscess caused by enteric organisms and cutaneous lesions mimicking pyoderma gangrenosum.[51]

Physical Findings

Patients presenting with acute diverticulitis will be tender to palpation in the left lower quadrant and left iliac region. There may be limited rigidity or localized guarding to deeper palpation. With resolution of the acute phase, palpation may reveal a mass in the left lower quadrant A positive psoas sign and/or obturator sign may reflect retroperitoneal and/or pelvic involvement of the inflammatory process.

In the event of a gross perforation with development of fecal or purulent peritonitis, the area of tenderness will spread throughout the abdomen. Guarding will become prominent and the abdominal wall will become rigid.

Complications

Bleeding

Bleeding is not recognized as a feature of diverticulitis. Bleeding related to diverticulosis is discussed in Chapter 20 (Lower Gastrointestinal Hemorrhage).

Perforation

Gross perforation can occur at two levels. If an abscess forms and then ruptures, purulent peritonitis is the result. If a large perforation occurs through the diverticulum directly into the peritoneum, fecal peritonitis is the result. Mixed fecal and purulent peritonitis may result from the rupture of an abscess which has an ongoing communication with the bowel lumen. Clinically, the presentation is that of either abrupt onset of abdominal pain for a free perforation or an abrupt exacerbation of progressive localized pain in the case of a ruptured abscess. A pneumoperitoneum is typically seen on abdominal films or computed tomographic (CT) scan. Rapid progression to diffuse abdominal pain and rigidity can be expected.

Abscess

An abscess most often results from the mechanism described above. Small abscesses less than 1 cm in diameter will frequently resolve with antibiotic therapy. Larger abscesses may require drainage. CT-guided percutaneous drainage is the preferred approach when possible because it can convert the high risks of an urgent operation to a much safer elective operation.

Fistula

The incidence of fistulization reported in the literature ranges from 5% to 33% depending largely on the type of referral center making the report.[52] Colovesical fistula is the most common fistula associated with diverticular disease and diverticular disease is the most common cause of colovesical fistula. Other relatively common fistulas associated with diverticular disease are colocutaneous, colovaginal, and coloenteric. Most patients who develop a colovaginal fistula have had a previous hysterectomy. Other fistulas have rarely been described and include colocolic, ureterocolic, colouterine, colosaphingeal, coloperineal, sigmoido-appendiceal, colovenous, and even fistulas to the thigh (a variant of a colocutaneous fistula).

The diagnosis of a diverticular fistula is generally clinical. Many fistulas will not be directly identifiable by imaging studies. Thus, excess efforts should not be undertaken to try to radiographically or otherwise demonstrate a fistula. Gas seen in the bladder on a CT scan in a patient who has not had their urethra or bladder instrumented is the most sensitive/common finding with a colovesical fistula. The primary aim of a diagnostic workup is not to see the fistula but to determine the etiology [diverticulitis, cancer, inflammatory bowel disease (IBD), etc.] so that appropriate therapy can be initiated.

Stricture

The development of a phlegmon with repeated attacks of acute disease or long-term persistent disease may result in a stricture. Although a relatively uncommon complication, patients will present with constipation, abdominal pain, and bloating. It is necessary to rule out carcinoma as the true cause of the stricture. Colonoscopy is the first choice to help make this distinction; however, it is not uncommon for associated bowel angulation and fixation to prevent endoscopic visualization. Contrast studies may assist the evaluation in such instances but resection may be necessary to make a diagnosis.

Obstruction

On rare occasions, complete obstruction may occur. If caused by diverticular disease, most patients will respond to initial medical management allowing an elective resection at a later date. Persistence of an obstruction may require a Hartmann's procedure or primary anastomosis with proximal diversion for management. The successful use of colonic stents to relieve obstruction secondary to diverticulitis has been described.[53,54] In this setting, the stent is used as a bridge to surgery with later elective resection. However, the use of stents in benign disease is controversial. Some investigators have found a high incidence of complications leading to emergency surgery for removal of the stent and management of complications when a stent is used in this setting.[55]

Ureteral Obstruction

The ureter is infrequently involved with diverticular disease. When involved, it is most frequently the left ureter. Rarely diverticular disease has been reported as fistulizing to the ureter. A stricture may occur but compression is more common. This can result from retroperitoneal fibrosis secondary to diverticular inflammation. Most often, this resolves with resolution of the underlying inflammatory process although rarely ureterolysis has been advised.[56]

Phlegmon

A phlegmon represents an inflammatory mass. It may or may not be associated with a central abscess. A phlegmon can significantly complicate the technical aspects of resection. Many phlegmons will resolve with antibiotic therapy. If resection is planned because of recurrent episodes of disease, it is best to treat the acute phlegmon, to resolution if possible, before resection. On occasion, operation becomes necessary in the face of an acute phlegmon. This situation may be the source of some descriptions of "malignant" diverticulitis as earlier described.

Saint's Triad

Saint's triad is a described association of diverticulosis, cholelithiasis, and hiatal hernia. Although it has been suggested that the triad occurs in 3%–6% of the general population,[47] it is of unknown clinical significance and likely represents the normal concomitant distribution of these common maladies.

Diagnostic Tests

Endoscopy

Endoscopy in the face of acute diverticulitis must be undertaken with extreme caution because of risk of gross perforation and decreased chance of success for complete colonic evaluation. It can provide important information before operation but will change acute management in less than 1% of cases.[57] Generally, in the absence of an urgent indication, colonoscopy should be delayed until resolution of the acute episode is complete.

In the case of elective colonoscopy, the unexpected finding of acute diverticulitis (manifested as erythema, edema, pus, or granulation tissue at a diverticula opening) is distinctly unusual, occurring in just 0.8% of patients. Treatment with antibiotic therapy for such findings is generally unnecessary because follow-up has shown that symptoms of diverticulitis do not develop after the colonoscopy.[58]

Abdominal X-rays

When used, plain films of the abdomen should be done supine and upright/left lateral decubitus because the primary value is to rule out pneumoperitoneum or to assess for a possible obstruction. However, either of these two complications can also be assessed with CT scan, so in many centers, the plain abdominal film is rarely used.

Contrast Studies

Barium or water-soluble contrast studies have proponents for their use but CT scan offers an examination of much broader scope in one evaluation making it the preferred imaging study in many centers. However, because of costs, some clinicians will use CT scan only if there is clinical suspicion of an abscess or other complicating feature for which an alternative to standard bowel rest and antibiotics might be applied. A water-soluble contrast study can evaluate the lumen of the bowel if there is concern about distal bowel obstruction. It may be an important part of the assessment for the possible use of a stent if malignant disease is suspected.

Contrast studies have been shown to identify fistulas, most often colovaginal or coloenteric. Some clinicians prefer the anatomic view of the entire colon provided by BE because it distinguishes the extent of diverticulosis throughout the colon and can assess for stricture and colonic length. In most centers, contrast studies, if used at all, are used in a limited manner to evaluate the anatomy of the colon before an operation.

CT Scan

An important advantage to a CT scan is the ability to document diverticulitis, even if uncomplicated, when the diagnosis is in doubt. Studies using CT scan as the initial diagnostic test have shown that up to 5% of patients admitted for acute diverticulitis have been hospitalized for the incorrect clinical diagnosis.[59]

It has been demonstrated that CT can recognize and stratify patients according to the severity of their disease. It can distinguish uncomplicated disease with predictably short length of stay from complicated disease as defined by abscess, fistula, peritonitis, or obstruction and a predictably long length of stay. It also provides information about extracolonic pathology and anatomic variation useful for surgical planning. Early CT-guided drainage of abscesses allows downstaging of complicated diverticulitis to convert an otherwise urgent or emergent operation with attendant increases in morbidity and mortality to the safety of an elective operation.[59] In some selected cases, there may be no need for elective resection.

Ultrasonography

Transrectal ultrasound (TRUS) has been used in the evaluation of diverticular disease in conjunction with transabdominal ultrasound (TAUS). Combining TRUS with TAUS reveals complications not visualized on TAUS alone including inflamed diverticula. TRUS may be an accurate adjunct for confirming clinically suspected acute colonic diverticulitis when the rectosigmoid or perirectal tissues are affected as one might see in the case of malignant diverticulitis. It helps avoid false-negative results and defines the severity of disease in the lower sigmoid colon better than TAUS alone. TRUS may prove to be a useful adjunct in selected cases of rectosigmoid diverticulitis and perirectal involvement by diverticular disease in centers where CT scanning is not readily available.[60]

Magnetic Resonance Imaging

Preliminary studies using magnetic resonance imaging colonography have shown a high correlation with CT findings in patients with diverticular disease without exposure to ionizing radiation. Three-dimensional rendered models and virtual colonoscopy can be performed only in the nonacute setting. These comprehensive three-dimensional models, rather than BE, may have a role in presurgical planning with concurrent assessment of the residual colon.[61]

Differential Diagnosis

The differential diagnosis for diverticular disease includes IBS, carcinoma, IBD, appendicitis, bowel obstruction, ischemic colitis, gynecologic disease, and urologic disease. Of these, IBS is perhaps the most difficult to differentiate in many patients.

Irritable Bowel Syndrome

In many ways, the distinction between chronic diverticulitis and noninflammatory diverticular disease relies on the pathologist whereas the distinction between noninflammatory diverticular disease and IBS relies on the diagnostic acumen of the clinician and the long-term outcomes of resection. Because of the prevalence of diverticular disease, many patients with IBS will have concomitant diverticular disease. However, because diverticular disease is usually asymptomatic, the presence of diverticulosis in these patients will often not be the source of their symptoms but rather just a source of confusion in the differential. It is helpful to be familiar with the Rome II criteria (Table 18-2) for the diagnosis of IBS in order to sort through this differential.

TABLE 18-2. The Rome II criteria for IBS

IBS can be diagnosed based on at least 12 weeks (which need not be consecutive) in the preceding 12 months, of *abdominal discomfort or pain that has two of three of these features*:
1. Relieved with defecation; and/or
2. Onset associated with a change in frequency of stool; and/or
3. Onset associated with a change in form (appearance) of stool.

Symptoms that cumulatively support the diagnosis of IBS:
1. Abnormal stool frequency (>3 stools per day or <3 stools per week)
2. Abnormal stool form (lumpy/hard or loose/watery stool)
3. Abnormal stool passage (straining, urgency, or feeling of incomplete evacuation);
4. Passage of mucus
5. Bloating or feeling of abdominal distension

Red Flag symptoms that are *not* typical of IBS:
1. Pain that often awakens/interferes with sleep
2. Diarrhea that often awakens/interferes with sleep
3. Blood in stool (visible or occult)
4. Weight loss
5. Fever
6. Abnormal physical examination

Colon Neoplasia

Distinguishing diverticular disease from cancer can be difficult. Imaging techniques can provide significant diagnostic assistance, but occasionally a resection is necessary to be certain. Several features of BE studies support a diagnosis of diverticular disease including preservation of the mucosa, long strictures, and the presence of diverticula. A BE is preferred by some clinicians to assess the extent of the diverticulosis and evaluate the length of the colon before resection. Although colonoscopy can frequently resolve this issue, it is not always successful because of acute angulations or narrowing of the lumen. CT evaluates the entire abdomen, can identify concurrent disease, and may give clues as to the underlying colonic pathology.

The increasing incidence of colonic neoplasia with increasing age parallels that of diverticular disease. Polyps and cancer must be considered whenever a diagnostic workup for diverticular disease is begun. Although unusual, cases of adenocarcinoma arising within a diverticulum have been reported.[62] Because colonic diverticula are thin walled, containing only mucosa and serosa, early penetration by cancer is likely, leading to advanced stages with small primary lesions.

Although historically diverticular disease is not believed to have an etiologic link to colon cancer, a causal association has been identified between left-sided colon cancer and diverticulitis. In a review of 7159 patients from the Swedish Cancer Registry, patients with diverticulitis had a long-term increased risk of left-sided colon cancer compared with patients with asymptomatic diverticulosis (odds ration = 4.2).[63–65]

Inflammatory Bowel Disease

Crohn's disease can be a particularly difficult differential to make. Both Crohn's and diverticular disease may present with similar complications including fistulas, phlegmons, and abscesses. Rectal involvement, anal disease, extracolonic signs, and bleeding suggest Crohn's. Recurrent "diverticulitis" requiring a repeat resection should always raise the question of possible Crohn's disease.[66] Ulcerative colitis is rarely a significant differential problem because bleeding is not a prominent symptom of diverticulitis and a simple endoscopic examination showing inflammation within the rectum should suffice to rule out diverticular disease. In the unusual circumstance in which diverticulitis and ulcerative colitis both exist, treatment should be targeted to both entities simultaneously.

Other Colitides, Appendicitis, Gynecologic and Urologic Disease

Endoscopy can be an important adjunct in differentiating IBD, ischemic colitis, and other forms of colitis although caution must be used in the acute setting. A major advantage of the CT scan is the ability to evaluate for many of the other potential differentials including appendicitis, gynecologic and urologic disease.

Associated Conditions

There is such a high incidence of diverticulosis among patients with autosomal dominant polycystic kidney disease that some consider it an extrarenal manifestation.[67] These patients undergoing renal transplantation are at particularly high risk for devastating infectious complications because of their immunocompromised state. Many transplant centers recommend prophylactic sigmoid resection in those polycystic kidney patients scheduled for transplantation with a documented history of diverticulitis.[67–70]

Uncommon Presentations

Diverticulitis in Young Patients

Young patients with diverticular disease are usually male,[45,71] obese,[72,73] and have a higher incidence of right-sided diverticulitis.[74,75] Young patients undergoing operation are frequently misdiagnosed preoperatively[72,73,76] with appendicitis being the most common misdiagnosis.[76] Historically, diverticular disease in patients younger than 50 years of age has been described as more virulent and with more serious complications.[45,72,77–79] Many recommend that patients younger than age 50 have an elective resection after a single episode of acute disease. Recent evidence is mixed.

In some series, young people present with more severe disease at first presentation[74,77–79] but less frequently have a resection at that time. Reasons for this include missed diagnoses and rapid response to therapy. With fewer resections for more complex disease, a higher percentage of young patients return with delayed complications and the appearance of more aggressive disease. Elective resection after the first episode of diverticulitis is thus advised.[77–79]

Others have recommended elective resections at a younger age to avoid the increased morbidity and mortality associated with urgent or emergent surgery in the elderly (0% versus 34.9%).[80] Some recommendations for elective resection in the young patient are based on cost savings related to definitive surgical management versus the higher costs of ongoing medical treatment for recurring disease.[81] These types of recommendations assume a high risk of recurrent disease.

There is evidence that diverticular disease in young patients is changing. It is not as rare as it used to be[72,82,83] and continues to become more common.[83] Recent evidence suggests there is not increased risk of complications from diverticular disease in the young.[73,75,76,82–86] Based on these findings, resection after a single episode of diverticulitis is not recommended.

Data are difficult to interpret because the presentations of diverticular disease are so varied and most studies are small and retrospective with risks of unrecognized selection bias. However, it does seem that diverticular disease is more common in young patients than generally recognized. Obesity may be a risk factor, probably related to diet. Diets high in fiber are less likely to result in obesity as well as diverticular disease.

The issue of male predominance could be a result of missed diagnoses in females. Young females frequently have a gynecologic focus of attention placed on causes of abdominal pain other than diverticular disease and accentuated by the general poor recognition of the prevalence of diverticular disease in younger patients.

Current recommendations for resection are based on the predicted risk of developing a serious complication that would lead to emergency surgery with increased morbidity and mortality and frequent use of colostomy in this setting. To improve management, we must become better at predicting who is at risk for recurrent disease. Age alone does not seem to be a reliable factor. The use of CT to identify "severe" or "complex" diverticular disease seems most promising.

The risk of complications within 5 years of a first attack of diverticulitis exceeds 50% if CT shows severe diverticulitis at the initial episode.[86] Mild findings on CT can be defined as localized thickening of colonic wall and inflammation of pericolic fat. Severe findings are defined as abscess and/or extraluminal air and/or extraluminal contrast. In a recent study, the incidence of remote complications was the highest (54% at 5 years) for young patients with severe diverticulitis on CT and the lowest (19% at 5 years) for older patients with mild disease. Young age and severe diverticulitis taken separately were both statistically significant factors of poor outcome (P = .007 and .003, respectively), although age was no longer significant after stratification for disease severity on CT (P = .07).[86] Other studies have shown similar risks associated with complex disease on CT.[85,87]

Rectal Diverticula

Rectal diverticula are rare. They are typically true diverticula because they include the muscular layer of the rectum in their wall, and are frequently solitary. Inflammation can generally be managed with antibiotics.

Cecal and Right-sided Diverticulitis

Right-sided diverticular disease is much more common in the Far East than in the West, representing 35%–84% of diverticula in that region. Patients present an average of 20 years younger than with sigmoid diverticulitis. Classically, cecal diverticula are described as true diverticula containing all layers of the bowel wall. However, most cecal diverticula actually are false and frequently not solitary.

It is estimated that 13% of patients with cecal diverticulosis develop diverticular inflammation. Cecal diverticulitis can be graded according to the extent of the inflammation. Grade I disease refers to an easily recognizable projecting inflamed cecal diverticulum. Grade II is an inflamed cecal mass. Grade III encompasses a localized abscess or fistula. Grade IV is a free perforation or ruptured abscess with diffuse peritonitis. Cecal diverticulitis is correctly diagnosed preoperatively only 5% of the time. Appendicitis is the preoperative diagnosis in more than two-thirds of cases.[88] Intraoperative diagnosis is relatively easy with Grade I and to a lesser extent with Grade II disease. Most episodes of cecal diverticulitis presenting with Grade III or Grade IV disease are misdiagnosed intraoperatively as perforated carcinoma.

If a correct diagnosis of uncomplicated cecal diverticulitis can be made preoperatively, then antibiotics and treatment similar to left-sided disease is appropriate. This is rare, however. When discovered intraoperatively, the options for treatment include: 1) appendectomy, nonresection of the diverticulum and postoperative antibiotic therapy; or 2) appendectomy with diverticulectomy for Grade I and identifiable Grade II disease. For not readily identifiable Grade II, Grade III, and Grade IV disease, failed treatment, or when cancer is a consideration, right hemicolectomy is the procedure of choice. Appendectomy should always accompany nonresection or diverticulectomy whenever the base of the appendix is not inflamed. This is to avoid confusion at a later date.[89,90]

Giant Colonic Diverticulum

Giant diverticula of the colon are rare entities associated with sigmoid diverticular disease. They are generally pseudodiverticula with inflammatory rather than colonic mucosal walls. They usually arise off of the antimesenteric border of the sigmoid colon. The mechanism of formation is unknown but they have been reported as large as 30–40 cm.[91,92] Twelve percent occur in patients younger than age 50.

Diagnosis is by plain film of the abdomen which shows a large, solitary, gas-filled cavity. Communication with the colon can be demonstrated with contrast enema. The differential includes congenital duplication of the colon, cholecystenteric fistula, colonic volvulus, emphysematous cholecystitis, infected pancreatic pseudocyst, pneumatosis cystoides intestinalis, Meckel's diverticulum, intraabdominal abscess, giant duodenal diverticulum, dilated intestinal loop, gastric dilatation, tuboovarian abscess, and mesenteric cyst.[93]

Most patients will present with vague symptoms of abdominal discomfort or pain and a soft, mobile abdominal mass. A few patients will present with one of the known complications which include perforation, sepsis, intestinal obstruction, or volvulus. The natural history is slow enlargement over time. The treatment of choice is resection of the diverticulum and adjacent colon at time of diagnosis if the patient is symptomatic.

Diverticular Disease of the Transverse Colon

This is an exceedingly rare condition. Clinical presentation most often mimics appendicitis, cholecystitis, or, less frequently, ischemic or Crohn's colitis. It is reported to occur in a younger age group than sigmoid disease and is more common in females. Treatment parallels that of sigmoid diverticulitis; however, resection is usually performed because a preoperative diagnosis is more difficult and a carcinoma frequently cannot be ruled out.

Treatment

Medical and Dietary Management

The primary management of asymptomatic diverticular disease is diet. The goal of dietary manipulation is to increase the bulkiness of stool thus increasing lumen size, decreasing transit time, and decreasing intraluminal pressures. This decreases segmentation which has been described as a significant factor in the development of diverticular disease. The ideal amount of fiber is not known; however, the recommended daily amount is 20–30 g. In general, fiber can be obtained by consuming foods high in fiber or through supplementation with one or more of a large variety of bulk laxatives. Epidemiologic evidence strongly suggests a diet high in fiber can reduce the risk of developing diverticulosis. What is less clear is whether a high fiber diet can prevent diverticulitis and its complications in patients who already have diverticulosis. Recent evidence is building in support of this concept.[94–97]

Acute Diverticulitis

In the absence of systemic signs and symptoms (high fever, marked leukocytosis, tachycardia, and hypotension), most patients experiencing symptoms of diverticulitis will respond to a regimen of bowel rest and antibiotics as outpatients. Diet is usually restricted to low residue or clear liquids during the acute illness but with resolution of the acute symptoms, a high fiber diet should be instituted. There is no need to restrict the ingestion of seeds or hulls because there are no data to substantiate this practice.

Appropriate antibiotics should be instituted to include coverage of Gram-negative and anaerobic bacteria. The most predominant organisms cultured from acute diverticular abscess and peritonitis include the aerobic and facultative bacteria *Escherichia coli* and *Streptococcus* spp. The most frequently isolated anaerobes include *Bacteroides* spp. (*B. fragilis* group), *Peptostreptococcus*, *Clostridium*, and *Fusobacterium* spp.[98]

The use of anticholinergics as adjunctive therapy is based on theoretically reducing pain related to spasm and hypermotility in the sigmoid colon. Efficacy has not been proven.

Signs of more advanced disease including marked leukocytosis, high fever, tachycardia, or hypotension as well as a physical examination demonstrating more advanced intraabdominal pathology, dictate a need for inpatient management. Patients admitted for inpatient care will usually undergo a baseline CT scan which can confirm the diagnosis, rule out potential alternative diagnoses, and evaluate for complicated disease that would require a change in initial management.[59]

Antibiotics should be administered via an intravenous route. Generally the patient will be placed NPO (nothing by mouth) until there is evidence that clinical progress is being made and surgery will not be necessary. The diet is then gradually advanced from clear liquids and then to low residue for a variable period of time before reinstituting a high fiber diet. Symptoms should improve within 24–72 hours. Failure to improve should prompt further diagnostic workup including repeat CT scan and reevaluation of the need for alternative interventions such as operation or abscess drainage. Worsening of the patient's clinical condition, particularly progression to generalized peritonitis, should prompt urgent operative management.

Surgical Management

The surgical management of diverticular disease is replete with varied options that allow for customizing an operation to meet the needs of the individual patient. A thorough knowledge of these options and the indications for each are necessary for the surgeon managing these cases. The goal should always be to manage a complex patient in a way that will maximize the opportunity to avoid emergency surgery in favor of an elective resection.

Surgical options include primary resection with anastomosis with or without proximal diversion, resection with proximal colostomy, and oversewing of the rectal remnant (Hartmann's procedure) or mucous fistula (Mikulicz operation), simple diversion with drainage of the affected segment, diversion with oversewing of the perforation site, and, rarely, subtotal colectomy. Adjunctive measures include on-table lavage and the option of a laparoscopic approach.

The historical discussion of these options would include the use of a three-stage approach with diversion and drainage followed by a second operation for resection and a third operation for reestablishment of intestinal continuity. A modification of this approach includes oversewing of a visible site of perforation with an omental patch as a part of the initial operation.[99] Alternatives include a two-stage approach consisting of a Hartmann's or Mikulicz procedure followed by a second operation for reestablishment of intestinal continuity and resection with primary anastomosis, with or without proximal diversion, as a single operation. For the most part, today's discussions revolve around the relative merits of a one-stage versus a two-stage approach in acute cases requiring urgent or emergent surgery.[100–102] The three-stage approach is unlikely to be used except in the most extreme cases of medical instability.[103,104]

The following sections will discuss the applications of these approaches to the various presentations of diverticular disease including both chronic and acute forms. Special consideration will be given to the management of intraabdominal abscess.

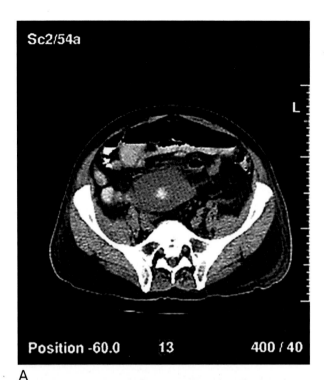

Intraabdominal Abscess

For a patient found to have an abscess, there is much clinical evidence supporting the advantages of percutaneous drainage and the conversion of an emergent operation with its attendant increased morbidity and mortality to the relative safety of elective operation.[59,105] An abscess not responding to medical management should be drained percutaneously or transrectally as appropriate to its location (Figure 18-2).

If drainage cannot be accomplished nonoperatively or if drainage is performed but fails to resolve systemic signs and symptoms, operation is indicated. Generally, the clinical scenario in this situation would be that of an advanced Hinchey class II. Although it is possible that intraoperative findings would support a resection with primary anastomosis with or without proximal diversion, it is more likely that a Hartmann's resection will be required.

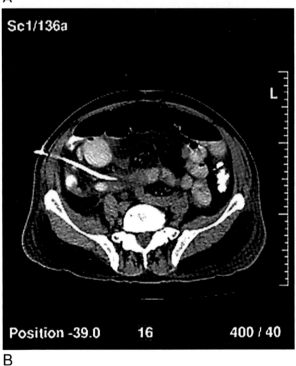

Indications for Surgery for Acute Disease

The indications for surgery of acute disease include: 1) failure to respond to nonoperative management including a persistent phlegmon, failure of percutaneous or transrectal drainage of an abscess or increasing fever, leukocytosis, tachycardia, hypotension, signs of sepsis, or a worsening physical examination; 2) free perforation with peritonitis; and 3) obstruction that does not resolve with conservative therapy. Perforation without peritonitis may not require operation (Figure 18-3).

FIGURE 18-2. **A** A centrally located pelvic diverticular abscess. **B** The same abscess after CT-guided percutaneous drainage.

Surgical Procedures

For acute disease, the choice of operation is highly dependent on the degree of inflammatory response encountered at the time of operation. Because most acute disease can be managed nonoperatively (including the percutaneous drainage of most abscesses), the fact that an operation has become necessary suggests rather advanced pathology and the need to be conservative. *In general*, most Hinchey class I and some class II disease can be managed with a one-stage procedure (resection and anastomosis) if the patient is stable, the extent of contamination is limited, and adequate bowel

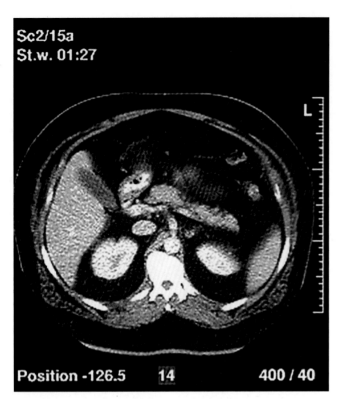

Sc2/15a
St.w. 01:27

Position -126.5   14   400 / 40

FIGURE 18-3. This CT scan shows a small pneumoperitoneum anteriorly. There was not physical evidence of peritonitis. This patient was managed nonoperatively with intravenous antibiotics.

preparation is possible,[100,106] recognizing, however, that the necessity of mechanical bowel preparation in elective colon resections has been recently questioned.[107] Proximal diversion may be appropriate. Most cases of Hinchey class III and IV disease will require a two-stage approach. Some recent evidence suggests a possible role for resection with primary anastomosis and proximal diversion in highly selected cases without gross fecal contamination.[100,103]

A major disadvantage of a two-stage procedure is that 35%–45% of patients never have their colostomy closed. Women are more likely than men to not have closure.[108,109] However, in patients with preexisting incontinence, a Hartman's pouch should be the procedure of choice. For patients who do not undergo closure of their stoma, it is critical that their rectal stump undergo scheduled surveillance for neoplasia as the remaining rectum has the same risk for neoplasia as the remainder of the colon.[110]

Complications

Predictors of complications from resection for diverticular disease include advanced age (older than 70–75 years), two or more comorbid conditions, obstipation at initial examination, the use of steroids, sepsis, obesity,[103,111,112] and emergent rather than elective resection. Complications of resection

include anastomotic leak and hemorrhage. The prevalence of leak from a low intraperitoneal anastomosis is generally considered to be between 2% and 5%.[113] Such leaks can lead to localized or systemic sepsis without an abscess, an abscess with or without sepsis, peritonitis, and stricture. The diagnosis is dependent on a high index of suspicion on the part of the surgeon and quick response to any unusual signs of sepsis. Fever, vague abdominal pain, diarrhea, obstructive symptoms, oliguria, prolonged postoperative ileus, and sepsis all should raise the concern of a leak. The diagnosis is usually confirmed by water-soluble contrast enema and/or CT scan with intravenous, oral, and rectal contrast.

A contained leak without an abscess can usually be managed with intravenous antibiotics and response assessed. Free extravasation of contrast failure to respond to treatment within 24–48 hours or initial severe sepsis or peritonitis requires exploration with resection of the anastomosis and proximal diversion. Repair of the anastomosis with proximal diversion is usually unsatisfactory because of the high risk for recurrent leak in this inflammatory setting. An exception would be a "pin-hole" leak with limited inflammatory response which may be managed with repair, colonic lavage, and proximal diversion.

A leak that results in an abscess can generally be managed with percutaneous or transrectal drainage. Again, failure to respond will require laparotomy, take down of the anastomosis, and proximal diversion.

A colocutaneous fistula related to a diverticular resection will usually respond to nonoperative measures. Provided that there is no distal obstruction or foreign body and that Crohn's was not the cause of the original symptoms, spontaneous closure should be anticipated. Important steps to take to facilitate this closure include drainage of any undrained abscess, attention to nutritional needs, and appropriate wound care.

Stricture is an unusual complication related to diverticular resections unless the underlying process is Crohn's disease. In the rare instance when stricture does occur, the likely etiologies include ischemia or localized sepsis caused by confined leak. Such strictures can usually be managed by dilatation with a hydrostatic balloon or rigid proctoscopy but occasionally will require a formal restapling or resection.

Ureteral injuries are reported to occur in 1%–10% of abdominal surgeries.[114] Early identification of any injury is the key to preventing significant morbidity. Although ureteral stents have not been shown to decrease the rate of injury, they do improve intraoperative identification of the ureters and the early identification of any ureteral injury.[115] The decision to place ureteral stents before operation should be a function of clinical suspicion and the extent of retroperitoneal inflammation on CT scan.

General postoperative complications related to colon and rectal surgery and specifics related to the recognition and management of the specific complications mentioned above are discussed more thoroughly in Chapter 10, Postoperative Complications.

Indications for Surgery for Recurring and Chronic Disease

Patients with multiple, recurrent episodes of acute diverticulitis documented by CT scan should be considered for resection. The practice parameters of the American Society of Colon and Rectal Surgeons states that elective resection should be considered after one or two well-documented attacks of diverticulitis depending on the severity of the attack and age and medical fitness of the patient. Patients with complicated diverticulitis should be considered for resection after one attack.[116] The ultimate goal is to perform an operation electively rather than as an emergency. This requires correctly predicting those patients that are most likely to end up with a serious complication as a result of their disease. One suggestion has been to resect after one episode of diverticulitis in young patients (generally younger than 40–50 years).

It is now doubtful that age itself should be a primary consideration in the decision to operate. The literature is mixed with proponents of a more aggressive approach to the disease in young patients[45,72,74,77–79,81] and those that believe age alone does not significantly increase risk.[71,73,75,76,80,82–84] Other factors apply, most of which are not age related.

CT evidence of complicated or "severe" disease has been one of those criteria that have shown some promise in predicting risk. Abscess, extraluminal air, and extraluminal contrast have been associated with an increased risk of poor outcome from medical management regardless of age.[85,87]

Another approach is to identify specific groups of patients (other than age) who are at increased risk. Immunocompromised patients are one group that is at particular risk for poor outcome.[33] The risk is attributable to a higher incidence of free perforation and more severe inflammatory complications when perforation does occur. Patients with autosomal dominant polycystic kidney disease undergoing renal transplant are a very high risk group.[67–70] Prophylactic resection in such patients with a history of any diverticulitis is recommended.

Recent data have suggested that the recommendation for resection after two episodes of diverticulitis treated as an inpatient may result in too many patients undergoing resection thereby increasing the total cost of health care. Performing resection after the third episode of diverticulitis results in significant cost savings.[117] Performing resection after four documented episodes rather than after two results in fewer deaths, fewer colostomies, and additional cost savings of more than $5000 per patient in those younger than 50.[118] Others question the role of elective resection at all because of the high success rate of nonoperative management and the large percentage of patients presenting with urgent surgical disease that have no previous history of diverticulitis.[119,120] This mirrors the experience of one of the authors (S.M.G.) in which it has *not* been found necessary to resect *all* patients with complicated disease, even after percutaneous drainage of diverticular abscesses.

Surgical Procedures

Patients undergoing resection for chronic disease will almost always be candidates for single-stage resection with primary anastomosis. Additionally, patients returning for closure of a colostomy after initial diversion and drainage, diversion with oversew of perforation, or diversion with resection via either Hartmann's or a Mikulicz procedure, can all typically be managed with one additional operation only.

Complications

The complications related to operation for chronic disease in many ways parallel those already discussed for acute disease. In addition, a noted complication of operating on chronic disease is failure to achieve symptomatic relief. This usually results from a missed diagnosis of Crohn's disease or IBS. Any "recurrence" of symptoms after resection for chronic diverticulitis should raise the suspicion of this possibility. The presence of functional bowel symptoms preoperatively in this group of patients has been associated with poorer functional results postoperatively.[121]

Management of Fistula

The general principle of management is resection of the colon, usually with primary anastomosis. Treatment of the other involved organ/site varies. For the bladder, simple drainage of the bladder with an indwelling urethral catheter for 5–7 days is advised. No treatment of the vagina is required in most circumstances. Cutaneous fistulas will usually close by delay or secondary intention. Enteric fistulas require repair or resection of the involved small bowel or colon. Ureteral drainage for fistulas to the ureter, observation or hysterectomy for uterine fistulas, salpingo-oophorectomy for fistulas to the tubes, and appendectomy would be the most common treatments for uncomplicated fistulas of the other less common varieties. If there is any question of cancer, an en bloc resection of a portion of the involved organ must accompany the resection.

Occasionally nonoperative management is appropriate when symptoms are minor or when the patient is at otherwise too great a risk for other health reasons. The use of long-term suppressive antibiotic therapy in selected patients with colovesical fistula has been shown to eliminate symptoms and prevent complications related to the fistula until death from other causes.[122]

Techniques for Appropriate Resection

The practice parameters of the American Society of Colon and Rectal Surgeons set out several general recommendations regarding resection of diverticular disease. For elective resections, all thickened, diseased colon, but not necessarily the entire proximal diverticula-bearing colon, should be removed. It may be acceptable to retain proximal diverticular colon as long as the remaining bowel is not hypertrophied. All of the sigmoid colon should be removed. When anastomosis is elected, it should be made to normal rectum and must be free of tension and well vascularized.[123] The single most important predictor of recurrence after sigmoid resection for uncomplicated diverticulitis is an anastomosis to the distal sigmoid colon rather than the rectum.[124]

Laparoscopic Surgery

The role of laparoscopy in the management of diverticular disease is evolving. Recent data suggest decreased overall costs associated with laparoscopic resections when compared with open resections.[125,126] Patients who are converted from laparoscopic to open procedures are a concern with regard to added costs but conversion rates are less than 20% in experienced centers, and are somewhat[125–131] predictable[128,131] and thus probably avoidable in many instances.[128] Higher conversion rates are associated with more complex disease.[132] Recurrence rates match those for open procedures,[129,131,132] and length of stay is shorter[125,126] and complications fewer.[126] As data continue to accumulate, it seems that laparoscopic surgery will have a significant role in the management of diverticular disease.

Appendix: Practice Parameters for the Treatment of Sigmoid Diverticulitis

Prepared by The Standards Task Force, The American Society of Colon and Rectal Surgeons.

The initial evaluation of a new patient with suspected acute diverticulitis should include a problem-specific history and physical examination; a complete blood count, urinalysis, and plain abdominal radiographs may be useful in selected clinical scenarios. Computerized tomography scan of the abdomen and pelvis is usually the most appropriate imaging modality in the assessment of suspected diverticulitis. Contrast enema x-ray, cystography, ultrasound, and endoscopy are sometimes useful in the initial evaluation of a patient with suspected acute diverticulitis.

Nonoperative treatment typically includes dietary modification and oral or intravenous antibiotics. Radiologically guided percutaneous drainage is usually the most appropriate treatment for patients with a large diverticular abscess.

After resolution of an initial episode of acute diverticulitis, the colon should be adequately evaluated to confirm the diagnosis. Colonoscopy or contrast enema x-ray (probably with flexible sigmoidoscopy) is appropriate to exclude other diagnoses, primarily cancer, ischemia, and inflammatory bowel disease.

Urgent sigmoid colectomy is required for patients with diffuse peritonitis or for those who fail nonoperative management of acute diverticulitis. The decision to recommend elective sigmoid colectomy after recovery from acute diverti-

culitis should be made on a case-by-case basis. Elective colon resection should typically be advised if an episode of complicated diverticulitis is treated nonoperatively. The resection should be carried proximally to compliant bowel and extend distally to the upper rectum. When a colectomy for diverticular disease is performed, a laparoscopic approach is appropriate in selected patients.

Reprinted from Dis Colon Rectum 2006; 49: 939–944. Copyright © 2006. All rights reserved. American Society of Colon and Rectal Surgeons.

References

1. Almy TP, Howell DA. Diverticula of the colon. N Engl J Med 1980;302:324–331.
2. Rankin FW, Brown PW. Diverticulitis of the colon. Surg Gynecol Obstet 1930;50:836–847.
3. Heller SN, Hackler LR. Changes in the crude fiber content of the American diet. Am J Clin Nutr 1978;31:1510–1514.
4. Parks TG. Natural history of diverticular disease of the colon. Clin Gastroenterol 1975;4:53–69.
5. Colcock BF. Diverticular Disease of the Colon. Philadelphia: WB Saunders; 1971.
6. Schoetz DJ Jr. Diverticular disease of the colon: a century-old problem. Dis Colon Rectum 1999;42:703–709.
7. Corman ML. Colon and Rectal Surgery. 5th ed. Philadelphia: Lippincott Williams & Wilkins; 2005.
8. Somasekar K, Foster ME, Haray PN. The natural history diverticular disease: is there a role for elective colectomy? J R Coll Surg Edinb 2002;47:481–484.
9. Roberts PL, Veidenheimer MC. Current management of diverticulitis. Adv Surg 1994;27:189–208.
10. Morris CR, Harvey IM, Stebbings WS, et al. Epidemiology of perforated colonic diverticular disease. Postgrad Med J 2002; 78:654–658.
11. Painter NS, Truelove SC, Ardran GM, et al. Segmentation and the localization of intraluminal pressures in the human colon, with special reference to the pathogenesis of colonic diverticula. Gastroenterology 1965;49:169–177.
12. Mann CV. Problems in diverticular disease. Proctology 1979;1:20–25.
13. Ryan P. Two kinds of diverticular disease. Ann R Coll Surg Engl 1991;73:73–79.
14. Floch MH, Bina I. The natural history of diverticulitis: fact and theory. J Clin Gastroenterol 2004;38(suppl):S2–S7.
15. Hinchey EJ, Schaal PG, Richards GK. Treatment of perforated diverticular disease of the colon. Adv Surg 1978;12:85–109.
16. Colecchia A, Sandri L, Capodicasa S, et al. Diverticular disease of the colon: new perspectives in symptom development and treatment. World J Gastroenterol 2003;9:1385–1389.
17. Huizinga JD, Waterfall WE, Stern HS. Abnormal response to cholinergic stimulation in the circular muscle layer of the

human colon in diverticular disease. Scand J Gastroenterol 1999;34:683–688.

18. Maselli MA, Piepoli AL, Guerra V, et al. Colonic smooth muscle responses in patients with diverticular disease of the colon: effect of the NK2 receptor antagonist SR48968. Dig Liver Dis 2004;36:348–354.

19. Golder M, Burleigh DE, Belai A, et al. Smooth muscle cholinergic denervation hypersensitivity in diverticular disease. Lancet 2003;361:1945–1951.

20. Tomita R, Fujisaki S, Tanjoh K, et al. Role of nitric oxide in the left-sided colon of patients with diverticular disease. Hepatogastroenterology 2000;47:692–696.

21. Aldoori WH, Giovannucci EL, Rimm EB, et al. A prospective study of diet and the risk of symptomatic diverticular disease in men. Am J Clin Nutr 1994;60:757–764.

22. Manousos O, Day NE, Tzonou A, et al. Diet and other factors in the aetiology of diverticulosis: an epidemiological study in Greece. Gut 1985;26:544–549.

23. Cummings JH, Stephen AM. The role of dietary fibre in the human colon. Can Med Assoc J 1980;123:1109–1114.

24. Edwards C. Physiology of the colorectal barrier. Adv Drug Deliv Rev 1996;28:173–190.

25. Anonymous. Dietary fibre: importance of function as well as amount [editorial]. Lancet 1992;340:1133–1134.

26. Mariadason JM, Catto-Smith A, Gibson PR. Modulation of distal colonic epithelial barrier function by dietary fibre in normal rats. Gut 1999;44:394–399.

27. Hirose Y, Sugie S, Yoshimi N, et al. Induction of apoptosis in colonic epithelium treated with 2-amino-1-methyl-6-phenylimidazo[4,5-b]pyridine (PhIP) and its modulation by a P4501A2 inducer, beta-naphthoflavone, in male F344 rats. Cancer Lett 1998;123:167–172.

28. Sesink AL, Termont DS, Kleibeuker JH, et al. Red meat and colon cancer: the cytotoxic and hyperproliferative effects of dietary heme. Cancer Res 1999;59:5704–5709.

29. McConnell EJ, Tessier DJ, Wolff BG. Population-based incidence of complicated diverticular disease of the sigmoid colon based on gender and age. Dis Colon Rectum 2003;46:1110–1114.

30. Hart AR, Kennedy HJ, Stebbings WS, et al. How frequently do large bowel diverticula perforate? An incidence and cross-sectional study. Eur J Gastroenterol Hepatol 2000;12:661–665.

31. Schwartz HA. Lower gastrointestinal side effects of nonsteroidal anti-inflammatory drugs. J Rheumatol 1981;8:952–954.

32. Day TK. Intestinal perforation associated with osmotic slow release indomethacin capsules. BMJ 1983;287:1671–1672.

33. Tyau ES, Prystowsky JB, Joehl RJ, et al. Acute diverticulitis. A complicated problem in the immunocompromised patient. Arch Surg 1991;126:855–858.

34. Painter NS, Truelove SC. The intraluminal pressure patterns in diverticulosis of the colon. Part II. The effect of morphine. Gut 1964;5:207–213.

35. Papagrigoriadis S, Macey L, Bourantas N, et al. Smoking may be associated with complications in diverticular disease. Br J Surg 1999;86:923–926.

36. Aldoori WH, Giovannucci EL, Rimm EB, et al. A prospective study of alcohol, smoking, caffeine, and the risk of symptomatic diverticular disease in men. Ann Epidemiol 1995;5:221–228.

37. Tonnesen H, Engholm G, Moller H. Association between alcoholism and diverticulitis. Br J Surg 1999;86:1067–1068.

38. Morganstern L, Weiner R, Michel SL. "Malignant" diverticulitis. A clinical entity. Arch Surg 1979;114:1112–1126.

39. Killingback M. Surgical treatment of diverticulitis. In: Fazio VW, Church JM, Delaney CP, eds. Current Therapy in Colon and Rectal Surgery. 2nd ed. Philadelphia: Elsevier/Mosby; 2005:284–295.

40. Breen RE, Corman ML, Robertson WG, et al. Are we really operating on diverticulitis? Dis Colon Rectum 1986;29:174.

41. Thorn M, Graf W, Stefansson T, Pahlman L. Clinical and functional results after elective colonic resection in 75 consecutive patients with diverticular disease. Am J Surg 2002;183:7–11.

42. Horgan AF, McConnell EJ, Wolff BG, et al. Atypical diverticular disease: surgical results. Dis Colon Rectum 2001;44:1315–1318.

43. Hughes ESR, Cuthbertson AM, Carden ABG. The surgical management of acute diverticulitis. Med J Aust 1963;1:780–782.

44. Hinchey EJ, Schaal PG, Richards GK. Treatment of perforated diverticular disease of the colon. Adv Surg 1978;12:85–109.

45. Makela J, Vuolio S, Kiviniemi H, et al. Natural history of diverticular disease: when to operate? Dis Colon Rectum 1998;41:1523–1528.

46. Chautems R, Ambrosetti P, Ludwig A, et al. Long-term follow-up after first acute episode of sigmoid diverticulitis: is surgery mandatory? Dis Colon Rectum 2001;44:A12.

47. Boles RS, Jordan SM. The clinical significance of diverticulosis. Gastroenterology 1958;35:579–581.

48. Fearnhead NS, Mortensen NJ. Clinical features and differential diagnosis of diverticular disease. Best Pract Res Clin Gastroenterol 2002;16:577–593.

49. Farmakis N, Tudor RG, Keighley MR. The 5-year natural history of complicated diverticular disease. Br J Surg 1994;81:733–735.

50. Horner JL. Natural history of diverticulosis of the colon. Am J Dig Dis 1958;3:343–350.

51. Polk HC, Tuckson WB, Miller FB. The atypical presentations of diverticulitis. In: Welch JP, Cohen JL, Sardella WV, Vignati PV, eds. Diverticular Disease, Management of the Difficult Surgical Case. Baltimore: Williams & Wilkins; 1998:384–393.

52. Gordon PH. Diverticular disease of the colon. In: Gordon PH, Nivatvongs S, eds. Principles and Practice of Surgery for the colon, Rectum and Anus. 2nd ed. St. Louis: Quality Medical Publishing; 1999:975–1043.

53. Davidson R, Sweeney WB. Endoluminal stenting for benign colonic obstruction. Surg Endosc 1998;12:353–354.

54. Tamim WL, Ghellai A, Counihan TC, et al. Experience with endoluminal colonic wall stents for the management of large bowel obstruction for benign and malignant disease. Arch Surg 2000;135:434–438.

55. Paul L, Pinto I, Gomez H, et al. Metallic stents in the treatment of benign diseases of the colon: preliminary experience in 10 cases. Radiology 2002;223:715–722.

56. Siminovitch JMP, Fazio VW. Obstructive uropathy secondary to sigmoid diverticulitis. Dis Colon Rectum 1980;23:504–507.

57. Sakhnini E, Lahat A, Melzer E, et al. Early colonoscopy in patients with acute diverticulitis: results of a prospective pilot study. Endoscopy 2004;36:504–507.

58. Ghorai S, Ulbright TM, Rex DK. Endoscopic findings of diverticular inflammation in colonoscopy patients without clinical acute diverticulitis: prevalence and endoscopic spectrum. Am J Gastroenterol 2003;98:802–806.

59. Hachigian MP, Honickman S, Eisenstat TE, et al. Computed tomography in the initial management of acute left-sided diverticulitis. Dis Colon Rectum 1992;35:1123–1129.

60. Hollerweger A, Rettenbacher T, Macheiner P, et al. Sigmoid diverticulitis: value of transrectal sonography in addition to transabdominal sonography. AJR Am J Roentgenol 2000;175: 1155–1160.

61. Schreyer AG, Furst A, Agha A, et al. Magnetic resonance imaging based colonography for diagnosis and assessment of diverticulosis and diverticulitis. Int J Colorectal Dis 2004;19: 474–480.

62. Cohn KH, Weimar JA, Fani K, et al. Adenocarcinoma arising within a colonic diverticulum: report of two cases and review of the literature. Surgery 1993;113:223–226.

63. Stefansson T, Ekbom A, Sparen P, et al. Association between sigmoid diverticulitis and left-sided colon cancer: a nested, population-based, case control study. Scand J Gastroenterol 2004;39:743–747.

64. Stefansson T, Ekbom A, Sparen P, et al. Increased risk of left sided colon cancer in patients with diverticular disease. Gut 1993;34:499–502.

65. Stefansson T, Ekbom A, Sparen P, et al. Cancers among patients diagnosed as having diverticular disease of the colon. Eur J Surg 1995;161:755–760.

66. Berman IR, Corman ML, Coller JA, et al. Late-onset Crohn's disease in patients with colonic diverticulitis. Dis Colon Rectum 1979;22:524.

67. Lederman ED, McCoy G, Conti DJ, et al. Diverticulitis and polycystic kidney disease. Am Surg 2000;66:200–203.

68. Dominguez FE, Albrecht KH, Heemann U, et al. Prevalence of diverticulosis and incidence of bowel perforation after kidney transplantation in patients with polycystic kidney disease. Transpl Int 1998;11:28–31.

69. Lederman ED, Conti DJ, Lempert N, et al. Complicated diverticulitis following renal transplantation. Dis Colon Rectum 1998;41:613–618.

70. Pirenne J, Lledo-Garcia E, Benedetti E, et al. Colon perforation after renal transplantation: a single-institution review. Clin Transplant 1997;11:88–93.

71. Acosta JA, Grebenc ML, Doberneck RC, et al. Colonic diverticular disease in patients 40 years old or younger. Am Surg 1992;58:605–607.

72. Schauer PR, Ramos R, Ghiatas AA, et al. Virulent diverticular disease in young obese men. Am J Surg 1992;164:443–446.

73. Schweitzer J, Casillas RA, Collins JC. Acute diverticulitis in the young adult is not "virulent." Am Surg 2002;68:1044–1047.

74. Minardi AJ Jr, Johnson LW, Sehon JK, et al. Diverticulitis in the young patient. Am Surg 2001;67:458–461.

75. Reisman Y, Ziv Y, Kravrovitc D, et al. Diverticulitis: the effect of age and location on the course of disease. Int J Colorectal Dis 1999;14:250–254.

76. Spivak H, Weinrauch S, Harvey JC, et al. Acute colonic diverticulitis in the young. Dis Colon Rectum 1997;40: 570–574.

77. Ambrosetti P, Robert JH, Witzig JA, et al. Acute left colonic diverticulitis: a prospective analysis of 226 consecutive cases. Surgery 1994;115:546–550.

78. Ambrosetti P, Robert JH, Witzig JA, et al. Acute left colonic diverticulitis in young patients. J Am Coll Surg 1994;179: 156–160.

79. Anderson DN, Driver CP, Davidson AI, et al. Diverticular disease in patients under 50 years of age. J R Coll Surg Edinb 1997;42:102–104.

80. Biondo S, Pares D, Marti Rague J, et al. Acute colonic diverticulitis in patients under 50 years of age. Br J Surg 2002;89: 1137–1141.

81. Cunningham MA, Davis JW, Kaups KL. Medical versus surgical management of diverticulitis in patients under age 40. Am J Surg 1997;174:733–735.

82. Guzzo J, Hyman N. Diverticulitis in young patients: is resection after a single attack always warranted? Dis Colon Rectum 2004;47:1187–1190.

83. West SD, Robinson EK, Delu AN, et al. Diverticulitis in the younger patient. Am J Surg 2003;186:743–746.

84. Vignati PV, Welch JP, Cohen JL. Long-term management of diverticulitis in young patients. Dis Colon Rectum 1995;38:627–629.

85. Poletti PA, Platon A, Rutschmann O, et al. Acute left colonic diverticulitis: can CT findings be used to predict recurrence? AJR Am J Roentgenol 2004;182:1159–1165.

86. Chautems RC, Ambrosetti P, Ludwig A, et al. Long-term follow-up after first acute episode of sigmoid diverticulitis: is surgery mandatory? A prospective study of 118 patients. Dis Colon Rectum 2002;45:962–966.

87. Ambrosetti P, Robert J, Witzig JA, et al. Prognostic factors from computed tomography in acute left colonic diverticulitis. Br J Surg 1992;79:117–119.

88. Lo CY, Chu KW. Acute diverticulitis of the right colon. Am J Surg 1996;171:244–246.

89. Komuta K, Yamanaka S, Okada K, et al. Toward therapeutic guidelines for patients with acute right colonic diverticulitis. Am J Surg 2004;187:233–237.

90. Thorson AG, Ternent CA. Cecal diverticulitis. In: Welch JP, Cohen JL, Sardella WV, Vignati PV, eds. Diverticular Disease, Management of the Difficult Surgical Case. Baltimore: Williams & Wilkins; 1998:428–441.

91. Scerpella PR, Bodensteiner JA. Giant sigmoid diverticula. Report of two cases. Arch Surg 1989;134:1244–1246.

92. Mainzer F, Minagi H. Giant sigmoid diverticulum. AJR Am J Roentgenol 1971;113:352–353.

93. de Oliveira NC, Welch JP. Giant diverticula of the colon. In: Welch JP, Cohen JL, Sardella WV, Vignati PV, eds. Diverticular Disease, Management of the Difficult Surgical Case. Baltimore: Williams & Wilkins; 1998:410–418.

94. Aldoori W, Ryan-Harshman M. Preventing diverticular disease. Review of recent evidence on high-fibre diets. Can Fam Physician 2002;48:1632–1637.

95. Aldoori WH, Giovannucci EL, Rockett HR, et al. A prospective study of dietary fiber types and symptomatic diverticular disease in men. J Nutr 1998;128:714–719.

96. Aldoori WH, Giovannucci EL, Rimm EB, et al. Prospective study of physical activity and the risk of symptomatic diverticular disease in men. Gut 1995;36:276–282.

97. Marlett JA, McBurney MI, Slavin JL. Position of the American Dietetic Association: health implications of dietary fiber. J Am Diet Assoc 2002;102:993–1000.

98. Brook I, Frazier EH. Aerobic and anaerobic microbiology in intra-abdominal infections associated with diverticulitis. J Med Microbiol 2000;49:827–830.

99. Kronborg O. Treatment of perforated sigmoid diverticulitis: a prospective randomized trial. Br J Surg 1993;80:505–507.

100. Bahadursingh AM, Virgo KS, Kaminski DL, et al. Spectrum of disease and outcome of complicated diverticular disease. Am J Surg 2003;186:696–701.

101. Schilling MK, Maurer CA, Kollmar O, et al. Primary vs. secondary anastomosis after sigmoid colon resection for perforated diverticulitis (Hinchey Stage III and IV): a prospective outcome and cost analysis. Dis Colon Rectum 2001;44: 699–703.

102. Farthmann EH, Ruckauer KD, Haring RU. Evidence-based surgery diverticulitis: a surgical disease? Langenbecks Arch Surg 2000;385:143–151.

103. Chandra V, Nelson H, Larson DR, et al. Impact of primary resection on the outcome of patients with perforated diverticulitis. Arch Surg 2004;139:1221–1224.

104. Zeitoun G, Laurent A, Rouffet F, et al. Multicentre, randomized clinical trial of primary versus secondary sigmoid resection in generalized peritonitis complicating sigmoid diverticulitis. Br J Surg 2000;87:1366–1374.

105. Rothenberger DA, Wiltz O. Surgery for complicated diverticulitis. Surg Clin North Am 1993;73:975–992.

106. Maggard MA, Chandler CF, Schmit PJ, et al. Surgical diverticulitis: treatment options. Am Surg 2001;67:1185–1189.

107. Guenaga KF, Matos D, Castro AA, et al. Mechanical bowel preparation for elective colorectal surgery. Cochrane Database Syst Rev 2003;2:CD001544.

108. Maggard MA, Zingmond D, O'Connell JB, et al. What proportion of patients with an ostomy (for diverticulitis) get reversed? Am Surg 2004;70:928–931.

109. Desai DC, Brennan EJ Jr, Reilly JF, et al. The utility of the Hartmann procedure. Am J Surg 1998;175:152–154.

110. Haas PA, Fox TA Jr. The fate of the forgotten rectal pouch after Hartmann's procedure without reconstruction. Am J Surg 1990;159:106–110.

111. Pessaux P, Muscari F, Ouellet JF, et al. Risk factors for mortality and morbidity after elective sigmoid resection for diverticulitis: prospective multicenter multivariate analysis of 582 patients. World J Surg 2004;28:92–96.

112. Elliott TB, Yego S, Irvin TT, Elliott TB, Yego S, Irvin TT. Five-year audit of the acute complications of diverticular disease. Br J Surg 1997;84:535–539.

113. Vernava AM III, Longo WE. Postoperative anastomotic complications. In: Hicks TC, Beck DE, Opelka FG, Timmcke AE, eds. Complications in Colon and Rectal Surgery. Baltimore: Williams & Wilkins; 1996:82–98.

114. Roach MB, Donaldson DS. Urologic complications of colorectal surgery. In: Hicks TC, Beck DE, Opelka FG, Timmcke AE, eds. Complications in Colon and Rectal Surgery. Baltimore: Williams & Wilkins; 1996:99–117.

115. Leff EI, Groff W, Rubin RJ, et al. Use of ureteral catheters in colonic and rectal surgery. Dis Colon Rectum 1982;25:457–460.

116. Practice parameters for the treatment of sigmoid diverticulitis. The Standards Task Force. The American Society of Colon and Rectal Surgeons. Dis Colon Rectum 2000;43:289.

117. Richards RJ, Hammitt JK. Timing of prophylactic surgery in prevention of diverticulitis recurrence: a cost-effectiveness analysis. Dig Dis Sci 2002;47:1903–1908.

118. Salem L, Veenstra DL, Sullivan SD, et al. The timing of elective colectomy in diverticulitis: a decision analysis. J Am Coll Surg 2004;199:904–912.

119. Sarin S, Boulos PB. Long-term outcome of patients presenting with acute complications of diverticular disease. Ann R Coll Surg Engl 1994;76:117–120.

120. Lorimer JW. Is prophylactic resection valid as an indication for elective surgery in diverticular disease? Can J Surg 1997; 40:445–448.

121. Thorn M, Graf W, Stefansson T, et al. Clinical and functional results after elective colonic resection in 75 consecutive patients with diverticular disease. Am J Surg 2002;183:7–11.

122. Moss RL, Ryan JA Jr. Management of enterovesical fistulas. Am J Surg 1990;159:514–517.

123. Wong WD, Wexner SD, Lowry A, et al. Practice parameters for the treatment of sigmoid diverticulitis: supporting documentation. The Standards Task Force. The American Society of Colon and Rectal Surgeons. Dis Colon Rectum 2000;43: 290–297.

124. Thaler K, Baig MK, Berho M, et al. Determinants of recurrence after sigmoid resection for uncomplicated diverticulitis. Dis Colon Rectum 2003;46:385–388.

125. Dwivedi A, Chahin F, Agrawal S, et al. Laparoscopic colectomy vs. open colectomy for sigmoid diverticular disease. Dis Colon Rectum 2002;45:1309–1314.

126. Senagore AJ, Duepree HJ, Delaney CP, et al. Cost structure of laparoscopic and open sigmoid colectomy for diverticular disease: similarities and differences. Dis Colon Rectum 2002;45:485–490.

127. Gervaz P, Pikarsky A, Utech M, et al. Converted laparoscopic colorectal surgery. Surg Endosc 2001;15:827–832.

128. Schlachta CM, Mamazza J, Seshadri PA, et al. Predicting conversion to open surgery in laparoscopic colorectal resections. A simple clinical model. Surg Endosc 2000;14:1114–1117.

129. Schwandner O, Farke S, Fischer F, et al. Laparoscopic colectomy for recurrent and complicated diverticulitis: a prospective study of 396 patients. Langenbecks Arch Surg 2004; 389:97–103.

130. Schwandner O, Farke S, Bruch HP. Laparoscopic colectomy for diverticulitis is not associated with increased morbidity when compared with non-diverticular disease. Int J Colorectal Dis 2005;20(2):165–172.

131. Vargas HD, Ramirez RT, Hoffman GC, et al. Defining the role of laparoscopic-assisted sigmoid colectomy for diverticulitis. Dis Colon Rectum 2000;43:1726–1731.

132. Thaler K, Weiss EG, Nogueras JJ, et al. Recurrence rates at minimum 5-year follow-up: laparoscopic versus open sigmoid resection for uncomplicated diverticulitis. Surg Laparosc Endosc Percutan Tech 2003;13:325–327.

19
Colonic Volvulus

Michael D. Hellinger and Randolph M. Steinhagen

Introduction/Historical Perspective

Volvulus of the bowel refers to a twisting or torsion of the intestine about its mesentery. The term volvulus, which may involve any segment of the intestinal tract from stomach to rectum, is a Latin word for twisted used by the Romans to signify this condition.[1] Volvulus of the colon usually occurs in the sigmoid or cecum, but may involve any segment of colon. In addition, synchronous volvulus of the sigmoid and cecum,[2] or sigmoid and ileum may occur.[3] In the United States, volvulus represents a rare cause of intestinal obstruction, encompassing less than 5% of large bowel obstructions. However, worldwide it is a much more common form of large bowel obstruction, representing more than 50% of the cases in some countries.[4–6]

The first record of colonic volvulus is found in the Ebers Papyrus from ancient Egypt. This record stated that either volvulus would spontaneously reduce or the segment of bowel would "rot in his belly." The writings further document that if this condition did not resolve, the patient should be prepared for remedies to induce detorsion. As early as 1500 BC, therefore, it was recognized that detorsion was crucial for resolution of this condition. Even in ancient times, a high fiber diet was believed to be contributory to the development of volvulus. At that time, treatment was directed at symptoms and relief of the obstruction. External manipulation combined with purgatives was the treatment of the times. Hippocrates advocated use of a 10-digit long suppository and air blown into the anus with a metal worker's bellows. This is perhaps the earliest predecessor to today's sigmoidoscopic decompression.[1,7]

During subsequent years, reports concerning colonic volvulus were infrequent. It was not until the 19th century, when investigators began attempting to determine causes of disease, that this entity was discussed further. Perhaps the fact that volvulus was not recognized as a cause of colonic obstruction was accounted for by the rarity of the diagnosis before the 1800s. In 1872, Crise reported 12 cases, and in 1884 Treves reported 34 cases of colonic volvulus. In 1894, Obalinski recognized regional variations in frequency of volvulus.[1,7,8]

Throughout most of the 19th century, management was nonoperative. Operative intervention was reserved for life-threatening situations. High mortality rates for intestinal operations in the face of obstruction were the reasons cited in avoiding surgery. With advances in anesthesia and antisepsis, surgical procedures were developed. In 1883, Atherton performed the first successful operative detorsion of a sigmoid volvulus in the United States. The next year, Treves recommended colectomy for volvulus complicated by gangrene. By 1889, in fact, all of the surgical options for volvulus, including detorsion, -pexy, and resection with or without stoma, had been described.[1,7]

Early in the 20th century, with improvements in early diagnosis and rapid therapy, mortality rates began to decrease and surgical therapy became the mainstay. Mortality rates decreased from 30%–60% to under 20%. Mortality for gangrenous bowel remained high (30%–40%), reflecting a delay in diagnosis and treatment. Moynihan's statement in 1905 that a mortality of greater than 10% is the mortality of delay had been confirmed in many series.[1,7] Until the mid-20th century, immediate surgical intervention was the standard of care.

In 1947, Bruusgaard, from Norway, challenged the routine surgical approach, and reported a success rate of 86% for nonoperative reduction of sigmoid volvulus with proctoscopic decompression and placement of a rectal tube.[9] This paved the way for today's therapeutic algorithms in the management of colonic and specifically sigmoid volvulus.[1,7] Finally, with widespread use of flexible endoscopy, many authors have reported successful detorsion and decompression of all forms of colonic volvulus using the colonoscope or flexible sigmoidoscope.[10–15] Because of high recurrence rates, these endoscopic methods are currently recommended as definitive treatment only for very high-risk individuals who are too ill to undergo surgery, and as a temporizing measure until eventual surgery under more controlled conditions for all other patients.[1,7,9,14–16]

The differential diagnosis of colonic volvulus encompasses any cause of colonic distention. This includes all of the mechanical as well as the nonobstructive causes. Mechanical causes include colonic and extracolonic neoplasms, as well as benign entities such as diverticulitis and inflammatory bowel disease. Nonobstructive causes include colonic pseudo-obstruction (Ogilvie's syndrome), and various intraabdominal processes that may result in an intestinal paralysis. In addition, Hirschsprung's disease must also be considered.[5,6,17]

Cecal Volvulus

Incidence and Epidemiology

Worldwide, cecal volvulus accounts for 40%–60% of all colonic volvuli. Originally described in 1837 by Rokitansky, it remains, however, an uncommon cause of intestinal obstruction. The worldwide incidence is estimated at 2.8–7.1 per million people per year. Most reported cases occur in younger individuals with a predilection for females.[18–20] In a review of the published literature between 1959 and 1989, Rabinovici et al.[19] found a mean age of 53 years and a female to male ratio of 1.4:1.

Pathogenesis/Etiology

True cecal volvulus is actually an axial torsion of the cecum, terminal ileum, and ascending colon about its mesentery (Figure 19-1A). A variant, cecal bascule (Figure 19-1B), occurs when the cecum folds anteriorly over the ascending colon without an axial twist. This represents approximately 10% of cases of cecal volvulus. Review of patient characteristics indicates that there is a high rate of prior abdominal operations in patients who subsequently develop cecal volvulus, and previous surgery has been considered to be a potential causative factor. A clear prerequisite is a mobile cecum and ascending colon. A congenital component involves lack of fixation of the right colon, which then assumes an intraabdominal position.[4,18–20] In fact, a cadaver study revealed an 11% incidence of freely mobile right colons, and a 26% incidence of cecal mobility sufficient to allow folding. The authors concluded that 37% had cecums mobile enough to allow for volvulus.[4]

However, because cecal volvulus is so rare, factors other than cecal mobility must be involved. Prior abdominal surgery with colonic mobilization, recent surgical manipulation, adhesion formation, congenital bands, distal colonic obstruction, pregnancy, pelvic masses, extremes of exertion, and hyperperistalsis have all been implicated.[4,18–20] During abdominal surgery, excessive mobilization or manipulation of the cecum and ascending colon or placement/withdrawal of packs may precipitate postoperative volvulus.[4] Previous reports of cecal volvulus reveal that 30%–70% of patients had undergone prior surgery.[19,20] In the long term, an adhesive band may act as a fulcrum for a previously mobilized ileum and right colon to rotate axially. Displacement of the cecum by an enlarged uterus or pelvic mass may also promote volvulus. In fact, several series report that 10% of patients with cecal volvulus are pregnant at the time of presentation.[4,20]

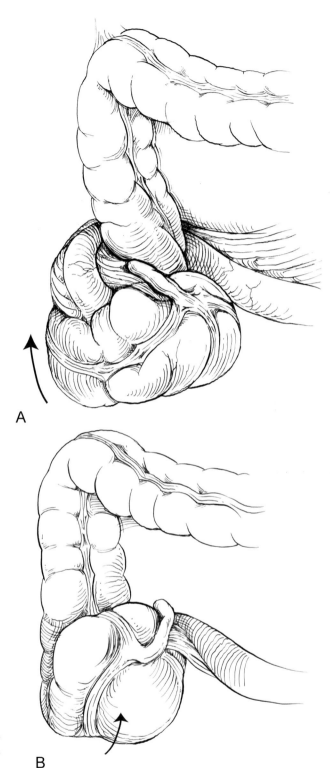

FIGURE 19-1. **A** Schematic illustration of a cecal volvulus. **B** Schematic illustration of a cecal bascule.

Clinical Presentation

Symptoms and signs of cecal volvulus are that of small bowel obstruction. The majority of patients present with abdominal pain, distention, constipation, nausea, and vomiting. Abdominal distention is less marked than with more distal forms of colonic volvulus. The presentation may be that of an acute obstruction or one of an intermittent or recurrent pattern. In the intermittent pattern, because duration of symptoms is brief, diagnosis may be quite difficult. Acute volvulus results in a closed loop cecal obstruction and distal small bowel obstruction. This may progress to a more fulminant presentation when ischemia and gangrene develop. At that point, the patient will present with peritoneal signs and systemic manifestations of an acute abdominal process. Before onset of gangrene, fever and leukocytosis are unreliable factors.[17–19,21]

Diagnosis

The diagnosis is most often made on the basis of the combination of clinical presentation and plain abdominal films or barium enema. Plain films may identify the classic coffee bean deformity directed toward the left upper quadrant (Figure 19-2A). If not, barium enema may reveal a "bird's beak" or column cut-off sign in the right colon (Figure 19-2B).[4,17–19] In the review by Rabinovici et al., 53% of cases were diagnosed preoperatively with clinical evaluation combined with radiologic investigation. The diagnosis was suspected in 46% of plain films, and barium enema was diagnostic in 88% of cases when obtained. However, 47% were not diagnosed until laparotomy.[18] Although barium enema is of clear value when the diagnosis is in question, in obvious cases, performance of this study may needlessly delay surgical therapy. It therefore should not be routinely used.[4]

Treatment/Outcome

Laparotomy remains the primary treatment modality for cecal volvulus. Many patients are not diagnosed until exploration, and nonoperative modalities have generally been unsuccessful. However, both radiographic and endoscopic reduction have been reported. Whereas radiographic attempts at reduction are generally believed to carry a high risk of perforation, other modalities have been used as temporizing measures.[4,5,16,18] Percutaneous decompression via computed tomographic scan guidance has been reported to be effective in decompressing a massively dilated colon in otherwise inoperable candidates.[22,23]

Although significantly less efficacious than in the treatment of distal volvulus, colonoscopic reduction of cecal volvulus (Figure 19-3) has been reported with some success. Reasons cited for limited use of this approach include difficulty traversing the extent of unprepared bowel to reach the right colon, difficulty performing the detorsion, the relative infrequency in which the diagnosis is made before laparotomy, and the higher rate of ischemic changes in cecal volvulus than in sigmoid volvulus. In fact, several authors have condemned this approach as only unnecessarily delaying definitive surgical intervention and potentially placing the patient at risk for perforation. However, if successfully used, there may be a

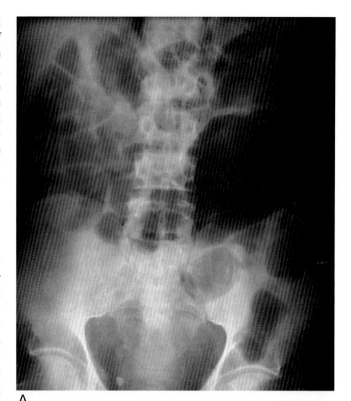

A

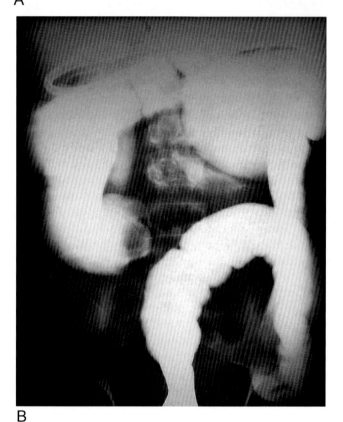

B

Figure 19-2. **A** Plain abdominal X-ray of a cecal volvulus with a "coffee bean" deformity evident in the left upper quadrant. **B** Barium enema study of a cecal volvulus revealing a bird's beak deformity.

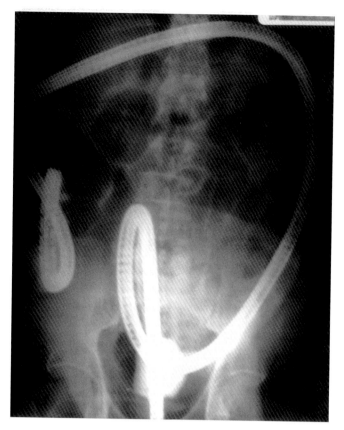

FIGURE 19-3. Colonoscopic reduction of a cecal bascule.

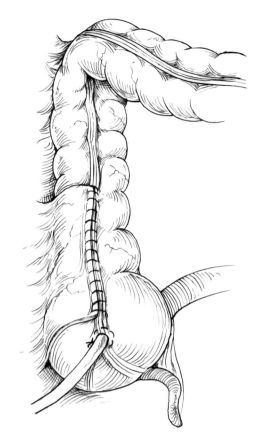

FIGURE 19-4. Colopexy and cecostomy for cecal volvulus.

relatively low rate of recurrence and the requirement for subsequent surgery is debated.[4,5,10,11,16,18,24,25]

In general, the majority of individuals undergo surgical intervention with a clear diagnosis of cecal volvulus, for complete bowel obstruction, or for an acute surgical abdomen. Obviously, in the face of gangrenous or ischemic bowel, resection is mandatory. When viable bowel is encountered, although resection is the preferred option, other alternatives exist. These include detorsion alone or combined with some fixation procedure. Fixation options include cecopexy and/or cecostomy. Appendicostomy has also been reported.[4,5,18,19,25,26]

Generally, fixation is accomplished by cecopexy and/or cecostomy. Cecopexy is performed by elevating a lateral peritoneal flap along the entire length of the ascending colon, and suturing the flap to the serosa of the anterior colonic wall, thereby placing the ascending colon in a partially retroperitoneal location, and eliminating the excess mobility (Figure 19-4). An advantage of tube cecostomy is that it not only anchors the cecum, but also provides a vent for the distended colon. Cecostomy is relatively simple to perform, and after removal of the tube, spontaneous closure is common.[4,5,18,25] In a review of the literature, Rabinovici et al.[19] found that detorsion, cecopexy, and cecostomy all carry similar recurrence rates of 12%–14%. Interestingly, they also noted a mortality for cecostomy triple that of either cecopexy or detorsion (32%

versus 10% and 13%, respectively). Other authors have reported recurrence rates ranging from 0% to 30%.[4,5,18,25]

Resection, however, carries virtually no risk of recurrence and is not associated with a higher rate of postoperative complications when compared with cecopexy alone.[18,25] After resection, primary anastomosis can usually be safely performed. However, in the face of gangrenous bowel, end ileostomy may be a safer procedure. The ultimate decision regarding intestinal anastomosis is one made at the time of surgery, taking into account degree of contamination, and the patient's overall status.[4,5,18,19,25,26] Overall mortality is independent of the procedure chosen, rather it is related to whether or not the surgery is elective or emergent and the presence or absence of gangrene. Literature documents no mortality in the elective situation. If viable bowel is found at the time of an emergency operation, mortality ranges from 7% to 15%. This increases to 33%–41% in the face of gangrenous bowel.[4,18,25]

Transverse Colon Volvulus

Incidence and Epidemiology

Volvulus of the transverse colon is an exceptionally rare finding. It is estimated to represent from 1% to 4% of all forms of colonic volvulus. However, in Eastern and Scandinavian countries, it may comprise 30%–40% of cases. This form of volvulus tends to occur more often in the young, with most series showing a peak incidence in the second through fourth decades of life. There is a two- to threefold female predominance.[4,18,20,27–29]

Pathogenesis/Etiology

Although anatomic factors are key to the development of transverse colon volvulus, physiologic, rather than congenital, factors seem to have a crucial role in the development. These patients frequently have a history of chronic constipation and/or laxative abuse, previous abdominal surgery, a diet high in fiber, recurrent distal obstruction, and institutionalization. There are also reports, however, of an association with malrotation, Hirschsprung's disease, and Chilaiditi's syndrome. Finally, adhesive bands, frequently reported in these patients, may act as a fulcrum around which the bowel can twist. Specific factors that may increase the risk of occurrence are a redundant or elongated transverse colon with narrow mesenteric attachments, narrowed distance between the flexures, and an absence or paucity of fixation of the mesentery. These factors increase the likelihood of an axial rotation of the transverse colon about its mesentery.[4,18,20,27–31]

Clinical Presentation

Transverse colon volvulus presents as a large bowel obstruction. Presentation may be as a subacute recurring process or may take a more fulminant course. The subacute form is associated with repetitive episodes, each with gradual onset. Although associated with significant abdominal distension, pain is mild to moderate, and vomiting is usually absent. Up to 50% of patients admit to previous episodes. The fulminant form is associated with less distension, but marked pain and vomiting. Clinical deterioration is rapid in these cases.[4,17,27–29,31]

Although diagnosis may be suspected on clinical presentation, plain films are rarely diagnostic. The diagnosis is therefore usually made at the time of exploration. Plain films may reveal a distended proximal colon with decompressed distal bowel and two distinct air-fluid levels representing two limbs of the volvulized transverse colon. This has been described as a bent inner-tube appearance with the apex pointing inferiorly. Barium contrast studies, if performed, will demonstrate a bird's beak deformity at the distal transverse colon. However, awaiting these studies only leads to a delay in definitive management.[4,17,27–30]

Treatment/Outcome

Although successful endoscopic decompression has been reported, surgical intervention is the recommended treatment modality. Based on literature from surgical detorsion, it is assumed that endoscopic treatment will lead to a high rate of

recurrence, and may therefore be best reserved for those high-risk individuals who show no signs of compromised bowel.[12,14,18] However, colonoscopy may serve to confirm intestinal viability and allow for a less emergent definitive procedure to be performed.[30]

Operative procedures include detorsion with or without colopexy, and resection. Most authors recommend either segmental transverse colectomy or extended right colectomy as definitive treatment. Clearly, in the presence of nonviable bowel, resection is mandatory.[12,14,18,30–32] As in cecal volvulus, the decision regarding primary anastomosis versus diversion is made during surgery, taking into account the severity of the disease process and the patient's overall condition. When viable bowel is encountered, several different colopexy procedures have been reported. These include suture of the greater omentum, transverse mesocolon, or transverse colon itself to the anterior abdominal wall and/or pelvis,[18,30,32] and the U colopexy reported by Mortensen.[31] In this procedure, after reduction and needle decompression of the volvulus, the redundant U-shaped loop of transverse colon is sutured to the adjacent limbs of ascending and descending colon (Figure 19-5).

Recurrence from either detorsion or colopexy has been reported to range from 30% to 75%, whereas resection eliminates virtually all risk of recurrence.[25,32] Mortality, however,

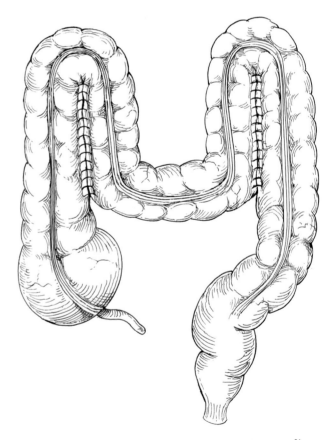

FIGURE 19-5. Parallel coloplasty as described by Mortensen.[31]

from resection has been reported to be as high as 33%. This is primarily in the setting of gangrene or perforation.[18,27] In these cases, mortality may be decreased by construction of an end stoma or extended resection with ileocolic anastomosis.[30]

Splenic Flexure Volvulus

Incidence and Epidemiology

Having been described in fewer than 50 patients in the English literature, volvulus of the splenic flexure of the colon is the rarest form of colonic volvulus. It is estimated to represent 1%–2% of all cases of colonic volvulus. It seems to be more common in women and occurs at a younger age than cecal or sigmoid volvulus.[4,13,25,33,34]

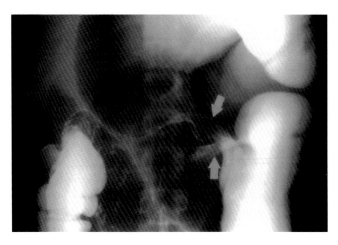

FIGURE 19-6. Barium enema study of a chronic splenic flexure volvulus. Arrows indicate the point of rotation and bird's beak deformity.

Pathogenesis/Etiology

The infrequency of this form of volvulus is believed to be the result of multiple attachments of the splenic flexure, and the retroperitoneal position of the descending colon. Three ligaments, the gastrocolic, splenocolic, and phrenocolic, are responsible for fixation of the splenic flexure. Congenital absence, laxity, or iatrogenic disruption of these ligaments may lead to excessive mobility of the splenic flexure. In addition, an intraperitoneal descending colon and adhesive bands from previous surgery may further predispose to the development of this form of volvulus. In fact, up to two-thirds of patients have had prior abdominal surgery. Finally, it has been speculated that chronic constipation may lead to redundancy of the colon and elongation of the mesentery. This may possibly create laxity of the ligamentous attachments.[4,13,25,33,34]

Clinical Presentation

As in transverse colon volvulus, the presentation may be acute and fulminant, or a more chronic or subacute event. Many patients have a history of severe chronic constipation, with longstanding laxative abuse. At presentation, the majority of patients have significant abdominal distention and pain. Although nausea and vomiting are common, obstipation is rare. Very few patients present with strangulation, gangrene, or findings of an acute surgical abdomen.[4,33,34]

Four features have been described radiographically that may suggest splenic flexure volvulus. They are: 1) a markedly dilated air-filled colon with an abrupt termination at the splenic flexure; 2) two widely spaced air-fluid levels, one in the cecum and the other in the transverse colon; 3) an empty descending and sigmoid colon; and 4) a bird's beak obstruction at the splenic flexure on contrast enema examination (Figure 19-6). An additional sign is a crescenteric gas shadow in the left upper quadrant of the abdomen.[13,33]

Treatment/Outcome

Although colonoscopic and fluoroscopic decompression have been reported, most reports have identified surgery as the primary mode of management. Surgical options include resection with or without stoma formation, or detorsion with or without colopexy. Segmental resection may be considered; however, the majority of these patients will have an associated redundant, dilated colon and a history of chronic constipation. Therefore, these patients may be better served by undergoing an extended resection with an ileosigmoid or ileorectal anastomosis. Stomas should be reserved for cases involving gangrenous bowel with perforation and peritoneal contamination, or for other high-risk cases.[4,13,25,34]

No mortality has been reported with either form of surgical management. The complication rate, excluding recurrence, is in the range of 10%. Resection carries a 0% recurrence rate. However, the recurrence rate after detorsion alone, whether performed surgically, endoscopically, or fluoroscopically, is approximately 20%–25%. As a result of these high recurrence rates, nonoperative decompression/detorsion should be reserved for extremely high-risk patients who are not candidates for surgical intervention, or as a temporizing measure before a semi-elective definitive resection.[4,13,34]

Sigmoid Volvulus

Incidence and Epidemiology

Although it is the most common form of volvulus seen, volvulus of the sigmoid colon is not very common in the United States and Western Europe, accounting for less than 10% of all cases of large bowel obstruction.[5,6,19,35] In some regions of Asia, Africa, and other less-developed portions of the world, however, the situation is significantly different. In these areas, sigmoid volvulus accounts for 20%–50% of the cases of intestinal obstruction. Overall, there is a substantial male predominance, especially in developing nations. However, sigmoid volvulus is the most common cause of intestinal obstruction in pregnancy, accounting for nearly 45% of all intestinal obstructions in this group of women.[3,4,5,19] The reasons for geographic differences in incidence are thought to be primarily related to diet. In the West, relatively lower amounts of fiber are consumed, resulting in a much higher incidence of colorectal cancer and diverticular disease, which are the more common etiologies for colonic obstruction in these areas. In less-developed regions of Asia and Africa, extremely high fiber diets result in significantly elongated colons, and lead to development of sigmoid volvulus, in relatively young patients.

Pathogenesis/Etiology

Any condition that results in an elongated colon predisposes to the development of volvulus. In order for volvulus of any part of the intestinal tract to occur, there must be a long redundant, mobile segment, with a relatively narrow mesenteric attachment, such that the sites of fixation at each end are relatively close together. The sigmoid colon is the ideal location for this configuration: the sigmoid can be extremely redundant and mobile and the sites of fixation at the descending-sigmoid junction and the rectosigmoid junction are often in close proximity to each other.[3,19]

Although a single etiology has not been identified, several theories do exist. In 1849, in his Manual of Pathological Anatomy, Von Rokitansky proposed that the primary causative factor was a "congenital or acquired long, loose, and floppy mesentery." Thirty-five years later, in his text of intestinal obstruction, Treves indicated that the loop in sigmoid volvulus "must be of considerable length, the mesocolon must be long and very narrow at its parietal attachment, so that two ends of the loop may be brought as close together as possible."[3]

In the West, the typical patient with sigmoid volvulus is an elderly institutionalized male, often receiving psychotropic medications, who is usually extremely constipated. Other factors that have been implicated are laxative abuse, previous abdominal surgery, and diabetes.[3,5,18] In other parts of the world, the patients are significantly younger.[24,36,37] Megacolon from any etiology, but especially Hirschsprung's disease or Chagas' disease, predisposes to volvulus.[3,8,19]

Gross features of the sigmoid colon include progressive widening and eventual loss of taenia coli, absence of appendices epiploicae, and a thickened narrowed fibrous mesentery. The scarring forms patches and bands coined "shrinking mesosigmoiditis" by Brusgaard, and is believed to be the result of previous episodes of volvulus.[9,19,38] The rotation may be either clockwise or counterclockwise. Once the rotation has reached 360 degrees, a closed loop obstruction occurs. Hyperperistalsis and fluid secretion into the closed loop add to increased pressure and tension. Eventually, as blood flow is compromised, ischemia and necrosis develop. Additionally, the diminished blood flow may lead to arterial and venous thrombosis. Three patterns of necrosis have been described: 1) at the neck of the volvulus, 2) any location within the closed loop, and 3) in the proximal descending colon or distal rectum because of retrograde mesenteric thrombosis. Because the sigmoid loop is usually chronically thickened, it is unlikely for a perforation to occur in this location. In the face of a competent ileocecal valve, perforation is more common in the cecum.[39]

Clinical Presentation

As previously described, the patient is typically a male nursing home resident, on psychotropic medications, with a history of chronic constipation. These patients may not complain of pain, but rather a caregiver notices an extremely long interval between bowel movements, associated with significant abdominal distension. In younger patients, constipation, distension, and abdominal pain are the predominant symptoms.[38] Before arrival at the hospital, the patient may have been given enemas or laxatives, without relief. This therapy may have, in fact, made the distension worse. There is often significant delay between onset and evaluation.[40,41] It has been reported that 40%–60% of patients will give a history of having had similar episodes.[4,38]

On presentation, the distension is often dramatic. Unlike the patient with fecal impaction, the rectal ampulla is empty. Plain abdominal films typically show massive colonic distension, with or without small bowel dilatation (depending on the competence of the ileocecal valve). The very large sigmoid loop will be orientated toward the right upper quadrant. The adjacent walls of the sigmoid will appear to be thickened, arising out of the left lower quadrant, giving the classical "bent inner tube" sign (Figure 19-7A).[38] In the majority of cases, plain radiographs are sufficient to establish the diagnosis.[40] In fact, plain abdominal X-rays alone are diagnostic in 60%–75% of cases.[39,42] However, the massive distension may, occasionally, make the diagnosis difficult to establish with certainty. In those cases, a contrast enema should be obtained. This study will show the obstruction at the rectosigmoid junction, with the classical bird's beak configuration (Figure 19-7B).[5,39] The addition of barium enema to the plain abdominal X-rays may increase the diagnostic yield to near 100%.[42]

The major diagnosis from which sigmoid volvulus must be distinguished is colonic obstruction caused by neoplasm. Usually the abdominal X-rays can distinguish one from the other; however, in the presence of truly massive distension, differentiation may be difficult. At the time of attempted sigmoidoscopic detorsion, the obstructing neoplasm will hopefully be visualized and the true diagnosis will be apparent. The other condition that may cause clinical confusion is colonic megacolon associated with abnormal colonic motility. This condition also presents in elderly, constipated nursing home patients. The X-rays can look remarkably similar.

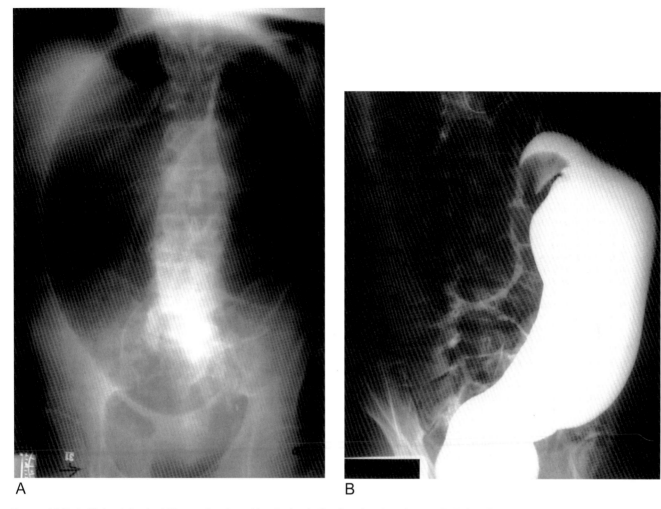

A   B

FIGURE 19-7. **A** Plain abdominal X-ray of a sigmoid volvulus indicating the "bent inner tube" sign. **B** Barium enema study of a sigmoid volvulus indicating the bird's beak deformity and complete obstruction to retrograde flow of contrast.

Because rectal tube decompression will generally rapidly and successfully relieve the distension associated with this form of megacolon, distinction from volvulus can be difficult. It is important to make the distinction, however, because this condition is also associated with a high incidence of recurrence, but will not be successfully treated by sigmoid resection. In one series, a 37% incidence of recurrent "volvulus" was seen after sigmoid resection and anastomosis. However, virtually all of these patients had megacolon-associated abnormal colonic motility.[43]

Treatment/Outcome

The patient with sigmoid colon volvulus should be hydrated and resuscitated. Since 1947, when Bruusgaard[9] reported a 90% success rate with sigmoidoscopic detorsion, the mainstay of emergency therapy has generally been detorsion and decompression. Detorsion of sigmoid volvulus has been described using several techniques, including rigid proctoscopy, flexible sigmoidoscopy or colonoscopy, blind

passage of a rectal tube, and use of a column of barium during barium enema examination.[7,9,10,14,15,24] Successful decompression using one of these techniques is generally reported in the range of 70%–80%.[18,39–41,44]

A significant concern is that the sigmoid may already be gangrenous. Several authors in Asia and Africa have noted an incidence of gangrene approaching 50%, as well as a significant incidence of double volvulus (ileosigmoid knotting) rarely seen in the West, and have therefore recommended emergency laparotomy without attempts at detorsion.[36,37,45–47] If ischemic mucosa is visualized, attempts at detorsion should be immediately abandoned and operative intervention should be undertaken emergently. For this reason, we strongly recommend using only those detorsion techniques that visualize the mucosa before detorsion. Attempts at detorsion via blind passage of a rectal tube should be avoided. Attempted detorsion of nonviable bowel will lead to a high incidence of perforation and peritonitis. The presence of nonviabilty should be suspected by the presence of signs and symptoms of compromised bowel and/or systemic sepsis, such as fever, leukocytosis, and especially localized tenderness over the sigmoid loop. If these are present, decompression should not even be attempted. The patient should be taken for emergent surgery. In approximately 25% of cases, the site of the twist will be more proximal than can be reached with a rigid proctoscope.[14] Use of flexible scopes can obviate this problem. The major complication associated with attempted detorsion is inadvertent perforation. This is more likely in the presence of gangrene, but can occur with viable bowel as well.

Once decompression has been accomplished, there is usually forceful evacuation of flatus and stool (frequently all over the clothes and shoes of an unsuspecting novice) and visible deflation of the patient's abdominal distension. A rectal tube should then be gently inserted into the colon to a point proximal to the site of the twist (which is usually within 20 cm of the anus). The tube should then be fixed in place, to allow continued decompression and prevention of recurrence. A plain abdominal film should be obtained to document decompression and the patient should be admitted to the hospital. Successful detorsion provides the advantage of converting a surgical emergency to an elective situation.

Over the next several days, bowel function is likely to return to normal. Medical conditions (cardiac, pulmonary, renal, etc.) should be addressed, electrolyte abnormalities should be corrected, and the patient's condition optimized. Colonoscopy, to rule out a proximal lesion, should be performed, and then a decision must be made. The rectal tube can be safely removed and the patient could be discharged from the hospital; however, it is well established that the rate of recurrent sigmoid volvulus is in excess of 25%.[48,49] In fact, most authors document a recurrence rate of greater than 50%, and some report recurrences as high as 80%–90%.[18,21] However, one report notes that 15 of 29 patients (52%) with sigmoid volvulus never required surgery. Twenty-three of 26 successfully decompressed patients were observed. Twelve recurred, six of whom were again decompressed and observed. Four of these patients had no further recurrence. Whereas none of the conservatively treated patients developed a complication, 43% of the surgical patients died.[35] The overall condition of the patient, the ease with which the volvulus was untwisted, and whether or not there were previous episodes of volvulus, are all factors that must be considered in the decision to perform definitive surgery.

The standard elective surgical procedure is sigmoid resection with primary anastomosis; however, a number of nonresective techniques have been described, including nonsurgical endoscopic sigmoidopexy with or without tube fixation,[17,50,51] extraperitoneal sigmoidopexy,[52] sigmoidopexy to the transverse colon and/or the parieties,[17] mesosigmoplasty,[53,54] colopexy with banding,[55] mesenteric fixation,[7] and laparoscopic fixation.[56] Although several authors have reported excellent results using pexy without resection,[52–54] others have reported recurrence rates in excess of 25%.[38] Whereas recurrence after resection approaches zero, resection with anastomosis was historically accompanied by relatively

substantial morbidity and mortality,[42] prompting a number of investigators to seek less risky alternatives.

Bhatnagar and Sharma[52] reported a series of 84 patients treated by sigmoidopexy with extraperitonealization. They reported a mortality of 9%. Patients were followed for a mean of 6.7 years with no evidence of recurrence (48 patients were followed for more than 5 years). Salim,[55] however, reported on a technique of percutaneous deflation, followed by tube detorsion and decompression, and finally intraperitoneal sigmoidopexy. He conducted a prospective, randomized trial of this nonresectional technique compared with resection and primary anastomosis. Of the initial 21 patients randomized to the decompression followed by surgical arm, six required emergency surgery. The remaining 15 were able to undergo an elective resection. Of note, he reported no recurrences and a mortality of 0% in the colopexy group as opposed to 13% in the group undergoing resection.[55]

Finally, the technique of mesosigmoidoplasty deserves discussion. This procedure is performed by incising the elongated sigmoid mesentery vertically along its axis. Peritoneal flaps are then created which are then approximated transversely (Figure 19-8). This procedure thereby creates a shortened, broad mesentery precluding future bowel rotation. Although one author has reported a recurrence of 28%, most report recurrences of less than 2%. Mortality ranges from 0% to 7%.[53,54]

Modern surgical and anesthetic techniques, including the use of surgical staplers, have reduced operative complications substantially. Resection with anastomosis, therefore, should currently be considered the standard of care for elective cases. However, in circumstances in which continence is an issue, an end stoma may be a better alternative. Colostomy via a

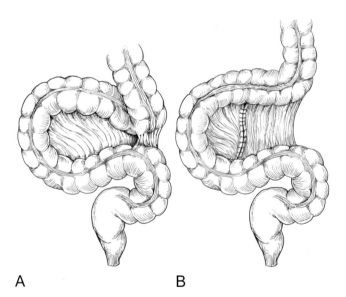

A   B

FIGURE 19-8. Mesosigmoidoplasty. **A** A longitudinal peritoneal incision is made in the elongated, narrow mesentery. **B** The incision is then closed transversely, broadening the mesenteric base and shortening the height of the sigmoid loop.

minimal left lower quadrant incision has been suggested for debilitated patients, too sick to undergo formal laparotomy.[57]

Laparoscopic techniques have also been applied,[58–60] but in general, because the redundant distended colon obscures the working space and the incision required to deliver the specimen is also large enough to exteriorize the redundant sigmoid colon and perform an adequate resection and anastomosis, there is little to be gained by the use of laparoscopy.[60] In fact, the entire resection and anastomosis can often be performed via a limited left lower quadrant muscle splitting incision, a very small midline incision, or via a Pfannenstiel incision.

If decompression is not possible, if the patient has signs and symptoms of peritonitis or colonic ischemia, or if gangrenous mucosa is visualized during attempted decompression, the situation becomes a surgical emergency. The patient should be rehydrated, electrolyte abnormalities and anemia should be corrected, the patient should be given intravenous antibiotics, and emergency surgery should be undertaken. The patient should be explored via a midline laparotomy, the volvulus should be manually reduced if the bowel is viable, and the redundant, twisted sigmoid should be resected. However, when gangrenous bowel is encountered during laparotomy, detorsion should not be performed. Accumulated toxins and bacteria may be released into the circulation, resulting in sepsis and cardiovascular collapse. Maintenance of the volvulus is therefore paramount as one obtains early vascular control. Inspection of the proximal colon must be performed, because in the face of a competent ileocecal valve, the closed loop obstruction produces rapid cecal ischemia and perforation.[21,38] Obviously, avoidance of fecal contamination is paramount. With the use of 90-mm linear staplers, even though the bowel proximal to the volvulus may be enormously dilated, resection without spillage is usually possible. Generally, an anastomosis should be avoided if the proximal colon is massively dilated and loaded with feces. Some authors have applied the technique of intraoperative colonic lavage to facilitate primary anastomosis.[61] In most cases, the proximal sigmoid should be exteriorized as an end-sigmoid colostomy; the distal end can be treated with a Hartmann-type closure, or a mucus fistula. A single prospective, randomized trial comparing primary anastomosis to the Hartmann's procedure in 14 patients with gangrenous bowel, revealed a 50% anastomotic leak rate. In addition, mortality was more than double in those patients in whom an anastomosis was performed (33% versus 13%).[36] Although the colostomy can generally easily be reversed in an elective manner, it must be recognized that because of the age and infirmity of many of these patients, in actual practice, the colostomy is often permanent.

Overall mortality rates for the treatment of sigmoid volvulus range from 14% to 45%. Emergency surgery without preoperative detorsion is associated with mortality rates of 20%–45%. If nonviable bowel is encountered, these rates may exceed 50%. In fact, several studies report mortality of 60%–80% in these cases.[9,17,21,35,36,38–41,62] Elective surgery,

after detorsion, is currently associated with mortality rates below 10%, despite the fact that these are generally patients with multiple comorbidities. However, older data reveal this mortality was as high as 25%.[7,9,17,21,35,36,38–41,62]

Paradoxically, outcomes in developed nations tend to be far worse than those in developing countries. This is presumed to be attributable to the older age and presence of significant comorbidities of the patients in the Western nations.[4,38] Ballantyne,[42] in a review of 67 series of sigmoid volvulus worldwide before 1981, compared mortality of nongangrenous and gangrenous bowel in the United States as compared with the rest of the world. He noted that the overall mortality in the United States was 25% and internationally 18%. When gangrenous bowel was present, the United States mortality further exceeded the international rate (80% versus 48%). However, for the nongangrenous, elective procedures, the United States mortality was somewhat less than the worldwide rate (10.6% versus 12.6%).

It has been suggested that a nonresectional approach may be safer in these ill patients. However, nonoperative decompression alone carries 0%–12% mortality. This may be related to attempted detorsion in the presence of ischemic bowel. Finally, operative detorsion with or without pexy carries a similar mortality to elective resection and anastomosis (8%–14%). Therefore, one must consider the overall risk of recurrence as well as the risk of mortality. As expected, any nonresectional procedure carries a substantial risk of recurrence. For decompression alone it ranges from 25% to 70%, whereas detorsion, with or without pexy, has been associated with recurrence rates of 23%–40%. Most authors indicate that the risk of recurrence after resection approaches zero; it has been reported to be as high as 5% in some series.[17,9,21,35,36,38–41,62] This is usually attributed to concomitant megacolon and/or megarectum.[48] The only prospective randomized trial comparing elective resection and primary anastomosis with mesosigmoidoplasty confirms these findings. None of the resected patients and 29% of the plastied patients experienced recurrence. However, there was no mortality in the plasty group as compared with 10% in the resection group.[36]

Ileosigmoid Knotting

Incidence and Epidemiology

Ileosigmoid knotting, also called compound volvulus, is a rare form of volvulus uncommon in the West. It is, however, comparatively more common in certain areas of Africa, Asia, and the Middle East. In particular, large series are reported from Turkey, Russia, Scandinavia, Uganda, and India. It is more common in males than females, and presents at a younger age than sigmoid volvulus. In fact, it has rarely been reported in individuals older than 50 years of age.[3,63–67]

The geographic distribution corresponds with regions of the world where diets high in bulk and carbohydrates are consumed with large volumes of liquid. The incidence is highest in groups in which one single large meal is consumed daily. It has been reported to peak in the followers of Islam during Ramzan when a single large meal is consumed at sunset after a full day's fast.[3,63-67]

Pathogenesis/Etiology

Theories of the pathogenesis of ileosigmoid knotting focus on a large volume diet high in bulk and carbohydrates, associated with large volumes of concomitant liquid ingestion. This may lead to an elongated abnormally mobile small intestinal mesentery, in addition to a long narrow pedicled sigmoid mesentery. The simultaneous consumption of a large meal combined with a large volume of fluid may then initiate an acute knot formation. As the bolus empties into the jejunum, the bowel becomes hyperperistaltic, and the weight acts to pull it into the left paracolic gutter. The empty distal loops of small bowel are then displaced around a narrow-based sigmoid. Continued peristalsis leads to further rotation of the loop, internal herniation, and knot formation (Figure 19-9). The fact that this entity usually occurs in the early morning hours lends further credence to the theory that dietary and dining habits of certain populations are causative.[3,63-67]

Alver et al.,[64] in a review of 68 cases, described four different patterns of ileosigmoid knot formation which differentiate between an active or passive segment of bowel and the direction of rotation. Usually, the ileum is the active component and wraps around the sigmoid in either a clockwise or counterclockwise manner. Alternatively, the sigmoid may wrap around a passive segment of ileum, either clockwise or counterclockwise.

Clinical Presentation

The presentation of ileosigmoid knotting is one of acute onset, often with a fulminant course. There is a dramatic absence of prior similar attacks that are frequently seen in other forms of volvulus. Patients usually present in shock with signs of an intraabdominal catastrophe. The patient may complain of severe colicky abdominal pain, which begins in the periumbilical region. Nausea and vomiting, as well as distension, are early findings. At surgery, gangrenous intestine is found in 70%–100% of cases. As the result of the severity of the condition at presentation, acidosis, hypovolemia, oliguria, hypotension, and tachycardia are common findings.[3,63-67]

Preoperative diagnosis is extremely difficult because of the confusing nature of the presentation and unfamiliarity with

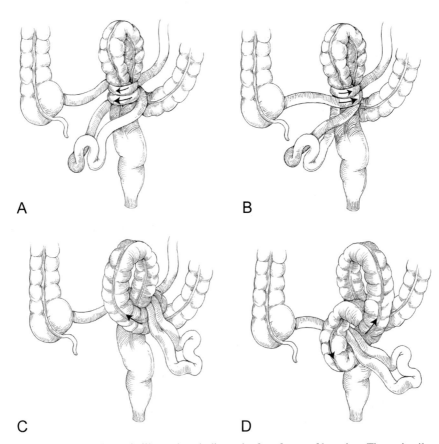

A   B

C   D

FIGURE 19-9. Ileosigmoid knotting: these schematic illustrations indicate the four forms of knotting. The active ileum may rotate around the sigmoid colon in either a clockwise **A** or counterclockwise **B** direction. Much more infrequently, the sigmoid colon may act as the active loop and rotate in either a clockwise **C** or counterclockwise **D** direction around the ileum.

this entity. Clinically, the patient's condition presents as a small bowel obstruction, but radiographic evaluation is more consistent with a large intestinal obstruction. In fact, X-rays are often atypical, and the diagnosis is correctly made in fewer than 20% of patients preoperatively. However, several characteristic radiographic features of ileosigmoid knotting have been identified. These include a double obstruction, with an obstructed distended sigmoid loop pulled to the right and a proximal small bowel obstruction on the left. A diagnostic triad has been proposed consisting of a clinical small bowel obstruction, a radiographic large bowel obstruction, and the inability to pass a sigmoidoscope to decompress a suspected sigmoid volvulus.[3,64–67]

Treatment/Outcome

Because of the high incidence of ischemia and gangrene at the time of presentation, after an initial period of rapid resuscitation and antibiotic administration, patients should be taken for emergent abdominal exploration. Controversy clearly exists regarding the preferred surgical approach. Treatment recommendations have ranged from simple detorsion to double resection. Because of the high likelihood of gangrenous bowel, most authors advocate en bloc resection of both segments of intestine without attempts to untwist the bowel. They state that untying the knot may be time consuming, difficult, hazardous, and may lead to systemic release of endotoxin and propagation of shock. Finally, perforation may ensue, leading to peritoneal contamination.[3,63–66] However, others have recommended detorsion if one or both segments of bowel are thought to be viable. Deflation of the torsed segments had been shown to assist in untying the knot and diminishing the risk of rupture. There are conflicting data on recurrence after detorsion alone.[3,63–66] Some authors advise resection of the sigmoid in all cases because of the possibility of recurrent knotting or eventual sigmoid volvulus.[62,64–66]

Although most perform a primary ileoileal or ileocolic anastomosis in patients with gangrenous small bowel, a Hartmann's procedure is usually performed when the sigmoid is found to be nonviable. When the sigmoid is viable, despite the lack of bowel preparation, some authors have reported safe colorectal anastomoses. Because of the risk of inferior mesenteric artery or superior rectal artery thrombosis, most authors also advocate resection of the sigmoid well past the areas of twisting and/or gangrene to ensure adequate blood supply.[3,63–67]

Overall surgical mortality generally ranges from 30% to 50%. One review of seven patients reported no mortality, despite finding gangrenous colon in all seven patients, and gangrenous ileum in three.[63–67] Mortality for nongangrenous bowel is generally less than that for gangrenous bowel. Reports range from 10% to 30% for nongangrenous intestine, and 40% to 50% for gangrenous bowel.[3,64–66] Alver et al.,[64] however, noted a paradoxic relationship between duration of symptoms and mortality. Those patients who presented within

24 hours had a mortality of 42%, whereas those that presented later had a much lower mortality rate of 20%. Additionally, he noted that the rate of gangrene was 91% in the early presenters but only 57% in the late presenters. This reflects the more rapid fulminant course of the patients that present earlier.[64] In addition, when extensive gangrene of the small bowel is found, leaving the patient with less than 60 cm of residual bowel, mortality has been shown to be 100%.[64]

References

1. Tan PY, Corman ML. History of colonic volvulus. Semin Colon Rectal Surg 1999;10:122–128.
2. Moore JH, Cintron JR, Duarte B, et al. Synchronous cecal and sigmoid volvulus: report of a case. Dis Colon Rectum 1992;35:803–805.
3. Puthu D, Rajan N, Shenoy GM, Pai SU. The ileosigmoid knot. Dis Colon Rectum 1991;34:161–166.
4. Ballantyne GH, Brandner MD, Beart RW, et al. Volvulus of the colon: incidence and mortality. Ann Surg 1985;202:83–92.
5. Frizelle FA, Wolff BG. Colonic volvulus. Adv Surg 1996;29:131–139.
6. Geer DA, Arnaud G, Beitler A, et al. Colonic volvulus: The army medical center experience 1983–1987. Am Surg 1991;57:295–300.
7. Ballantyne GH. Review of sigmoid volvulus: history and results of treatment. Dis Colon Rectum 1982;25:494–501.
8. Ballantyne GH. Review of sigmoid volvulus: clinical patterns and pathogenesis. Dis Colon Rectum 1982;25:823–830.
9. Bruusgaard C. Volvulus of the sigmoid colon and its treatment. Surgery 1947;22:466–478.
10. Orchard JL, Mehta R, Khan AH. The use of colonoscopy in the treatment of colonic volvulus: three cases and review of the literature. Am J Gastroenterol 1984;77:543–545.
11. Anderson MJ, Okoke N, Spencer RJ. The colonoscope in cecal volvulus: report of three cases. Dis Colon Rectum 1978;21:71–74.
12. Joergensen K, Kronborg O. The colonoscope in volvulus of the transverse colon. Dis Colon Rectum 1980;23:357–358.
13. Sanderson AJ, Elford J, Hayward SJ. Case report: volvulus of the splenic in a patient with systemic sclerosis. Br J Radiol 1995;68:537–539.
14. Brother TE, Strodel WE, Eckhauser FE. Endoscopy in colonic volvulus. Ann Surg 1987;206:1–4.
15. Ghazi A, Shinya H, Wolff WI. Treatment of volvulus of the colon by colonoscopy. Ann Surg 1976;183:263–265.
16. Stamos MJ, Hicks T. Nonoperative management of colonic volvulus. Semin Colon Rectal Surg 1999;10:145–148.
17. Tsushima GK, Fleshner PR. Colonic volvulus: imaging, diagnosis, and differential diagnosis. Semin Colon Rectal Surg 1999;10:139–144.
18. Friedman JD, Odland MD, Bubrick MP. Experience with colonic volvulus. Dis Colon Rectum 1989;32:409–416.
19. Rabinovici R, Simansky DA, Kaplan O, et al. Cecal volvulus. Dis Colon Rectum 1990;33:765–769.
20. Margolin DA, Whitlow CB. The pathogenesis and etiology of colonic volvulus. Semin Colon Rectal Surg 1999;10:129–138.
21. Nivatvongs S, Bubrick MP. Volvulus of the colon. In: Nivatvongs S, Gordon P, eds. Principles and Practice of Surgery for the

Colon, Rectum, and Anus. 2nd ed. St Louis, MO: Quality Medical Publishing; 1999:1046–1063.

22. Casola G, Withers C, van Sonnenberg E, et al. Percutaneous cecostomy for decompression of the massively distended cecum. Radiology 1986;158:793–794.

23. Patel D, Ansai E, Berman MD. Percutaneous decompression of cecal volvulus. Am J Radiol 1987;148:747.

24. Arigbabu AO, Badejo OA, Akinola DO. Colonoscopy in the emergency treatment of colonic volvulus in Nigeria. Dis Colon Rectum 1985;28:795–798.

25. Halverson AL, Orkin BA. Operative therapy for colonic volvulus. Semin Colon Rectal Surg 1999;10:149–153.

26. Singh JL, Wexner SD. Colonic volvulus: a treatment algorithm. Semin Colon Rectal Surg 1999;10:158–163.

27. Loke KL, Chan CS. Case report: transverse colon volvulus—unusual appearance on barium enema and review of the literature. Clin Radiol 1995;50:342–344.

28. Plorde JJ, Raker EJ. Transverse colon volvulus and associated Chilaiditi's syndrome: case report and literature review. Am J Gastroenterol 1996;91:2613–2616.

29. Eisenstat TE, Raneri AJ, Mason GR. Volvulus of the transverse colon. Am J Surg 1977;134:396–399.

30. Gumbs MA, Kashan F, Shumofsky F, Yerubandi SR. Volvulus of the transverse colon: report of cases and review of the literature. Dis Colon Rectum 1983;26:825–828.

31. Mortensen NJ. Volvulus of the transverse colon. Postgrad Med J 1979;55:54–57.

32. Anderson R, Lee D, Taylor RV, Ross HM. Volvulus of the transverse colon. Br J Surg 1981;68:179–181.

33. Cho YU, Sohn SK, Chi HS, Kim KW. Volvulus of the splenic flexure of the colon. Yonsei Med J 1994;35:97–100.

34. Hellinger MD, Ferrara A, Martini M, et al. Volvulus of the splenic flexure of the colon: report of two cases and review of the literature. Contemp Surg 1995;46:309–315.

35. Theuer C, Cheadle WG. Volvulus of the colon. Am Surg 1991;57:145–150.

36. Bagarabi M, Conde AS, Longo R, Italiano A, et al. Sigmoid volvulus in West Africa: a prospective study on surgical treatments. Dis Colon Rectum 1993;36:186–190.

37. Khanna AK, Kumar P, Khanna R. Sigmoid volvulus. Study from a North Indian Hospital. Dis Colon Rectum 1999;42:1081–1084.

38. Gibney EJ. Volvulus of the sigmoid colon. Surg Obstet Gynecol 1991;173:243–255.

39. Mangiante EC, Croce MA, Fabian TC, et al. Sigmoid volvulus. A four decade experience. Am Surg 1989;55:41–44.

40. Grossman EM, Longo WE, Stratton MD, et al. Sigmoid volvulus in Department of Veteran Affairs Medical Centers. Dis Colon Rectum 2000;43:414–418.

41. Hiltunen KM, Syrja H, Matikainen M. Colonic volvulus. Diagnosis and results of treatment in 82 patients. Eur J Surg 1992;158:607–611.

42. Ballantyne GH. Sigmoid volvulus: high mortality in county hospital patients. Dis Colon Rectum 1981;24:515–520.

43. Morrissey TB, Deitch EA. Recurrence of sigmoid volvulus after surgical intervention. Am Surg 1994;60:329–331.

44. Wertkin MG, Aufses AH Jr. Management of volvulus of the colon. Dis Colon Rectum 1978;21:40–45.

45. Kuzu MA, Aslar AK, Soran A, et al. Emergent resection for acute sigmoid volvulus. Results of 106 consecutive cases. Dis Colon Rectum 2002;45:1085–1090.

46. Naaeder SB, Archampong EQ. One-stage resection of acute sigmoid volvulus. Br J Surg 1995;82:1635–1636.

47. Tiwary N, Prasad S. Mesocoloplasty for sigmoid volvulus: a preliminary report. Br J Surg 1976;63:961–962.

48. Chung YFA, Eu KW, Nyam DCNK, et al. Minimizing the recurrence after sigmoid volvulus. Br J Surg 1999;86:231–233.

49. Hines JR, Geurkink RE, Bass RT. Recurrence and mortality rates in sigmoid volvulus. Surg Obstet Gynecol 1967;124:567–570.

50. Chiulli RA, Swantkowski TM. Sigmoid volvulus treated with endoscopic sigmoidopexy. Gastrointest Endosc 1993;39:194–196.

51. Pinedo G, Kirberg A. Percutaneous endoscopic sigmoidopexy in sigmoid volvulus with T-fasteners. Report of two cases. Dis Colon Rectum 2001;44:1867–1870.

52. Bhatnagar BNS, Sharma CLN. Nonresective alternatives for the cure of nongangrenous sigmoid volvulus. Dis Colon Rectum 1998; 441:381–388.

53. Akgun Y. Mesosigmoidoplasty as a definitive operation in treatment of acute sigmoid volvulus. Dis Colon Rectum 1996;39:579–581.

54. Subrahmanyam M. Mesosigmoidoplasty as a definitive operation for sigmoid volvulus. Br J Surg 1992;79:683–684.

55. Salim AS. Management of acute volvulus of the sigmoid colon: a new approach by percutaneous deflation and colopexy. World J Surg 1991;15:68–73.

56. Miller R, Roe AM, Eltringham WK, Espiner HJ. Laparoscopic fixation of sigmoid volvulus. Br J Surg 1992;79:435.

57. Caruso DM, Kassir AA, Robles RA, et al. Use of trephine stoma in sigmoid volvulus. Dis Colon Rectum 1996;39:1222–1226.

58. Chung CC, Kwok SPY, Leung KL, et al. laparoscopic-assisted sigmoid colectomy for volvulus. Surg Laparosc Endosc 1997;7:423–425.

59. Chung RS. Colectomy for sigmoid volvulus. Dis Colon Rectum 1997;40:363–365.

60. Fleshman JL. Laparoscopic management of colonic volvulus. Semin Colon Rectal Surg 1999;10:154–157.

61. Gurel M, Alic B, Bac B, et al. Intraoperative colonic irrigation in the treatment of acute sigmoid volvulus. Br J Surg 1989;76:957–958.

62. Pahlman L, Enblad P, Rudberg C, Krog M. Volvulus of the colon. A review of 93 cases and current aspects of treatment. Acta Chir Scand 1989;155:53–56.

63. Akgun Y. Management of ileosigmoid knotting. Br J Surg 1997;84:672–673.

64. Alver O, Durkaya OM, Mustafa T, et al. Ileosigmoid knotting in Turkey: review of 68 cases. Dis Colon Rectum 1993;36:1139–1147.

65. Gibney EJ, Mock CN. Ileosigmoid knotting. Dis Colon Rectum 1993;36:855–857.

66. Raveenthiran V. The ileosigmoid knot: new observations and changing trends. Dis Colon Rectum 2001;44:1196–1200.

67. Young WS, White A, Grave GF. The radiology of ileosigmoid knot. Clin Radiol 1978;29:211–216.

20
Lower Gastrointestinal Hemorrhage

Frank G. Opelka, J. Byron Gathright, Jr., and David E. Beck

Lower gastrointestinal hemorrhage refers to a spectrum of intestinal bleeding that arises distal to the ligament of Treitz. It may range from occult bleeding or occasional spotting of blood to massive lower intestinal hemorrhage. Massive lower intestinal hemorrhage is difficult to define. Patients often describe massive bleeding into their commode even when a small amount of blood discolors the water. True massive intestinal hemorrhage typically involves hemodynamic compromise or symptomatic anemia. Multiple sources define massive bleeding to include patients with a hematocrit less than 30%, patients with transfusion requirements (up to 3–5 units of blood/blood products), or orthostasis requiring resuscitation.

Primarily, lower intestinal hemorrhage arises from within the colon. Billingham[1] described lower gastrointestinal hemorrhage as a conundrum with five key concerns. First, the condition may arise from bleeding throughout the gastrointestinal tract. Second, intermittent bleeding precludes a prompt identification of the site of hemorrhage. Third, patients requiring surgery may undergo a procedure without a specific preplanned site of resection and with considerable morbidity and mortality. Fourth, despite aggressive surgical management, persistent bleeding may occur. And finally, there is no consensus about the precise diagnostic and therapeutic pathways for patients.

From the perspective of the emergency room care, massive lower gastrointestinal hemorrhage is a relatively uncommon emergency. Longstreth[2] studied a large health maintenance organization (HMO)-based population in San Diego, California, noting an annual incidence rate of 20.5/100,000 patients with a male predominance. His study reflected a retrospective survey and chart review defining incidence. The incidence of significant bleeding increases with age. The association with aging may suggest senescent changes associated with the small intestine and colon. Certainly aging reflects the surging prevalence of colonic diverticulosis and intestinal angiodysplasia in the elderly. It is of interest to note that the California HMO group had a high incidence of diverticulosis (41.6%) and infrequent angiodysplasia (2.7%).

However, Longstreth admits the limitations of the study design may not precisely determine the true etiologies of lower gastrointestinal hemorrhage.

Lower gastrointestinal bleeding presents with varying degrees of hemorrhage. Patients may experience minor bleeding when they describe the passage of 100–250 mL of blood, possibly a few clots, and often mixed with mucous. Other patients experience brisk, copious bleeding with major, self-limited hemorrhage. Finally, certain patients present with massive and continuous hemorrhage associated with hypovolemia. The hemorrhage may present as melena or hematochezia. Melena typically suggests bleeding from a more proximal source in the colon or small intestine. Hematochezia suggests left colonic, rectal, or anal sources. It is wise to note that upper gastrointestinal hemorrhage may present with the rectal bleeding given blood's cathartic effect and rapid intestinal transit. Jensen and Machicado[3] outlined the safety of emergency panendoscopy in patients with hematochezia and negative nasogastric lavage. His 1988 study provided additional insights in demonstrating an upper source for bleeding in 11% of patients.[4] Overall, it is believed that upper sources may present with lower gastrointestinal bleeding symptoms in 10%–15% of cases.

Most often the intestinal bleeding resolves spontaneously with supportive hospital care. Once it resolves, investigations should begin to identify the potential sources. Actual bleeding sources are not so frequently identified by the current limitations of our diagnostic tools. In clinical scenarios in which the bleeding resolved spontaneously, the diagnostic evaluation may only unmask potential sources. Without associated attached clot or active bleeding, the true site of hemorrhage may never be elucidated. On occasion, the intestinal hemorrhage does not resolve. It continues, creating hemodynamic compromise. Ongoing hemorrhage demands aggressive medical and surgical management. Oftentimes, patients with massive hemorrhage are plagued with significant comorbidities that complicate their individual resuscitation. Their comorbidities must be considered in the diagnostic and therapeutic phases of the care plan.

History and physical examination fall short of an adequate classification system to ultimately predict patient needs or clinical outcome. A patient may portray a worrisome history of massive hemorrhage and still resolve spontaneously with simple, supportive measures. Other patients may sequester blood in large volume and seem to have stopped bleeding. While under observation their scenario promptly changes with ongoing, massive hemorrhage. They require prompt therapy. Still other patients may bleed aggressively, stop for a few days, and then repeat their massive exsanguinations. In addition, diagnostic studies often are invasive procedures with limited sensitivities and specificities.

More and more, physicians witness special patient groups with massive lower gastrointestinal hemorrhage. Current disease managements call for concurrent care with anticoagulants or antiplatelet agents for underlying cardiovascular conditions. Current treatment regimens incorporate long-term anticoagulants and antiplatelet agents. Hemorrhage in these patients proves more life-threatening. Landefeld and Goldman[5] noted a 22% long-term risk of bleeding on anticoagulant therapy with warfarin. Gastrointestinal hemorrhage is one of five independent risk factors. Current increased patient exposure to antiplatelet therapy associated with treatment of cardiovascular conditions may increase the comorbid challenges in patients with lower gastrointestinal massive hemorrhage.

Etiologies

Common causes for lower gastrointestinal hemorrhage include colonic diverticula, angiodysplasia, ischemic colitis, and inflammatory bowel disease. Hemorrhage also stems from intestinal tumors or malignancies. Unusual causes include nonsteroidal antiinflammatory drug (NSAID)-related nonspecific colitis, Meckel's diverticulum, and anorectal diseases. The reported mortality with varying etiologies is summarized in Table 20-1.

Diverticular Disease

Diverticulosis is a common malady in Western civilization. Approximately 50% of the population by age 60 years has evidence of diverituclosis.[10] Most diverticula represent pulsion diverticula or pseudodiverticula that are actually outpouchings of the mucosa and submucosa through defects in the muscular layer of the bowel at sites of penetration of the vasa recta. It is theorized that slow intestinal transit and increased intraluminal pressure within the segmentation process promote the development of the diverticula.

The precise mechanism of diverticular hemorrhage is unknown. In the late 1800s, Kebs outlined the vascular anatomy of the vasa recta and the mucosal blood supply. Further, Drummond,[11] in 1916, displayed the relationship between the vasa recta and the neck of the diverticulum. In 1976, Meyers et al.[12] defined the bleeding sites as the ruptured vasa recta in the diverticulum. He noted structural changes located eccentrically in the vasa recta at the site of rupture, intimal thickening with thinning of the media, the absence of any acute or chronic inflammation, and stated that these vascular changes were typically the result of focal injury. It is generally accepted that thinning of the media in the vasa recta predisposes to intraluminal rupture: focal injury may occur from trauma related to a fecalith.

It is unclear how frequently diverticula are the true cause of hemorrhage. The incidence spans a range of 15% to 48%. Oftentimes, authors attribute the condition to diverticula after the hemorrhage has ceased despite a lack of proof of actual cause, a presumptive diagnosis. Diagnostic evaluations, such as colonoscopy, do not identify a precise source for the hemorrhage without the presence of witnessed bleeding or an adherent clot. Oftentimes, for lack of a more precise etiology, diverticula are present and, therefore, become the primary culprit. Despite being considered a major source for colonic hemorrhage, bleeding from diverticula is a relatively rare event affecting only 4%–17% of patients with diverticulosis.[13]

In most cases, bleeding ceases spontaneously, but in 10%–20% of cases, the bleeding continues unabated in the absence of intervention.[14] Once bleeding has occurred, the natural history and risk of rebleeding are poorly understood. Finne[15] comments that the risk of rebleeding after an episode of bleeding is approximately 25% but increases to 50% among patients who have had two or more prior episodes of diverticular bleeding. Right sided colonic diverticula occur less frequently than left sided or sigmoid diverticula but are thought to be responsible for a disproportionate incidence of diverticular bleeding. This finding is not well established, however, and there is often difficulty distinguishing between bleeding from an arteriovenous malformation or angiodysplasias and bleeding from diverticulosis. The overall high prevalence of diverticulosis in the population at risk for lower gastrointestinal hemorrhage makes the exact diagnosis of many bleeding episodes equivocal.

TABLE 20-1. Mortality of lower gastrointestinal bleeding by etiology

Investigator	Diverticulosis (%)	Angiodysplasia (%)	Cancer/polyp (%)	Colitis/ulcer (%)	Anorectal (%)	Other (%)	Mortality (%)
Jensen and Machicado,[3] 1997	23	40	15	12	5	4	NA
Longstreth,[2] 1997	41	3	9	16	5	14	3.6
Bramley et al.,[6] 1996	24	7	10	21	9	4	5.1
Richter et al.,[7] 1995	48	12	11	6	3	6	2
Rossini et al.,[8] 1989	15	4	30	22	0	11	NA
Jensen and Machicado,[9] 1988	20	37	14	11	5	5	NA

Operative management of diverticular bleeding is indicated when bleeding continues unabated and is not amenable to angiographic or endoscopic therapy. It also should be considered in patients with recurrent bleeding localized to the same colonic segment. In a stable healthy patient, the operation consists of a segmental bowel resection (usually a right colectomy or sigmoid colectomy) followed by a primary anastomosis. One additional note about diverticular hemorrhage focuses on recurrence for patients who stopped bleeding and required no operative intervention. In Longstreth's San Diego study,[2] the author noted that 9% of patients returned within 1 year with another episode. At 2 years, there was little change, 10%; 19% at 3 years; and 25% at 4 years.

Angiodysplasia

Angiodysplasia was described by Margolis et al.[16] in 1960 when they noted the radiographic features during an intraoperative angiogram performed for colonic bleeding. Angiodysplasias are thin-walled arteriovenous communications located within the submucosa and mucosa of the intestine. Angiodysplasias may be congenital or, more typically, acquired. They could be isolated or multiple. In the acquired form, distortions of the postcapillary venules may arise as a degenerative lesion associated with increases in intraluminal pressure. The intraluminal pressure occurs from loss of the precapillary sphincter and a resultant increased pressure transmitted through the capillary bed into the venules. As these vessels respond to the arterial flow, it results in thickening and ectasia. The vessels eventually entangle as tufts within the submucosa and erode into the mucosa proper.

No one is quite certain precisely why angiodysplasias occur. Current hypotheses suggest a loss of vascular integrity related to loss of transforming growth factor (TGF) β signaling cascade or from a deficiency in mucosal type IV collagen. McAllister et al.[17] suggest that a genetic error in endoglin production alters TGF β and, thus, the integrity of the vascular endothelial cells. Roskell et al.[18] noted the loss of mucosal type IV collagen in pathologic specimens of angiodysplasia.

Angiodysplasias are uncommon before age 60, increase with age, and are associated with aortic stenosis (Heyde's syndrome), chronic renal failure, and von Willebrand's disease. Osler-Weber-Rendu (hereditary hemorrhagic telangiectasias) is a hereditary condition with telangiectasias of the lung, nervous system, skin, and intestine. These patients present with multiple lesions. In 1995, Christopher Gostout[19] editorialized in questioning the association of angiodysplasias with aortic stenosis.

When angiodysplasias are noted during angiography or colonoscopy, unless a hemorrhagic blush is seen during the angiogram or colonoscopy, it is difficult to accurately accuse this malady as the source of hemorrhage.[20] In the past, angiodysplasia was the diagnosis chosen when no bleeding source could be identified and the abnormal vessels were present. In addition, many drew an association between the angiodysplasias and aortic stenosis. The association between the ecstatic vascular tufts and aortic stenosis was dispelled by Imperiale and Ransohoff[21] in the late 1980s. However, the association persisted in anecdotes until Bhutani and colleagues[20] reviewed 37 patients and found no greater incidence of aortic valvular disease than the control group.

Angiography remains the gold standard for the diagnosis of angiodysplasia. After injection of contrast, a series of images are collected in three phases. In the arterial phase, the radiographic findings of angiodysplasia demonstrate early venous filling which normally occurs in later phases. During the next phase, capillary phase, small, tortuous tufts are seen entangled and filled with contrast. Finally, the late phase study demonstrates a persistent of this arteriovenous tuft and a persistent of a slow, emptying vein.[22] When angiography identifies a bleeding angiodysplasia, treatment with embolization therapy or directed infusion of vasopressin will decrease or stop the bleeding.

Colonoscopy has increased as a screening agent for colorectal cancers as well as during the investigation for colorectal bleeding. Expectantly, more angiodysplasias are seen during endoscopy than in the past. In contrast to the angiographic findings described by Boley et al., Bhutani et al.[20] highlighted the colonoscopic criteria in describing these lesions. The mucosal surface contains a cherry red lesion that is typically flat. The lesions are greater than 2 mm in size and have a "fern-like" appearance. A central feeding vessel is not always visible. It is important to identify these lesions during scope insertion. Occasionally, the inexperienced endoscopists may attribute colonoscopic suction trauma to an angiodysplastic area. By searching for the vascular muscular lesions during scope insertion, the endoscopist will avoid misnaming scope mucosal trauma as angiodysplasia. Initial experience in identifying these lesions related to a few angiographic studies. The early evidence suggested the lesions were predominantly right sides. Since colonoscopy has become more available, both left and right sided lesions are thought to occur.

Other Causes of Lower Gastrointestinal Hemorrhage

Multiple other etiologies cause lower gastrointestinal bleeding and most are not associated with a massive hemorrhage or acute symptomatic anemia. Colonic ischemia, inflammatory bowel disease, and colonic malignancies occur frequently. Each presents in a different manner. Typically, ischemic colitis presents with the abrupt onset of abdominal pain, followed by colic and a mucoid, bloody diarrhea. Inflammatory bowel disease, Crohn's, and ulcerative colitis present with a change in stool patterns. Patients develop diarrhea followed by hematochezia or melena. Localized transmural involvement or colic could add pain-related symptoms. Colorectal carcinomas are associated with exophytic, ulcerative lesions that may bleed insidiously. Only rarely does the malignant process proceed to acute, symptomatic hemorrhage.

More unusual causes of hemorrhage involve small intestinal tumors, known also as gastrointestinal stromal tumors (GIST). These lesions enlarge and surpass their blood supply. In that event, the ischemia in the tumor will ulcerate and may cause a localized hemorrhage. Meckel's diverticulum represent another atypical cause of bleeding. These lesions occur in the distal ileum. Ectopic gastric mucosa leads to localized acidic contents and resultant ulcerations of the contralateral intestinal wall. Finally, NSAID-associated intestinal hemorrhage occurs most frequently in the terminal ileum and cecum. Long-acting NSAIDS cause a localized mucosal injury. These remnants from the agents have been noted at the site of perforating ulcers. It seems that the terminal ileum and cecum may serve as a reservoir and harbor these agents long enough to establish the mucosal defects. Diaphragm-like strictures are pathognomonic for NSAID injuries and may result from a healing ridge related to repeated injuries from the agents.

Occult Hemorrhage

Obscure or occult gastrointestinal bleeding is a condition that frustrates the patient and the physicians. The hemorrhage is often massive and intermittent. The traditional tests of nuclear scintigraphy, colonoscopy, and angiography provide no solution. It occurs infrequently. One study noted occult bleeding in no more than 5% of all patients admitted with lower gastrointestinal massive hemorrhage. Frequent recurrences create chronic anemic states in patients and require occasional admissions for transfusions. These patients may harbor angiodysplasias in the small intestine or right colon. Patients in this situation may benefit from small bowel contrast radiography or capsule endoscopy.[23–26] Additionally, elective angiography with cecal magnification may reveal small angiodysplasias.

If the occult hemorrhage recurs and investigations fail to reveal the source, a variety of provocative diagnostic angiographic studies have been described. Most studies prefer to incite bleeding using either heparin or thrombolytics. Once the site of bleeding is identified, it may be difficult to control without an operation. In these instances, the surgeon should prepare and hold an operating room. Once the location is identified, a superselective catheter is left in the distal artery. During the conduct of surgery, the surgeon can palpate the catheter within the vessel and direct the surgical resection.

Initial Assessment, Resuscitation, and Stabilization

Massive lower gastrointestinal hemorrhage requires prompt clinical attention. Patients who present with symptoms secondary to the bleeding have urgent resuscitation needs. These symptoms further define the significance of the hemorrhage. Patients may demonstrate pallor, fatigue, angina, tachypnea, cardiac palpitations, postural hypotension, and syncope.

Prompt attention requires placement of vascular access with large bore intravenous fluids. Further hemodynamic monitoring requires cardiac rhythm monitoring and placement of a urinary catheter. A nasogastric tube placed will screen for the presence of upper gastric sources for bleeding. Kovacs and Jensen[27] noted 17.9% of lower gastrointestinal hemorrhage presentations involved an upper gastrointestinal source. The nasogastric tube is effective in detecting prepyloric hemorrhage. The nasogastric decompression need not be continued after an appropriate period of observation to exclude upper intestinal sources.

The treatment goals for resuscitation are to restore volume and, replete red blood cell deficiencies and their impact on oxygen delivery. In addition, all coagulopathies require reversal. Patients require laboratory profiles that include a complete blood count, serum electrolytes, a coagulation profile, and a type and crossmatch for packed red blood cells.

The initial specific diagnostic evaluation begins with a digital anorectal examination and anoscopy. A rigid proctosigmoidoscopy will allow the examiner to evacuate the rectum of blood and clots. A complete mucosal assessment serves to exclude internal hemorrhoids, anorectal solitary ulcers, neoplasms, and colitis. If nothing is found and subsequent surgery becomes necessary, the evaluation of the rectum and anorectal function greatly aids in surgical decisions. A normal anorectal examination allows the surgeon to consider a primary rectal anastomosis as a treatment possibility. In the event that the physician discovers a source for bleeding during the examination, oftentimes therapy can immediately control the hemorrhage.

Once the resuscitation demonstrates a stable patient, the next phase of the diagnostic evaluation ensues. What is the first test to evaluate the cause of bleeding? Currently, three tests are considered for the initial evaluation. These tests include colonoscopy, nuclear scintigraphy, and angiography. Colonoscopy and angiography offer therapeutic intervention whereas nuclear scanning is purely diagnostic. Decisions as to which test to use depend on the clinical judgment, local expertise, severity of the event, and the current activity of the hemorrhage.

It may be helpful to subdivide patients into three general clinical categories based on the history, physical, and the initial laboratory data. Is the hemorrhagic event 1) minor and self-limited, 2) major and self-limited, or 3) major and ongoing? Major ongoing hemorrhage requires prompt intervention with angiography or surgery. Minor, self-limited may undergo a colonic lavage and colonoscopy within 24 hours. Major, self-limited may be more difficult to define. Within the spectrum of these three clinical groups, the major, self-limited hemorrhage patients create the current controversy. These patients need a diagnostic test to determine if they require prompt therapy or observation. Should these patients undergo nuclear imaging or colonoscopy?

Radionuclide imaging (Figure 20-1) detects the slowest bleeding rates. It is able to detect rates of 0.1–0.5 mL/min.

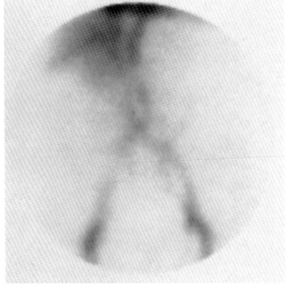

A

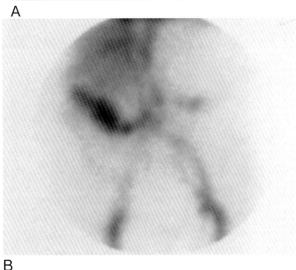

B

FIGURE 20-1. Selected images from a 99mTc-labeled RBC gastrointestinal bleeding study in a patient with known diureticulosis. Images acquired at 1 minute (A) and 14 minutes (B). Abnormal increased isotopic activity developed in the proximal transverse colon, which progressed antegrade to the descending colon.

Thus, it is a technique that is more sensitive than angiography. Unfortunately, the nuclear scanning cannot reliably localize the site of hemorrhage. The specificity (precise origin) using radionuclide scans of small bowel versus large intestine bleeding does not reliably compare with angiography.[28] Two general techniques are used for nuclear imaging, technetium sulfur colloid scans and 99mTc pertechnetate-tagged red blood cells (RBCs). Sulfur colloid scans have a short half-life and detect very low rates of hemorrhage (0.1 mL/min). It is effective to detect brisk hemorrhage but cannot detect sporadic bleeding. The more frequently preferred agent for lower gastrointestinal hemorrhage radionuclide scanning is the pertechnetate-tagged RBC scans. The tagged RBC scans may cover a period of hours

and allow for reimaging within 24 hours. Nuclear scintigraphy has variable results, suggesting that scan timing, technical skills, and experience may increase accuracy. Current reports suggest accuracies ranging from 24% to 91%.[29]

Ng et al.[30] recommend nuclear imaging for the patients with a major, self-limited hemorrhage. Their data suggest that the timing of the blush predicts the success of angiography. In other words, if the nuclear scan demonstrates an immediately positive blush (within the first 2 minutes of scanning), it is highly predictive of a positive angiogram (60%). The data of Ng et al. seemed predictive for surgery in 24% of patients if the first blush was positive. Just as important, if the initial images in the Ng et al. study did not demonstrate a blush, the study is highly predictive of a negative angiogram (93%) and the need for surgery decreased to 7%. Thus, if the nuclear scan is negative, it provides objective evidence that the patient is not actively bleeding and may be evaluated by colonoscopy.

Colonoscopy

Many authors believe that colonoscopy has clearly demonstrated the highest efficacy and should be the first study in patients with major bleeding that appears self-limited.[31] In general, this may be true if efficacy of the study includes a broad array of the common etiologies for properly defined massive hemorrhage. Controversy abounds with colonoscopy as the preferred first study if the etiologies for hemorrhage are unlikely sources for major hemorrhage. Whether colonoscopy should be undertaken emergently depends on the general ability to maintain a stable patient. If the hemodynamic profile continues to drift toward hypotension and the massive hemorrhage continues unabated during the resuscitation process, the rate of hemorrhage may require more prompt attention. Patients with extremely brisk hemorrhage require a prompt angiogram. Colonoscopy in such patients proves difficult to prep with lavage and the acute exsanguinations may limit intraluminal visualization to deploy all the therapeutic options except for only the most experienced endoscopists.

If the patient appears stable with self-limited hemorrhage, colonoscopy is the preferred diagnostic study. Jensen et al.[3,4,9] have long been proponents of "emergency colonoscopy." This group and others have demonstrated high cecal intubation rates (95%) and a diagnostic accuracy of 72% and 86%. On a cautious note, the Jensen diagnostic studies demonstrated atypical etiologies for massive hemorrhage including ischemic colitis, inflammatory bowel disease, and cancer. The rate of bleeding in these conditions may be more amenable to urgent colonoscopy (within 24 hours) rather than emergent colonoscopy in patients diverticular or angiodysplastic, hemorrhagic rates.

Should the patient undergo a colonic lavage before colonoscopy? Longstreth[2] reported that 80.8% of patients had colonoscopy after electrolyte-polyethylene glycol solution purge, usually within 24 hours of admission. His report reflects the more typical approach to patients. Once the patient undergoes observation and stabilization, the need for acute intervention seems avoided. Then the endoscopist may plan for a more controlled, stable, urgent colonoscopy with a lavage which occurs within the first 24 hours. The Longstreth Kaiser Permanente study demonstrated a broad scope of etiologies (see Table 20-2).

The major benefit of colonoscopy depends on the ability to provide a definitive localization of ongoing active bleeding and the potential for therapy. Many landmarks for colonoscopy may be obscured during hemorrhage. Because of the inability to appreciate all intraluminal landmarks and locate the segment that is bleeding, once the endoscopist highlights a bleeding source, the region of the intestine requires a tattoo to mark the site with India ink. In such patients, if the hemorrhage continues and fails medical management, the tattoo greatly assists the surgeon in localizing the hemorrhage.

The endoscopist has many therapeutic options to control the bleeding. Kovacs and Jensen[27] have described several therapeutic tools to control bleeding in upper and lower gastrointestinal hemorrhage. Therapeutic armamentarium for the colon includes thermal agents such as heater probes, bipolar coagulation, and laser therapy. Injection therapy primarily uses topical and intramucosal epinephrine. Mechanical therapy includes endoscopically applied clips (Figure 20-2).[27]

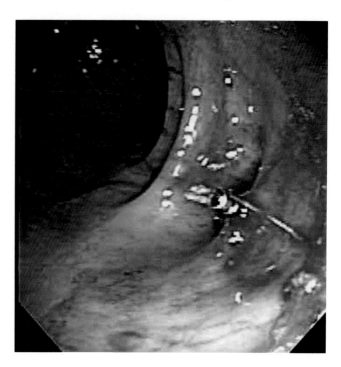

FIGURE 20-2. Clip applied to bleeding diverticular vessel.

Angiography

Angiography is diagnostic and therapeutic in the treatment of intestinal hemorrhage. The clinical judgment for choosing angiography involves three different types of hemorrhage. First, acute, major hemorrhage with ongoing bleeding requires emergency angiography. Second, patients with an early blush during nuclear scintigraphy may benefit from therapeutic angiography. Finally, angiograms may define a potential source for hemorrhage in occult and recurrent gastrointestinal hemorrhage. To appreciate an angiographic blush of contrast, the study requires a hemorrhage rate of at least 1 mL/min.[32] Positive yields with angiography vary greatly. Patient selection will increase yields and avoid overuse of angiograms. Generally, reports demonstrate yields that range from 40% to 78%.[33–36]

TABLE 20-2. Final diagnosis in patients hospitalized for acute lower gastrointestinal hemorrhage[31]

	n (%)
Colonic diverticulosis	91 (41.6)
Colorectal malignancy	20 (9.1)
Ischemic colitis	19 (8.7)
Acute colitis, unknown cause	11 (5.0)
Hemorrhoids	10 (4.6)
Postpolypectomy hemorrhage	9 (4.1)
Colonic angiodysplasia	6 (2.7)
Crohn's disease	5 (2.3)
Other	22 (10.1)
Unknown	26 (11.9)
Total	219 (100)

Angiography provides highly accurate localization of the site of bleeding (Figure 20-3) and the angiographic blush may suggest a specific etiology, but it lacks the accuracy of colonoscopy. Highly accurate localization provides for focused therapy. Hemorrhagic site may receive highly selective, intraarterial vasopressin infusion. The potent arterial contraction may reduce or halt the hemorrhage. Infusion rates of vasopressin are at concentrations of 0.2 U/min and may progress to 0.4 U/min. The systemic effects and cardiac impact of vasopressin may limit maximizing the dosage. Vasopressin controls bleeding in as many as 91% of patients. Bleeding may recur in as many as 50% of patients once the vasopressin is tapered.

Angiographic technology also allows for arterial embolization to control hemorrhage. Superselective mesenteric angiography with current microcatheters allows for embolization of the vasa recta of the intestine, vessels as small as 1 mm. In the past, arterial embolization of larger vessels risked intestinal ischemia or infarction. The risk of intestinal infarctions of larger selective vessels may exceed 20%. Arteriography also has complication rates related to angiography, separate from the therapy delivered at the site of bleeding. These include arterial thrombosis, distant arterial emboli, and renal toxicity from the angiographic dye.

Embolization therapy provides immediate arrest of the bleeding. Embolization uses a combination of agents to control bleeding including Gelfoam pledgets, coils, and polyvinyl alcohol particles. In 2001, Funaki et al.[37] reported experience with microcoil embolization in 27 patients. They succeeded in 93% and had reasonable long-term

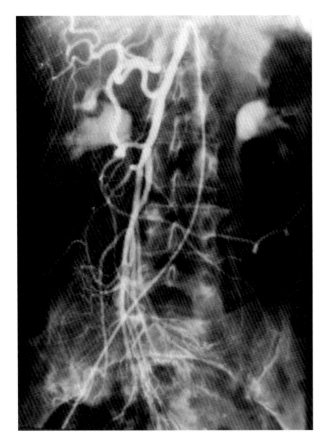

Figure 20-3. Angiogram demonstrating extravasation (hemorrhage) in cecum.

results—81%. Most of his patients had diverticular hemorrhages. His recurrent bleed patients had angiodysplasias. In a similar experience, Peck et al.[38] reported rebleeding in three of four patients with cecal angiodysplasias. The data suggest that angiodysplasias have multiple feeding vessels and may contribute to the recurrence.

Operative Therapy

Surgical therapy for massive lower intestinal bleeding is rare, often definitive, and associated with significant mortality. Most sources of bleeding spontaneously resolve or are controlled with the current therapeutic interventions. Few patients currently require surgical treatment. If the patient is hemodynamically unresponsive to the initial resuscitation, then radiographic, radionuclide, and endoscopic evaluations are usurped by the need for urgent surgery. Other patients may have the site of hemorrhage localized, yet the available therapeutic interventions fail to control the bleeding. Patient mortality increases with their transfusion requirements, suggesting the severity of the hemorrhage. Bender noted a reduced mortality (7%) for patients requiring less than 10 units of blood. The mortality increased to 27% for patients in excess of 10 units.[39] Therefore, once a patient reaches 6–7 units during the resuscitation and the hemorrhage remains ongoing, surgical intervention becomes eminent.

The surgeon tailors the approach to the patient and depends on the diagnostic information gathered before the operation. All patients require an open laparotomy with a thorough examination of the entire intestine. The first objective in surgery focuses on the location of the intraluminal blood with the hope of segmentally isolating the possible sources of bleeding. If the colon visually appears filled with blood and the small intestine remains spared, the surgeon must still examine the entire abdomen and then focus on colonic sources of bleeding. If the small bowel contains blood, then the operative team has a larger area of concern and close inspection.

Once the surgeon completes the initial visual inspection, a complete exploration ensues. The exploration begins in the stomach, duodenum, and considers possible missed upper gastrointestinal sources. Next, the small intestine must undergo examination from the ligament of Treitz to the ileocecal valve. Palpation of the intestine may demonstrate such etiologies as a Meckel's diverticulum, ileitis, colitis, or a GIST.

Upon completion of the exploration phase, if no source appears obvious, the surgeon may consider intestinal enteroscopy. The enteroscope or colonoscope will expose the luminal surface and transilluminate the intestinal wall for occult lesions. Transillumination may identify vascular anomalies, small ulcers or tumors. Endoscopic access to the intestine may require upper enteroscope, a transgastric approach, a transcolonic approach, or insertion through the anus. Once a hemorrhage site is identified, the surgeon can perform an appropriate segmental resection. Intraoperative endoscopy is a technically difficult endeavor. A team approach with two surgeons or the availability of an experienced endoscopist is important to identify the elusive lesions causing the hemorrhage.

If the source of bleeding cannot be found, and it appears to arise from the colon, the surgeon should perform a subtotal or total colectomy. Stable patients will tolerate a primary ileosigmoid or ileorectal anastomosis in this circumstance. Unstable patients require an end ileostomy with closure of the rectal stump or a mucous fistula. Once stable, the patient may return for ileostomy closure. The rectum and sigmoid colon require reexamination endoscopically to assure no bleeding persists. Before the endoscopy, a simple saline "washout" with a transanal catheter or via the rigid proctosigmoidoscope may provide for safe passage and careful examination of the remaining mucosa.

The key concerns with operative management are, first, a delay in the decision to operate until the hemorrhage reaches a critical point beyond 10 units of blood. This seems to contribute to the high mortality rate. Second, mortality rates for patients requiring urgent surgery consistently reach a range hovering between 10% and 35%.[40] Few authors note mortalities less than 10% or greater than 40%. Third, notable recurrence rates of 10% are attributable to the limits of isolating the precise cause of the bleeding. The rates of recurrence increase if a surgeon elects to perform a limited right or left colectomy without precise localization of the hemorrhage. Limited segmental colectomies continue to have high mortality rates and excessive persistent bleed rates of 20%.[41] A total colectomy offers the same mortality with a lower chance of recurrent or persistent hemorrhage.

New Frontiers

Horton and Fishman[42] commented about the advanced imaging within computerized tomography. Current thinly sliced, fast image acquisition combined with three-dimensional software packages has revolutionized the imaging of the vascular tree. Abdominal, and specifically intestinal vascular imaging now details smaller than "named" vessels. Current use focuses on chronic conditions such as mesenteric ischemia and inflammatory bowel disease. Case reports and animal modeling note it is a feasible study for gastrointestinal hemorrhage. New scanners promise even more with 16 0.5-mm slices acquired in 0.4 seconds. Image acquisition synchronized with intravascular contrast may outline a site of contrast extravasation or blush. The detail available may define intestinal hemangiomas, arteriovenous malformations, and angiodysplasias. The sensitivity and specificity of computed tomographic angiography in patients with gastrointestinal hemorrhage are unknown and require further comparison studies to current diagnostic studies.

Anderson[43] noted magnetic resonance angiogram creates images using the bright signal from blood. The three-dimensional images are reconstructed using computerized imaging to project a two-dimensional image that mimics a conventional angiogram. Further improvement develops from contrast-enhanced magnetic resonance angiography (CEMRA). With current techniques, the resultant images are not as specific or as refined as an angiogram. The technique may detect the extravasation of blood pooling in various segments of the intestine. In addition to localizing the side, the study may distinguish small intestine versus large intestine. These studies may prove an enhancement when compared with nuclear scintigraphy.

Wireless capsular endoscopy is an ideal diagnostic adjunct for patients with occult hemorrhage.[24,25] The first generation of capsules are 11 × 30 mm. The capsules are easily swallowed and tolerated. The current system captures two images per second and transmits the images to a recording apparatus secured to a belt the patient wears. Transmitted images are later reviewed by the endoscopist.

Lewis and Swain[44] reported the results from the first clinical trial. They noted a source of occult hemorrhage in 7 of 11 patients. The sites noted included angiodysplasia, ileal ulcers, and a tumor. Rossini et al.[45] corroborated their work in noting success in 7 of 10 patients.

The evaluation and management of lower gastrointestinal hemorrhage remains a challenge for surgeons. An algorithm summarizing the management is provided in Figure 20-4.

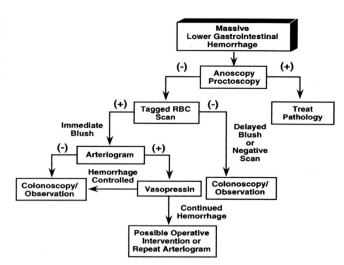

FIGURE 20-4. Algorithm for the management of lower gastrointestinal hemorrhage.

References

1. Billingham RP. The conundrum of lower gastrointestinal bleeding. Surg Clin North Am 1997;77(1):241–252.
2. Longstreth GF. Epidemiology and outcome of patients hospitalized with acute lower gastrointestinal hemorrhage: a population-based study. Am J Gastroenterol 1997;92:419–424.
3. Jensen DM, Machicado GA. Colonoscopy for diagnosis and treatment of severe lower gastrointestinal bleeding. Routine outcomes and cost analysis. Gastrointest Endosc Clin North Am 1997;7(3):477–498.
4. Jensen DM. Diagnosis and treatment of severe hematochezia. The role of urgent colonoscopy after purge. Gastroenterology 1988;95(6):1569–1574.
5. Landefeld CS, Goldman L. Major bleeding in outpatients treated with warfarin: incidence and prediction by factors known at the start of outpatient therapy. Am J Med 1989;87(2):144–152.
6. Bramley PN, Masson JW, McKnight G, et al. The role of an open-access bleeding unit in the management of colonic haemorrhage. A 2-year prospective study. Scand J Gastroenterol 1996; 31(8):764–769.
7. Richter JM, Christensen MR, Kaplan LM, Nishioka NS. Effectiveness of current technology in the diagnosis and management of lower gastrointestinal hemorrhage. Gastrointest Endosc 1995;41(2):93–98.
8. Rossini FP, Ferrari A, Spandre M, et al. Emergency colonoscopy. World J Surg 1989;13(2):190–192.
9. Jensen DM, Machicado GA. Diagnosis and treatment of severe hematochezia: the role of urgent colonoscopy after purge. Gastroenterology 1988;95:1569–1574.
10. McGuire HW, Haynes BW. Massive hemorrhage from diverticular disease of the colon: guidelines for therapy based on bleeding pattern in fifty cases. Ann Surg 1972;175:847.
11. Drummond H. Sacculi of the large intestine. Br J Surg 1916; 4:407–413.
12. Meyers MA, Alonso DR, Gray GF, Baer JW. Pathogenesis of bleeding colonic diverticulosis. Gastroenterology 1976;71: 577–583.

13. Ure T, Vernava AM, Longo WE. Diverticular bleeding. Semin Col Rect Surg 1994;5:32.

14. McGuire HW, Haynes BW. Massive hemorrhage from diverticular disease of the colon: guidelines for therapy based on bleeding pattern in fifty cases. Ann Surg 1972;175:847.

15. Finne CO III. The aggressive management of serious lower gastrointestinal bleeding. Probl Gen Surg 1992;9:597.

16. Margolis AR, Heinbecker P, Bernard HR. Operative mesenteric angiography in the search for the site of bleeding in unexplained gastrointestinal hemorrhage. A preliminary report. Surgery 1960;48:534–537.

17. McAllister K, Grogg K, Johnson D, et al. Endoglin, a TGF-beta binding protein of endothelial cells, is the gene for hereditary hemorrhagic telangiectasia type 1. Nat Genet 1994;8:345–351.

18. Roskell DE, Biddolph SC, Warren BF. Apparent deficiency of mucosal vascular collagen type IV associated with angiodysplasia of the colon. J Clin Pathol 1998;51:18–20.

19. Gostout CJ. Angiodysplasia and aortic valve disease: let's close the book on this association. Gastrointest Endosc 1995;42:491–493.

20. Bhutani MS, Gupta SC, Markert RJ, Barde CJ, Donese R, Gopalswamy N. A prospective controlled evaluation of endoscopic detection of angiodysplasia and its association with aortic valve disease. Gastrointest Endosc 1995;42:398–402.

21. Imperiale TF, Ransohoff DF. Aortic stenosis, idiopathic gastrointestinal bleeding and angiodysplasia: is there an association? Gastroenterology 1988;95:1670–1676.

22. Boley SJ, Sprayregen S, Sammartano RJ, et al. The pathophysiologic basis for the angiographic signs of vascular ectasias of the colon. Radiology 1977;125:615–621.

23. Beck DE. Diagnostic imaging. In: Beck DE, ed. Handbook of Colorectal Surgery. 2nd ed. New York: Marcel Dekker; 2003: 43–77.

24. Iddan G, Meron G, Glukhovsky A, et al. Wireless capsule endoscopy. Nature 2000;405:417.

25. Appleyard M, Fireman Z, Glukhovsky A, et al. A randomized trial comparing wireless capsule endoscopy with push enteroscopy for the detection of small-bowel lesions. Gastroenterology 2000;119:1431–1438.

26. Appleyard M, Glukhousky A, Swain P. Wireless-capsule diagnostic endoscopy for recurrent small-bowel bleeding. N Engl J Med 2001;344:232–233.

27. Kovacs TO, Jensen DM. Recent advances in the endoscopic diagnosis and therapy of upper gastrointestinal, small intestinal, and colonic bleeding. Med Clin North Am 2002;86:1319–1356.

28. Dusold R, Burke K, Carpentier W, et al. The accuracy of technetium-99m-labeled red cell scintigraphy in localizing gastrointestinal bleeding. Am J Gastroenterol 1994;89:345–348.

29. Imbembo AL, Bailey RW. Diverticular disease of the colon. In: Sabiston D, ed. Textbook of Surgery. Philadelphia: WB Saunders; 1991:910–920.

30. Ng DA, Opelka FG, Beck DE, et al. Predictive value of technetium Tc 99m-labeled red blood cell scintigraphy for positive angiogram in massive lower gastrointestinal hemorrhage. Dis Colon Rectum 1997;40:471–477.

31. Bounds BC, Friedman LS. Lower gastrointestinal bleeding. Gastroenterol Clin 2003;32:1107–1125.

32. Zuckerman DA, Bocchini TP, Birnbaum EH. Massive hemorrhage in the lower gastrointestinal tract in adults: diagnostic imaging and intervention. AJR Am J Roentgenol 1993;161:703–711.

33. Koval G, Benner KG, Rosch J, et al. Aggressive angiographic diagnosis in acute lower gastrointestinal hemorrhage. Dig Dis Sci 1987;32:248–253.

34. Browder W, Cerise EJ, Litwin MS. Impact of emergency angiography in massive lower gastrointestinal bleeding. Ann Surg 1986;204:530–536.

35. Britt LG, Warren L, Moore OF III. Selective management of lower gastrointestinal bleeding. Am Surg 1983;49:121–125.

36. Gomes AS, Lois JF, McCoy RD. Angiographic treatment of gastrointestinal hemorrhage: comparison of vasopressin infusion and embolization. AJR Am J Roentgenol 1986;146:1031–1037.

37. Funaki B, Kostelic JK, Lorenz J, et al. Superselective microcoil embolization of colonic hemorrhage. AJR Am J Roentgenol 2001;177(4):829–836.

38. Peck DJ, McLoughlin RF, Hughson MN, Rankin RN. Percutaneous embolotherapy of lower gastrointestinal hemorrhage. J Vasc Interv Radiol 1998;9:747–751.

39. Bender JS, Wiencek RG, Bouwman DL. Morbidity and mortality following total abdominal colectomy for massive lower gastrointestinal bleeding. Am Surg 1991;57:536–540; discussion 540–541.

40. Corman ML. Vascular diseases. In: Corman ML, ed. Colon and Rectal Surgery. Philadelphia: JB Lippincott; 1993:860–900.

41. Finne CO III. The aggressive management of serious lower gastrointestinal bleeding. Probl Gen Surg 1992;9:597.

42. Horton KM, Fishman EK. CT angiography of the GI tract. Gastrointest Endosc 2002;55:S37–41.

43. Anderson CM. GI magnetic resonance angiography. Gastrointest Endosc 2002;55:S42–48.

44. Lewis BS, Swain P. Capsule endoscopy in the evaluation of patients with suspected small intestinal bleeding: the results of the first clinical trial. Gastrointest Endosc 2001;53:AB70.

45. Rossini FP, Pennazio M, Santui R, et al. Early experience with wireless capsule diagnostic endoscopy in patients with small bowel bleeding. Am J Gastroenterol 2000;96:S111–112.

21
Endometriosis

Michael J. Snyder and Steven J. Stryker

Endometriosis is a disease characterized by the presence of endometrial glands and stroma outside the uterine cavity. It is one of the most common conditions requiring surgery for women during their reproductive years. Endometriosis, although not fatal, may be associated with disabling pain and intractable infertility. The degree of symptoms varies widely and does not always correspond to the extent of pathology encountered at surgery. Small lesions may cause severe pain and infertility whereas larger lesions may be asymptomatic and found only incidentally during surgery for other diagnoses. Diagnosis is typically made or confirmed at laparoscopy or during laparotomy. Colon and rectal surgeons often become involved in the management of patients with intestinal endometriosis. This involvement may occur as a result of a combined procedure with a gynecologist or in management of an endometrioma masquerading as a neoplastic or inflammatory lesion. Treatment for endometriosis is usually multimodal and may include an operation in those patients with infertility, pelvic pain, obstruction, or a poor response to hormonal suppression. Although advances in diagnostic tests and therapy have been made, endometriosis remains a frustrating and incompletely understood disease for both patients and physicians.

Epidemiology

The true prevalence of endometriosis is unknown. There is no noninvasive screening test for endometriosis, and its diagnosis depends on the visual or pathologic identification of implants during laparoscopy or laparotomy. Various authors have estimated that up to 15% of all women of reproductive age and one-third of infertile women have endometriosis.[1,2] A study by Houston et al.[3] is the only population-based study of endometriosis. After reviewing the medical records for Caucasian women in Rochester, Minnesota, during the 1970s, they estimated that 6.2% of premenopausal women have endometriosis.

Although endometriosis is primarily a disease of the reproductive years, the widespread use of exogenous estrogens and increasing obesity in our society have made it more prevalent in postmenopausal women. Conversely, there is a decrease in the incidence of the disease when women use oral contraceptives or experience multiple pregnancies.[4] These observations, coupled with the fact that the incidence of endometriosis increases over time after a woman's last childbirth, suggest that uninterrupted menstrual cycles predispose susceptible individuals to the development of endometrial implants.[5] There is no racial predilection for endometriosis other than in Japanese women, who have double the incidence of the disease compared with Caucasian women.[6]

Etiology

The precise etiology that completely explains the cause and pathogenesis of endometriosis is unknown. The two most popular theories as to etiology are coelomic metaplasia and the implantation of viable endometrial cells from retrograde menstruation through the fallopian tubes. Coelomic metaplasia, postulated by Meyers, suggests that under the correct hormonal milieu, the coelomic epithelium will undergo metaplastic changes and transform into endometrial tissue.[7] He bases his theory on studies demonstrating that the peritoneum and uterine endometrium both originate from embryonic coelomic epithelium. Although this theory offers a good explanation for endometriosis in men and nonmenstruating women, it does not adequately address the anatomic distribution and clinical pattern of endometriosis. The vast majority of endometriosis occurs in the pelvis, but the peritoneum at risk with this theory is evenly distributed throughout the abdominal cavity. In addition, metaplasia should worsen with age and endometriosis clearly does not.

Retrograde menstruation, first proposed by Sampson[8] in 1921, remains the most plausible explanation for the distribution of endometrial implants. This theory postulates that endometriosis arises from retrograde menstruation through the fallopian tubes and into the peritoneal cavity. Viable endometrial tissue has been demonstrated in menstrual effluent, and endometriosis has been induced both in primates, with artificially produced retrograde menstruation,[9] and in women volunteers who permitted injection of menstrual tissue into their peritoneum.[10] This theory, however, is probably only part of the answer.

Whereas retrograde menstruation is very common, occurring in virtually all women, endometriosis affects only a small minority. Clearly, other factors must be involved to permit the implantation and growth of endometrial tissue. Several studies indicate a possible genetic aspect to endometriosis. Simpson et al.[11] demonstrated that the disease seems to occur more frequently within families. He found a 7% relative risk for blood relatives of affected individuals as opposed to a 1% relative risk for nonblood controls. Additionally, the clinical manifestations of the disease were more severe among the related group. It seems that the inheritance pattern is polygenic or a combination of genetic and environmental factors. This conclusion is consistent with the clinical associations with delayed childbearing and uninterrupted cyclic menstruation.

Dmowski et al.[12] have theorized that the genetic factor may involve the immune system. They demonstrated depressed cellular immunity in monkeys with spontaneous endometriosis. Other investigators have confirmed alterations in both cellular and humoral immunity in women with endometriosis.[13,14] The most striking change observed in cellular immunity is the high concentration of activated macrophages and decreased functional capacity of natural killer cells. The most significant abnormality in humoral immunity is the presence of autoantibodies against different cellular components. These changes have been observed in both the peritoneal cavity and the systemic circulation, suggesting that endometriosis may be a systemic disease. It is still unclear whether these changes represent manifestations of the disease or a subsequent reaction to it. This research, however, suggests that mild subclinical immunosuppression may subsequently lead to endometriosis many years later.

Clinical Manifestations

The most common sites where endometriosis occurs are summarized in Table 21-1. The most frequent of these are in the pelvis. Potential sites of implantation in the abdomen include the appendix, small bowel, and diaphragm. Rarely, implantation may occur in the inguinal canal (in patients with hernias), surgical incisions, the vulva, vagina, cervix, or systemically in the lungs, bronchi, or kidneys.

TABLE 21-1. Sites and incidence of endometriosis

Common	Less common	Rare
Ovaries 60%–75%	Appendix 2%	Diaphragm
Uterosacral ligaments 30%–65%	Ureter 1%–2%	Inguinal canal
Cul-de-sac 20%–30%	Terminal ileum 1%	Liver
Uterus 4%–20%	Bladder <1%	Spleen
Rectosigmoid colon 3%–10%	Abdominal scars < 1%	Kidney

Because the majority of women have disease confined to the pelvis, the most common presenting complaints relate to menstrual irregularities, pelvic pain, and infertility. Many women with endometriosis may be completely asymptomatic and the natural history of the disease in these patients has never been well defined. In studies with placebo arms, a few interesting observations have been made. A trial involving infertile women with otherwise asymptomatic endometriosis revealed that laparoscopic scoring of the severity of the disease increased over the length of the study in almost 50% of the placebo group.[15] Another study compared pain scores in women receiving placebo versus gonadotropin-releasing hormone (GnRH) analogs.[16] The cumulative dysmenorrhea rate and severity of pain were significantly lower in the treatment group suggesting a progressive course of the disease when untreated. Other studies on infertile women revealed that mild endometriosis can spontaneously resolve and that medical therapy may only suppress the disease until hormonal stimulation resumes.[17]

Ovarian hormones to varying degrees influence all endometrial tissue, and many of the clinical manifestations of endometriosis reflect the changing concentration of these hormones during a typical menstrual cycle. Under the influence of pituitary-stimulating hormones, the ovary begins to secrete estrogen at the beginning of the menstrual cycle. This stimulates endometrial mitosis with cellular proliferation in concert with neovascularization. At the midpoint of the cycle, progesterone production by the corpus luteum begins and promotes secretory changes in the endometrium in anticipation of implantation. The loss of progesterone at the end of the menstrual cycle from involution of the corpus luteum destabilizes the endometrium and induces menstruation.

Pelvic Pain and Dysmenorrhea

Pain is the most common symptom of endometriosis, affecting up to 80% of patients subsequently diagnosed with the disease. Endometriosis has been discovered in 30%–50% of women undergoing laparoscopy for pelvic pain.[18] Pelvic pain associated with endometriosis presents as dysmenorrhea, dyspareunia, or chronic noncyclic pelvic pain. There are women, however, with extensive endometriosis and little or no pain. Total lesion volume does seem to correlate directly to the degree of pain.[19] Symptoms are related to the depth of penetration of the lesion, the type of lesion, and its location. Implants involving the uterosacral ligaments and rectovaginal septum are most frequently implicated. The pain is typically most intense just before menstruation and lasts for the duration of menstruation. The pain is often associated with back pain, dyschezia, and levator muscle spasm, and is more severe with advanced stages of endometriosis.

Dysmenorrhea occurs in most women with endometriosis. The association is not well understood, and some have hypothesized that high uterine pressures cause dysmenorrhea with retrograde menstruation, a consequence of these increased pressures.[20] Other investigators, however, have failed to show an increase in the prevalence of dysmenorrhea with early-stage endometriosis.[21]

Dyspareunia, deep pelvic pain with vaginal penetration, is usually a symptom of advanced endometriosis. Dyspareunia is most pronounced just before menstruation and is associated with specific coital positions. The presence of dyspareunia is often indicative of the degree of fixation of the pelvic organs, especially in the cul-de-sac of Douglas and the rectovaginal septum.

Chronic noncyclic pelvic pain is pain present for longer than 6 months, and may be intermittent or continuous. The pain is often associated with both perineural inflammation and uterosacral ligament involvement with endometriosis.[22] Gastrointestinal and urinary complaints may accompany the pain.

Pain in the shoulder during or just preceding menstruation may be attributable to endometrial implants involving the diaphragm. The diaphragm should always be viewed during laparoscopy, so these diaphragmatic deposits can possibly be treated with laser vaporization. Differentiation from adhesions associated with pelvic inflammatory disease (Fitz-Hugh and Curtis syndrome) is usually not difficult unless the two pathologies coexist.

The pathophysiology of pain arising from endometriosis is not completely clear. Pain may occur from the cyclic growth and subsequent increase in pressure within the capsule surrounding the implant. Alternatively, extravasation of menstrual debris into the surrounding tissue may occur with subsequent edema and release of inflammatory mediators. As the implant matures with surrounding unyielding scar tissue, the stretching of this scar by the products of the endometrial glands may produce pain. This scenario is probably particularly true for deeper implants. A study by Cornillie et al.[22] discovered that all women with implants deeper than 1 cm experienced severe pelvic pain.

Adhesions, very common in endometriosis, may also be associated with pain. Adherence of the colon and small bowel along with retroflexion of the uterus from extensive posterior adhesions may occur. Such retroflexion and fixation of the rectosigmoid can result in pressure on the sacrum with consequent back and rectal pain.

Since the 1960s, multiple investigators have attempted to define the role of prostaglandins in the pathogenesis of pelvic pain.[23,24] Macrophages are responsible for the removal of foreign material such as the endometrial implants. They are present around the endometrial implants and are potent producers of inflammatory mediators such as the prostaglandins. Both prostacyclin (PGI-2) and prostaglandin E-2 are able to sensitize pain receptors to chemical mediators. Leukotriene B-4, another macrophage product, is a potent chemotactic agent and leukocyte activator. These factors are thought to explain some of the pelvic pain, but not all studies agree.[24] The relative transient nature of prostaglandin action and the inherent difficulty in measuring pain complicates attempts to quantify the impact of chemical mediators.

Infertility

The relationship between endometriosis and infertility is also unclear. Some studies have demonstrated a high percentage of infertile patients with endometriosis.[25] Certainly, those reports comparing rates of endometriosis for women undergoing elective laparoscopic sterilization versus laparoscopy for infertility have demonstrated a fourfold or greater increase in the infertile group. In women with known endometriosis, the infertility rate is 30%–50%. Whether endometriosis causes infertility or is the product of uninterrupted menstruation is still hotly debated.

There is little disagreement that moderate to severe disease with mechanical distortion of the fallopian tubes, ovaries, and peritoneum can potentiate infertility. Pelvic endometriosis and the resulting inflammatory response can produce dense, fibrotic adhesions that may significantly interfere with both the oocyte release from the ovary and the ability of the fallopian tube to pick up and transmit the oocyte to the uterus. Blockage of the tube may produce a hydrosalpinx, and in one recent study, endometriosis was the etiology in 14% of patients undergoing tubal reconstruction for occlusion.[26] In moderate or severe endometriosis, the pregnancy rates after surgery are 50% and 40%, respectively, compared with only 7% when expectant management is practiced.[27,28] Surgical treatment of these patients is clearly beneficial.

Treatment of infertile patients with mild endometriosis is more problematic. A study by Inoue et al.[29] on 2000 infertile women with mild endometriosis did not reveal any improvement in fertility with either medical or surgical therapy when compared with expectant management. Other studies have demonstrated a lower pregnancy per cycle rate in patients with endometriosis compared with those free of the disease.[30]

Intestinal Symptoms

Although some women with intestinal endometriosis may be asymptomatic, some degree of intestinal complaints is typically found in those women with moderate to severe disease. Bowel involvement occurs in 12%–37% of cases of endometriosis, and depending on the site of involvement, the symptoms of endometriosis may vary somewhat. In patients with intestinal endometriosis, the rectosigmoid is involved in more than 70%, followed by the small bowel and appendix. Rectosigmoid disease often results in alterations in bowel habits such as constipation, diarrhea, a decreased caliber of the stool, tenesmus, or, rarely, rectal bleeding. Such symptoms appear more often around the time of menses. Colonic endometriosis can present with obstruction and may be difficult to differentiate from other causes of large bowel obstruction, such as Crohn's disease or neoplasm. This difficulty is of particular concern in the postmenopausal woman on hormone replacement therapy.

Intestinal perforation may occur with endometriosis. Colonic perforation has been reported during pregnancy from endometriosis.[31] Perforation also occurs with transmural appendiceal endometriosis.

For those patients with asymptomatic intestinal endometriosis, the natural history seems to be benign. Prystowsky et al.,[32] who followed 44 patients with known intestinal endometriosis for a period of 1–12 years, found that only one patient developed clinically significant gastrointestinal symptoms. Consequently, intestinal resection in these asymptomatic patients is probably unwarranted.

Confusion between small bowel endometriosis and Crohn's disease is common, because both can produce similar endoscopic and even histologic findings (Figure 21-1). Small bowel implants involving the terminal ileum are often noted incidentally at the time of laparoscopy and may often be asymptomatic. When symptoms occur, they are usually nonspecific such as recurrent abdominal pain and bloating. Occasionally, acute or chronic small bowel obstruction develops from extensive fibrotic adhesions which are caused by endometriosis.

The next most frequent site of intestinal endometriosis is the appendix. Endometrial implants are not infrequently found when the appendix is removed incidentally. The clinical significance of appendiceal endometriosis is less than that involving the small bowel and colon. Although endometrial implants may produce acute appendicitis with right lower quadrant abdominal pain, nausea, fever, and leukocytosis, historically most abdominal explorations for presumed acute appendicitis with a subsequent diagnosis of endometriosis have been attributable to ruptured endometrial cystic implants involving the ovary. Endometriosis of the appendix may also produce a chronic obstruction of the intestinal lumen with formation of a mucocele or periappendiceal inflammatory mass that is difficult to distinguish from a neoplasm. Finally, endometrial implants of the appendix and cecum may serve as lead points for an intussusception.

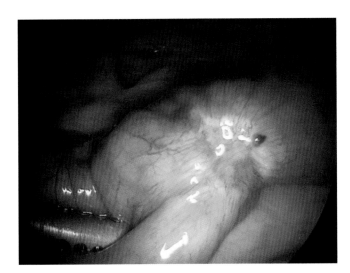

FIGURE 21.1. Endometriosis involving the small intestine.

Malignant Transformation

Malignant transformation of endometriosis is an uncommon complication of the disease. Almost 80% of the tumors are ovarian and two-thirds are endometrioid carcinomas. Patients with ovarian neoplasms arising from endometriosis are younger than the typical ovarian cancer patient, with most tumors occurring in the fourth decade of life.[33] Symptoms of pelvic pain and an enlarging pelvic mass are the most common symptoms. In women with known endometriosis, a cyst larger than 10 cm, cyst rupture, or a change in the nature of the chronic pelvic pain are potential signs of malignancy.

The rectosigmoid colon is the most common site for extragonadal tumors arising from endometriosis. Prolonged unopposed estrogen exposure is a significant risk factor, and rectal bleeding is the most common symptom. Recurrent symptoms of pelvic endometriosis after hysterectomy and bilateral salpingo-oophorectomy can be possible signs of malignant degeneration. Endometrial carcinoma is the most common tumor type. Histologically, the tumor must be shown to arise from the colon rather than invading it from another source. The diagnosis also requires that endometriosis or premalignant changes in endometrial glands be found contiguous with the invasive neoplasm.[34]

Treatment of both ovarian and extragonadal tumors is based on the particular stage of the tumor. The prognosis is generally good with tumors confined to the ovary or an extragonadal site having 5-year survivals greater than 60%. Even if a locally extensive tumor is encountered, there may be a benefit from aggressive local resection.

Diagnosis

Physical Examination

Patients with mild cases of endometriosis may have a normal physical examination and the diagnosis may not even be suspected unless the patient undergoes laparoscopy. For patients with pelvic pain, careful bimanual and rectal examination may reveal nodularity or induration especially in the uterosacral ligaments or cul-de-sac of Douglas. Fixed tender retroversion of the uterus in a patient without previous pelvic surgery may raise suspicion for endometriosis. Palpation of the ovaries may reveal an ovarian mass. Because these ovarian masses are generally soft and cystic, those less than 5 cm in diameter may be difficult to palpate. Cyclical pain or bleeding from any location, especially coinciding with menses, should be adequately investigated for endometriosis. The inguinal canal, previous incisions, umbilicus, and lungs can all be potentially involved with endometrial implants.

Laboratory Evaluation

CA-125, an antigen expressed on tissues derived from human coelomic epithelium, is increased in women with moderate to severe endometriosis. However, the sensitivity and specificity of this test is poor because the antigen may be mildly increased in other diseases and within the normal range in women with mild endometriosis. The concentration of CA-125 does correlate with the severity of the disease and is probably most useful in gauging response to medical therapy. It may also be of value in following women after resection who had increased levels preoperatively and are again exhibiting symptoms of endometriosis. No other serum markers are commercially available, but assays of antiendometrial antibodies and endometrial secretory protein PP14 are currently being evaluated for clinical relevance.[35]

Endoscopy

Because the lesions begin on the outside of the intestine, endoscopic evaluation of the large bowel is often normal except in severe disease or infiltrating nodular endometrial implants. Occasionally, serosal involvement with adhesions can lead to obstruction. Endoscopically, the mucosa is generally intact, occasionally associated with significant luminal narrowing. Infiltration of the submucosa, although uncommon, may produce nodularity and distortion of the overlying mucosa (Figure 21-2). These findings may be difficult to visually differentiate from Crohn's disease, ischemia, or malignancy. Pressure against these areas of distorted bowel may produce pain that suggests the diagnosis of endometriosis. In addition, biopsies of the mucosa, taken in areas of endometriosis, can resemble solitary rectal ulcer or prolapse syndromes. Rarely is the diagnosis of endometriosis definitively confirmed by endoscopy or from endoscopic biopsies. Colonoscopy is, however, useful in excluding colon cancer from the differential diagnosis, especially in older patients presenting with a rectosigmoid mass while on hormone replacement.

Rigid proctoscopy is very helpful in predicting the depth of rectosigmoid involvement in patients with severe endometriosis of the cul-de-sac of Douglas. After two enemas are given to remove any fecal debris, the rigid proctoscope is deployed above the rectosigmoid and slowly withdrawn with care to maintain adequate insufflation. The mucosa is often fixed over area of submucosal or deep muscular involvement with tethering or puckering and loss of the normal mucosal mobility. In our experience, these mucosal findings have correlated with significant intestinal wall invasion by the endometrial implant and often a need for intestinal resection.

Imaging Techniques

Imaging techniques used to facilitate the diagnosis of endometriosis include ultrasonography, barium enema, computed tomography (CT), magnetic resonance imaging (MRI), and immunoscintigraphy. Many of these tests are obtained for the evaluation of chronic pelvic pain and/or bleeding from the reproductive tract or colon. They are primarily used to rule out more common conditions, but there are some findings that may strongly suggest the diagnosis of endometriosis before visual or pathologic confirmation by laparoscopy or laparotomy.

Transvaginal ultrasound has been used for several years to evaluate ovarian endometriomas. It is a sensitive test and in experienced hands provides specificity greater than 90% for ovarian endometriosis. Ultrasound of the pelvis, however, is not very sensitive in detecting focal nonovarian endometrial implants. Endometriosis has been termed "the great mimicker" because the appearance on ultrasound is highly variable with some lesions being nearly sonolucent and others quite echogenic.

Endorectal ultrasound is a potentially valuable tool to determine rectal wall invasion by endometrial implants in the cul-de-sac. Chapron and colleagues[36] studied the reliability of endorectal ultrasound in assessing the depth of bowel invasion with rectovaginal endometriosis. In 17 patients with proven deep pelvic endometriosis, the ultrasound revealed infiltration of the bowel wall and suggested the need for intestinal resection. The ultrasound findings were subsequently confirmed at laparoscopy and evaluation of the pathologic specimen in 16 patients. Twenty-one other patients with endometriosis of the cul-de-sac of Douglas whose ultrasounds did not show infiltration of the rectal wall did not require intestinal resection and were able to have complete removal of the endometriosis with laparoscopic techniques without complications. The accuracy of ultrasound was recently confirmed by Doniec and colleagues[37] who determined both the sensitivity and specificity of preoperative staging of rectal wall involvement by endometriosis to be 97%. The only real concern in evaluating patients having cul-de-sac endometriosis by endorectal ultrasound is the significant discomfort experienced by the patient when rectal distention from the balloon probe compresses the implant.

Barium enema examination is another imaging technique often obtained by gynecologists for the intestinal complaints associated with deep pelvic endometriosis. The lateral and

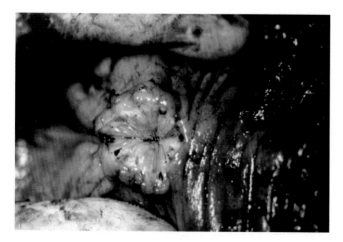

FIGURE 21.2. Polypoid endometrial implant of the colon.

prone cross-table views of the rectum offer excellent evaluation of the cul-de-sac of Douglas as long as care is taken in ensuring that the balloon is kept in the distal rectum (Figure 21-3). Studies in patients without bowel wall involvement are either normal or reveal smooth extrinsic compression with normal mucosa. Deep invasion of the bowel wall by endometriosis produces a variety of appearances on barium enema. Irregularities of the rectal wall such as tethering or even polypoid lesions may be difficult to distinguish from inflammatory bowel disease or neoplasm. Strictures of the rectosigmoid may also be identified on barium enema.

CT is the imaging technique probably used most frequently for the evaluation of abdominal and pelvic pain. Unfortunately, there is no standard CT appearance for a mass caused by endometriosis to clearly differentiate it from pelvic masses attributable to other causes. Cystic lesions are more often seen on the ovaries, whereas deeper pelvic disease usually consists of either solid lesions or mixed cystic/solid lesions. CT evaluation of the pelvic sidewall for endometrial implants is better than ultrasound, but there is still significant overlap between endometriosis and infectious or malignant pathology. CT scanning is probably most useful for patients with pelvic pain and a negative ultrasound to assess the musculoskeletal boundaries of the pelvis and the rectosigmoid colon.

When pelvic endometriosis is strongly suspected, MRI is more useful than CT scanning because of the benefit of imaging in multiple planes and the lack of ionizing radiation. MRI

is rarely used, however, as an initial study in women with pelvic pain because of the higher cost, patient discomfort (claustrophobia), the length of the scanning, and, until recently, the relative inaccessibility of scanners outside major medical centers. Sagittal images are particularly valuable in imaging the cul-de-sac of Douglas. MRI is superior to CT scanning for extraperitoneal lesions and the evaluation of pelvic masses.[38] Identification of endometrial implants is dependent on the hemorrhage that occurs in these lesions. The time between imaging and the most recent hemorrhage may determine in which weighted images the masses are most intensely seen.

Immunoscintigraphy with radioactive iodine-labeled CA-125 monoclonal antibodies has been studied to clarify the extent of pelvic endometriosis, particularly in the face of severe pelvic adhesive disease.[39] In such a study of 28 women, 22 had a positive test with 16 confirmed to have endometriosis. Two of five women had a negative test despite having histologically confirmed endometriosis. As such, immunoscintigraphy is not currently recommended for screening and remains primarily a research tool.

Laparoscopy

The diagnosis of endometriosis usually requires direct visual and/or tactile assessment of the abdomen and pelvis. Laparoscopy is currently the initial approach to many patients suspected of having endometriosis, and has revolutionized both its diagnosis and treatment. Most patients with severe pelvic pain and many patients with refractory infertility undergo laparoscopy. The timing of laparoscopy in relation to the menstrual cycle is unimportant except in patients being evaluated for infertility. In these patients, the procedure is performed in the luteal phase to provide additional valuable information concerning ovarian function.

The technique of diagnostic laparoscopy has become widespread in both the surgical and gynecologic literature. A camera, often attached to a video monitoring system with photographic and recording capabilities, is introduced at the level of the umbilicus or upper abdomen, and a second instrument is placed in a suprapubic location to allow manipulation of the pelvic and abdominal viscera. A thorough examination of the entire abdomen and especially the pelvis is critical to enable complete assessment of the disease. Both ovaries should be mobilized to evaluate the pelvic peritoneum, and the uterus should be manipulated to allow complete visualization of the cul-de-sac of Douglas, uterosacral ligaments, sigmoid colon, and ureters. It is important to view the base of the appendix as well as the distal small bowel and surface of the diaphragm.

Obtaining a complete assessment of the abdominal and pelvic viscera can be technically demanding. The accuracy of laparoscopy is completely dependent on the surgeon's visual evaluation of the abdomen and pelvis. The findings of endometriosis can be very subtle, and several studies have

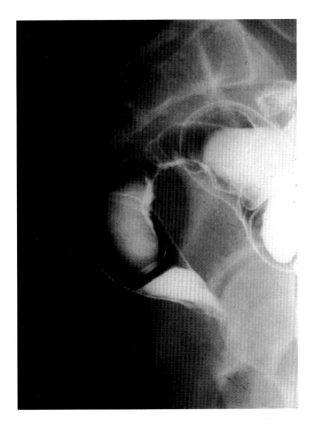

FIGURE 21.3. Barium enema demonstrating a rectosigmoid stricture.

demonstrated that visually normal peritoneum may have microscopic evidence of endometriosis.[40] The extent of endometriosis should be carefully documented and staged. The current staging system has been formulated primarily for infertility and was revised by the American Society for Reproductive Medicine in 1998 (Figure 21-4).[41] This revision is certainly an improvement over previous staging systems that were more concerned with adhesions than with implants. Virtually all patients with intestinal lesions requiring resection are Stage IV, especially if they have cul-de-sac involvement.

Patient's Name _____ Date_____

Stage I (Minimal) - 1–5
Stage II (Mild) - 6–15
Stage III (Moderate) - 16–40
Stage IV (Severe) - > 40

Laparoscopy _____ Laparotomy _____ Photography_____
Recommended Treatment _____

Total _____

Prognosis _____

PERITONEUM	ENDOMETRIOSIS	< 1cm	1–3cm	> 3cm
	Superficial	1	2	4
	Deep	2	4	6
OVARY	R Superficial	1	2	4
	Deep	6	16	20
	L Superficial	1	2	4
	Deep	4	16	20

	POSTERIOR CUL-DE-SAC OBLITERATION	Partial		Complete	
		4		40	

	ADHESIONS	< 1/3 Enclosure	1/3–2/3 Enclosure	<2/3 Enclosure
OVARY	R Filmy	1	2	4
	Dense	4	8	16
	L Filmy	1	2	4
	Dense	4	8	16
TUBE	R Filmy	1	2	4
	Dense	4•	8•	16
	L Filmy	1	2	4
	Dense	4•	8•	16

•If the fimbriated end of the fallopian tube is completely enclosed, change the point assignment to 16.
Denote appearance of superficial implant types as red [(R), red, red-pink, flamelike, vesicular blobs, clear vesicles], white [(W), opacifications, peritoneal defects, yellow-brown], or black [(B) black, hemosiderin deposits, blue]. Denote percent of total described as R___ %,W___ % and B___%. Total should equal 100%.

Additional Endometriosis: _____

Associated Pathology:_____

To Be Used with Normal Tubes and Ovaries
L   R

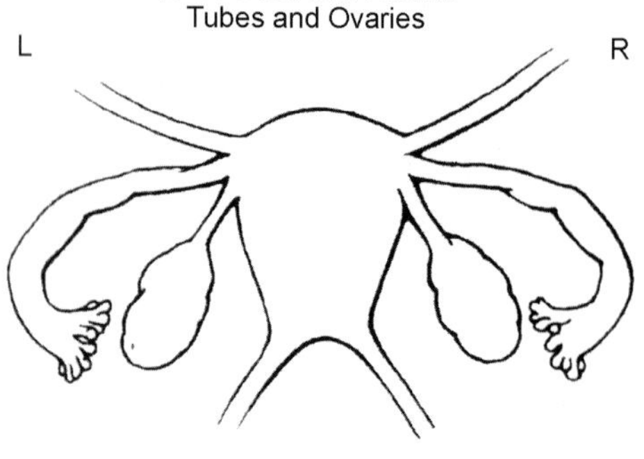

To Be Used with Abnormal Tubes and/or Ovaries
L   R

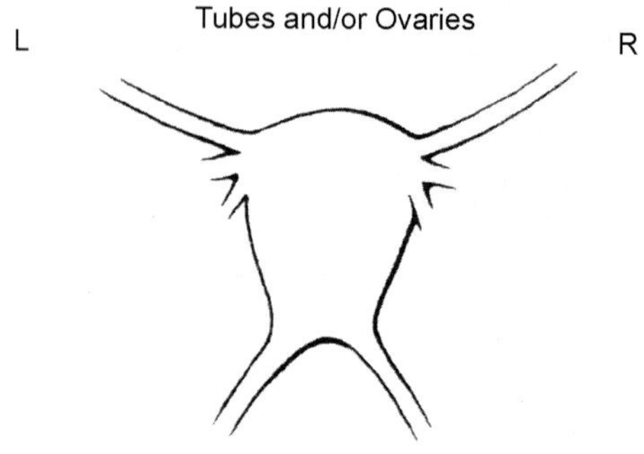

FIGURE 21.4. Revised American Society for Reproductive Medicine 1996 classification of endometriosis.[41]

The current classification system, however, is often not useful for the gastrointestinal surgeon. The more critical information for the surgeon is the identification and location of intestinal lesions. There is no uniform type of endometrial lesion. The classic implant is nodular with a variable degree of fibrosis and pigmentation. The color may be black, white, brown, blue, or even red. The appearance of the lesion may be vesicular, papular, or hemorrhagic (Figure 21-5). Glandular tissue is found in the great majority of these lesions. Lesions may change color or consistency over time, with red lesions noted early in the course of the disease and blue/black ones typical of older implants. Healed implants appear as fibrotic nodules. There are also a wide variety of atypical lesions occasionally associated with positive biopsies. The inability to definitively identify endometriosis through purely visual means necessitates pathologic confirmation of the disease before a definitive diagnosis can be made, especially in mild disease.

Implants in the cul-de-sac of Douglas, which occur in nearly 20% of women with endometriosis, were initially described by Cullen in 1920. Ninety percent of these represent an important variant that is especially relevant for the intestinal surgeon. Unlike endometriomas found at other sites, these lesions are histologically characterized by desmoplastic tissue composed of fibrous and smooth muscle cells with strands of endometrial glands and stroma. The major component of the lesion is the fibromuscular tissue and not the endometrial tissue typical of other locations. These implants are both proliferative and infiltrating and more than 25% extend at least 5 mm in depth.[42] The depth of invasion may be difficult to assess laparoscopically, and the full extent of the implant may not be appreciated until laparotomy. The progressive fibrosis leads to narrowing of the intestinal lumen and occasionally to bowel obstruction.

These rectovaginal implants also behave differently during the menstrual cycle. There are poor to absent secretory changes during the luteal phase. Vasodilatation and not necro-

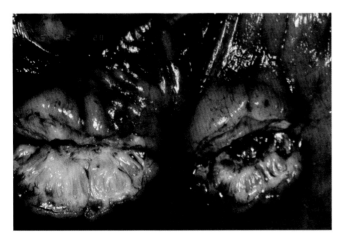

FIGURE 21.5. Endometrial implants with hemorrhagic centers and fibrosis.

sis and bleeding occur at menstruation. Resistance to medical therapy is common with several studies demonstrating no significant decrease in mitotic activity in rectovaginal endometriosis after GnRH agonist (GnRH-a) treatment.[43] This resistance is thought to be attributable to estrogen receptor inactivity, inadequate drug access, or genetic programming that is only secondarily affected by estrogen.

Treatment

Treatment options for women with endometriosis are currently based on the severity and type of symptoms. Currently, prevention of endometriosis is not yet possible, and therefore treatment is primarily begun to ameliorate symptoms. Some women with endometriosis are completely asymptomatic and the implants are found incidentally at the time of surgery for other reasons. A study by Martin et al.[44] in 1989 revealed that 25% of women undergoing elective tubal ligation had asymptomatic endometrial implants. This finding strongly suggests that not all women with endometriosis require treatment. Other authors have analyzed the prevalence of endometriosis in these asymptomatic women with regard to the time from their last pregnancy. They discovered that the odds of having endometrial implants increased significantly at 10 years after the last pregnancy.[5,45] Consequently, as the natural history seems unclear, long-term follow-up of these patient cohorts may demonstrate late development of symptoms and the need for more aggressive medical or surgical management. Even menopause, either surgical or natural, is not completely protective. The widespread use of hormone replacement therapy has revealed that up to 20% of these patients will have recurrent endometriosis. Not surprisingly, the majority of these patients had deep pelvic or intestinal disease.[46]

Before the introduction of diagnostic laparoscopy in the 1960s, exploratory laparotomy was the only modality available for the diagnosis and treatment of endometriosis. Laparoscopy revolutionized the diagnostic evaluation of these women and allowed patients with limited disease to undergo medical therapy. With improvements in laparoscopic techniques and equipment in the past decade, notably the development of laparoscopic laser techniques, many if not most early endometrial lesions can now be ablated at the time of diagnosis. Even complex excisional surgery involving the bowel and ureter can be occasionally performed safely via a laparoscopic approach in many patients. As advanced laparoscopic techniques have become more widespread, the indications and use of medical therapy is also evolving.

Medical Management

Medical therapy is designed to treat the symptoms of endometriosis, notably pelvic pain. Because pelvic pain may have causes other than the endometriosis seen during laparoscopy, a trial of ovarian suppression with a 3-month course of either danazol or a GnRH-a is often used to help determine the contribution of the pain from the endometrial implants. Most patients will have cessation of pain from endometriosis in the first month of amenorrhea. In those patients with infertility, with or without pelvic pain, the primary goal is an intrauterine pregnancy. After other causes of infertility have been excluded, ovarian suppression may allow for laparoscopic removal of downsized, smaller endometrial lesions with optimal preservation of ovarian tissue.

Despite the many advances in the surgical treatment of endometriosis, there are still some significant advantages to medical therapy. Surgery can remove only lesions that are both visible and accessible. Microscopic disease or disease on vital structures is often left behind. Subsequent recurrence is not surprising. Additionally, there are complications associated with ablative surgery in the pelvis, especially if the woman requires multiple attempts at control of her disease. For infertile women, the adhesions that can form after any pelvic surgery may further impair the ability to conceive. In addition, laser destruction of ovarian implants may destroy germinal tissue and conceivably limit the reproductive potential from the involved ovary. In limited disease, medical therapy is comparable with surgery in terms of relief of symptoms, recurrence of disease, and subsequent pregnancy rates. Finally, medical therapy does not require specialized training or equipment, and is much less costly than surgery.

Medical therapy alone also has significant potential disadvantages. All the hormonal therapies subsequently discussed have side effects and often require prolonged treatment. Medical therapies manipulate the hormonal environment to suppress the cyclic secretion of ovarian estrogen and progesterone, and this suppression induces atrophy of the ectopic endometrium so that over several months the implants regress. Advanced lesions, especially those with a nodular, proliferative histology will often only partially regress. No current hormonal regimen can completely eradicate these lesions, and upon cessation of therapy, the lesions may again become symptomatic.

Oral Contraceptives

The first effective medical therapy for endometriosis was introduced by Kistner. He proposed the administration of high-dose, continuous estrogen/progestens in 1958. These agents result in the induction of pseudo-pregnancy with hyperhormonal amenorrhea. Pituitary and ovarian function is thereby suppressed, and in the later stages of the treatment regimen, endometrial implants resorb and resolve. The usual treatment regimen consists of daily administration of a tablet for 6–9 months. When Vercellini and colleagues[47] compared oral contraceptives with GnRH-a, they found that deep dyspareunia and pelvic pain were reduced in both groups, with fewer side effects experienced by the oral contraceptive women. Pain relief appeared similar in the two groups at 1 year. Side effects rarely cause cessation of treatment, but

exacerbation of endometriotic symptoms may occur early in the course of treatment.

Another drug regimen used for the treatment of endometriosis involves administration of synthetic progestens alone. This may induce a pseudo-pregnancy by acting in concert with endogenous estrogens. Ovarian suppression is often inconsistent. Both oral and depot preparations are available. In patients who do not desire pregnancy and in whom surgery is contraindicated, depot progestens have been effective in ameliorating pelvic pain with equivalent efficacy to danazol.[48] Side effects include breakthrough vaginal bleeding, weight gain, and fluid retention.

Danazol

Danazol was first used extensively for endometriosis in the mid-1970s, and until the introduction of GnRH-a, was the most widely used drug for suppression of the ectopic endometrium. Danazol lowers peripheral estrogen and progesterone levels by a direct effect on ovarian steroidogenesis and pituitary production of follicle-stimulating hormone (FSH) and luteinizing hormone (LH). Danazol also binds directly to endometrial cellular receptors leading to atrophy and suppression of proliferation. In addition, danazol is a potent immunomodulator with beneficial effects on both humoral and cellular immunity.[49]

The side effects of danazol necessitate discontinuation in less than 5% of patients for short courses,[50] but is poorly tolerated for long-term suppression. Predictable manifestations of menopause are most common. Danazol also raises free testosterone levels and produces a hyperandrogenic state, especially at lower doses. Hirsutism, acne, weight gain, and deepening voice changes may occur. In addition, because danazol alters lipid metabolism and liver function, it should not be used in women with increased liver enzymes, liver disease, or complications of atherosclerosis.

Gonadotropin-releasing Hormone Agonists

The introduction of GnRH-a as a new treatment modality for endometriosis has improved results, primarily by a reduction in side effects. GnRH-a are synthetic molecules derived from the 10 peptide long GnRH. Continuous administration of GnRH-a completely suppresses pituitary release of FSH and LH. Administered either by injection or intranasally beginning in the mid-luteal phase of the menstrual cycle, the current recommended length of therapy is 6 months. Pain relief is complete in more than 50% of women and significantly decreased in more than 90%. Laparoscopic evaluation after 6 months of treatment indicates resolution or a significant decrease in size of the lesions in the majority of patients. Studies comparing danazol and GnRH-a indicate similar clinical efficacy.[51]

Side effects of GnRH-a are predictably attributable to the sometimes profound hypoestrogenic state many of these women experience. Up to 90% of patients will experience hot flashes, night sweats, vasomotor instability, atrophic vaginitis, migraines, or depression. Cessation of therapy for side effects is uncommon. The degree of bone loss that can occur with the typical 6-month treatment regimen is unclear, but GnRH-a is not recommended for women with osteoporosis. Interestingly, a potentially serious complication can result when GnRH-a is inadvertently administered at the wrong point in the menstrual cycle, and a brief period of hypersecretion of FSH and LH occurs. Rarely, this upsurge in gonadotropin activity may precipitate an acute exacerbation in endometriotic symptoms, occasionally necessitating emergency surgical intervention.[52]

Surgical Management

Surgical treatment of endometriosis has evolved significantly over time. Before the advent of laparoscopy and suppressive medical therapy, most operations were performed for advanced disease and consisted of radical removal of the uterus and ovaries. Although the most effective treatment of pelvic pain still consists of surgical castration along with resection of the endometrial implants, many of these young patients strongly desire to maintain their options for pregnancy. Currently, surgery is considered conservative only when reproductive potential is preserved. Therefore, the major goal of surgical therapy for endometriosis is to completely excise or ablate the endometrial implants. Secondary goals include preservation of ovarian function and minimizing postoperative adhesion formation. Currently, we approach these patients in concert with gynecologists experienced with treating ovarian endometriosis to completely remove all gross disease, restore normal anatomy, and optimize fertility.

General Principles

Endometriosis is an invasive disease that can extend deeply into the retroperitoneum, and is often surrounded by a rim of fibrosis that may make it difficult to completely assess the true extent of the implant. Removal of the lesions requires sharp excision or vaporization with electrocautery and/or the CO_2 laser. Both techniques have the potential for iatrogenic injury to the intestinal or urinary tracts. Recognizing when a lesion is completely ablated is highly dependent on surgical technique and the expertise of the surgeon. Utilizing techniques that minimize injury to the surrounding tissue, such as a cutting current to outline lesions to be removed by electrocautery and high-power density settings with the CO_2 laser are desirable. Laparoscopic hydrodissection is also very useful in identifying normal surrounding tissue.

Meticulous hemostasis and frequent irrigation is critical to maintaining good visualization of the operative field in both open and laparoscopic surgery. Tissue planes are often distorted, especially in the cul-de-sac of Douglas, and intraoperative instrumentation of the vagina or proctoscopic evaluation of the rectum may help avoid iatrogenic injury to these structures. Finally, minimizing tissue trauma with gentle handling will decrease adhesions and maximize potential fertility.

All patients undergoing surgery for advanced endometriosis, either by an open or laparoscopic approach, should have a full mechanical and antibiotic bowel preparation. Prophylactic antibiotics and other appropriate practices for patients undergoing major abdominal or pelvic surgery are standard. Patients are positioned in the low lithotomy position with access to both the vagina and rectum for instrumentation. Ureteral stents are liberally used and are especially useful in women with severe obliterative disease in the cul-de-sac and in reoperative pelvic surgical procedures.

Provided that complete removal of the endometriosis is performed, no specific technique or approach has been proven to be superior. With endometriosis, the surgeon's experience and skill are paramount. In experienced hands, laparoscopic removal of extensive endometriosis can be accomplished. However, removal of deep lesions in the rectovaginal septum necessitating bowel resection still often requires open laparotomy to safely and completely excise the endometrial implant with restoration of intestinal continuity.

The management and techniques concerning the surgical treatment of ovarian and ureteral endometriosis are extensively discussed in the appropriate gynecologic and urologic literature. This discussion on surgical therapy will concentrate on management of intestinal lesions.

Rectovaginal Endometriosis

Endometriosis of the cul-de-sac of Douglas that extends into the rectovaginal septum is the most common site of intestinal involvement and may require intestinal resection. These lesions are often deep fibrotic nodules that extend from the posterior vagina and anterior rectum to the uterosacral ligaments (Figure 21-6). Small superficial lesions involving the intraperitoneal rectum may be vaporized with the CO_2 laser or

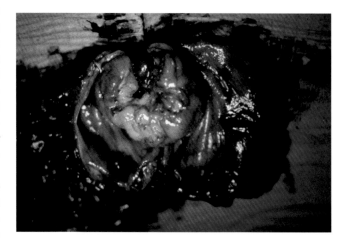

FIGURE 21.6. Deep infiltrating endometrial implant of the rectosigmoid.

electrocautery. When using either technique, it is critical to initially outline the lesion to be removed to ensure complete extirpation because distortion of the planes and tissue can otherwise make it difficult to assess the completeness of excision. Cutting current as opposed to coagulating current is preferred. The former technique minimizes carbonization that can make it challenging to recognize when an adequate depth has been achieved by the appearance of normal tissue. After the lesion is removed, the bowel wall is carefully assessed. Because most of these superficial lesions can be removed without entering the mucosa, the defects can be closed with interrupted transversely placed Lembert stitches.

Surgical treatment of the deeper lesions is more controversial. Removal of the rectosigmoid with reanastomosis is technically demanding and should be performed by skilled intestinal surgeons to minimize complications in these young patients. As experience has grown, there has been a shift to more aggressive therapy, usually in conjunction with gynecologists who remove endometrial deposits on the ovaries and fallopian tubes. Medical treatment has not proven adequate for these infiltrating lesions, so it is no surprise that castration alone has also proven ineffective.[53] Many of these women have chronic pain or partial colonic obstructive symptoms after bilateral salpingo-oophorectomy when the endometrial implant is not resected. As a result, excision of the implant either with a disc of rectal wall or a formal anterior resection is recommended for women with symptoms related to the endometriosis. Both procedures can occasionally be performed laparoscopically if the endometriosis is completely removed. Unfortunately, laparoscopy often misses lesions that are not visually apparent and discernible only by palpation. It should be noted, however, that for severe disease, laparoscopic ablation, when possible, had similar crude pregnancy rates in comparison to laparotomy, and both techniques were clearly superior to medical management alone.[54]

The infiltrating nodular endometrial implants involving the rectovaginal portion of the cul-de-sac often invade both the vagina and rectum. Because removal of the implant will require resection of a portion of the rectal wall, dissection of the lesion from the vagina allows for en bloc removal of the lesion with the rectal wall. There is often no discernible plane between these lesions and the walls of the rectum or vagina. Care must be taken to avoid penetration of the vaginal wall with possible injury to the cervix, especially in women desiring eventual pregnancy. Often it is advantageous to mobilize the rectum in the posterior and lateral tissue planes to adequately define the lesion before attempting the anterior dissection. Blunt dissection of the rectovaginal plane below the area of involvement may help clarify the distorted anatomy and avoid inadvertent entry into the bowel lumen. After careful dissection of the lesion from the vagina, the normal rectovaginal plane is reached, and the fixed, hard mass may suddenly become mobile and amenable to resection.

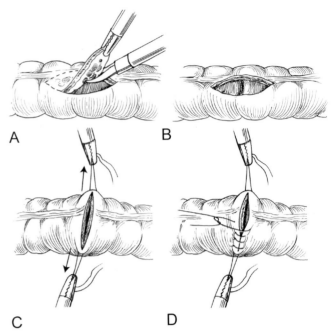

FIGURE 21.7. Disc excision of an endometrial implant.

Disc excision of the anterior rectal wall, by either laparoscopic or open technique, is performed for single lesions usually less than 3 cm in diameter (Figure 21-7). After marking the lesions circumferentially with electrocautery, stay sutures are placed on either side of the endometrial implant. Full-thickness bowel wall excision is then performed with the cutting current electrocautery. Interrupted transverse absorbable sutures are subsequently placed to close the resulting defect.

Segmental resection of the rectosigmoid is performed for larger lesions or when neoplasia is a concern. Margins are to grossly normal bowel, and unless there are multiple lesions, an extensive colonic resection is not required. High ligation of the sigmoid vessels is also unnecessary, and the anastomosis may be either hand-sewn or stapled. When resection is performed laparoscopically, the involved segment may be removed by extending one of the port sites. Nezhat et al.[55] have described a technique of prolapsing the lesion outside the anus for resection. Redwine et al.[56] have described a transvaginal approach for specimen removal. Open or laparoscopic excision of these deeply infiltrating rectovaginal lesions is very technically demanding. The lack of discernible tissue planes, the intimate association of the rectum and vagina, and the frequent occurrence of distal infiltration of endometriosis down to the mid to lower rectum makes laparoscopic resection possible in only a small minority of these patients and only by surgeons very experienced in complex intestinal laparoscopy. Even in the hands of experienced laparoscopists, rectovaginal fistula requiring ileostomy has been reported to occur after these resections.[54] Proctoscopic insufflation to assess for leak is practiced routinely by the authors with all rectal anastomoses, whether performed open or laparoscopically.

Small Bowel and Appendiceal Endometriosis

Although endometriosis involving the small bowel or appendix is much less common than rectosigmoid disease, careful inspection of these organs is critical in patients with advanced endometriosis to ensure complete removal of all gross disease and to minimize recurrence. Superficial small bowel implants may be treated with sharp excision, electrocautery, or the laser, as described above. Deeper implants may require small bowel resection, and, if within 5 cm of the ileocecal valve, may need an ileocecectomy. Appendiceal endometriosis is treated with appendectomy. Occasionally, a surgeon will encounter a patient with an endometrial implant while operating for another condition. Although the lesion may exhibit a classic visual appearance consistent with endometriosis, a biopsy to confirm the diagnosis and exclude malignancy is important. Several studies have suggested that few patients with small asymptomatic endometrial implants of the appendix will become symptomatic, but no study has yet defined the natural history of these lesions. As a result, for those patients with asymptomatic endometriosis, observation is probably sufficient, but hormone replacement therapy should be avoided to avoid stimulation of the implants.

Results After Surgical Therapy

Recurrence of endometriosis after surgical excision is difficult to assess because of a wide variability in the operative approach to endometriosis by various authors and the obvious need for postoperative laparoscopy to document asymptomatic recurrence. Although there are no long-term prospective studies to date, the larger studies suggest a histologically confirmed rate of recurrent endometriosis of approximately 19%.[57] Gauging the response to surgery by the resolution of preoperative pelvic pain or infertility is easier to measure. The largest series of intestinal resections for advanced intestinal endometriosis by Bailey et al.[58] found that 86% of patients had complete or near complete relief of their preoperative pelvic pain. In addition, a 50% crude pregnancy rate was achieved which was comparable with rates found when treating much lower stages of disease. These results in more than 130 cases with a median follow-up of 5 years were achieved with minimal morbidity, no anastomotic leaks, and no documented instance of recurrent colorectal endometriosis. Laparoscopic series of intestinal resections performed for extensive endometriosis have reported similar pregnancy rates albeit with smaller number of cases, higher complication rates, and shorter long-term follow-up.[59]

Combined Medical and Surgical Therapy

Both medical and surgical therapies for endometriosis have potential reasons why each treatment alone may not be successful in eradicating the disease and minimizing recurrence. Medical therapy affects endometrial implants variably, and there is a high instance of recurrence after cessation of therapy. Surgery may not remove microscopic disease, and postsurgical adhesions may contribute to postoperative pelvic pain and infertility. For these reasons, combination therapy either pre- or postoperatively has been used for several years, although with a paucity of prospective, randomized data to conclusively prove long-term improvement in recurrence and symptoms.

The rationale for preoperative medical therapy conducted over a period of 3–6 months is principally to decrease the inflammation and possibly the size of the endometrial implants. Presumably, this therapy will allow easier excision with diminished adhesion formation. Medical therapy may also reduce the vascularity of endometrial implants. A prospective study by Buttram[60] in 1985 revealed an improvement in pregnancy rates with 6 months of danazol given preoperatively with all stages of endometriosis. The optimal length of therapy and long-term (and not just delayed) recurrence rates must still be elucidated. Postoperative treatment with danazol and oral contraceptive pills has not been shown to have durability, and the initial excitement over improved recurrence rates at 12 months has not been duplicated after longer follow-ups.[60] Our current use of combined therapy, after laparoscopic confirmation of advanced pelvic endometriosis, is a 3- to 6-month course of a GnRH-a before definitive surgery for virtually all patients able to tolerate the medical therapy.

Conclusion

The diagnosis and management of intestinal endometriosis has evolved tremendously over the last 20 years with the widespread availability of laparoscopy and a clear understanding of the necessity to remove all endometrial implants in symptomatic patients. With the advent of stapling devices that facilitate low pelvic anastomoses, the intestinal surgeon should be able to resect the endometrial implants and restore bowel continuity in virtually all patients with minimal morbidity and preserved fertility, when desired. Further improvements in outcomes will probably not occur until a better understanding of the precise etiology and growth of the endometrial implant is discovered.

References

1. Hasson HM. Incidence of endometriosis in diagnostic laparoscopy. J Reprod Med 1976;16:135–138.
2. Drake TS, Grunert GM. The unsuspected pelvic factor in the infertility evaluation. Fertil Steril 1980;34:27–31.
3. Houston DE, Noller KL, Melton J III, Selwyn BJ. The epidemiology of pelvic endometriosis. Clin Obstet Gynecol 1988;31(4): 787–800.

4. Halme J, Stovall D. Endometriosis and its medical management. In: Walch EE, Zacur HA, eds. Reproductive Medicine and Surgery. St. Louis: Mosby; 1995:695–710.

5. Moen MH. Is a long period without childbirth a risk factor for endometriosis? Hum Reprod 1991;6:1404–1407.

6. Miyazawa K. Incidence of endometriosis among Japanese women. Obstet Gynecol 1976;48:407–409.

7. Ridley JH. The histogenesis of endometriosis. A review of facts and fancies. Obstet Gynecol Surv 1968;20:1–35.

8. Sampson JA. Perforating hemorrhagic (chocolate) cysts of the ovary, their importance and especially their relation to pelvic adenomas of endometrial type. Arch Surg 1921;3:245–323.

9. Telinde RW, Scott RB. Experimental endometriosis. Am J Obstet Gynecol 1950;60:1147–1173.

10. Ridley JH, Edwards KI. Experimental endometriosis in the human. Am J Obstet Gynecol 1958;76:783–790.

11. Simpson JL, Elias S, Malinak LR, Buttram VC. Heritable aspects of endometriosis. 1. Genetic studies. Am J Obstet Gynecol 1980; 137:327–331.

12. Dmowski WP, Steele RW, Baker GF. Deficient cellular immunity in endometriosis. Am J Obstet Gynecol 1981;141:377–383.

13. Vigano P, Vercellini P, DiBlasio AM, et al. Deficient anti-endometrium lymphocyte mediated cytotoxicity in patients with endometriosis. Fertil Steril 1991;56:894–899.

14. Oosterlynck DJ, Cornillie FJ, Waer M, et al. Women with endometriosis show a defect in natural killer activity resulting in a decreased cytotoxicity to autologous endometrium. Fertil Steril 1991;56:45–51.

15. Thomas EJ, Cooke ID. Impact of gestrinone on the course of asymptomatic endometriosis. Br Med J 1987;294:272–274.

16. Bergqvist A, Thorbjorn B, Hogstrom L, et al. Effects of triptorelin versus placebo on the symptoms of endometriosis. Fertil Steril 1998;69:702–708.

17. Evers JLH. The second-look laparoscopy for evaluation of the result of medical treatment of endometriosis should not be performed during ovarian suppression. Fertil Steril 1987;47:502–504.

18. Vercillini P, Fedele L, Molteni P, et al. Laparoscopy in the diagnosis of gynecologic chronic pelvic pain. Int J Gynaecol Obstet 1990;32:261–265.

19. Koninckx PR, Meuleman C, Demeyere S, et al. Suggestive evidence that pelvic endometriosis is a progressive disease, whereas deeply infiltrating endometriosis is associated with pelvic pain. Fertil Steril 1991;55:759–765.

20. Schulman H, Duvivier R, Blattner P. The uterine contractility index: a research and diagnostic tool in dysmenorrhea. Am J Obstet Gynaecol 1983;145:1049–1058.

21. Liu DTY, Hitchcock A. Endometriosis: its association with retrograde menstruation, dysmenorrhea and tubal pathology. Br J Obstet Gynaecol 1986;93:859–862.

22. Cornillie FJ, Oosterlynck DJ, Lauweryns J, et al. Deeply infiltrating pelvic endometriosis: histology and clinical significance. Fertil Steril 1990;53:978–993.

23. Badaway S, Marshall L, Gabal A, et al. The concentration of 13,14-dihydro-15-keto-prostaglandin F2alpha and prostaglandin E2 in peritoneal fluid of infertile patients with and without endometriosis. Fertil Steril 1982;38:166–170.

24. Dawood M, Khan-Dawood F, Wilson L. Peritoneal fluid prostaglandins and prostanoids in women with endometriosis, chronic pelvic inflammatory disease, and pelvic pain. Am J Obstet Gynecol 1984;148:391–395.

25. Hull MGR, Glazener CMA, Kelly NJ, et al. Population study of causes, treatment, and outcome of infertility. Br Med J 1985;291: 1693–1697.

26. Fortier KJ, Haney AF. The pathologic spectrum of uterotubal junction obstruction. Obstet Gynecol 1985;65:93–98.

27. Buttram VC Jr, Reiter RC. Endometriosis. In: Buttram VC Jr, Reiter RC, eds. Surgical Treatment of the Infertile Female. Baltimore: Williams & Wilkins; 1985:89–148.

28. Garcia CR, David SS. Pelvic endometriosis: infertility and pelvic pain. Am J Obstet Gynecol 1977;129:740–747.

29. Inoue M, Kobayshi Y, Honda I, et al. The impact of endometriosis on the reproductive outcome of infertile patients. Am J Obstet Gynecol 1992;167:278–282.

30. Jansen RPS. Minimal endometriosis and reduced fecundability: prospective evidence from an artificial insemination by donor program. Fertil Steril 1986;46:141–143.

31. Floberg J, Backdahl M, Silfersward C, et al. Postpartum perforation of the colon due to endometriosis. Acta Obstet Gynecol Scand 1984;63:183–184.

32. Prystowsky JB, Stryker SJ, Ujiki GT, Poticha SM. Gastrointestinal endometriosis. Arch Surg 1988;123:855–858.

33. Aure JC, Hoeg K, Kolstad P. Carcinoma of the ovary and endometriosis. Acta Obstet Gynecol Scand 1971;50:63–67.

34. Yantiss RK, Clement PB, Young RH. Neoplastic and pre-neoplastic changes in gastrointestinal endometriosis. Am J Surg Pathol 2000;24:513–524.

35. Kennedy SH, Starkey PM, Sargent I, et al. Anti-endometrial antibodies in endometriosis measured by an enzyme-linked immunosorbent assay before and after treatment with danazol and nafarelin. Obstet Gynecol 1990;75:914–917.

36. Chapron C, Dumontier I, Dousset B, et al. Results and role of rectal endoscopic ultrasonography for patients with deep pelvic endometriosis. Hum Reprod 1998;13:2266–2270.

37. Doniec JM, Kahlke V, Peetz F, et al. Rectal endometriosis: high sensitivity and specificity of endorectal ultrasound with an impact for the operative management. Dis Colon Rectum 2003; 46:1667–1673.

38. Kinkel K, Chapron C, Balleyguier C, et al. Magnetic resonance imaging characteristics of deep endometriosis. Hum Reprod 1999;14:1080–1086.

39. Kennedy SH, Soper ND, Mojiminiyi OA. Immunoscintigraphy of endometriosis. A preliminary study. Br J Obstet Gynaecol 1988;95:693–697.

40. Vasquez G, Cornillie FJ, Brosens IO. Peritoneal endometriosis: scanning electron microscopy in visually normal peritoneum. Fertil Steril 1986;42:696–703.

41. American Society for Reproductive Medicine. Revised American Society for Reproductive Medicine classification of endometriosis: 1996. Fertil Steril 1997;67:817–821.

42. Donnez J, Nisolle M, Casanas-Roux F, et al. Stereometric evaluation of peritoneal endometriosis and endometriotic nodules of the rectovaginal septum. Hum Reprod 1995;11:224–228.

43. Koninckx PR. Deeply infiltrating endometriosis. In: Brosens I, Donnez J, eds. Endometriosis: Research and Management. Carnforth, UK: Parthenon Publishing; 1993:437–446.

44. Martin DC, Hubert GD, Vander Zwaag R, et al. Laparoscopic appearances of peritoneal endometriosis. Fertil Steril 1989;51: 63–67.

45. Koninckx PR, Martin DC. Deep endometriosis: a consequence of infiltration or retraction or possibly adenomyosis externa? Fertil Steril 1992;58:924–928.

46. Gray LA. Endometriosis of the bowel: role of bowel resection, superficial excision, and oophorectomy in treatment. Ann Surg 1973;177:580–587.

47. Vercellini P, Aimi G, Panazza S, et al. A gonadotropin-releasing hormone agonist versus a low-dose oral contraceptive for pelvic pain associated with endometriosis. Fertil Steril 1992;60: 75–79.

48. Dmowski WP, Radwanska E, Rana N. Recurrent endometriosis following hysterectomy and oophorectomy: the role of residual ovarian fragments. Int J Obstet 1988;26:93–103.

49. Dmowski WP, Gebel H, Braun DP. The role of cell mediated immunity in pathogenesis of endometriosis. Acta Obstet Gynecol Scand 1994;159(S):7–14.

50. Noble AD, Letchworth AT. Medical treatment of endometriosis: a comparative trial. Postgrad Med J 1979;55:37–39.

51. Wheeler JM, Knitte JD, Miller JD. Depot Leuprolide versus danazol in treatment of women with symptomatic endometriosis. Am J Obstet Gynecol 1992;167:1367–1371.

52. Hall LH, Malone JM, Ginsburg KA. Flare-up of endometriosis induced by gonadotropin-releasing hormone agonist leading to bowel obstruction. Fertil Steril 1995;64:1204–1206.

53. Redwine DB. Endometriosis persisting after castration: clinical characteristics and results of surgical management. Obstet Gynecol 1994;83:405–413.

54. Olive DL, Lee KL. Analysis of sequential treatment protocols for endometriosis-associated infertility. Am J Obstet Gynecol 1986;154:613.

55. Nezhat C, Pennington E, Nezhat F, Silfen SL. Laparoscopically assisted anterior rectal wall resection and reanastomosis for deeply infiltrating endometriosis. Surg Laparosc Endosc 1991;1: 106–108.

56. Redwine DB, Koning M, Sharpe DR. Laparoscopically assisted transvaginal segmental resection of the rectosigmoid colon for endometriosis. Fertil Steril 1996;65:193–197.

57. Wheeler JM, Malinak LR. Recurrent endometriosis. Contrib Gynecol Obstet 1987;16:13–21.

58. Bailey HR, Ott MT, Hartendorp P. Aggressive surgical management for advanced colorectal endometriosis. Dis Colon Rectum 1994;37:747–753.

59. Jerby BL, Kessler H, Falcone T, Milsom JW. Laparoscopic management of colorectal endometriosis. Surg Endosc 1999;13: 1125–1128.

60. Buttram VC, Reiter RC, Ward SM. Treatment of endometriosis with danazol: report of a six year prospective study. Fertil Steril 1985;43:353.

22
Colon and Rectal Trauma and Rectal Foreign Bodies

Demetrios Demetriades and Ali Salim

Colon Injuries

The management of colon injuries has been one of the most controversial issues in trauma and has undergone many radical changes in the last few decades. Despite the dramatic reduction of colon-related mortality from about 60% during World War I to about 40% during World War II to about 10% during the Vietnam War and to lower than 3% in the last decade, the colon-related morbidity remains unacceptably high. The abdominal sepsis rate has remained at about 20% in most prospective studies in the last decade (Table 22-1).[1–6] No other organ injury is associated with a higher septic complication rate than colon. In some subgroups of patients with colon injuries in the presence of Penetrating Abdominal Trauma Index (PATI) >25 or with multiple blood transfusions, the incidence of intraabdominal sepsis has been reported to be as high as 27%.[7] In patients with destructive colon injuries requiring resection, the reported incidence of abdominal complications is about 24%.[6] Many studies have attempted to identify risk factors for complications and optimize the treatment.

Epidemiology

The vast majority of colon injuries are caused by penetrating trauma. In American urban centers, firearms are by far the most common cause of injury. In anterior or posterior abdominal gunshot wounds, the colon is the second most frequently injured organ after the small bowel and it is involved in about 27% of cases undergoing laparotomy.[8,9] In anterior abdominal stab wounds, the colon is the third most frequently injured organ after the liver and small bowel and an injury is found in about 18% of patients undergoing laparotomy. In posterior stab wounds, the colon is the most frequently injured organ and is injured in about 20% of patients undergoing laparotomy.[10] In gunshot wounds, the transverse colon is the most frequently affected segment. In stab wounds, the left colon is the most frequently injured segment, probably because of the predominance of right-handed assailants.

Blunt trauma to the colon is uncommon and is diagnosed in about 0.5% of all major blunt trauma or in 10.6% of patients undergoing laparotomy.[11,12] Most of these injuries are partial thickness and only 3% of patients undergoing laparotomy have full-thickness colon perforations.[11,13] Traffic trauma is the most common cause of blunt colon injury. Deceleration injuries may cause avulsion of the colon from the mesentery resulting in ischemia but blowout perforations caused by transient closed loop formation may occur as well. Seatbelts increase the risk of hollow viscous perforations and the presence of a seatbelt mark sign is a predictor of hollow viscous injury. In rare cases, colonic wall hematoma or contusion may result in delayed perforation several days after the injury. The left colon is the most frequently injured segment followed by the right colon and the transverse colon.[11]

Diagnosis

The diagnosis of colon injury is almost always made intraoperatively. However, with the introduction of selective nonoperative management of penetrating abdominal trauma, there has been a concern of missing colon injuries. This is particularly important in penetrating injuries of the back because small retroperitoneal colon injuries may not give early clinical signs. A rectal examination may show blood in the stool, especially in cases with distal colon or rectal injuries. A preoperative erect chest film may show the nonspecific presence of free air under the diaphragm. The colon can reliably be evaluated by soluble enema studies or abdominal computed tomography (CT) scan with soluble rectal contrast. Retroperitoneal gas or contrast extravasation are diagnostic and an exploratory laparotomy should be performed. Other investigations, such as ultrasound or diagnostic peritoneal lavage have no role in the evaluation of suspected colon injuries.

The preoperative diagnosis of colon injury after blunt trauma can be a major challenge, especially if the patient is unevaluable because of severe associated head injuries. The diagnosis may be suspected by the presence of free gas or thickened colonic wall on the routine abdominal CT scan. In

TABLE 22-1. Incidence of abdominal septic complications in colon injuries (prospective studies)

Author	No. of patients	Abdominal sepsis (%)
George et al.,[1] 1989	102	33
Chappuis et al.,[2] 1991	56	20
Demetriades et al.,[3] 1992	100	16
Ivatury et al.,[4] 1993	252	17
Gonzalez et al.,[5] 1996	114	24
Demetriades et al.,[6] 2001	297	24
Overall	921	22

some cases, the diagnosis may be delayed by many days with catastrophic consequences.

Intraoperatively, every paracolic hematoma caused by penetrating trauma should be explored and the underlying colon should be evaluated carefully. Failure to adhere to this important surgical principle is a serious error with medical and legal implications. Paracolic hematomas caused by blunt trauma should not undergo routine exploration unless there is evidence of colon perforation.

Colon Injury Scale

The American Association for the Surgery of Trauma (AAST) developed a grading system for organ injuries in order to have objective criteria for the classification of the severity of the injury and enable reliable comparisons of results. On the basis of the injury grade, an Abbreviated Injury Score is assigned and may be used for the calculation of the Injury Severity Score (ISS). The AAST Colon Injury Scale is shown in Table 22-2.

Operative Management

Historical Perspective

The first guidelines regarding the management of colon injuries were published by the United States Surgeon General and mandated proximal diversion or exteriorization of all colon wounds.[14] This unusual directive was initiated because of the very high mortality of colorectal injuries during the early years of World War II. The mortality in both civilian and military reports exceeded 50%.[15,16] Although these guidelines were not based on any scientific evidence, they were credited

TABLE 22-2. AAST Colon Injury Scale

Grade	Injury description
I	a) Contusion or hematoma without devascularization
	b) Partial thickness laceration
II	Laceration ≤50% of circumference
III	Laceration >50% of circumference
IV	Transection of the colon
V	Transection of the colon with segmental tissue loss

for the significant reduction of mortality in the last years of the war. However, during this period, many other major changes in trauma care took place. Faster evacuation from the battlefield and early definitive care, improved resuscitation protocols, and introduction of penicillin and sulfadiazine could all have contributed to the reduction of mortality. The policy of mandatory colostomy for all colon injuries remained the unchallenged standard of care until the late 1970s. Stone and Fabian[17] reported the first major scientific challenge of this policy in 1979. In a prospective, randomized study, which excluded patients with hypotension, multiple associated injuries, destructive colon injuries, and delayed operations, the authors concluded that primary repair was associated with fewer complications than colostomy. The exclusion criteria were perceived as risk factors for anastomotic leak and were absolute indications for diversion.

With mortality rates attributable to colon-related complications improving over the next few years, surgeons challenged the validity of the "standard" contraindications for primary repair or resection and anastomosis. A few prospective randomized studies with no exclusion criteria (class I evidence) confirmed the safety of primary repair, at least in nondestructive colon injuries. Another alternative to primary repair or colostomy was exteriorized repair, which was introduced in the 1970s. With this technique, the sutured colon was exteriorized and observed for 4–5 days. If the repair remained intact during this period of observation, the colon was returned to the abdominal cavity. If the repair leaked, it was converted to a loop colostomy.[18,19] The enthusiasm for this approach waned in the 1980s because of the overwhelming evidence of the superiority of primary repair.

In the 1990s and 2000s, primary repair became the standard of care in most cases although there is still some skepticism by many surgeons, especially in the presence of certain risk factors such as destructive colon injuries, severe contamination, multiple injuries, and delays in treatment.

Nondestructive Colon Injuries

There is now enough class I evidence (prospective, randomized studies) supporting primary repair in all nondestructive colon injuries (injuries involving <50% of the bowel wall and without devascularization) irrespective of risk factors. Chappuis et al.[2] in a randomized study of 56 patients with no exclusionary criteria concluded that primary repair should be considered in all colon injuries irrespective of risk factors. In another landmark study, Sasaki et al.[20] randomized 71 patients with colon injuries to either primary repair or diversion, without any exclusionary criteria. The overall complication rate was 19% in the primary repair group and 36% in the diversion group. In addition, the complication rate for colostomy closure was 7%. The authors concluded that primary repair is the method of choice of treatment of all penetrating colon injuries in the civilian population despite any associated risk factors for adverse outcome.

Gonzalez et al.[5] published another important prospective, randomized study in 1996. The authors randomized 109 patients to primary repair on diversion, independent of any risk factors. The sepsis-related complication rate was 20% in the primary repair group and 25% in the diversion group. In the presence of certain risk factors, such as severe fecal contamination, shock on admission, blood loss 1000 mL, or more than two associated organ injuries, the diversion group had a higher complication rate, although this difference did not reach statistical significance. Gonzalez et al.[21] continued their study and the series increased to 176 patients with penetrating colon injury. The study concluded again that in civilian trauma, all penetrating colon injuries should be primarily repaired.

Overall, collective review of all available prospective, randomized studies (class I evidence) identified 160 patients with primary repair and an incidence of 13.1% of abdominal sepsis complications. In the group of 143 patients treated with diversion, the abdominal sepsis complication rate was 21.7% (Table 22-3). In addition to the available class I evidence, numerous prospective observational studies (class II evidence) demonstrated the superiority of primary repair over diversion in nondestructive injuries.[1,3,4,22] In conclusion, there is sufficient class I and II data to support routine primary repair of all nondestructive colon injuries, irrespective of risk factors for abdominal complications. No study has ever shown that colostomy is associated with better results than primary repair.

Despite the available scientific evidence, there is still some skepticism about liberal primary repair and many surgeons still consider colostomy as the procedure of choice in many colon injuries. In a survey of 317 Canadian surgeons in 1996, 75% of them chose colostomy in low-velocity gunshot wounds to the colon.[23] In another survey of 342 American Trauma Surgeons, members of the AAST, a colostomy was the procedure of choice in 3% of colon perforations with minimal spillage, in 43% of perforations with gross spillage, in 18% of colon injuries involving >50% of the wall, and in 33% of cases with colon transection.[24] It is obvious that old traditions still have a significant role in modern trauma surgery.

Destructive Colon Injuries

Until recently, there was no sufficient class I or II data regarding the management of destructive colon injuries requiring resection (loss of >50% of bowel wall or devascularization). The available prospective, randomized studies included only 36 patients with colon resection and anastomosis. The overall

incidence of anastomotic leak was 2.5% and no deaths occurred. All these studies recommended primary anastomosis irrespective of the presence of any risk factors for abdominal complications.[2,20,21] In a recent prospective but not randomized study on colon injuries by Cornwell et al.,[7] there were 25 patients with destructive colon injuries treated by resection and anastomosis and two patients treated by resection and colostomy. All patients had a PATI >25 or were transfused with >6 units of blood or the operation was delayed by >6 hours from the time of injury. There were two anastomotic leaks (8%) and both were fatal. The study concluded that some high-risk patients with destructive colon injuries might benefit from diversion. Unfortunately, the study did not include enough patients with diversion for comparison with the primary anastomosis group. There are two retrospective studies, which included only destructive colon injuries requiring resection: Stewart et al.[25] analyzed 60 patients, 43 of whom were managed by resection and anastomosis and 17 by diversion. The overall anastomotic leak rate was 14% and in the subgroup of patients with blood transfusion >6 units, the leak rate was 33%. The authors suggested that primary anastomosis should not be performed in patients receiving massive blood transfusions or in the presence of underlying medical illness. Another retrospective study from Los Angeles analyzed the complications in a series of 140 patients with destructive colon injuries requiring resection.[26] The incidence of intraabdominal sepsis was similar in the groups with primary anastomosis or diversion. Univariate analysis identified Abdominal Trauma Index >25 or hypotension in the emergency room to be associated with increased risk of anastomotic leak. The study suggested that a diversion procedure might be appropriate in these high-risk subgroups of patients.

In summary, the available prospective, randomized studies, which include only a small number of cases, recommend resection with anastomosis irrespective of risk factors. Two large retrospective studies advocate diversion in the subgroups of patients with certain risk factors such as PATI >25, multiple blood transfusions, or associated medical illness.[25,26] The guidelines of the Eastern Association for the Surgery of Trauma published in 1998[27] supported resection and primary anastomosis in the subgroups of patients with destructive colon injuries if they are a) hemodynamically stable intraoperatively, b) have minimal associated injuries (PATI <25, ISS <25), c) have no peritonitis, and d) have no underlying medical illness. The guidelines suggest that patients with shock, significant associated injuries, peritonitis, or underlying disease should be managed with resection and colostomy.[27] However, these

TABLE 22-3. Primary repair versus diversion: prospective, randomized studies with no exclusion criteria

Study	Primary Repair		Diversion	
	No. of patients	Abdominal septic complications (%)	No. of patients	Abdominal complications (%)
Chappuis et al.[2]	28	4(14.3)	28	5(17.9)
Sasaki et al.[20]	43	1(2.3)	28	8(28.6)
Gonzalez et al.[21]	89	16(18)	87	18(21)
Total	160	21(13.1)	143	31(21.7)

guidelines were based on class III evidence. In their review of the literature, there were only 40 patients in class I studies with resection and anastomosis and the anastomotic leak rate was 2.5% and without mortality. In class II studies, there were only 12 patients who underwent resection and anastomosis and the leak rate was 8.3% without mortality. In class III retrospective studies, there were 303 patients with a leak rate of 5.2% and three deaths (1%) as a result of the leak.

In view of the lack of large prospective studies in the literature, the AAST sponsored a prospective multicenter study to evaluate the safety of primary anastomosis or diversion and identify independent risk factors for colon-related complications in patients with destructive colon injuries requiring resection.[6] The study included 297 patients with penetrating injuries requiring colon resection (rectal injuries were excluded) that survived at least 72 hours. The overall colon-related mortality was 1.3% (four deaths) and all deaths occurred in the diversion groups ($P = .01$). The overall incidence of abdominal complications was 24% and the most common complication was an intraabdominal abscess (19% of patients) followed by fascia dehiscence (9%). The incidence of anastomotic leaks was 6.6%. Multivariate analysis identified three independent risk factors for abdominal complications: severe fecal contamination, >4 units of blood transfusions within the first 24 hours, and single-agent antibiotic prophylaxis. If all three risk factors were present, the incidence of abdominal complications was about 60%, if any two factors were present the complications rate was 34%, if only one factor was present this figure was about 20%, and with no risk factors it was 13%. The method of colon management, delay of operation >6 hours, shock at admission, site of colon injury, PATI >25, ISS >20, or associated intraabdominal injuries were not found to be independent risk factors. In a second analysis, the group of patients with primary anastomosis was compared with the group with diversion, using multivariate analysis which controlled for PATI >25, transfusion >6 units of blood, >6 hours' delay of operation, shock at admission, and severe fecal contamination. These factors have been described in previous studies as significant risks for abdominal complications. With colon diversion serving as reference (RR 1.00) for comparison, the adjusted relative risk of primary anastomosis was exactly the same (1.00).

In a similar analysis according to subgroups with ileo-colostomy, colocolostomy, ileostomy, and colostomy, the adjusted relative risk of abdominal complications was similar. In another analysis, all patients were classified into either a high-risk group (if any of the following factors was present: hypotension at admission, blood transfusions >6 units, delay of operation >6 hours, severe peritoneal contamination, or PATI >25) or a low-risk group if the above factors were not present. These risk factors are considered by many surgeons as strong indications for diversion. The colon-related mortality in the high-risk patients was 4.5% (4 of 88 patients) in the diversion group and no deaths in the 121 patients who underwent primary anastomosis ($P = .03$). Multivariate analysis showed that the adjusted relative risk of abdominal complication in patients with primary anastomosis or diversion was similar, in both the low-risk and high-risk patients (Table 22-4). There was a trend toward shorter intensive care unit and hospital stay in the primary anastomosis group. The study concluded that "In view of these findings and the fact that colon diversion is associated with worse quality of life and requires an additional operation for closure, colon injuries requiring resection should be managed by primary repair, irrespective of risk factors."[6] Damage control procedures with abdominal packing and temporary closure of the abdominal wall with a prosthetic material pose a special dilemma regarding the management of destructive colon injuries. No studies have ever addressed this issue and the existing practices are based on personal beliefs and experience. The authors advocate primary anastomosis because of the theoretical disadvantages of having a colostomy, which is an open source of fecal material, near an open abdomen. The only conditions for which there is agreement for colostomy are the presence of severe colon edema or a questionable blood supply of the colon. In these situations, at least theoretically, a diversion procedure might be a safe option.

Risk Factors for Abdominal Complications

The abdominal complication rate in colon injuries is very high, with a sepsis rate of about 20% (Table 22-1). In destructive colon injuries requiring resection, the prospective AAST colon resection study of 298 patients recorded an overall incidence of 24% of abdominal complications. Many studies attempted to identify risk factors for complications and on the basis of these risks to modify the treatment.

Left Versus Right Colon Injuries

For many years and until recently, there was an anecdotal perception that left colon injuries are associated with a higher risk of anastomotic leaks and septic complications than right

TABLE 22-4. AAST colon resection study: comparison of abdominal complications between primary anastomosis and diversion in high- and low-risk patients[6]

Patient population	Primary anastomosis: abdominal complications (%)	Diversion: abdominal complications (%)	Adjusted relative risk (95% CI)	P value
All patients	22	27	0.81 (0.55–1.41)	.69
Low-risk patients*	13	8	1.26 (0.21–8.39)	.82
High-risk patients*	28	30	0.90 (0.53–1.40)	.67

*High-risk patients were those with PATI >25 or severe fecal contamination or 6 hours from injury to operation or transfusion of >6 units of blood pre-/intra-operatively systolic blood pressure ≤90 mm Hg. Low-risk patients were those without any of the above risk factors.

colon injuries. This perception was based on theoretical reasons (different anatomy and blood supply, higher concentration of bacteria, and poorer healing properties in the left colon) rather than clinical evidence. This perception led surgeons to advocate liberal primary repair of right colon wounds and colostomy in left colon wounds. However, no clinical or experimental study has ever demonstrated any healing differences between the two sides of the colon or any evidence that the two anatomic sides should be treated differently. Experimental work in baboons, which have very similar anatomy and bacteriology with humans, showed no difference of the healing properties between the right and left colon.[28] The study involved resection of a 10-cm segment of right colon and a 10-cm segment of left colon and primary anastomosis, without any mechanical or chemical preparation of the colon. The healing of the anastomosis was assessed at autopsy 7 days postoperatively (leak, local abscess), mechanically by measuring the breaking strength of the anastomosis, and biochemically by measuring the hydroxyproline concentrations at the anastomotic site. The study showed identical healing properties of the two sides of the colon.[28]

In another study using the same model, one of the authors evaluated the effect of hypovolemia (blood loss of 20 mL/kg) on healing of the left and right sides of the colon and again no differences were found[29] (Figures 22-1 and 22-2).

Associated Abdominal Injuries

Earlier studies suggested that multiple or severe associated intraabdominal injuries (PATI >25) are associated with a high incidence of septic complications and they were considered as contraindications for primary repair of the colon.[4,7] This factor was considered even more critical in destructive colon injuries and was suggested as indication for diversion.[26,27] However, class I and II studies have shown that although multiple associated intraabdominal injuries are significant risk factors for intraabdominal sepsis, the method of colon management does

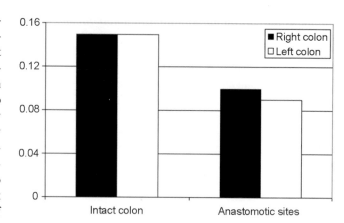

FIGURE 22-2. Breaking strengths of the right and left colon are similar (values in N/mm^2).

not affect the incidence of abdominal sepsis.[3,5–7,30] Some studies have suggested that the creation of an ostomy in these high-risk patients may independently contribute to abdominal sepsis.[30] The current class I and II literature supports primary repair or resection and anastomosis in patients with severe or multiple associated abdominal injuries.

Shock

There is now sufficient class I and II evidence that preoperative or intraoperative shock is neither an independent risk factor for abdominal sepsis nor a contradiction for primary colon repair or anastomosis.[3,5,6]

Blood Transfusions

Multiple blood transfusion (>4 units of blood within the first 24 hours) has been shown to be a major independent risk factor for abdominal septic complications.[6,30] In a large prospective AAST study of 297 patients with penetrating destructive colon injuries requiring resection, blood transfusion was the most critical independent factor for abdominal sepsis [adjusted relative risk (RR), 2.0; 95% confidence interval (CI), 1.31–2.83; $P = .001$].[6] However, the method of colon management did not influence the complication rate in this group of patients and primary anastomosis was recommended.[6]

Injury Severity Score

The ISS is not an independent risk factor for abdominal sepsis and high ISS (>15) is not a contraindication for primary repair or anastomosis.[3,6]

Fecal Contamination

Severe fecal contamination of the peritoneal cavity is a major independent risk factor for abdominal sepsis.[1,6,11,26,30,31] This finding led some studies to suggest that the presence of severe contamination should be a contraindication for primary repair

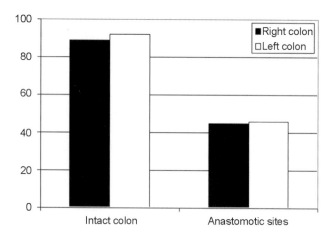

FIGURE 22-1. Hydroxyproline concentrations (biochemical marker of wound healing) are similar in both sides of the colon (values in µg/mg).

or anastomosis.[1,11,31,32] However, all prospective, randomized studies and recent large prospective observational studies have shown that the method of colon management in this group of patients does not influence the septic complication rate and recommended primary repair or anastomosis.[2,5,6]

Specific Associated Abdominal Injuries

There is class III evidence that the combination of colon injuries with pancreatic or ureteric injuries is associated with an increased incidence of septic complications.[33,34] However, there is no evidence that the presence of any of these injuries is a contraindication for primary repair or anastomosis.[6]

Time from Injury to Operation

The length of delay of surgical repair over which the septic complication rate increases is not well defined. Some studies suggest >6 hours whereas others >12 hours as the critical delays associated with an increased risk of infections.[7,22,26,35] It seems that the degree of contamination is much more important than the delay in surgical management and the time delay in itself should not be used as a criterion for primary repair or diversion. In a prospective study of 297 destructive colon injuries, the incidence of abdominal complication was 11.4% (4/35) in the group of patients with preoperative time >6 hours and 26.1% in patients with times <6 hours. Multivariate analysis failed to identify time delay as an independent risk factor.[6]

Retained Missiles

Missiles, which passed through the colon and remained lodged in the tissues, are not associated with increased risk of local sepsis and they should be removed only if it is technically easy and does not prolong the operation. In a study of 84 patients with gunshot wounds of the colon, the bullet remained in the body in 40 and was removed in 44. The incidence of local septic complications was 5% in patients with retained bullets and 7% in those without.[36]

Anatomic Location of Colon Injury

There is a plethora of classes I, II, and III evidence that the incidence of complications is similar in right and left colon injuries.

Temporary Abdominal Wall Closure

Damage control laparotomy and temporary abdominal wall closure with prosthetic material seem to be associated with increased incidence of abdominal septic complications. The crude relative risk of abdominal sepsis in patients with temporary abdominal wall closure has been reported to be 2.12 (1.32–3.40) ($P = .005$) in a study of 297 of destructive colon injuries requiring resection. However, multivariate analysis failed to identify this method as independent risk factor.[6] There is no literature addressing the optimal management of colon injuries in this group of patients. The authors prefer primary repair or resection and anastomosis, to avoid a colostomy near an open abdomen.

Anastomotic Leaks

Colon leaks remain the most serious complication in repaired or anastomosed colons. The overall incidence of suture line failures is fairly low. In a collective review of 35 prospective or retrospective studies with 2964 primary repairs, Curran reported 66 (2.2%) leaks.[6,37] In prospective studies including 534 patients with colon repair or resection and anastomosis, there were 17 (3.2%) leaks.[6,37] The leak rate after resection and anastomosis is significantly higher than in simple repairs. In a collective review of 362 patients with resection and anastomosis, the overall incidence of anastomotic leak was 5.5%.[37] In another large retrospective study of 112 patients with penetrating or blunt colonic injuries treated by resection and primary anastomosis, Murray et al.[26] reported a leak rate of 9%. In a more recent multicenter prospective study of 197 patients with penetrating colon injuries who underwent resection and primary anastomosis, the leak rate was 6.6%.[6]

The risk factors for anastomotic leak are not well defined. It seems that colocolostomies are associated with a higher incidence of anastomotic leaks than ileocolostomies. Murray et al.[26] reported a leak rate of 4% in 56 patients with ileocolostomies and 13% in 56 colocolostomies. Univariate analysis identified PATI >25, >6 units of blood transfusion, and hypotension in the emergency room as risk factors for anastomotic leak. A multicenter prospective AAST study reported a leak rate of 4.2% for ileocolostomies and 8.9% in colocolostomies.[6] The leaks occurred in patients with or without multiple blood transfusions, severe contamination, and multiple associated injuries. No significant independent risk factors could be identified.

The prognosis of anastomotic leaks is usually good and most of the patients can safely be managed nonoperatively with low-residue diet. In most cases, the leak results in a fecal fistula, which heals spontaneously within a few days. In other cases, the leak results in a local abscess, which can be drained percutaneously. However, in some patients, the colonic leak causes severe intraabdominal sepsis and a proximal diversion procedure may be required. Curran and Borzotta[37] reported no deaths in a collective series of 66 patients with repair leaks. However, Murray et al. reported two colon-related deaths in a group of 10 patients with anastomotic leak. The AAST multicenter study reported no deaths in the 13 patients with anastomotic leaks. The overall mortality attributable to colon leak-related complications in a collective review of 3161 trauma patients treated with primary repair or resection and anastomosis was only 0.1%.[6,37]

In summary, colonic leaks occur more often in patients with colocolostomies than patients with ileocolostomies. External fecal fistulas can safely be managed nonoperatively with low-residue diet. Localized abscesses are best drained percutaneously by interventional radiology and the ensuing fecal fistula almost always closes spontaneously. Reexploration of the abdomen and creation of fecal diversion with or without resection of the leaking colon should be reserved only for patients with generalized peritonitis or failed percutaneous drainage.

Technique of Colon Repair

In nondestructive injuries, repair of the injured colon should be performed after debridement of the perforation. This step is critical in gunshot wounds and failure to debride may result in breakdown of the suture line. In destructive injuries, resection to normal and well-perfused edges should be performed and the anastomosis should be tension free. The method of anastomosis, hand-sewn or stapled, does not influence the incidence of abdominal complications or leak rate and it should be surgeon's preference. In a prospective AAST study of 207 patients with penetrating destructive injuries who underwent resection and anastomosis, 128 cases were managed by hand-sewn and 79 cases by stapled anastomosis. The incidence of anastomotic leak was 7.8% and 6.3%, respectively. Multivariate analysis adjusting for blood transfusions, degree of fecal contamination, and antibiotic coverage showed identical complication rates (stapled anastomosis adjusted RR = 0.99).[38] Application of fibrin glue around the anastomosis may be beneficial although no study has ever evaluated its role in colonic anastomosis in trauma. Further protection of the anastomosis with adjacent omentum is recommended whenever possible. It is the practice of the authors to apply fibrin glue and cover the anastomosis with omentum in all cases with resection and anastomosis.

Rectal Injuries

The management of rectal trauma has undergone many changes in the same manner as colon injuries, with many of the principles of management evolving from wartime experiences. The mortality related to rectal trauma has decreased dramatically from 67% during World War I down to today's civilian reports of 0%–10%.[39-44] Likewise, the morbidity, which was as high as 72% during the Vietnam War, is now as low as 10%.[44,45] The mainstay of management, developed from lessons learned from combat experiences, has remained controversial and includes: 1) diversion of fecal stream, 2) distal rectal washout, 3) presacral drainage, and 4) debridement and closure of wounds when possible. Because of the paucity of class I and class II data, no consensus has been achieved with respect to the optimal management of rectal trauma.

Anatomy

The anatomy of the rectum makes it difficult to apply the principles of colon trauma management. The majority of the rectum is completely surrounded by the bony pelvis, making

injuries infrequent, and exposure difficult. The rectum varies in length from 12 to 15 cm, with only the upper two-thirds anteriorly and the upper one-third laterally covered by peritoneum (intraperitoneal rectum). The lower third of the rectum completely lacks peritoneal covering (extraperitoneal rectum) which makes exposure and repair of injuries difficult. Finally, the rectum is easily accessible from the anus, with the anterior peritoneal reflection only approximately 6 cm from the anal verge. This results in a not uncommon finding of intraperitoneal injury from rectal foreign bodies.

Epidemiology

For the various anatomic reasons, injuries to the rectum occur infrequently, and are usually the result of penetrating trauma. In most series, gunshot and shotgun wounds account for 80%–85% of injuries, and stab wounds for 3%–5%.[39,46,47] The incidence of rectal trauma is low, with most series describing relatively few injuries. In a series of 59 patients with gunshot wounds to the buttocks, only 3.4% had rectal injuries.[48] In another series of 192 patients with gunshot wounds to the back, 2.6% had a rectal injury.[9] Interestingly, in a series of 309 anterior abdominal gunshot wounds, and a series of 37 transpelvic gunshot wounds, no rectal injuries were identified, reiterating the infrequency of this injury.[8,49]

Other causes include iatrogenic injuries from urologic and endoscopic procedures, sexual misadventure, and anorectal foreign bodies. Blunt trauma accounts for 5%–10% of cases, and is usually the result of pelvic fractures or impalement.[39,42,46,47,50] Rectal injuries have been reported in nearly 2% of all pelvic fractures.[51]

Diagnosis

The diagnosis of intraperitoneal rectal injury, similar to colonic injuries, is almost always made intraoperatively. Extraperitoneal rectal injuries may not always be as obvious. A high index of suspicion is necessary with both blunt and penetrating mechanisms to avoid missing an injury. The cornerstone for diagnosing an extraperitoneal injury is the combination of a digital rectal examination and rigid proctoscopy. In most series, the diagnostic accuracy of the digital rectal examination and rigid proctoscopy ranges from 80% to 95%.[39,44,47,52-54] However, the false-negative rate of the two has been reported to be as high as 31%.[40] For this reason, any suggestion of a rectal injury, even with a normal rectal and proctoscopic examination, should prompt further evaluation. In hemodynamically stable patients with a mechanism suspicious for a rectal injury (gluteal, perineal, and transpelvic gunshot wounds, pelvic fractures, and foreign body insertion), a digital rectal examination and a rigid proctoscopy must be performed and in the appropriate cases further evaluation by means of a contrast study should be considered.

Rectal Organ Injury Scale

The grading system developed by the AAST for rectal injuries (Table 22-5) is similar to that of colonic injuries (Table 22-2).

TABLE 22-5. AAST Rectal Organ Injury Scale

Grade	Injury description
I	a) Contusion or hematoma without devascularization
	b) Partial-thickness laceration
II	Laceration ≤50% of circumference
III	Laceration >50% of circumference
IV	Full-thickness laceration with extension into the perineum
V	Devascularized segment

Operative Management

Historical Perspective

The history of rectal trauma parallels that of colon trauma with much of the early management principles evolving from lessons learned from wartime experiences. Mortality from rectal gunshot wounds was as high as 67% in World War I and the early part of World War II, until the Army Surgeon General mandated colostomy for fecal diversion for all colon and rectal injuries.[14,39,55] Subsequently, the mortality decreased to 35%.[55] Retrorectal drainage was added in 1943, which appeared to bring the mortality down further to approximately 5%.[39,56] Shortly after World War II, several civilian series demonstrated satisfactory results with colostomy and presacral drainage.[57,58] During the Vietnam War, in which more destructive injuries were encountered, colostomy and presacral drainage alone was found to be inadequate. Rectal repair and distal rectal washout were added to the management and was associated with improved results.[45] Early postwar civilian studies demonstrated acceptable results when colostomy, rectal repair, presacral drainage, and distal irrigation were all used.[40,59] Interestingly, there were other studies that also demonstrated acceptable results when only colostomy and presacral drainage were used.[42,56,60] Presently there is no acceptable gold standard for the treatment of rectal injuries, because most studies have been unable to demonstrate any advantage of the various treatment options.

Intraperitoneal Injuries

With no class I or class II data present regarding the management of intraperitoneal rectal injuries and limited class III data that combines both extraperitoneal and intraperitoneal injuries, it is difficult to make a conclusion regarding management. However, several studies do indicate that injuries to the intraperitoneal rectum can be managed similar to left colon injuries with primary repair without the need for colostomy.[43,47,52,54,61] No increase in abdominal complications was found in these series when primary repair without colostomy was performed. The authors' program advocates primary repair in this group of patients.

Extraperitoneal Injuries

As previously mentioned, there is no agreement in terms of the optimal management of extraperitoneal rectal injuries, but the mainstay of treatment has included four main components: 1) fecal diversion with colostomy, 2) presacral drainage, 3) distal rectal washout, and 4) repair of the injury when possible. Each will be addressed separately below.

Fecal Diversion with Colostomy

Since World War II, the mainstay of management of extraperitoneal injuries has been proximal colostomy.[39,42,43,50,52–54] The only controversial aspect has been whether to perform a loop colostomy versus an end colostomy. Some argue that a loop colostomy does not offer complete fecal diversion, whereas proponents of loop colostomy argue that a properly constructed loop colostomy will function as a true diverting colostomy with the benefit of simple construction and rapid closure.[39,52] In fact, Rombeau et al.[62] demonstrated that a properly constructed loop colostomy, supported by a solid rod above the level of the skin, achieves complete fecal diversion. The authors believe that the type of colostomy should be dictated by the operative findings. Extensive destruction of the rectum that requires a resection may best be served with a Hartmann's procedure, whereas injuries that are not repaired or require limited dissection may be addressed by a loop colostomy.

Recently, there have been reports of primary repair without fecal diversion in selected extraperitoneal rectal injuries.[46,47,52,54,63] In a series of 30 patients with extraperitoneal rectal injuries, five were transanally repaired without fecal diversion and no subsequent morbidity.[47] Similarly, injuries right at the peritoneal reflection, or injuries encountered with minimal dissection, may also be primarily repaired without the need for colostomy.[54]

Presacral Drainage

Presacral drainage was added to the armamentarium in World War II, because it was thought to decrease the pelvic sepsis rate.[52,64] It has remained controversial, with many studies showing a benefit with its use,[39,40,42,52,65] whereas other studies failing to show any benefit.[43,46,53,54,66] In a series of 30 consecutive patients with extraperitoneal injuries from the authors' institution, no benefit with the use of presacral drains was found.[53] Despite the conflicting data, many authors still recommended its use for most injuries.[54] This was challenged recently by a randomized, prospective trial evaluating the importance of presacral drainage.[67] In a series of 48 patients, 23 randomized to presacral drainage and 25 randomized to no drainage, no difference in pelvic sepsis was encountered. This represents the first and only class I study involving rectal injuries. Although it was a study with relatively few patients, it convincingly demonstrated that the addition of presacral drainage is unnecessary. The authors have completely abandoned the use of presacral drainage several years ago. It involves an additional procedure and dissection into an uninvolved space. The drains that are placed often become malpositioned or malfunction. Most importantly, there is no proof that it improves outcome.

Distal Rectal Washout

Distal rectal irrigation was added to the management of rectal injuries during the Vietnam War, when Lavenson and Cohen[45] reported a decrease in morbidity from 72% to 10% with its use. Since then, there have been supporters of rectal washout[46,41,43,59] as well as nonsupporters.[39,42,46,52,66] The overall value of distal washout is questionable. It has been suggested that there may be a benefit in patients with high velocity wounds,[39,44] and in patients with rectal injuries from pelvic fractures.[68,69] However, this remains controversial. The authors do not recommend distal bowel irrigation. There is no proven benefit, and it may be associated with a high risk of infection because of spillage of intraluminal contents out of unrepaired rectal injuries.[56]

Rectal Repair

The addition of rectal repair to colostomy was also introduced during the Vietnam War.[45] However, rectal repair with or without a diverting colostomy is infrequently performed for extraperitoneal injuries.[53] In the majority of cases, repair is not technically feasible, with some series reporting successful repair in only 20%–37% of cases.[39,43,52] Even when repair is performed, no outcome advantage has been proven.[39,42,43] Attempts at repair are associated with extensive dissection and unnecessary contamination of the peritoneal cavity. Attempts at repair should only be made when the rectal injury is encountered during the exposure of an associated injury such as bladder or iliac vessel, or if the injury is easily accessible at the peritoneal reflection. As previously mentioned, injuries that are easily accessible from the transanal route may also be repaired with excellent results.[47]

Miscellaneous Options

Although extremely rare, abdominoperineal resection has been described for patients with severe bleeding, massive tissue loss, or devascularizing injuries.[40,63,70] Recent reports have introduced laparoscopy in the management of rectal injuries.[71,72] In a prospective study of 20 patients with extraperitoneal rectal injuries, laparoscopy (to rule out an intraperitoneal injury), followed by a diverting loop sigmoid colostomy without laparotomy yielded excellent results.[72]

Associated Injuries

Associated injuries are often seen with rectal injuries and have been reported to occur in as many as 77% of cases.[39,53] Genitourinary, and in particular bladder injuries, are usually the most frequently seen associated injuries, occurring in 30%–64% of cases.[39,42,46] Every effort should be made to close both injuries and separate both sites with well-vascularized tissue such as omentum. This should reduce the high incidence of rectovesical fistula, which can occur in up to 24% of patients with combined bladder and rectal injuries[52,73] (Figure 22-3).

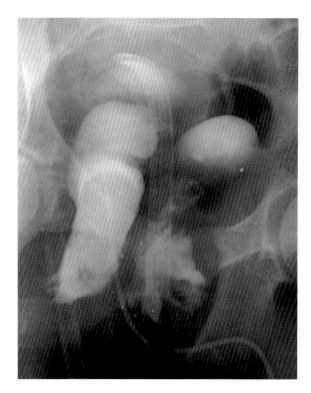

FIGURE 22-3. Rectovesical fistula after repair of a gunshot wound involving the rectum and the bladder. Every effort should be made to separate the two organs with vascularized tissue such as omentum, to reduce the risk of this complication.

Wound Management

The incidence of wound sepsis in patients with colon or rectal injury is high. In a prospective study of 100 patients with gunshot wounds and routine skin closure, the wound infection rate was 11%.[3] Primary wound closure in the presence of severe fecal spillage is a significant risk factor for wound sepsis and fascia dehiscence. This high-risk group of patients is best managed by delayed primary closure of the skin 3–5 days postoperatively.

Antibiotic Prophylaxis

In view of the high incidence of septic complications in patients with colon injuries, appropriate antibiotic prophylaxis is critical. It is a standard practice to cover against both aerobes and anaerobes. In early studies, the combination of penicillin/aminoglycoside/metronidazole was a popular antibiotic choice. Subsequent studies showed that in penetrating abdominal trauma, single agents were as good as combination antibiotics.[74,75] However, practically all available studies included a large number of fairly minor or moderately severe abdominal injuries and only a small number of severe colon injuries with extensive fecal spillage. The reported overall incidence of intraabdominal abscess in abdominal trauma series is about 3%[75] whereas in severe colon injuries is about 19%.[6] The AAST destructive colon injury study identified single-antibiotic-agent prophylaxis as an independent risk factor for abdominal sepsis. The overall incidence of abdominal septic complications was 31% in patients who received single-agent prophylaxis and 16% in patients who received combination antibiotics (adjusted RR, 1.78; 95% CI, 1.12–2.67; P = .02). Further comparison of the two agents used for single antibiotic prophylaxis (cephalosporin versus ampicillin/sulbactam) showed an abdominal infection rate of 37% in the cephalosporin group and 22% in the ampicillin/sulbactam group (crude RR, 1.67; 95% CI, 0.93–2.99; P = .07). It is possible that although single agents may be effective in minor or moderate trauma, they might be suboptimal in severe colon injuries. It is also possible that it might be necessary to cover against *Enterococcus*. Weigelt et al.[76] in a prospective, randomized study of 595 abdominal trauma patients compared ampicillin/sulbactam with cefoxitin. The wound infection rate was significantly lower with ampicillin/sulbactam. The study suggested that the lower infection rate with ampicillin/sulbactam was attributable to better *Enterococcus* coverage. The issue of antibiotic coverage in colon injuries merits further investigation. The authors' current choice is ampicillin/sulbactam prophylaxis in all suspected abdominal hollow viscous injury.

The duration of antibiotic prophylaxis has been a controversial issue. There is now class I evidence that 24-hour prophylaxis is at least as effective as prolonged prophylaxis for 3–5 days, even in the presence of major risk factors for abdominal sepsis, such as colon injury, multiple blood transfusions, and high Abdominal Trauma Index. In a prospective, randomized study of 63 patients with penetrating colon injuries and associate Abdominal Trauma Index >25 or >6 units of blood transfusions or delay of operation >6 hours, Cornwell et al.[7] reported an abdominal infection complication rate of 19% in patients who received 24 hours' antibiotic prophylaxis and 38% in patients who received 5 days' prophylaxis.

With respect to rectal injuries, no study has addressed the type or length of antibiotic therapy. In the available studies that have even mentioned antibiotics, length of therapy has been at least 2 days using single or double agents covering both aerobes and anaerobes.[39,67,72] It is the authors' preference to use ampicillin/sulbactam for prophylaxis in all patients with rectal injuries.

Trauma Ostomy Complications

When deciding about the method of management of a colon or rectal injury, the surgeon should take into account the problems related to the creation of a stoma and later on the complications associated with the subsequent operation for colostomy closure. The presence of an ostomy is in itself a significant emotional trauma, especially in an image-conscious young person. In addition, the incidence of complications directly related to the ostomy construction is a significant one. The most common serious complications include necrosis, retraction, prolapse, parastomal abscess, and parastomal hernia. Less serious complications include troublesome skin irritation and poor location with difficulties in the application of the collection bag. Park et al.[77] in a series of 528 stomas created for trauma reported an incidence 22% of severe or minor early complications and 3% of late complications directly related to the stoma.

The morbidity of colostomy closure is significant (Figure 22-4). In a collective review of 809 colostomy closures in trauma patients during the period 1970–1990, the overall incidence of colon-related complications was 13.1% (major complications 5.3%; minor complications 7.8%).[37] Another study of 110 colostomy closures reported an overall local complication rate of 14.5%, including 2.7% colon leaks.[78] In a more recent collective review of 1085 colostomy closures, the overall complication rate was 14.8%.[79]

The timing of colostomy closure does not seem to have an important role in the incidence of complications. Early studies had suggested colostomy closure should be performed after 3 months from the original operation to allow time for the colostomy to "mature."[80,81] Subsequent studies showed that closure of the stoma earlier than 3 months is safe and not associated with increased complication rates.[78,82] More recent studies even recommended closure during the same admission of the injury, which is usually within 2 weeks of the colostomy construction.[83] The optimal time for colostomy closure should be individualized and time should be allowed for wound healing and nutritional recovery. This might

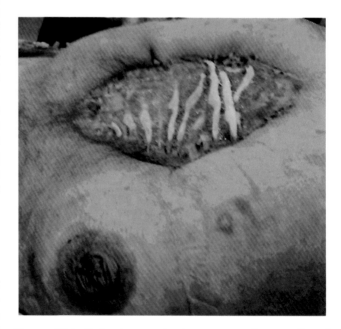

FIGURE 22-4. End colostomy in the presence of a complicated abdominal wound with protruding mesh. Closure of this colostomy is a high-risk procedure.

require only a few weeks for some patients or many months in severely injured patients.

Rectal Foreign Bodies

Rectal foreign bodies represent an uncommon cause of rectal injury, accounting for <5% of cases[39,42,52] (see Figure 22-5). More often, patients present to the hospital with a retained foreign body. These patients present an unusual, yet surprisingly common management dilemma.[84] Most objects can be safely removed in the emergency department; however, a small percentage of patients will require general anesthesia and operative management with or without laparotomy. In a review of 87

patients presenting with a retained foreign body at the authors' institution, 75% were successfully retrieved at the bedside whereas 8% required laparotomy with colotomy for foreign body extraction.[85] The only independent risk factor for operative intervention was if the foreign body was located in the sigmoid colon (odds ratio, 2.25; 95% CI, 1.1–4.4; $P = .04$).

Patients with a history of retained foreign body who present with peritonitis should be taken directly to the operating room. Without peritonitis, patients should have an attempt at retrieval at the bedside. If unsuccessful, patients should be taken to the operating room with an attempt at transanal extraction under intravenous sedation. As mentioned previously, patients most likely to require operative intervention are those with the foreign body located in the sigmoid colon.[85] The use of grasping

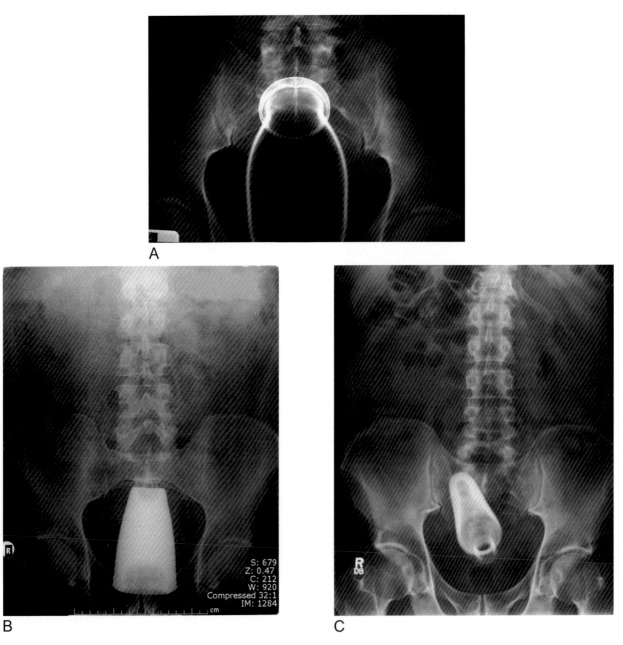

FIGURE 22-5. **A–C** Rectal foreign bodies of various shapes and sizes.

forceps should be avoided because it may lead to rectal mucosal injury. If transanal extraction is unsuccessful, then a laparotomy should be performed to maneuver the foreign body into the rectum for transanal removal.[86] If this is unsuccessful, then a colotomy may be necessary for foreign body retrieval.

References

1. George SM, Fabian TC, Voeller GR, et al. Primary repair of colon injuries: a prospective trial in nonselected patients. Ann Surg 1989;209:728–734.

2. Chappuis CW, Frey DJ, Dietzen CD, Panetta TP, Buechter KJ, Cohn I. Management of penetrating colon injuries. A prospective randomized trial. Ann Surg 1991;213:492–497.

3. Demetriades D, Charalambides D, Pantanowitz D. Gunshot wounds of the colon: role of primary repair. Ann R Coll Surg Engl 1992;74:381–384.

4. Ivatury RR, Gaudino J, Nallathambi MN, Simon RJ, Kazigo ZJ, Stahl WM. Definitive treatment of colon injuries: a prospective study. Am Surg 1993;59:43–49.

5. Gonzalez RP, Merlotti GJ, Holevar MR. Colostomy in penetrating colon injury: is it necessary? J Trauma 1996;41:271–275.

6. Demetriades D, Murray JA, Chan L, et al. Penetrating colon injuries requiring resection: Diversion or primary anastomosis? An AAST prospective multicenter study. J Trauma 2001;50: 765–773.

7. Cornwell EE, Velmahos GC, Berne TV, et al. The fate of colonic suture lines in high-risk trauma patients: a prospective analysis. J Am Coll Surg 1998;187:58–63.

8. Demetriades D, Velmahos G, Cornwell E, et al. Selective nonoperative management of gunshot wounds of the anterior abdomen. Arch Surg 1997;132:178–183.

9. Velmahos G, Demetriades D, Foianini E, et al. A selective approach to the management of gunshot wounds of the back. Am J Surg 1997;174:342–346.

10. Demetriades D, Rabinowitz B, Sofianos C, et al. The management of penetrating injuries of the back. A prospective study of 230 patients. Ann Surg 1988;207:72–74.

11. Ross SE, Cobean RA, Hoyt DB, et al. Blunt colonic injury: a multicenter review. J Trauma 1992;33:379–384.

12. Ciftci AO, Tanyel FC, Salman AB, et al. Gastrointestinal tract perforation due to blunt abdominal trauma. Pediatr Surg Int 1998;13:259–264.

13. Munns J, Richardson M, Hewett P. A review of intestinal injury from blunt abdominal trauma. Aust N Z Surg 1995;65: 857–860.

14. Moore EE, Cogbill TH, Malangoni MA, et al. Organ injury scaling. II. Pancreas, duodenum, small bowel, colon, and rectum. J Trauma 1990;30:1427–1429.

15. Elkin DC, Ward WC. Gunshot wounds of the abdomen: survey of 238 cases. Ann Surg 1943;118:780–787.

16. Ogilvie WH. Abdominal wounds in the Western desert. Surg Gynecol Obstet 1944;78:225–238.

17. Stone HH, Fabian TC. Management of perforating colon trauma: randomization between primary closure and exteriorization. Ann Surg 1979;190:430–436.

18. Schrock TR, Christensen N. Management of perforating injuries of the colon. Surg Gynecol Obstet 1972;135:65–68.

19. Kirkpatrick JR. Management of colonic injuries. Dis Colon Rectum 1974;17:319–321.

20. Sasaki LS, Allaben RD, Golwala R, Mittal VK. Primary repair of colon injuries: a prospective randomized study. J Trauma 1995; 39:895–901.

21. Gonzalez RP, Falimirsky ME, Holevar MR. Further evaluation of colostomy in penetrating colon injury. Am Surg 2000;66:342–347.

22. Baker LW, Thomson SR, Chadwick SJ. Colon wound management and prograde colonic lavage in large bowel trauma. Br J Surg 1990;77:872–876.

23. Pezin ME, Vestrup JA. Canadian attitudes toward use of primary repair in management of colon trauma: a survey of 317 members of the Canadian Association of General Surgeons. Dis Colon Rectum 1996;39:40–44.

24. Eshraghi N, Mallins R, Mayberry JC, Brand DM, Crass RA, Trunkey DD. Surveyed opinion of American Trauma Surgeons in management of colon injuries. J Trauma 1998;44:93–97.

25. Stewart RM, Fabian TC, Groce MA, Pritchard FE, Minord G, Kadsk KA. Is resection with primary anastomosis following destructive colon wound always safe? Am J Surg 1994;168: 316–319.

26. Murray JA, Demetriades D, Colson M, et al. Colon resection in trauma: colostomy versus anastomosis. J Trauma 1999;46: 250–254.

27. Pasquale M, Fabian TC. EAST Ad Hoc Committee. Practice management guidelines for trauma from the Eastern Association for the Surgery of Trauma. J Trauma 1998;44:941–947.

28. Demetriades D, Lawson HH, Sofianos C, Oosthuizen MM, Kurstjens S, Frolich J. Healing of the right and left colon. An experimental study. S Afr Med J 1988;73:657–658.

29. Sofianos C, Demetriades D, Oosthuizen MM, Becker PJ, Hunter S. The effect of hypovolemia on healing of the right and left colon. An experimental study. S Afr J Surg 1992;30:42–43.

30. Deute CJ, Tyburski J, Wilson RF, Collinge J, Steffies C, Coerlin A. Ostomy as a risk factor for posttraumatic infection in penetrating colonic injuries: univariate and multivariate analyses. J Trauma 2000;49:628–637.

31. Burch JM, Martin RR, Richardson RJ, et al. Evolution of the treatment of the injured colon in the 1980's. Arch Surg 1991; 126:979–984.

32. Flint LM, Vitale GC, Richardon JD, et al. The injured colon: relationships of management to complications. Ann Surg 1981;193:619–623.

33. Ivatury RR, Nallathambi M, Rao P, Stahl WM. Penetrating pancreatic injuries. Analysis of 103 consecutive cases. Am Surg 1990;56:90–95.

34. Velmahos GC, Degiannis E, Wells M, Souter I. Penetrating ureteral injuries: the impact of associated injuries on management. Am Surg 1996;62:461–468.

35. Morgado PJ, Alfaro R, Morgado PJ Jr, et al. Colon trauma: clinical staging for surgical decision making. Analysis of 119 cases. Dis Colon Rectum 1992;35:986–990.

36. Demetriades D, Charalambides D. Gunshot wounds of the colon: role of retained bullets in sepsis. Br J Surg 1993;80:772–773.

37. Curran TJ, Borzotta AP. Complications of primary repair of colon injury: literature review of 2,964 cases. Am J Surg 1999; 177:42–47.

38. Demetriades D, Murray JA, Chan LS, et al. Handsewn versus stapled anastomosis in penetrating colon injuries requiring resection: a multicenter study. J Trauma 2002;52:117–121.

39. Burch JM, Feliciano DV, Mattox KL. Colostomy and drainage for civilian rectal injuries: is that all? Ann Surg 1989;209: 600–611.

40. Grasberger RC, Hirsch EF. Rectal trauma: a retrospective analysis and guidelines for therapy. Am J Surg 1983;145:795–799.

41. Shannon FL, Moore EE, Moore FA, McCroskey BL. Value of distal colon washout in civilian rectal trauma: reducing gut bacterial translocation. J Trauma 1988;28:989–994.

42. Tuggle D, Huber PJ. Management of rectal trauma. Am J Surg 1984;148:806–808.

43. Mangiante EC, Graham AD, Fabian TC. Rectal gunshot wounds: management options in penetrating rectal injuries. Am Surg 1986;52:37–40.

44. Morken JJ, Kraatz JJ, Balcos EG, et al. Civilian rectal trauma: a changing perspective. Surgery 1999;126:693–700.

45. Lavenson GS, Cohen A. Management of rectal injuries. Am J Surg 1971;122:226–231.

46. Thomas DD, Levison MA, Dykstra BJ, Bender JS. Management of rectal injuries: dogma versus practice. Am Surg 1990;56:507–510.

47. Levine JH, Longo WE, Pruitt C, et al. Management of selected rectal injuries by primary repair. Am J Surg 1996;172:575–579.

48. Velmahos GC, Demetriades D, Cornwell EE, et al. Gunshot wounds to the buttocks: predicting the need for operation. Dis Colon Rectum 1997;40:307–311.

49. Velmahos GC, Demetriades D, Cornwell EE. Transpelvic gunshot wounds: routine laparotomy or selective management? World J Surg 1998;22:1034–1038.

50. Brunner RG, Shatney CH. Diagnostic and therapeutic aspects of rectal trauma: blunt versus penetrating. Am Surg 1987;53:215–219.

51. Aihara R, Blansfield JS, Millham FH, et al. Fracture locations influence the likelihood of rectal and lower urinary tract injuries in patients sustaining pelvic fractures. J Trauma 2002;52:205–209.

52. Ivatury RR, Licata J, Gunduz Y, et al. Management options in penetrating rectal injuries. Am Surg 1991;57:50–57.

53. Velmahos GC, Gomez H, Falabella A, Demetriades D. Operative management of civilian rectal gunshot wounds: simpler is better. World J Surg 2000;24:114–118.

54. McGrath V, Fabian TC, Croce MA, et al. Rectal trauma: management based on anatomic distinctions. Am Surg 1998;64:1136–1141.

55. Ogilvie WH. Abdominal wounds in the Western desert. Surg Gynecol Obstet 1944;78:225–238.

56. Trunkey D, Hays RJ, Shires GT. Management of rectal trauma. J Trauma 1973;13:411–415.

57. Taylor ER, Thompson JE. The early treatment, and results thereof, of injuries of the colon and rectum. Int Abstr Surg 1948;87:209–228.

58. Woodhall JP, Ochsner A. The management of perforating injuries of the colon and rectum in civilian practice. Recent Adv Surg 1949;20:305–321.

59. Vitale GC, Richardson JD, Flint LM. Successful management of injuries to the extraperitoneal rectum. Am Surg 1983;49:159–162.

60. Bartizal JF, Boyd DR, Folk FA, et al. A critical review of management of 392 colonic and rectal injuries. Dis Colon Rectum 1974;17:313–318.

61. Maxwell RA, Fabian TC. Current management of colon trauma. World J Surg 2003;27:632–639.

62. Rombeau JL, Wilk PJ, Turnbull RB, Fazio VW. Total fecal diversion by the temporary skin-level loop transverse colostomy. Dis Colon Rectum 1978;21:223–226.

63. Haas PA, Fox TAJ. Civilian injuries of the rectum and anus. Dis Colon Rectum 1979;22:17–23.

64. Armstrong RG, Schmitt HJ, Patterson LT. Combat wounds of the extraperitoneal rectum. Surgery 1983;74:570–583.

65. Weil PH. Injuries of the retroperitoneum portions of the colon and rectum. Dis Colon Rectum 1983;26:19–21.

66. Levy RD, Strauss P, Aladgem D, et al. Extraperitoneal rectal gunshot injuries. J Trauma 1995;38:274–277.

67. Gonzalez RP, Falimirski ME, Holevar MR. The role of presacral drainage in the management of penetrating rectal injuries. J Trauma 1998;45:656–661.

68. Maull KI, Sachatello CR, Ernst CB. The deep perineal laceration: an injury frequently associated with open pelvic fractures—a need for aggressive surgical management. J Trauma 1977;17:685–696.

69. Richardson JD, Harty J, Amin M, et al. Open pelvic fractures. J Trauma 1982;22:533–538.

70. Getzen LC, Pollack EG, Wolfman EF. Abdominoperineal resection in the treatment of devascularizing rectal injuries. Surgery 1977;82:310–313.

71. Navsaria PH, Graham R, Nicol A. A new approach to extraperitoneal rectal injuries: laparoscopy and diverting loop sigmoid colostomy. J Trauma 2001;51:532–535.

72. Navsaria PH, Shaw JM, Zellweger R, et al. Diagnostic laparoscopy and diverting sigmoid loop colostomy in the management of civilian extraperitoneal rectal gunshot injuries. Br J Surg 2004;91:460–464.

73. Franko ER, Ivatury RR, Schwalb DM. Combined penetrating rectal and genitourinary injuries: a challenge in management. J Trauma 1993;34:347–353.

74. Hooker KD, Dipiro JT, Wynn JJ. Aminoglycoside combinations versus beta-lactams alone for penetrating abdominal trauma: a meta-analysis. J Trauma 1991;31:1155–1160.

75. Sims EH, Thadepalli H, Ganesan K, Mandal AK. How many antibiotics are necessary to treat abdominal trauma victims? Am Surg 1997;63:525–535.

76. Weigelt JA, Easley SM, Thal ER, Palmer LD, Newman VS. Abdominal surgical wound infection is lowered with improved perioperative enterococcus and bacteroides therapy. J Trauma 1993;34:579–585.

77. Park JJ, Del Pino A, Orsay CP, et al. Stoma complications: the Cook County Hospital experience. Dis Colon Rectum 1999;42:1575–1580.

78. Demetriades D, Pezikis A, Melissas J, Parekh D, Pickles G. Factors influencing the morbidity of colostomy closure. Am J Surg 1988;155:594–596.

79. Berne JD, Velmahos GC, Chan LS, Asensio JA, Demetriades D. The high morbidity of colostomy closure after trauma: further support for the primary repair of colon injuries. Surgery 1998;123:157–164.

80. Frend H, Raniel J, Maggia-Sulaw W. Factors affecting the morbidity of colostomy closure. Dis Colon Rectum 1982;25:712–715.

81. Parks S, Hastings P. Complications of colostomy closure. Am Surg 1985;149:672–675.

82. Renz BM, Feliciano DV, Sherman R. Same admission colostomy closure (SACC): a new approach to rectal wounds—a prospective study. Ann Surg 1993;3:279–283.

83. Velmahos GC, Degiannis E, Weels M, Souter I, Saadia R. Early closure of colostomies in trauma patients: a prospective randomized trial. Surgery 1995;118:815–820.

84. Barone JE, Yee J, Nealon TF. Management of foreign bodies and trauma of the rectum. Surg Gynecol Obstet 1983;156:453–457.

85. Lake JP, Essani R, Petrone P, et al. Management of retained colorectal foreign bodies: predictors of operative intervention. Dis Colon Rectum 2004;47:1694–1698.

23
Colorectal Cancer: Epidemiology, Etiology, and Molecular Basis

Nancy N. Baxter and Jose G. Guillem

Epidemiology

Colorectal cancer (CRC) is a disease with a major worldwide burden. It is the fourth most frequently diagnosed malignancy in both sexes with almost 1 million people developing CRC annually.[1] CRC is the third most common cause of cancer death in the world, responsible for 630,000 deaths annually.[2] In the United States, CRC is the third most common cancer in men and women and the second most common cause of cancer death overall. CRC accounts for 11% of cancers diagnosed.[3] It is estimated that 147,000 cases will be diagnosed in the United States in 2004 and that there will be 57,000 deaths from the disease.[3]

The worldwide incidence of CRC is increasing; in 1975, the worldwide incidence of CRC was only 500,000.[4] In Western countries, some of the increase is attributable to the aging of the population; however, in countries with a low baseline rate of CRC, an increase in incidence after adjustment for age has been found. Before 1985, the age-adjusted incidence of CRC in the United States had been increasing; however, since this time, the rates have declined an average of −1.6% per year[5] (Figure 23-1). This reduction has been mainly confined to the Caucasian race and is largely limited to a decrease in the incidence of distal cancers. Therefore, the recent decrease in incidence in the United States may be attributable to screening, specifically screening with flexible sigmoidoscopy,[6] although other factors are likely to have influenced this trend. The incidence of proximal cancers has remained relatively stable over the same time period.[5,6] Currently, the overall probability of an individual developing CRC in United States over a lifetime is almost 6%.[3]

From a population perspective, age is the most important risk factor for CRC. CRC is predominantly a disease of older individuals; 90% of cases are diagnosed over the age of 50.[3] The risk of CRC continues to increase with age (Figure 23-2). The incidence per 100,000 people aged 80–84 is more than 7 times the incidence in people aged 50–54. However, CRC can occur at any age and the incidence of CRC occurring in patients younger than age 40 may be increasing.[7]

In the United States the risk of CRC differs by gender. The incidence of CRC is more than 40% higher in men than women.[5] Overall, the incidence of CRC in men is 64 per 100,000 males as compared with 46 per 100,000 females.[3] In addition, the ratio of colon to rectal cancer differs in the United States by gender; the ratio of colon to rectal cases for women is 3:1 as compared with 2:1 for males.[3]

Race and ethnicity influence CRC risk; Ashkenazi Jewish individuals seem to be at a slightly increased risk of CRC.[8] At least part of this increased incidence may be attributable to a higher prevalence of the *I1307K* mutation of the adenomatous polyposis gene, a mutation that confers an increased risk of CRC development. The *I1307K* mutation is found in 6.1% of unselected Ashkenazi Jewish individuals and 28% of Jewish individuals with CRC[9] whereas the mutation is rare in other populations.[10] In the United States, the incidence of CRC is higher in African-Americans of either gender as compared with Caucasians. Asian American/Pacific Islanders, Native Americans, and Hispanic Americans experience a lower incidence of CRC than Caucasians[3,11] (Table 23-1). African-Americans have not experienced the substantial reduction in incidence of CRC found to have occurred in Caucasians; before 1980, incidence in African-Americans was actually lower than in Caucasians. In African-Americans, the increased rate of cancer is predominantly attributable to a higher rate of proximal cancers.[12–14]

The Surveillance Epidemiology and End Results registry (a National Cancer Institute population-based cancer registry representing 14% of the population in the United States) reports cancer incidence and stage over time (Table 23-2). Between 1992 and 1999 for all patients diagnosed with CRC, 38% of patients were diagnosed with localized disease, 38% with regional disease, and 19% with metastatic disease. Five percent of patients were unstaged. As a proportion of total cases, African-Americans were more likely to present with advanced disease; 24% of African-Americans have metastatic

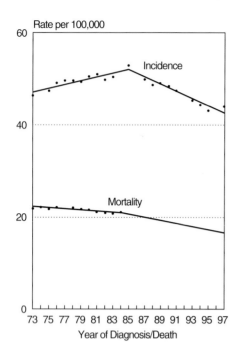

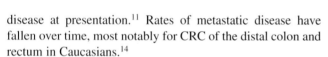

FIGURE 23-1. CRC incidence and death rates in the United States 1973–1997. (From Ries et al.[5] Copyright © 2000 American Cancer Society. Reprinted by permission of Wiley-Liss, Inc., a subsidiary of John Wiley & Sons, Inc.)

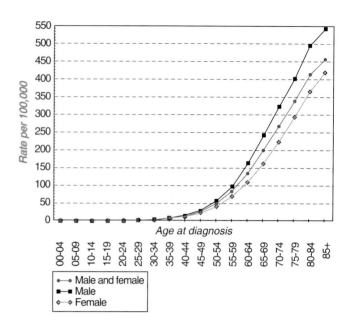

FIGURE 23-2. Age-specific incidence rates in the United States. Age-specific incidence both genders—circles. Age-specific incidence in males—squares. Age-specific incidence in females–diamonds. [Generated from the Surveillance, Epidemiology, and End Results (SEER) Program (www.seer.cancer.gov) SEER*Stat Database: Incidence—SEER 9 Regs Public-Use, Nov 2002 Sub (1973–2000), National Cancer Institute, DCCPS, Surveillance Research Program, Cancer Statistics Branch, released April 2003, based on the November 2002 submission.]

disease at presentation.[11] Rates of metastatic disease have fallen over time, most notably for CRC of the distal colon and rectum in Caucasians.[14]

There is substantial geographic variation in the incidence of CRC, with relatively high rates in North America, Western Europe, and Australia and relatively low rates in Africa and Asia[15] (Figure 23-3). Such observations led to Burkitt's[16] hypothesis—that dietary differences, specifically fiber and fat intake, between populations were responsible for the marked variation in rates of CRC found around the world. Burkitt observed that populations in low-risk areas of the third world had greater stool bulk, a faster colonic transit time, and higher dietary fiber intake than populations in high-risk westernized regions. Although such ecologic studies are confounded by numerous factors (for example, variations in average life expectancy, cancer detection methods, etc.), environmental factors (most prominently dietary factors) are still considered

to have a major role in this disease. This argument is supported by studies of migrants from low prevalence areas to high prevalence areas. Such studies generally demonstrate that the incidence of CRC in the migrants increases rapidly to become similar and in some cases to exceed the incidence of the high-risk area.[17] Interestingly, there is less variation in the incidence of rectal cancer between countries as compared with the incidence of colon cancer.[18,19]

Mortality from CRC is declining in the United States as age-adjusted CRC death rates peaked in the 1940s at 35 per 100,000. Rates in women have steadily decreased since this time and in 1998, the CRC death rate in women was 18.6 per 100,000. In men, death rates changed little until the 1980s and 1990s then decreased significantly; in 1998, the CRC death rate was 26.1 per 100,000 for men.[19] Improvements in surgical and medical treatments likely explain some of the change particularly that identified before 1985. More recently, the

TABLE 23-1. Incidence and mortality rates* for CRC by site, race, and ethnicity, United States 1996–2000

		Caucasian	African-American	Asian American and Pacific Islander	American Indian/Alaska Native	Hispanic/Latino
Incidence	Male	64.1	72.4	57.2	37.5	49.8
	Female	46.2	56.2	38.8	32.6	32.9
Mortality	Male	25.3	34.6	15.8	18.5	18.4
	Female	17.5	24.6	11.0	12.1	11.4

*Per 100,000 age-adjusted to the 2000 United States standard population.
Source: Adapted from Jemal et al.,[11] with permission from Lippincott Williams & Wilkins.

TABLE 23-2. Stage at diagnosis

	Caucasians	African-Americans
Localized	38	34
Regional	38	36
Distant	19	24
Unstaged	5	7

reduced mortality rate is likely secondary to the reduced incidence of CRC. In fact, no improvement in case fatality has been identified since 1986[20] indicating the trends in mortality are likely complex, particularly given the gender differences. African-Americans have the highest mortality rate from CRC in the United States (Table 23-1). The reasons for the higher mortality rate are likely multifactorial including the higher incidence of CRC, and the differences in stage distribution. However, African-Americans had worse 5-year survival for all stages of disease, and the difference in 5-year survival rates between Caucasians and African-Americans has actually increased over time; from an absolute difference of 5% in the 1970s (51% versus 46%) to an absolute difference of 13%

in the 1990s (63% versus 53%).[11,21] Differences in incidence, stage distribution, and survival of CRC between Caucasians and African-Americans are in part attributable to differences in socioeconomic status, screening rates, and treatment[22]; however, the differences may also be attributable to genetic and environmental factors that have yet to be elucidated.[23]

Because CRC is a survivable cancer, with 5-year survival rates adjusted for life expectancy of 63%,[3] the prevalence of people living with a diagnosis of CRC in the population is substantial. In 1996, more than 380,000 Americans older than 65 years of age received some type of CRC care (treatment or follow-up).[24] In total in 2004, more than 1 million living Americans have had a diagnosis of CRC.[25]

Etiology

Dietary Constituents and Supplements

The colon is constantly exposed to the substances we ingest and the byproducts of ingestion. Thus, the role of diet in the pathogenesis of CRC has long been speculated. However, the relationship between diet and CRC risk is at best unclear. Studies in this area are difficult to conduct, because exposures tend to be multifactorial and change over time with our diet. In addition, because colorectal carcinogenesis is a multistep process, a number or combination of exposures may be necessary, and genetic susceptibility is likely to have a role. In addition, in most cases, randomized trials are not feasible, and therefore studies must be observational in nature. When intervention studies are possible, follow-up is relatively short term (compared with the long-term exposure that may be necessary for cancer development), and single dietary components are generally selected for evaluation although the influence of diet may depend on complex interactions between dietary constituents. In addition, to reduce sample size, some studies are conducted on patients with a history of adenomatous polyps. Some interventions in these patients may not be effective, because such patients may have already acquired numerous genetic alterations in normal-appearing colonic mucosa. Some interventions may need to be instituted before development of polyps. Although it can be stated that an individual with no other risk factors for CRC who ingests a diet that is high in fiber, fruits, and vegetables and low in animal fat and red meat will be on average at lower risk of CRC than an individual who eats a diet low in fiber, fruits, and vegetables and high in animal fat and red meat, it is difficult to determine with certainty which dietary components or combinations are responsible for the decreased risk.

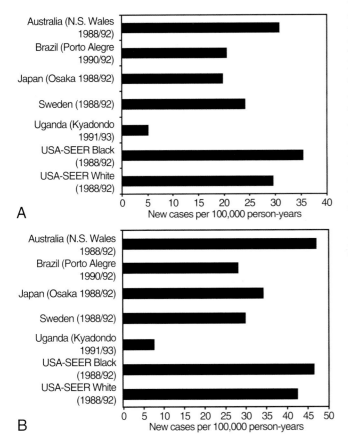

FIGURE 23-3. **A** Age-standardized (to the world population) incidence rates of cancer of the large bowel among females. **B** Age-standardized (to the world population) incidence rates of cancer of the large bowel among males. (Reprinted from Lagiou.[15] Copyright © 2002 by Oxford University Press, Inc. Used by permission of Oxford University Press, Inc.)

Dietary Fat

Dietary fat, particularly saturated animal fat has been implicated in carcinogenesis in the colon and rectum. Early research using animal models demonstrated a carcinogenic effect of dietary fat on colonic mucosa,[26–28] and ecologic studies found parallels between CRC rates and dietary fat consumption. Countries with populations eating a high fat diet had higher CRC rates than countries with populations eating a lower fat diet.[29] However, dietary fat consumption is related to a number of other factors that may influence cancer risk, including other dietary factors such as dietary fiber and micronutrient consumption, as well as life-style factors such as exercise and alcohol consumption. Therefore, ecologic comparisons between countries are subject to a substantial risk of confounding.[30]

More than 13 case-control studies have been conducted to evaluate the relationship between dietary fat intake and the risk of CRC. These have been quantitatively summarized by Howe et al.[31] and include 5287 cases with CRC and 10,470 controls. Although positive associations were identified for total energy intake and CRC in almost all of the studies, there was no energy-independent relationship between dietary fat intake and CRC risk. After controlling for total energy intake, the odds of development of CRC in subjects with the highest dietary fat intake as compared with those with the lowest intake was 0.90 [95% confidence interval (CI), 0.72–1.13]. Overall, there was no evidence for any association of total dietary fat intake and development of CRC. A small but consistent relationship between cholesterol intake and CRC was identified.

At least six cohort studies have been conducted to evaluate the relationship between dietary fat and CRC.[32–37] Only one study[36] identified an association between dietary animal fat and development of CRC, with a twofold increase in CRC in the highest consumers of animal fat as compared with the lowest consumers. A separate analysis of this same cohort indicated that regular intake of red meat was associated with a 2.5-fold increase in CRC risk as compared with infrequent consumption.[38] In fact, the evidence that red meat consumption is associated with CRC is in general more compelling than the evidence of an association with dietary fat. Given the lack of evidence for an independent association of dietary fat with CRC, it is unlikely that the animal fat in red meat is responsible for the association between red meat and CRC.

Red Meat

There are a number of potential carcinogenic mechanisms unrelated to fat content that may result in a causal relationship between red meat ingestion and CRC. Red meat is high in iron, a prooxidant. Dietary iron may increase free-radical production in the colon, and these free radicals may cause chronic mucosal damage or promote other carcinogens. In humans, red meat ingestion stimulates production of N-nitroso compounds in a dose-response manner.[39] Because many N-nitroso compounds are known carcinogens, this is a potential mechanism for an association between red meat and CRC. Formation of heterocyclic amines and polycyclic aromatic hydrocarbons in meat by cooking over an open flame or cooking until well done may be an important factor because these compounds are carcinogenic in animal models.[40]

Many epidemiologic studies have been conducted to determine the effect of ingestion of red meat on CRC risk. Two metaanalyses have been published,[41,42] one combining the results of 13 cohort studies,[41] the other combining 21 case-control studies and six cohort studies.[42] In the two studies, the pooled estimate for the increase in the risk of CRC caused by meat consumption was similar; the pooled estimate for the odds of development of CRC in the highest meat-consuming groups as compared with the lowest was 1.14. A daily increase of 100 g of red meat (3.5 ounces) was associated with a 12%–17% increased risk of CRC. The risk was substantially higher with the ingestion of processed meat. Of note, individuals that consume diets high in red meat generally consume diets low in other dietary factors,[43] such as antioxidants that may themselves be important in colorectal carcinogenesis. It is therefore difficult to rule out the possibility that the apparent effect of red meat on development of CRC may be confounded or modified by other dietary or lifestyle factors.

Fruit and Vegetable Intake

The effect of dietary intake of fruit and vegetables on CRC risk has been extensively evaluated. Fruits and vegetables are a source of antioxidants, including carotenoids and ascorbate. Other bioactive constituents in fruits and vegetables that may protect against carcinogenesis include the indoles and isothiocyanates. Previous research, including results from 22 case-control studies and four prospective cohort studies, has provided substantial support for the hypothesis that vegetable intake reduces the risk of CRC, whereas intake of fruit did not seem to have an effect.[44] More recent data, however, have not demonstrated a convincing link between vegetable or fruit intake and a reduced risk of CRC. In four large prospective cohort studies (the Nurse's Health Study of 121,700 women, the Health Professionals Follow-up Study of 51,529 men, the Netherlands Cohort Study on Diet and Cancer including 120,852 men and women, and the Cancer Prevention Study II Nutrition Cohort, including 133,163 men and women),[45–47] fruit and vegetable intake was not statistically significantly associated with a reduced risk of CRC. Of note, participants in the Nurse's Health Study and the Health Professionals Follow-up Study had a higher consumption of fruits and vegetables and a higher prevalence of multivitamin use than the general United States population.[48] The Netherlands study did show a trend toward a reduced risk of colon cancer in women eating large amounts of fruit and vegetables, particularly the brassica vegetables (cabbages, kale, broccoli, Brussels sprouts, and cauliflower) and cooked leafy vegetables. The Cancer Prevention Study II[47] also demonstrated a non–statistically significant trend for a higher colon cancer risk in men with the lowest vegetable consumption and women with the lowest fruit consumption.

Two additional studies have recently evaluated the effect of fruit and vegetable consumption in cohorts of women enrolled in breast cancer screening studies.[48,49] In the first study[48] of 61,463 women enrolled in the Swedish Two Counties randomized trial of screening mammography, fruit and vegetable consumption was associated with a decreased risk of CRC. Individuals consuming greater than 5.0 servings per day had a relative risk (RR) of CRC of 0.73 compared with individuals consuming less than 2.5 servings. The second study[49] included 45,490 women who participated in the Breast Cancer Detection Demonstration Project, a National Cancer Institute–sponsored breast cancer screening program. These women completed a food frequency questionnaire and were followed for 386,142 person-years. No association between fruit and vegetable intake and CRC risk was identified, even after adjustment for other potential confounders. In addition, a dietary intervention trial has been conducted; the Polyp Prevention Trial, randomized 2079 people with colorectal adenomas to either intensive dietary counseling with assignment to a diet low in fat and high in fruits, vegetables, and fiber or control.[50] No difference in adenoma recurrence rate was found in the intervention group as compared with the control group.

Overall, the evidence for an association between fruit and vegetable intake and the risk of CRC is inconsistent. Given this lack of concordant data, it is unlikely that a large number of cases of CRC can be attributed directly to a lack of fruit or vegetables, or that major additional interventions to increase consumption would lead to a substantial reduction in the incidence of CRC.

Fiber

Dietary fiber was one of the first dietary components thought to have a protective role in carcinogenesis. An association of a high fiber diet with a decreased risk of CRC was first theorized in 1969 by Burkitt[16]; however, the data regarding the association between fiber and CRC risk are conflicting. Several mechanisms have been proposed for the protective effects of fiber: fiber may increase intestinal transit and therefore reduce the length of exposure of the colon to carcinogens, and fiber may dilute or absorb various potential carcinogens, particularly bile salts. In addition, products of fiber degradation and fermentation in the colon (such as butyrate) may also have a role.[51] Overall, there has been little consistent evidence that a high fiber intake is associated with a decreased risk of CRC.[51] Two large American cohort studies, the Nurses Health study[52] and the Health Professionals' Follow-up Study,[35] found no evidence of benefit of fiber on CRC risk.

However, two recent studies have reopened the debate. In the Prostate, Lung, Colorectal and Ovarian Screening Trial,[53] a nested case-control study of more than 37,508 people undergoing flexible sigmoidoscopy was performed using food frequency questionnaires. People who reported the highest amounts of fiber in their diets had the lowest risk of colorectal adenomas, 27% less than people who ate the least amount of fiber. The strongest association was found for fiber from

grains, cereals, and fruits but not for fiber from legumes and vegetables. When colonic and rectal adenomas were evaluated separately, the effect of fiber was seen only in colonic adenoma. In a second study, a prospective cohort study comparing the diet of more than 500,000 people in 10 European countries, investigators in the European Prospective Investigation into Cancer and Nutrition[54] found that people who ate the most fiber had a 25% lower incidence of CRC than those who ate the least fiber. Again, the protective effect was highest for colon and least for rectum.

Dietary interventions to increase fiber intake have proven unsuccessful in reducing the risk of colorectal neoplasia. A metaanalysis has evaluated the effect of five intervention trials.[55] These studies randomized a total of 4349 individuals to some form of fiber supplementation or high fiber dietary intervention.[50,56–59] When the data were combined, there was no difference between the intervention and control groups for the number of subjects developing at least one adenoma [RR = 1.04 (95% CI, 0.95–1.13)]. The authors concluded that there is currently no evidence from randomized studies to suggest that increased dietary fiber intake will reduce the incidence or recurrence of adenomatous polyps within a 2- to 4-year period.

Currently there is no single accepted definition of fiber. Many different types of fiber exist (soluble/nonsoluble, polysaccharides/nonpolysaccharides) and these differences may influence CRC risk. In addition, fiber intake itself may not be protective but may be correlated with other healthy lifestyle choices as well as other components of a healthy diet (for example, high vegetable, low fat, and low meat). The lack of effect found in randomized trials as compared with observational studies indicates this may be the case. However, the intervention trials may have been too short in duration to be able to demonstrate an effect.

Calcium

Substantial epidemiologic and experimental evidence exists to support the beneficial effect of calcium on the prevention of colorectal neoplasia. Calcium has the capacity to bind and precipitate bile acids and may directly influence mucosal cell proliferation. Most, although not all, of the observational studies evaluating the influence of dietary calcium have demonstrated a protective effect of calcium on risk of CRC. Particularly compelling, two randomized double-blind placebo-controlled intervention trials of calcium for the prevention of adenoma recurrence that included a total of 1346 subjects[57,60] have demonstrated that the use of calcium supplementation (1200 mg daily for a mean duration of 4 years or 2000 mg daily for a mean duration of 3 years) was associated with a reduction in the recurrence of colorectal adenoma, although only one study[60] achieved statistical significance. In a metaanalysis of the two studies, the overall odds of developing recurrent adenomas was 0.74 for patients randomized to receive calcium as compared with placebo.[61]

The effect of calcium on a non–high-risk cohort is less clear. A metaanalysis of available studies conducted in 1996[62] concluded that the evidence to support the benefit of calcium intake on reduction of colorectal neoplasia was not consistent with a substantial effect. More recently, large observational studies have supported a modest effect of calcium in the prevention of CRC, particularly calcium supplementation. In a study of 87,998 women from the Nurses' Health Study and 47,344 men from the Health Professionals Follow-up Study, an RR of distal CRC of 0.73 was found for those ingesting more than 700 mg of calcium per day. No association was found for proximal cancers.[63] In the Cancer Prevention Study II, Nutrition Cohort Study, 60,866 men and 66,883 women completed a detailed dietary questionnaire and were followed for 5 years. Total calcium intake (from diet and supplements) was associated with marginally lower CRC risk in men and women (RR = 0.87; 95% CI, 0.67–1.12, highest versus lowest quintiles, P trend = .02).[64] A pooled analysis of 10 cohort studies including 534,536 individuals[65] evaluating the influence of dairy foods and calcium on CRC confirms a consistently decreased risk of CRC for those with the highest intake of dietary calcium as compared with those with the lowest intake. Although the effect of calcium may be modest, given that CRC is a common disease, the overall impact of optimizing calcium intake from a population standpoint could be substantial.

Folate

Folate, a B vitamin, is important for normal DNA methylation. Methylation is important in the regulation of cellular gene expression. Folate deficiency may lead to cancer through disruption of DNA synthesis and repair, or loss of control of proto-oncogene activity.[66] In 15 retrospective epidemiologic[67] studies evaluating the association between folate and CRC risk, most demonstrate a statistically significant or trend toward a significant relationship between higher intake of folate and a reduced risk of CRC or adenoma formation. There are 11 prospective studies that have evaluated the influence of folate on CRC risk in North American and European populations.[67] In an unpublished metaanalysis of these data, a 20% reduction in the risk of CRC was found in those with the highest folate ingestion as compared with those with the lowest level of ingestion.[68] Although the relationship between folate and CRC in epidemiologic studies is generally consistent, it is not uniform, and there are no large-scale randomized trials evaluating the effect of folate supplementation on CRC or adenoma risk in the general population. Of note, since 1998, the United States Food and Drug Administration has required folate fortification of all flour and cereal grain products in the United States,[69] and thus folate consumption in the population is likely increasing.

Alcohol

Alcohol ingestion has a possible role in colorectal carcinogenesis. Alcohol may alter folate absorption, increasing CRC through reduction of folate bioavailability. Acetaldehyde, a product of alcohol metabolism may have a role, and alcohol may also contribute to abnormal DNA methylation directly. A metaanalysis of five follow-up studies and 22 case-control studies published in 1990[70] demonstrated only a weak association between alcohol and CRC, although the effect was stronger when only rectal cancer was considered. A more recent pooled analysis[71] of eight cohort studies examining the relationship between alcohol intake and CRC including a total of 489,979 people in five countries has been conducted. An increased risk of CRC was identified in persons with an alcohol intake of two or more drinks per day (an amount consumed by only 4% of women and 13% of men in these studies). For those individuals who drank two to three drinks per day, the RR of CRC as compared with nondrinkers was 1.16. For those people who drank three or more drinks per day, the RR (1.41) was greater. The association was found for all sites in the colon and rectum and for both women and men. No clear difference was seen in the risk attributable to specific types of alcohol (beer versus wine versus spirits). Of note, these cohort studies were limited to a single measure of alcohol consumption at baseline and thus could not assess duration of alcohol use or lifetime alcohol exposure. However, the findings of an association with alcohol intake are consistent, and there are no studies that demonstrate a protective effect of higher alcohol consumption.[72] Thus, the totality of the evidence indicates that a high level of alcohol intake (two or more drinks per day) is associated with an increased risk of CRC.

Aspirin and Nonsteroidal Antiinflammatory Drugs

There is considerable observational evidence that the use of aspirin or other nonsteroidal antiinflammatory drugs (NSAIDs) has protective effects at all stages of colorectal carcinogenesis (aberrant crypt foci, adenoma, carcinoma, and death from CRC).[73] The mechanism of antineoplastic action of NSAIDs is incompletely understood but it is believed that both cyclooxygenase (COX)-dependent and COX-independent pathways may be important.

At least 30 observational studies have been conducted to evaluate the influence of NSAID (primarily aspirin) use on development of CRC and colorectal adenoma. A consistent reduction in the risk of colorectal neoplasia in NSAID users is identified in these studies of various design, that use various methods of controlling for potential confounders.[73] In a pooled analysis of studies evaluating the effect on colorectal adenoma, the summary RR for colorectal adenoma in aspirin users was 0.7 and in NSAID users was 0.6, indicating a statistically significant reduction in risk in aspirin and NSAID users.[74] In the pooled analysis of the effect of aspirin and NSAIDs on CRC risk, the results were virtually the same.[75] Overall, the data evaluating the effect of nonaspirin NSAIDs is more limited than that for aspirin.[76]

Several intervention studies have been conducted, and a Cochrane review of the results of the randomized controlled intervention trials has been published.[77,78] The authors of this metaanalysis reviewed one population-based prevention trial (including 22,071 people),[79] three secondary prevention trials in people with sporadic polyps (including 2028 patients),[80–82] and four trials in 150 patients with familial adenomatous polyposis (FAP).[83–86] The authors conclude based on data from these high-quality trials that there is some evidence for the effectiveness of intervention strategies using NSAIDs for the prevention of colorectal adenoma. However, the single primary prevention trial reviewed[79] did not demonstrate a decreased incidence of CRC in the intervention group. Therefore, the results of ongoing trials evaluating the effects of NSAIDs on CRC development are necessary before the widespread usage of NSAIDs as a chemopreventive agent for this disease. Serious gastrointestinal complications occur in regular users of aspirin and NSAIDs. Although events are rare, hospitalizations for gastrointestinal complications occur in 7 to 13 per 1000 chronic users of NSAIDs per year.[87,88] Because chemopreventive agents must be used in the general population to substantially reduce the burden of disease, the risks of chemoprophylaxis with aspirin or NSAIDs may outweigh the benefits. Some recent studies have evaluated the role of COX-2 inhibitors in the prevention of CRC.[89,90] However, in comparison to aspirin, the research evaluating COX-2 inhibitors is limited. In addition, because there are potential cardiotoxic effects of COX-2 inhibitors, their use in chemoprevention cannot be supported.[91] A number of authors have evaluated the cost-effectiveness of chemoprevention of CRC with NSAIDs[92,93] or COX-2 inhibitors[94,95] and found that chemoprophylaxis with these compounds is not cost effective.

Hormone Replacement Therapy

Observational studies have demonstrated an association between hormone replacement therapy (HRT) in women and a reduction in both incidence and mortality from CRC. Possible mechanisms for the effect of HRT include a reduction in bile acid secretion (a potential promoter or initiator of CRC), as well as estrogen effects on colonic epithelium, both directly and through alterations in insulin-like growth factor with the use of estrogens. A metaanalysis of 18 observational studies of postmenopausal HRT demonstrated a 20% reduction in incidence of CRC in women who had taken HRT as compared with those that had never taken HRT.[96] The Women's Health Initiative was a randomized trial of estrogen plus progestin in postmenopausal women including 16,608 women. The study was discontinued early, because after a mean of 5.2 years of follow-up, it was determined that the relative risk of breast cancer in the treatment group exceeded the predefined stopping boundary and the overall risk of adverse outcomes exceeded the benefits.[97] At that time, there seemed to be a protective effect of HRT on incidence of CRC. With further follow-up, a total of 122 cases of CRC developed in this cohort[98]: 43 cases in the group receiving HRT and 72

cases in the group receiving placebo, indicating that relatively short-term HRT was associated with a significantly decreased risk of CRC. Interestingly, the women who developed CRC while on HRT were more likely to present at an advanced stage than women who developed CRC when on placebo. The frequency of screening for CRC was similar between the two groups.

Overall, there seems to be a consistent reduction in the risk of CRC with the use of HRT. However, given the potential adverse effect of HRT, this should not be used as a primary preventive strategy for CRC.[99] Interestingly, some authors have found that the influence of estrogen on CRC risk is related to microsatellite instability (MSI)—the presence of estrogen seems to protect against MSI whereas lack of estrogen in older women increases the risk of development of an MSI-positive tumor.[100]

Obesity

Obesity seems to increase the risk of colon cancer in men and premenopausal women. Case-control studies[101,102] and cohort studies[103–105] have demonstrated a strong association between a high body mass index and incidence of CRC, with a twofold increased risk of CRC found in the obese. One of the proposed mechanisms for the association is the relative insulin resistance found in many obese patients. Insulin resistance results in hyperinsulinemia and increased activity of IGF (insulinlike growth factor) peptides. High IGF-1 levels are associated with cell proliferation[103] and may increase the risk of colonic neoplasia. In the past, most studies have demonstrated a stronger association between obesity and CRC risk in men than in women. More recent evidence has demonstrated that in women, the association between obesity and CRC risk may be modified by estrogen. Several observational studies have demonstrated an increased risk of CRC in obese women; however, the association was limited to premenopausal women.[104,106,107] In postmenopausal women, the increased estrogen production associated with obesity was thought to mitigate the risk. Of note, not all observational studies have confirmed this relationship.[103]

Physical Activity

More than 50 studies have been conducted to evaluate the influence of physical activity on CRC risk. Overall, the literature is relatively consistent with respect to the effect: greater physical activity (occupational, leisure, or total activity) is associated with a reduced risk of CRC. The effect is relatively small; the estimated increased risk of colon cancer in the sedentary ranges from 1.6 to 2.0. (Of note, this figure compares to the increased risk of heart disease attributable to a sedentary lifestyle of 1.3 to 1.4.) The effect of physical activity on colon cancer is consistent in both case-control studies and cohort studies.[108] Although physical activity may be associated with a number of other healthy lifestyle factors, studies controlling for such factors (diet, smoking, nonsteroidal use, body mass) show an independent protective effect of physical activity. The effect of physical activity on the risk of rectal cancer is somewhat less consistent; some studies demonstrate no effect, and in studies that do demonstrate an effect, it is weaker. The amount of physical activity required to have an effect is substantial—risk reduction is estimated to occur with 3.5–4 hours of vigorous activity (running) per week but requires 7–35 hours of moderate activity (walking at a brisk pace) per week.[108]

The biologic mechanisms that explain the relationship between physical activity and CRC risk are unclear. Increased physical activity leads to changes in insulin sensitivity and IGF levels, and both insulin and IGF have been demonstrated to potentially be involved with colorectal carcinogenesis.[109–111] Additional proposed mechanisms include effects of physical activity on prostaglandin synthesis, effects on antitumor immune defenses, and the reduction in percent body fat associated with exercise.[112] The mechanism is almost certainly multifactorial. Nonetheless, for a host of health-related reasons, frequent moderate to vigorous physical activity can be recommended to most patients without hesitation.

Smoking

Consistent with a 35- to 40-year time lag between exposure and induction of cancer, early studies did not demonstrate an association between cigarette smoking and colorectal neoplasia. More recent studies are more consistently positive. In a review of the literature conducted in 2001,[113] 21 of 22 studies evaluating the relationship between cigarette smoking and colorectal adenoma were positive, smokers demonstrating a two- to threefold increase of adenoma risk as compared with nonsmokers. Twenty-seven epidemiologic studies have been conducted that demonstrate an association between tobacco and risk of CRC.[113] Of studies conducted in the United States, conducted after 1970 in men, and 1990 in women (studies with adequate induction time—35 to 40 years after smoking became prevalent), most demonstrated an association between heavy smoking and increased CRC risk. Most studies demonstrated an effect at relatively high levels of smoking (20 or more cigarettes per day). In the studies reviewed, the CRC risk was 1.4- to 2-fold higher in smokers than in nonsmokers.

Smoking may modify the effect of micronutrients on CRC risk. In a randomized, controlled trial of antioxidants including β-carotene, or vitamin C and E supplementation in the prevention of recurrence of colorectal adenomas, among subjects who neither smoked nor drank alcohol, β-carotene was associated with a substantial reduction in the risk of recurrent adenoma (RR = 0.56). This effect was significantly attenuated in participants who were either smokers or drinkers. For participants who were both smokers and drank alcohol, β-carotene supplementation actually resulted in a doubling of the risk of recurrent adenoma formation.[114] A large study[115] found that patients with MSI-positive tumors were more

likely to smoke more than 20 cigarettes a day, and had smoked for longer period of times than controls or patients with MSI-negative tumors. In this study, other factors such as physical activity, NSAID use, and body mass index were less consistently associated with MSI-positive tumors. The authors postulate that cigarette smoke may generate replication errors, overwhelming the DNA mismatch repair (MMR) mechanism, or may affect MMR directly.

Cholecystectomy

Abnormal bile acid metabolism may predispose both to CRC and cholelithiasis. After cholecystectomy, increased quantities of secondary bile acids have been detected in the feces and may have a role in colonic carcinogenesis. Studies in this area are difficult, because dietary and lifestyle factors related to cholelithiasis may confound the relationship between gallbladder disease and CRC risk. A metaanalysis of studies evaluating the effect of cholecystectomy on CRC risk published in 1993[116] demonstrated conflicting results. Analysis of the 33 case-control studies generated a pooled RR for CRC after cholecystectomy of 1.34 (95% CI, 1.14–1.57), limited to the proximal colon. However, no significant effect was found when the results of six cohort studies were evaluated.

Two recent large prospective cohort studies have been conducted to evaluate this relationship. In a long-term follow-up study of 278,460 patients after cholecystectomy followed for up to 33 years,[117] a significantly increased risk of small bowel malignancies and proximal colonic malignancies was found as compared with the general population. No association was found with more distal bowel cancer. In a study using data from the Nurses' Health Study,[118] a significant positive association between cholecystectomy and the risk of CRC was found (RR 1.21, 95% CI 1.01–1.46, after adjusting for important CRC risk factors including diet, family history, calcium intake, body mass index, and use of hormone replacement therapy). In this study, the risk of CRC after cholecystectomy was increased both for proximal bowel and rectal cancers. A history of gallstones was associated with similar risks. No increase in the risk of colorectal adenoma was identified in those patients having had a cholecystectomy.

Inflammatory Bowel Disease

Patients with long-standing inflammatory bowel disease (IBD) are known to be at an increased risk of CRC, although it is difficult to precisely estimate the risk. The magnitude of the risk has been studied extensively in ulcerative colitis (UC); however, rates vary among studies, particularly those performed in referral centers versus population-based studies. In addition, treatment and surveillance may influence the risk and thus more recent studies may have a lower risk than in studies before surveillance was common. A metaanalysis[119] of 116 studies evaluating the risk of CRC in UC patients found the overall prevalence of CRC in UC patients was 3.7% (95% CI, 3.2%–4.2%). In 19 of the studies reviewed, the duration of colitis was reported by decade. In the first 10 years after onset of colitis, the incidence rate of CRC was 2/1000 per year of disease, for the second decade the incidence rate of CRC was estimated to be 7/1000 per year of disease, and in the third decade the incidence rate of CRC was 12/1000 per year of disease. This corresponds to a cumulative probability of CRC of 2% after 10 years of disease, 8% after 20 years, and 18% after 30 years. The risk of CRC geographically varied and was higher in studies conducted in the United States. The metaanalysis did not evaluate extent of disease (pancolitis versus left-sided disease versus proctitis).

Extent of disease does seem to have a significant influence on CRC risk in UC. In a Swedish population-based cohort of 3117 patients with UC,[120] less extensive disease was associated with a lesser risk of CRC. As a ratio of the observed incidence and expected incidence, the increased risk of CRC in this cohort was 1.7 for those with ulcerative proctitis (95% CI, 0.8–3.2); 2.8 for those with left-sided colitis (95% CI, 1.6–4.4); and 14.8 for those with pancolitis (95% CI, 11.4–18.9). Other studies have supported these findings.[121]

Other factors that may modify the risk of CRC in patients with UC but are currently not proven include age at onset of UC, family history of CRC, and the related diagnosis of primary sclerosing cholangitis.[121] For patients with long-standing extensive UC, colectomy is an effective (albeit aggressive) strategy for prevention of CRC. Other strategies include endoscopic surveillance for dysplasia and/or the use of chemopreventive agents. Overall, the evidence for the effectiveness of surveillance colonoscopy is weak[122]; there are no randomized, controlled trials or cohort studies that have been conducted to evaluate surveillance colonoscopy in the prevention of CRC in UC.[123] In addition, neither of the two published case-control studies[124,125] has demonstrated a clear statistically significant benefit for endoscopic surveillance (although there was a trend toward benefit). Nevertheless, endoscopic surveillance is usually performed in patients with pancolitis for more than 10 years' duration who wish to avoid colectomy. There is also some evidence that chemoprevention of CRC in patients with UC may be possible. There is some evidence that 5-ASA products may decrease the rate of dysplasia in patients with UC.[126] Other promising agents include folate, calcium, and in patients with primary sclerosing cholangitis, ursodiol.[126]

The relationship between Crohn's disease and the development of CRC has been less consistently demonstrated. In studies using data from referral-based practices, the risk of development of CRC seems to be significantly increased in patients with extensive Crohn's colitis.[121] The magnitude of increased risk seems similar to that of UC[127]; however, in population-based studies, particularly those more recently published, a less dramatic effect is seen. The two largest studies have conflicting results. In a Canadian population-based cohort study, the risk of CRC in 2857 patients with

Crohn's disease was compared with a randomly selected group of controls matched 10:1 for age, gender, and geographic location. Patients with Crohn's disease were found to have an increased risk of colon cancer [incidence rate ratio (IRR) = 2.6; 95% CI, 1.69–4.12] but not rectal cancer (IRR = 1.08; 95% CI, 0.43–2.70). Patients with Crohn's disease also had an increased risk of cancer of the small intestine (IRR = 17.4; 95% CI, 4.16–72.9), and lymphoma (IRR = 2.40; 95% CI, 1.17–4.97). Some of these results are similar to those data from a population-based study in Denmark of 2645 patients hospitalized for Crohn's disease[128] and followed for up to 17 years. The rate of CRC in this group was not substantially increased as compared with the expected rate of CRC in the Danish population, the standardized incidence ratio for CRC was 1.1 (95% CI, 0.6–1.9). However, similar to the Canadian study, the risk of small intestinal cancer was increased 18-fold in the Crohn's disease group. Of note, in both studies, relatively few cases of CRC developed in Crohn's patients. Still, it is difficult to explain the dramatically different findings of the studies. It is possible that the pattern of disease or treatment differs between these two populations in a way that influenced CRC risk. Regardless, the effect of Crohn's disease on development of CRC requires further investigation.

Family History

Individuals with a family history of CRC are at an increased risk of themselves developing CRC. In a metaanalysis[129] of 27 observational studies that have evaluated the risk of family history on development of CRC, individuals with a first-degree relative with CRC had a 2.25 RR (95% CI, 2.00–2.53) of developing CRC as compared with those without a family history. The risk was slightly higher with a first-degree relative with colon cancer (RR = 2.42) than with rectal cancer (RR = 1.89). The risk increased if more than one first-degree relative had CRC (RR = 4.25) or if a relative was diagnosed before the age of 45 (RR = 3.87). The RR of CRC was also increased if a first-degree relative had a history of a colorectal adenoma (RR = 1.99). The clustering of risk in families may be attributed to an inherited susceptibility, common environmental exposures, or a combination of both factors. The influence of a more distant family history of CRC on individual risk has not been determined with certainty.

Some of the increased risk attributed to family history is due to inheritance of known susceptibility genes, such as mutations in the adenomatous polyposis coli gene, *p53* gene, or in MMR genes, particularly *MSH2*, *MLH1*, and *MSH6*[130] and these are discussed in detail elsewhere in this text. Importantly, the majority of cases of CRC cannot be attributed to known genetic defects even when associated with a family history of CRC. Recognized genetic syndromes account for only a small proportion of all cases of CRC. Additional autosomal dominant genetic defects conferring a high risk of CRC will almost certainly be found; however, at least some of the increased risk of CRC associated with a family history is likely attributable to other genetic factors, such as recessive susceptibility genes, autosomal dominant genes with low penetrance, or complex interactions between an individual's genetic makeup and environmental factors.

Despite the importance of family history on risk of CRC, up to 25% of individuals with a first-degree relative with confirmed CRC do not report having such a family history,[131] and even those that do report a history may not be aware of the increased risk associated with this.[132] This fact has important implications for assessment of family history as well as patient and family counseling.

Other Risk Factors

Radiation

Cases of rectal carcinoma have been reported in individuals who have undergone radiation for pelvic malignancies, primarily cervical cancer[133] and prostate cancer.[134] Because rectal cancer is relatively common, these cases may represent sporadic rectal cancers developing after long-term survival from other pelvic malignancies. However, the cancers occur in the radiated field, tend to be associated with radiation changes to the adjacent rectal mucosa, and are more likely to be of mucinous histology[135,136] than typical sporadic cancers, thereby strengthening the likelihood of a causal association. Nevertheless, the vast majority of individuals undergoing radiation for pelvic malignancies will not develop rectal cancer.

Ureterosigmoidostomy

Formation of a ureterosigmoidostomy has been associated with an increased risk of carcinoma in the area of the ureterosigmoid anastomoses. It is difficult to estimate the increase in risk of colon cancer attributable to ureterosigmoidostomy—many were fashioned for malignant diseases that may themselves be associated with an increased risk of colon cancer, nevertheless the risk seems to be high. The estimated increase ranges from 100 to 7000 times the risk in the normal population[137] and up to 24% of patients with a ureterosigmoidostomy will develop neoplasia at the anastomosis. The average latency period from formation of the ureterosigmoidostomy to development of malignancy is 26 years.[138] Patients who have undergone conversion to another form of urinary diversion remain at risk of neoplasia if the ureterosigmoid anastomoses were not resected in their entirety. Although the cause of this dramatic increased risk is not known, it seems to require the exposure of colonic mucosa to the mixture of urine and feces.[137]

Fortunately, with several options for urinary diversion, this procedure is now rarely performed. Those individuals living with a functional ureterosigmoidostomy should be counseled regarding their heightened risk and undergo regular sigmoidoscopic surveillance.[137]

Acromegaly

Acromegaly, a rare endocrine syndrome resulting from secretion of excess growth hormone from a pituitary neoplasm has been found to be associated with an increased risk of CRC in several studies.[139–141] The magnitude of the risk is unclear, with reports ranging from nonsignificant increases in risk to an RR of 18.3.[141] In a population-based cohort study performed in Sweden and Denmark, the standardized incidence ratio of colon cancer in patients with acromegaly as compared with the general population was 2.6 (95% CI, 1.6–2.7).[139] Patients with acromegaly have increased levels of circulating IGF-1, and this may be responsible for the increased risk of colorectal neoplasia identified in these patients.[142]

Molecular Basis

All cancer, at its root, has a genetic basis. Carcinogenesis is a multistep process, requiring an accumulation of acquired and inherited genetic alterations. With this succession of genetic alterations, cells acquire a growth advantage over surrounding cells, and in a Darwinian-type process normal cells evolve into cancer cells.[143] In normal cells, growth and replication is a highly regulated process, and disruption of this regulation at multiple levels is required for clinically relevant cancer to develop. Defects in genes that code for important proteins in the regulation of the cell cycle seem to be critical for carcinogenesis. Hanahan and Weinberg[143] have described six alterations in regulatory mechanisms that seem constant in most cancers from the several hundred genetic mutations that have been identified in cancer cells (Figure 23-4):

1. Self-sufficiency in growth signals. Ordinarily, cells must receive growth signals to actively proliferate, assuring that cellular proliferation occurs only when necessary to maintain homeostasis. To proliferate autonomously, cancer cells must lose this need for exogenous growth signal.
2. Insensitivity to antigrowth signals. Normally, there are numerous growth-inhibitory signals that function within a cell to maintain the cell in a quiescent and/or differentiated state. Cells with neoplastic potential must develop mechanisms to evade these antigrowth signals, enabling proliferation and dedifferentiation.
3. Evading apoptosis. Development of cancer requires not only a loss of control over cellular proliferation, but also a loss of control over programmed cell death (apoptosis). Apoptosis normally occurs in response to the cellular environment and is likely a major mechanism whereby cells that have acquired significant genetic mutations are destroyed. Tumor cells must circumvent apoptosis (either at a regulatory level or at an effector level) to continue to develop and proliferate.
4. Limitless replicative potential. Many cells are able to replicate only a finite number of times preventing clonal expansion of any given cell. Even after acquiring independence

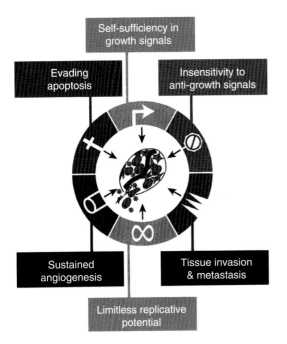

FIGURE 23-4. Alterations in regulatory mechanisms important for carcinogenesis. (Reprinted from Hanahan and Weinberg,[143] copyright © 2000, with permission from Elsevier.)

from normal signals for cellular growth and death to develop into clinically significant cancer, cancer cells must gain unlimited capacity for replication. Intrinsic limits to proliferation must be evaded.

5. Sustained angiogenesis. Virtually all cells must reside within 100 μm of a capillary to supply the cell with oxygen and nutrients required for functioning. Angiogenesis in normal tissue is closely regulated, and balancing of inducers and inhibitors of angiogenesis is an essential component of homeostasis. For neoplastic cells to develop into clinically significant cancer, they must develop the ability to induce and sustain angiogenesis, circumventing these homeostatic mechanisms to provide an adequate blood supply to support their ongoing growth.

6. Development of ability to invade and metastasize. For cancer cells to develop the ability to invade other tissue and metastasize, a number of changes must occur. Normally, cells in tissue adhere to each other. A loss of this normal cell to cell adhesion must occur in the cancer microenvironment to permit metastasis to occur. In addition, the cancer cells must develop methods of modifying new environments to support continued growth.

Although all six alterations in cell regulation are required for the development of clinically significant cancer, the sequence of events and mechanisms are variable. The sequence of genetic mutations (or alterations) is less important than the accumulation of mutations, although some mutations tend to occur early in the neoplastic process and are termed initiators, whereas others tend to occur later and are termed

promoters. In addition, certain genetic mutations (somatic or inherited) may be particularly critical and affect cell regulation in several important ways. Many such critical genes belong to two broad categories of genes involved in carcinogenesis: oncogenes and tumor suppressor genes. Additionally, caretaker genes that function to prevent the accumulation of somatic mutations are also critical to colorectal carcinogenesis. Abnormalities in caretaker genes greatly increase the risk of cancer development, independent of environmental influence. Of note, although the role of genes in carcinogenesis is described, in reality it is the protein products of the genes that are directly involved in changes in cell regulation.

Mutations in oncogenes result in an abnormal gain or excess of a particular protein function. An oncogene product when expressed in a given cell (or when the product is expressed at the wrong time in the cell cycle, expressed with an enhanced function, or expressed in larger quantities than normally present) contributes to development of critical alterations in the mechanisms of cell regulation. Mutations causing such expression behave in a dominant manner, i.e., mutation of only one of the two alleles present is required to produce activation and phenotypic expression and promote carcinogenesis. The *ras* oncogene is the most frequently mutated oncogene identified in CRCs. The *K-ras* proto-oncogene, located on the short arm of chromosome 12 (12p) is mutated in approximately half of all CRCs.[144] The *K-ras* gene product seems to be involved in the transduction of exogenous growth signals. Point mutations in the *K-ras* gene lead to a function gain, conferring a growth advantage to the cells, although the role of *K-ras* in carcinogenesis is incompletely understood. Other oncogenes that are frequently identified in sporadic colon cancer include *c-myc* and *c-erbB2*.[145]

Tumor suppressor genes normally inhibit cellular proliferation or promote apoptosis. When gene expression is lost, there is a loss of this normal inhibitory control of the cell cycle. In general, gene expression is lost only when both alleles of the gene are inactivated [Knudson's two-hit theory of carcinogenesis[146] (Figure 23-5)], either through inherited mutation, somatic mutations, or both.

There are a number of tumor suppressor genes that have been found to have an important role in CRC carcinogenesis, including the *APC*, *DCC*, *p53*, and *MCC* genes.

The adenomatous polyposis coli (*APC*) gene located on the long arm of chromosome 5 (5q), is considered a gatekeeper gene of colorectal carcinogenesis as mutations in the *APC* gene seem to be initiators of this disease. Mutations in the *APC* gene have been found in 50% of sporadic adenomas and in 75% of sporadic cases of CRC.[144] FAP, discussed in detail elsewhere in this text, results from inheritance of a germline mutation in the *APC* gene. Mutations involve base-pair mutations, insertions or deletions that result in the formation of a stop codon, halting protein synthesis leading to formation of a truncated or shortened protein product that affects the function of the protein. The location of the germline mutation in the *APC* gene varies between families with FAP, and results

Germline Mutation (Inherited Disease)

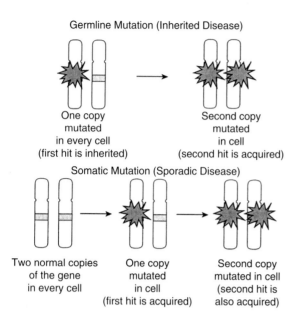

One copy
mutated
in every cell
(first hit is inherited)

Second copy
mutated
in cell
(second hit is acquired)

Somatic Mutation (Sporadic Disease)

Two normal copies
of the gene
in every cell

One copy
mutated
in cell
(first hit is acquired)

Second copy
mutated in cell
(second hit is
also acquired)

FIGURE 23-5. Loss of suppressor-gene function. (Reprinted from Calvert and Frucht[145] with permission from Annals of Internal Medicine.)

in the varying phenotypic expression of FAP found between families. Although only a single abnormal allele is inherited in FAP, sporadic mutations are always acquired resulting in the formation of hundreds to thousands of colonic adenomas and ultimately carcinoma. A specific germline mutation of the *APC* gene, the *I1307K* mutation, although not resulting in FAP, is found primarily in persons of Ashkenazi Jewish origin,[147] and results in an increased predisposition to CRC,[148] although the risk is much lower than for individuals with FAP. An additional mutation, *E1317Q*, may also result in an increased predisposition to CRC.[149]

The APC protein normally regulates the *Wnt* (wingless signaling pathway), an important pathway in cell regulation and development, through modulation of beta-catenin—a critical protein in the *Wnt* pathway. Normally, the protein product of the *APC* gene binds beta-catenin intracellularly forming a multiprotein complex that inhibits beta-catenin function. The increased functional levels of beta-catenin that result from alterations in APC protein product function leads to cell proliferation, and enhances cell to cell adhesion, limiting cell migration. Thus, hyperproliferating cells accumulate and aberrant crypt foci, the earliest phase of colorectal neoplasia.[150]

The *p53* gene, located on the short arm of chromosome 17 (17p) is an important gatekeeper gene for carcinogenesis—it is the most frequently mutated gene in human cancers.[151] Normally, by slowing the cell cycle, *p53* facilitates DNA repair during replication When repair is not feasible, *p53* induces apoptosis. Inactivation of *p53* is found in up to 75% of sporadic colorectal tumors[145]; however, the mutation seems to occur late in the tumorigenic sequence. Thus *p53* gene mutations do not seem to be initiators of carcinogenesis but act as key limiting factors for malignant transformation. This

thought is supported by the finding that patients with Li Fraumeni syndrome (an inherited defect in *p53*) do not have an increased risk of CRC.[152] In addition, *p53* expression may be an independent prognostic marker in patients with CRC.[153,154] Most studies demonstrate a lower survival rate in patients with advanced cancers that are *p53* negative as compared with those whose tumors express *p53* gene product particularly in those who receive chemotherapy.[155]

The "deleted in colorectal cancer" (*DCC*) gene was identified on the long arm of chromosome 18 (18q) in 1989.[156] Mutations in this gene have been found in the majority of CRCs. The gene product of *DCC* is a transmembrane protein that is important in cell–cell adhesion, and therefore inactivation of *DCC* may enhance the metastatic potential of CRC through changes in adhesion. Similar to *p53*, patients who have *DCC*-positive tumors may have a better prognosis than those with *DCC*-negative (mutated) tumors.[157]

Located in close proximity to the *DCC* gene, mutations in a group of genes termed *SMADs* (*SMAD2* and *SMAD4*) have been reported in CRCs. The protein products of these genes are components of the transforming growth factor (TGF)-β signaling pathway, which mediates growth inhibitory signals from cell surface to nucleus.

Because millions of base-pairs must be replicated during mitosis, errors in DNA replication occur and must be corrected by caretaker genes. The MMR system has a critical function in the detection and correction of errors in DNA replication, maintaining DNA integrity. MMR genes function as spell checkers—base-pair mismatches are identified, excised, and the correct sequence is synthesized and replaced.[72] Lack of MMR function results in an accumulation in errors in DNA replication, increasing the probability that a mutation in an important gene in cell regulation will occur, will be preserved, and carcinogenesis will thus be initiated or promoted. Defects in the MMR system are identified by the detection microsatellite instability. Microsatellites are small regions of DNA located throughout the genome that do not code for individual genes. They consist of small base sequences that are repeated in a highly polymorphic manner—the number of repeats may range from dozens to hundreds and the number of repeats varies from allele to allele, and from individual to individual. Microsatellites are particularly susceptible to MMR gene defects, thus in cases of CRC attributable to MMR gene mutations, microsatellite replication errors accumulate, leading to detectable differences in the pattern of microsatellites in the tumor and in normal tissue; this is termed microsatellite instability (MSI). When testing CRC for MSI, laboratories evaluate a number of microsatellite loci. The National Cancer Institute recommends the testing of five microsatellite sequences[158] to determine the MSI status of a tumor. If two or more of the five sequences demonstrate MSI, the tumor is designated MSI-high (MSI-H). If only one of the five sequences demonstrates changes in tumor microsatellite markers, the tumor is designated MSI-low (MSI-L). If no markers are changed, the tumor is microsatellite stable.

Approximately 15% of CRC is MSI.[158] MSI-H tumors are more likely to be high-grade, right-sided,[159] mucinous, and have tumor-infiltrating lymphocytes.[160,161] In addition, MSI tumors may have a better prognosis than microsatellite stable tumors,[162] but may be less responsive to chemotherapy.[163]

A number of MMR genes (*MLH1*, *MSH2*, *MSH3*, *MSH6*, and *PMS1*) have been identified. Germline mutations in the *MLH1* and *MSH2* genes are responsible for the majority (>90%)[164,165] of cases of the hereditary nonpolyposis colorectal cancer (HNPCC) syndrome (discussed fully elsewhere in the text), whereas approximately 5%–10% of HNPCC cases are attributable to mutations in the *MSH6* gene. Germline mutations in other MMR genes are rare.[166] Similar to tumor suppressor genes, both alleles of an MMR gene must be mutated or inactivated for MMR function to be lost. Sporadic tumors that demonstrate an MSI-H phenotype generally have a loss of *MLH1* function, attributable not to mutation but to aberrant methylation of the promoter region of the *MLH1* gene.[167] Methylation of cytosines in cytosine–guanosinedinucleotide repeats (termed CpG islands) results in the silencing of transcription, without an actual change in the nucleotide sequence of the gene.[168] The cause of the methylation is unknown, although it is associated with increasing age[169] and is not limited to MMR genes.

MYH is an additional DNA repair gene specifically active for adenine-guanine mismatches.[170] This gene has been found to be responsible for some cases of *APC* mutation-negative FAP. This defect is inherited in an autosomal recessive manner, i.e., defects must be inherited from both parents to result in phenotypic expression of the disease.[171]

In their landmark article, Vogelstein et al.[172] (Figure 23-6) described the pathogenesis of colon cancer as one that follows a predictable sequence of events, from adenoma to carcinoma, with histologic changes developing as genetic mutations are acquired over time. Initially, a mutation in a gatekeeper gene such as the *APC* gene occurs resulting in proliferation of the colorectal mucosa and leads to the first histologically detectable event, the aberrant crypt focus. In aberrant crypt foci, the crypts have larger diameters than normal and stain more darkly with methylene blue[150] and can be detected in rats as soon as 2 weeks after carcinogen exposure.[173] With additional genetic changes, cells within the aberrant crypt become dysplastic and an adenoma forms. Further genetic alterations are acquired, resulting in an increase in the size of the adenoma. However, the majority of adenomas do not develop into carcinoma. Therefore, additional genetic alterations are required before the severity of dysplasia increases, and eventually, particularly with mutations in tumor promoters such as *p53*, carcinoma develops. This pathway to carcinogenesis is termed the chromosomal instability pathway. Tumors forming through this pathway demonstrate extensive cytogenetic abnormalities, such as aneuploidy, and visible chromosomal losses and gains.[174]

CRC most frequently demonstrates chromosomal instability, indicating this is the most common genetic cause of colorectal carcinogenesis.[175] However, tumors that are MSI-H appear to develop through a separate pathway, termed the microsatellite mutator or microsatellite unstable pathway. These tumors are diploid and tend not to demonstrate gross chromosomal abnormalities. MMR defects in these tumors

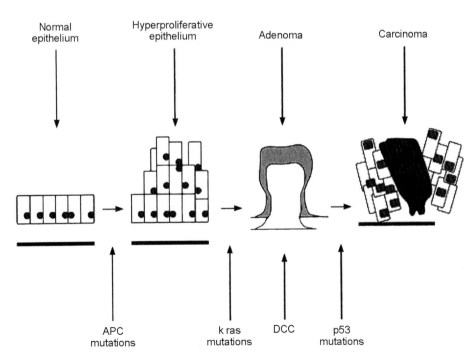

FIGURE 23-6. The adenoma to carcinoma sequence of colorectal carcinogenesis. (Reprinted from Hardy RG, Meltzer SJ, Jankowski JA. ABC of CRC. Molecular basis for risk factors. Br Med J 2000;321:886–889, with permission of the BMJ Publishing Group.)

lead to genetic mutations in key cell regulator genes, particularly the TGF-β pathway. Although MSI-H tumors may arise from adenomas, there is increasing evidence that sporadic MSI-H tumors also arise from hyperplastic polyps and serrated adenomas.[176] Serrated adenomas are polyps that in the past would have been classified as hyperplastic polyps but have architectural features both of hyperplastic polyps and cytologic features of classic adenomas. Because only 70% of all colorectal carcinomas are believed to arise from classic adenomas, serrated adenomas may be the precursor lesion for a substantial number of cancers.[177] However, the risk associated with serrated adenomas, in terms of progression to cancer, is unknown and currently under investigation.

Development of CRC in UC represents a third pathway to the carcinogenesis in the colon. Most cancers develop in UC without a precursor polyp and therefore a direct dysplasia to carcinoma sequence is postulated.[72] Genetically, cancers associated with UC seem to be heterogenous; aneuploidy and disruption of *p53* may occur as early events, however MMR genes may also be affected.

References

1. Parkin DM, Bray FI, Devesa SS. Cancer burden in the year 2000. The global picture. Eur J Cancer 2001;37(suppl 8):S4–66.
2. Shibuya K, et al. Global and regional estimates of cancer mortality and incidence by site. II. Results for the global burden of disease 2000. BMC Cancer 2002;2(1):37.
3. American Cancer Society Website Cancer Facts and Figures. 2004. Available at: http://www.cancer.org/downloads/STT/CAFF2004PWSecured.pdf.
4. Boyle P, Langman JS. ABC of colorectal cancer: epidemiology. BMJ 2000;321(7264):805–808.
5. Ries LA, et al. The annual report to the nation on the status of cancer, 1973–1997, with a special section on colorectal cancer. Cancer 2000;88(10):2398–2424.
6. Rabeneck L, Davila JA, El-Serag HB. Is there a true "shift" to the right colon in the incidence of colorectal cancer? Am J Gastroenterol 2003;98(6):1400–1409.
7. O'Connell JB, et al. Rates of colon and rectal cancers are increasing in young adults. Am Surg 2003;69(10):866–872.
8. Feldman G. Do Ashkenazi Jews have a higher than expected cancer burden? Implications for cancer control prioritization efforts. Isr Med Assoc J 2001;3(5):341–346.
9. Laken SJ, et al. Familial colorectal cancer in Ashkenazim due to a hypermutable tract in APC. Nat Genet 1997;17(1):79–83.
10. Prior TW, et al. The I1307K polymorphism of the APC gene in colorectal cancer. Gastroenterology 1999;116(1):58–63.
11. Jemal A, et al. Cancer statistics, 2004. CA Cancer J Clin 2004; 54(1):8–29.
12. Cheng X, et al. Subsite-specific incidence rate and stage of disease in colorectal cancer by race, gender, and age group in the United States, 1992–1997. Cancer 2001;92(10):2547–2554.
13. Nelson RL, et al. The relation of age, race, and gender to the subsite location of colorectal carcinoma. Cancer 1997;80(2):193–197.
14. Troisi RJ, Freedman AN, Devesa SS. Incidence of colorectal carcinoma in the U.S.: an update of trends by gender, race, age, subsite, and stage, 1975–1994. Cancer 1999;85(8):1670–1676.
15. Lagiou P. Burden of cancer. In: Adami HO, Hunter D, Trichopoulos D, eds. Textbook of Cancer Epidemiology. Oxford: Oxford University Press; 2002:3–28.
16. Burkitt DP. Related disease—related cause? Lancet 1969;2(7632):1229–1231.
17. Flood DM, et al. Colorectal cancer incidence in Asian migrants to the United States and their descendants. Cancer Causes Control 2000;11(5):403–411.
18. Parkin DM, Pisani P, Ferlay J. Global cancer statistics. CA Cancer J Clin 1999;49(1):33–64, 1.
19. Wingo PA, et al. Long-term trends in cancer mortality in the United States, 1930–1998. Cancer 2003;97(12 suppl):3133–3275.
20. Rabeneck L, et al. Outcomes of colorectal cancer in the United States: no change in survival (1986–1997). Am J Gastroenterol 2003;98(2):471–477.
21. Anderson WF, Umar A, Brawley OW. Colorectal carcinoma in black and white race. Cancer Metastasis Rev 2003;22(1):67–82.
22. Morris AM, et al. Racial disparities in rectal cancer treatment: a population-based analysis. Arch Surg 2004;139(2):151–155; discussion 156.
23. Carethers JM. Racial and ethnic factors in the genetic pathogenesis of colorectal cancer. J Assoc Acad Minor Phys 1999; 10(3):59–67.
24. Mariotto A, et al. The prevalence of patients with colorectal carcinoma under care in the U.S. Cancer 2003;98(6):1253–1261.
25. National Cancer Society Cancer Control and Population Sciences Estimated US Cancer Prevalence. Available at: http://cancercontrol.cancer.gov/ocs/prevalence. Accessed March 17, 2005.
26. Nigro ND, et al. Effect of dietary beef fat on intestinal tumor formation by azoxymethane in rats. J Natl Cancer Inst 1975;54(2):439–442.
27. Reddy BS, et al. Effect of quality and quantity of dietary fat and dimethylhydrazine in colon carcinogenesis in rats. Proc Soc Exp Biol Med 1976;151(2):237–239.
28. Broitman SA, et al. Polyunsaturated fat, cholesterol and large bowel tumorigenesis. Cancer 1977;40(5 suppl):2455–2463.
29. Hursting SD, Thornquist M, Henderson MM. Types of dietary fat and the incidence of cancer at five sites. Prev Med 1990;19(3):242–253.
30. Willett WC. Dietary fat intake and cancer risk: a controversial and instructive story. Semin Cancer Biol 1998;8(4):245–253.
31. Howe GR, et al. The relationship between dietary fat intake and risk of colorectal cancer: evidence from the combined analysis of 13 case-control studies. Cancer Causes Control 1997;8(2):215–228.
32. Stemmermann GN, Nomura AM, Heilbrun LK. Dietary fat and the risk of colorectal cancer. Cancer Res 1984;44(10):4633–4637.
33. Goldbohm RA, et al. A prospective cohort study on the relation between meat consumption and the risk of colon cancer. Cancer Res 1994;54(3):718–723.
34. Bostick RM, et al. Sugar, meat, and fat intake, and non-dietary risk factors for colon cancer incidence in Iowa women (United States). Cancer Causes Control 1994;5(1):38–52.
35. Giovannucci E, et al. Intake of fat, meat, and fiber in relation to risk of colon cancer in men. Cancer Res 1994;54(9):2390–2397.
36. Willett WC, et al. Relation of meat, fat, and fiber intake to the risk of colon cancer in a prospective study among women. N Engl J Med 1990;323(24):1664–1672.

37. Flood A, et al. Meat, fat, and their subtypes as risk factors for colorectal cancer in a prospective cohort of women. Am J Epidemiol 2003;158(1):59–68.

38. Kushi L, Giovannucci E. Dietary fat and cancer. Am J Med 2002;113(suppl 9B):63S–70S.

39. Bingham SA, et al. Does increased endogenous formation of N-nitroso compounds in the human colon explain the association between red meat and colon cancer? Carcinogenesis 1996;17(3):515–523.

40. de Kok TM, van Maanen JM. Evaluation of fecal mutagenicity and colorectal cancer risk. Mutat Res 2000;463(1):53–101.

41. Sandhu MS, White IR, McPherson K. Systematic review of the prospective cohort studies on meat consumption and colorectal cancer risk: a meta-analytical approach. Cancer Epidemiol Biomarkers Prev 2001;10(5):439–446.

42. Norat T, et al. Meat consumption and colorectal cancer risk: dose-response meta-analysis of epidemiological studies. Int J Cancer 2002;98(2):241–256.

43. Elmstahl S, et al. Dietary patterns in high and low consumers of meat in a Swedish cohort study. Appetite 1999;32(2):191–206.

44. World Cancer Research Fund/American Institute for Cancer Research. Food, nutrition and the prevention of cancer: a global perspective. Washington DC: American Institute for Cancer Research; 1997.

45. Michels KB, et al. Prospective study of fruit and vegetable consumption and incidence of colon and rectal cancers. J Natl Cancer Inst 2000;92(21):1740–1752.

46. Voorrips LE, et al. Vegetable and fruit consumption and risks of colon and rectal cancer in a prospective cohort study: The Netherlands Cohort Study on Diet and Cancer. Am J Epidemiol 2000;152(11):1081–1092.

47. McCullough ML, et al. A prospective study of whole grains, fruits, vegetables and colon cancer risk. Cancer Causes Control 2003;14(10):959–970.

48. Terry P, et al. Fruit, vegetables, dietary fiber, and risk of colorectal cancer. J Natl Cancer Inst 2001;93(7):525–533.

49. Flood A, et al. Fruit and vegetable intakes and the risk of colorectal cancer in the Breast Cancer Detection Demonstration Project follow-up cohort. Am J Clin Nutr 2002;75(5):936–943.

50. Schatzkin A, et al. Lack of effect of a low-fat, high-fiber diet on the recurrence of colorectal adenomas. Polyp Prevention Trial Study Group. N Engl J Med 2000;342(16):1149–1155.

51. Sengupta S, Tjandra JJ, Gibson PR. Dietary fiber and colorectal neoplasia. Dis Colon Rectum 2001;44(7):1016–1033.

52. Fuchs CS, et al. Dietary fiber and the risk of colorectal cancer and adenoma in women. N Engl J Med 1999;340(3):169–176.

53. Peters U, et al. Dietary fibre and colorectal adenoma in a colorectal cancer early detection programme. Lancet 2003;361 (9368):1491–1495.

54. Bingham SA, et al. Dietary fibre in food and protection against colorectal cancer in the European Prospective Investigation into Cancer and Nutrition (EPIC): an observational study. Lancet 2003;361(9368):1496–1501.

55. Asano T, McLeod RS. Dietary fibre for the prevention of colorectal adenomas and carcinomas. Cochrane Database Syst Rev 2002(2):CD003430.

56. Alberts DS, et al. Lack of effect of a high-fiber cereal supplement on the recurrence of colorectal adenomas. Phoenix Colon Cancer Prevention Physicians' Network. N Engl J Med 2000; 342(16):1156–1162.

57. Bonithon-Kopp C, et al. Calcium and fibre supplementation in prevention of colorectal adenoma recurrence: a randomised intervention trial. European Cancer Prevention Organisation Study Group. Lancet 2000;356(9238):1300–1306.

58. MacLennan R, et al. Randomized trial of intake of fat, fiber, and beta carotene to prevent colorectal adenomas. The Australian Polyp Prevention Project. J Natl Cancer Inst 1995; 87(23):1760–1766.

59. McKeown-Eyssen GE, et al. A randomized trial of a low fat high fibre diet in the recurrence of colorectal polyps. Toronto Polyp Prevention Group. J Clin Epidemiol 1994;47(5): 525–536.

60. Baron JA, et al. Calcium supplements for the prevention of colorectal adenomas. Calcium Polyp Prevention Study Group. N Engl J Med 1999;340(2):101–107.

61. Weingarten MA, Zalmanovici A, Yaphe J. Dietary calcium supplementation for preventing colorectal cancer and adenomatous polyps. Cochrane Database Syst Rev 2004(1):CD003548.

62. Bergsma-Kadijk JA, et al. Calcium does not protect against colorectal neoplasia. Epidemiology 1996;7(6):590–597.

63. Wu K, et al. Calcium intake and risk of colon cancer in women and men. J Natl Cancer Inst 2002;94(6):437–446.

64. McCullough ML, et al. Calcium, vitamin D, dairy products, and risk of colorectal cancer in the Cancer Prevention Study II Nutrition Cohort (United States). Cancer Causes Control 2003;14(1):1–12.

65. Cho E, et al. Dairy foods, calcium, and colorectal cancer: a pooled analysis of 10 cohort studies. J Natl Cancer Inst 2004; 96(13):1015–1022.

66. Kim YI. Folate, colorectal carcinogenesis, and DNA methylation: lessons from animal studies. Environ Mol Mutagen 2004;44(1):10–25.

67. Kim YI. Role of folate in colon cancer development and progression. J Nutr 2003;133(11 suppl 1):3731S–3739S.

68. Hunter DJ. In: Environmental Mutagen Society Colon Cancer Conference, 2003, Miami Florida.

69. U.S. Food and Drug Administration. Food standards: amendment of standards of identity for enriched grain products to require addition of folic acid. Final rule. 21 DFR Parts 136, 137, and 139. Fed Regist 1996;61:8781–8807.

70. Longnecker MP, et al. A meta-analysis of alcoholic beverage consumption in relation to risk of colorectal cancer. Cancer Causes Control 1990;1(1):59–68.

71. Cho E, et al. Alcohol intake and colorectal cancer: a pooled analysis of 8 cohort studies. Ann Intern Med 2004;140(8):603–613.

72. Potter JD. Colorectal cancer: molecules and populations. J Natl Cancer Inst 1999;91(11):916–932.

73. Hawk ET, Umar A, Viner JL. Colorectal cancer chemoprevention: an overview of the science. Gastroenterology 2004; 126(5):1423–1447.

74. Garcia Rodriguez LA, Huerta-Alvarez C. Reduced incidence of colorectal adenoma among long-term users of nonsteroidal anti-inflammatory drugs: a pooled analysis of published studies and a new population-based study. Epidemiology 2000;11(4):376–381.

75. Garcia-Rodriguez LA, Huerta-Alvarez C. Reduced risk of colorectal cancer among long-term users of aspirin and nonaspirin nonsteroidal antiinflammatory drugs. Epidemiology 2001; 12(1):88–93.

76. Gwyn K, Sinicrope FA. Chemoprevention of colorectal cancer. Am J Gastroenterol 2002;97(1):13–21.

77. Asano TK, McLeod RS. Nonsteroidal anti-inflammatory drugs and aspirin for the prevention of colorectal adenomas and cancer: a systematic review. Dis Colon Rectum 2004;47(5):665–673.

78. Asano TK, McLeod RS. Non steroidal anti-inflammatory drugs (NSAID) and aspirin for preventing colorectal adenomas and carcinomas. Cochrane Database Syst Rev 2004(2):CD004079.

79. Gann PH, et al. Low-dose aspirin and incidence of colorectal tumors in a randomized trial. J Natl Cancer Inst 1993;85(15): 1220–1224.

80. Baron JA, et al. A randomized trial of aspirin to prevent colorectal adenomas. N Engl J Med 2003;348(10):891–899.

81. Sandler RS, et al. A randomized trial of aspirin to prevent colorectal adenomas in patients with previous colorectal cancer. N Engl J Med 2003;348(10):883–890.

82. Benamouzig R, et al. Daily soluble aspirin and prevention of colorectal adenoma recurrence: one-year results of the APACC trial. Gastroenterology 2003;125(2):328–336.

83. Giardiello FM, et al. Treatment of colonic and rectal adenomas with sulindac in familial adenomatous polyposis. N Engl J Med 1993;328(18):1313–1316.

84. Giardiello FM, et al. Primary chemoprevention of familial adenomatous polyposis with sulindac. N Engl J Med 2002;346 (14):1054–1059.

85. Labayle D, et al. Sulindac causes regression of rectal polyps in familial adenomatous polyposis. Gastroenterology 1991;101 (3):635–639.

86. Steinbach G, et al. The effect of celecoxib, a cyclooxygenase-2 inhibitor, in familial adenomatous polyposis. N Engl J Med 2000;342(26):1946–1952.

87. Singh G, Triadafilopoulos G. Epidemiology of NSAID induced gastrointestinal complications. J Rheumatol Suppl 1999;56:18–24.

88. Wolfe MM, Lichtenstein DR, Singh G. Gastrointestinal toxicity of nonsteroidal antiinflammatory drugs. N Engl J Med 1999;340(24):1888–1899.

89. Rahme E, et al. The cyclooxygenase-2-selective inhibitors rofecoxib and celecoxib prevent colorectal neoplasia occurrence and recurrence. Gastroenterology 2003;125(2):404–412.

90. Gupta RA, Dubois RN. Colorectal cancer prevention and treatment by inhibition of cyclooxygenase-2. Nat Rev Cancer 2001;1(1):11–21.

91. Bresalier RS, et al. Cardiovascular events associated with rofecoxib in a colorectal adenoma chemoprevention trial. N Engl J Med 2005;352(11):1092–1102.

92. Suleiman S, Rex DK, Sonnenberg A. Chemoprevention of colorectal cancer by aspirin: a cost-effectiveness analysis. Gastroenterology 2002;122(1):78–84.

93. Ladabaum U, et al. Aspirin as an adjunct to screening for prevention of sporadic colorectal cancer. A cost-effectiveness analysis. Ann Intern Med 2001;135(9):769–781.

94. Hur C, Simon LS, Gazelle GS. The cost-effectiveness of aspirin versus cyclooxygenase-2-selective inhibitors for colorectal carcinoma chemoprevention in healthy individuals. Cancer 2004;101(1):189–197.

95. Arguedas MR, Heudebert GR, Wilcox CM. Surveillance colonoscopy or chemoprevention with COX-2 inhibitors in average-risk post-polypectomy patients: a decision analysis. Aliment Pharmacol Ther 2001;15(5):631–638.

96. Grodstein F, Newcomb PA, Stampfer MJ. Postmenopausal hormone therapy and the risk of colorectal cancer: a review and meta-analysis. Am J Med 1999;106(5):574–582.

97. Rossouw JE, et al. Risks and benefits of estrogen plus progestin in healthy postmenopausal women: principal results from the Women's Health Initiative randomized controlled trial. JAMA 2002;288(3):321–333.

98. Chlebowski RT, et al. Estrogen plus progestin and colorectal cancer in postmenopausal women. N Engl J Med 2004;350 (10):991–1004.

99. Rymer J, Wilson R, Ballard K. Making decisions about hormone replacement therapy. BMJ 2003;326(7384):322–326.

100. Slattery ML, et al. Estrogens reduce and withdrawal of estrogens increase risk of microsatellite instability-positive colon cancer. Cancer Res 2001;61(1):126–130.

101. Caan BJ, et al. Body size and the risk of colon cancer in a large case-control study. Int J Obes Relat Metab Disord 1998;22(2): 178–184.

102. Kune GA, Kune S, Watson LF. Body weight and physical activity as predictors of colorectal cancer risk. Nutr Cancer 1990;13(1–2):9–17.

103. Lin J, et al. Body mass index and risk of colorectal cancer in women (United States). Cancer Causes Control 2004;15(6): 581–589.

104. Terry PD, Miller AB, Rohan TE. Obesity and colorectal cancer risk in women. Gut 2002;51(2):191–194.

105. Murphy TK, et al. Body mass index and colon cancer mortality in a large prospective study. Am J Epidemiol 2000;152(9): 847–854.

106. Terry P, et al. Body weight and colorectal cancer risk in a cohort of Swedish women: relation varies by age and cancer site. Br J Cancer 2001;85(3):346–349.

107. Slattery ML, et al. Body mass index and colon cancer: an evaluation of the modifying effects of estrogen (United States). Cancer Causes Control 2003;14(1):75–84.

108. Slattery ML. Physical activity and colorectal cancer. Sports Med 2004;34(4):239–252.

109. Woodson K, et al. Loss of insulin-like growth factor-II imprinting and the presence of screen-detected colorectal adenomas in women. J Natl Cancer Inst 2004;96(5):407–410.

110. Slattery ML, et al. Associations among IRS1, IRS2, IGF1, and IGFBP3 genetic polymorphisms and colorectal cancer. Cancer Epidemiol Biomarkers Prev 2004;13(7):1206–1214.

111. Sandhu MS, et al. Association between insulin-like growth factor-I: insulin-like growth factor-binding protein-1 ratio and metabolic and anthropometric factors in men and women. Cancer Epidemiol Biomarkers Prev 2004;13(1):166–170.

112. Friedenreich CM, Orenstein MR. Physical activity and cancer prevention: etiologic evidence and biological mechanisms. J Nutr 2002;132(11 suppl):3456S–3464S.

113. Giovannucci E. An updated review of the epidemiological evidence that cigarette smoking increases risk of colorectal cancer. Cancer Epidemiol Biomarkers Prev 2001;10(7):725–731.

114. Baron JA, et al. Neoplastic and antineoplastic effects of beta-carotene on colorectal adenoma recurrence: results of a randomized trial. J Natl Cancer Inst 2003;95(10):717–722.

115. Slattery ML, et al. Associations between cigarette smoking, lifestyle factors, and microsatellite instability in colon tumors. J Natl Cancer Inst 2000;92(22):1831–1836.

116. Giovannucci E, Colditz GA, Stampfer MJ. A meta-analysis of cholecystectomy and risk of colorectal cancer. Gastroenterology 1993;105(1):130–141.

117. Lagergren J, Ye W, Ekbom A. Intestinal cancer after cholecystectomy: is bile involved in carcinogenesis? Gastroenterology 2001;121(3):542–547.

118. Schernhammer ES, et al. Cholecystectomy and the risk for developing colorectal cancer and distal colorectal adenomas. Br J Cancer 2003;88(1):79–83.

119. Eaden JA, Abrams KR, Mayberry JF. The risk of colorectal cancer in ulcerative colitis: a meta-analysis. Gut 2001;48(4): 526–535.

120. Ekbom A, et al. Ulcerative colitis and colorectal cancer. A population-based study. N Engl J Med 1990;323(18):1228–1233.

121. Sharan R, Schoen RE. Cancer in inflammatory bowel disease. An evidence-based analysis and guide for physicians and patients. Gastroenterol Clin North Am 2002;31(1):237–254.

122. Mpofu C, Watson AJ, Rhodes JM. Strategies for detecting colon cancer and/or dysplasia in patients with inflammatory bowel disease. Cochrane Database Syst Rev 2004(2):CD000279.

123. Loftus EV Jr. Does monitoring prevent cancer in inflammatory bowel disease? J Clin Gastroenterol 2003;36(5 suppl):S79–83; discussion S94–96.

124. Eaden J, et al. Colorectal cancer prevention in ulcerative colitis: a case-control study. Aliment Pharmacol Ther 2000;14(2): 145–153.

125. Karlen P, et al. Is colonoscopic surveillance reducing colorectal cancer mortality in ulcerative colitis? A population based case control study. Gut 1998;42(5):711–714.

126. Croog VJ, Ullman TA, Itzkowitz SH. Chemoprevention of colorectal cancer in ulcerative colitis. Int J Colorectal Dis 2003;18(5):392–400.

127. Gillen CD, et al. Ulcerative colitis and Crohn's disease: a comparison of the colorectal cancer risk in extensive colitis. Gut 1994;35(11):1590–1592.

128. Mellemkjaer L, et al. Crohn's disease and cancer risk (Denmark). Cancer Causes Control 2000;11(2):145–150.

129. Johns LE, Houlston RS. A systematic review and meta-analysis of familial colorectal cancer risk. Am J Gastroenterol 2001;96(10):2992–3003.

130. Lynch HT, de la Chapelle A. Hereditary colorectal cancer. N Engl J Med 2003;348(10):919–932.

131. Glanz K, et al. Underreporting of family history of colon cancer: correlates and implications. Cancer Epidemiol Biomarkers Prev 1999;8(7):635–639.

132. Jacobs LA. Health beliefs of first-degree relatives of individuals with colorectal cancer and participation in health maintenance visits: a population-based survey. Cancer Nurs 2002;25(4):251–265.

133. Tamai O, et al. Radiation-associated rectal cancer: report of four cases. Dig Surg 1999;16(3):238–243.

134. Brenner DJ, et al. Second malignancies in prostate carcinoma patients after radiotherapy compared with surgery. Cancer 2000;88(2):398–406.

135. Shirouzu K, et al. Clinicopathologic characteristics of large bowel cancer developing after radiotherapy for uterine cervical cancer. Dis Colon Rectum 1994;37(12):1245–1249.

136. Jao SW, et al. Colon and anorectal cancer after pelvic irradiation. Dis Colon Rectum 1987;30(12):953–958.

137. Woodhouse CR. Guidelines for monitoring of patients with ureterosigmoidostomy. Gut 2002;51(suppl 5):V15–16.

138. Husmann DA, Spence HM. Current status of tumor of the bowel following ureterosigmoidostomy: a review. J Urol 1990;144(3):607–610.

139. Baris D, et al. Acromegaly and cancer risk: a cohort study in Sweden and Denmark. Cancer Causes Control 2002;13(5): 395–400.

140. Orme SM, et al. Mortality and cancer incidence in acromegaly: a retrospective cohort study. United Kingdom Acromegaly Study Group. J Clin Endocrinol Metab 1998;83(8):2730–2734.

141. Jenkins PJ, Besser M. Clinical perspective: acromegaly and cancer—a problem. J Clin Endocrinol Metab 2001;86(7): 2935–2941.

142. Jenkins PJ, et al. Insulin-like growth factor I and the development of colorectal neoplasia in acromegaly. J Clin Endocrinol Metab 2000;85(9):3218–3221.

143. Hanahan D, Weinberg RA. The hallmarks of cancer. Cell 2000;100(1):57–70.

144. Robbins DH, Itzkowitz SH. The molecular and genetic basis of colon cancer. Med Clin North Am 2002;86(6):1467–1495.

145. Calvert PM, Frucht H. The genetics of colorectal cancer. Ann Intern Med 2002;137(7):603–612.

146. Knudson AG Jr. Mutation and cancer: statistical study of retinoblastoma. Proc Natl Acad Sci USA 1971;68(4):820–823.

147. Niell BL, et al. Genetic anthropology of the colorectal cancer-susceptibility allele APC I1307K: evidence of genetic drift within the Ashkenazim. Am J Hum Genet 2003;73(6): 1250–1260.

148. Rozen P, et al. Clinical and screening implications of the I1307K adenomatous polyposis coli gene variant in Israeli Ashkenazi Jews with familial colorectal neoplasia. Evidence for a founder effect. Cancer 2002;94(10):2561–2568.

149. Frayling IM, et al. The APC variants I1307K and E1317Q are associated with colorectal tumors, but not always with a family history. Proc Natl Acad Sci USA 1998;95(18): 10722–10727.

150. Takayama T, et al. Aberrant crypt foci of the colon as precursors of adenoma and cancer. N Engl J Med 1998;339(18): 1277–1284.

151. Kirsch DG, Kastan MB. Tumor-suppressor p53: implications for tumor development and prognosis. J Clin Oncol 1998;16(9):3158–3168.

152. Birch JM, et al. Cancer phenotype correlates with constitutional TP53 genotype in families with the Li-Fraumeni syndrome. Oncogene 1998;17(9):1061–1068.

153. Rosati G, et al. Thymidylate synthase expression, p53, bcl-2, Ki-67 and p27 in colorectal cancer: relationships with tumor recurrence and survival. Tumour Biol 2004;25(5–6):258–263.

154. Resnick MB, et al. Epidermal growth factor receptor, c-MET, beta-catenin, and p53 expression as prognostic indicators in stage II colon cancer: a tissue microarray study. Clin Cancer Res 2004;10(9):3069–3075.

155. Iacopetta B. TP53 mutation in colorectal cancer. Hum Mutat 2003;21(3):271–276.

156. Fearon ER, et al. Identification of a chromosome 18q gene that is altered in colorectal cancers. Science 1990;247(4938): 49–56.

157. Shibata D, et al. The DCC protein and prognosis in colorectal cancer. N Engl J Med 1996;335(23):1727–1732.

158. Umar A, et al. Revised Bethesda guidelines for hereditary nonpolyposis colorectal cancer (Lynch syndrome) and microsatellite instability. J Natl Cancer Inst 2004;96(4):261–268.

159. Ward R, et al. Microsatellite instability and the clinicopathological features of sporadic colorectal cancer. Gut 2001;48(6): 821–829.

160. Smyrk TC, et al. Tumor-infiltrating lymphocytes are a marker for microsatellite instability in colorectal carcinoma. Cancer 2001;91(12):2417–2422.

161. Jass JR, et al. Morphology of sporadic colorectal cancer with DNA replication errors. Gut 1998;42(5):673–679.

162. Gryfe R, et al. Tumor microsatellite instability and clinical outcome in young patients with colorectal cancer. N Engl J Med 2000;342(2):69–77.

163. Ribic CM, et al. Tumor microsatellite-instability status as a predictor of benefit from fluorouracil-based adjuvant chemotherapy for colon cancer. N Engl J Med 2003;349(3):247–257.

164. Peltomaki P. Deficient DNA mismatch repair: a common etiologic factor for colon cancer. Hum Mol Genet 2001;10(7):735–740.

165. Lynch HT, de la Chapelle A. Genetic susceptibility to non-polyposis colorectal cancer. J Med Genet 1999;36(11):801–818.

166. Liu B, et al. Analysis of mismatch repair genes in hereditary non-polyposis colorectal cancer patients. Nat Med 1996;2(2):169–174.

167. Cunningham JM, et al. Hypermethylation of the hMLH1 promoter in colon cancer with microsatellite instability. Cancer Res 1998;58(15):3455–3460.

168. Toyota M, et al. Distinct genetic profiles in colorectal tumors with or without the CpG island methylator phenotype. Proc Natl Acad Sci USA 2000;97(2):710–715.

169. Kakar S, et al. Frequency of loss of hMLH1 expression in colorectal carcinoma increases with advancing age. Cancer 2003;97(6):1421–1427.

170. Al-Tassan N, et al. Inherited variants of MYH associated with somatic G:C–>T:A mutations in colorectal tumors. Nat Genet 2002;30(2):227–232.

171. Sieber OM, et al. Multiple colorectal adenomas, classic adenomatous polyposis, and germ-line mutations in MYH. N Engl J Med 2003;348(9):791–799.

172. Vogelstein B, et al. Genetic alterations during colorectal-tumor development. N Engl J Med 1988;319(9):525–532.

173. Bird RP, Good CK. The significance of aberrant crypt foci in understanding the pathogenesis of colon cancer. Toxicol Lett 2000;112–113:395–402.

174. Lengauer C, Kinzler KW, Vogelstein B. Genetic instability in colorectal cancers. Nature 1997;386(6625):623–627.

175. Grady WM. Genomic instability and colon cancer. Cancer Metastasis Rev 2004;23(1–2):11–27.

176. Higuchi T, Jass JR. My approach to serrated polyps of the colorectum. J Clin Pathol 2004;57(7):682–686.

177. Jass JR. Pathogenesis of colorectal cancer. Surg Clin North Am 2002;82(5):891–904.

24
Screening for Colorectal Neoplasms

Thomas E. Read and Philip F. Caushaj

Cancer of the colon and rectum is the second leading cause of cancer-related death in the United States. In 1997, it was estimated that 131,000 Americans were diagnosed with colorectal cancer, and 55,000 died from this disease.[1] Without undergoing screening or preventive action, approximately 1 in every 17 people in this country will develop colorectal cancer at some point in life. However, evidence is mounting that colorectal adenocarcinoma can be prevented by detecting and removing adenomatous polyps, and that detecting early-stage cancers reduces mortality from the disease.[2-6] Both polyps and early-stage cancers are usually asymptomatic; cancers that have grown large enough to cause symptoms have a much worse prognosis. This contrast highlights the need for screening in asymptomatic persons.

Most people will be of average risk and require screening for colorectal cancer and polyps beginning at age 50.[7] However, a substantial number of people are at increased risk because of an inherited predisposition to the disease and need screening or treatment as early as puberty. By virtue of their practice, colon and rectal surgeons, gastroenterologists, and medical oncologists have contact with many patients with colorectal carcinoma as well as at-risk family members. These specialists have the opportunity to guide the evaluation of at-risk persons and be advocates for appropriate screening examinations.

The explosion of genetic research in the last 15 years has enabled us to better understand inherited forms of colorectal cancer, and has helped to define high-risk populations that need endoscopic or genetic screening for these diseases early in life. The adenomatous polyposis coli gene is thought to function as a gatekeeper of colorectal neoplasia. Germline and somatic truncating mutations of the adenomatous polyposis coli gene are thought to initiate colorectal tumor formation in familial adenomatous polyposis (FAP) and sporadic colorectal carcinogenesis, respectively. Genetic testing for FAP can help guide surveillance and treatment of patients at risk for the disease. Hereditary nonpolyposis colorectal cancer (HNPCC) is thought to be the result of DNA mismatch repair deficiency, and genetic testing for HNPCC may ultimately prove to have clinical value for patients in HNPCC families.

The effectiveness of screening for colorectal cancer has been a subject of controversy. In 1995, the United States Preventive Task Force reversed earlier position statements and endorsed screening of asymptomatic average-risk persons, using fecal occult blood testing and sigmoidoscopy.[8,9] In 1996, the federal Agency for Health Care Policy and Research (AHCPR) convened a collaborative group of experts representing the American College of Gastroenterology, American Gastroenterological Association, American Society of Colon and Rectal Surgeons, American Society for Gastrointestinal Endoscopy, and Society of American Gastrointestinal Endoscopic Surgeons to critically evaluate the available evidence on colorectal cancer screening and to develop appropriate clinical practice guidelines.[10] The panel studied 3500 peer-reviewed publications to assess the performance, effectiveness, acceptability to patients, cost-effectiveness, and outcome of different screening examinations. The AHCPR guidelines[7] were, in essence, endorsed by the American Cancer Society[11] and are virtually identical to the Practice Parameters for the Detection of Colorectal Neoplasms published by the Standards Committee of the American Society of Colon and Rectal Surgeons.[12] They provide the framework for this review.

Classification of Risk and Screening Recommendations

The cornerstone in determining a patient's risk for developing colorectal cancer is the family history. Failure to properly investigate a patient's family history of colorectal neoplasia can lead to inappropriate and inadequate treatment of both the patient and at-risk family members.

TABLE 24-1. Patients with colorectal cancer

75%	Average risk (sporadic)
15%–20%	Family history of colorectal cancer
3%–8%	HNPCC
1%	FAP
1%	Ulcerative colitis

Average Risk

As can be seen in Table 24-1, the majority of patients who develop colorectal cancer have no identifiable risk factors. Persons considered to be at average risk for colorectal cancer do not fit any of the higher risk categories. Specifically, average-risk persons have no symptoms associated with colorectal cancer, no personal history of colorectal cancer or adenomatous polyps, no family history of colorectal neoplasia, no inflammatory bowel disease, and no unexplained anemia.

Screening recommendations (Table 24-2): The AHCPR panel recommended that average-risk persons should undergo one of the following screening regimens, beginning at age 50:

1. Fecal occult blood testing annually
2. Flexible sigmoidoscopy every 5 years
3. Fecal occult blood testing annually and flexible sigmoidoscopy every 5 years
4. Air contrast barium enema every 5–10 years
5. Colonoscopy every 10 years

Although the panel stated that all of the screening strategies are acceptable options,[7] each strategy has unique strengths and weaknesses. The fecal occult blood test (FOBT) is a guaiac-based test for peroxidase activity that is nonspecific and will fail to detect many small cancers and precancerous lesions.[13] Nevertheless, several large randomized controlled trials have shown that annual or biannual testing for fecal occult blood with complete diagnostic evaluation of the colon (primarily with colonoscopy) for patients with a positive FOBT reduces mortality from colorectal cancer.[3,14,15] The AHCPR panel listed FOBT alone as an option for colorectal cancer screening. However, because of the lack of sensitivity of FOBT, the American Cancer Society recommends combining annual FOBT with flexible sigmoidoscopy every 5 years rather than using FOBT alone as a screening method.[11]

A major drawback to using FOBT as a screening technique is poor compliance. Only 38%–60% of the patients in prospective trials completed all the planned FOBT tests,[3,14,15] and use of FOBT in the general population is estimated to be lower than in the research environment.[16] The steps necessary for adequate sample collection, combined with dietary restrictions to avoid agents that can cause false-positive and false-negative results may also hinder compliance with FOBT. Proper performance of FOBT involves the sampling of atraumatically obtained stool from three consecutive bowel movements in a patient who has not ingested red meat, aspirin, nonsteroidal inflammatory medications, turnips, melons, salmon, sardines, horseradish, or vitamin C for the 2 days preceding the test and throughout the test period.[7,17] The restriction of frequently ingested foods and medications, combined with the natural aversion to stool sampling, makes annual FOBT unappealing to many persons.

FOBT should not be confused with random stool guaiac testing, which is the analysis of stool found on digital rectal examination for blood. The lack of adequate diet and medication restriction before the test, potential for trauma to the anal canal during digital rectal examination, and the inability to reliably obtain stool from the distal rectum make the test unreliable.[18] To date, random stool guaiac examination has not been demonstrated to have benefit in screening for colorectal cancer.

TABLE 24-2. Screening for colorectal cancer and polyps

Risk category	Screening method	Age to begin screening
Average risk	Choose one of the following: FOBT annually* Flexible sigmoidoscopy every 5 yr* FOBT annually + flexible sigmoidoscopy every 5 yr Air contrast barium enema every 5–10 yr† Colonoscopy every 10 yr	50 yr
Family history	Choose one of the following: 1. Colonoscopy every 10 yr 2. Air contrast barium enema every 5 yr†	40 yr, or 10 yr before diagnosis of the youngest affected family member, whichever is earliest
HNPCC	Colonoscopy every 1–3 yr Genetic counseling Consider genetic testing	21 yr
FAP	Flexible sigmoidoscopy or colonoscopy every 1–2 yr Genetic counseling Consider genetic testing	Puberty
Ulcerative colitis	Colonoscopy with biopsies for dysplasia every 1–2 yr	7–8 yr after the diagnosis of pancolitis; 12–15 yr after the diagnosis of left-sided colitis

*The American Cancer Society recommends the combination of yearly FOBT and flexible sigmoidoscopy as preferable to either examination alone.
†Rigid proctoscopy is recommended as an adjunctive examination to allow adequate visualization of the distal rectum. Furthermore, flexible sigmoidoscopy may be necessary to more completely evaluate a tortuous or spastic sigmoid colon.

In some settings, FOBT test slides are rehydrated, which contributes to the high incidence of false-positive tests and is not recommended by the manufacturer. Hemoccult SENSA, which seems to be as sensitive as the original Hemoccult test, is the guaiac technique currently recommended for use.[19] In the future, immunochemical techniques or genetic analysis of cellular material in stool may prove to be more effective than current FOBT technology in detecting occult colorectal neoplasms via stool sampling.[20,21]

The effectiveness of *sigmoidoscopy* as a screening tool depends on its ability to detect cancers and adenomatous polyps in the distal colon. If adenomatous polyps are found at flexible sigmoidoscopy, colonoscopy should be strongly considered because almost one-third of such patients will have neoplastic lesions in the proximal colon.[22] The effectiveness of sigmoidoscopy in reducing mortality from colorectal cancer has never been proven by a randomized, controlled trial, although case-control studies have shown a benefit.[2,6,23] There was only a trend toward limited benefit of one-time screening sigmoidoscopy, followed by colonoscopy for patients found to have polyps, in the Telemark study from Norway.[24,25] The Prostate, Lung, Colon and Ovary Trial supported by the National Cancer Institute is evaluating flexible sigmoidoscopy in a randomized, controlled setting, but mortality data are not expected until 2008.[7] A multicenter prospective trial examining the potential benefit of one-time screening flexible sigmoidoscopy at age 60 is currently underway in the United Kingdom and Italy.[26]

The AHCPR panel listed flexible sigmoidoscopy alone as an option for colorectal cancer screening, although such a strategy will fail to detect neoplasms in the proximal colon unless adenomatous polyps or cancer are found in the distal colon that prompt colonoscopy. For this reason, The American Cancer Society recommends combining flexible sigmoidoscopy every 5 years with annual FOBT, rather than using flexible sigmoidoscopy alone as a screening method.[11] Although this combined approach may detect more proximal neoplasms than flexible sigmoidoscopy alone, 15%–25% of patients with negative flexible sigmoidoscopy and negative FOBT will have neoplastic lesions in the proximal colon at colonoscopy, calling the rationale for this approach into question.[27–31]

The efficacy of *barium enema* in preventing colorectal cancer mortality has never been evaluated in a controlled trial, but can be inferred from the fact that detecting polyps and early-stage cancers by other methods reduces the incidence and mortality from colorectal cancer. Air contrast barium enema will detect 50%–80% of polyps <1 cm, 70%–90% of polyps >1 cm, and 50%–80% of Stage I and II adenocarcinomas.[32–35] Single column barium enema is less sensitive and should be combined with flexible sigmoidoscopy if used as a screening tool.[7] Rigid proctoscopy should be considered as an adjunct examination because the balloon on the enema catheter often prevents adequate imaging of the distal rectum. Another major limitation of barium enema as a screening method is

that patients usually require colonoscopy if lesions are detected.

Colonoscopy is the only screening technique that allows the detection and removal of premalignant lesions throughout the colon and rectum, and is the final common pathway for any positive screening test. Although its effectiveness depends on the skill and experience of the endoscopist to both reach the cecum and to identify small lesions, it remains the gold standard to evaluate the colonic mucosa.[7] The ability of colonoscopy to reduce colorectal cancer mortality has been demonstrated indirectly through studies showing that detecting and removing polyps reduces the incidence of colorectal cancer and that detecting early cancers lowers the mortality from the disease.[2–6] Compliance with screening colonoscopy may be superior to that of other methods because no confirmatory examinations are required, and thus, patients are subjected to a single bowel preparation.

CT colography (*virtual colonoscopy*) was developed in an attempt to increase compliance with colorectal cancer screening, based on the impression that persons would be more inclined to have a "scan" than a "scope." The technique involves thin-section computed tomography (CT) with three-dimensional computer reconstructions to examine the colonic mucosa (Figure 24-1A,B).[36,37] Although the technique has the advantages of being noninvasive and not requiring sedation, a vigorous oral laxative preparation is required, because adherent stool cannot be differentiated from neoplasia on CT. In addition, a rectal catheter and air insufflation is used to distend the colon. CT colography cannot be assumed to be more appealing to all patients who are reluctant to undergo colonoscopy, because many patients are deterred more by the laxative preparation beforehand than by the endoscopic procedure itself, and find rectal air insufflation in the absence of sedation uncomfortable.[38] Initial trials demonstrated that CT colography was not as sensitive as colonoscopy in the detection of small polyps,[39] although with improvements in technology and with greater experience with interpretation, CT colography may ultimately prove to be as reliable as colonoscopy in detecting colorectal neoplasia.[40] Regardless of its accuracy, CT colography suffers (as does contrast enema) from the disadvantage that biopsies cannot be obtained and positive findings require endoscopic confirmation.

The Office of Technology Assessment of the United States Congress found that FOBT, flexible sigmoidoscopy, air contrast barium enema, and colonoscopy are equally cost effective as screening strategies, with an estimated cost of less than $20,000 per year of life saved (assuming screening begins at age 50 and is discontinued at age 85).[7,41,42] Although cost-benefit analyses such as these are exceedingly complex, this estimate is well within the acceptable range of cost effectiveness by United States health standards and compares favorably to screening mammography for women older than age 50. As of January 1, 1998, Medicare has reimbursed screening examinations for colorectal cancer in average-risk persons older than the age of 50.[43] In 2001,

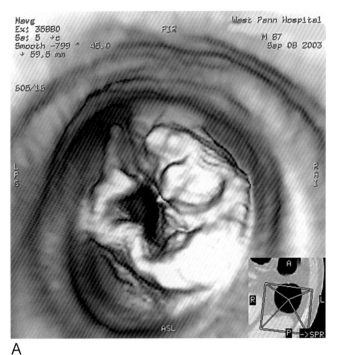

A

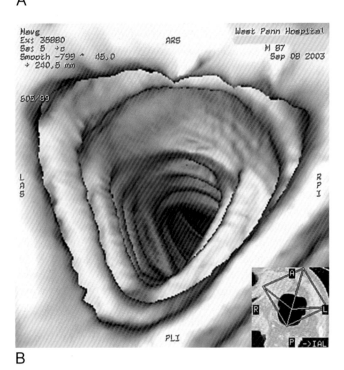

B

FIGURE 24-1. **A** CT colography of an 87-year-old patient with a large tumor of the splenic flexure who could not undergo colonoscopy. The circumferential cancer can be seen occupying the lumen of the colon. **B** This image is of the transverse colon proximal to the cancer.

Medicare authorized reimbursement for screening colonoscopy for average-risk persons. As of January 2004, the Centers for Medicare and Medicaid Services guidelines for reimbursement for colorectal cancer screening are as follows (excerpted from their Web site, http://www.cms.hhs. gov/medlearn/refcolcn.asp):

- FOBT: once every 12 months
- Flexible sigmoidoscopy: once every 48 months
- Colonoscopy: once every 24 months if the patient is at high risk for colon cancer; and once every 10 years (but not within 48 months of a screening sigmoidoscopy) if the patient is not at high risk for colon cancer
- Double contrast barium enema: physician can decide to use instead of a sigmoidoscopy or colonoscopy

At present, the choice of screening strategy for average-risk persons is made with influence from primary care physicians, patients, and third-party payers. Although the AHCPR panel's recommendation of five different screening strategies may offer flexibility, it may also cause confusion and uncertainty.[44] Two of the five strategies depend on compliance with yearly FOBT, which has been extremely difficult to achieve even in the setting of controlled trials. Only air contrast barium enema and colonoscopy provide total colonic evaluation, and contrast enema suffers from the necessity of performing colonoscopy if a lesion is detected. Screening colonoscopy every 10–15 years beginning at age 50 may ultimately prove to be the most cost-effective method of screening average-risk persons for colorectal cancer. Hopefully, future technologic advances will allow for total colonic evaluation with minimal patient discomfort and embarrassment, at reasonable cost. If a simple stool-labeling technique is developed that allows for reliable differentiation of stool from mucosa on CT without the need for cathartic bowel preparation, CT colography may fit these criteria.

Personal History of Adenomatous Polyps or Adenocarcinoma

A personal history of adenomatous polyps or colorectal adenocarcinoma places a person at higher than average risk for the development of metachronous neoplasms. Surveillance colonoscopy is thus recommended by virtually all consensus groups.[12,45] The interval between colonoscopies has been the subject of some debate, and no blanket recommendation can be given for all patients. A rational surveillance strategy should take into account the patient's age, comorbid conditions, life expectancy, completeness of prior examinations, pattern of neoplastic growth, and histologic features of previously resected neoplasms. For instance, a 60-year-old patient in good health who undergoes colonoscopic polypectomy of a single small tubular adenoma should probably undergo surveillance colonoscopy in 3–5 years.[45] A patient in good health who is found to have adenomas that are multiple, large, or dysplastic on initial screening colonoscopy should be considered for colonoscopy at an earlier interval, such as 6–12 months. However, a 90-year-old patient with severe comorbidities and limited life expectancy would not benefit as much from early surveillance, because removal of premalignant lesions will probably not alter lifespan or quality of life.

Patients who undergo curative resection of colorectal adenocarcinoma should undergo regular surveillance colonoscopy to detect new metachronous primary neoplasms. The recommendation of the Standards Task Committee of the American Society of Colon and Rectal Surgeons is for initial postresection colonoscopy at 1 year, followed by colonoscopy every 3–5 years thereafter, depending on the pathology found at the preceding colonoscopic examination. Obviously, all the considerations made for the selection of postpolypectomy surveillance intervals, as noted above, apply in this situation as well. The purpose of the colonoscopy is not specifically to look for tumor recurrence at the anastomotic suture line, because suture line recurrence in the absence of unresectable extraluminal disease is extremely uncommon,[46] but rather to search for new primary neoplasms.

Family History of Colorectal Cancer or Adenomatous Polyps

A family history of colorectal cancer or adenomatous polyps increases the risk of developing colorectal cancer. In general, closer familial relationships to affected relatives, younger age of onset, and larger numbers of affected relatives increase the risk.[7,47,48] A careful family history should always be obtained to exclude one of the better-defined inherited colorectal cancer syndromes, such as HNPCC or FAP.

As a greater understanding of the molecular genetics of colorectal cancer is gained, many patients with familial colorectal cancer may eventually be categorized as having distinct inherited syndromes. Recently, a germline mutation of the adenomatous polyposis coli gene (I1307K variant) was identified in persons of Ashkenazi Jewish descent that predisposes to the development of colorectal adenomas and carcinoma.[10,49–54] The mutation causes hypermutability of the adenomatous polyposis coli gene and is thought to contribute to carcinogenesis independent of mismatch repair deficiency.[51] In the future, genetic testing for this mutation in at-risk persons may have clinical utility.

Screening recommendations: The AHCPR panel recommended that patients with first-degree relatives with colorectal cancer or adenomatous polyps begin screening for colorectal neoplasia at age 40, or 10 years before the age at diagnosis of the affected relative, whichever is earliest.[7] Those patients whose first-degree relatives developed colorectal cancer before age 50 may be at higher risk, and complete colonic evaluation with colonoscopy should be strongly considered.[7] Patients with a second-degree relative with colorectal cancer, or relative with adenomatous polyps diagnosed over age 60, may be screened as an average-risk person.[7] As of January 1, 1998, Medicare will reimburse for screening colonoscopy for high-risk patients when performed at least 2 years after the last screening colonoscopy or barium enema.[43]

Hereditary Nonpolyposis Colorectal Cancer

HNPCC is an inherited disorder that predisposes patients to the development of colorectal cancer, with up to 75% of patients developing the disease by age 65.[55–58] HNPCC is inherited in an autosomal dominant manner, and is thought to be the result of germline mutations in mismatch repair genes (genes that code for proteins responsible for correcting errors during DNA replication). Patients with HNPCC typically develop cancer between age 40 to 50 and most tumors occur proximal to the splenic flexure. "Nonpolyposis" refers to the distinction between HNPCC and FAP (in which patients have hundreds of polyps), but is somewhat misleading because patients with HNPCC develop adenomatous polyps. The progression from adenoma to carcinoma seems to be accelerated in HNPCC patients as compared with patients with sporadic cancers, and there is a tendency to develop multiple colorectal cancers in HNPCC.[55,59–61] Patients with HNPCC are also at high risk for cancers of other organs, especially the ovary and uterus.

The ability to conclusively identify gene carriers is not yet fully developed, thus the penetrance of colorectal cancer in gene carriers can only be estimated (about 90%). In addition, some patients in HNPCC families who do not have identifiable germline mismatch repair gene mutations will develop colorectal cancer.[62] For these reasons, the diagnosis of HNPCC in a family remains clinical. The Amsterdam criteria (colorectal cancer in three or more family members; two generations affected; one affected person a first-degree relative of another; and one cancer diagnosed before age 50) are the strictest criteria and have the highest concordance with known mismatch repair gene mutations.[62] These criteria were originally developed for research purposes, to standardize the definition of HNPCC. However, they fail to identify patients who may be affected with HNPCC but do not fit the strict criteria because of unknown or abbreviated family histories, as well as patients with a personal or family history of extracolonic malignancies associated with HNPCC. A recent National Cancer Institute working group acknowledged the shortcomings of the Amsterdam criteria as clinical guidelines and published recommendations to expand the clinical suspicion of HNPCC to a broader range of patients.[58] The International Collaborative Group on Hereditary Non-Polyposis Colorectal Cancer has also proposed similar criteria.[62]

Microsatellite instability has been reported in 85%–90% of HNPCC colorectal cancers.[56] Detection of this phenotype has been proposed as a screening method to trigger germline mutational analysis in kindreds with uncertain family histories.[58] However, microsatellite instability is also found in approximately 15% of sporadic cancers, and has not been universally found to be predictive of familial cancer.[62,63]

At present, the "true" definition of HNPCC remains uncertain. Neither refined clinical criteria nor germline mutational analysis has provided a model of the syndrome that is predictive of phenotype in all cases. Clinically, the absence of microsatellite instability or mismatch repair gene mutation does not negate a family history that suggests an autosomal dominant predisposition to developing colorectal cancer. At-risk family members still require aggressive screening.

Screening recommendations: Expert panels convened by the AHCPR[7] and the Cancer Genetics Studies Consortium[55] recommend that persons who are members of a family that fits clinical criteria for HNPCC undergo colonoscopy at age 20–25, and repeat colonoscopy every 1–3 years. The short time interval between colonoscopies results from the accelerated adenoma to carcinoma progression thought to occur in HNPCC. Patients and their family members should be referred for genetic counseling. Germline testing for mismatch repair gene mutations can be considered,[64] but because the predictive value of such testing is only 30%–50%,[62] colonoscopy should be performed regardless.

Familial Adenomatous Polyposis

FAP is caused by a defect in the adenomatous polyposis coli gene, which is inherited in an autosomal dominant manner.[65] Patients with FAP develop hundreds of adenomatous polyps as early as puberty, and will ultimately develop colorectal cancer, usually by age 40.[66,67] Patients with FAP are also prone to develop a variety of extracolonic tumors, notably duodenal adenomas and carcinomas, and desmoid tumors.[66] FAP mutations do occur spontaneously, accounting for patients who are diagnosed with the disease without a family history of FAP.[68] Attenuated FAP is a rare variant of the disease, with polyps and cancers developing later in life.[69]

The most frequently used genetic test for FAP is an assay for a truncated protein product of the mutated adenomatous polyposis coli gene. Because only about 80% of families with FAP will have a mutation that produces a truncated protein, the predictive value of testing at-risk family members is greatest if the proband (affected relative) has a positive test.[70]

Screening recommendations: Patients with a family history of FAP should undergo flexible sigmoidoscopy or colonoscopy at puberty.[7,71] Lower endoscopy should be repeated every 1–2 years. Genetic testing should be considered, especially in large pedigrees where genotyping might be more cost effective than repeated endoscopy.[71] If the proband has a positive truncated protein assay, at-risk relatives who test negative may be screened as average-risk persons.[71]

Because of the socioeconomic, medicolegal, and emotional issues surrounding genetic testing, it cannot be emphasized enough that genetic testing for FAP should be done after genetic counseling and informed consent.[70] Trained genetic counselors can guide patients through the testing process and help interpret results. Giardiello et al.[70] found that 32% of physicians ordering genetic tests for FAP misinterpreted the results of the test, and that less than 20% of patients tested had received pretest genetic counseling or written informed consent. These numbers are sobering when one considers that FAP has 100% mortality if left untreated. Patients should also undergo screening upper endoscopy for duodenal adenomas.[72]

Inflammatory Bowel Disease

Patients with ulcerative colitis have an increased risk of developing colorectal cancer. This risk begins approximately 7–8 years after diagnosis in patients with pancolitis, and 12–15 years after diagnosis in patients with limited left-sided colitis.[7] There may be an increased risk of colorectal cancer in patients with Crohn's colitis, although this is less well defined.[73–78]

Screening recommendations: It is common practice for patients with ulcerative colitis to undergo screening colonoscopy with multiple random biopsies looking for dysplasia every 1–2 years, beginning 7–8 years after diagnosis in patients with pancolitis and 12–15 years after diagnosis in patients with left-sided colitis.[7,79,80] However, evidence that surveillance reduces mortality, or is better than timing a colectomy according to extent and duration of disease, is weak.[7,79,80]

Future Directions

It is troubling that so much energy and expense is devoted to the cure of advanced or recurrent colorectal cancer in the United States, while so little is devoted to screening for polyps and early-stage cancers. It is estimated that only 10%–30% of adults older than the age of 50 in this country undergo any regular screening for colorectal neoplasia.[16,81,82] In a report issued in 2002, the United States General Accounting Office found that colorectal cancer screening is the least utilized preventive health benefit available to Medicare beneficiaries (General Accounting Office, Medicare–Beneficiary Use of Clinical Preventive Services, Report No. GAO-22-422; April 2002). As is the case in the general population, only 25% of Medicare beneficiaries are screened each year with FOBT, compared with much higher rates for other regular cancer screening tests such as mammography (75%) or Pap smear testing (66%). Until recently, screening for colorectal cancer has not received much publicity in the United Sates, despite colorectal cancer being the second leading cause of cancer-related death in this country, and despite having a well-defined, identifiable, and treatable precursor lesion (the adenomatous polyp). Both health care professionals and the public need to become more aware of the potential benefits of colorectal cancer screening.

As the genetics of inherited colorectal cancer syndromes become better understood, it will be possible to conclusively identify high-risk populations. It is of paramount importance that screening efforts be directed toward these populations. Genetic counselors are invaluable resources, both to counsel family members and to help direct genetic testing.

References

1. Parker SL, Tong T, Bolden S, Wingo PA. Cancer statistics, 1997. CA Cancer J Clin 1997;47:5–27.
2. Newcomb P, Norfleet R, Storer B, Surawicz T, Marcus P. Screening sigmoidoscopy and colorectal cancer mortality. J Natl Cancer Inst 1992;84:1572–1575.
3. Kronborg O, Fenger C, Olsen J, Jorgensen OD, Sondergaard O. Randomised study of screening for colorectal cancer with faecal-occult-blood test. Lancet 1996;348:1467–1471.
4. Winawer SJ, Flehinger BJ, Schottenfeld D, Miller DG. Screening for colorectal cancer with fecal occult blood testing and sigmoidoscopy. J Natl Cancer Inst 1993;85:1311–1318.
5. Winawer SJ, Zauber AG, Ho MN, et al. Prevention of colorectal cancer by colonoscopic polypectomy. The National Polyp Study Workgroup. N Engl J Med 1993;329:1977–1981.
6. Muller AD, Sonnenberg A. Protection by endoscopy against death from colorectal cancer. A case-control study among veterans. Arch Intern Med 1995;155:1741–1748.
7. Winawer SJ, Fletcher RH, Miller L, et al. Colorectal cancer screening: clinical guidelines and rationale. Gastroenterology 1997;112:594–642.
8. Frame PS, Berg AO, Woolf S. U.S. Preventive Services Task Force: highlights of the 1996 report. Am Fam Physician 1997;55:567–576, 581–582.
9. Levin B, Bond JH. Colorectal cancer screening: recommendations of the U.S. Preventive Services Task Force. American Gastroenterological Association. Gastroenterology 1996;111:1381–1384.
10. Laken SJ, Petersen GM, Gruber SB, et al. Familial colorectal cancer in Ashkenazim due to a hypermutable tract in APC. Nat Genet 1997;17:79–83.
11. Byers T, Levin B, Rothenberger D, Dodd GD, Smith RA. American Cancer Society guidelines for screening and surveillance for early detection of colorectal polyps and cancer: update 1997. American Cancer Society Detection and Treatment Advisory Group on Colorectal Cancer. CA Cancer J Clin 1997;47:154–160.
12. Simmang CL, Senatore P, Lowry A, et al. Practice parameters for detection of colorectal neoplasms. The Standards Committee, The American Society of Colon and Rectal Surgeons. Dis Colon Rectum 1999;42:1123–1129.
13. Rockey DC, Koch J, Cello JP, Sanders LL, McQuaid K. Relative frequency of upper gastrointestinal and colonic lesions in patients with positive fecal occult-blood tests. N Engl J Med 1998;339:153–159.
14. Hardcastle JD, Chamberlain JO, Robinson MH, et al. Randomised controlled trial of faecal-occult-blood screening for colorectal cancer. Lancet 1996;348:1472–1477.
15. Mandel JS, Bond JH, Church TR, et al. Reducing mortality from colorectal cancer by screening for fecal occult blood. Minnesota Colon Cancer Control Study. N Engl J Med 1993;328:1365–1371.
16. Anderson LM, May DS. Has the use of cervical, breast, and colorectal cancer screening increased in the United States? Am J Public Health 1995;85:840–842.
17. Ransohoff DF, Lang CA. Screening for colorectal cancer with the fecal occult blood test: a background paper. American College of Physicians. Ann Intern Med 1997;126:811–822.
18. Nakama H, Fattah AS, Zhang B, Kamijo N. Digital rectal examination sampling of stool is less predictive of significant colorectal pathology than stool passed spontaneously. Eur J Gastroenterol Hepatol 2000;12:1235–1238.
19. Colorectal Cancer Screening: Clinical Practice Guidlines in Oncology. JNCCN 2003;1:72–93.
20. Traverso G, Shuber A, Levin B, et al. Detection of APC mutations in fecal DNA from patients with colorectal tumors. N Engl J Med 2002;346:311–320.
21. Limburg PJ, Devens ME, Harrington JJ, Diehl NN, Mahoney DW, Ahlquist DA. Prospective evaluation of fecal calprotectin as a screening biomarker for colorectal neoplasia. Am J Gastroenterol 2003;98:2299–2305.
22. Read TE, Read JD, Butterly LF. Importance of adenomas 5 mm or less in diameter that are detected by sigmoidoscopy. N Engl J Med 1997;336:8–12.
23. Selby J, Friedman G, Quesenberry C, Weiss N. A case-control study of screening sigmoidoscopy and mortality from colorectal cancer. N Engl J Med 1992;326:653–657.
24. Thiis-Evensen E, Hoff GS, Sauar J, Langmark F, Majak BM, Vatn MH. Population-based surveillance by colonoscopy: effect on the incidence of colorectal cancer. Telemark Polyp Study I. Scand J Gastroenterol 1999;34:414–420.
25. Thiis-Evensen E, Hoff GS, Sauar J, Majak BM, Vatn MH. The effect of attending a flexible sigmoidoscopic screening program on the prevalence of colorectal adenomas at 13-year follow-up. Am J Gastroenterol 2001;96:1901–1907.
26. Atkin WS, Edwards R, Wardle J, et al. Design of a multicentre randomised trial to evaluate flexible sigmoidoscopy in colorectal cancer screening. J Med Screen 2001;8:137–144.
27. Lieberman D, Smith F. Screening for colon malignancy with colonoscopy. Am J Gastroenterol 1991;86:946–951.
28. Achkar E, Carey W. Small polyps found during fiberoptic sigmoidoscopy in asymptomatic patients. Ann Intern Med 1988;109:880–883.
29. Brady PG, Straker RJ, McClave SA, Nord HJ, Pinkas M, Robinson BE. Are hyperplastic rectosigmoid polyps associated with an increased risk of proximal colonic neoplasms? Gastrointest Endosc 1993;39:481–485.
30. Rex DK, Smith JJ, Ulbright TM, Lehman GA. Distal colonic hyperplastic polyps do not predict proximal adenomas in asymptomatic average-risk subjects. Gastroenterology 1992;102:317–319.
31. Mehran A, Jaffe P, Efron J, Vernava A, Liberman A. Screening colonoscopy in the asymptomatic 50- to 59-year-old population. Surg Endosc 2003;17(12):1974–1977.
32. Steine S, Stordahl A, Lunde OC, Loken K, Laerum E. Double-contrast barium enema versus colonoscopy in the diagnosis of neoplastic disorders: aspects of decision-making in general practice. Fam Pract 1993;10:288–291.
33. Hixson LJ, Fennerty MB, Sampliner RE, McGee D, Garewal H. Prospective study of the frequency and size distribution of polyps missed by colonoscopy. J Natl Cancer Inst 1990;82:1769–1772.
34. Hixson LJ, Fennerty MB, Sampliner RE, Garewal HS. Prospective blinded trial of the colonoscopic miss-rate of large colorectal polyps. Gastrointest Endosc 1991;37:125–127.

35. Fork FT. Double contrast enema and colonoscopy in polyp detection. Gut 1981;22:971–977.

36. Fenlon HM, Nunes DP, Clarke PD, Ferrucci JT. Colorectal neoplasm detection using virtual colonoscopy: a feasibility study. Gut 1998;43:806–811.

37. Rex DK. CT and MR colography (virtual colonoscopy): status report. J Clin Gastroenterol 1998;27:199–203.

38. Akerkar GA, Yee J, Hung R, McQuaid K. Patient experience and preferences toward colon cancer screening: a comparison of virtual colonoscopy and conventional colonoscopy. Gastrointest Endosc 2001;54:310–315.

39. Fenlon HM, Nunes DP, Schroy PC 3rd, Barish MA, Clarke PD, Ferrucci JT. A comparison of virtual and conventional colonoscopy for the detection of colorectal polyps. N Engl J Med 1999;341:1496–1503.

40. Pickhardt PJ, Choi JR, Hwang I, et al. Computed tomographic virtual colonoscopy to screen for colorectal neoplasia in asymptomatic adults. N Engl J Med 2003;349:2191–2200.

41. Wagner JL. Cost-effectiveness of screening for common cancers. Cancer Metastasis Rev 1997;16:281–294.

42. Wagner J. From the Congressional Office of Technology Assessment. JAMA 1990;264:2732.

43. Bull Am Coll Surg 1998;83:13.

44. Walsh JM, Terdiman JP. Colorectal cancer screening: scientific review. JAMA 2003;289:1288–1296.

45. Winawer SJ, Zauber AG, O'Brien MJ, et al. Randomized comparison of surveillance intervals after colonoscopic removal of newly diagnosed adenomatous polyps. The National Polyp Study Workgroup. N Engl J Med 1993;328:901–906.

46. Read TE, Mutch MG, Chang BW, et al. Locoregional recurrence and survival after curative resection of adenocarcinoma of the colon. J Am Coll Surg 2002;195:33–40.

47. Winawer SJ, Zauber AG, Gerdes H, et al. Risk of colorectal cancer in the families of patients with adenomatous polyps. National Polyp Study Workgroup. N Engl J Med 1996;334:82–87.

48. Fuchs CS, Giovannucci EL, Colditz GA, Hunter DJ, Speizer FE, Willett WC. A prospective study of family history and the risk of colorectal cancer. N Engl J Med 1994;331:1669–1674.

49. Frayling IM, Beck NE, Ilyas M, et al. The APC variants I1307K and E1317Q are associated with colorectal tumors, but not always with a family history. Proc Natl Acad Sci USA 1998;95: 10722–10727.

50. Gryfe R, Di NN, Lal G, Gallinger S, Redston M. Inherited colorectal polyposis and cancer risk of the APC I1307K polymorphism. Am J Hum Genet 1999;64:378–384.

51. Prior TW, Chadwick RB, Papp AC, et al. The I1307K polymorphism of the APC gene in colorectal cancer. Gastroenterology 1999;116:58–63.

52. Rozen P, Shomrat R, Strul H, et al. Prevalence of the I1307K APC gene variant in Israeli Jews of differing ethnic origin and risk for colorectal cancer. Gastroenterology 1999;116:54–57.

53. Woodage T, King SM, Wacholder S, et al. The APCI1307K allele and cancer risk in a community-based study of Ashkenazi Jews. Nat Genet 1998;20:62–65.

54. Gryfe R, Di NN, Gallinger S, Redston M. Somatic instability of the APC I1307K allele in colorectal neoplasia. Cancer Res 1998;58:4040–4043.

55. Burke W, Petersen G, Lynch P, et al. Recommendations for follow-up care of individuals with an inherited predisposition to cancer. I. Hereditary nonpolyposis colon cancer. Cancer Genetics Studies Consortium. JAMA 1997;277:915–919.

56. Lynch HT, Smyrk T. Hereditary nonpolyposis colorectal cancer (Lynch syndrome). An updated review. Cancer 1996;78: 1149–1167.

57. Myrhoj T, Bisgaard ML, Bernstein I, Svendsen LB, Sondergaard JO, Bulow S. Hereditary non-polyposis colorectal cancer: clinical features and survival. Results from the Danish HNPCC register. Scand J Gastroenterol 1997;32:572–576.

58. Rodriguez-Bigas MA, Boland CR, Hamilton SR, et al. A National Cancer Institute Workshop on Hereditary Nonpolyposis Colorectal Cancer Syndrome: meeting highlights and Bethesda guidelines. J Natl Cancer Inst 1997;89:1758–1762.

59. Box JC, Rodriguez-Bigas MA, Weber TK, Petrelli NJ. Clinical implications of multiple colorectal carcinomas in hereditary nonpolyposis colorectal carcinoma. Dis Colon Rectum 1999;42: 717–721.

60. Fitzgibbons RJ Jr, Lynch HT, Stanislav GV, et al. Recognition and treatment of patients with hereditary nonpolyposis colon cancer (Lynch syndromes I and II). Ann Surg 1987;206:289–295.

61. Watson P, Lin KM, Rodriguez-Bigas MA, et al. Colorectal carcinoma survival among hereditary nonpolyposis colorectal carcinoma family members. Cancer 1998;83:259–266.

62. Park JG, Vasen HF, Park KJ, et al. Suspected hereditary nonpolyposis colorectal cancer: International Collaborative Group on Hereditary Non-Polyposis Colorectal Cancer (ICG-HNPCC) criteria and results of genetic diagnosis. Dis Colon Rectum 1999;42:710–715.

63. Samowitz WS, Slattery ML, Kerber RA. Microsatellite instability in human colonic cancer is not a useful clinical indicator of familial colorectal cancer. Gastroenterology 1995;109:1765–1771.

64. Vasen HF, van BM, Buskens E, et al. A cost-effectiveness analysis of colorectal screening of hereditary nonpolyposis colorectal carcinoma gene carriers. Cancer 1998;82:1632–1637.

65. Leppert M, Dobbs M, Scambler P, et al. The gene for familial polyposis coli maps to the long arm of chromosome 5. Science 1987;238:1411–1413.

66. Arvanitis ML, Jagelman DG, Fazio VW, Lavery IC, McGannon E. Mortality in patients with familial adenomatous polyposis. Dis Colon Rectum 1990;33:639–642.

67. Vasen HF, Griffioen G, Offerhaus GJ, et al. The value of screening and central registration of families with familial adenomatous polyposis. A study of 82 families in The Netherlands. Dis Colon Rectum 1990;33:227–230.

68. Rustin RB, Jagelman DG, McGannon E, Fazio VW, Lavery IC, Weakley FL. Spontaneous mutation in familial adenomatous polyposis. Dis Colon Rectum 1990;33:52–55.

69. Spirio L, Olschwang S, Groden J, et al. Alleles of the APC gene: an attenuated form of familial polyposis. Cell 1993;75:951–957.

70. Giardiello FM, Brensinger JD, Petersen GM, et al. The use and interpretation of commercial APC gene testing for familial adenomatous polyposis. N Engl J Med 1997;336:823–827.

71. Cromwell DM, Moore RD, Brensinger JD, Petersen GM, Bass EB, Giardiello FM. Cost analysis of alternative approaches to colorectal screening in familial adenomatous polyposis. Gastroenterology 1998;114:893–901.

72. Marcello PW, Asbun HJ, Veidenheimer MC, et al. Gastroduodenal polyps in familial adenomatous polyposis. Surg Endosc 1996;10:418–421.

73. Fireman Z, Grossman A, Lilos P, et al. Intestinal cancer in patients with Crohn's disease. A population study in central Israel. Scand J Gastroenterol 1989;24:346–350.

74. Gollop JH, Phillips SF, Melton LD, Zinsmeister AR. Epidemiologic aspects of Crohn's disease: a population based study in Olmsted County, Minnesota, 1943–1982. Gut 1988;29:49–56.

75. Kvist N, Jacobsen O, Norgaard P, et al. Malignancy in Crohn's disease. Scand J Gastroenterol 1986;21:82–86.

76. Gyde SN, Prior P, Macartney JC, Thompson H, Waterhouse JA, Allan RN. Malignancy in Crohn's disease. Gut 1980;21:1024–1029.

77. Greenstein AJ, Sachar DB, Smith H, Janowitz HD, Aufses AJ. Patterns of neoplasia in Crohn's disease and ulcerative colitis. Cancer 1980;46:403–407.

78. Weedon DD, Shorter RG, Ilstrup DM, Huizenga KA, Taylor WF. Crohn's disease and cancer. N Engl J Med 1973;289:1099–1103.

79. Provenzale D, Kowdley KV, Arora S, Wong JB. Prophylactic colectomy or surveillance for chronic ulcerative colitis? A decision analysis. Gastroenterology 1995;109:1188–1196.

80. Lennard JJ, Melville DM, Morson BC, Ritchie JK, Williams CB. Precancer and cancer in extensive ulcerative colitis: findings among 401 patients over 22 years. Gut 1990;31:800–806.

81. Screening for colorectal cancer—United States, 1992–1993, and new guidelines. MMWR 1996;45:107–110.

82. Brown ML, Potosky AL, Thompson GB, Kessler LG. The knowledge and use of screening tests for colorectal and prostate cancer: data from the 1987 National Health Interview Survey. Prev Med 1990;19:562–574.

25
Polyps

Marcus J. Burnstein and Terry C. Hicks

The word polyp refers to a macroscopically visible lesion or mass projecting from an epithelial surface. Polyp is a descriptive and nonspecific term—the specific diagnosis of a polyp is made by histopathologic examination. Polyps may be classified as neoplastic or nonneoplastic. Neoplastic polyps encompass epithelial tumors such as adenomas, polypoid adenocarcinomas, and carcinoid tumors, as well as nonepithelial lesions such as lipomas, leiomyomas, and lymphomatous polyps. Nonneoplastic polyps include hamartomas, hyperplastic polyps, and inflammatory polyps. Colorectal polyps may be further classified on the basis of clinical information as sporadic or hereditary, the latter category making up the polyposis syndromes discussed in Chapter 26.

Adenomas

The adenoma, a benign neoplasm of the epithelium, is the most common and most important colorectal polyp. Adenomas may be single or multiple, sporadic or hereditary. Adenomas are dysplastic and premalignant. Most adenocarcinomas arise from adenomas, and the removal of adenomas has been shown to be effective in decreasing the incidence of colorectal cancer.[1] It is the relationship between adenomas and adenocarcinomas that confers upon adenomas their tremendous clinical significance.

Clinical Presentation

Most adenomas are clinically silent and are found by screening or by investigation of symptoms unrelated to the adenoma. Large colonic adenomas may cause gross bleeding or may cause anemia secondary to occult blood loss. Large rectal adenomas, in addition to bleeding, may cause mucus discharge, tenesmus, and urgency. Mucus production in sufficient volume to cause electrolyte disturbances has been described. Distal rectal adenomas may rarely prolapse through the anus.

Colonoscopy is the most accurate test for polyps. The US National Polyp Study showed conclusively that colonoscopy is more accurate than double contrast barium enema for the diagnosis of colorectal polyps.[2] Barium enema detected a polyp in only 39% of cases in which one was subsequently found at colonoscopy. Even when a patient had a polyp ≥1 cm in diameter, the barium enema was negative in 52% of cases. The false-positive rate for barium enema was 14%. Computed tomography (CT) colonography (virtual colonoscopy) has a sensitivity for adenomas >1 cm of approximately 90% and for adenomas 0.6–0.9 cm of approximately 80%. The false-positive rate is 17%. CT colonography is an evolving technology and its role in screening is being defined. Virtual colonoscopy may be particularly useful in the evaluation of patients with incomplete colonoscopy.[3,4]

Pathology

Small adenomas are usually sessile (broad-based) and redder than the background mucosa. As polyps enlarge, some become pedunculated (attached to the bowel wall by a stalk of submucosa lined by normal mucosa) and some remain sessile, diffusely carpeting the bowel wall. The distribution of adenomas in the National Polyp Study was cecum 8%, ascending colon 9%, hepatic flexure 5%, transverse colon 10%, splenic flexure 4%, descending colon 14%, sigmoid 43%, and rectum 8%.[5] The likelihood of synchronous sporadic adenomas when one adenoma was found approached 40%.[6]

There are three main histologic subtypes of adenomas: tubular, villous, and tubulovillous. Tubular adenomas exhibit dysplastic tubules in ≥80% of the lesion. Villous adenomas have dysplastic villous fronds in ≥80% of the lesion. The finger-like villi are actually elongated crypts with a length that is more than twice the length of normal crypts. Tubulovillous adenomas have >20% tubular and <80% villous formation.[7] In the National Polyp Study, of 3358 sporadic colorectal adenomas, 87% were tubular, 5% villous, and 8% tubulovillous.[5]

In adenomas, cellular proliferation is not limited to the lower half of the tubule, as in normal colonic epithelium, and the normal process of cellular maturation and differentiation from the basal zone of the crypt to the surface of the lesion does not occur. Adenomas can be graded by the degree to which epithelial growth is disturbed. Mild dysplasia is characterized by tubules that are lined from top to bottom by epithelium that is morphologically similar to the normal basal proliferative zone. The nuclei are enlarged, oval, hyperchromatic, and normally oriented. There is a slight excess of mitotic figures but the architecture is not disrupted. In moderate dysplasia, the nuclear features are more advanced, cellular polarity is less preserved, there is nuclear stratification, and glands are more crowded. In severe dysplasia, there are large vesicular nuclei, irregular, and conspicuous nucleoli, scalloped nuclear membranes, and increased nuclear to cytoplasmic ratio. Nuclear polarity is disrupted and marked cellular pleomorphism and aberrant mitoses are present. Structural alterations include budding and branching tubules, back-to-back arrangement of glands, and cribriform growth of epithelial cells in clusters and sheets; mitotic figures are numerous. The terms carcinoma in situ and intramucosal carcinoma are often used to describe these severely dysplastic adenomas, but these terms are potentially misleading because these lesions do not have metastatic potential. Although the lymphatics of the colon and rectum are closely associated with the muscularis mucosa, only lesions that have invaded through the muscularis mucosa have the potential to metastasize. The dominant risk factors for invasive carcinoma, that is, cancer cells invading beyond the muscularis mucosa, are polyp size and villous histology.[8,9]

Dysplastic epithelium may become misplaced within the submucosa of a polyp and may mimic invasive cancer. This situation, called pseudo-invasion, is usually seen in pedunculated sigmoid polyps and is believed to be the result of torsion, ischemia, and architectural distortion. Pseudo-invasion is distinguished from invasive cancer by retention of lamina propria around the displaced glands, a lack of morphologic features of malignancy in the epithelium, and the presence of hemosiderin, indicating mucosal ischemia and hemorrhage.[10]

Epidemiology

Adenoma prevalence, the percentage of the population bearing one or more adenomas at a given point in time, is largely a function of age, gender, and family history.[11] Colonoscopy-determined prevalence rates in asymptomatic average risk individuals older than 50 years range from 24% to 47%.[12–15] Prevalence rates determined by colonoscopy are approximately double the rates determined by flexible sigmoidoscopy.[11] The prevalence rate approximately doubles from age 50 to 60, but does not clearly continue to increase with age, unlike the incidence of colorectal cancer. Higher prevalence rates have been identified in men, with a 1.5 relative risk compared with age-matched women.[12,13,15] A multicentered screening colonoscopy study examined the risk of colorectal adenomas in a cohort of individuals with one affected first-degree relative with sporadic colorectal cancer and found the odds ratio to be 1.5 for adenomas, 2.5 for large adenomas, 1.2 for small adenomas, and 2.6 for high-risk adenomas (see below).[16] The prevalence of adenomas is higher in relatives of individuals with colorectal cancer or adenoma at a young age, and in individuals with multiple relatives with cancer or adenomas.[17]

The incidence of adenomas is the rate at which individuals develop colorectal adenomas over a specified time interval.[11] The incidence of adenomas at intervals ranging from 6 months to 4 years in postpolypectomy surveillance colonoscopy studies varies from 30% to 50%.[18–21] Most incident polyps are small, and a higher incidence has been associated with polyp multiplicity at the index colonoscopy, increased size of the index polyp, older age, and a family history of a parent with colorectal cancer.[1,18,22–24]

The incidence rate after a clearing colonoscopy is actually the sum of the true incidence rate of new adenoma formation plus the miss rate at the initial colonoscopy, plus the recurrence rate of incompletely removed polyps.[11] Judged by repeat endoscopy, including studies with same-day back-to-back colonoscopies, the miss rate for adenomas ≥1 cm is approximately 5%, for adenomas 6–9 mm is approximately 10%, and for adenomas ≤5 mm approaches 30%.[25–28] The high miss rates for small lesions suggest that most adenomas detected on surveillance colonoscopy are actually lesions that were missed during the index examination. Incident polyps are distributed more proximally, consistent with the observation that miss rates for adenomas are higher in the proximal colon.[25] The miss rates must be kept in perspective; in postpolypectomy surveillance studies, the cancer incidence is low and in the National Polyp Study, colonoscopic surveillance was associated with a 76%–90% reduction in the cancer incidence compared with reference populations.[1]

More important than the overall incidence rate is the incidence rate for advanced adenomas, defined as polyps ≥1 cm in size or containing high-grade dysplasia, or containing appreciable villous tissue.[29] The incidence rate for advanced adenomas ranges from 6% to 9%[29] and is closely related to the findings at initial colonoscopy. Three or more polyps at the initial colonoscopy has been shown to increase the risk of subsequent advanced adenomas, and in the National Polyp Study, age >60 years plus a family history of a parent with colorectal cancer was also a predictor of incident advanced adenomas.[30] The cumulative incidence of advanced adenomas at 3 and 6 years of follow-up in the National Polyp Study in the highest risk group (three or more adenomas at baseline, or age ≥60 years plus a parent with colorectal cancer) were 10% and 20%, respectively.[30] The lowest risk group (only one adenoma and age <60 years at baseline) had an incidence of advanced adenomas of <1% at both 3- and 6-year follow-up. The 5-year incidence of advanced adenomas in individuals with a previously negative colonoscopy is also <1%.[31]

The appearance of incident cancers at short intervals in patients who have had a clearing colonoscopy suggests that either a neoplasm was missed or that cancer developed rapidly. Aggressive adenomas have been recognized in hereditary non-polyposis colorectal cancer, a condition in which patients may go from a normal colonoscopy to an established cancer in 1–3 years.[18,32,33] These cancers show a phenotype called microsatellite instability (MSI), a feature that is also present in 15% of sporadic cancers. Sporadic cancers with high-frequency MSI (MSI-H) may have developed rapidly.[11]

Adenoma-carcinoma Sequence

The prevalence of sporadic adenomas in the general population ≥60 years is approximately 30%–40% but the lifetime risk of developing colorectal cancer in Western countries is 6% by age 85; this observation suggests that only a few adenomas become adenocarcinomas. The likelihood that a diminutive tubular adenoma will progress to become an adenocarcinoma is difficult to determine. One longitudinal study showed that over a 3- to 5-year period, only 4% of 213 adenomas measuring 2–15 mm increased in size.[34] Slow transformation of adenomas is suggested by the fact that the mean age of adenoma patients precedes the mean age of cancer patients by 7 years. A mathematical model suggested that it takes 2–3 years for an adenoma ≤5 mm to grow to 1 cm, and another 2–5 years for the 1-cm adenoma to progress to cancer.[35] For a lesion ≥1 cm, the cancer probability is 3%, 8%, and 24% after 5, 10, and 20 years, respectively.[36] Overall, the yearly rate of conversion from adenoma to carcinoma has been estimated to be 0.25%, but the risk is higher for polyps >1 cm (3%) for villous adenomas (17%) and for adenomas with high-grade dysplasia (37%).[37]

In a study that analyzed 7590 adenomatous polyps to determine risk factors for high-grade dysplasia or invasion, size was the strongest predictor.[9] The percent of adenomas with high-grade dysplasia or invasive cancer based on the size of the polyp was: <5 mm, 3.4%; 5–10 mm, 13.5%; and >10 mm, 38.5%. Villous change, left-sided lesions, and age ≥60 years were also associated with advanced histologic features; no invasive cancer was found in polyps ≤5 mm.

On a molecular level, a simplified view of the traditional pathway from adenoma to adenocarcinoma is as follows: adenoma development is dependent on an individual epithelial cell having both copies of the *APC* gene deactivated.[38] This feature seems to allow for mutations in additional oncogenes, the key targets being *K-ras, DCC, P53*.[39] The accumulation of molecular abnormalities is associated with the development of invasive cancer. This pathway is the predominant pathway of colorectal carcinogenesis and is what is seen in familial adenomatous polyposis. Not all colorectal cancer follows the adenoma-carcinoma pathway, and alternate pathways to colorectal cancer are increasingly recognized. These pathways may involve polypoid lesions such as the hyperplastic polyp, the mixed polyp, and the serrated adenoma.

In hereditary nonpolyposis colorectal cancer (HNPCC), patients inherit a mutated copy of a DNA mismatch repair (MMR) gene. When the second copy is inactivated, loss of MMR function results in the development of mutations throughout the gene. The accumulation of mutations is associated with the rapid evolution of adenocarcinoma, often without a recognizable precursor lesion. When there is a precursor lesion for an HNPCC cancer, it is often a typical adenoma, but hyperplastic polyps and mixed polyps with distinct components of hyperplastic and adenomatous polyps have been implicated in some HNPCC cancers.[40–42]

Management

When an adenoma is found, every effort should be made to do a complete colonoscopy to the cecum because of the high rate of synchronous neoplasms in patients with adenomas and adenocarcinomas. However, the significance of a single, small (<1 cm) tubular adenoma on a screening flexible sigmoidoscopy is controversial. Most studies of screening flexible sigmoidoscopy suggest that patients with no distal polyps, distal hyperplastic polyps, or single small tubular adenomas have a similar low risk of proximal advanced adenomas, in the range of 0%–4%. Multiple studies support the recommendation that villous polyps regardless of size and adenomas >1 cm are important markers for the presence of advanced adenomas and carcinoma in the proximal colon.[43]

The majority of colorectal polyps are treated by endoscopic snare polypectomy; polyp removal is performed using electrocautery snare. As current is delivered to the snare, heat is generated in the encircled tissue which is cut and coagulated. The polyp is transected as the snare is tightened. The degree of thermal damage must balance the need for vessel coagulation with the need to avoid full-thickness injury to the bowel wall. The colon wall is thin, varying from 1.7 to 2.2 mm.[44] The mucosa, submucosa, and muscularis propria each contribute approximately one-third to the thickness of the wall. Injection of saline solution (with or without epinephrine) into the submucosa, increases the distance between the mucosa and the muscularis propria and increases the safety of endoscopic polypectomy.[45] Submucosal injection is most often used for sessile polyps in the right colon, especially those >1.5 cm in diameter. The addition of dye, such as methylene blue, to the injected solution may make it easier to recognize the edges of the polyp. Injection volumes range from a few milliliters to 30 mL. Sessile polyps >2 cm are often best dealt with by a piecemeal approach. Tissue is retrieved for histologic analysis which should include the histologic type of polyp, degree of dysplasia, and status of the margins. Even small polyps should be removed. For some small polyps, a specimen for histologic examination may be most efficiently obtained and the lesion most safely eradicated by cold biopsy or cold snare, that is, without current.

The technical aspects of colonoscopy, including the potential complications of this procedure, are reviewed in Chapter 5. Some technical tips in polypectomy include[45]:

- Aspiration of gas and decreasing wall tension may facilitate placing the snare around the polyp.
- Position the polyp at 5–6 o'clock; the snare enters the field at this orientation and makes it easier to capture the polyp.
- Perform polypectomy on withdrawal when the scope is "straight"—this method increases the effectiveness of tip deflection and scope rotation.
- Use submucosal injection of saline for large (>1.5–2 cm) sessile lesions; begin the injection on the proximal aspect of the polyp, thereby tilting the lesion toward the scope.
- In piecemeal polypectomy, start on the proximal aspect; a spike-tip snare allows the snare to be anchored so that pushing the sheath causes the snare loop to widen for more effective placement.
- Retrieval of proximal lesions is best accomplished with a device such as a Roth basket (US Endoscopy Group, Mentor, OH); smaller polyps may be suctioned into a trap; distal lesions may be suctioned onto the end of the scope.

Almost all polyps can be safely endoscopically removed, but if the polyp appears to be malignant, snare polypectomy may not be possible, and is generally inadvisable. Malignancy should be suspected in the setting of irregular surface contour, ulceration, friability, firm or hard consistency, thickening of the stalk, and nonlifting with submucosal injection (a feature of submucosal invasion or fibrosis from previous attempts at polypectomy).[45,46] It is particularly important that if polypectomy is performed for a suspicious polyp, the site of the polyp should be precisely localized by tattooing the bowel wall with India ink or similar dye.

Some large polyps may not be amenable to polypectomy and are treated by colon resection; in these instances, a conventional oncologic resection should be done.

Rectal Adenomas

Sessile villous adenomas are usually encountered in the rectum and the larger lesions may not be amenable to snare polypectomy. Local excision or rectal resection may be required. For lesions in the lower half of the rectum, endoanal excision is generally performed. For more proximal lesions, transanal endoscopic microsurgery (TEM) may be appropriate. Larger lesions that extend too proximally for endoanal excision will usually be best managed by anterior resection. If the lesion extends into the anal canal, anterior resection with endoanal mucosectomy and hand-sewn coloanal anastomosis may be needed to restore intestinal continuity.

Preoperatively, the lesion should be evaluated with respect to the risk of containing invasive cancer. The best clinical clue to the presence of invasion is firmness on digital rectal examination, although previous attempts at removal can produce fibrosis.[47] Endoanal ultrasound and magnetic resonance imaging may be helpful, but sensitivity with respect to a small focus of submucosal invasion is low.

When invasive cancer is present, treatment will be determined primarily by the level and size of the lesion, the depth of mural penetration, and by any evidence of lymphatic metastases. More proximal rectal lesions will usually be treated by anterior resection. Selected small proximal lesions may be managed by TEM. More distal lesions will need either resection or local excision. If biopsy of a hard area reveals a poorly differentiated cancer, a resectional approach is recommended. Even small rectal cancers that are not poorly differentiated carry a risk of lymph node metastases. A study from Memorial Sloan-Kettering Cancer Center evaluated whether standard pathologic factors predicted lymph node metastases from small rectal cancers.[48] Of 318 patients with T1 or T2 rectal cancers who underwent rectal resection, 159 patients were considered potentially eligible for local excision. Even in the absence of poor pathologic factors (advanced T stage, poorly differentiated histology, lymphatic or vascular invasion), 15% of patients had lymph node metastases.

The technical aspects of TEM and endoanal excision are discussed in Chapter 30.

Surveillance

After polypectomy of large or multiple adenomas (three or more) or advanced adenomas, cancer risk is increased three- to fivefold.[49] The risk of subsequent cancer is not measurably increased in patients with only one or two small tubular adenomas.[22,50] The National Polyp Study determined that colonoscopy performed 3 years after initial polypectomy protects patients as well as more frequent examinations.[1] Recommendations for surveillance postpolypectomy are based on the estimated risk of metachronous neoplasia[51,52]:

- After colon clearance, first follow-up colonoscopy in 3 years (for most patients).
- First follow-up colonoscopy in 5 years for low-risk patients [fewer than three small (<1 cm) tubular adenomas, no significant family history of colorectal cancer or adenomas].
- If first follow-up examination is negative, second follow-up colonoscopy in 5 years.
- Earlier follow-up colonoscopy for selected patients with multiple or large sessile adenomas.
- Individualize for age and comorbidity. (After removal of a small tubular adenoma, no follow-up may be indicated in elderly patients, or for those individuals with significant comorbidity, or the first follow-up can be delayed for 5 years.)

For large sessile polyps (>3 cm), there is a significant recurrence rate after endoscopic polypectomy. Even when the endoscopist believes that the entire polyp has been removed, follow-up examination reveals residual polyp in approximately 50%. There should be close follow-up, for example, every 3–6 months in the first year, every 6–12 months in the second year, and yearly to the fifth year. Treating the base and edge of the polypectomy defect with the argon plasma coagulator has been shown to decrease the incidence of residual polyp.[53]

The Malignant Polyp

Polyps with cancer cells penetrating the muscularis mucosa are malignant polyps. Invasion is invariably limited to the submucosa. In terms of TNM classification, these are T1NxMx lesions. Malignant polyps (T1 lesions) account for 2%–12% of polyps in colonoscopic polypectomy series.[54–56] The risk of malignancy related to adenoma size in one large series was 0.6–1.5 cm, 2%; 1.6–2.5 cm, 19%; 2.6–3.5 cm, 43%; and >3.5 cm, 76%.[54]

The clinical decision to proceed with further treatment, such as resection or local excision, depends on the estimated risk of lymph node metastases and the patient's general condition.[57] The main determinant of the risk of lymph node metastasis is the depth or level of invasion of cancer within the polyp. Haggitt's classification[58] of malignant polyps (Figure 25-1) is based on the level of invasion:

Level 0: noninvasive (severe dysplasia)
Level 1: cancer invading through the muscularis mucosa but limited to the head of a pedunculated polyp
Level 2: cancer invading the neck of a pedunculated polyp
Level 3: cancer invading the stalk of a pedunculated polyp
Level 4: cancer invading into the submucosa of the bowel wall below the stalk of a pedunculated polyp. All sessile polyps with invasive cancer are level 4.

The stalk of a pedunculated polyp is covered by normal mucosa and has a central core of submucosa. A line drawn at the junction of normal and adenomatous epithelium is the transition between the stalk and the head of the polyp. The junction zone is called the neck.

Kudo[59] has stratified the depth of submucosal invasion into three levels (Figure 25-2):

SM1: invasion into the upper third of the submucosa
SM2: invasion into the middle third of the submucosa
SM3: invasion into the lower third of the submucosa

Haggitt levels 1, 2, and 3 are SM1; Haggitt level 4 may be SM1, SM2, or SM3.

The risk of lymph node metastases is <1% for pedunculated polyps with Haggitt level 1, 2, or 3.[58,60,61] The risk of lymph node metastases for Haggitt level 4 lesions, pedunculated or sessile, ranges from 12% to 25%.[62–64] Factors reported to be associated with an increased risk of lymph node metastases include lymphovascular invasion,[48,63] poor differentiation,[48,65,66] gender,[48] extensive budding, microaci-

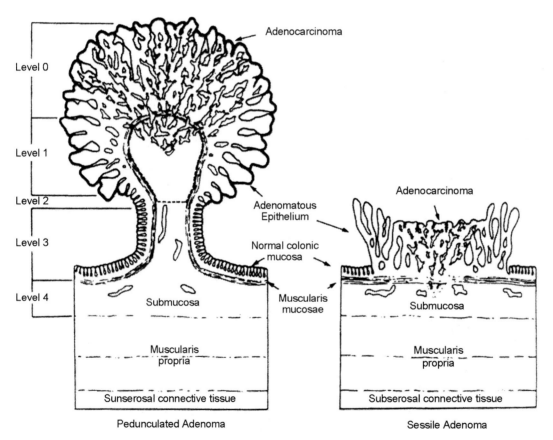

FIGURE 25-1. Anatomic landmarks of pedunculated and sessile malignant polyps. (Reprinted from Haggitt et al.,[58] copyright 1985, with permission from the American Gastroenterological Association.)

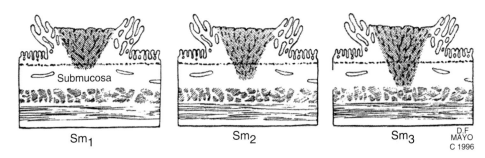

FIGURE 25-2. Depth of submucosal invasion in sessile malignant polyps. Sm_1: invasion into upper third; Sm_2: invasion into middle third; Sm_3: invasion into lower third. (Reprinted from Nivatvongs S. Surgical management of early colorectal cancer. Surg Clin North Am 2000;82:1052–1055, copyright 2000, with permission from Elsevier.)

nar structure,[67] flat or depressed lesions,[66] and SM3 level of invasion.[57,62,68] In a series of 353 T1 sessile cancers, the risk factors for lymph node metastasis that were statistically significant on multivariate analysis were SM3 level of invasion, lymphovascular invasion, and location in the lower third of the rectum.[62] In another study, only SM3 invasion was an independent risk factor for lymph node metastases.[68]

The rate of lymph node metastases from rectal lesions is not different than from colon lesions. However, T1 lesions in the distal third of the rectum have been found to have a higher risk of lymph node metastases than more proximal rectal lesions.[62] This finding is consistent with the high local recurrence rates, in the range of 5% to 28%, which have been observed after full-thickness local excision of T1 lesions of the distal rectum.[48,65,69,70]

A positive polypectomy margin should not be considered an adverse risk factor for recurrence—in general, this should be regarded as inadequate treatment. A distance of 2 mm beyond the deepest level of invasion is needed to consider the margin clear.[57]

In view of the risk of lymph node metastases of <1%, pedunculated polyps with invasion to Haggitt levels 1 to 3 are safely treated by snare polypectomy. Level 4 pedunculated lesions are treated as sessile lesions. Sessile lesions that are snared in one piece and have a margin of at least 2 mm are considered adequately treated.[57] If a piecemeal polypectomy was performed, margins cannot be adequately assessed and further treatment is needed. High-risk sessile lesions such as lesions with SM3, lymphovascular invasion, poor differentiation, and those in the lower third of the rectum should have an oncologic resection. For lower rectal lesions, full-thickness endoanal excision with adjuvant chemoradiation is an alternative approach. Nivatvongs's summary of the indications for oncologic resection are presented in Table 25-1.

Close endoscopic follow-up is required to look for local recurrence. A reasonable schedule is to examine the polypectomy site in 2–3 months and then every 6 months for the first 2 years; complete colonoscopy is done in the third year, and then at 3-year intervals.

Chemoprevention after polypectomy to inhibit adenoma recurrence cannot yet be recommended. Prospective randomized intervention trials have not been supportive of this approach. The role of chemoprevention is reviewed in Chapter 23.

Specific Adenomas

Flat and Depressed Adenomas

Some adenomas display a flat or depressed growth pattern and are not elevated above the mucosal surface; they are not "true polyps."[71] These lesions are recognized by color and textural changes, and by interruption of the capillary network pattern.[71,72] They are most readily identified by chromoendoscopy, a technique in which the mucosa is sprayed with indigo carmine dye.[73] The incidence of flat and depressed adenomas in three Western population studies was approximately 20%, and these lesions contained cancer more often

TABLE 25-1. Summary of malignant colorectal polyps that should have an oncologic bowel resection

A. Lesions in colon
  a) Pedunculated Haggitt level 4 with invasion into distal third of submucosa, or pedunculated lesions with lymphovascular invasion
  b) Lesions removed with margin <2 mm
  c) Sessile lesions removed piecemeal
  d) Sessile lesions with depth of invasion into distal third of submucosa (Sm_3)
  e) Sessile lesions with lymphovascular invasion
B. Lesions in middle third and upper third rectum
  Same as lesions in colon
C. Lesions in distal third rectum
  a) Pedunculated Haggitt level 4 with invasion into distal third of submucosa, or pedunculated lesions with lymphovascular invasion
  b) All sessile lesions
An alternative may be a per anal full-thickness excision plus chemoradiation.

Source: Reprinted from Nivatvongs S. Surgical management of early colorectal cancer. Surg Clin North Am 2000;82:1052–1055, copyright 2000, with permission from Elsevier.

than polypoid adenomas.[74–76] In a large United Kingdom study of 1000 patients in which chromoendoscopy was used to search for small flat lesions, 36% of the 321 detected adenomas were flat or depressed.[74] The overall risk of a polypoid lesion containing early cancer was 8%, but was 14% for the flat lesions. Flat or depressed lesions that were >1 cm were about twice as likely as protruding lesions of a similar size to contain high-grade dysplasia or cancer. Twenty-nine percent of flat lesions >1 cm contained either high-grade dysplasia or cancer. The average size of advanced flat and depressed adenomas is smaller than that of their polypoid counterparts. Because of the risk of cancer, these small lesions should be removed, either by endoscopic polypectomy or by operative resection. It has been suggested that using special dyes and magnifying colonoscopy should be incorporated into general endoscopic practice.[71]

Serrated Adenomas

The serrated adenoma is a more recently recognized histologic phenotype of sporadic adenoma.[77] Serrated adenomas are uncommon, accounting for approximately 0.5%–1.3% of colorectal polyps.[78,79] Initially, serrated adenomas were described as hyperplastic polyps that contained adenomatous features. The serrated adenoma has serrated crypts that are longer and broader than in hyperplastic polyps. The crypts contain cells with enlarged hyperchromatic and stratified nuclei (as in adenomas) as well as cells with normally arranged, small, basal nuclei (as in hyperplastic polyps).[80,81]

It is unclear whether serrated adenomas develop in association with hyperplastic polyps or develop de novo. Both types of polyps are primarily found in the rectosigmoid region, and they have similar mucin characteristics. Endoscopically, most serrated adenoma look like hyperplastic polyps—pale, slightly protruding lesions, and most are in the range of 0.2–7.5 mm in diameter. Some serrated adenomas are larger and may resemble villous adenomas.

A pathway to colorectal cancer called the "serrated pathway" has been postulated, in which colorectal cancer develops through precursor lesions that have serrated glandular architecture. The serrated polyps include the mixed polyp, in addition to the hyperplastic and serrated adenoma. The mixed polyp is recognized by distinct areas of hyperplastic and adenomatous morphology.

The relationship between hyperplastic polyps, serrated adenomas, and cancer is not clear. In one report, 5.8% of colorectal cancers were associated with an adjacent serrated adenoma and some serrated adenomas harbor high-grade dysplasia.[79,82] A review concluded that the risk of high-grade dysplasia was the same in serrated adenomas as in the more common adenomatous phenotypes.[79] The serrated adenoma pathway may be a separate route to colon cancer characterized by methylation of promoter regions leading to switching off MMR genes, resulting in replication errors and ultimately to cancer. Hyperplastic polyps and serrated

adenomas show MSI in the absence of *APC* mutations. Individuals with sporadic colorectal cancer with high-level MSI cancers (MSI-H) are 4 times more likely to harbor at least one serrated polyp than individuals with low MSI cancers.[74]

Nonneoplastic Polyps

Hyperplastic Polyps

Hyperplastic polyps are the result of a failure of programmed cell death.[33,38,80,81] The epithelial cells differentiate and mature normally but accumulate on the mucosal surface producing small sessile elevations. Cellular crowding results in the characteristic microscopic appearance of tubules with a saw-tooth or serrated pattern. Mature goblet cells are the main cellular component of hyperplastic polyps, whereas adenomatous crypts have reduced numbers of goblet cells. The cytoplasm of hyperplastic polyps is eosinophilic on hematoxylin and eosin staining and the nuclei remain at the base with minimal stratification.

Hyperplastic polyps are the most common polyps found on flexible sigmoidoscopy. The true ratio of hyperplastic polyps to adenomas approximates 1:1. In a study of 1964 diminutive (≤5 mm) polyps, 41% were adenomas, 37% hyperplastic polyps, and 18% nonneoplastic. Combining histologic data from several studies of diminutive polyps revealed that 53% were adenomas and that approximately 0.5% had high-grade dysplasia; <0.1% contained invasive cancer.[43]

Most hyperplastic polyps are small (<3–5 mm in diameter), pale, usually located in the rectosigmoid region, and are almost always asymptomatic. Hyperplastic polyps are often multiple. Although hyperplastic and adenomatous polyps have characteristic appearances, biopsy is needed to make a diagnosis. Endoscopic diagnosis has a sensitivity of 80% and a specificity of 71%.[82] Chromoendoscopy can improve the endoscopist's ability to distinguish hyperplastic from adenomatous polyps. Hyperplastic polyps have a characteristic star-like pit pattern when stained with indigo carmine and assessed with a magnifying colonoscopy. Adenomatous polyps have surface grooves. The sensitivity and specificity of this technique in discriminating between adenomatous and nonadenomatous polyps was found to be 93% and 95%, respectively.[83]

Data conflict as to whether hyperplastic polyps found on a screening examination represent an increased risk of future neoplasia. Whereas some authors have suggested that left-sided hyperplastic polyps are predictors of proximal adenomas, the National Polyp Study found no association between left-sided hyperplastic polyps and synchronous adenomas. A report using data from two large chemoprevention studies demonstrated that hyperplastic polyps were not predictive of an increased risk of developing adenomatous polyps on follow-up colonoscopy.[84] The American College of Gastroenterology states that hyperplastic polyps found on flexible sigmoidoscopy are not an indication for colonoscopy.[85] There are no specific recommendations for treatment and follow-up of right-sided hyperplastic polyps.

Hyperplastic polyps have been implicated in some colorectal cancers, especially in HNPCC. HNPCC cancers arise through mutations in one of several MMR genes; sporadic colon cancer with defective MMR occurs as a result of deactivation of a single gene—*hMLH1*. Inactivation occurs through methylation of the *hMLH1* gene promoter. The molecular phenotype of abnormal MMR is MSI. MSI has been used to distinguish these high-level MSI cancers (MSI-H) from cancers with low or no level of MSI, as seen in *APC*-related cancers.[86] A strong association of MSI-H cancers with residual adenomas has not been observed.[87] Sporadic adenocarcinomas arising through the defective MMR pathway (MSI-H adenocarcinoma) occur in older patients (>70 years), have a female gender bias, and are predominantly located in the right colon.[88] The vast majority lack *APC* mutations. These MSI-H cancers can be associated with large hyperplastic polyps, and analysis of these combined lesions demonstrates that both the cancer component and the hyperplastic polyp epithelial cells lack *hMLH1* expression. This suggests that hyperplastic polyps may serve as fertile soil for gene-specific hypermethylation leading to knockout of *hMLH1* and loss of DNA MMR function.[33,38]

Carriers of hyperplastic polyps clearly at increased risk for colorectal cancer are those with the hereditary syndrome of hyperplastic polyposis. This syndrome is diagnosed if multiple (>30) or large (>10 mm) hyperplastic polyps are found, especially in the proximal colon, with a positive family history of hyperplastic polyposis. The syndrome is thought to be very rare. Reports of patients with hyperplastic polyposis syndrome showed an average age of 52 years, >100 polyps in half the cases, and an average polyp diameter of 16 mm (range, 5–45 mm), and half the reported patients also had a cancer (half of these in the right colon).There are no general guidelines for the management of hyperplastic polyps or the hyperplastic polyposis syndrome.[80,81] (see Chapter 26).

Hamartomas

Juvenile polyps are hamartomas, localized overgrowths of normal mature cells. Most juvenile polyps are round, pink, smooth, and pedunculated, although some are small and sessile. Juvenile polyps are composed of dilated mucus-filled cystic spaces surrounded by lamina propria which has a mesenchymal appearance with inflammatory cells and eosinophils. The muscularis mucosa does not participate in the formation of a juvenile polyp, and the unique potential of these lesions to twist and "auto-amputate" has been ascribed to the absence of supporting muscle fibers. Most juvenile polyps present in childhood, but they may present in infancy or in adulthood. Usually, only one or two polyps are found. Up to three polyps may be seen in nonfamilial conditions. Symptoms include rectal bleeding, mucus discharge, diarrhea, and abdominal pain, intussusception and prolapse of a polyp through the anus. Treatment is snare polypectomy.

Numerous hamartomatous polyps are present in juvenile polyposis syndrome, Peutz-Jeghers syndrome, Cowden disease, and Cronkhite-Canada Syndrome. Although sporadic hamartomatous polyps are not dysplastic and are not believed to be premalignant, the syndromes of hamartomatous polyposis have a significant rate of cancer development. These syndromes are discussed in Chapter 26.

Inflammatory Polyps

Inflammatory or pseudopolyps (a misnomer) are associated with colitis, most often ulcerative colitis and Crohn's disease, but can result from any form of severe colonic inflammation. The inflammatory polyp is a remnant or island of normal or minimally inflamed mucosa. The presence of inflammatory polyps in inflammatory bowel disease is not associated with dysplasia or cancer risk. Inflammatory polyps are almost always multiple. Treatment is directed at the underlying bowel disease.

Lymphoid Polyps

Benign enlargements of lymphoid follicles may produce polyps that are usually seen in the rectum. The overlying mucosa is normal. The lesions are typically multiple; their cause is unknown. Histologic criteria for establishing the benign nature of lymphoid polyps have been described: lymphoid tissue is entirely within the mucosa and submucosa; there is no invasion of the muscularis propria; at least two germinal centers must be seen; if the specimen does not include the muscle coat and no germinal centers are seen, then the diagnosis of lymphoid polyp cannot be made.

Lipomas, leiomyomas, lymphoma, hemangiomas, and carcinoid tumors are discussed in Chapter 37.

References

1. Winawer SJ, Zauber AG, Ho MN, et al. Prevention of colorectal cancer by colonoscopic polypectomy. The National Polyp Study Workgroup. N Engl J Med 1993;329:1977–1981.
2. Winawer SJ, Stewart ET, Zauber AG, et al. A comparison of colonoscopy and double-contrast barium enema for surveillance after polypectomy. National Polyp Study Work Group. N Engl J Med 2000;342:1766–1772.
3. Fenlon HM, Nunes DT, Schroy PC III, et al. A comparison of virtual and conventional colonoscopy for the detection of colorectal polyps. N Engl J Med 1999;341:1496–1503.
4. Hara AK. The future of colorectal imaging: computed tomographic colonography. Gastroenterol Clin North Am 2002;31:1045–1060.
5. Winawer SJ, Fletcher RH, Miller L, et al. Colorectal cancer screening: clinical guidelines and rationale. Gastroenterology 1997;112:594–642.
6. Bond JH. Polyp guideline: diagnosis, treatment, and surveillance for patients with nonfamilial colorectal polyps. The Practice

Parameters Committee of the American College of Gastroenterology. Ann Intern Med 1993;119:836–843.

7. Rubio CA, Jaramillo E, Lindblom A, et al. Classification of colorectal polyps: guidelines for the endoscopist. Endoscopy 2002; 34:226–236.

8. Simons BD, Morrison AS, Lev R, et al. Relationship of polyps to cancer of the large intestine. J Natl Cancer Inst 1992;84: 962–966.

9. Gschwantler M, Kriwanek S, Langner E, et al. High-grade dysplasia and invasive carcinoma in colorectal adenomas: a multivariate analysis of the impact of adenoma and patient characteristics. Eur J Gastroenterol Hepatol 2002;14:183–188.

10. Muto T, Bussey HJR, Morson BC. Pseudo-carcinomatous invasion in adenomatous polyps of the colon and rectum. J Clin Pathol 1973;26:25–31.

11. Villavicencio RT, Rex DK. Colonic adenomas: prevalence and incidence rates, growth rates, and miss rates at colonoscopy. Semin Gastrointest Dis 2000;11:185–193.

12. Lieberman DS, Smith FW. Screening for colon malignancy with colonoscopy. Am J Gastroenterol 1991;86:946–951.

13. Foutch PG, Mai H, Pardy K, et al. Flexible sigmoidoscopy may be ineffective for secondary prevention of colorectal cancer in asymptomatic, average-risk men. Dig Dis Sci 1991;36:924–928.

14. Johnson DA, Gurney MS, Volpe RJ, et al. A prospective study of the prevalence of colonoscopic neoplasms in asymptomatic patients with an age-related risk. Am J Gastroenterol 1990;85: 969–974.

15. Rex DK, Lehman GA, Ulbright TM, et al. Colonic neoplasia in asymptomatic persons with negative fecal occult blood tests: influence of age, gender and family history. Am J Gastroenterol 1993;88:825–831.

16. Pariente A, Milan C, Lafon J, et al. Colonoscopic screening in first-degree relatives of patients with "sporadic" colorectal cancer: a case-control study. The Association Nationale des Gastro-enterologues des Hopitaux and Registre Bourguinon des Cancers Digestifs (INSERM CRI 9505). Gastroenterology 1998;115: 7–12.

17. Gaglia P, Atkin WS, Whitelaw S, et al. Variables associated with the risk of colorectal adenomas in asymptomatic patients with a family history of colorectal cancer. Gut 1995;36:385–390.

18. Rex DK. Colonoscopy: a review of its yield for cancers and adenomas by indication. Am J Gastroenterol 1995;90:353–365.

19. Schatzkin A, Lanza E, Corle D, et al. Lack of effect of a low-fat, high-fiber diet on the recurrence of colorectal adenomas. Polyp Prevention Trial Study Group. N Engl J Med 2000;342: 1149–1155.

20. Triantafyllou K, Papatheodoridis GV, Paspatis GA, et al. Predictors of the early development of advanced metachronous colon adenomas. Hepatogastroenterology 1997;44:533–538.

21. Alberts DS, Martinez ME, Roe DJ, et al. Lack of effect of a high-fiber cereal supplement on the recurrence of colorectal adenomas. Phoenix Colon Cancer Prevention Physicians' Network. N Engl J Med 2000;342:1156–1162.

22. Noshirwani KC, van Stolk RU, Rybicki LA, et al. Adenoma size and number are predictive of adenoma recurrence: implications for surveillance colonoscopy. Gastrointest Endosc 2000;51(4 pt 1): 433–437.

23. Holtzman R, Poulard JB, Bank S, et al. Repeat colonoscopy after endoscopic polypectomy. Dis Colon Rectum 1987;30: 185–188.

24. Woolfson IK, Eckholdt GJ, Wetzel CR, et al. Usefulness of performing colonoscopy one year after endoscopic polypectomy. Dis Colon Rectum 1990;33:389–393.

25. Rex DK, Cutler CS, Lemmel GT, et al. Colonoscopic miss rates of adenomas determined by back-to-back colonoscopies. Gastroenterology 1997;112:24–28.

26. Hoff G, Vatn M. Epidemiology of polyps of the rectum and sigmoid colon. Endoscopic evaluation of size and localization of polyps. Scand J Gastroenterol 1985;20:356–360.

27. Kronborg O, Hage E, Deichgraeber E. A prospective, partly randomized study of the effectiveness of repeated examination of the colon after polypectomy and radical surgery for cancer. Scand J Gastroenterol 1981;16:879–884.

28. Hixson LS, Fennerty MB, Sampliner RE, et al. Prospective study of the frequency and size distribution of polyps missed by colonoscopy. J Natl Cancer Inst 1990;82:1769–1772.

29. Leiberman DA, Weiss DG, Bond JH, et al. Use of colonoscopy to screen asymptomatic adults for colorectal cancer. Veterans Affairs Cooperative Study Group 380. N Engl J Med 2000;343: 162–168.

30. Winawer SJ. Appropriate intervals for surveillance. Gastrointest Endosc 1999;49(3 pt 2):S63–S66.

31. Rex DK, Cummings OW, Helper DJ, et al. Five-year incidence of adenomas after negative colonoscopy in asymptomatic average-risk persons. Gastroenterology 1996;111:1178–1181.

32. Jarvinen HJ, Aarnio M, Mustonen H, et al. Controlled 15-year trial on screening for colorectal cancer in families with hereditary nonpolyposis colorectal cancer. Gastroenterology 2000;118: 829–834.

33. Jass JR. Pathogenesis of colorectal cancer. Surg Clin North Am 2002;82:891–904.

34. Knoernschild HE. Growth rate and malignant potential of colonic polyps: early results. Surg Forum 1963;14:137–138.

35. Carroll RLA, Klein M. How often should patients be sigmoidoscoped? A mathematical perspective. Prev Med 1980;9:741–746.

36. Stryker SJ, Wolff BG, Culp CE, et al. Natural history of untreated colonic polyps. Gastroenterology 1987;93:1009–1013.

37. Eide TJ. Risk of colorectal cancer in adenoma-bearing individuals within a defined population. Int J Cancer 1986;38:173–176.

38. Lamlum H, Papadopoulou A, Ilyas M, et al. APC mutations are sufficient for the growth of early colorectal adenomas. Proc Natl Acad Sci USA 2000;97:2225–2228.

39. Konishi M, Kikuchi-Yanoshita R, Tanaka K, et al. Molecular nature of colon tumors in hereditary nonpolyposis colon cancer, familial polyposis, and sporadic colon cancer. Gastroenterology 1996;111:307–317.

40. Burgart LJ. Colorectal polyps and other precursor lesions. Need for an expanded view. Gastroenterol Clin North Am 2002;31: 959–970.

41. Hawkins NJ, Ward RL. Sporadic colorectal cancers with microsatellite instability and their possible origin in hyperplastic polyps and serrated adenomas. J Natl Cancer Inst 2001;93: 1307–1313.

42. Jass JR, Kottier DS, Pokos V, et al. Mixed epithelial polyps in association with hereditary non-polyposis colorectal cancer providing an alternative pathway of cancer histogenesis. Pathology 1997;29:28–33.

43. Farraye FA, Wallace M. Clinical significance of small polyps found during screening with flexible sigmoidoscopy. Gastrointest Endosc Clin North Am 2002;12:41–51.

44. Tsuga K, Haruma K, Fujimura J, et al. Evaluation of the colorectal wall in normal subjects and patients with ulcerative colitis using an ultrasonic catheter probe. Gastrointest Endosc 1998; 48:477–484.

45. Waye JD. Endoscopic mucosal resection of colonic polyps. Gastrointest Endosc Clin North Am 2001;11:537–548, vii.

46. Uno Y, Munakata A. The non-lifting sign of invasive colon cancer. Gastrointest Endosc 1994;40:485–489.

47. Nivatvongs S, Nicholson JD, Rothenberger DA, et al. Villous adenomas of the rectum: the accuracy of clinical assessment. Surgery 1980;87:549–551.

48. Blumberg D, Paty PB, Guillem JG, et al. All patients with small intramural rectal cancers are at risk for lymph node metastases. Dis Colon Rectum 1999;42:881–885.

49. Atkin WS, Morson BC, Cuzick J. Long-term risk of colorectal cancer after excision of rectosigmoid adenomas. N Engl J Med 1992;326:658–662.

50. Spencer RJ, Melton LJ III, Ready RL, et al. Treatment of small colorectal polyps: a population based study of risks of subsequent carcinoma. Mayo Clin Proc 1984;59:305–310.

51. Bond JH. Colorectal cancer update. Prevention, screening, treatment and surveillance for high-risk groups. Med Clin North Am 2000;84:1163–1182, viii.

52. Bond JH. Colon polyps and cancer. Endoscopy 2003;35:27–35.

53. Zlatanic J, Waye JD, Kim PS, et al. Large sessile colonic adenomas: use of argon plasma coagulator to supplement piecemeal snare polypectomy. Gastrointest Endosc 1999;49:731–735.

54. Nusko G, Mansmann U, Partzsch U, et al. Invasive carcinoma in colorectal adenomas: multivariate analysis of patient and adenoma characteristics. Endoscopy 1997;29:626–631.

55. Hermanek P, Gall FP. Early (microinvasive) colorectal carcinoma: pathology diagnosis surgical treatment. Int J Colorectal Dis 1986;1:79–84.

56. Nivatvongs S. Complications in colonoscopic polypectomy: an experience with 1,555 polypectomies. Dis Colon Rectum 1986;29:825–830.

57. Nivatvongs S. Surgical management of malignant colorectal polyps. Surg Clin North Am 2002;82:959–966.

58. Haggitt RC, Glotzbach RE, Soffer EE, et al. Prognostic factors in colorectal carcinomas arising in adenomas: implications for lesions removed by endoscopic polypectomy. Gastroenterology 1985;89:328–336.

59. Kudo S. Endoscopic mucosal resection of flat and depressed types of early colorectal cancer. Endoscopy 1993;25:455–461.

60. Kyzer S, Begin LR, Gordon PH, et al. The care of patients with colorectal polyps that contain invasive adenocarcinoma: endoscopic polypectomy or colectomy. Cancer 1992;70:2044–2050.

61. Nivatvongs S, Rojanasakul A, Reiman ME, et al. The risk of lymph node metastases in colorectal polyps with invasive adenocarcinoma. Dis Colon Rectum 1991;34:323–328.

62. Nascimbeni R, Burgart LG, Nivatvongs S, et al. Risk of lymph node metastases in T1 carcinoma of colon and rectum. Dis Colon Rectum 2002;45:200–206.

63. Cooper HS, Deppisch LM, Gourley WK, et al. Endoscopically removed malignant colorectal polyps: clinical pathologic correlations. Gastroenterology 1995;108:1657–1665.

64. Coverlizza S, Risio M, Ferrari A, et al. Colorectal adenomas containing invasive carcinoma: pathologic assessment of lymph node metastatic potential. Cancer 1989;64:1937–1947.

65. Brodsky JT, Richard GK, Cohen AM, et al. Variables correlated with the risk of lymph node metastases in early rectal cancer. Cancer 1992;69:322–326.

66. Tanaka S, Harouma K, Teixeira CR, et al. Endoscopic treatment of submucosal invasive colorectal carcinoma with special reference to risk factors for lymph node metastases. J Gastroenterol 1995;30:710–717.

67. Goldstein NS, Hart J. Histologic features associated with lymph node metastases in stage T1 and superficial T2 rectal adenocarcinomas in abdominoperineal resection specimens. Identifying a subset of patients for whom treatment with adjuvant therapy or completion abdominoperineal resection should be considered after local excision. Am J Clin Pathol 1999;111:51–58.

68. Kikuchi R, Takano M, Takagi K, et al. Management of early invasive colorectal cancer: risk of recurrence and clinical guidelines. Dis Colon Rectum 1995;38:1286–1295.

69. Garcia-Aguilar J, Mellgren A, Sirivongs P, et al. Local excision of rectal cancer without adjuvant therapy: a word of caution. Ann Surg 2000;231:345–351.

70. Chakravarti A, Compton CC, Shellito PC, et al. Long-term follow-up of patients with rectal cancer managed by local excision with and without adjuvant irradiation. Ann Surg 1999;230: 49–54.

71. Reinacher-Schick A, Schmiegel W. Surveillance strategies in patients after polypectomy. Dig Dis 2002;20:61–69.

72. Muto T, Kamiya J, Sawada T, et al. Small "flat adenoma" of the large bowel with special reference to its clinicopathologic features. Dis Colon Rectum 1985;28:847–851.

73. Jaramillo E, Watanabe M, Slezak P, et al. Flat neoplastic lesions of the colon and rectum detected by high-resolution video endoscopy and chromoscopy. Gastrointest Endosc 1995;42:114–122.

74. Rembacken BJ, Fujii T, Cairns A, et al. Flat and depressed colonic neoplasms: a prospective study of 1000 colonoscopies in the UK. Lancet 2000;355:1211–1214.

75. Saitoh Y, Waxman I, West AB, et al. Prevalence and distinctive biologic features of flat colorectal adenomas in the North American population. Gastroenterology 2001;120:1657–1665.

76. Smith GA, Oien KA, O'Dwyer PJ. Frequency of early colorectal cancer in patients undergoing colonoscopy. Br J Surg 1999;86: 1328–1331.

77. Estrada RG, Spjut HJ. Hyperplastic polyps of the large bowel. Am J Surg Pathol 1980;4:127–133.

78. Longacre TA, Fenoglio-Preiser CM. Mixed hyperplastic adenomatous polyps/serrated adenomas. A distinct form of colorectal neoplasia. Am J Surg Pathol 1990;14:524–537.

79. Matsumoto T, Mizuno M, Shimizu M, et al. Clinicopathological features of serrated adenoma of the colorectum: comparison with traditional adenoma. J Clin Pathol 1999;52:513–516.

80. Hawkins NJ, Bariol C, Ward RL. The serrated neoplasia pathway. Pathology 2002;34:548–555.

81. Rembacken BJ, Trecca A, Fujii T. Serrated adenomas. Dig Liver Dis 2001;33:305–312.

82. Norfleet RG, Ryan ME, Wyman JB. Adenomatous and hyperplastic polyps cannot be reliably distinguished by their appearance through the fiberoptic sigmoidoscope. Dig Dis Sci 1988;33:1175–1177.

83. Axelrad AM, Fleischer DE, Geller AJ, et al. High resolution chromoendoscopy for the diagnosis of diminutive colon polyps: implications for colon cancer screening. Gastroenterology 1996;110:1253–1258.

84. Bensen SP, Cole BF, Mott LA, et al. Colorectal hyperplastic polyps and risk of recurrence of adenomas and hyperplastic polyps. Polyp Prevention Study (Letter). Lancet 1999;354: 1873–1874.

85. Bond JH. Polyp guidelines: diagnosis, treatment, and surveillance for patients with colorectal polyps: Practice Parameters Committee of the American College of Gastroenterology. Am J Gastroenterol 2000;95:3053–3063.

86. Bowland CR, Thibodeau SN, Hamilton SR, et al. A National Cancer Institute Workshop on Microsatellite Instability for cancer detection and familial pre-disposition: development of international criteria for the determination of microsatellite instability in colorectal cancer. Cancer Res 1998;58:5248–5257.

87. Young J, Leggett B, Gustafson C, et al. Genomic instability occurs in colorectal carcinomas but not in adenomas. Hum Mutat 1993;2:351–354.

88. Cunningham JM, Kim CY, Christenson ER, et al. The frequency of hereditary defective mismatch repair in a prospective series of unselected colorectal carcinomas. Am J Hum Genet 2001;69: 780–790.

26
Polyposis Syndromes

Robin K.S. Phillips and Susan K. Clark

Multiple colorectal polyps occur in a number of conditions, including the inflammatory polyps of inflammatory bowel disease, intestinal lipomatosis, and neurofibromatosis. Usually these can all be identified histopathologically, and will not be discussed further in this chapter, but biopsy is always essential in polyposis syndromes or mistakes will be made.

Familial Adenomatous Polyposis

Familial adenomatous polyposis (FAP) is an autosomal dominantly inherited condition caused by mutation of the *APC* gene, which occurs with a frequency of about 1:10,000.[1] Mutation of this tumor suppressor gene results in a generalized disorder of tissue growth regulation and a range of clinical manifestations, principally the formation of multiple gastrointestinal adenomas and carcinomas, but also a variety of extraintestinal abnormalities.

In the past, FAP accounted for about 1% of all colorectal cancers, but an understanding of its inheritance, surveillance of at-risk family members, and the introduction of prophylactic large bowel resection have resulted in this contribution now being in the region of 0.05% in countries where such services are available.[2] Patients with a firm diagnosis of FAP or in whom it is suspected, together with their family, should be referred to a polyposis registry.

Polyposis Registries

The aim of polyposis registries is to provide counseling, support, and clinical services for families with FAP.[3] This includes thorough pedigree analysis and identification of at-risk family members, who are offered clinical surveillance and genetic testing so that those affected can be offered prophylactic surgery. Some registries also coordinate postoperative surveillance and provide a focal point for audit and research.

Observational studies suggest that the introduction of registries, together with the use of prophylactic surgery, has led to increased life expectancy and a dramatic reduction in the incidence of colorectal cancer in FAP.[2]

Features of FAP

The Large Bowel

The cardinal manifestation of FAP is the development of more than 100 colorectal adenomatous polyps, which inevitably progress to carcinoma if not removed (Figure 26-1). Polyps usually appear in adolescence, with colorectal cancer diagnosed at an average age of about 40 years. Although most patients have a family history of FAP, about 25% do not, their disease being attributable to a new mutation.[1] These individuals usually present with a symptomatic colorectal cancer or, more rarely, with anemia, rectal bleeding, or mucous discharge caused by benign polyps.

Extracolonic Manifestations

The extracolonic manifestations of FAP are shown in Table 26-1. Two of these, duodenal cancer and desmoid disease, have now emerged as the major sources of morbidity and mortality, exceeding colorectal cancer as cause of death[6] (Figure 26-2).

Other features may be a useful clue in diagnosis. Congenital hypertrophy of the retinal pigment epithelium (CHRPE), a patchy fundus discoloration, was considered a potential screening tool before advances in genetics. Isolated CHRPE is seen in normal people, but the presence of more than four is a specific phenotypic marker present in two-thirds of FAP families.[7]

Genetics

The APC Gene

APC is a large gene situated on chromosome 5q21. A genetic basis underlying the adenoma-carcinoma sequence in colorectal carcinogenesis has been elucidated,[8] and subsequent studies have confirmed that in both FAP and the majority of

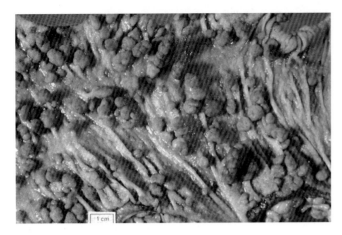

FIGURE 26-1. The large bowel in classical familial adenomatous polyposis.

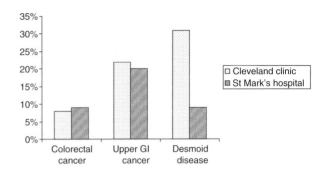

FIGURE 26-2. FAP-related cause of death in patients after prophylactic colectomy.

sporadic colorectal cancers, mutation of the *APC* gene is one of the earliest events.

More than 500 germline mutations causing FAP have been identified, almost all resulting in truncation of the APC protein product.[9] Mutations have been found between codons 168 (exon 4) and 2839 (exon 15), but most are between codons 168 and 1640 (exon 15) in the 5' half of the coding region, with a particular concentration at two "hotspots," codons 1061 and 1309.

The APC Protein

APC is ubiquitously expressed, but the mRNA is found at particularly high levels in normal colonic mucosa[10] and in many epithelia is only found when cell replication has ceased and terminal differentiation is established.[11]

The 300-kDa APC protein is found in the cytoplasm and has sites of interaction with a range of other proteins including β-catenin and the cytoskeleton. It has a central role in the highly conserved Wnt signaling pathway, which has functions in the normal development of three-dimensional structures and is abnormally activated in some malignancies. APC binds and down-regulates cytoplasmic β-catenin, preventing its translocation to the nucleus. Abnormal APC protein fails to do this, so that β-catenin is free to enter the nucleus and form a complex which results in specific transcription of cell cycle stimulating DNA sequences, and hence proliferation.[12]

Genotype-phenotype Correlation in FAP

There is evidence of correlation between the position of the germline *APC* mutation (genotype) and some aspects of the phenotype in patients with FAP (Figure 26-3). Mutation at codon 1309 is associated with particularly large numbers of colonic polyps,[13] and between codon 1250 and 1464 with earlier onset of, and death from, colorectal cancer. Mutations located 5' of codon 160 and 3' of codon 1597 have been identified in a form of FAP with attenuated colonic polyposis,[14] which accounts for about 10% of those affected.

Some extracolonic manifestations have also been associated with mutation at certain sites, but this is not clear for upper gastrointestinal polyposis.[15] CHRPE occurs only with mutation between codons 450 (exon 9) and 1444,[16] and desmoids occur in individuals with any mutation, but the presence of a germline mutation 3' of codon 1444 can be associated with highly penetrant desmoid disease.[17]

TABLE 26-1. Extracolonic features of FAP

System	Feature	Frequency (%)
Upper gastrointestinal tract	Upper gastrointestinal adenomas	95
	Upper gastrointestinal carcinoma	5
	Fundic gland polyps	40
Connective tissue	Osteomas (especially jaw)	80
	Desmoids	15
Dental	Unerupted and supernumerary teeth	17
Cutaneous	Epidermoid cysts	50
Endocrine	Adrenocortical adenomas[4]	5
	Papillary thyroid carcinoma[5]	1
Hepatobiliary	Biliary tract carcinoma	<1
	Hepatoblastoma	<1
Central nervous system	CHRPE	75
	Tumors (especially medulloblastoma)	<1

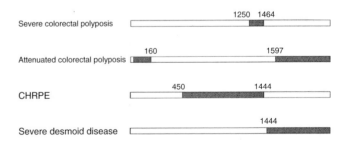

FIGURE 26-3. Schematic representation of the *APC* gene showing genotype-phenotype correlations.

However, identical *APC* mutations may be associated with diverse phenotypes, suggesting that other genetic modifiers are involved[18] and that environment probably also has some influence.

MYH Polyposis

An autosomal recessive form of familial adenomatous polyposis, caused by mutation in the MutY homolog (*MYH*) gene, has recently been described.[19] Whereas many of the individuals identified with biallelic *MYH* mutations had fewer than 100 polyps, some had many hundreds, and thus a genuine clinical diagnosis of FAP. Colonic microadenomas and duodenal adenomas have also been reported in this group, but desmoids and fundic gland polyps have not been described to date, and CHRPE status remains uncertain. This discovery has major implications for genetic counseling, because, for the first time, an autosomal recessive form of FAP has been identified. This diagnosis should be considered in families in which no *APC* mutation has been identified, the mode of inheritance is not clearly autosomal dominant, or polyp numbers are low.

Clinical Variants of FAP

Attenuated FAP

A group of patients have been described who develop fewer than 100 colorectal polyps (usually between one and 50), at a greater age (34–44 years) than in "classical" FAP, but who may still exhibit extracolonic manifestations and carry a germline *APC* mutation.[20] Colorectal cancers also occur correspondingly later (mean 56 years) in this group, and with incomplete penetrance. The polyps have a rather different distribution, being more frequently found proximal to the splenic flexure, and their number varies significantly between family members, some of whom may have hundreds of adenomas.

This can result in diagnostic confusion because the clinical picture is very similar to HNPCC, and indeed the first kindreds described were thought to have a form of HNPCC before they were identified as carrying *APC* mutations.[21] A number of distinct mutations has been identified in individuals with attenuated FAP (AFAP); the mutations are clustered in exons 3 and 4, at the 5′ end of the gene, and also at the 3′ end of exon 15. Fundic gland polyps and duodenal adenomas are frequent, but CHRPEs are unusual in this group, as are desmoids in those with a 5′ mutation. In contrast, families with 3′ mutations (beyond about codon 1444) seem to have a high risk of desmoid disease together with attenuated large bowel disease. The missense *APC* mutation I1307K has been identified in Ashkenazi Jews with multiple adenomas and E1317Q[22] has also been found in association with an AFAP whereas *MYH* mutations have been found in up to 30% of cases of multiple (15–100) colorectal adenomas.[19]

The main consequence of the attenuated phenotype is that it causes diagnostic difficulty. Because the polyps are predominantly right sided, the disease may be missed by flexible sigmoidoscopy. A careful search (including upper gastrointestinal endoscopy) for extracolonic features of FAP, dye-spray colonoscopy to confirm polyp number, and testing of tumor or polyp tissue for microsatellite instability and mismatch repair immunohistochemistry may be helpful.

Once diagnosis is confirmed, management is essentially the same as for FAP with a more classic phenotype,[23] although ileorectal anastomosis (IRA) is probably reasonable in most patients. The only exceptions to this situation might be in the small group with a strongly inherited tendency to develop severe desmoid disease, potentially triggered by surgery, and a very mild colonic phenotype, where meticulous surveillance with endoscopic polypectomy might be justified.

Gardner's Syndrome

Gardner described the association between FAP and epidermoid cysts, osteomas and "fibromas," later found to be desmoid tumors in 1953. The term "Gardner's syndrome" was only later used to describe colorectal polyposis occurring with these extracolonic manifestations. Gardner's syndrome is now considered to be genetically indistinct from FAP, and systematic examination[24] has revealed that most patients with FAP have at least one extraintestinal feature. Although it is of historical interest, the term Gardner's syndrome is no longer considered a genetic or clinically entity and should be regarded as obsolete.[25]

Turcot's Syndrome

This syndrome is the association between colorectal adenomatous polyposis and central nervous system tumors. Recent molecular genetic investigation[26] has shown that about two-thirds of families have mutations in the *APC* gene, with cerebellar medulloblastoma as the predominant brain tumor. Most of the other third, including Turcot's original family, seem to be variants of HNPCC with glioblastoma as the predominant brain tumor, and multiple (but fewer than 100) colorectal adenomas. This illustrates how one syndrome can be caused by mutations in more than one gene, the phenomenon of genetic heterogeneity.

Diagnosis

Genetic Testing

Genetic testing should be preceded by thorough counseling, with the provision of written information about the process and consequences, and should only be done once informed consent has been obtained. The implications with respect to confidentiality, employment, insurance, and other financial issues vary from country to country, but must be discussed before testing.

The first step in the process is mutation detection. DNA from an individual with FAP is analyzed to identify a mutation in *APC*, which is successful in about 80% of cases. Failure to detect an *APC* mutation does not exclude a diagnosis of FAP, and may occur for a variety of reasons including gene deletion and some missense mutations. Such results have been misinterpreted as ruling out the diagnosis of FAP,[27] with potentially serious consequences.

If mutation detection has been successful, at-risk family members can be offered predictive testing with a high degree of accuracy. This testing is generally done between the ages of 12 and 15 years, when the individual is old enough to take part in genetic counseling. There is no need for testing to be done earlier, because the disease does not usually become clinically manifest and treatment is rarely indicated before the mid-teens.

From time to time colorectal surgeons will encounter very young children with a positive genetic test that has been organized, not because of symptoms but as simple screening, often by a pediatrician; finding this can cause great management difficulty. There is understandable parental concern, yet the phenotype is not developed to guide surgical choice, cyclooxygenase (COX)-2 inhibitors have not been tested in a pediatric age group, and the chance of cancer is vanishingly slight. Yet abdominal pain, frequent in small children, creates a parental and even pediatrician pressure for colonoscopy and sometimes surgery earlier than is usually desirable.

In the event of negative predictive testing (i.e., an individual does not possess the family mutation), that person can be discharged from further surveillance and be reassured that they do not have FAP. This approach reduces the costs and risks associated with endoscopic surveillance, as well as removing the anxiety of living with a potential diagnosis of FAP. A positive test result allows optimal surveillance and prophylaxis to be targeted to those individuals who need it, and knowledge of the site of mutation can aid decision making with regard to prophylactic surgery.

Clinical Surveillance

In kindreds in whom mutation detection has not been performed or has not been informative, at-risk individuals should be offered regular clinical surveillance. This surveillance starts at the age of 12–14 years, when adenomas would be expected to develop. Although there have been reports of polyps and even cancers occurring earlier than this, they are very rare. Clearly, anyone at risk of FAP should undergo colonoscopy if they become symptomatic.

Surveillance is initially by flexible sigmoidoscopy, because it is well tolerated and most polyps are in the left colon and rectum. If this continues, colonoscopy should then be performed from around the age of 20, alternating with flexible sigmoidoscopy so that one or other is done each year. The vast majority of individuals with FAP will develop polyps by the age of 30, but there is no consensus regarding the age at which surveillance can cease. It should certainly continue until the age of 40 years, and longer in families in which the disease tends to manifest late.

There are various pitfalls in endoscopy in these patients. In the young, lymphoid follicles may have a dramatic appearance, mimicking adenomatous polyposis. Biopsy is therefore mandatory. Conversely, small polyps are easy to miss. The use of a dye-spray technique, together with multiple biopsies to identify microadenomas, can be very helpful in identifying FAP and avoiding an underestimate of the polyp burden.[28]

Management of the Large Bowel

Timing of Prophylactic Surgery

Once FAP has been diagnosed, the aim is to perform prophylactic surgery. Invasive cancer is very rare in patients younger than the age of 18 years, and usually causes symptoms.[29] Patients with severe polyposis (more than 1000 colonic or more than 20 rectal polyps), or those people who are symptomatic, should have surgery as soon as possible. In those individuals with milder disease, it can usually be delayed until an educationally and socially convenient time (e.g., a long school vacation). In these circumstances, annual colonoscopy is recommended to monitor disease, but the aim should be to avoid delay, so that most will have surgery between the ages of 16 and 20, which is well before invasive disease usually develops.

Choice of Operation

The surgical options for the management of this condition are proctocolectomy with end ileostomy (with or without Koch pouch), colectomy with IRA or proctocolectomy with ileoanal pouch (IPAA). Because few patients desire a permanent ileostomy, proctocolectomy is rarely done, although it remains an option that should be considered in some circumstances, and may be necessary if a low rectal cancer encroaches on the anal canal, if ileoanal pouch formation is impossible (e.g., because of mesenteric desmoid) or ill advised (e.g., in the presence of poor sphincter function). In most cases, however, the choice is between the latter two options, and is a matter of considerable ongoing debate, the essence of which is the balance between functional results and morbidity of surgery on the one hand and prevention of cancer on the other. Both procedures can be performed with laparoscopic mobilization, so that a midline laparotomy is not essential, a merely cosmetic improvement but with potentially great appeal to essentially healthy young people undergoing this surgery. Both the IRA and the IPAA can be performed by laparotomy, laparoscopy, laparoscopic or hand-assisted procedures. The only proven benefit of the minimally invasive approaches is superior cosmesis as compared with laparotomy.

IRA is more straightforward to perform, and requires only one procedure, with a shorter hospital stay and fewer complications.[30] The risks of erectile and ejaculatory dysfunction caused by nerve damage during pelvic dissection are avoided, as is the significant reduction in fecundity observed in women after IPAA.[31] In addition, bowel frequency and soiling are less.[32] In a teenager facing prophylactic surgery, these functional factors are of great significance, particularly when most cancer risk is a few decades away and later conversion to a pouch is usually possible.

The main disadvantage of IRA is that follow-up studies have shown a 12%–29% risk of developing a cancer in the retained rectum within 20–25 years,[33] the risk being dependent on age, rather than time since surgery. High-density (more than 1000) colonic polyposis is associated with a cancer risk double that in milder disease,[34] and also with severe polyposis in the rectum after IRA, leading to frequent need for completion proctectomy. FAP attributable to mutation in exon 15G, which includes the frequently mutated codon 1309, consistently results in this severe colorectal phenotype.[35] In this group, there is a high rate of subsequent proctectomy if IRA is done as the first-line procedure.[36]

IPAA has the attraction of removing the colon and rectum entirely, and complication rates and functional results have improved with experience. There has been controversy over the need for mucosectomy to remove the anorectal transition zone, which theoretically prevents cuff neoplasia, but results in more complications and perhaps poorer function. Dysplasia in the transition zone occurs after both double-stapled and mucosectomy techniques, and the latter technique is probably only rarely indicated in individuals with extensive severe low rectal polyposis.

Surveillance of ileoanal pouches from various centers has shown adenomas in up to 53%,[37,38] and even some cancers.[39] Because IPAA has only been available for approximately 20 years, and has only been performed frequently for FAP in the last 15 years, the full significance of this will not be clear for some time. However, the cases reported to date confirm that neoplasia can occur in these pouches, which is of considerable concern; thus, careful follow-up is essential.

Much of the data on outcome after IRA follow surgery done before IPAA was introduced, when IRA was the only way to avoid a permanent stoma. It was almost certainly done in circumstances when IPAA would now be considered preferable (i.e., more advanced age, high-density polyposis, codon 1309 mutation). There is some evidence to suggest that rectal cancer rates and the need for completion proctectomy in patients having IRA since IPAA has been practiced are much lower than previously thought.[40] Other factors contributing to high rectal cancer rates in historical studies include inadequate postoperative surveillance, and the fact that in many cases the operation performed was a subtotal colectomy with ileosigmoid anastomosis, leaving a long rectosigmoid segment, inherently more difficult to visualize.

IRA is a reasonable and safe option today in young patients, particularly children and teenagers without 1309 mutation or severe polyposis,[23,36] and is strongly indicated if there are fewer than five rectal polyps. Most individuals presenting over the age of 25 years and those with severe polyposis or known to carry a mutation in codon 1309 should be advised to undergo IPAA. But there are other issues: pouch surgery in young men has an approximately 1% risk of damage to erection, ejaculation, and bladder function; in women fertility is compromised. In addition, some families prefer a certain operation, regardless of the medical advice they have received.

Postoperative Surveillance

After IRA, the retained rectum should be examined, ideally using a flexible sigmoidoscope, every 6–12 months, the interval depending on the severity of disease. In about two-thirds of patients, rectal adenoma regression is seen in the first few years after IRA.[41] Polyps larger than 5 mm should be removed; repeated fulguration can result in scarring, making future surveillance difficult and unreliable. If severe dysplasia or uncontrolled polyposis develops, completion proctectomy with or without ileoanal pouch formation is indicated.

In patients who have had IPAA, the pouch should be examined by flexible endoscopy annually, and a careful digital examination of the anorectal transition zone should be performed.

Chemoprevention

A range of chemopreventive agents have been studied in FAP, in part because of the problems of managing the retained rectum after IRA, but also because this disease provides a useful experimental model of colorectal carcinogenesis. In placebo controlled trials, both the nonsteroidal antiinflammatory drug (NSAID) sulindac[42] and the COX-2 inhibitor celecoxib[43] have reduced the number and size of colorectal adenomas. It would be inappropriate, however, to regard such treatment as an alternative to prophylactic surgery, because no benefit in terms of cancer reduction has been demonstrated, and there have been reports of rectal carcinoma occurring in patients on sulindac despite a good response in terms of reduction in polyp number and size. But there are circumstances, for example, when completion proctectomy is impossible because of desmoid disease, or while awaiting surgery that must otherwise unavoidably be delayed, or in patients with a very high family risk of desmoid disease, when the use of such agents has a definite place.

Upper Gastrointestinal Polyposis

Fundic gland polyps, which are areas of cystic hyperplasia,[44] are found in about 50% of individuals with FAP. These have a very low malignant potential, but gastric adenomas, dysplasia, and invasive carcinoma have been described.[45] There is an increase in gastric cancers in patients with FAP in Japan[46] and Korea, but this finding is not seen in the West. An excess of gallbladder and bile duct adenomas and carcinoma has also been reported.[47,48]

Prospective studies have demonstrated that more than 95% of individuals with FAP have duodenal adenomas,[49] which tend to occur about 15 years later than large bowel polyps.[50] Adenomas are found throughout the small intestine, but most are at or just distal to the ampulla of Vater. Duodenal or periampullary cancer occurs in approximately 5% overall, at an average age of 50 years.

Surveillance of the Duodenum

Duodenal adenomas may be clearly defined polyps or more confluent areas, and biopsies of macroscopically normal mucosa may reveal microadenomas. In contrast to the situation in the large bowel, only a minority of these will progress to invasive carcinoma, but when they do the prognosis is very poor. To stratify the severity of duodenal polyposis, the Spigelman staging was developed[51] and has been widely adopted (Tables 26-2 and 26-3). A prospective 10-year follow-up of Spigelman's original cohort has identified a 36% risk of developing invasive carcinoma in those with stage IV disease at the start of the study, and a 2% risk in those with stage II or III disease. Several carcinomas were missed on endoscopy, and all of those who developed cancer died as a result, despite surgery.[15]

Regular endoscopic surveillance is recommended, so that individuals at high risk of developing carcinoma can be identified and offered intervention, although there is currently no evidence that this approach decreases the rate of invasive disease.[52,53] Examination of the duodenum using both forward- and side-viewing scopes, together with multiple biopsies,[15] starting at the age of 25 years, is recommended.

Management

Management of severe duodenal polyposis is difficult, but the outcome once invasive carcinoma has developed is poor. Duodenotomy and open polypectomy are associated with 100% recurrence just a year after surgery.[54] Endoscopic mucosal resection seems a more attractive option, but is made difficult by the frequently plaque-like morphology of the polyps and involvement of the ampulla. Even simple biopsy of the ampulla can result in acute pancreatitis,[55] and repeated diathermy in this region can lead to scarring and stricturing. Argon plasma coagulation is of some use. Photodynamic therapy has been tried, but photosensitization and the need for multiple treatments[56] means that it is not currently a practical option.

The use of chemoprevention to prevent progression of earlier stage disease has attracted great interest. Calcium, starch, vitamin C, and ranitidine have been tried, with no effect. Sulindac can result in regression of small polyps,[57] but has little effect on larger ones. A randomized trial of the COX-2 inhibitor celecoxib showed significant improvement in the Spigelman stage for those with mild to moderate disease.[58]

Duodenectomy, whether by a classical Whipple's procedure or using pylorus or pancreas preserving techniques, has been considered a last resort because of its significant morbidity and mortality. However, given the very poor prognosis once neoplasia becomes frankly invasive, the high rate of diagnosis of invasive disease which was preoperatively thought to be benign,[59] and the limitations of other options, it should be seriously considered for advanced premalignant disease.[15,59]

Desmoid Disease

Desmoids are locally invasive, nonmetastasizing clonal proliferations of myofibroblasts.[60] Their etiology, pathogenesis, and natural history are not clearly understood. The importance of desmoid disease lies in its significant contribution to disease-related mortality in FAP.[6] Overall mortality ranges from 10% to 50%,[61] and desmoids can also contribute to death from other causes by making surgery for rectal or upper gastrointestinal malignancy difficult or even impossible.[62,63]

Ten to fifteen percent of patients with FAP develop desmoid,[64] with a peak incidence at around 30 years, 2–3 years after surgery. Whereas sporadic desmoids are considerably more common in females than males, this difference is less marked in the setting of FAP.

Clinical Features

Desmoids occurring in association with FAP typically arise within the abdomen (70%), especially in the small bowel mesentery, and in the abdominal wall (15%), although many other sites have been described. Mesenteric desmoids (Figure 26-4) can be either well-defined mass lesions, or a more diffuse fibromatous infiltration. Encasement or compression of the mesenteric blood vessels can result in ischemia and perforation of the bowel, and makes resection hazardous. A desmoid tumor can also cause direct compression of bowel and ureters. The presence of a desmoid may preclude adequate mesenteric length to fashion an IPAA.

Trauma (particularly in the form of surgery) and estrogens have both been implicated in the etiology of these lesions, although they can occur spontaneously. There is evidence for some degree of genotype-phenotype correlation. Desmoids have been reported to occur more frequently in patients with germline mutations located toward the 3′ end of the gene.[16,65]

TABLE 26-3. Derivation of Spigelman stage from scores

Total points	Spigelman stage	Suggested interval to next duodenoscopy (yr)
0	0	5
1–4	I	3–5
5–6	II	3
7–8	III	1
9–12	IV	1

TABLE 26-2. Scoring of polyp features in Spigelman staging for duodenal adenomas

Points allocated	No. of polyps	Size of polyps (mm)	Histology	Dysplasia
1	1–4	1–4	Tubular	Mild
2	5–20	5–10	Tubulovillous	Moderate
3	>20	>10	Villous	Severe

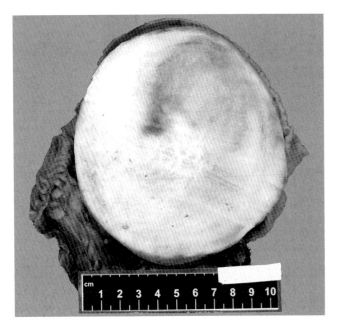

FIGURE 26-4. Desmoid tumor arising in the small bowel mesentery.

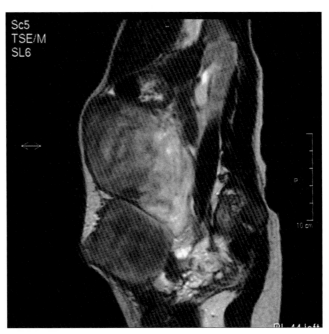

FIGURE 26-5. MRI scan showing intraabdominal desmoid tumor.

Some mutations in this region are associated with severe desmoid disease inherited with high penetrance, but individuals with such mutations do not always develop this manifestation. However, many patients with desmoid have mutations in the 5′ half of the gene so modifier genes may well also delay a part.

There is disputed evidence whether desmoid formation starts with the development of a desmoid precursor lesion, a plaque-like area of thickened peritoneum, which may progress to a more diffuse mesenteric fibromatosis and then to a desmoid mass.[66,67] Desmoid natural history is very variable, about 10% resolving spontaneously, 10% growing rapidly and relentlessly, and the remainder either showing cycles of growth and resolution or remaining stable.[68]

Investigation

Computed tomographic scanning is the mainstay of investigation, allowing imaging and measurement of the desmoid itself, as well as demonstrating the relationship to other structures such as the ureters and bowel.[69] Early mesenteric fibrosis appears as ill-defined soft tissue infiltration of the mesenteric fat, with a characteristic, whorled appearance.[67] Magnetic resonance imaging (Figure 26-5) may have a place, and there is some evidence that T2-weighted signal intensity correlates with subsequent growth.[70] Because only a small proportion of desmoids grow and cause significant clinical problems, the ability to predict such progression might be very useful. Because desmoid disease frequently causes ureteric compression, regular ultrasound monitoring of the kidneys permits timely intervention.

Management

The treatment of desmoids is controversial, empirical, and often difficult. Surgery is widely accepted as the first-line treatment for troublesome extraabdominal and abdominal wall desmoids. Recurrence is common (20%–50%), but complications are few. Within the abdomen the situation is very different, because the majority lie in the small bowel mesentery, encasing the mesenteric vasculature. The result is a high perioperative mortality rate (usually from hemorrhage)[71] and substantial morbidity, particularly because of extensive loss of small bowel. Ureteric obstruction is best managed with stents, and proximal defunctioning may be required in some patients with bowel obstruction or perforation.

Various medical treatments have been reported, the most widely used being NSAIDs (particularly Sulindac) and anti-estrogens (tamoxifen or toremifene). There have been no prospective controlled trials, and particularly in view of the unpredictable and variable behavior of desmoids, the small retrospective series reported are difficult to interpret. Cytotoxic chemotherapy has been used in irresectable or aggressive desmoid disease, and objective remissions have been noted with a variety of different agents. There have been several encouraging reports of an anti-sarcoma regimen consisting of doxorubicin and dacarbazine in the treatment of life-threatening intraabdominal desmoid disease[72,73] and more recently a less toxic combination of vinblastine and methotrexate has produced some responses.[74,75]

One proposed treatment protocol[23] for intraabdominal desmoid suggests initial treatment with sulindac 150–200 mg twice daily. If growth continues, tamoxifen (80–120 mg per day) is added. If progression is rapid or relentless, chemotherapy is considered. Treatment of desmoids preferably should take place in the setting of an international study.

Peutz-Jeghers Syndrome

This syndrome, which has an incidence in the region of 1 in 200,000, consists of perioral, buccal, and occasionally genital melanin pigmentation together with gastrointestinal hamartomatous polyposis. Pigmentation can also be seen on the lips and sometimes on the eyelids, hands and feet, or be absent altogether. It usually appears in early childhood and tends to fade in the late twenties. The polyps occur predominantly in the small intestine (78%), but are also found in the stomach (38%), colon (42%), and rectum (28%).[76] They are hamartomas with a characteristic branching morphology, containing smooth muscle. Adenomatous change with dysplasia and progression to invasive adenocarcinoma has been observed.[77]

Inheritance

Peutz-Jeghers is autosomal dominantly inherited with high penetrance, and is caused by mutation of *LKB1* (also known as *STK11*) on chromosome 19p13.3,[78] which encodes a serine-threonine kinase of unknown function. Mutation of *LKB1* is only found in about 50% of cases, and has been formally excluded in some,[79] suggesting that other genes are responsible in a proportion of cases. Although a family history is frequently evident, new mutations are responsible for a significant number of cases.

Clinical Issues

Polyp-related Complications

The most common clinical problems in Peutz-Jeghers syndrome are anemia caused by chronic blood loss from large polyps and small bowel obstruction, caused by intussusception with a polyp at the apex. Repeated emergency bowel resections can lead to increasing operative difficulty and even short-bowel syndrome.

Risk of Malignancy

Follow-up studies have shown that individuals with this syndrome are at increased risk of developing a range of malignancies at a particularly young age.[80] Indeed, by the age of 57 years, approximately half of all patients in one series had died of cancer, of which about half were gastrointestinal.[81] It is estimated that there is a 50-fold excess of gastrointestinal cancer in Peutz-Jeghers syndrome, resulting in a lifetime risk of approximately 20% of colorectal cancer and about 5% of gastric cancer, as well as breast, pancreatic (30% lifetime risk), ovarian sex-cord tumors (10% of females), feminizing Sertoli

cell testicular tumors in prepubertal boys, and cervical malignancies.

Management

Gastrointestinal Surveillance

Two or three yearly gastroduodenoscopy and colonoscopy with polypectomy are recommended, with barium study (and increasingly capsule endoscopy) of the small intestine at the same interval. Hemoglobin should be checked annually. Small bowel polyps causing symptoms or anemia, or measuring more than 1.5 cm, should be removed at laparotomy with intraoperative enteroscopy.

Laparotomy in Peutz-Jeghers Syndrome

The technique of laparotomy with intraoperative enteroscopy was introduced to reduce the repeated emergency laparotomies and small bowel resections undertaken on these patients. At laparotomy an enterotomy is made, usually at the site of the largest polyp, and a flexible endoscope is passed through a sterile laparoscope sheath to the proximal and distal ends of the small bowel. During scope withdrawal, polyps are excised using a snare or electrocautery biopsy forceps, and then retrieved via the enterotomy. This approach identifies many more polyps than conventional palpation and transillumination of the bowel, permitting removal without multiple enterotomies and increasing obstruction-free interval.[82] This procedure may be amenable to performance in a laparoscopically assisted method.

Extraintestinal Surveillance

Mammography in premenopausal woman lacks sensitivity, but there is little evidence to support ultrasound or MRI as alternatives. Testicular tumors tend to occur in prepubertal boys, and it would seem sensible to encourage regular examination. Women should undergo standard cervical and breast screening according to nationally agreed protocols. Although in some centers regular ultrasound scanning of the pancreas and ovaries is performed, there is no evidence that such measures have any impact on prognosis. Indeed, even in rare cases of familial pancreatic cancer, an appropriate screening method remains controversial. It is important that clinicians caring for these patients are aware of the high cancer risk, and maintain a high index of suspicion.

Juvenile Polyposis

Juvenile polyps are hamartomas that lack smooth muscle histologically, having poor anchorage to the bowel wall, and not infrequently becoming detached and being passed anally. Solitary juvenile polyps may affect up to 2% of children and adolescents, but have little or no malignant potential.[83]

Juvenile polyposis is characterized by the finding of multiple juvenile polyps in the large bowel, although the stomach (and perhaps small intestine) is affected as well in about 50%.[84] The precise number of juvenile polyps needed to make the diagnosis varies among authors, with numbers between three and five being suggested. Most affected individuals develop 50–200 polyps, but some have very few. One juvenile polyp in a patient with a family history of juvenile polyposis is sufficient to diagnose juvenile polyposis.

It is a rare condition, with a frequency of about 1 per 100,000, and presents with rectal bleeding, anemia, or polyp prolapse, at an average age of approximately 9 years. The polyps are hamartomas, with a characteristic hyperplastic stroma, abundant lamina propria, cystic glands, and inflammation. Adenomatous dysplasia occurs in up to half of these, which may then progress to invasive adenocarcinoma.

Other morphologic abnormalities including macrocephaly, mental retardation, cleft lip or palate, congenital heart disease, genitourinary malformations, and malrotations are found in 10%–20%.[85]

Genetics

This syndrome is genetically heterogeneous, with three separate genes currently implicated. Mutations have been identified in affected individuals in *SMAD4* which lies on chromosome 18q21 and is a known tumor suppressor gene, implicated in sporadic colorectal carcinogenesis. It codes for a protein involved in the transforming growth factor-β signaling pathway, and germline mutations have been found in 35%–60% of juvenile polyposis patients in the United States, but rather fewer (3%–28%) in Europe.[86] Recently, germline mutations of *BMPR1A* on 10q22, which encodes a protein involved in the same signaling pathway, have been found in a further 15%.[87] *PTEN* mutations have also been reported in so-called "juvenile polyposis,"[85] but it is as yet unclear whether these are genuine cases, or in fact Cowden syndrome, or even whether this syndrome is simply a clinical variant of juvenile polyposis.[88]

Cancer Risk and Management

The cumulative risk of colorectal cancer has been estimated at 30%–50%, and 10%–20% in the upper gastrointestinal tract.[86]

First-degree relatives of affected individuals should be screened by colonoscopy from around the age of 12 years if asymptomatic[89] and five yearly thereafter. In most cases, the polyps can be controlled by regular endoscopic polypectomy, with both upper gastrointestinal endoscopy and colonoscopy recommended at least every 2 years. In cases in which polyps are either too numerous or too large to be managed in this way, colectomy and IRA or restorative proctocolectomy is advised.[90] It is not clear whether endoscopic surveillance and polypectomy are adequate to prevent malignancy, but there are insufficient data to justify purely prophylactic colectomy.

Affected individuals should also undergo upper gastrointestinal surveillance from the age of 25 years.

Other Juvenile Polyposes

Several very rare dominantly inherited conditions have been described in which juvenile-type hamartomatous colorectal polyps occur together with other features. In these syndromes, the juvenile polyps seem to be of low malignant potential.[91]

Cowden Syndrome

This is autosomal dominantly inherited and attributable to mutation of the *PTEN* gene,[92] which encodes a protein tyrosine phosphatase involved in inhibiting cell growth. It is characterized by macrocephaly (30%), trichilemmomas (which are considered pathognomonic), and both benign and malignant neoplasms of the thyroid, breast, uterus, and skin. The hamartomas occur in the mouth as well as other parts of the gastrointestinal tract, resulting in a nodular appearance of the buccal mucosa.

Bannayan-Riley-Ruvalcaba Syndrome

Here the juvenile polyps (50%) are associated with characteristic pigmented penile macules, macrocephaly, mental retardation (50%), lipomatosis, and hemangiomas. *PTEN* mutations have also been identified in this syndrome.[93] It seems likely as Cowden and Bannayan-Riley-Ruvalcaba syndromes are caused by mutation of the same gene that they are slightly different forms of the same disorder,[87] and families have been identified in which both phenotypes are evident.[94] The risk of colorectal cancer is not clear.

Metaplastic Polyposis

Metaplastic (hyperplastic) polyps are the most common lesions observed in the large bowel, being found in 40% at the age of 50 years. Their significance is unclear and there is much controversy surrounding their potential as precursors of adenomas and carcinoma. There is increasing evidence of correlation between numbers of metaplastic polyps and adenomas and cancer risk.[95] In addition, metaplastic polyposis, a loosely defined entity in which multiple hyperplastic polyps are seen, does appear to be associated with an increased risk of colorectal cancer, often with microsatellite instability.[96] There are at present, however, insufficient data to allow clear guidance on clinical management.

Cronkhite-Canada Syndrome

This is a very rare condition with onset in adulthood and no evidence of an inherited predisposition. The disease is characterized by gastrointestinal hamartomatous polyposis together with ectodermal abnormalities including alopecia, onychodystrophy, and hyperpigmentation of the skin of the face and eyelids. The gastric mucosa resembles Ménétrier's disease, and malabsorption and protein loss can lead to anemia, diarrhea, weight loss, edema, and tetany. Hypokalemia can also be a feature.

Multiple juvenile-type polyps, with marked inflammatory features, are found in the duodenum in 75% of cases, the small intestine in 50%, and occasionally in the stomach and large bowel. Adenomatous change is seen and gastrointestinal cancer has been reported in about 10%.

The pathogenesis of this condition is unknown, and there is no established treatment. Management is essentially supportive, with aggressive fluid resuscitation and nutrition. Tetracycline can help, and corticosteroids have also been used.[97]

References

1. Bisgaard ML, Fenger K, Bulow S, et al. Familial adenomatous polyposis (FAP): frequency, penetrance and mutation rate. Hum Mutat 1994;3:121–125.
2. Bulow S. Results of national registration of familial adenomatous polyposis. Gut 2003;52:742–746.
3. Church JM, McGannon E. A polyposis registry: how to set one up and make it work. Semin Colon Rectal Surg 1995;6:48–54.
4. Johnson Smith TGP, Clark SK, Katz DE, et al. Adrenal masses are associated with familial adenomatous polyposis. Dis Colon Rectum 2000;43:1739–1742.
5. Cetta F, Olschwang S, Petracci M. Genetic alterations in thyroid carcinoma associated with familial adenomatous polyposis: clinical implications and suggestions for early detection. World J Surg 1998;22:1231–1236.
6. Belchez LA, Berk T, Bapat BV, et al. Changing causes of mortality in patients with familial adenomatous polyposis. Dis Colon Rectum 1996;39:384–387.
7. Olschwang S, Tiret A, Laurent-Puig P, et al. Restriction of ocular fundus lesions to a specific subgroup of APC mutations in adenomatous polyposis coli patients. Cell 1993;75:959–968.
8. Fearon ER, Vogelstein B. A model for colorectal tumourigenesis. Cell 1990;61:759–767.
9. Van der Luijt RB, Khan PM, Vasen HFA, et al. Molecular analysis of the APC gene in 105 Dutch kindreds with familial adenomatous polyposis. Hum Mutat 1997;9:7–16.
10. Schnitzler M, Dwight T, Marsh DJ, et al. Quantitation of APC messenger RNA in human tissues. Biochem Biophys Res Commun 1995;217:385–392.
11. Midgley CA, White S, Howitt R, et al. APC expression in normal human tissues. J Pathol 1997;181:426–433.
12. Fodde R. The APC gene in colorectal cancer. Eur J Cancer 2002;20:905–911.
13. Nugent KP, Phillips RKS, Hodgson SV, et al. Phenotypic expression in familial adenomatous polyposis: partial prediction by mutation analysis. Gut 1994;35:1622–1623.
14. Friedl W, Caspari R, Senteller M, et al. Can APC mutation analysis contribute to therapeutic decisions in familial adenomatous polyposis? Experience in 680 FAP families. Gut 2001;48:515–521.
15. Groves CJ, Saunders BP, Spigelman AD, Phillips RKS. Duodenal cancer in patients with familial adenomatous polyposis (FAP): results of a 10 year prospective study. Gut 2002;50:636–641.
16. Caspari R, Olschwang S, Friedl W, et al. Familial adenomatous polyposis: desmoid tumours and lack of ophthalmic lesions (CHRPE) associated with APC mutations beyond codon 1444. Hum Mol Genet 1995;4:337–340.
17. Eccles DM, van der Luijt R, Breukel C, et al. Hereditary desmoid disease due to a frameshift mutation at codon 1924 of the APC gene. Am J Hum Genet 1996;59:1193–1201.
18. Crabtree MD, Tomlinson IPM, Hodgson SV, et al. Explaining variation in familial adenomatous polyposis: relationship between genotype and phenotype and evidence for modifier genes. Gut 2002;51:420–423.
19. Sieber OM, Lipton L, Crabtree M, et al. Multiple colorectal adenomas, classic adenomatous polyposis and germ-line mutations in MYH. N Engl J Med 2003;348:791–799.
20. Hernegger GS, Moore HG, Guillem JG. Attenuated familial adenomatous polyposis: an evolving and poorly understood entity. Dis Colon Rectum 2002;45:127–134.
21. Lynch HT, Smyrk T, McGinn T, et al. Attenuated familial adenomatous polyposis. Cancer 1995;76:2427–2433.
22. Lamlum H, Al Tassan N, Jaeger E, et al. Germline APC variants in patients with multiple colorectal adenomas, with evidence for the particular importance of E1317Q. Hum Mol Gene 2000;9:2215–2221.
23. Church J, Simmang C. Practice parameters for the treatment of patients with dominantly inherited colorectal cancer (familial adenomatous polyposis and hereditary nonpolyposis colorectal cancer). Dis Colon Rectum 2003;46:1001–1012.
24. Davies DR, Armstrong JG, Thakker N, et al. Severe Gardner syndrome in families with mutations restricted to a specific region of the APC gene. Am J Hum Genet 1995;57:1151–1158.
25. Parks TG. Extracolonic manifestations associated with familial adenomatous polyposis. Ann R Coll Surg Engl 1990;72:181–184.
26. Paraf F, Jothy S, Van Meir EG. Brain tumour-polyposis syndrome: two genetic diseases? J Clin Oncol 1997;15:2744–2758.
27. Giardiello FM, Brensinger JD, Petersen GM, et al. The use and interpretation of commercial APC gene testing for familial adenomatous polyposis. N Engl J Med 1997;336:823–827.
28. Wallace MH, Frayling IM, Clark SK, et al. Attenuated adenomatous polyposis coli: the role of ascertainment bias through failure to dye-spray at colonoscopy. Dis Colon Rectum 1999;42:1078–1080.
29. Church JM, McGannon E, Burke C, et al. Teenagers with familial adenomatous polyposis: what is their risk for colorectal cancer? Dis Colon Rectum 2002;45:127–129.
30. Madden MV, Neale KF, Nicholls RJ, et al. Comparison of the morbidity and function after coloectomy and ileorectal anastomosis or restorative proctocolectomy for familial adenomatous polyposis. Br J Surg 1991;78:789–792.
31. Olsen KO, Juul S, Bulow S, et al. Female fecundity before and after operation for familial adenomatous polyposis. Br J Surg 2003;90:227–231.
32. Soravia C, Klein L, Berk T, et al. Comparison of ileal pouch-anal anastomosis and ileorectal anastomosis in patients with familial adenomatous polyposis. Dis Colon Rectum 1999;42:1028–1034.
33. Nugent KP, Phillips RKS. Rectal cancer risk in older patients with familial adenomatous polyposis and an ileorectal anastomosis: a cause for concern. Br J Surg 1992;79:1204–1206.

34. Debinsky HS, Love S, Spigelman AD, et al. Colorectal polyp counts and cancer risk in familial adenomatous polyposis. Gastroenterology 1996;110:1028–1030.

35. Bertario L, Russo A, Radice P, et al. Genotype and phenotype factors as determinants for rectal stump cancer in patients with familial adenomatous polyposis. Ann Surg 2000;231:538–543.

36. Bulow C, Vasen H, Jarvinen H, et al. Ileorectal anastomosis is appropriate for a subset of patients with familial adenomatous polyposis. Gastroenterology 2000;119:1454–1460.

37. Groves CJ, Beveridge IG, Swain DJ, et al. Adenoma prevalence and ileal mucosa in pouch vs neoterminal ileum. Gut 2002;50(suppl 2):A22–23.

38. Parc YR, Olschwang S, Desaint B, et al. Familial adenomatous polyposis: prevalence of adenomas in the ileal pouch after restorative proctocolectomy. Ann Surg 2001;233:360–364.

39. Heuschen UA, Heuschen G, Autscbach F, et al. Adenocarcinoma in the ileal pouch: late risk after restorative proctocolectomy. Int J Colorectal Dis 2001;16:126–130.

40. Church J, Burke C, McGannon E, et al. Risk of rectal cancer after colectomy and ileorectal anastomosis for familial adenomatous polyposis: a function of available options. Dis Colon Rectum 2003;46:1175–1181.

41. Nicholls RJ, Springall RG, Gallagher P. Regression of rectal adenomas after colectomy and ileorectal anastomosis for familial adenomatous polyposis. Br Med J 1988;296:1707–1708.

42. Giardello FM, Hamilton SR, Krush AJ, et al. Treatment of colonic and rectal adenomas with sulindac in familial adenomatous polyposis. N Engl J Med 1993;328:1313–1316.

43. Steinbach LT, Lynch P, Phillips RKS, et al. The effect of Celecoxib, a cyclo-oxygenase inhibitor, in familial adenomatous polyposis. N Engl J Med 2000;342:1946–1958.

44. Wallace MH, Phillips RKS. Upper gastrointestinal disease in patients with familial adenomatous polyposis. Br J Surg 1998;85:742–750.

45. Zwik A, Munir M, Ryan CK, et al. Gastric adenocarcinoma and dysplasia in fundic gland polyps of a patient with attenuated adenomatous polyposis coli. Gastroenterology 1997;113:659–663.

46. Iwama T, Mishima Y, Utsunomiya J. The impact of familial adenomatous polyposis on the tumorigenesis and mortality at the several organs. Ann Surg 1993;217:101–108.

47. Nugent KP, Spigelman AD, Talbot IC, et al. Gallbladder dysplasia in patients with familial adenomatous polyposis. Br J Surg 1994;81:291–292.

48. Jarvinen HJ, Nyberg M, Peltokallio P. Biliary involvement in familial polyposis coli. Dis Colon Rectum 1983;26:525–528.

49. Heiskanen I, Kellokumpu I, Jarvinen H. Management of duodenal adenomas in 98 patients with familial adenomatous polyposis. Endoscopy 1999;31:412–416.

50. Sanabria JR, Croxford R, Berk TC, et al. Familial segregation in the occurrence and severity of periampullary neoplasms in familial adenomatous polyposis. Am J Surg 1996;171:136–140.

51. Spigelman AD, Williams CB, Talbot IC, et al. Upper gastrointestinal cancer in patients with familial adenomatous polyposis. Lancet 1989;2:783–785.

52. Burke CA, Beck GJ, Church JM, van Stolk RU. The natural history of untreated duodenal and ampullary adenomas in patients with familial adenomatous polyposis followed in an endoscopic surveillance program. Gastrointest Endosc 1999;49:358–364.

53. Vasen HFA, Bülow S, Nyrhoj T, et al. Decision analysis in the management of duodenal adenomatosis in familial adenomatous polyposis. Gut 1997;40:716–719.

54. Penna C, Bataille N, Balladur P, et al. Surgical treatment of severe duodenal polyposis in familial adenomatous polyposis. Br J Surg 1998;85:665–668.

55. Nugent KP, Spigelman AD, Williams CB, et al. Iatrogenic pancreatitis in familial adenomatous polyposis. Gut 1993;34:1269–1270.

56. Mlkvy P, Messman H, Debinsky H, et al. Photodynamic therapy for polyps in familial adenomatous polyposis: a pilot study. Int J Colorectal Dis 1995;31A:1160–1165.

57. Wallace MH, Phillips RK. Preventative strategies for periampullary tumours in FAP. Ann Oncol 1999;10(suppl 4):201–203.

58. Phillips RKS, Wallace MH, Lynch PM, et al. A randomised, double blind, placebo controlled study of celecoxib, a selective cyclooxygenase 2 inhibitor, on duodenal polyposis in familial adenomatous polyposis. Gut 2002;50:857–860.

59. de Vos tot Nederveen Cappel WH, Jarvinen JH, Bjork J, et al. Worldwide survey among polyposis registries of surgical management of severe duodenal adenomatosis in familial adenomatous polyposis. Br J Surg 2003;90:705–710.

60. Middleton SB, Frayling IM, Phillips RK. Desmoids in familial adenomatous polyposis are monoclonal proliferations. Br J Cancer 2000;82:827–832.

61. Clark SK, Phillips RKS. Desmoids in familial adenomatous polyposis. Br J Surg 1996;83:1494–1504.

62. Penna C, Kartheuser A, Parc R, et al. Secondary proctectomy and ileal pouch-anal anastomosis after ileorectal anastomosis for familial adenomatous polyposis. Br J Surg 1993;80:1621–1623.

63. Mao C, Huang Y, Howard JM. Carcinoma of the ampulla of Vater and mesenteric fibromatosis (desmoid tumour) associated with Gardner's syndrome: problems in management. Pancreas 1995;10:239–245.

64. Church JM. Desmoid tumours in familial adenomatous polyposis. Surg Oncol Clin North Am 1994;3:435–448.

65. Dobbie Z, Spycher M, Mary JL, et al. Correlation between the development of extracolonic manifestations in FAP patients and mutations beyond 1403 in the APC gene. J Med Genet 1996;33:274–280.

66. Clark SK, Smith TG, Katz DE, et al. Identification and progression of a desmoid precursor lesion in patients with familial adenomatous polyposis. Br J Surg 1998;85:970–973.

67. Middleton SB, Clark SK, Matravers P, et al. Stepwise progression in the development of desmoids in familial adenomatous polyposis. Dis Colon Rectum 2003;46:481–485.

68. Church JM. Desmoid tumours in patients with familial adenomatous polyposis. Semin Colorectal Surg 1995;6:29–32.

69. Brooks AP, Reznek RH, Nugent KP, et al. CT appearances of desmoid tumours in familial adenomatous polyposis: further observations. Clin Radiol 1994;49:601–607.

70. Healy JC, Reznek RH, Clark SK, et al. MR appearances of desmoid tumours in familial adenomatous polyposis. AJR Am J Roentgenol 1997;169:465–472.

71. Clark SK, Neale KF, Landgrebe JC, Phillips RKS. Desmoid tumours complicating familial adenomatous polyposis. Br J Surg 1999;86:1185–1189.

72. Lynch HT, Fitzgibbons R Jr, Chong S, et al. Use of doxorubicin and dacarbazine for the management of unresectable

intra-abdominal desmoid tumours in Gardner's syndrome. Dis Colon Rectum 1994;37:260–267.

73. Poritz LS, Blackstein M, Berk T, et al. Extended follow-up of patients treated with cytotoxic chemotherapy for intra-abdominal desmoid tumours. Dis Colon Rectum 2001;44:1268–1273.

74. Skapek SX, Hawk BJ, Hoffer FA, et al. Combination chemotherapy using vinblastine and methotrexate for the treatment of progressive desmoid tumour in children. J Clin Oncol 1998;16:3021–3027.

75. Azzarelli A, Gronchi A, Bertulli R, et al. Low-dose chemotherapy with methotrexate and vinblastine for patients with advanced aggressive fibromatosis. Cancer 2001;92:1259–1264.

76. McGarrity TJ, Kulin HE, Zaino RJ. Peutz-Jeghers syndrome. Am J Gastroenterol 2000;95:596–604.

77. Gruber SB, Entius EM, Petersen GM, et al. Pathogenesis of adenocarcinoma in Peutz-Jeghers syndrome. Cancer Res 1998;58:p5267–5270.

78. Hemminki A, Markie D, Tomlinson I, et al. A serine/threonine kinase gene defective in Peutz-Jeghers syndrome. Nature 1998;391:184–187.

79. Boardman LA, Couch FJ, Burgart LJ, et al. Genetic heterogeneity in Peutz-Jeghers syndrome. Hum Mutat 2000;16:23–30.

80. Giardello FM, Bresinger JD, Tersmette AC, et al. Very high risk of cancer in familial Peutz-Jeghers syndrome. Gastroenterology 2000;119:1447–1453.

81. Spigelman AD, Murday V, Phillips RKS. Cancer and the Peutz-Jeghers syndrome. Gut 1989;30:1588–1590.

82. Edwards DP, Khosraviani K, Stafferton R, et al. Long-term results of polyp clearance by intraoperative enteroscopy in the Peutz-Jeghers syndrome. Dis Colon Rectum 2003;46:48–50.

83. Nugent KP, Talbot IC, Hodgson SV, et al. Solitary juvenile polyps: not a marker for subsequent malignancy. Gastroenterology 1993;105:698–700.

84. Desai DC, Murday V, Phillips RKS, et al. A survey of phenotypic features in juvenile polyposis. J Med Genet 1998;35:476–481.

85. Olschwang S, Serova-Sinilnikova AM, Lenoir GM, et al. PTEN germ-line mutations in juvenile polyposis coli. Nat Genet 1998;18:1214.

86. Howe JR, Mitros FA, Summers RW. The risk of gastrointestinal carcinoma in familial juvenile polyposis. Ann Surg Oncol 1998;5:751–756.

87. Zhou XP, Woodford-Richens K, Lehtonen R, et al. Germline mutations in BMPR1A/ALK3 cause a subset of juvenile polyposis syndrome and of Cowden and Bannayan Riley-Ruvalcaba syndrome. Am J Hum Genet 2001;69:704–711.

88. Lynch ED, Ostermeyer EA, Lee MK, et al. Inherited mutations in PTEN that are associated with breast cancer, Cowden disease and juvenile polyposis. Am J Hum Genet 1997;61:1254–1260.

89. Hoffenberg EJ, Sauaia A, Malttzman T, et al. Symptomatic colonic polyps in childhood: not so benign. J Pediatr Gastroenterol Nutr 1999;28:175–181.

90. Jarvinen H. Juvenile gastrointestinal polyposis. Probl Gen Surg 1993;10:749–757.

91. Murday V, Slack J. Inherited disorder associated CRC. Cancer 1989;8:139–157.

92. Liaw D, Marsh DJ, Li J, et al. Germline mutations of the PTEN gene in Cowden disease, an inherited breast and thyroid cancer syndrome. Nat Genet 1997;16:64–67.

93. Marsh DJ, Coulon V, Lunetta KL, et al. Mutation spectrum and genotype-phenotype analyses in Cowden disease and Bannayan-Zonana syndrome, two hamartoma syndromes with germline PTEN mutation. Hum Mol Genet 1998;7:507–515.

94. Zori RT, March DJ, Graham GE, et al. Germline PTEN mutation in a family with Cowden syndrome and Bannayan-Riley-Ruvalcaba syndrome. Am J Med Genet 1998;80:399–402.

95. Liljegren A, Lindblom A, Rotstein S, et al. Prevalence and incidence of hyperplastic polyps and adenomas in familial colorectal cancer: correlation between the two types of colon polyps. Gut 2003;52:1140–1147.

96. Leggett BA, Deveraux B, Biden K, et al. Hyperplastic polyposis. Am J Surg Pathol 2001;25:177–184.

97. Hanzawa M, Yoshikawa N, Tezuka T, et al. Surgical treatment of Cronkhite-Canada syndrome associated with protein loosing enteropathy. Dis Colon Rectum 1998;41:932–934.

27
Colon Cancer Evaluation and Staging

Eric G. Weiss and Ian Lavery

Colorectal cancer is the third most common cancer affecting persons in the United States. In 2004, there were an estimated 146,940 new cases of colon and rectal cancer with colon cancer making up the majority of new cases at 106,370.[1] Overall, approximately 38% of newly diagnosed patients with colorectal cancer in the United States will die of their disease.

Clinical Presentation

Most importantly, colon cancers are diagnosed in patients who are asymptomatic, who undergo surveillance, or who are investigated for other problems such as amenia. In symptomatic patients, the most common presenting symptoms are abdominal pain, change in bowel habits, rectal bleeding, and occult blood in the stool.[2] These symptoms frequently mean that the tumor is more advanced than in asymptomatic patients.

Abdominal pain is the most common presenting symptom of colon cancer. The pain can vary in type, location, and intensity. In the early phases or stages of colon cancer without evidence of obstructive symptoms, the pain can be vague, dull, and poorly localized. With progression of the disease with a larger growing mass or a mass causing obstruction, symptoms of intestinal obstruction will eventually occur. This type of pain is characterized by crampy, colicky pain, often associated with meals, and occurring after meals. The location of the pain is often periumbilical or midabdominal but can be located at the site of obstruction.

A change in bowel habits is the second most common symptom of colon cancer. The changes seen can be very subtle or very significant. In early lesions the change may be minor, with only a change in stool frequency. There can be changes in size, shape, and/or consistency of bowel movements. Characteristic changes include narrowing of the stool, irregular shape, and typically looser or diarrheal stool. The symptoms will depend on the location of the tumor. Right-sided tumors occur where the bowel lumen is larger and the stool is liquid. Symptoms occur later, but on the left side where the stool is more solid and the lumen narrower, symptoms occur at an earlier stage.

Rectal bleeding may be present in as many as 25% of patients with colon cancer.[3,4] The bleeding may be of varying intensity and color. Bright red rectal bleeding is more consistent with a more distal location of a cancer. The mistake of attributing rectal bleeding to hemorrhoids even in a young population can lead to serious and at times fatal delays in the diagnosis of a colon cancer. Almost all patients regardless of age who present with rectal bleeding should undergo colonoscopic evaluation. In a series of 570 patients, 50 years of age or younger with rectal bleeding who underwent endoscopic evaluation, there was a 17.5% incidence of colorectal neoplasm.[5]

Patients undergoing stool guaiac tests for occult blood in the stool for routine screening with a positive result have a 5.1% chance of having an invasive cancer and a 24% chance of having a benign polyp.[6]

As mentioned previously, some of the symptoms that occur may be early or late based on the distribution of cancer within the colon. There has been a more proximal shift overall of colon cancers with more tumors being in the proximal colon. The Lahey Clinic reported a 10-year representative anatomic site distribution in which the cancer was located in the right colon in 18%, the transverse colon in 9%, the descending colon in 5%, the sigmoid colon in 25%, and the rectum in 43%.[7]

Staging and Prognostic Factors

Evolution of Staging Systems

The original staging system for colorectal cancer was reported by Cuthbert Dukes in 1930 and then revised by him in 1932.[8] This classification had three stages: A, B, and C. Stage A had the cancer limited to the bowel wall, Stage B had cancer that spread by direct extension to extrarectal tissues, and Stage C had cancer with regional lymph node metastasis. Dukes further revised the classification in 1944 to subdivide the Stage C group into those with positive regional lymph nodes below a ligature (C1) and at a ligature (C2). In addition a more advanced stage, Stage D was added for distant metastases.

Others have subsequently modified the Dukes' staging system in an attempt to further stratify, prognosticate, and treat patients with a more useful system. The most common modification is know as the Astler Coller Modification.[9] In this modification, the Dukes' B and Dukes' C tumors are subdivided into two groups, each with Dukes' B having depth of tumor invasion into but not through the colonic wall with (B2) or without (B1) lymph node involvement. Similarly, Dukes' C tumors with full-thinness tumor invasion involving lymph nodes, Stage C2, and when they are not C1. Although both the Dukes' and modified Dukes' staging systems are still used, the TMN staging system is the preferred method of colorectal cancer staging.

Current Staging Systems

The TNM classification is the system developed by the American Joint Committee on Cancer (AJCC) and the International Union Against Cancer (UICC). It utilizes three descriptors based on each letter in the name, T for tumor depth, N for nodal involvement, and M for metastases. Based on a combination of T, N, and M for any given tumor, an overall stage from Stage I to IV can be determined. The most recent AJCC/UICC definitions were published in 2002.[10]

The T stage can be divided into seven possible categories based on the depth of invasion. Tis, carcinoma in situ, represents a nonmalignant tumor, T1 has invasion into the submucosa, T2 has invasion into the muscularis propria, T3 has invasion into the subserosa or nonperitonealized pericolonic or rectal tissue (through the bowel wall). T4 has invasion of other organs or structures. The T3 category can be further subdivided by the depth of penetration into the muscularis propria. The N stage can be divided into three categories. N0, with no lymph node involvement, N1 with 1–3 lymph nodes involved, and N2 with 4 or more lymph nodes involved. The M stage is only divided into two categories, either no metastases (M0) or distant metastases (M1).

Typically, the combination of T, N, and M will lead to one of four stages based on the combination of findings. Stage 0 is Tis, N0, and M0. Stage 1 is T1 or T2, N0, M0. Stage 2 is T3 or T4, N0, M0. Stage 3 is Any T, N1 or N2, and M0. Stage 4 is Any T, Any N, and M1. In the most recent AJCC/UICC Definitions, Stage II and III are subdivided into two Stage II categories: Stage IIA (T3, N0, M0) and Stage IIB (T4, N0, M0); and three Stage III categories: Stage IIIA (T1 or T2, N1, M0), Stage IIIB (T3 or T4, N1, M0), and Stage IIIC (Any T, N2, M0).

The importance of staging is for treatment planning and prognosis.

Clinical Prognostic Factors

Age

As with many cancers, colon cancer incidence increases with increasing age. Most series report a mean age in the sixth decade for nonhereditary colon cancer. Patients with familial adenomatous polyposis (FAP) will present with colon cancer in their mid to late 30s if colectomy is not performed before this age. Patients with hereditary nonpolyposis colorectal cancer (HNPCC) can present at any age but tend to have colon cancer between the ages of 40 and 60, significantly younger than individuals with nonhereditary colon cancers.

It has been reported that younger patients present with worse tumors being of more advanced stage and grade. However, recent studies refute this claim. O'Connell et al.[11] recently reported using SEER data a comparison of two groups of patients with colon cancer. The SEER database is a prospectively entered database of the National Cancer Institute in the United States and stands for Surveillance, Epidemiology, and End Results. They compared outcome in patients 20–40 years of age to those 40–60 years of age. Although there was an increased incidence of higher stage tumors, stage for stage they had an equivalent or improved 5-year survival.

Symptoms

Obstruction and perforation are poor prognostic signs often associated with advanced disease. In addition, because patients are operated on in an urgent manner, their operative morbidity and mortality is increased. Chen and Sheen-Chen[12] reported on outcome in patients with obstructing and/or perforated colon cancer. Perforated cancers had a 9% operative mortality compared with obstructed cancers of 5%. Overall 5-year survival was 33% in each group, approximately 2 times the expected rate based on similar stages in noncomplicated cases.

Blood Transfusion

Blood transfusions can cause immunosuppression in the postoperative period which may allow for an inability to combat tumor cells shed at the time of surgery and theoretically lead to a worse prognosis. Sibbering et al.[13] reported on 266 patients with colon cancer, some of whom received blood transfusions and others that did not. There was no difference in survival comparing the two groups. However, Chung et al.[14] reviewed 20 papers, representing 5236 patients supporting the hypothesis that perioperative blood transfusions are associated with an increased recurrence and death from colon carcinoma.

Adjacent Organ Involvement

Local extension of colon carcinoma can involve any structure or organ adjacent to the primary tumor. It occurs in 5%–12% of colorectal cancers. All tumors with local extension would be considered T4. For right colon cancers, the most frequently involved structures are the liver, duodenum, pancreas, and abdominal wall. Kama et al.[15] reported a 75% disease-free survival of 14–41 months after en bloc pancreaticoduodenectomy and right colectomy. Similarly, Izbicki et al.[16] reported on 83 patients with colorectal cancer undergoing extended en bloc resections. Comparing extended to nonextended resections; mean survival of both groups was around 45 months conferring the benefit of extended resections when necessary to achieve R0 resections. These data were supported by Kroneman et al.[17] who found 4-year survival was 33% after en bloc resection compared with those receiving noncurable resections of 6 months.

Histologic/Biochemical/Genetic Factors

Histologic Grade

Broders described classifying adenocarcinomas by the degree of differentiation. He described four grades based on how much of the tumor had differentiated cells within it. Today three grades are used and include Grade 1 with well-differentiated features, Grade 2 moderately differentiated, and Grade 3 poorly differentiated. The vast majority of colon cancers are moderately differentiated (Grade 2) with preservation of gland-forming architecture. However, the amount of preservation of this architecture is variable and when absent leads to sheets of invasive cells classified as poorly differentiated. The degree of differentiation corresponds to prognosis. Poorly differentiated tumors have a worse prognosis stage for stage compared with better differentiated tumors.[18]

Mucin Production and Microsatellite Instability

Microsatellite instability, known as MSI, is associated with HNPCC. MSI is an alteration in mismatch repair genes which are important to repairing errors in replication. When altered, they can lead to colorectal cancer. Because there is loss of one of the two alleles in HNPCC, these patients tend to present earlier in life, with multiple colonic and extracolonic cancers. Many HNPCC cancers are mucin producing which when present have a better prognosis compared with non–mucin-producing tumors in these patients.

Signet-cell Histology

Signet-ring or signet-cell tumors have a worse prognosis in many intestinal cancers. Signet-cell tumors tend to be of a more advanced stage when discovered. In a comparison between signet-ring and non–signet-ring colon cancers, it was noted that patients with signet-ring cancers were younger, had more advanced stages, and an increased incidence of liver metastases.[19] In addition, the rate of curative resection was lower at 35% compared with 79%. This rate was similar to poorly differentiated tumors at 46% at 5 years. In another study, the risk of peritoneal seeding was higher in signet-cell tumors leading to a high incidence of palliative resections and a mean survival of 16 months.[20]

Venous Invasion

Blood vessel invasion has been linked with poor prognosis both independently as well as with its association with lymph node metastasis. Blood vessel invasion can occur intramurally within the wall of the colon itself or in the surrounding tissue. Although arterial invasion occurs, most series define and describe vascular invasion based on venous invasion. Venous invasion in colon cancer occurs in 42% of patients and increases with increasing grade and stage.[21] Patients with blood vessel invasion had a 74% survival compared with those without it at 85%. In those patients with both intramural and extramural vascular invasion, the prognosis was even worse at 32%.

Perineural Invasion

The growth of tumor along perineural spaces is known as perineural invasion and, similar to venous invasion, it increases with increasing grade and stage of the tumor. It occurs in 14%–32% of colorectal cancers and can extend to as far away as 10 cm from the primary tumor. Numerous studies have confirmed poorer prognosis when perineural invasion is noted.[22,23]

Lymph Node Involvement

Lymph node metastasis has been long understood to be one of, if not the most, important prognostic factors in colon cancer outcome. All currently utilized staging systems as described above for colon cancer use and rely on the presence or absence of lymph node metastases. It is therefore important to adequately remove the lymph node bearing tissue associated with the underlying colon cancer. It has been reported by Scott and Grace[25] that, if 13 lymph nodes are not recovered, adequate staging cannot be performed. The main determinant for an adequate lymph node harvest is surgical but a variety of means to enhance the yield have been developed and include fat clearance with xylene, other chemicals, and polymerase chain reaction techniques.[26] Using these techniques, more lymph nodes, or lymph nodes not found by standard techniques, can be discovered, improving the accuracy of staging and allowing for better prognosis and application of adjuvant treatment.

Carcinoembryonic Antigen

Carcinoembryonic antigen (CEA), a glycoprotein absent in normal colonic mucosa but present in 97% of patients with colon cancer, was discovered in 1965.[27] CEA increase correlates with either disease that has metastasized to the liver or with very large tumors. Patients with disease confined to the colonic mucosa or submucosa will have increased CEA in 30%–40% of cases. It is therefore not useful for screening but can be used to follow patients with colon cancer. In patients with increased CEA preoperatively and localized disease that is resectable, the CEA should decrease after surgery. If the CEA level does not decrease, then occult metastases may be present and may be an indication for adjuvant therapy. The absolute level of CEA is also important. A CEA of greater than 15 mg/mL predicts an increased risk of metastases in otherwise apparently curable colon cancer.[28] A normal preoperative CEA may become increased with metastatic disease. Controversy exists as to the utility of following CEA postoperatively because it may not allow any advantage to salvage or treatment when compared with symptomatic recurrences.[29] Despite that, the routine periodic CEA measurement is endorsed by the American Society of Colon and Rectal Surgeons in their Practice Parameters.[30]

Sentinel Node

The idea of a sentinel lymph node being present and if identified be able to predict lymph node metastases has become standard of care in breast cancer and melanoma. Its application to colon cancer is in its infancy and may be less important in colon cancer than these others. The idea that the lymphatic drainage can be mapped and the first node identified has significance in oncologic surgery. In colon cancer, resecting the associated lymphovascular pedicle with the primary cancer is considered paramount to performing an adequate operation; this adds little to no morbidity unlike excising level 3 nodes in breast cancer patients. In an attempt to validate the sentinel lymph node theory in colon cancer, Paramo et al.[31] reported on their experience with 45 patients who underwent intraoperative sentinel lymph node mapping using isosulfan blue dye. Sentinel lymph nodes were identified 82% of the time and predicted regional metastases in 98% of cases, with only a single case of a false-negative sentinel lymph node. Others have agreed that its utility may be marginal in colon cancer.[32]

DNA Ploidy

Normal cells are made up of diploid cells. Tumors can maintain normal diploid cells or can be aneuploid. Numerous studies show that nondiploid tumors have a worse prognosis and correlate with more advanced Dukes' stage.[33]

Spreading Patterns

Colon cancer can spread via a variety of pathways. Spread can be local or distant based on these pathways.

Intramural Spread

Intramural spread is the tumor spreading along the bowel wall either proximally or distally in one of the bowel wall layers. Like rectal cancers, colon cancer rarely spreads this way. In a study of 42 colorectal cancers of which 64% were colonic, the maximum extent of intramural spread was 2 cm.[34] This supports the practice of excising 5 cm or more of colon on either side of a tumor to decrease the risk of anastomotic recurrence.[36]

Transmural Spread

As they become more advanced, colon cancers invade the colonic wall. Almost all colon cancers start as a mucosal lesion and then penetrate a variable degree into deeper layers of the colonic wall. This colonic wall invasion is the basis of many of the currently used staging systems including the Dukes' and TNM. Transmural spread is the mechanism that produces T4 tumors. T4 tumors penetrate full thickness into the colonic wall and then by direct extension or adherence, invade into other structures in proximity to the primary tumor. When present, en bloc resection is mandatory for an R0 resection. Preoperative evaluation can sometimes predict adjacent organ involvement but often it is an intraoperative finding.

Margins

The acceptable bowel wall margins are dictated by three issues: first, thickness of penetration of the bowel wall margin and the risk based on the distance of local tumor spread intramurally. As described above, colon cancer rarely invades proximally or distally along the bowel wall for more than 2 cm. Convention has led to the recommendation that proximal and distal margins be a minimum of 5 cm. It has been stated that the "ideal extent of a bowel resection is defined by removing the blood supply and the lymphatics at the level of the origin of the primary feeding arterial vessel."[35] These other two factors may modify the length of the proximal and/or distal margins because further resections may be required because of these issues.

Radial Margins

The circumferential margins are important to both colon and rectal cancer, but most series and studies have been confined to rectal cancers. It has been shown that positive circumferential margins in rectal cancer are associated with local recurrence rates as high as 85%.[36] In colon cancer, the radial margins are less important with the exception of T4 tumors where en bloc resection is required. Typically for colon cancer, the only radial margin that may be involved in a tumor less than T4 are those tumors with serosal involvement. In 279 patients with colon cancer, serosal involvement was not associated with a poorer outcome, and outcome was related only to tumor stage.[37]

Transperitoneal/Implantation

Tumors with serosal involvement can shed viable tumor cells which can spread throughout the peritoneal cavity and implant on a variety of structures. Usually, tumors will implant on the ovaries, omentum, serosal, or peritoneal surfaces. When widespread, this is known as carcinomatosis. When localized to the ovaries which occurs in 3%–5% of patients, bilateral oophorectomy should be performed. In a recent series, 86% of patients with ovarian metastases had transmural extension of the primary colon cancers.[38]

Lymphatic

Lymphatic invasion is the most common mechanism leading to metastatic disease. Lymphatics exist within the colonic wall and lymphatic invasion correlates with the depth of penetration of colon cancers. T1 tumors have a risk of lymph node involvement up to 9%, T2 up to 25%, and T3 up to 45%. Most currently used staging systems assign increased stage to increasing T stage and lymph node involvement and prognosis correlates with the overall stage. The lymphatic drainage goes along the venous drainage of the colon, ultimately coursing through the portal vein and into the liver. Metastatic liver disease is believed to occur typically as a result of lymphatic spread.

Hematogenous

Hematogenous spread of colon cancer is less common than lymphatic spread. Hematogenous spread will bypass the liver and allow tumor cells to go peripherally into the systemic circulation. This is thought to be the mechanism for the development of pulmonary metastases.

Metastatic Evaluation

Once diagnosed with colon carcinoma, a search for metastatic disease is often performed. This assessment includes a variety of imaging studies, laboratory tests, and endoscopic procedures.

Detection and Management of Synchronous Lesions

Synchronous polyps and cancers occur in patients with colon cancer. Most colon cancers are diagnosed by colonoscopy and the remainder of the colon is evaluated at the same time by colonoscopy. However, if an obstructing lesion is noted that will not allow a colonoscope to pass, evaluation of the more proximal colon may be jeopardized. Alternatives to evaluating the remainder of the colon in these instances include contrast enemas, virtual colonoscopy, or intraoperative colonoscopy at the time of resection. In a series of 158 patients with incomplete colonoscopies, barium enema was used to examine the remainder of the colon. Six lesions greater than 1 cm were identified with five of six being proximal cancers or advanced adenomas.[40] Virtual colonoscopy was used in 34 patients suspected of colon cancer with incomplete colonoscopies. Virtual colonoscopy identified all primary and three synchronous tumors proximal to the primary tumor.[40] When a colon cancer is diagnosed by colonoscopy, synchronous cancers occur in 6% or fewer of patients. When present, it should raise the suspicion of possibly HNPCC which is associated with synchronous colon cancer. When synchronous colon cancer is diagnosed, the treatment should consider a subtotal colectomy.

Distant Metastatic Disease

Distant metastatic disease associated with colon cancer is almost always either liver or lung metastases. Although bone, brain, and other organ involvement can occur, it is rare and therefore the search for these metastases in an asymptomatic patient is unwarranted. The search for liver and lung metastases can be accomplished by a variety of imaging studies including ultrasound, computed tomography (CT) scan, magnetic resonance imaging (MRI), chest X-ray, and positron emission tomography (PET) scans. Each test has different abilities, availabilities, and costs.

Liver Metastases

The first available test for the evaluation of the liver for metastases is surface ultrasound. Surface ultrasound is available in almost all institutions; however, its accuracy compared with newer modalities is lower in comparative studies comparing it with CT and liver scans.[41,42]

CT scan is the most frequently used method to preoperatively and postoperatively determine the presence or absence of liver metastases associated with colon cancer. There are numerous advantages to cross-sectional imaging such as CT over ultrasound and include the ability to find abdominal wall or contiguous organ invasion as well as liver metastases. Standard CT scan is 64% sensitive in identifying liver lesions larger than 1 cm. MRI of the liver has been poorly studied and is not typically used in the evaluation of liver metastases.

Lung Metastases

Lung metastases occur in 3.5 % of patients with colon cancer[43]; there are limited data on the utility of plain chest radiographs or CT scans in the initial evaluation of the lungs for metastatic disease. CT scan clearly has advantages over plain radiographs and can identify and characterize lung pathology better than plain X-rays. Given that most patients will undergo CT imaging of the abdomen before surgical intervention, the addition of imaging of the chest via CT seems reasonable. One must be careful about the amount of intravenous contrast when simultaneously scanning multiple regions such as chest, abdomen, and pelvis.

PET Scans

PET scans are currently approved only for patients with suspected metastatic disease and not for the use in primary staging of colon cancer. However, based on the data from studies looking at patients with metastatic disease, PET scans may have a role in determining if any metastatic disease exists at the time of initial diagnosis.

Appendix: Practice Parameters for the Detection of Colorectal Neoplasms

Prepared by The Standards Committee, The American Society of Colon and Rectal Surgeons

Drs. Clifford L. Simmang and Peter Senatore, Project Directors; Ann Lowry, Chair; Terry Hicks, Council Representative; Marcus Burnstein, Frederick Dentsman, Victor Fazio, Edward Glennon, Neil Hyman, Bruce Kerner, John Kilkenny, Richard Moore, Walter Peters, Theodore Ross, Paul Savoca, Anthony Vernava, W. Douglas Wong

Colorectal cancer is the most preventable visceral cancer, and its incidence makes it one of the most important. The lifetime probability of an individual developing colorectal cancer is 5%–6%, translating into an estimated 133,500 new cancers of the colon and rectum diagnosed annually. It is further estimated that 54,900 people will die of their cancer each year. Although the incidence was relatively stable during the last half of the 20th century, there seems to have been a decrease during the past decade. Mortality is also decreasing, which suggests greater awareness of the disease and improved detection. Nevertheless, 65% of patients present with advanced disease. It is also reported that when the disease is localized, the 5-year survival rate is approximately 90% for colon cancer and 80% for cancer of the rectum. Most cases are diagnosed after 50 years of age. Although the results of some investigations have not demonstrated a reduction in mortality with screening, those statistics do not reflect the number of patients who are spared from death by early detection and endoscopic removal of polyps, which blunts the adenoma-to-carcinoma sequence.

A consortium of five medical societies (American College of Gastroenterology, American Gastroenterological Association, The American Society of Colon and Rectal Surgeons, American Society for Gastrointestinal Endoscopy, and Society of American Gastrointestinal Endoscopic Surgeons) responded to a request for a proposal from the Agency for Health Care Policy and Research to develop national guidelines for colorectal cancer screening. An interdisciplinary panel of 16 health care professionals from the fields of medicine, nursing, consumer advocacy, health care economics, behavioral sciences, and radiology evaluated the currently available evidence for colorectal cancer screening and made recommendations for physicians and the public. The panel studied 3500 peer-reviewed published articles and analyzed 350 articles in detail specifically assessing the following: 1) performance of screening tests; 2) effectiveness of screening tests; 3) acceptability to patients; 4) cost effectiveness; and 5) outcome. A computer simulation of the consequences of conducting the various screening strategies in the population was done to determine the risks and benefits of each test. The guidelines made recommendations for people in two groups: average individuals and individuals at increased risk for developing colorectal cancer. All screening strategies, including annual fecal occult blood testing, screening sigmoidoscopy every 5 years, screening by both annual fecal occult blood testing and flexible sigmoidoscopy (every 5 years), double contrast barium enema every 5–10 years, and colonoscopy every 10 years were found to have a net benefit. The panel analyzed an Office of Technology Assessment study for screening average-risk individuals, which demonstrated that costs associated with colorectal cancer screening are within the range of cost effectiveness frequently accepted for other tests, such as mammography.

Recently revised colorectal cancer screening guidelines from the American Cancer Society have been announced. The new guidelines divide the population into three categories—average, moderate, and high risk—with specific recommendations for each. The American Society of Colon and Rectal Surgeons endorses the colorectal cancer screening guidelines by the American Cancer Society, which were based in part on "Colorectal Cancer Screening and Surveillance Clinical Guidelines and Rationale" published by the consortium and specialty societies and discussed above. Guidelines governing the detection of colorectal neoplasms as set forth by The American Society of Colon and Rectal Surgeons Task Force are presented in Table 27-1.

Low-Risk Individuals

For low-risk asymptomatic persons, screening should begin at the age of 50. Low-risk or average-risk patients are those who are asymptomatic, age 50 or older, have a family history of colorectal cancer limited to non–first-degree relatives, and no other risk factors (65%–75% of people). Annual digital rectal examination should be performed. In addition, fecal occult blood testing (FOBT) should be performed annually. Yearly testing is chosen because the randomized trials show that yearly testing is more effective for decreasing mortality than testing every 2 years. Rehydration improves the sensitivity of the test at the expense of specificity. Dietary avoidance of rare meat, turnips, melons, horseradish, salmon, and sardines can decrease the rate of false-positive test results. Aspirin and other nonsteroidal drugs should also be avoided. Diagnostic workup of positive FOBT results should include an evaluation of the entire colon. Double-contrast barium enema can examine the entire colon with relatively high sensitivity and specificity for large polyps (>1 cm) and cancers and is less expensive than colonoscopy. However, it is not possible to biopsy or remove neoplasms during the same procedure, so

TABLE 27-1. Screening guidelines

Risk	Procedure	Onset (age, yr)	Frequency
I. Low or average: 65%75%	Digital rectal exam *and* one of the following:	50	Yearly
A. Asymptomatic: no risk factors	Fecal occult blood testing and flexible sigmoidoscopy	50	FOBT yearly, flex-sig every 5 yr
B. Colorectal cancer in no first-degree relatives	Total colon exam (colonoscopy or double contrast barium enema and proctosigmoidoscopy	50	Every 5–10 yr
II. Moderate risk: 20%–30% of people			
A. Colorectal cancer in first-degree relative, age 55 or younger, or two or more first-degree relatives of any age	Colonoscopy	40 or 10 yr before the youngest case in the family, whichever is earlier	Every 5 yr
B. Colorectal cancer in a first-degree relative older than age 55	Colonoscopy	50 or 10 yr before the age of the case, whichever is earlier	Every 5–10 yr
C. Personal history of large (>1 cm) or multiple colorectal polyps of any size	Colonoscopy	1 yr after polypectomy	If recurrent polyps, 1 yr If normal, 5 yr
D. Personal history of colorectal malignancy, surveillance after resection for curative intent	Colonoscopy	1 yr after resection	If normal, 3 yr If still normal, 5 yr If abnormal, as above
III. High risk (6%–8% of people)			
A. Family history of hereditary adenomatous polyposis	Flexible sigmoidoscopy; consider genetic counseling; consider genetic testing	12–14 (puberty)	Every 1–2 yr
B. Family history of hereditary nonpolyposis colon cancer	Colonoscopy; consider genetic counseling; consider genetic testing	21–40 40	Every 2 yr Every yr
C. Inflammatory bowel disease			
1. Left-side colitis	Colonoscopy	15th	Every 1–2 yr
2. Pancolitis	Colonoscopy	8th	Every 1–2 yr

FOBT, fecal occult blood testing; Flex-sig, flexible sigmoidoscopy.

that patients with abnormalities must undergo an additional examination by colonoscopy to establish the diagnosis and provide treatment. Adding flexible sigmoidoscopy to double-contrast barium enema increases sensitivity, but the magnitude in clinical importance of the additional sensitivity is uncertain. For these reasons, colonoscopy, which can examine the entire colon with few false-negative or false-positive findings and can provide definitive treatment of polyps and some cancers during the same procedure, is usually chosen. For patients who have negative FOBT results, flexible sigmoidoscopy performed every 5 years is recommended. A 5-year interval is chosen because of the observation that few polyps arise and progress to advanced cancer in a 5-year period. If a polyp is identified, it should be biopsied. If the pathologic diagnosis is a hyperplastic polyp, then no additional evaluation is required. If the pathologic diagnosis is an adenoma, then colonoscopy should be recommended.

Colonoscopy permits visualization of the entire colon directly, along with detection and removal of polyps and biopsy of cancers throughout the colon. It can be considered for screening of average-risk individuals. An interval of 10 years has been chosen for asymptomatic, average-risk people because of strong direct evidence that few clinically important lesions are missed by this examination and that it takes an average of approximately 10 years for an adenomatous polyp, particularly one <1 cm in diameter, to transform into invasive cancer. In addition, a controlled trial has shown a very low incidence of advanced adenomas during surveillance follow-up colonoscopy after an initial examination with negative results.[20] Indirect evidence from the National Polyp Study indicates that few polyps will arise and progress to advanced cancer in less time in patients with no special risk factors.

Moderate-Risk Individuals

Patients at moderate risk for cancer are those who have one or more first-degree relatives with colorectal cancer or personal history of colorectal neoplasia (20%–30% of people).

Colorectal Neoplasia in a Close Relative

People with a first-degree relative (sibling, parent, or child) who has a colorectal cancer or adenomatous polyp should be offered the same options as average-risk people, but with several important differences. Those people with two or more affected close relatives or with an affected close relative younger than age 55 are at even further increased risk, and surveillance should begin at the age of 40 years or 10 years before the youngest case in the family, whichever is earlier. Colonoscopy is the recommended procedure of choice in this situation. If colorectal cancer is detected in a close relative older than age 55, then screening should begin with colonoscopy at the age of 50 or 10 years before the age of the case, whichever is earlier.

Patients with Other Risk Factors

Patients with prior endometrial, ovarian, or breast cancer and those who have had pelvic radiation, could be followed up according to the guidelines established for patients with a family history of colon cancer. Patients with a ureterocolonic anastomosis should be followed up yearly with flexible sigmoidoscopy as a minimum and colonoscopy if the area of anastomosis cannot be visualized by sigmoidoscopy. Total colonic examination may be recommended for patients with acromegaly, *Streptococcus bovis*, *Streptococcus sanguis*, or a *Clostridium septicum* bacteremia, schistosomiasis, extramammary perianal Paget's disease, and dermatomyositis.

Polyp Surveillance

For patients who have had a neoplasm identified by sigmoidoscopic examination, a biopsy should be performed. If the pathologic finding is an adenoma, then a colonoscopy should be performed. For a polyp detected during a barium enema examination, a colonoscopy is the recommended procedure. Colonoscopy can directly inspect the entire colon for the presence of synchronous lesions and allow the removal of polyps or biopsy of a larger neoplasm. If a large (>1 cm) polyp is removed, or if multiple polyps of any size are identified and removed, colonoscopy should be repeated 1 year later. If a single, small (<1 cm), tubular adenoma is identified and removed, colonoscopy should be repeated in 3–5 years. If the results of this examination are normal, then colonoscopy should be repeated every 5 years. The finding of an adenoma at any of the follow-up examinations may prompt yearly colonoscopy until the colon is again cleared of polyps. Studies may need to be repeated when the entire colon is not visualized, when there is poor preparation or spasm, when polypectomy is deemed incomplete or complications ensue that require intervention, when there is diagnostic uncertainty, or when tumor debulking is necessary. If the pathologic diagnosis of the initial polyp is a hyperplastic polyp, no diagnostic studies are required at this time and the patient should continue appropriate screening evaluation.

If a polypectomy is performed for curative intent of an invasive cancer, follow-up colonoscopy should be performed in 6–12 months. If these examination results are normal, colonoscopy should be repeated every 3–5 years as long as the colon remains clear. If, between total colonoscopic examinations, it is necessary to visualize high-risk sites, such as those from which a large, sessile polyp has been removed from the rectum in a piecemeal manner, sigmoidoscopy is a viable alternative.

Personal History of Colorectal Malignancy

When the colon has been cleared by barium enema or colonoscopy before resection for cancer, colonoscopy or barium enema is performed again approximately 1–3 years after surgical resection. If the colon was not cleared before surgical resection, colonoscopy or barium enema is recommended in 3–6 months. If the follow-up examination results are normal, it is repeated in 3 years and if they are still normal, the interval between colonic surveillance can be extended to every 5 years.

High-risk Individuals

Patients at high risk for developing colorectal cancer are those with a hereditary or genetic predisposition for development of colorectal cancer, and those patients with inflammatory bowel disease (6%–8% of people).

Family History of FAP

FAP is characterized by the development of multiple (more than 100) adenomatous polyps in the colon and rectum. Inheritance is by an autosomal dominant manner with high penetrance.

It is recommended that endoscopic examination of the rectum and sigmoid colon be performed every 12 months beginning at the age of puberty (12–14 years). For those patients with familial adenomatous polyposis who have undergone a total abdominal colectomy with an ileorectal anastomosis, it may be desirable to examine the rectum every 6–12 months.

Definitive data regarding appropriate duration of screening is not available. As a general guideline, intense surveillance could change to routine screening at age 40 in families with uniformly severe disease. In families with variability in the severity of polyposis, screening should continue until age 60, although the interval might be increased to 2 years after age 40.

People with a family history of FAP should also be considered for genetic counseling and consider genetic testing to see if they are gene carriers. A negative genetic test result rules out FAP only if an affected family member has an identified mutation. Gene carriers or indeterminate cases should be offered flexible sigmoidoscopy as recommended above. If polyposis is present, colonoscopy is not a reliable screening test for malignancy and prophylactic surgery is indicated, preferably before the patient is 20 years old. If genetic test results are negative, screening should be the same as for low-risk individuals.

Family History of HNPCC

HNPCC is an autosomal dominant disease characterized by early-onset colorectal tumors, primarily in the right colon, that are frequently associated with other cancers. A common standard for the diagnosis of HNPCC, referred to as the Amsterdam criteria, is the existence of three or more relatives with colorectal cancer, one of whom is a first-degree relative and involves at least two generations, with one or more cases diagnosed before the age of 50. The Amsterdam criteria have been criticized as being too rigid, failing to take into account small families where a dominant pattern of inheritance may not be obvious and extracolonic cancers that make up the syndrome of HNPCC. When a strong family history is present, the possibility of HNPCC must be considered.

People with a family history of colorectal cancer in multiple close relatives and across generations, especially if the cancers occurred at a young age, should receive genetic counseling and consider genetic testing for HNPCC. When performed, genetic test results are positive in approximately 80% of these families. It is recommended that individuals considering genetic testing be counseled regarding the unknown efficacy of measures to reduce risks and associated issues and that care for individuals with cancer-predisposing mutations be provided whenever possible within the context of research protocols designed to evaluate clinical outcomes.

Endoscopic examination should begin between the ages of 20 and 25 years or at least 10 years younger than the family member who had colorectal cancer. The endoscopic procedure of choice is colonoscopy and this should be performed every 2 years until the age of 40 years. After the age of 40 years, colonoscopy should be performed annually. Unless genetic testing results are negative, surveillance should be performed as long as the patient's overall medical condition warrants it. Colonoscopy is selected because the cancers and precursor adenomatous polyps are both predominantly proximal to the splenic flexure.

Inflammatory Bowel Disease

Ulcerative Colitis

The increased risk of developing colorectal cancer in patients with inflammatory bowel disease is well established, with a lifetime incidence of 6% in patients with ulcerative colitis (UC). Up to 1% of all cases of colorectal cancers seen in the general population may be associated with inflammatory bowel disease. The risk of developing colorectal cancer is low until 8 years of disease duration, after which the risk increases exponentially to reach as high as 56 times that of the general population by the fourth decade of disease. The degree of risk also depends on extent of involvement and age of onset. The strongest predisposing factor for cancer is the anatomic extent of the inflammation, with patients at most risk if they have pancolitis or ulceration extending proximally to the splenic flexure and least risk if the disease is limited to the rectum and sigmoid colon. Because the risk of developing dysplasia or cancer increases with longer disease duration, efficient surveillance calls for more frequent testing as the risk increases with duration. It is common practice to perform surveillance colonoscopy every 1–2 years after 8 years of disease in patients with pancolitis or after 15 years in patients with colitis limited to the left colon.[6] Ulcerative proctitis does not need extraordinary cancer surveillance.

Crohn's Disease

Patients with Crohn's disease have a 20-fold increased risk of colon carcinoma over the general population; however, less than the increased risk seen with UC. Compared with sporadic colorectal cancer, colorectal cancers in Crohn's disease occur at an earlier age (48 versus 60 years), are more often located in the right colon, and are more frequently multiple. In particular, sites of stricture and fistula formation seem particularly prone to the development of carcinomas. It is clear that Crohn's disease warrants attention to risk of cancer; however, evidence for the most appropriate surveillance program is lacking. We recommend a moderate program, such as recommended for left-sided UC with surveillance colonoscopy every 1–2 years after 15 years of disease.

Reprinted from Dis Colon Rectum 1999;42(9):1123–1129. Copyright © 2003. All rights reserved. American Society of Colon and Rectal Surgeons.

References

1. Cancer Facts and Statistics 2004. Atlanta: American Cancer Society.
2. Beart RW, Steele GD, Merck HR, et al. Management and survival of patients with adenocarcinoma of the colon and rectum: a national survey of the Commission on Cancer. J Am Coll Surg 1995;181:225–236.
3. Ferraris R, Senore C, Fracchia M, et al. Predictive value of rectal bleeding for distal colonic neoplastic lesions in a screened population. Eur J Cancer 2004;40:245–252.
4. Helfand M, Marton KI, Zimmer-Gembeck MJ, et al. History of visible rectal bleeding in a primary care population: initial assessment and 10-year follow-up. JAMA 1997;277:44–48.
5. Lewis JD, Shih CE, Blecker D. Endoscopy for hematochezia in patients under 50 years of age. Dig Dis Sci 2001;46:2660–2665.
6. Gilbertsen VA, Williams SE, Schuman L, et al. Paper presentation at the International Symposium on Colorectal Cancer. New York, March 1979.

7. Corman ML, Veidenheimer MC, Coller JA. Colorectal carcinoma: a decade of experience at the Lahey Clinic. Dis Colon Rectum 1979;22:477–479.

8. Dukes CE. The spread of cancer of the rectum. Br J Surg 1930; 17:643.

9. Astler VB, Coller FA. Prognostic significance of direct extension of carcinoma of the colon and rectum. Ann Surg 1954;139:846.

10. Greene Fl, Page DL, Fleming ID, et al. Cancer Staging Manual. 6th ed. New York: Springer; 2002.

11. O'Connell JB, Maggard MA, Liu JH, et al. Do young colon cancer patients have worse outcomes? World J Surg 2004;28:558–562.

12. Chen HS, Sheen-Chen SM. Obstruction and perforation in colorectal adenocarcinoma: an analysis of prognosis and current trends. Surgery 2000;127:370–376.

13. Sibbering DM, Locker AP, Hardcastle JD, et al. Blood transfusion and survival in colorectal cancer. Dis Colon Rectum 1994; 37:358–363.

14. Chung M, Steinmetz OK, Gordon PH. Perioperative blood transfusion and outcome after resection for colorectal carcinoma. Br J Surg 1993;80:427–432.

15. Kama NA, Reis E, Doganay M, et al. Radical surgery of colon cancers directly invading the duodenum, pancreas and liver. Hepatogastroenterology 2001;48:114–117.

16. Izbicki JR, Hosch SB, Knoefel WT, et al. Extended resections are beneficial for patients with locally advanced colorectal cancer. Dis Colon Rectum 1995;38:1251–1256.

17. Kroneman H, Castelein A, Jeekel J. En bloc resection of colon carcinoma adherent to other organs: an efficacious treatment? Dis Colon Rectum 1991;34:780–783.

18. Cooper HS, Slemmer JR. Surgical pathology of carcinoma of the colon and rectum. Semin Oncol 1991;18:367–380.

19. Bittorf B, Merkel S, Matzel KE, et al. Primary signet-ring cell carcinoma of the colorectum. Langenbecks Arch Surg 2004;389: 178–183.

20. Psathakis D, Schiedick TH, Krug F, et al. Ordinary colorectal adenocarcinoma vs primary colorectal signet-ring cell carcinoma: study matched for age, gender, grade and stage. Dis Colon Rectum 1999;42:1618–1625.

21. Minsky BD, Mies C, Recht A, et al. Resectable adenocarcinoma of the rectosigmoid and rectum. II. The influence of blood vessel invasion. Cancer 1988;61:1417–1424.

22. Knudsen JB, Nilsson T, Sprechler M, et al. Venous and nerve invasion as prognostic factors in postoperative survival of patients with respectable cancer of the rectum. Dis Colon Rectum 1983;26:613–617.

23. Compton CC. Pathology report in colon cancer: what is prognostically important. Dig Dis 1999;17:67–79.

24. Scott KW, Grace RH. Detection of lymph node metastases in colorectal carcinoma before and after fat clearance. Br J Surg 1989;76:1165–1167.

25. Herrera L, Luna P, Villarreal JR. Lymph-node clearance techniques. Dis Colon Rectum 1991;34:513–514.

26. Koren R, Seigal A, Klein B, Halpern M, et al. Lymph node revealing solution: simple new method for detecting minute lymph nodes in colon cancer. Dis Colon Rectum 1997;40:407–410.

27. Gold P, Freedman SO. Demonstration of tumor-specific antigens in human colonic carcinomata by immunological tolerance and absorption techniques. J Exp Med 1965;121:439.

28. Wiratkapun S, Kraemer M, Seow-Choen F, et al. High preoperative serum carcinoembryonic antigen predicts metastatic recurrence in potentially curative colonic cancer: results of a five-year study. Dis Colon Rectum 2001;44:231–235.

29. Moertel CG, Fleming TR, MacDonald JS, et al. An evaluation of the carcinoembryonic antigen (CEA) for monitoring patients with resected colon cancer. JAMA 1993;270:943–947.

30. The Standards Practice Task Force, The American Society of Colon and Rectal Surgeons. Practice parameters for the surveillance and follow up of patients with colon and rectal cancer. Dis Colon Rectum 2004;47:807–817.

31. Paramo JC, Summerall J, Poppiti R, Mesko TW. Validation of sentinel node mapping in patients with colon cancer. Ann Surg Oncol 2002;9:550–554.

32. Fazio VW, Kirian RP. Surgical treatment of colon cancer: does sentinel node technology have a role? Adv Surg 2003;37:71–94.

33. Scott NA, Rainwater LM, Weiand HS, et al. The relative prognostic value of flow cytometric DNA analysis and conventional clinicopathologic criteria in patients with operable cancer. Dis Colon Rectum 1987;30:513–520.

34. Hughes TG, Jenevein EP, Poulos E. Intramural spread of colon carcinoma. A pathologic study. Am J Surg 1983;146: 697–699.

35. Nelson H, Petrelli N, Carlin A, et al. Guidelines 2000 for colon and rectal cancer surgery. J Natl Cancer Inst 2001;93:583–596.

36. de Haas-kock DF, Baeten CG, Jager JJ, et al. Prognostic significance of radial margins of clearance in rectal cancer. Br J Surg 1996;83:781–785.

37. Tominaga T, Sakabe T, Koyama Y, et al. Prognostic factors for patients with colon or rectal carcinoma treated with resection only. Five-year follow-up report. Cancer 1996;78:403–408.

38. Wright JD, Powell MA, Mutch DG, et al. Synchronous ovarian metastases at the time of laparotomy for colon cancer. Gynecol Oncol 2004;92:851–855.

39. Chong A, Shah JN, Levine MS, et al. Diagnostic yield of barium enema examination after incomplete colonoscopy. Radiology 2002;223:620–624.

40. Neri E, Giusti P, Battolla L, et al. Colorectal cancer: role of CT colonography in the preoperative evaluation after incomplete colonoscopy. Radiology 2002;223:615–619.

41. Alderson PO, Adams DF, McNeil BJ, et al. Computed tomography, ultrasound, and scintigraphy of the liver in patients with colon or breast carcinoma: a prospective comparison. Radiology 1983;149:225–230.

42. Glover C, Douse P, Kane P, et al. Accuracy of investigations for asymptomatic colorectal liver metastases. Dis Colon Rectum 2002;45:476–484.

43. Pihl E, Hughes ES, McDermott FT, et al. Lung recurrence after curative surgery for colorectal cancer. Dis Colon Rectum 1987;30:417–419.

28
Surgical Management of Colon Cancer

Anthony J. Senagore and Robert Fry

All colorectal adenocarcinomas develop from a single transformed cell which through numerous cell divisions unimpeded by cell death forms a macroscopic lesion involving the lumen of the bowel. The staging of colorectal cancer assesses the depth of penetration of the bowel wall, the involvement of regional lymph nodes, the involvement of adjacent organs, and the presence or absence of distant metastases. An increasingly wide variety of putative molecular markers for aggressiveness and metastatic potential have been analyzed; however, the most accurate prognostic indicator remains the true stage of the cancer. This fact is the basis for recognizing adequate locoregional oncologic principles when performing curative resections of colon cancer. The purpose of this chapter is to primarily address issues directly related to the safe and oncologically sound methods of performing a curative resection of a colonic carcinoma. Important and related issues, such as clinicopathologic staging systems, the role of adjuvant or neoadjuvant treatments, and molecular markers are addressed in detail in other sections of this text.

Preoperative Preparation

Planning an operation for a patient with colon cancer requires the surgeon to have as much understanding as possible of the tumor's location in the bowel, the stage of the cancer, and the patient's physiologic status.

A variety of scoring systems are available for grading operative risk of surgical patients. The most widely applied scoring system is the American Society of Anesthesia score (1–4); however, this tool only provides information regarding the risk of an anesthesia complication given a certain physiologic status.[1,2] A more recent tool is the POSSUM and the modified p-POSSUM which include the additional risks related to underlying nutritional status and the performance of a colectomy.[3–5] These tools, although of limited specificity for the individual patient, do provide an estimation of the relative risks for both the patient and the entire surgical team.

Localization of the tumor and the histopathology are important data elements that allow preoperative selection of an operative plan and selection of the optimal resection margins. The presence of a lesion at watershed areas of vascular supply such as the hepatic and splenic flexures may require more extensive resection of colonic length for a safe and complete oncologic procedure. An extended right or left colectomy may be indicated to remove all contributing vascular supplies. In addition, information consistent with the hereditary nonpolyposis colon cancer (HNPCC) (right-sided lesion, Crohn's-like inflammatory response, young patient, and positive family history) would support the resection of the abdominal colon rather than a simple segmental resection. This diagnosis may also be supported by special stains of the biopsy specimen which demonstrate microsatellite instability, the hallmark of the disease which develops from mutations in the DNA mismatch repair system.

Colonoscopy is widely used today and represents the optimal means of diagnosing the lesion, identifying location, providing histopathologic material, and tattooing for intraoperative localization when required. Contrast enema is another means of localizing the lesion anatomically which should be considered to localize a lesion when colonoscopy fails to clearly define the portion of bowel involved. Computed tomography (CT) allows the localization of larger lesions, identification of local organ invasion, and provides important staging information regarding the presence of extracolonic disease, particularly liver involvement. Although intraoperative ultrasound may provide this information, most surgeons will obtain a CT as a screening tool (see Practice Parameters). Although positron emission tomography has recently been approved for colon cancer staging, in isolation its role in assessing the majority of primary, curable lesions remains speculative. It may be very useful for recurrent cancer, where it is essential to determine the presence of disease outside the scope of resection and may provide evidence of widely metastatic disease when planning a radical resection. Thus, an unnecessary noncurative operation with high morbidity may be avoided.

Bowel preparation has historically been considered an essential component of the preoperative preparation of the patient with colon cancer. The performance of mechanical cleansing combined with oral antibiotics reduces the concentration of aerobic and anaerobic bacteria within the colon and has been shown to decrease the incidence of wound infection from 35% to 9%.[6–8] However, more recent prospective, randomized studies have questioned the additional benefit of luminal preparation, compared with the use of appropriate intravenous antibiotics administered in a timely manner. A recent metaanalysis by Bucher et al.[9] reviewed 565 patients with a mechanical bowel preparation versus 579 without a preparation. Interestingly, all but one study demonstrated a higher anastomotic leak rate in the mechanical preparation group with an odds ratio of 1.8.[10,11] Other surgical site infectious complications were also more frequent in the mechanical preparation group. However, most of these studies included high-volume polyethylene glycol in the preparation group. Similar conditions may or may not apply to bowel preparation with the lower volume sodium phosphate preparation. Selective use of mechanical bowel preparation in combination with systemic antibiotics may be justified. A mechanical bowel preparation is still advantageous for laparoscopic colectomy because the reduction in stool volume within the colon makes manipulation of the bowel easier with the small instruments and reduces the size of the extraction site.

Surgical Technique

There are many approaches to the technical performance of each segmental colonic resection. This description will provide general technical methods and document standard anatomic landmarks that should be common to all patients.

Right Colectomy

The patient is placed supine on the operating table. The modified lithotomy position may be useful in cases in which intraoperative endoscopy is necessary. A vertical midline incision is made sufficiently long to allow complete visualization of the operative field. A self-retaining retractor should be placed so as to allow the entire surgical team free hands to conduct the procedure. Thorough examination of the abdominal and pelvic contents should be performed. Particular attention should be given to potential metastatic sites, especially the liver. The increasing use of intraoperative ultrasound has demonstrated the superiority of liver assessment of this modality compared with clinical examination or CT. In the female patient, the ovaries should be examined not only for the risk of metastatic deposits, but also for primary neoplasms. The resectability of the tumor should be assessed with minimal manipulation of the lesion. It is important to determine the presence of disease adherent to adjacent viscera

which should be included with an en bloc resection. It is rare for cancer of the right colon to be unresectable; however, extensive involvement of the vena cava, superior mesenteric artery, or the pancreas may necessitate a palliative resection or bypass procedure.

The key to an oncologically safe and effective resection of a colon cancer requires clear lateral margins, resection of the locoregional lymph node bearing mesentery for both cure and staging, and fashioning of an accurate and well-vascularized anastomosis. Therefore, a right colectomy is required for a tumor at any location in the ascending colon. The author prefers the medial to lateral "no touch" technique. However, the section senior editor prefers the lateral to medial technique. Thus, as can be seen, both approaches are acceptable alternatives.

The Medial Approach

The resection begins with exposure of the right colon mesentery by reflecting the small bowel to the left side of the abdomen. The right colic artery (present in 50% of cases) and the ileocolic vessels can be elevated from the retroperitoneum. A vertical incision is made at the root of the right colon mesentery just caudal to the third portion of the duodenum to the right of the superior mesenteric artery (see Figure 28-1). The vessel(s) is elevated off the retroperitoneum and a proximal ligation is performed at the origin off the superior mesenteric

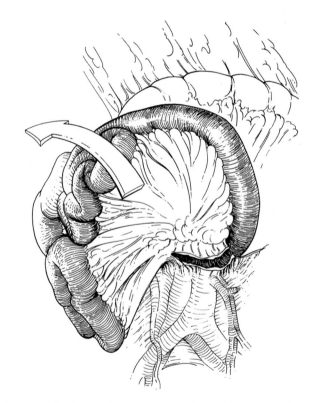

FIGURE 28-1. The drawing demonstrates the incision made at the root of the right colon mesentery just caudal to the third portion of the duodenum to the right of the superior mesenteric artery.

artery (see Figure 28-2). The right colon mesentery is then dissected off the retroperitoneum. This will allow identification of the hepatic branch of the middle colic artery (MCA) as the transverse colon is approached rostrally. Dissection caudally toward the terminal ileum permits ligation of the ileal vascular branches. The right colon can then be released from its peritoneal attachments laterally along the right gutter and transversely over the right iliac artery and brought to the midline. The hepatic flexure suspensory ligaments should be carefully divided to avoid injury to the common bile duct and should be secured with energy or ligatures because of large veins in the ligament. The terminal ileum should be divided 5–15 cm proximal to the ileocecal valve to ensure good vascular supply (see Figure 28-3 for extent of resection). The transverse colon is divided just to the right of the main trunk of the MCA. The right branch of the MCA may be taken, if required. The attached omentum over the right side of the transverse colon should be resected with the specimen. The ileocolic anastomosis can be fashioned according to the desire of the operating surgeon. The author prefers to divide the ileum and colon with linear staplers and perform a functional end-to-end anastomosis by anastomosing the antimesenteric surfaces of the bowel segments with a linear cutting stapler and closing the remaining colotomy with a transverse application of the linear stapler. Closure of the mesenteric defect is optional but may be appropriate to prevent trusion of the small intestine around the terminal ileal vascular pedicle.

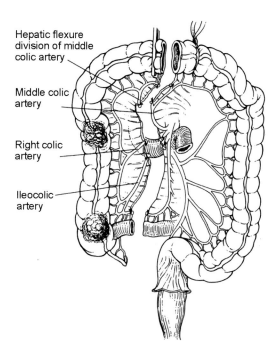

FIGURE 28-3. The drawing demonstrates the appropriate levels for vascular ligation and colonic transition for a right hemicolectomy. Notably, the transverse colon is divided just to the right of the main trunk of the MCA, although the right branch of the MCA may be taken, if required. The middle colic vessels are demonstrated and may be ligated during the performance of an extended right hemicolectomy. This leaves the descending colon in place supported by the left colic artery.

Lateral Approach

Dissection of the right colon may begin laterally along the peritoneal reflection fold which attaches colon to retroperitoneum. The avascular plane between mesentery and retroperitoneum should lead the dissection over the kidney and duodenum from the lateral aspect to make the right colon a midline structure. Vascular ligation can be performed as the final step in the same sites as for the medial approach.

Extended Right Colectomy

An extended right colectomy should be performed for any lesion involving the transverse colon including the hepatic and splenic flexure. This procedure requires proximal ligation of the middle colic vessels which are preserved in a standard right hemicolectomy (see Figure 28-3). Once again this accomplishes complete resection, lymph node clearance, and most importantly two well-vascularized bowel segments for anastomosis.

The operation proceeds in similar manner as the right colectomy described above. However, rather than proceeding through the transverse colon mesentery to ligate and divide the right branch of the MCA, dissection continues in the retroperitoneal plane to identify the main middle colic arterial trunk anterior to the pancreas. This vessel is ligated and

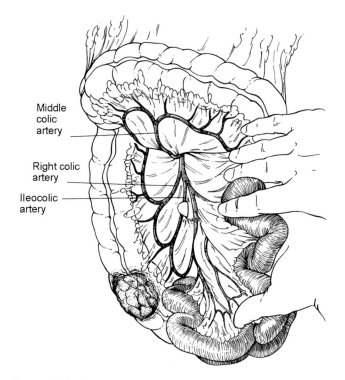

FIGURE 28-2. The vessel(s) is elevated off the retroperitoneum and a proximal ligation is performed at the origin off the superior mesenteric artery. The surgeon's finger is used to demonstrate the vascular origin for accurate placement of the ligation.

divided. The right colon is then mobilized medially as before and then the lesser sac is entered through the gastrocolic ligament outside the gastroepiploic artery so that the omentum can be resected with the transverse colon. The splenic flexure is released from the tail of the pancreas, tip of the spleen, and anterior surface of the left kidney. The left colon and mesentery are divided just proximal to the left colic artery which is preserved for right-sided lesions. The left ascending colic may be sacrificed for left transverse colon lesions preserving the left descending and sigmoid vessels, where a more distal colonic (ileosigmoid) anastomosis is desired. The ileocolic anastomosis is then constructed based on surgeon preference with functional end-to-end/side-to-side technique or end-to-end technique.

Left Colectomy

The Medial Approach

The small bowel mesentery is mobilized to the right upper quadrant to expose the origin of the inferior mesenteric artery (IMA) (Figure 28-4) located just caudal to the third portion of the duodenum (see Figure 28-4). An incision running along the base of the left colic and sigmoid mesentery from the sacral promontory to the ligament of Treitz, exposes the aorta, bifurcation of the common iliac arteries, and IMA vein. The IMA is ligated and divided proximal to the origin of the left colic artery and the inferior mesenteric vein (IMV) is ligated at the base of the pancreas. The avascular plane filled with areolar tissue is developed beneath mesentery and left colon along the entire left gutter. The left ureter is easily identified at this stage and should be freed from overlying mesentery to avoid injury before vascular ligation. The mesentery is elevated off the retroperitoneum and the sigmoid colon mobilized from the pelvic ileum. The left colon is finally mobilized medially from its lateral abdominal wall attachments and the splenic flexure is released. The attachments to the left kidney, tail of the pancreas, and tip of the spleen can be released bloodlessly. Once again, the omentum should be taken with the left transverse colon. The left MCA in the base of the transverse colon mesentery is divided to preserve blood flow to the right transverse colon from the right MCA. Occasionally, it may be necessary to divide the right MCA to allow the right transverse colon to reach the sigmoid for an anastomosis. However, an extended right colectomy and ileosigmoid or ileorectal anastomosis may be preferable if there is any concern related to the blood supply of the distal right colon as the proximal component of the anastomosis. Another alternative is to perform a retroileal right colon to rectum anastomosis if maintenance of the right colon is desired. This is performed by swinging the fully mobilized colon in a counterclockwise direction down into the pelvis to place the cut edge of the right colon mesentery across the pelvic brim (Figure 28-5). Once again the anastomosis is left to the discretion of the surgeon.

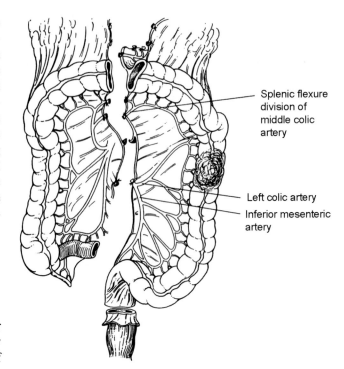

FIGURE 28-4. The small bowel mesentery is mobilized to the right upper quadrant to expose the origin of the IMA located just caudal to the third portion of the duodenum (see Figure 28-4). An incision running along the base of the left colic and sigmoid mesentery from the sacral promontory to the ligament of Treitz, exposes the aorta, bifurcation of the common ilial arteries, and IMA vein. The IMA is ligated and divided proximal to the take-off of the left colic artery. The left branch of the middle colic vessels will require ligation and division for a formal left colectomy.

The Lateral Approach

An incision is made first at the attachments of the sigmoid colon at the pelvic brim and then along the left gutter medial to the white line of Toldt. An areolar tissue plane is found between the mesentery of the left colon and retroperitoneal structures which can be bluntly dissected as far as the midline. The splenic flexure is mobilized with this plane as the guide. Finally, the medial incision is made along the base of the left colon mesentery to expose the IMA and IMV as described above. The procedure proceeds as for the medial approach.

Sigmoid Colectomy

High ligation of the IMA (Figure 28-4) is necessary when performing a sigmoid colectomy to remove all of the lymphatic drainage, and more importantly to ensure construction of a tension-free anastomosis. The ascending branch of the left colic artery should be preserved to allow retrograde blood flow via the marginal artery from the middle colic arterial supply. The splenic flexure should be released to avoid anastomotic

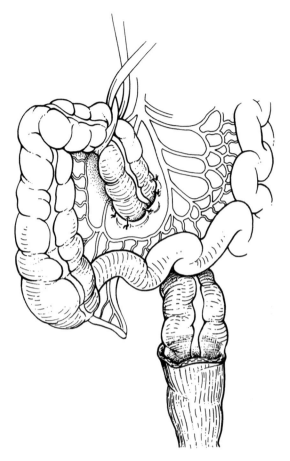

FIGURE 28-5. An alternative method of reconstruction that preserves the right colon is a retroileal right colon to rectum anastomosis. This is performed by swinging the fully mobilized colon in a counterclockwise direction down into the pelvis to place the cut edge of the right colon mesentery across the pelvic brim.

tension. The sigmoid colon is mobilized to the level of the middle colic vessels medial to lateral or lateral to medial and the proximal rectum is mobilized from the sacral promontory. The patient is always in modified lithotomy position to allow transanal access for the anastomosis. An end-to-end circular stapled anastomosis can be performed between proximal left colon and rectum, after dividing the rectosigmoid junction with a transverse linear stapler. A leak test with air insufflation of a submerged anastomotic segment should be performed in all cases using either an endoscope or bulb syringe.

Total Abdominal Colectomy with Ileorectal Anastomosis

This procedure may be required for circumstances in which the patient has been diagnosed with HNPCC, attenuated familial adenomatous polyposis, metachronous cancers in separate colon segments, and frequently in acute malignant distal colon obstructions with unknown status of the proximal bowel. The access to vascular supply and mesenteric dissection has been

described above. The terminal ileum should be sufficiently mobilized to allow easy reach to the rectum. A circular stapled end-to-end anastomosis or functional end-to-side/side-to-side anastomosis are both appropriate. Proper sizing of the circular stapler is needed to avoid ischemia and stricture.

Special Circumstances

Acute Obstruction

Acute colonic obstruction produces dilated bowel with a large amount of fecal loading proximal to the blockage. The associated bacterial overgrowth coupled with possible impairment of blood flow in the proximal bowel, have been the primary factors that have classically dictated resection and proximal diversion. Lee et al.[12] compared left- and right-sided resections managed by primary anastomosis and found similar leak rates (left 6.9% versus right 5.2%) and mortality rates (left 8.9% versus right 7.3%) when compared with historical nonobstructed controls (<2% and <1%, respectively).[12–16] On-table colonic lavage has been advocated as an alternative means of dealing with the obstructed colon. Several cohort studies have demonstrated the safety and efficacy of this approach for avoiding a colostomy without increasing leak rates (<5%) or sepsis.[14–16] Another approach at attempting to protect at-risk anastomoses has been omental wrapping. A large prospective randomized trial by Merad et al.[17] did not demonstrate any significant difference in anastomotic leak rates or the sequelae of those leaks. A complete resection of the tumor and obstructed proximal bowel with primary ileocolic anastomosis has been shown to be safe and carry low leak rates.[18]

Prophylactic Oophorectomy

The debate continues regarding the relative risks and benefits of a prophylactic bilateral oophorectomy in women with colon cancer. The potential benefits are removal of an ovary seeded by colon cancer cells which will manifest as a delayed metastatic site and reduction in the risk of primary ovarian cancer in this age group. The data are limited for both issues. A randomized trial of prophylactic oophorectomy has shown no benefit to survival.[19] The risk of micrometastatic implants in the ovary increases with Dukes' stage and approaches 10%.[20,21] A comparison of cohorts of women with and without prophylactic oophorectomy could not demonstrate a survival advantage but a 3.2% versus 0% risk of primary ovarian cancer in survivors with ovaries not resected.[22] In general, prophylactic oophorectomy is not performed.

Colon Cancer and Abdominal Aortic Aneurysm

The simultaneous presence of a colorectal cancer and abdominal aortic aneurysm which requires surgical management causes a clinical dilemma in many situations. A survey of general surgery program directors revealed that vascular surgeons preferred to repair the aneurysm first, whereas the nonvascular surgeons preferred colectomy.[23] The primary risk is that performing either operation first may cause complications that significantly delay the second procedure. The risk of performing a colectomy synchronously with placement of graft material is a graft infection; however, this risk does not seem excessive based on the small data sets available.[23–27] In all likelihood, the best guidance suggests that any aneurysm >6 cm should be repaired first or synchronously in the face of an associated colon cancer to avoid the risk of rupture.[25] Endoluminal grafting of an appropriate aneurysm may eliminate the majority of these quandaries in the future.[25]

Synchronous Management of Colon Cancer and Liver Metastases

The potential benefit of simultaneous colectomy and hepatectomy is the avoidance of two laparotomies and possible reduction in operative risk. Conversely, delayed management of colonic hepatic metastases offers the ability to accurately stage patients and avoid the risk of hepatectomy in a group of patients who will prove to have more widely metastatic disease in several months. Selection of patients who have limited hepatic involvement and who are positron emission tomography negative for distant disease has resulted in increased resectability and 5-year survival after hepatectomy.[28] The risks of simultaneous colectomy and hepatectomy do not seem to be excessive in select patients operated by expert groups.[29–31] However, the risks may be less with smaller nonanatomic liver resections coupled with right colectomy. Radiofrequency ablation will be discussed in Chapter 34.[32,33]

Sentinel Node Assessment

Sentinel node assessment was first described as a means of improving staging and treatment for melanoma patients and is currently considered standard of care for breast cancer patients.[34,35] Saha described the application of sentinel node identification for colorectal cancer patients with proposed benefits of a high rate of node identification and pathologic upstaging.[36] The technique involves either in vivo injection of 0.5–1 cc of isosulfan blue dye subserosally at the periphery of the tumor (node visualization within 30–60 seconds), or ex vivo injection of 1–2 cc in a similar manner after the bowel has been resected.[35] Subsequent evaluation of the technique, including some modifications, has demonstrated false-negative rates approaching 60%, and limitations in rectal cancers.[36–38]

There are several concerns that restrict routine implementation of sentinel node assessment in colorectal cancer. First, there is no consensus of opinion regarding the prognostic significance of micrometastatic lymph nodes in colorectal cancer, particularly those identified by immunohistochemistry

or polymerase chain reaction.[39–45] Second, the relatively high false-negative rates and/or lack of node visualization mentioned previously, limit the confidence in restricting microsectioning and use of special stains to the group with stained nodes. Finally, there is insufficient evidence that the technique is sufficiently accurate to alter the extent of surgical resection.[46] Before sentinel node assessment can be routinely recommended, two hurdles must be overcome: 1) provision of incontrovertible evidence that micrometastatic disease identified by any technique correlates with survival; and 2) that the survival rates can be favorably impacted by an adjuvant chemotherapy regimen. Therefore, at the present time, routine lymph node mapping cannot be recommended.

Outcome of Colectomy for Colon Cancer

In general, the operative outcome and long-term survival after resection of curable colon cancer parallels the TNM and Dukes' stage (A1, well above 90%; B2, 65%–90%; C3, 45%–75%) which may be modulated by adjuvant chemotherapy.[47,48] The risk of locoregional recurrence after colectomy is a rare occurrence and should be less than 5%.[49–51] However, the impact of the surgeon's experience and the associated expertise of the institution have recently been found to have a profound effect on outcome. High-volume surgeons, particularly those at high-volume institutions, have demonstrated significantly lower perioperative complications and an improved survival after colectomy for colon cancer.[52–55] A colectomy for palliation should rarely be performed and only in patients with life-threatening comorbidities or advanced incurable disease. Local extension of colon cancer may be treated with chemoradiation initially to allow eventual resection and primary anastomosis.

In addition to experience, the overall surgical approach to management of margins and extent of resection has a significant effect on outcome after colon cancer resection. The margins to be considered included proximal and distal bowel margins, radial margins, and extent of mesenteric resection which encompasses the nodal resection and proximal vascular ligation. The adequacy of proximal and distal bowel margins is primarily defined by the vascular ligation and hence the adequacy of vascular supply to the intended anastomotic segments. Although not clearly defined, it is generally agreed that 5 cm proximal and distal bowel margins are sufficient to allow resection of mural tumor spread. Grinnell originally evaluated the patterns of mural spread of tumor in the colon via lymphatics and found no instance of spread greater than 4 cm in the most advanced cases.[56] More recent data would suggest that mural tumor migration is rarely greater than 2 cm either proximal or distal to the palpable tumor edge.[57] Similarly, there is no need to resect any specific amount of terminal ileum, other than defined by vascular supply because mural spread to the ileum is a very rare event. Vascular ligation is generally performed at the origin of the primary feeder vessel to a colonic segment. For resection of the right colon and transverse colon, the debate is relatively moot because of the constraints of the arterial origin of the right colic and middle colic arteries. Ligation for left-sided resections has been debated, primarily in sigmoid or anterior resections because ligation of the IMA may be performed at the aorta, or just distal to the left colic artery takeoff. A report from St. Marks assessed this issue in 1370 patients and found that survival was equivalent for all stages for the ligation options except for the most advanced node positive cases who fared worse with ligation at the aorta.[58] This counter-intuitive finding was more likely related to the higher stage of patients identified by the wider lymphatic resection. A comparison of left hemicolectomy and segmental colectomy (ligation of the IMA versus more distal) by the French Association for Surgical Research could not discern either a different survival rate or pattern based on the ligation or resection performed.[59] Jagoditsch et al.[47] demonstrated the benefits of careful surgical technique which resulted in a complete resection of all tumor (R0).[49] Their data demonstrated an operative mortality of 1.3% and a 5-year survival rate of 71.8% for curative operations in Stage I–III disease.

Summary

Surgery for colonic cancer has been increasingly better defined and the data clearly support the benefits of wide mesenteric resection, clear radial margins, and resection of adherent adjacent organs. Although the precise level of proximal vascular ligation may remain debatable, it is equally clear that the major trunk vessel and the entire supporting mesentery should comprise the specimen. Attention to surgical detail coupled with improved perioperative care strategies are essential to minimizing operative morbidity and mortality.

Appendix: Practice Parameters for Colon Cancer

Prepared by The Standards Practice Task Force, The American Society of Colon and Rectal Surgeons
Daniel Otchy, MD, Neil H. Hyman, MD, Clifford Simmang, MD, Thomas Anthony, MD, W. Donald Buie, MD, Peter Cataldo, MD, James Church, MD, Jeffrey Cohen, MD, Frederick Dentsman, MD, C. Neal Ellis, MD, John W. Kilkenny III, MD, Clifford Ko, MD, Richard Moore, MD, Charles Orsay, MD, Ronald Place, MD, Janice Rafferty, MD, Jan Rakinic, MD, Paul Savoca, MD, Joe Tjandra, MD, Mark Whiteford, MD
I. Diagnostic evaluation
II. Preoperative assessment
Guideline—Preoperative, carcinoembryonic antigen level should be obtained. Level of evidence (Class II, Grade A)

Guideline—Evaluation with preoperative CT scanning of selected patients is indicated and routine preoperative CT scanning is optional. Level of evidence (Class II, Grade B)
Guideline—Routine performance of preoperative chest X-rays is acceptable. Level of evidence (Class III, Grade C)
III. Preparation for operation
A. Informed consent
Guideline—Informed consent should be obtained preoperatively. Level of evidence (Class III, Grade C)
B. Mechanical bowel preparation
Guideline—Mechanical bowel preparation is nearly universally used in elective surgery. Level of evidence (Class II, Grade A)
Guideline—Outpatient bowel preparation is generally safe and cost effective. Level of evidence (Class II, Grade A)
C. Prophylactic antibiotics
Guideline—Prophylactic antibiotics are recommended for patients undergoing colon resection. Level of evidence (Class I, Grade A)
D. Blood cross-match and transfusion
Guideline—Blood transfusion should be based on physiologic need. Level of evidence (Class III, Grade C)
E. Thromboembolism prophylaxis
Guideline—All patients undergoing surgery for colon cancer should receive prophylaxis against thromboembolic disease. Level of evidence (Class I, Grade A)
IV. Operative issues
A. Operative technique
Guideline—The extent of resection of the colon should correspond to the lymphovascular drainage of the site of the colon cancer. Level of evidence (Class II, Grade B)
B. Synchronous colon cancer
Guideline—Synchronous colon cancers can be treated by two separate resections or subtotal colectomy. Level of evidence (Class II, Grade B)
C. Contiguous organ attachment
Guideline—Colon cancers adherent to adjacent structures should be resected en bloc. Level of evidence (Class II, Grade A)
D. Synchronous resection of liver metastases
Guideline—Resection of synchronous liver metastases may be reasonable to perform at the time of the initial colon resection. Level of evidence (Class III, Grade B)
E. Role of oophorectomy
Guideline—Bilateral oophorectomy is advised when one or both ovaries are grossly abnormal or involved with contiguous extension of the colon cancer. However, prophylactic oophorectomy is not recommended. Level of evidence (Class II, Grade B)
F. Role of laparoscopic resection
Guideline—Relative merits of laparoscopic versus open resection for colon cancer remain unproved at this time. Level of evidence (Class II, Grade B)
V. Operative issues—emergent
A. Obstructing colon cancer

Guideline—Patients with an obstructing right or transverse colon cancer should undergo a right or extended right colectomy. A primary ileocolic anastomosis can be performed in the appropriate clinical setting. Level of evidence (Class II, Grade C)

Guideline—For the patient with a left-sided colonic obstruction, the procedure selected should be individualized from a variety of appropriate operative approaches. Level of evidence (Class II, Grade C)

B. Colonic perforation

Guidelines—The site of a colonic perforation caused by colon cancer should be resected, if at all possible. Level of evidence (Class III, Grade C)

C. Massive colonic bleeding

Guideline—Acutely bleeding colon cancers that require emergent resection should be removed following the same principles as in elective resection. Level of evidence (Class III, Grade C)

VI. Staging of colon cancer

Guideline—Colon cancers should be staged using the TNM staging system. Level of evidence (Class II, Grade B)

Guideline—To be properly evaluated, one should strive to have a minimum of 15 lymph nodes examined microscopically. Level of evidence (Class II, Grade B)

VII. Adjuvant therapy

A. Chemotherapy

Guideline—Postoperative adjuvant systemic chemotherapy has a proven benefit in Stage III colon cancer and may be beneficial in certain high-risk Stage II patients. Level of evidence (Class I, Grade A)

B. Immunotherapy

Guideline—The value of immunotherapy for colon cancer is undetermined. Its use is recommended within the setting of a clinical trial. Level of evidence (Class II, Grade C)

C. Intraperitoneal/Intraportal Chemotherapy

Guideline—Intraperitoneal and intraportal infusions of chemotherapy are recommended only in the confines of a clinical trial. Level of evidence (Class II, Grade C)

D. Radiation therapy

Guideline—The role for radiation therapy in colon cancer is limited. Level of evidence (Class II, Grade C)

References

1. Keats A. The ASA classification of physical status: a recapitulation. Anaesthesiology 1978;49:233–236.
2. Menke H, Klein A, John KD, Junginger T. Predictive value of ASA classification for the assessment of perioperative risk. Int Surg 1993;78:266–270.
3. Copeland GP, Jones D, Walters M. POSSUM: a scoring system for surgical audit. Br J Surg 1991;78(3):355–360.
4. Jones DR, Copeland GP, de Cossart L. Comparison of POSSUM with APACHE II for prediction of outcome from a surgical high-dependency unit. Br J Surg 1992;79(12):1293–1296.
5. Prytherch DR, Whiteley MS, Higgins B, Weaver PC, Prout WG, Powell SJ. POSSUM and Portsmouth POSSUM for predicting mortality. Physiological and Operative Severity Score for the Enumeration of Mortality and Morbidity. Br J Surg 1998;85(9):1217–1220.
6. Matheson DM, Arabi Y, Baxter-Smith D, et al. Randomised multicentre trial of oral bowel preparation and antimicrobials for elective colonic operations. Br J Surg 1978;65:597–600.
7. Clarke JS, Condon RE, Bartlett JG, et al. Preoperative oral antibiotics reduce septic complications of colon operations. Ann Surg 1977;186:251–259.
8. Solla JA, Rothenberger DA. Preoperative bowel preparation. A survey of colon and rectal surgeons. Dis Colon Rectum 1990;33:154–159.
9. Bucher P, Mermillod B, Morel P, Soravia C. Does mechanical bowel preparation have a role in preventing postoperative complications in elective colorectal surgery? Swiss Med Wkly 2004;134(5–6):69–74.
10. Guenaga KF, Matos D, Castro AA, Atallah AN, Wille-Jorgensen P. Mechanical bowel preparation for elective colorectal surgery. Cochrane Database Syst Rev 2003;(2):CD001544.
11. Zmora O, Mahajna A, Bar-Zakai B, et al. Colon and rectal surgery without mechanical bowel preparation: a randomized prospective trial. Ann Surg 2003;237(3):363–367.
12. Lee YM, Law WL, Chu KW, Poon RT. Emergency surgery for obstructing colorectal cancers: a comparison between right-sided and left-sided lesions. J Am Coll Surg 2001;193(6):717.
13. Murray JJ, Schoetz DJ Jr, Coller JA, Roberts PL, Veidenheimer MC. Intraoperative colonic lavage and primary anastomosis in nonelective colon resection. Dis Colon Rectum 1991;34(7):527–531.
14. Kressner U, Antonsson J, Ejerblad S, Gerdin B, Pahlman L. Intraoperative colonic lavage and primary anastomosis—an alternative to Hartmann procedure in emergency surgery of the left colon. Eur J Surg 1994;160(5):287–292.
15. Biondo S, Jaurrieta E, Jorba R, et al. Intraoperative colonic lavage and primary anastomosis in peritonitis and obstruction. Br J Surg 2001;88(10):1419.
16. Torralba JA, Robles R, Parrilla P, et al. Subtotal colectomy vs. intraoperative colonic irrigation in the management of obstructed left colon carcinoma. Dis Colon Rectum 1998;41(1):18–22.
17. Merad F, Hay JM, Fingerhut A, Flamant Y, Molkhou JM, Laborde Y. Omentoplasty in the prevention of anastomotic leakage after colonic or rectal resection: a prospective randomized study in 712 patients. French Associations for Surgical Research. Ann Surg 1998;227(2):179–186.
18. Fry RD, Fleshman JW, Kodner IJ. Abdominal colectomy with ileorectal anastomosis. South Med J 1984;77(6):711–714.
19. Young-Fadok TM, Wolff BG, Nivatvongs S, Metzger PP, Ilstrup DM. Prophylactic oophorectomy in colorectal cancer: preliminary results of a prospective randomized trial. Dis Colon Rectum 1998;41:277–283.
20. MacKeigan JM, Ferguson JA. Prophylactic oophorectomy and colorectal cancer in premenopausal patients. Dis Colon Rectum 1979;22(6):401–405.

21. Graffner HO, Alm PO, Oscarson JE. Prophylactic oophorectomy in colorectal carcinoma. Am J Surg 1983;146(2):233–235.

22. Schofield A, Pitt J, Biring G, Dawson PM. Oophorectomy in primary colorectal cancer. Ann R Coll Surg Engl 2001;83(2):81–84.

23. Lobbato VJ, Rothenberg RE, Laraja RD, Georgiou J. Coexistence of abdominal aortic aneurysm and carcinoma of the colon: a dilemma. J Vasc Surg 1985;2:724–726.

24. Bachoo P, Cooper G, Engeset J, Cross KS. Management of synchronous infrarenal aortic disease and large bowel cancer: a North-east of Scotland experience. Eur J Vasc Endosvasc Surg 2000;19(6):614–618.

25. Tilney HS, Trickett JP, Scott RA. Abdominal aortic aneurysm and gastrointestinal disease: should synchronous surgery be considered? Ann R Coll Surg Engl 2002;84(6):414–417.

26. Luebke T, Wolters U, Gawenda M, Brunkwall J, Hoelscher AH. Simultaneous gastrointestinal surgery in patients with elective abdominal aortic reconstruction: an additional risk factor? Arch Surg 2002;137(2):143–147; discussion 148.

27. Robinson G, Hughes W, Lippey E. Abdominal aortic aneurysm and associated colorectal carcinoma: a management problem. Aust N Z J Surg 1994;64(7):475–478.

28. Fernandez FG, Drebin JA, Linehan DC, Dehdashti F, Siegel BA, Strasberg SM. Five-year survival after resection for hepatic metastases from colorectal cancer in patients screened by positron emission tomography with F-18 fluorodeoxyglucose (FDG-PET). Ann Surg 2004;240:438–450.

29. Weber JC, Bachellier P, Oussoultzoglou E, Jaeck D. Simultaneous resection of colorectal primary tumour and synchronous liver metastases. Br J Surg 2003;90(8):956–962.

30. Martin R, Paty P, Fong Y, et al. Simultaneous liver and colorectal resections are safe for synchronous colorectal liver metastasis. J Am Coll Surg 2003;197(2):233–241; discussion 241–242.

31. De Santibanes E, Lassalle FB, McCormack L, et al. Simultaneous colorectal and hepatic resections for colorectal cancer: postoperative and long-term outcomes. J Am Coll Surg 2002;195(2):196–202.

32. Chapius PH, Dent OF, Fisher R, et al. A multivariate analysis of clinical and pathological variables in prognosis after resection of large bowel cancer. Br J Surg 1985;72:698–702.

33. Steinberg SM, Barkin JS, Kaplan RS, Stablein DM. Prognostic indicators of colon tumors. The Gastrointestinal Tumor Study Group Experience. Cancer 1986;57:1866–1870.

34. Morton DL, Wen DR, Wong JH, et al. Technical details of intraoperative lymphatic mapping for early stage melanoma. Arch Surg 1992;127:392–399.

35. Guiliano AE, Jones RC, Brennan M, et al. Sentinel lymphadenectomy in breast cancer. J Clin Oncol 1997;15:2345–2350.

36. Saha S, Wiese D, et al. Technical details of sentinel lymph node mapping in colorectal cancer and its impact on staging. Ann Surg Oncol 2000;7:120–124.

37. Wood TF, Saha S, Morton DL, et al. Validation of lymphatic mapping in colorectal cancer: in vivo, ex vivo, and laparoscopic techniques. Ann Surg Oncol 2000;8(2):150–157.

38. Joosten JJA, Strobble LJA, Wauters CAP, et al. Intraoperative lymphatic mapping and the sentinel lymph node concept in colorectal carcinoma. Br J Surg 1999;86:482–486.

39. Feig BW, Curley S, Berger DH, et al. A caution regarding lymphatic mapping in patients with colon cancer. Am J Surg 2001;182:707–712.

40. Broderick-Villa G, Ko A, O'Connell TX, Guenther JM, Daniel T, Difronzo LA. Does tumor burden limit the accuracy of lymphatic mapping and sentinel lymph node biopsy in colorectal cancer? Cancer J 2002;8:445–450.

41. Cutait R, Alves VA, Lopes LC, et al. Restaging of colorectal cancer based on the identification of lymph node micrometastases through immunoperoxidase staining of CEA and cytokeratins. Dis Colon Rectum 1991;34:917–920.

42. Jeffers MD, O'Dowd GM, Mulcahy H, et al. The prognostic significance of immunohistochemically detected lymph node micrometastases in colorectal carcinoma. J Pathol 1994;172:183–187.

43. Hayashi N, Ito I, Yanagisawa A, et al. Genetic diagnosis of lymph node metastasis in colorectal carcinoma. Lancet 1995;345:1257–1259.

44. Greenson JK, Isenhart CE, Rice R, et al. Identification of occult micrometastases in pericolic lymph nodes of Dukes B colorectal cancer patients using monoclonal antibodies against cytokeratin and CC49. Correlation with long term survival. Cancer 1994;1994:563–569.

45. Read TE, Fleshman JW, Caushaj PF. Sentinel lymph node mapping for adenocarcinoma of the colon does not improve staging accuracy. Dis Colon Rectum 2005;48:80–85.

46. Bertagnoli M, Miedema B, Redston M, et al. Sentinel node staging of respectable colon cancer: results of a multicenter trial. Ann Surg 2004;240:624–630.

47. Jagoditsch M, Lisborg PH, Jatzko GR, et al. Long term prognosis for colon cancer related to consistent radical surgery: multivariate analysis of clinical, surgical, and pathologic variables. World J Surg 2000;24:1264–1270.

48. Mcdermott FT, Hughes ESR, Pihl E, et al. Comparative results of surgical management of single carcinomas of the colon and rectum: a series of 1939 patients managed by one surgeon. Br J Surg 1981;68:850.

49. Read TE, Mutch MG, Chang BW, et al. Locoregional recurrence and survival after curative resection of adenocarcinoma of the colon. J Am Coll Surg 2002;195:33–40.

50. Harris GJ, Church JM, Senagore AJ, et al. Factors affecting local recurrence of colonic adenocarcinoma. Dis Colon Rectum 2002;45(8):1029–1034.

51. Angelopoulos S, Kanellos I, Christophoridis E, Tsachalis T, Kanellou A, Betsis D. Five-year survival after curative resection for adenocarcinoma of the colon. Tech Coloproctol 2004;8(suppl 1):s152–154.

52. Dimick JB, Cowan JA Jr, Upchurch GR Jr, Colletti LM. Hospital volume and surgical outcomes for elderly patients with colorectal cancer in the United States. J Surg Res 2003;114(1):50–56.

53. Gordon TA, Bowman HM, Bass EB, et al. Complex gastrointestinal surgery: impact of provider experience on clinical and economic outcomes. J Am Coll Surg 1999;189(1):46–56.

54. Dimick JB, Cowan JA Jr, Colletti LM, Upchurch GR Jr. Hospital teaching status and outcomes of complex surgical procedures in the United States. Arch Surg 2004;139(2):137–141.

55. Schrag D, Cramer LD, Bach PB, Cohen AM, Warren JL, Begg CB. Influence of hospital procedure volume on outcomes

following surgery for colon cancer. JAMA 2000;284(23): 3028–3035.

56. Grinnell RS. Distal intramucosal spread of carcinoma of the rectum and rectosigmoid. Surg Gynecol Obstet 1965;121: 1031–1035.

57. Quirke P, Dixon MF, Dundey P, et al. Local recurrence of rectal adenocarcinoma due to inadequate surgical resection: histopathologic study of lateral tumor spread and surgical excision. Lancet 1986;2:996–998.

58. Pezim ME, Nichols RJ. Survival after high or low ligation of the inferior mesenteric artery during curative surgery for rectal cancer. Ann Surg 1984;200:729–733.

59. Rouffet F, Hay J-M, Vacher B, et al. Curative resection for left colonic carcinoma: hemicolectomy vs segmental colectomy. A prospective, controlled, multicenter trial. Dis Colon Rectum 1994;37:651–659.

29
The Preoperative Staging of Rectal Cancer

Jonathan E. Efron and Juan J. Nogueras

The classification of cancers of the rectum into a staging system with both therapeutic and prognostic applications has been the goal of pathologists and clinicians for the greater part of the last century. Different staging systems for colorectal cancer are in use today; however, the majority are modifications of a common framework using similar nomenclature with the unfortunate results of inconsistencies and confusion. Most staging systems rely on examination of the pathologic specimen as well as information gained during surgery. Thus, they are useful only in the postoperative setting and have little use for the purpose of preoperative therapy. Cuthbert Dukes[1] declared in 1932 "if it would be possible to decide the category of the case before operating, this would be very useful information." As the therapeutic options available for the treatment of rectal cancer increase, the ability to accurately stage a rectal tumor preoperatively takes on greater importance. Accurate and reproducible preoperative staging provides uniformity among numerous investigative centers; specifically those involved in adjuvant preoperative therapy trials. Finally, the ability to stage the tumor preoperatively permits the physician to convey more accurate information to the patient and the family with regard to therapeutic options and prognosis.

The tumor-related factors of prognostic significance that are most useful in the preoperative staging of rectal cancers include the depth of penetration of the tumor through the rectal wall, the presence or absence of metastasis to the regional lymph nodes, and the presence of distant metastases. Clinicians have a variety of diagnostic tools at their disposal that can aid in delineating these aforementioned factors. The most frequently used modalities for the preoperative staging of rectal tumors available today are clinical examination, computed tomography (CT), magnetic resonance imaging (MRI), endorectal ultrasonography (ERUS), and positron emission tomography (PET).

At the time of history and physical examination, other initial evaluations are ordered. Laboratory tests including CEA (carcinoembryonic antigen) levels and liver function tests may also provide useful information in patients with rectal cancer. There is a small risk of metastatic spread of rectal cancer to the lung, bypassing the liver, therefore a baseline chest X-ray should also be obtained.

Clinical Evaluation

Because of its anatomic location, clinical examination of the rectum can be performed with minimal discomfort to the patient. Careful digital assessment of the rectal tumor may yield valuable information. Table 29-1 lists some of the important parameters that should be recorded during the physical examination of a rectal tumor. A clinical staging system based on tumor mobility was first established by York-Mason[2] in 1976 and subsequently modified in 1982.[3] In this clinical staging system, tumor mobility is correlated with the level of tumor penetration in the different layers of the rectal wall (Table 29-2). Nicholls et al.[3] evaluated this clinical staging system and discovered that senior examiners had an 80% accuracy in distinguishing CS1 and CS2 tumors from CS3 and CS4 tumors, but only a 50% accuracy in detecting lymph node metastasis. The accuracy was directly proportional to the experience of the examiner. Factors that facilitated clinical assessment were the number of quadrants involved, the mobility of the tumor, and palpable extrarectal growths. This study clearly showed that useful information can be obtained from digital examination of rectal tumors. However, certain limitations of a digital examination must be recognized. The accurate assessment of early invasion into the rectal wall has been disappointing, especially in selecting patients for local excision of such a tumor. Clinical staging is more accurate in correctly assessing the stage of more advanced lesions where local excision is not an option. Finally, only tumors of the mid and distal rectum can be assessed by digital examination.

TABLE 29-1. Tumor characteristics to assess on digital examination

Location
Morphology
Number of quadrants involved
Degree of fixation
Mobility
Extrarectal growths
Direct continuity
Separate

TABLE 29-2. Clinical staging system

Clinical stage	Mobility	Pathologic correlation (level of invasion)
CS1	Freely mobile	Submucosa
CS2	Mobile with rectal wall	Muscularis propria
CS3	Tethered mobility	Perirectal fat
CS4	Fixed/tethered fixation	Adjacent tissues

Local and Regional Staging

CT Scan

CT scan is helpful in providing an image of the entire pelvis and the relationship of the tumor to surrounding pelvic structures especially for advanced tumors. However, CT scan has not proven to be very accurate in determining the depth of penetration of the tumor through rectal wall or assessing involved perirectal lymph node metastasis.

Table 29-3 summarizes the results of several studies in which CT scan was used to delineate the penetration of the tumor through the rectal wall and the presence or absence of involved perirectal lymphadenopathy.[4–13]

The reported accuracy rate of CT scan in determining tumor penetration through the rectal wall ranges from 52% to 100%. CT scan is unable to depict the layers of the rectal wall. Thus, for tumors that are confined to the rectal wall, CT scan cannot distinguish tumors that are confined to the submucosa from those that have breached the submucosa and involve the muscularis propria. In cases of advanced tumor growth, CT scan

TABLE 29-3. Accuracy of CT scan in preoperative staging of rectal cancer

	No. of patients	T staging (%)	N staging (%)
Dixon et al., 1981[4]	47	78	49
Grabbe et al., 1983[5]	54	79	56
Freeny et al., 1986[7]	80	62	35
Thompson et al., 1986[6]	25	70	35
Holdsworth et al., 1988[8]	17	94	70
Goldman et al., 1991[9]	30	52	64
Zerhouni et al., 1996[10]	365	74	62
Matsuoka et al., 2002[11]	20	100	70
Chiesura-Corona et al., 2001[12]	105	82	79
Harewood et al., 2002[13]	80	71	76

does provides valuable information about the relationship of the tumor to the surrounding viscera and pelvic structures.

The accuracy of CT scan in determining lymph node involvement ranges from 35% to 70%. One drawback of CT scan is its inability to detect lymph nodes smaller than its resolution threshold of 1 cm. A second drawback of CT scan for the assessment of perirectal lymph node metastasis is its inability to differentiate between tumor metastasis and inflammation in enlarged lymph nodes.

New technology such as the multidetector-row CT (MDRCT) may significantly improve the ability of CT scans to accurately determine the depth of invasion and lymph node metastasis in rectal cancer. MDRCT utilizes four detectors which result in a much higher resolution and better multiplanar reformation of the images. Matsuoka et al.[14] compared 21 patients who had MDRCT with 21 patients that had MRI evaluations of the pelvis for rectal cancer. They reported an accuracy rate of 95% on depth of invasion for MDRCT versus 100% for MRI, whereas lymph node accuracy was 70% versus 61% for MDRCT and MRI, respectively.

Magnetic Resonance Imaging

MRI is a relatively new modality for the staging of rectal cancer. Since its original description in 1986,[15,16] multiple studies have compared the accuracy of MRI in staging rectal cancers with other imaging modalities such as CT scan and ERUS. Accuracy rates for MRI in the preoperative staging of rectal cancer have varied according to technique.

The traditional body coil MRI studies have ranged in accuracy from 55% to 95%.[15–35] The addition of an endorectal coil to this technique resulted in T stage accuracy rates of 66%–91%.[17,30,32,33,36] These results are listed in Table 29-4. Kim et al.,[27] in the largest published trial to date examining the accuracy of MRI staging of rectal cancer, compared the histopathologic staging with the preoperative staging in 217 patients. The accuracy for the depth of invasion was 81% and for regional lymph node metastasis was 63%. Their technique involved injection of intravenous contrast material and examining T1-weighted spin-echo images and T2-weighted turbo spin-echo images. Brown et al.[28] examined preoperative prognostic factors in 98 patients with rectal cancer using high-resolution MRI with a thin section technique. A whole body scan was performed and only T2 weighted images were examined. The accuracy rate in assessing the T stage was 94%, for lymph node involvement was 84%. In their article, Brown et al.[28] introduced new criteria to define MRI T staging (Table 29-5). MRI identification of metastatic lymph node involvement has not been standardized, which may explain the great variation in accuracy. Kim et al.[27] considered lymph node involvement if they demonstrated heterogeneous texture, irregular margins, or were enlarged to greater than 10 mm. However, Brown et al.[36] demonstrated that lymph node size was not an accurate predictor of metastatic disease and, therefore, they relied on mixed signal intensity and irregular or

TABLE 29-4. Accuracy of MRI in the preoperative staging of rectal cancer

	Year	No. of patients	T staging (%)	N staging (%)
de Lange et al.[18]	1990	29	89	65
Chan et al.[17*]	1991	12	91	75
Okizuka et al.[21]	1993	33	88	88
Thaler et al.[25]	1994	34	82	60
Schnall et al.[30*]	1994	36	81	72
Joosten et al.[32*]	1995	15	66	
Indinnimeo et al.[34*]	1996	23	78	79
Hadfield et al.[35]	1997	38	55	76
Zagoria et al.[33*]	1995	10	80	
Kim et al.[27]	2000	217	81	63
Gagliardi et al.[29]	2002	28	86	69
Brown et al.[28]	2003	94	85	84
Low et al.[31]	2003	48	85	68

*Endorectal coil used in MRI.

ill-defined borders of the lymph nodes. Further studies need to be performed to determine the accurate predictors of lymph node metastasis on MRI.

In recent years, tumor involvement of the circumferential resection margin (CRM) has been identified as an important predictor of locoregional recurrence in rectal cancer patients undergoing a radical proctectomy with total mesorectal excision (TME).[37–40] Postoperative radiation is not effective in reducing the risk of local recurrence in patients with a positive CRM,[41] and a curative operation in these patients will require either tumor downstaging by preoperative chemoradion, an extended resection, or both. Consequently, the preoperative assessment of the relationship of the tumor with the fascia propria of the rectum, the CRM in patients treated with TME, has become of utmost importance in deciding the type of neoadjuvant therapy and planning the surgical resection. The fascia propria of the rectum is well visualized by phased-array coil or endorectal coil MRI and several studies have suggested that MRI can predict with high degree of accuracy the distance of the tumor to the fascia propria of the rectum.[42–44] Furthermore, because of its multiplanar capabilities, MRI is the most accurate imaging technique in assessing the relationship of the tumor with the levator plate and the sphincter complex. This information may be useful in selecting patients with low rectal

TABLE 29-5. MRI T staging as proposed by Brown et al.[28]

MRI T stage

T1: Low signal in the submucosal layer or replacement of the submucosal layer by abnormal signal not extending into circular muscle layer.

T2: Intermediate signal intensity within muscularis propria. Outer muscle coat replaced by tumor of intermediate signal intensity that does not extend beyond the outer rectal muscle into perirectal fat.

T3: Broad-based bulge or nodular projection (not fine speculation) of intermediate signal intensity projecting beyond outer muscle coat.

T4: Extension of abnormal signal into adjacent organ; extension of tumor signal through the peritoneal reflection.

Source: Brown et al.[28] Copyright British Journal of Surgery Society Ltd. Reproduced with permission from John Wiley & Sons Ltd. on behalf of the BJSS Ltd.

cancer for a sphincter-saving procedure. Therefore, MRI with a surface coil provides useful information in patients with locally advanced rectal cancer.

Endorectal Ultrasound

Recently, there has been much interest in the technique of ERUS for the preoperative staging of rectal tumors. This approach is proving to be safe, reliable, and relatively inexpensive. It is an outpatient procedure requiring only enema preparation and no sedation or anesthesia. The frequency of the ultrasound transducer determines its focal range and ultrasonographic resolution. Complete circular imaging of the rectal wall can be obtained with the 360-degree rotating endorectal probe. Most investigators are now using a 7.0- or a 10-mHz transducer which provides a five-layer anatomic model of the rectal wall with three hyperechoic circles and two hypoechoic concentric circles (see Chapter 7).[45] Hildebrandt and Feifel[46,47] proposed a preoperative staging classification based on the ultrasonographically determined depth of penetration to the TMN classification system (see Chapter 7).

Table 29-6 lists the results of ERUS in the preoperative staging of rectal cancer.[9,13,25,47–57] The accuracy of the ultrasound in determining the depth of penetration of the tumor through the layers of the rectal wall varied from 60% to 93%. As with all modalities, there is a significant learning curve associated with the interpretation of the ERUS image. Orrom et al.[51] at the University of Minnesota demonstrated an accuracy of 75% in the overall group; however, when they looked at their last 6 months of the study, the authors showed an improvement with a 95% accuracy in determining depth of invasion. Overall, 5% of the tumors were overstaged. This tendency to overstage tumors was a common finding throughout this series because of the inability to differentiate perirectal inflammation from tumor infiltration in the perirectal fat. Orrom et al. also point out some of the pitfalls in performing this examination.[51] These authors routinely use a proctoscope to introduce the ultrasound probe, thereby ensuring that a

TABLE 29-6. Accuracy of ERUS in preoperative staging of rectal cancer

	No. of patients	T staging (%)	N staging (%)
Hildebrandt and Feifel, 1990[47]	137	88	73
Beynon et al., 1989[48]	100	93	83
Jochem et al., 1990[49]	50	80	72
Milson et al., 1990[50]	52	83	70
Orrom et al., 1990[51]	77	75	82
Goldman et al., 1991[9]	32	81	68
Thaler et al., 1994[25]	37	88	80
Starck et al., 1995[52]	34	88	71
Nielsen et al., 1996[53]	100	85	66
Massari et al., 1998[54]	75	91	76
Harewood et al., 2002[13]	80	91	82
Garcia-Aguilar et al., 2002[55]	545	69	64
Marusch et al., 2002[56]	422	63	—
Hull et al., 2004[57]	411	60	—

complete image of the tumor is obtained. This eliminates the possibility of error in the situation whereby a tumor is less invasive distally and more invasive proximally. A blind insertion of the endorectal probe has the potential to inadequately visualize the entire tumor and miss a proximal level of deeper invasion.

A longer-term follow-up of the Minnesota series was published in 2002 by Garcia-Aguilar et al.[55] These investigators reported their experience with 1184 patients with rectal carcinoma or villous adenoma that underwent endorectal ultrasonography. Histopathologic correlation was available for the 545 patients who had no prior radiotherapy. The accuracy of ERUS in assessing level of penetration was 69%, with 18% overstaged and 13% understaged. The accuracy for nodal involvement in the 238 patients who had radical surgery was 64% with 25% overstaged and 11% understaged. The overall accuracy in this large series is lower than previously reported. However, in this series, patients with locally advanced tumors that received preoperative radiation were eliminated from the analysis. The accuracy was higher for benign lesions, and for full-thickness lesions. Lower accuracy rates occurred for T1 and T2 lesions.

Preoperative radiation of rectal cancer causes various degrees of tumor regression resulting in scarring and fibrosis that impairs ultrasound imaging interpretation. Napoleon et al.[58] examined the results in determining depth of wall invasion in patients who had received radiotherapy and compared them with a group of patients with no previous radiotherapy. These authors determined that depth of wall invasion was correctly determined in 86% of patients without radiotherapy, but in only 47% of those patients in whom previous radiotherapy had been administered. Therefore, endorectal ultrasonography should be performed in the patient before receiving radiotherapy in order to increase its accuracy rate.

The accuracy in determining lymph node involvement with the ERUS varies from 68% to 83% (Table 29-6). Normal mesorectal nodes are not visualized with ERUS;

visible nodes are considered pathologic. However, ERUS cannot differentiate between inflammatory or neoplastic nodes. Hildebrandt et al.[59] have described different echogenic parameters in nodes that were replaced by tumor as compared with inflammatory lymph nodes. They determined that hypoechoic lymph nodes represented tumor metastases whereas hyperechoic lymph nodes represented inflammatory changes. They reported an overall accuracy rate of 78% and they attributed their errors to micrometastases, mixed lymph nodes, and changing echo patterns within inflammatory nodes.

Andersson and Aus[60] reported a case in which a transrectal ultrasound–guided biopsy of a hypoechoic perirectal lymph node was performed in order to verify metastatic growth in a patient who had already undergone a local excision of a rectal cancer. Harewood et al.[13] investigated the impact of ERUS-guided fine-needle aspiration of perirectal nodes in the preoperative staging of 80 consecutive patients with rectal cancer. In this series, fine-needle aspiration did not significantly improve nodal staging over ERUS.[13] Based on these results, and the potential risk of spreading cancer cells into the mesorectum in patients with metastatic lymph nodes, ultrasound-guided biopsy of enlarged perirectal nodes is not routinely used in clinical practice.

Several prospective studies have compared ERUS and MRI in the preoperative staging of rectal cancer. Surface coil MRI is less accurate than ERUS in assessing rectal wall invasion and is primarily used for the staging of locally advanced rectal cancers. MRI with endorectal coil allows visualization of the different layers of the rectal wall, and can potentially be used for the preoperative staging of early rectal cancers. Kwok et al.[61] performed a systematic review of the literature to compare the accuracy of several imaging techniques in the preoperative staging of rectal cancer. They concluded that ERUS has the highest sensitivity and specificity in assessing wall penetration, but MRI with endorectal coil had higher accuracy than ERUS in assessing nodal metastasis. However, MRI with endorectal coil is cumbersome to the patient, technically difficult, and not widely available.

Three-dimensional ultrasound is a new technique that has recently been developed. Kim et al.[62] compared the accuracy of conventional ultrasound to three-dimensional ultrasound in the staging of rectal cancer. They found no significant difference in accuracy of either depth of invasion or lymph node metastasis. Their study was small and there was a trend to higher accuracy with the three-dimensional ultrasound. Further investigation is required for the evaluation of three-dimensional ultrasound on rectal cancer staging.

Distant Metastases

The detection of distant metastasis is of prime importance for the accurate staging of rectal cancer. The most common site of distant spread of rectal cancer is the liver.

The most frequently used imaging modalities used today to detect liver metastasis are abdominal ultrasound and CT scans. MRI and intraoperative ultrasound are now used with increasing frequency, particularly in patients with known metastasis that are considered candidates for surgical resection.

Studies that have investigated the use of preoperative ultrasonography and CT in the detection of liver metastases have reported an overall accuracy ranging from 66% to 90%.[63–66] Table 29-7 lists some of the results of these earlier studies. Clarke et al.[67] investigated the accuracy on intraoperative ultrasonography in detecting liver metastasis according to their location by anatomic liver segments. Both techniques were similar in detecting liver metastasis except for lesions located in the lateral segment of the left lobe of the liver where preoperative ultrasonography was accurate (76%) compared with CT scan (29%). The lower resolution of CT scan in the left lateral segment lesions was attributed to artifacts from the stomach and cardiac motion.

Ward et al.[68] from the National Institute of Health reported the results of a study evaluating preoperative CT with various enhancement techniques and MRI of the liver. All patients eventually underwent laparotomy with intraoperative ultrasonography in some cases. Correlation of the imaging techniques with surgical findings was performed to determine the specificity and sensitivity of each test. The authors concluded that the MRI examination had the lowest false-positive rate and proved to be the best hepatic imaging study in the detection of colorectal metastases.

Despite refinements in enhancement techniques of CT[69] and external ultrasounds, along with the addition of MRI, the resolution threshold for liver metastases remains at approximately 1 cm. For lesions in the left lateral segment of the liver, this threshold is larger. Even after preoperative imaging, up to one-third of colorectal cancer patients are found at the time of surgery to have unsuspected additional liver lesions or extrahepatic metastases. Other modalities used to detect metastatic disease not seen with conventional imaging techniques are PET scan and radioimmunoscintigraphy.

PET scans have been shown to have higher sensitivity and specificity in detecting recurrent rectal cancer than both CT and MRI.[70–73] Although sensitivity and specificity in diagnosing tumor recurrence are higher for PET scans, its spacial resolution is not very accurate and therefore other studies such as MRI and/or CT scans are required to define the precise location of the tumor to important anatomic landmarks. Current scanners are available that fuse CT or MR images with the PET scan images. The ability of these fused images to increase sensitivity or specificity is being investigated. Cohade et al.[74] compared PET scan and PET/CT images in a series of 45 patients with colorectal cancer. They found that the overall staging accuracy increased from 78% to 89% with PET/CT. PET scans when coupled with other studies are also being used to assess the extent of pathologic response of rectal cancers that receive neoadjuvant therapy.[75,76] Further studies are required on this use of PET scans before any definitive conclusions can be drawn.

The impact of PET in the preoperative staging and management of rectal cancer patients has been studied by Heriot et al.[77] in a series of 46 patients who were assessed with PET scans at the time of their initial diagnosis. The surgical management was changed for 17% of the patients because of positive PET scan findings that upstaged the disease. These changes in management included canceling surgery and changing the field of administered radiation.

At the present time, PET scan is primarily used for the diagnosis of local and distant recurrence after curative surgery for colorectal cancer. It is also being used with increased frequency to detect distant metastasis of the time of the primary diagnosis of rectal cancer.

Immunoscintigraphy refers to the use of radiolabeled monoclonal antibodies that bind specifically to tumors to aid in detection and diagnosis. Most studies have primarily examined patients with colon cancer or either colon and rectal cancer. Few have examined primarily rectal cancer. The clinical application of this technique has been limited. Different monoclonal antibodies have been used, making it difficult to compare studies. The accuracy rate of immunoscintigraphy in detecting primary or metastatic colorectal cancers ranges from 63% to 96%.[78–85]

There has not been a defined role for the use of preoperative or intraoperative radiolabeled immunoscintigraphy when dealing with a primary rectal cancer. Likewise, its role in management of recurrent rectal cancer has yet to be well defined. Intraoperatively, it may enhance the surgeon's ability to assess both local and metastatic spread.

Conclusion

The accurate preoperative tumor staging is essential to select the best therapy for the rectal cancer patient. Presently, the depth of invasion and evidence of perirectal lymph node involvement is best assessed with ERUS. Abdominal and pelvic CT scanning or MRI are also important to detect extrarectal tumor spread and liver metastasis. A chest X-ray is also important to exclude pulmonary metastasis. The role of new imaging modalities such as PET in the staging of rectal cancer patients is currently under investigation.

TABLE 29-7. Accuracy of ultrasound and CT scan in the preoperative diagnosis of liver metastasis from colorectal cancer

	Ultrasound (%)	CT (%)
Sheur et al., 1985[63]	90	85
Gunven et al., 1985[64]	66	80
Castaing et al., 1986[65]	68	74
Gozzetti et al., 1986[66]	80	74

References

1. Dukes C. The classification of cancer of the rectum. J Pathol Bacteriol 1932;35:323–332.

2. York-Mason A. Rectal cancer. The spectrum of selective surgery. Proc R Soc Med 1976;69:237–244.

3. Nicholls RJ, York-Mason A, Morson BC, et al. The clinical staging of rectal cancer. Br J Surg 1982;69:404–409.

4. Dixon AK, Frye IK, Morson BC, et al. Pre-operative computed tomography of carcinoma of the rectum. Br J Radiol 1981;54: 655–659.

5. Grabbe E, Lierse W, Winkler R. The perirectal fascia: morphology and use in staging of rectal carcinoma. Radiology 1983;149:241–246.

6. Thompson WM, Halvorsen RA, Foster WL Jr, et al. Pre-operative and post-operative CT staging of rectosigmoid carcinoma. AJR Am J Roentgenol 1986;146:703–710.

7. Freeny PC, Marks WM, Tyan JA, et al. Colorectal carcinoma evaluation with CT: pre-operative staging and detection of postoperative recurrence. Radiology 1986;158:347–353.

8. Holdsworth PJ, Johnston D, Chalmers AG, et al. Endoluminal ultrasound and computed tomography in the staging of rectal cancer. Br J Surg 1988;75:1019–1022.

9. Goldman S, Arvidsson H, Norming U, et al. Transrectal ultrasound and computed tomography in preoperative staging of lower rectal adenocarcinoma. Gastrointest Radiol 1991;16: 259–263.

10. Zerhouni EA, Rutter C, Hamilton SR, et al. CT and MR imaging in the staging of colorectal carcinoma: report of the Radiology Diagnostics Oncology Group II. Radiology 1996;200:443–451.

11. Matsuoka H, Nakamura A, Masaki T, et al. Preoperative staging by multidetector-row computed tomography in patients with rectal carcinoma. Am J Surg 2002;184:131–135.

12. Chiesura-Corona M, Muzzio PC, Giust G, et al. Rectal cancer: CT local staging with histopathologic correlation. Abdom Imaging 2001;26:134–138.

13. Harewood GC, Wiersema MJ, Nelson H, et al. A prospective, blinded assessment of the impact of preoperative staging on the management of rectal cancer. Gastroenterology 2002;123:24–32.

14. Matsuoka H, Nakamura A, Masaki T, et al. A prospective comparison between multidetector-row computed tomography and magnetic resonance imaging in the preoperative evaluation of rectal carcinoma. Am J Surg 2003;185(6):556–559.

15. Hodgman CG, MacCarty RL, Wolff BG, et al. Preoperative staging of rectal carcinoma by computed tomography and 0.15T magnetic resonance imaging. Preliminary report. Dis Colon Rectum 1986;29:446–450.

16. Butch RJ, Stark DD, Wittenberg J, et al. Staging of rectal cancer by MR and CT. AJR Am J Roentgenol 1986;146:1155–1160.

17. Chan TW, Kressel HY, Milestone B, et al. Rectal carcinoma: staging at MR imaging with endorectal surface coil. Work in progress. Radiology 1991;181:461–467.

18. de Lange EE, Fechner RE, Edge SB, Spaulding CA. Preoperative staging of rectal carcinoma with MR imaging: surgical and histopathological correlation. Radiology 1990;176:623–628.

19. Waizer A, Powsner E, Russo I, Hadar S, Cytron S, et al. Prospective comparative study of magnetic resonance imaging versus transrectal ultrasound for preoperative staging and follow up of rectal cancer. Preliminary report. Dis Colon Rectum 1991;34: 1068–1072.

20. Ou YH. Value of MR imaging in the staging of rectal carcinoma. Zhonghua Zhong Liu Za Zhi 1992;13:442–445.

21. Okizuka H, Sugimura K, Ishida T. Preoperative local staging of rectal carcinoma with MR imaging and a rectal balloon. J Magn Reson Imaging 1993;3:329–335.

22. Golfieri R, Giampalma E, Leo P, et al. Comparison of magnetic resonance (0.5 T), computed tomography, and endorectal ultrasonography in the preoperative staging of neoplasms of the rectum-sigma. Correlation with surgical and anatomopathological findings. Radiol Med (Torino) 1993;85:773–783.

23. McNicholas MM, Joyce WP, Dolan J, Gibney RG, MacErlaine DP, Hyland J. Magnetic resonance imaging of rectal carcinoma: a prospective study. Br J Surg 1994;81:911–914.

24. Cova M, Frezza F, Pozzi-Mucelli RS, et al. Computed tomography and magnetic resonance in the preoperative staging of the spread of rectal cancer. A correlation with the anatomicopathological aspects. Radiol Med 1994;87:82–89.

25. Thaler W, Watzka S, Martin F, La Guardia G, et al. Preoperative staging of rectal cancer by endoluminal ultrasound vs. magnetic resonance imaging. Preliminary results of a prospective, comparative study. Dis Colon Rectum 1994;37:1189–1193.

26. Kusunoki M, Yanagi H, Kamikonya N, et al. Preoperative detection of local extension of carcinoma of the rectum using magnetic resonance imaging. J Am Coll Surg 1994;179:653–656.

27. Kim NK, Kim MJ, Park JK, Park SIL, Min JS. Preoperative staging of rectal cancer with MRI: accuracy and clinical usefulness. Ann Surg Oncol 2000;7(10):732–737.

28. Brown G, Radcliffe AG, Newcombe RG, Dallimore NS, Bourne MW, Williams GT. Preoperative assessment of prognostic factors in rectal cancer using high-resolution magnetic resonance imaging. Br J Surg 2003;90(3):355–364.

29. Gagliardi G, Bayar S, Smith R, Salem R. Preoperative staging of rectal cancer using magnetic resonance imaging with external phase-arrayed coils. Arch Surg 2002;137:447–451.

30. Schnall MD, Furth EE, Rosato EF, et al. Rectal tumor stage: correlation of endorectal MR imaging and pathologic findings. Radiology 1994;190:709–714.

31. Low RN, McCue M, Barone R, Saleh F, Song T. MR staging of primary colorectal carcinoma: comparison with surgical histopathological findings. Abdom Imaging 2003;28(6): 784–793.

32. Joosten FB, Jansen JB, Joosten HJ, et al. Staging of rectal carcinoma using MR double surface coil, MR endocoil and intra rectal ultrasound: correlation with histopathologic findings. J Comput Assist Tomogr 1995;19:752–758.

33. Zagoria RJ, Schlarb CA, Ott DJ, et al. Assessment of rectal tumor infiltration utilizing endorectal MR imaging and comparison with endoscopic rectal sonography. J Comput Assist Tomogr 1995;19:752–758.

34. Indinnimeo M, Grasso RF, Chicchini C, et al. Endorectal magnetic resonance imaging in the preoperative staging of rectal tumors. Int Surg 1996;81:419–422.

35. Hadfield MB, Nicholson AA, MacDonald AW, et al. Preoperative staging of rectal carcinoma by magnetic resonance imaging with a pelvic phased-array coil. Br J Surg 1997;84: 529–531.

36. Brown G, Richards CJ, Bourne MW, et al. Morphologic predictors of lymph node status in rectal cancer using high spatial resolution magnetic resonance imaging with histopathologic comparison. Radiology 2003;227:371–377.

37. Quirke P, Durdey P, Dixon MF, Williams NS. Local recurrence of rectal adenocarcinoma due to inadequate surgical resection: histopathological study of lateral tumor spread and surgical excision. Lancet 1986;2:996–999.

38. Adam IJ, Mohamdee MO, et al. Role of circumferential margin involvement in the local recurrence of rectal cancer. Lancet 1994;344:707–711.

39. Hall NR, Finan PJ, et al. Circumferential margin involvement after mesorectal excision of rectal cancer with curative intent: predictor of survival but not local recurrence? Dis Colon Rectum 1998;41(8):979–983.

40. Nagtegaal ID, Marijnen CA, et al. Circumferential margin involvement is still an important predictor of local recurrence in rectal carcinoma: not one millimeter but two millimeters is the limit. Am J Surg Pathol 2002;26(3):350–357.

41. Marijnen CA, Nagtegaal ID, et al. Radiotherapy does not compensate for positive resection margins in rectal cancer patients: report of a multicenter randomized trial. Int J Radiat Oncol Biol Phys 2003;55(5):1311–1320.

42. Beets-Tan RG. MRI in rectal cancer: the T stage and circumferential resection margin. Colorectal Dis 2003;5(5):392–395.

43. Branagan G, Chave H, et al. Can magnetic resonance imaging predict circumferential margins and TNM stage in rectal cancer? Dis Colon Rectum 2004;47(8):1317–1322.

44. Brown G, Daniels IR. Preoperative staging of rectal cancer: the MERCURY research project. Recent Results Cancer Res 2005; 165:58–74.

45. Nogueras JJ. Endorectal ultrasonography: technique, image interpretation, and expanding indications in 1995. Semin Colon Rectal Surg 1995;6:70–77.

46. Hildebrandt U, Feifel G. Preoperative staging of rectal cancer by intrarectal ultrasound. Dis Colon Rectum 1985;28:42–46.

47. Hildebrandt U, Feifel G. Endorectal sonography. Surg Annu 1990;22:169–183.

48. Beynon J, Mortensen NJ, Foy DM, et al. Preoperative assessment of mesorectal lymph node involvement in rectal cancer. Br J Surg 1989;76:276–279.

49. Jochem RJ, Reading CC, Dozois RR, et al. Endorectal sonographic staging of rectal carcinoma. Mayo Clinic Proc 1990;65: 1571–1577.

50. Milson JW, Graphner H. Intrarectal ultrasonography in rectal cancer staging and in the evaluation of pelvic disease: clinical uses of intrarectal ultrasound. Ann Surg 1990;212: 602–606.

51. Orrom WJ, Wong WD, Rothenberger DA, et al. Endorectal ultrasound in the preoperative staging of rectal tumors: a learning experience. Dis Colon Rectum 1990;33:654–659.

52. Starck M, Bohe M, Fork FT, et al. Endoluminal ultrasound and low-field magnetic resonance imaging are superior to clinical examination in the preoperative staging of rectal cancer. Eur J Surg 1995;161:841–845.

53. Nielsen MB, Qvitzau S, Pedersen JF, Christiansen J. Endosonography for preoperative staging of rectal tumors. Acta Radiol 1996;37:799–803.

54. Massari M, De Simone M, Cioffi U, et al. Value and limits of endorectal ultrasonography for preoperative staging of rectal carcinoma. Surg Laparosc Endosc 1998;8(6):438–444.

55. Garcia-Aguilar J, Pollack J, Lee SH, et al. Accuracy of endorectal ultrasonography in preoperative staging of rectal tumors. Dis Colon Rectum 2002;45:10–15.

56. Marusch F, Koch A, Schmidt U, et al. Routine use of transrectal ultrasound in rectal carcinoma: results of a prospective multicenter study. Endoscopy 2002;34:385–390.

57. Hull TL, Lavery I, et al. Inaccuracy of preoperative endolumen ultrasound (ELUS) for rectal adenocarcinoma and consequences. Dis Colon Rectum 2004;47(4):574.

58. Napoleon B, Pujol B, Berger F, et al. Accuracy of endosonography in the staging of rectal cancer treated by radiotherapy. Br J Surg 1991;78:785–788.

59. Hildebrandt U, Klein T, Feifel G, et al. Endosonography of pararectal lymph nodes: in vitro and in vivo evaluation. Dis Colon Rectum 1990;33:863–868.

60. Andersson R, Aus G. Transrectal ultrasound-guided biopsy for verification of lymph-node metastasis in rectal cancer. Acta Chir Scand 1990;156:659–660.

61. Kwok H, Bissett IP, Hill GL. Preoperative staging of rectal cancer. Int J Colorectal Dis 2000;15:9–20.

62. Kim JC, Cho YK, Kim SY, et al. Comparison study of three-dimensional and conventional endorectal ultrasonography used in rectal cancer staging. Surg Endosc 2002;16(9):1280–1285.

63. Sheur JC, Lee CS, Sung JL, et al. Intraoperative hepatic ultrasonography: an indispensable procedure in resection of small hepatocellular carcinomas. Surgery 1985;97:97–103.

64. Gunven P, Makuuchi M, Takayasu K, et al. Preoperative imaging of liver metastases: comparison of angiography, CT scan, and ultrasonography. Ann Surg 1985;202:573–579.

65. Castaing D, Emond J, Bisimeth IT, Kuntslinger F. Utility of operative ultrasound in the surgical management of liver tumors. Ann Surg 1986;204:600–605.

66. Gozzetti G, Mazziotti A, Bolondi L, et al. Intraoperative ultrasonography in surgery for liver tumors. Surgery 1986;99: 523–530.

67. Clarke MP, Kane RA, Steele G, et al. Prospective comparison of preoperative imaging and intraoperative ultrasonography in the detection of liver tumors. Surgery 1989;106:849–855.

68. Ward BA, Miller DL, Frank JA, et al. Prospective evaluation of hepatic imaging studies in the detection of colorectal metastases: correlation with surgical findings. Surgery 1989;106:180–187.

69. Yamaguchi A, Ishida T, Nishimura G, et al. Detection by CT during arterial portography of colorectal cancer metastases to liver. Dis Colon Rectum 1991;34:37–40.

70. Gupta N, Boman B, Frank A, et al. PET FDG imaging for the follow-up evaluation of treated colorectal cancer. Radiology 1991;181(suppl):199.

71. Ito K, Kato T, Tadokoro M, et al. Recurrent rectal cancer and scar: differentiation with PET and MR imaging. Radiology 1992;182(2):549–552.

72. Takeuchi O, Saito N, Koda K, et al. Clinical assessment of positron emission tomography for the diagnosis of local recurrence in colorectal cancer. Br J Surg 1999;85:932–937.

73. Whiteford MH, Whiteford HM, Yee LF, et al. Usefulness of FDG-PET scan in the assessment of suspected metastatic or recurrent adenocarcinoma of the colon and rectum. Dis Colon Rectum 2000;43(6):759–767.

74. Cohade C, Osman MM, Leal J, Wahl RL. Direct comparison of (18)F-FDG PET and PET/CT in patients with colorectal carcinoma. J Nucl Med 2003;44(11):1804–1805.

75. Guillem JG, Puig-La Calle J Jr, Akurst T, et al. Prospective assessment of primary rectal cancer response to preoperative radiation and chemotherapy using 18-flourodeoxyglucose

positron emission tomography. Dis Colon Rectum 2000;43(1): 18–24.

76. Delrio P, Lastoria S, Avallone A, et al. Early evaluation using PET-FDG of the efficiency of neoadjuvant radiochemotherapy treatment in locally advanced neoplasia of the lower rectum. Tumori 2003;89(4 suppl):50–53.

77. Heriot AG, Hicks RJ, Drummond EGP, et al. Does positron emission tomography change management in primary rectal cancer? A prospective assessment. Dis Colon Rectum 2004;47(4): 451–458.

78. Cohen AM, Martin EW Jr, Lavery I, et al. Radioimmunoguided surgery using iodine 125 B723 in patients with colorectal cancer. Arch Surg 1991;126(3):349–352.

79. Collier BD, Abdel-Nabi H, Doerr RI. Immunoscintigraphy performed with In-111 labeled CYT-103 in the management of colorectal cancer: comparison with CT. Radiology 1992;185: 179–186.

80. Bischo-Delaoye A, Delaloye B, Buchegger F, et al. Clinical value of immunoscintigraphy in colorectal carcinoma patients: a prospective study. J Nucl Med 1989;34:573–581.

81. Beatty JD, Williams LE, Yamauchi D, et al. Presurgical imaging with indium-labelled anti-carcinoembryonic antigen for colon cancer staging. Cancer Res 1990;50(suppl 3):922–926s.

82. Doerr R, Abel-Nabi H, Krag D, et al. Radiolabeled antibody imaging in the management of colorectal cancer. Results of a multicenter clinical study. Ann Surg 1991;214:118–124.

83. Corbisiero RM, Yamauchi DM, Williams LE, et al. Comparison of immunoscintigraphy and computerized tomography in identifying colorectal cancer: individual lesion analysis. Cancer Res 1991;51:5704–5711.

84. Lechner P, Lind P, Bitner G, et al. Anticarcinoembryonic antigen immunoscintigraphy with a 99m Tc-Fab [prime] fragment (Immu 4) in primary and recurrent colorectal cancer. A prospective study. Dis Colon Rectum 1993;36:930–935.

85. Steinstasseer A, Oberhausen E. Anti-CEA labeling kit BW 431/26: results of the European multicenter trial. Nuklearmedizin 1995;34:232–242.

30
Surgical Treatment of Rectal Cancer

Ronald Bleday and Julio Garcia-Aguilar

Approximately 42,000 patients each year are diagnosed with rectal cancer in the United States. Approximately 8500 die of this disease. Despite remarkable recent advances in new oncologic agents for the treatment of colon and rectal cancer, cure is almost never achieved without surgical resection. However, the current management of rectal cancer is now more varied and complex because of the new approaches with multimodality therapy and the refinements in surgical techniques. For example, small distal rectal cancers with minimal invasion can be treated with a local excision with or without adjuvant therapy. More proximal or more invasive tumors require a "radical" resection. The two most common procedures are the low anterior resection (LAR) and the abdominoperineal resection (APR). Extended resections are occasionally required for patients with cancers that invade or adhere to adjoining structures such as the sacrum, pelvic sidewalls, prostate, or bladder.

This Chapter discusses the surgical management of rectal cancer including a basic review of the preoperative evaluation and how it pertains to surgical planning, the preoperative preparation, the surgical procedures, the biology of rectal cancer as it relates to surgery, the issue of margins, and the technical nuances that need to be appreciated for a successful resection.

Evaluation of the Patient with Rectal Cancer

History

The patient with rectal cancer usually presents to the surgeon after a definitive endoscopic diagnosis. The patient's initial complaint may have been rectal bleeding, a change in bowel habits, or a sense of rectal pressure. However, with the increase in surveillance colonoscopy, many patients are completely asymptomatic on presentation. During the initial history, the surgeon should ask about certain symptoms because it will aid in selecting the best therapy for the patient. For example, tenesmus (the constant sensation of needing to move the bowels) is often indicative of a large cancer. Constant anal pain or pain with defecation suggests invasion of the anal sphincters or pelvic floor. Preemptive procedures such as a diverting colostomy may be required in patients with these distal painful cancers. Also, cancers growing into the anal sphincter are not candidates for a sphincter-sparing procedure. Questions concerning a patient's fecal continence should also be discussed before any therapy. Sphincter-sparing procedures can put a tremendous stress on even the most normal of pelvic floors and anal sphincters. A history of significant continence problems should prompt a discussion with the patient concerning quality of life issues. Sphincter-sparing surgery in these patients, even if technically possible, often leads to significant fecal soiling and the patient may be better served with a resection and permanent colostomy.

Physical Examination and Rigid Sigmoidoscopic Examination

A digital rectal examination (DRE) and a rigid sigmoidoscopy are essential to the surgical decision-making process. Both a proper examination and rigid sigmoidoscopy should be performed on the initial patient visit unless the patient has a painful invasive lesion. On DRE, fixation of the lesion to the anal sphincter, its relationship to the anorectal ring (the collection of muscles that make up the sphincters), and possible fixation to both the rectal wall and the pelvic wall can be evaluated. For mid rectal or upper rectal lesions, the DRE and rigid sigmoidoscopy can help determine how much normal rectum lies distal to the lower border of the tumor. With the combination of DRE and sigmoidoscopy at the initial visit, the surgeon can often determine whether a patient is a candidate for sphincter-sparing surgery, whether a temporary diverting ostomy is likely, and what anorectal function will be like post-treatment.

Colonoscopy

A colonoscopy should be performed before surgical resection of a rectal cancer. Colonoscopy allows for confirmation of a malignancy through biopsy and the diagnosis and possible removal of synchronous colonic lesions. Synchronous benign polyps have been reported in 13%–62% of cases and synchronous cancers have been reported in 2%–8% of cases.[1-6] Even if a colonoscopy has been recently performed on a patient, the surgeon should still perform a rigid sigmoidoscopy because estimates of the location of the lesion are often misleading. For example, because of the flexibility of the colonoscope, a lesion that is described as 15 cm from the anal verge can sometimes be a close as 5 cm from the anal verge when evaluated with the rigid scope. Finally, both with a colonoscope and rigid sigmoidoscope, one should describe the distance from the lower border of the lesion to a standard distal landmark. The National Cancer Institute (NCI) consensus group recommends the use of the "anal verge" as the starting point for measuring distance; however, this anatomic landmark is variable. An alternative is to use the dentate line as the zero point and measure the distance from the lower border of the lesion to the proximal border of the anorectal ring. This distance is essentially a measure of the maximal amount of rectum that one can resect before considering an APR.

Preoperative Staging

Preoperative staging of a patient with a rectal cancer is becoming essential in the decision-making process as adjuvant modalities become increasingly used preoperatively. Also, the range of surgical procedures that can be offered to a patient is in part dependent on the preoperative imaging. For a basic evaluation, all patients should receive a chest X-ray or chest computed tomography (CT) scan to exclude pulmonary metastases. One can obtain a carcinoembryonic antigen (CEA) level. If increased preoperatively, the CEA level should decrease to the normal range after treatment. CEA can then be followed postoperatively to detect a recurrence. Most other laboratory evaluations obtained preoperatively are useful for determining pertinent medical problems but are not very helpful in staging. By far, the most useful staging for rectal cancer is abdominal/pelvic imaging with CT, magnetic resonance imaging (MRI), or ultrasound (US)

Imaging for Rectal Cancer

Pretreatment abdominal and pelvic imaging of the patient with rectal cancer is necessary in this era because of the increasing value of preoperative adjuvant therapies. Therapy differs depending on stage, depth of invasion into the rectal wall within a stage, size of lesion, and location of the tumor. In particular, distal and mid rectal cancer treatment management will differ depending on the preoperative staging and

imaging. For upper rectal cancers, imaging to determine stage will often not influence the treatment plan. Many of these patients with upper rectal tumors will benefit from an LAR regardless of the stage and may not require neoadjuvant therapy as often as low and mid rectal cancers.

CT Scans

Differing opinions exist as to whether a CT scan is a useful routine assessment modality in a patient diagnosed with a rectal cancer. Some would argue that for routine, uncomplicated malignancies, a CT scan is generally not necessary, because the information obtained will not usually affect the treatment plan. This concept is probably more applicable to patients with colon cancers versus patients with rectal cancers. For rectal cancer, there may be some merit to a baseline preoperative CT scan for advanced lesions. CT scanning is quite accurate in assessing rectal tumors that have invaded adjacent organs. However, for assessment of small primary lesions, CT scanning has many limitations. CT scans do not effectively visualize the layers of the rectal wall and so do not help in evaluating the extent of rectal wall invasion of an early cancer. The overall accuracy of CT scanning in determining depth of invasion is approximately 70%. Additionally, CT scanning is limited in its ability to determine the presence or absence of lymph node metastases. Overall accuracy with CT scanning for assessing lymph nodes in rectal cancer is only 45%.[7-11]

The most current CT scanning, especially with dynamic contrast infusion, has a high accuracy rate in detecting liver metastases. However, abdominal US, similar to CT scan, can also detect occult liver metastases and should be used when the information obtained would alter therapeutic decisions.[12] MRI is also very useful in evaluating the liver before resection.

Endoluminal Imaging

Endoluminal imaging in the form of endoluminal US and endoluminal MRI has become extremely useful in the accurate preoperative staging of a rectal cancer. These modalities allow for more precise determination of the depth of invasion and the presence or absence of mesorectal lymph node metastasis. The knowledge of these factors is critical in determining the sequence and type of therapy for any given rectal cancer.

Endoscopic US is performed with a probe that is inserted into the rectum via the anus. The patient usually has taken a small preparation to clear the rectum of stool. A water-filled balloon is inflated and pressed against the rectal lesion. A 7.0- to 10.0-MHz transducer is then used to delineate the layers of the bowel wall into five distinct lines. Localized cancers involving only the mucosa and submucosa can therefore be distinguished from those tumors that penetrate the muscularis propria or extend through the rectal wall into the perirectal fat.[13] A modified TNM classification has been proposed,[14,15] in which a US stage T1 lesion (uT1) denotes a malignancy confined to the mucosa and submucosa, a uT2 lesion implies penetration of the muscularis propria, but confinement to the rectal wall, a uT3 lesion indicates invasion into the perirectal fat, and a uT4 lesion denotes a primary rectal malignancy that invades an adjacent organ. Studies have compared endorectal US (ERUS)[16,17] to DRE[17] and have found the US much more accurate. In a recent metaanalysis review, endoluminal US was found to be 95% accurate in distinguishing whether a tumor was confined to the rectal wall (T1, T2) versus invasion into the perirectal fat (T3 or greater).[18]

ERUS is less useful in predicting lymph node metastases with 80%–85% accuracy.[19] Endosonographically identified malignant lymph nodes are generally more hypoechoic in perirectal tissues.[20] However, these results are only seen with experienced operators.

Two methods of MRI can be used for the evaluation of rectal cancer. One can use the endorectal coil (ecMRI) or the surface coil MRI. The use of the MRI, either the endorectal or the surface coil, may offer some advantages compared with ERUS. First, it permits a larger field of view. Second, it may be less operator and technique dependent. And third, using the MRI may allow for the study of stenotic tumors.[21–24] Similar to ERUS, endorectal MRI (eMRI) can stage small-volume nodal disease and subtle transmural invasion. In general, eMRI has been more helpful in the assessment of perirectal nodal involvement than T stage. One reason is that MRI can identify involved nodes on the basis of characteristics other than size.[25] Reported accuracy rates of MRI for nodal staging range from 50% to 95%.[24-27]

Several series have compared the preoperative staging accuracy of ecMRI to ERUS in patients with rectal cancer.[24,26–28] In a report of 89 patients, the overall accuracy for T staging was similar (81%) for ecMRI and ERUS compared with only 65% for CT.[29] The accuracy for N staging was equally poor among the three modalities (63%, 64%, and 57% for ecMRI, ERUS, and CT, respectively). Somewhat similar results were noted in a series of 49 patients.[28] Transmural penetration was predicted by ecMRI with equal sensitivity (89%), but higher specificity (65% versus 33%) than ERUS. With both techniques, the predicted N stage had a relatively low correlation with pathologic N stage (45% versus 53%). In one report of 21 patients, ERUS seemed to be superior to ecMRI for determination of pathologic T stage (accuracy 83% versus 40%) because of better differentiation between T1 and T2 tumors. The accuracy for detecting perirectal tumor infiltration was 80% for ecMRI versus 100% for ERUS.[27]

The ecMRI is less operator dependent and in answering the critical question of whether a patient has Stage I versus Stage II or Stage III disease, ecMRI was 88% accurate. Those patients who were not staged correctly were usually overstaged and not understaged.

Double contrast MRI may permit more accurate T staging of rectal cancer by allowing better distinction among mucosa, muscularis, and perirectal tissues.[30,31] The specificity and sensitivity of ecMRI to predict infiltration of the anal sphincter was 100% and 90%, respectively. However, N staging was not improved with this approach; the sensitivity and specificity for nodal disease being 68% and 24%, respectively.

Phased-array surface coil MRI may prove to be the option of choice for staging of more advanced rectal cancers. The technique has been useful in predicting the likelihood of a tumor-free resection margin by visualizing tumor involvement of the mesorectal fascia.[32]

Preparation of the Rectal Cancer Patient for Surgery

After the diagnosis and staging of a rectal cancer, a decision needs to be made regarding optimal method of treatment. The surgical approach is dependent on the location of the tumor, its depth of invasion, and whether, in the preoperative evaluation, metastases have been discovered. Whether the patient is a candidate for a local excision or for a radical resection, the patient needs to be prepared for the procedure and the anesthetic so as to minimize perioperative and postoperative complications. Particular attention needs to be given to the patient's medical comorbidities. Unique to colon and rectal surgery is the need for a bowel preparation.

Bowel Preparation

Before the use of mechanical preparations and perioperative antibiotics, infection rates after colorectal surgery ranged as high as 60%.[33,34] Currently, there are several methods used to mechanically cleanse the large intestine. These include a diet of clear liquids 1–3 days before surgery combined with one of the following: laxatives, enemas, wholegut irrigation with saline via a nasogastric tube, mannitol solutions, polyethylene glycol (PEG) electrolyte lavage solutions, or PEG-based tablets. In a survey of colon and rectal surgeons in 1990, almost two-thirds preferred the PEG solutions for their patients because of the reliability of the cleansing results.[35] Many surgeons today continue to use these PEG solutions as a bowel preparation. There have been two recent metaanalyses that have concluded that mechanical bowel cleansing before colorectal surgery has no significant impact on perioperative infection rates.[36,37] Despite these recent studies, we would still recommend that some type of colonic cleansing occur before surgery because it is easier to manipulate the bowel if it is not filled with stool. It should be emphasized that one should not force a preparation on a patient because the benefits may be minimal. Furthermore, the choice of preparation should be selected depending on the individual. For instance, large-volume lavage solutions should not be used in patients with gastric emptying problems such as gastroparesis caused by diabetes. Saline laxatives are often phosphate- or magnesium-based and should not be used in patients with renal failure.

Antibiotic Prophylaxis

After mechanical cleansing of the large intestine, antibiotic prophylaxis is used to decrease the incidence of postoperative septic complications, because mechanical cleansing decreases the total volume of stool in the colon but does not affect the concentration of bacteria per milliliter of effluent.[38] Traditional prophylaxis uses an oral regimen known as the Nichols/Condon preparation. This regimen consists of neomycin 1 g and erythromycin base 1 g by mouth at 1:00 PM, 2:00 PM, and 11:00 PM on the day before surgery.[39] Many surgeons have substituted metronidazole 500 mg for the erythromycin base because it is bacteriocidal against a greater percentage of gut anaerobes.

Most surgeons use perioperative systemic antibiotics instead of oral antibiotics for antibiotic prophylaxis. Regimens need to include coverage for both aerobic and anaerobic gut bacteria. For long procedures, redosing should be considered depending on the serum half-life of the antibiotics used. Some have argued that double prophylaxis with both oral and intravenous antibiotics is of benefit in immunocompromised patients or in patients in whom the dissection is below the peritoneal reflection.

Other Perioperative Issues

Besides the mechanical and antibiotic preparation of the bowel, all patients are prepared in the usual manner for major surgery. Blood loss is usually quite minimal for most elective colorectal surgery and typically patients are not asked to donate autologous blood. Cardiac, pulmonary, and nutritional evaluations are performed when necessary. Perioperative systemic antibiotic coverage is expanded in patients with high-risk cardiac lesions such as prosthetic heart valves, a history of endocarditis, or a surgically constructed systemic-pulmonary shunt, and with intermediate-risk cardiac lesions such as mitral valve prolapse, valvular heart disease, or idiopathic hypertrophic subaortic stenosis.[38] Intravenous ampicillin 2 g and gentamicin 1.5 mg/kg are given 1/2–1 hour before the procedure and for at least one postoperative dose. Oral anticoagulation is stopped, and patients are placed on intravenous anticoagulation or on Lovenox approximately 5 days before surgery. The heparin or Lovenox is then stopped at the appropriate time before surgery (8 or 12 hours, respectively). Depending on the individual risk of the patient and the extent of the operative dissection, anticoagulation is restarted as early as 8 hours postoperatively, but without a bolus. Careful monitoring of the patient's hematocrit and partial thromboplastin time are necessary if early reheparinization is instituted.

Anatomic and Biologic Issues

Surgical Anatomy

The type of operation that can be offered to a patient with rectal cancer depends not only on tumor stage, but also on the location of the tumor in relation to the surgical anatomy. Surgical anatomy refers to the anatomic landmarks that determine resectability and sphincter preservation. The NCI consensus on rectal cancer recommended localizing the tumor relative to the anal verge which is defined as starting at the intersphincteric groove. Another important landmark defining the upper limit of the anal canal is the anorectal ring. From the surgeon's perspective, the top of the anorectal ring is the lower limit of a distal resection margin. A large, full-thickness cancer needs to be located high enough above the top of the anorectal ring to allow for an adequate distal margin if sphincter preservation is contemplated. If the dissection is to be carried lower toward the dentate line, then the tumor must be confined to the mucosa, submucosa, and superficial layer of the internal sphincter.

Biologic Issues

It is important to understand the clinical biology of rectal cancer. "Clinical" biology, means the typical pattern of growth and natural history of the spread of the disease. Studies have shown that colon cancer frequently arises in adenomatous polyps of the colon or rectum. Also, there is a 13%–62% incidence of polyps in patients with carcinoma of the colon or rectum.[40–43] The variation observed in the incidence of coexisting adenomas with carcinoma of the colon or rectum depends in part on the method of study.[1,2] Whatever method used to study the issue, one can clearly say that the vast majority of carcinomas arise in preexisting adenomas.[44–46] In preparing a patient for surgery, the surgeon should have the colon completely evaluated preoperatively so as to be able to operatively treat any synchronous disease that cannot be removed endoscopically.

The biology of lymph node metastases with invasive rectal cancer is important to note and is somewhat different from that of other solid tumors such as breast cancer. Gabriel et al.[47] reported in 1935 that colorectal cancers tend not to have "skip" metastases. Rectal cancers usually proceeded in an orderly march from the adjacent mesorectal nodes up the lymphatic chain to the upper extent of the mesentery along the inferior mesenteric artery (IMA) and vein systems. From the surgeon's perspective, this means that early intervention along with proper locoregional resection will cure most cancers. As part of a multimodality team that now treats most solid tumors, it must be emphasized to our medical colleagues that a rectal cancer is not a systemic disease from the first abnormal cell division. Aggressive local therapy in the form of an adequate resection is still the "anchor" to any therapy.

Surgical therapy may need to be customized in patients with certain polyposis syndromes or in cancers associated with inflammatory bowel disease. With both of these conditions, a total proctocolectomy needs to be performed. Sphincter preservation can be considered in certain patients but one needs to recognize that any mucosa left intact is at an increased risk of developing cancer. The anal transitional zone needs to be biopsied to identify dysplasia. If dysplasia is present, then a proctocolectomy with end ileostomy needs to be performed.

Surgical Procedures: Principles

Resection of the bowel with primary anastomosis was not a common phenomenon until the late 1940s. Before that time, surgery of the colon and rectum usually meant a permanent stoma.[48] Recent advances have been made in the surgical techniques for rectal cancer. The result is that primary resection and anastomosis without a colostomy or ileostomy is now the rule rather than the exception.

Palliation should be the goal in a patient for whom curative resection is not possible. If the patient is a reasonable operative risk and the extent of metastatic disease is minimal, then complete but palliative resection of the primary tumor leads to a better quality of life and prevents many of the distressing symptoms of an advanced primary lesion such as obstruction, bleeding, and pain. If the primary lesion is not resectable, then diversion of the fecal stream can significantly improve the patient's immediate status. Nonoperative therapy should be considered when there is significant metastatic disease and the primary tumor is relatively small and uncomplicated. In this situation, it is likely that the patient will die of metastatic disease before a complication from the primary tumor.

Variability in Outcome Based on Surgeon and Hospital Volume

The cancer resection margin in the extraperitoneal rectum is limited by the bony confines of the pelvis as well as by the proximity of adjacent anterior organs. In some cases, locoregional recurrence may be inevitable. However, locoregional failure may also result from incomplete surgery. There is accumulating evidence of variability among surgeons in local recurrence rates for stage-matched rectal cancers. McArdle and Hole[49] presented a review of 645 patients undergoing colorectal cancer resection at the Royal Infirmary in Glasgow. They observed significant variability in patients' postoperative morbidity, mortality, and ultimate survival, depending on the surgeon. The proportion of patients undergoing a curative resection varied from 40% to 76%, operative mortality from 8% to 30%, local recurrence from 0% to 21%, and anastomotic leak rates from 0% to 25%.

Hospital volume can also have an impact on colostomy rates, postoperative mortality, and overall survival as shown in a series of 7257 patients diagnosed with Stage I–III rectal cancer between 1994 and 1997.[50] When hospitals with the highest quartile of volume (more than 20 procedures annually) were compared with those with volumes in the lowest quartile (fewer than seven procedures annually), there were statistically significant differences in colostomy rates (29.5% versus 36.6%), 30-day postoperative mortality (1.6% versus 4.8%), and in overall 2-year survival (83.7% versus 76.6%).

The ability to perform sphincter-sparing surgery is also affected by hospital volume. In the United States Intergroup 0114 trial of 1330 patients with Stage II or III rectal cancer participating in an adjuvant treatment trial, APR rates were significantly higher in low-volume hospitals (46% versus 32% at lowest and highest volume hospitals, respectively).[51] Low hospital surgical volume was only an important predictor of inferior overall or recurrence-free survival in patients who did not complete their planned adjuvant chemoradiotherapy.

Total Mesorectal Excision

Total mesorectal excision in conjunction with an LAR or an abdominal perineal resection involves precise sharp dissection and removal of the entire rectal mesentery, including that distal to the tumor, as an intact unit.[52] Unlike conventional blunt dissection, the rectal mesentery is removed sharply under direct visualization emphasizing autonomic nerve preservation, complete hemostasis, and avoidance of violation of the mesorectal envelope. Its rationale is underscored by the hypothesis that the field of rectal cancer spread is limited to this envelope and its total removal encompasses virtually every tumor satellite. The reduction of positive radial margins can be reduced from 25% in conventional surgery to 7% in cases resected by TME. Furthermore, Adam et al.[53] showed that patients with positive radial margins were 3 times more likely to die and 12 times more likely to have local recurrence than patients without radial margin involvement.

Conventional surgery violates the circumference of the mesorectum during the blunt dissection along undefined planes. This leaves residual mesorectum in the pelvis. The higher rate of pelvic recurrence in conventional surgery is a reflection of inadequate resection and residual viable tumor burden within the pelvis. Several surgical teams using the TME technique have reported local failure rates ranging from 5% to 7% for Stage II and Stage III cancers.[52–56] By contrast, the North Central Cancer Treatment Group, NCCTG, control arm consisting of surgery plus radiotherapy had a local failure rate of 25% and the addition of chemotherapy only decreased the local failure rate to half that value.[57]

Of greater importance is the fact that improved local control seems to be translatable into improved overall survival. Survival ranges from 68% to 78% are observed among large published series when this technique is applied.

The meticulous dissection, however, is not without consequence. Prolonged operative time and increased anastomotic leak rates are noted. Anastomoses 3–6 cm from the anal verge have led up to 17% leak rates. Some centers are now routinely fashioning a protective diverting ostomy.

Conventional rectal surgery is associated with a significant incidence of sexual and urinary dysfunction. Presumably, this is related to damage to the pelvic autonomic parasympathetic and sympathetic nerves by blunt dissective forces.[58] Postoperative impotence and retrograde ejaculation or both have been observed in 25%–75% of cases particularly if lateral wall lymphadenectomy and splanchnic nerve resection are performed. By contrast, after TME with its careful nerve-sparing dissection, impotence has been reported in only 10%–29% of cases. A recent prospective study confirms that autonomic nerve preservation yields good results in terms of morbidity and functional outcome.[59]

There are well-recognized points during the rectal dissection where nerve injury can occur. The most proximal is the sympathetic nerve plexus surrounding the aorta. These sympathetic nerve trunks are also prone to injury near the pelvic brim as the bifurcate to each side of the pelvis. Intact nerves should look like a "wishbone" near the sacral promontory after a proper dissection. The clinical consequence of an isolated sympathetic nerve injury is retrograde ejaculation. If one proceeds with a dissection beneath the presacral or pelvic fascia from the sacral promontory around to the lateral pelvic sidewall, then one can injure both parasympathetic and sympathetic nerves which can result in impotence and bladder dysfunction. In the lower part of the mid rectum, the hypogastric plexus and nervi erigentes can be injured in the anterolateral pelvis. A radial dissection well outside the lymphovascular bundle which lies adjacent to the nerve and nerve plexus can also lead to a mixed parasympathetic and sympathetic injury. This bundle and the nerve structure are typically located just lateral to the seminal vesicles in a man or the cardinal ligaments in a woman. Finally, a dissection anterior to both layers of Denonvillier's fascia in a man can also put at risk the nerve and nerve plexus.

To date, all data are from prospectively gathered series and comparisons with historical controls. There are no randomized control data clearly showing benefits in terms of disease-specific and overall survival in patients undergoing TME as opposed to more conventional resection.

Adjuvant therapy has recently been shown to improve the results of TME surgery. In a two-arm, randomized study comparing TME with or without preoperative radiotherapy for resectable rectal cancer, patients receiving the combined therapy had a lower rate of local recurrence at 2 years. Subset analysis showed the most significant benefit in node-positive cancers.[60] The "completeness" of the TME also correlated with prognosis.[61] Adjuvant therapy should therefore be considered in patients undergoing TME surgery with Stage II and Stage III disease.

Figure 30-1 demonstrates schematically how the dissection should proceed. Figure 30-2 shows a cross-section of the rectum, the mesorectal fat, and the associated fascia.

Distal Margins and Radial Margins

The extent of resection margins in rectal cancer remains controversial. Although the first line of rectal cancer spread is upward along the lymphatic course, tumors below the peritoneal reflection also spread distally by intramural or

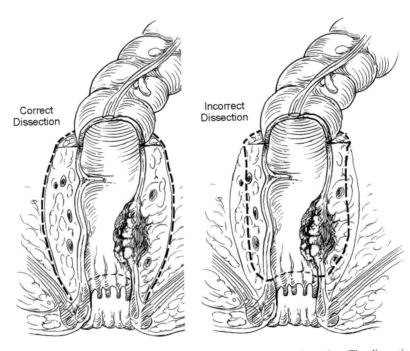

FIGURE 30-1. Schematic representation of the correct TME dissection versus an incorrect dissection. The dissection should proceed between the mesorectal fascia and the pelvic wall fascia to ensure a "complete" TME.

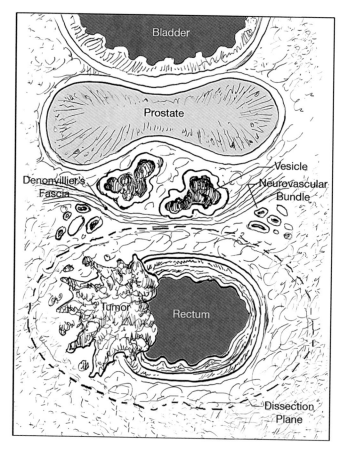

FIGURE 30-2. Transverse diagram of the structures of the mid rectum. The proper dissection proceeds just outside the mesorectal fat and fascia but with sparing of the neurovascular bundle and hypogastric plexus that is located anterolaterally along the pelvic sidewall. One or both layers of Denonvillier's fascia should be included in males and the equivalent fascial dissection along the back of the vagina in females.

extramural lymphatic and vascular routes. When distal intramural spread occurs, it is usually within 2.0 cm of the tumor, unless the lesion is poorly differentiated or widely metastatic.[62–64] Williams et al,[65] in 1983 reported distal intramural spread in 12 of 50 resected rectal cancer surgical patients. It was observed that 10 of the 12 had Stage III lesions. Only 6% had distal intramural spread greater than 2 cm. They concluded a "wet" margin of 2.5 cm was adequate in 94% of the patients. They noted that only five patients (10%) had tumor beyond a 1.5-cm margin, and all five of these had poorly differentiated, node-positive cancers. Also, the mortality in this group of patients was attributable to distant metastases, not local recurrence. All these patients had undergone an APR and had distal margins of greater than 5 cm. Grinnell[62] reported five cases of extramural retrograde lymphatic spread within 1.5 cm in 93 rectal cancers. He also reviewed 28 patients with atypical retrograde lymphatic dissemination. All these patients died within 5 years. He concluded retrograde lymphatic spread was a poor prognostic sign and more radical operations were not advantageous. Pollett and Nicholls[66] observed no differ-

ence in local recurrence rates whether distal margins of <2 cm, 2–5 cm, or >5 cm were achieved. Finally, in two early studies from the British literature, surgical pathology of rectal and rectosigmoid cancer demonstrated the clinical biology of extramural lymphatic spread. In the series by Goligher et al.[67] from 1951, only 6.5% of patients had metastatic glands below the primary tumor, whereas 93.5% had no retrograde spread. Approximately two-thirds of patients with retrograde spread had metastasis limited to within 6 mm of the distal tumor edge, and only 2% had metastasis beyond 2 cm. Dukes[68] published similar results in a study of more than 1500 patients with abdominoperineal cancer.

Further data from a randomized, prospective trial conducted by the National Surgical Adjuvant Breast and Bowel Project demonstrated no significant differences in survival or local recurrence when comparing distal rectal margins of <2 cm, 2–2.9 cm, and >3 cm.[69] As a result, a 2-cm distal margin has become acceptable for resection of rectal carcinoma, although a 5-cm proximal margin is still recommended.[70] The radial margin is more critical for local control.

It seems reasonable to conclude that a 2-cm distal margin is justified over a 5-cm distal margin. Even smaller distal margins may be acceptable in certain patients for whom there is no other option for sphincter preservation. In these cases, a frozen section analysis of the distal margin must be performed to confirm a cancer-free margin.

The discussion concerning the distal margin should not be confused with the issues regarding a TME and the radial margin. It is now clear that the status of the radial margin is perhaps the most critical in determining prognosis. Quirke et al.[71] in 1986 demonstrated tumor spread to the radial margins of 14 of 52 rectal cancers on whole mount specimens (27%). Twelve of these 14 patients subsequently developed local recurrence suggesting that local recurrence is largely a result of radial spread. Cawthorn et al.[55] also documented that tumor involvement of the lateral resection margin correlated with poor prognosis; however, it seemed to correlate more with distant spread and it was not a useful indicator of local recurrence.

Selection of Appropriate Therapy for Rectal Cancer

The management of rectal cancer has become increasingly complex. Presently, a surgeon has three major curative options: local excision, sphincter-saving abdominal surgery, and APR. Ideal candidates for local therapy that preserves anal sphincter anatomy and function include small T1 lesions (invasion only into the submucosa) and T2 lesions (invasion into the muscularis propria). As will be discussed, patients with T2 lesions probably should not have surgery alone. Recurrence is high. Preoperative or postoperative adjuvant chemoradiation is of benefit. At present, patients with T3 lesions (invasion into the perirectal fat) are not suitable candidates for local therapy and should be treated with an appropriate major resection as well as adjuvant therapy in most cases.

Certain clinical features also may have an impact on decisions about the appropriate therapy. Patients with physical handicaps may have significant difficulty in managing a stoma. Body habitus and patient gender influence the surgeon's ability to perform a sphincter-saving operation because of pelvic anatomy. Whereas a sphincter-saving procedure in a multiparous thin female can be straightforward, performing a low anastomosis in an obese male with a narrow pelvis can be extremely difficult. A history of pelvic irradiation or nonrectal pelvic malignancy can make a rectal resection and sphincter preservation more difficult.

In summary, each patient with rectal cancer should be viewed individually and a technical plan for their resection customized to their stage, gender, age, and body habitus (Figure 30-3). With these issues in mind, the technical choices for a radical resection are discussed below. In all of these resections, a TME should be performed. Local treatments are then described in detail.

Techniques of Rectal Excision

Abdominoperineal Resection

The APR was the first radical resection described by Miles in 1908 (reprinted in 1971).[72] Miles set out several principles to be achieved with any radical resection. These principles included:

- Removal of the whole pelvic mesocolon
- Removal of the "zone of upward spread" in the rectal mesentery
- Wide perineal dissection
- An abdominal anus
- Removal of the lymph nodes along the iliacs

Four of five of these principles are the anchor of our technique even today (the dissection along the iliacs is not done routinely).

Candidates for an APR are patients whose tumors are either into the anal sphincter or are so close to the anal sphincter that a safe distal margin cannot be obtained. Also, there is a small subset of patients with mid rectal tumors but with poor continence that benefit from an APR even though they are technically sphincter-preservation candidates. There have been recent reports that obturator/pelvic sidewall lymph nodes are more often involved in patients with very low rectal cancers. It has been suggested that these patients should undergo an extrafascial TME dissection.[73] Although there is some merit to this concept, we describe herein the typical APR with TME, excision of the sphincter and levators, and creation of a permanent colostomy.

Position

Usually a patient is placed in the lithotomy position. We often elevate the mid and upper sacrum off the bed with a blanket or a towel so that the coccyx is away from the bed and therefore able to be more easily prepped into the field.

Incision and Exploration

The abdomen is usually entered through a midline incision. In thin patients, the incision can often be kept below the umbilicus. Low transverse incisions can also be performed as long as the ostomy site is not compromised. The APR is also a good application of laparoscopic-assisted surgery. The abdominal portion of the procedure can be performed using laparoscopic techniques with extraction of the specimen through the perineum. It has yet to be shown, however, whether there is any value added with the laparoscopic-assisted approach.

The exploration of the abdomen and pelvis should be the first step after accessing the abdomen. The liver, aortic lymph nodes, superior hemorrhoidal lymph nodes, iliac lymph nodes, and the pelvis should all be examined. A large tumor burden, particularly multiple peritoneal implants, should lead to a reassessment of the need for resection and perhaps only a colostomy should be performed.

Mobilization

To excise the whole pelvic mesocolon and "zone of upward spread," the sigmoid colon and left colon need to be mobilized. The mobilization begins along the left pelvic brim. The gonadal vessels, ureter, and iliacs are reflected toward the retroperitoneum and the colon and mesocolon are pulled toward the midline. The left colon is mobilized but the splenic flexure rarely needs to be taken down. The dissection then is started on the right pelvic brim. Often, one can identify the sympathetic nerve trunks behind the superior hemorrhoidal artery (SHA) as one mobilizes the rectal mesocolon away from the sacral promontory.

Resection and Ligation

After mobilization of the mesentery, the bowel is divided near the sigmoid colon/left colon junction at right angles to the blood supply (Figure 30-4). Because a high ligation of the SHA or of the IMA is planned, the blood supply to most of the sigmoid colon will be compromised. For most cases, a ligation of the SHA flush with the left colic artery should be performed. A higher ligation of the IMA should be performed if there is any question of lymph node involvement outside the pelvis (e.g., palpable nodes along the SHA up to or above the left colic artery). The IMA should be ligated flush with the aorta and the inferior mesenteric vein should be ligated near the ligament of Treitz. A high ligation may also be required for additional colonic mobilization.

After dividing the bowel, sequential clamps of the sigmoid vessels are placed and the mesentery is ligated and divided. A high ligation is performed of the SHA with care being taken

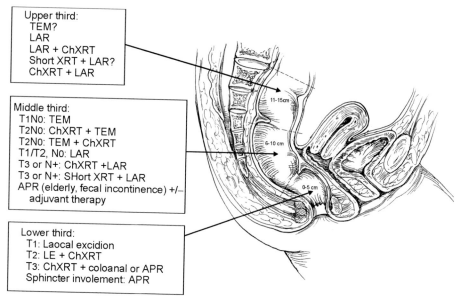

Upper third:
TEM?
LAR
LAR + ChXRT
Short XRT + LAR?
ChXRT + LAR

Middle third:
T1N0: TEM
T2N0: ChXRT + TEM
T2N0: TEM + ChXRT
T1/T2, N0: LAR
T3 or N+: ChXRT +LAR
T3 or N+: SHort XRT + LAR
APR (elderly, fecal incontinence) +/–
   adjuvant therapy

Lower third:
T1: Laocal excidion
T2: LE + ChXRT
T3: ChXRT + coloanal or APR
Sphincter involement: APR

FIGURE 30-3. Treatment options for rectal cancer depending on stage and location.

Stage I (T1N0, T2N0—The cancer is confined to the rectal wall and no nodes are involved)
- Distal rectal cancers: T1 (invasion into the submucosa only)
  - Local excision
  - Radical resection, often an APR
  - Adjuvant therapy is usually not recommended.
- Distal rectal cancers: T2 (invasion into the muscularis propria)
  - Local excision with preoperative or postoperative adjuvant therapy
  - Radical resection without adjuvant therapy, often an APR
- Mid rectal cancer: T1
  - TEM
  - Radical resection, usually an LAR with low anastomosis. A temporary proximal diverting ostomy is often required.
  - Adjuvant therapy is usually not recommended.
- Mid rectal cancer: T2
  - TEM with either preoperative or postoperative adjuvant therapy
  - Radical resection similar to a T1 cancer
  - Adjuvant therapy is not recommended if a radical resection is performed but is recommended after a TEM resection.
- Upper rectal cancers: T1 and T2
  - LAR

Stage II and Stage III cancers [Stage II cancers have invasion into the mesorectal fat (T3) but no involved mesorectal lymph nodes. Stage III cancers are any rectal cancer (T1, T2, or T3) but with involved lymph nodes.]
- Distal rectal cancers
  - Preoperative adjuvant therapy is most often recommended followed by a radical resection, usually an APR.
  - If preoperative imaging does not clearly define the stage of the cancer, resection can be done first followed by postoperative adjuvant therapy.
- Mid rectal cancers
  - Same as above for distal rectal cancers except an LAR is usually performed instead of an APR.
- Upper rectal cancers
  - LAR, with either preoperative or postoperative adjuvant therapy

Stage IV cancers
- Treatment for any cancer is dependent on the extent of metastasis. With better surgical and medical treatments for metastatic disease, locoregional control of the primary should be aggressive and similar to the above recommendations except in the most advanced cases.

(Key: LE, local excision; short XRT, short-course radiation therapy given 2 times a day for 5 days in larger fractions; ChXRT, long-course therapy given in 30 smaller fractions over 6 weeks in combination with chemotherapy)

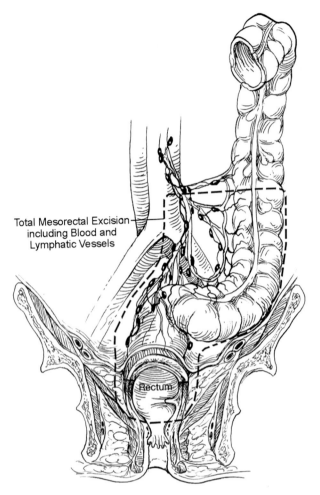

FIGURE 30-4. The vascular supply of the sigmoid and rectum. A typical ligation is performed at the junction of the SHA and left colic artery. In patients with a clinical suspicion of positive nodes at the level of the IMA or if vascular mobilization is needed for the left and transverse colon, then a ligation of the IMA is performed at the aorta.

to not injure the ureters, and also to make sure that the sympathetic nerve trunks are preserved.

The TME

A successful TME starts with the proper ligation of the SHA or IMA. As one dissects down toward the sacral promontory, the sympathetic nerve trunks are identified. The dissection plane is just anterior or medial to these nerves. Using the cautery or scissors, the nerves are reflected toward the pelvic sidewall while the mesorectal fascia surrounding the mesorectal fat is kept as an intact unit. The dissection starts posteriorly and then at each level proceeds laterally and then anteriorly. In the mid rectal area along the lateral sidewalls, one can sometimes see the parasympathetic nerves tracing anteriorly toward the hypogastric plexus. The plexus is usually on the anterolateral sidewall of the pelvis, just lateral to the seminal vesicles in the man and the cardinal ligaments in the woman. There is

often a tough "ligament" that traverses the mesorectum at this point. It theoretically contains the middle rectal artery. However, in a study by Jones et al.,[74] this artery is only present to any significance about 20% of the time.

The anterior dissection is perhaps the most difficult. In men, one should try to include the two layers of Denonvillier's fascia. This fascia is composed of peritoneum that has been entrapped between the seminal vesicles and prostate anterior and the rectum posterior (Figure 30-5). In woman, the peritoneum at the base of the pouch of Douglas is incised and the rectovaginal septum is then separated.

If done properly, the mesorectum begins to appear as a bulky bilobed structure. As one progresses distally beyond the mid rectum, the mesorectal fat begins to attenuate. At the pelvic floor there is often only a thin layer of mesorectal fat around the bowel.

The Perineal Dissection

As the abdominal procedure proceeds distally, the perineal dissection can commence. Before the preparation and draping of the patient, the position of the perineum is ensured so as to allow a wide elliptical incision around the anus. The rectum is usually cleared of any stool or residual preparation and the anus is sewn closed. The incision for the perineal dissection starts anteriorly at the perineal body, goes laterally to the ischiorectal spines, and then finishes posteriorly at the tip of the coccyx. After incising the skin and subcutaneous ischiorectal membrane and fat, the levators are then encountered. The perineal surgeon then coordinates their dissection with the abdominal team in the posterior precoccygeal plane. A pair of long scissors is used to divide the ligaments in the

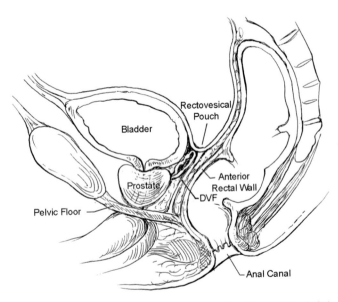

FIGURE 30-5. Sagittal view of the rectum, bladder, Denonvillier's fascia, and the prostate. The dissection should proceed anterior to one or both layers of Denonvillier's fascia.

posterior midline behind the rectum. Once a connection has been opened, the perineal surgeon places their finger above the levators and "hooks" them down toward the perineal field. The levators are then divided with the cautery. The dissection starts posteriorly and then proceeds laterally and anteriorly. Often it is best to complete the anterior dissection after the proximal portion of the specimen has been everted out to the perineal surgeon. The remaining attachments in the anterior plane are then divided with the cautery. Once the specimen is removed, hemostasis is ensured with the cautery or absorbable figure-of-8 sutures. Typically there are vessels that need to be ligated in the crease between the lateral prostate and the pelvic floor.

After irrigating the pelvis, one reapproximates the residual levators with absorbable sutures and then the subcutaneous fat, ischiorectal fat, and skin are closed in several layers. Drains in the pelvis can be brought out through the pelvis or via the abdomen.

Closure

With the specimen removed, attention is turned to creating an ostomy. Ideally, the patient has been marked by a certified ostomy therapist preoperatively. The end of the colon is carefully cleaned of any fat. The skin is divided in a circular shape at the ostomy site. A core of fat is removed from the subcutaneous tissues. The fascia is divided in a cruciate manner. The muscle is split but not divided, and then the peritoneum is incised. The hole is made wide enough to accommodate the bowel and the accompanying mesentery. The bowel should then be brought up through the opening so that it is 1–3 cm higher than the skin.

After creating the ostomy, pelvic drains are placed. These keep fluid from leaking through the perineal closure and allow for better healing and a reduced risk of a perineal hernia. The midline fascial opening is then closed and the skin approximated. After skin closure and placement of the dressing, the ostomy is then matured.

LAR with Sphincter Preservation

Sphincter-sparing procedures for resection of mid and some distal rectal cancers have become increasingly prevalent as their safety and efficacy have been established. The advent of circular stapling devices is largely responsible for their increasing popularity and utilization. An LAR involves dissection and anastomosis below the peritoneal reflection with ligation of the superior and middle hemorrhoidal arteries. An extended LAR indicates complete mobilization of the rectum down to the pelvic floor with division of the lateral ligaments and posterior mobilization through Waldeyer's fascia to the tip of the coccyx. Additionally, there is dissection of the plane between the anterior rectal wall and the vagina in a female patient and dissection of the plane between the rectum and the prostate in a male patient to a level distal to the

inferior margin of the prostate gland. As long as the surgeon can obtain a distal margin of at least 2 cm, an anastomosis can be considered appropriate if technically feasible. Body habitus, adequacy of the anal sphincter, encroachment of the tumor on the anal sphincters, and adequacy of the distal margin are all factors in determining the applicability of a sphincter-sparing operation.

Coloanal Anastomosis

The ultimate procedure in sphincter-saving operations is the ultra LAR with coloanal anastomosis. This operation preserves the sphincter mechanism in patients with very low-lying rectal cancer in whom the distal margin is at the minimally acceptable level yet adequate for cancer clearance. These operations are reserved for patients who have a distal rectal cancer that does not invade the sphincter musculature and in whom a standard extended LAR is technically not possible. After an adequate distal margin is achieved, the rectum is transected at the level of the pelvic floor musculature. The remaining anal mucosa between the dentate line and the level of transection of the pelvic floor can then be "stripped" and an anastomosis between the colon and the anus is performed to restore continuity. Alternatively, the procedure can be started at the dentate line with a tubular mobilization of the distal rectum in the intersphincteric groove. This perineal resection can proceed up to the superior margin of the puborectalis muscle before dissecting into the pelvis and connecting with the pelvic and abdominal dissection. The procedure usually requires full mobilization of the splenic flexure, such that the vascular supply of the left colon now based on the middle colic vessels can reach the distal pelvis. The coloanal anastomosis can also be done with a colonic J pouch. Because of the larger capacity of the J pouch construction, anorectal function is thought to be improved, especially early after the surgery. The J pouch is created by folding the distal end of the colon back on itself approximately 5–8 cm and then creating a common channel (Figure 30-6). The actual anastomosis to the anus is then done from the apex of the J in side to end manner. An alternative to the colonic J pouch is the coloplasty. This technique is similar in concept to a stricturoplasty. The distal colon is divided in a longitudinal direction for 8–10 cm starting 4–6 cm from the distal edge of the pedicle. The longitudinal incision is then approximated transversely making a larger reservoir capacity (Figure 30-7). The technique can decrease frequency in the early postoperative period but it has been associated with an increased number of anastomotic leaks. A proximal diverting stoma is advisable because of the potential for an anastomotic leak or vascular compromise of the left colon. Contraindications to the procedure include baseline fecal incontinence from deteriorated anal sphincter muscles; tumor invasion of the anal sphincter musculature or rectovaginal septum; tenesmus; and technical factors such as body habitus, tumor location, and tumor size.

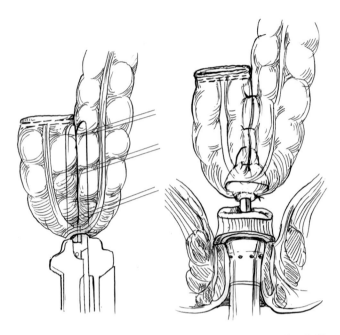

FIGURE 30-6. Construction of a colonic J pouch after an ultra LAR. The distal colon pedicle is folded back on itself to make a "J." A common channel is then created using a stapling device that will staple and divide. A larger reservoir is then created. The J pouch is then anastomosed to the anus using a circular stapler or in a hand-sewn manner.

Local Excision

Although the LAR and the APR are the mainstays of therapy for many distal rectal cancers, the radical resection is associated with significant morbidity and mortality. A review of the literature showed that mortality rates for the APR range from 0% to 6.3%,[75,76] with some studies having a 61% incidence of postoperative complications.[77] The majority of these complications are urinary dysfunction and perineal wound infections, with rates as high as 50% and 16%, respectively.[78] In our experience, the incidence of major wound complications was

10%.[79] Radical surgery, especially the APR, leads to a significant change in body image and social habits. In a patient survey performed in 1983 by Williams and Johnston,[80] 66% of patients complained of significant leaks from their stoma appliances, 67% experienced sexual dysfunction, and only 40% of patients who were working preoperatively returned to their jobs after their operation. Also, radical surgery does not guarantee a recurrence-free survival. The 5-year survival rate in the National Cancer Data Base for Stage I disease is 78%.[81] The complication rates, the change in body image with a colostomy, and the improvements in patient selection secondary to innovations in preoperative imaging modalities have led to a renewed interest in local excision of rectal cancers.

History

The first descriptions of local excision for rectal cancer date back to the late 1800s. At this time, there was little knowledge of the natural history of rectal cancer, and local excisions were viewed as the safest approach. In 1908, Miles[72] noted a high recurrence rate associated with local excision and developed a radical resection that was in keeping with the oncologic principles of the time. It was believed that radical resections such as Miles' APR provided the best opportunity for cure, and this radical resection quickly became the standard of care despite its increased morbidity and mortality over local excisions.

The first significant series published describing the use of local excision for rectal cancer was by Morson and colleagues[82] at St. Marks Hospital in London. Local excision had been used on patients who had either refused a colostomy or were deemed medically unfit for a radical operation secondary to comorbidities. In this series, they reported at the time of excision 91 patients with negative margins, and in the patients with negative margins only two had local recurrence whereas one had a distal recurrence. However, for the 69 patients with positive margins, 13 had a local recurrence and

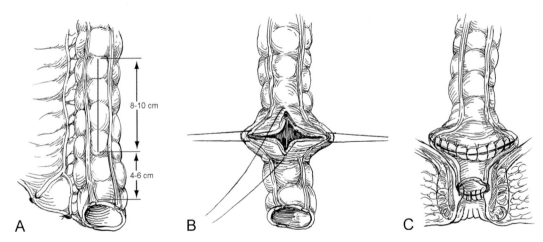

FIGURE 30-7. Construction of a coloplasty. The bowel is divided in a longitudinal manner as shown and resutured transversely to create a larger reservoir capacity.

one had distant recurrence. Most of the patients who underwent a local excision had T1 lesions. With these results, a "policy" was proposed to offer local excision to carefully selected patients with early small distal rectal cancers with well or moderately differentiated tumors.[82] These results prompted a renewed interest in local excision because they showed that local recurrence and survival rates were similar to those of APR for these small distal cancers, whereas the morbidity was greatly reduced.

Preoperative Evaluation

Proper patient selection remains the key to successful local excision of rectal cancers. The retrospective literature shows that there is a direct correlation between local recurrence and specific pathologic tumor features including depth of invasion, lymphatic invasion, histologic grade, and most importantly clear negative margins at the time of resection. In the past, preoperative evaluation relied solely on the DRE, which was found to have some success in demonstrating depth of invasion.[83,84] Recent studies have refuted this evidence,[85] and there are currently a number of imaging studies that can aid in the preoperative staging of rectal cancers, including ERUS and eMRI.

Preoperative evaluation begins with a thorough history and physical, taking care to note sphincter function, because local excision in the setting of poor preoperative sphincter function may be inappropriate. A digital rectal examination should be performed to assess the distance of the tumor from the anal verge, as well as its size and mobility. Tumors amenable to local excision should be <4 cm in diameter and occupy <40% of the bowel circumference. The distance of the tumor from the dentate line is important, because it will dictate which approach should be taken. Tumors <5 cm from the dentate are amenable to resection via a transanal procedure, whereas tumors in the middle third of the rectum may require a transcoccygeal approach or transanal endoscopic microsurgery (TEM). Immobile tumors are likely transmural, and thus not candidates for local excision. The overall health of the patient must be taken into account, because patients who are considered medically unfit for a major resection are often good candidates for local excision.

Imaging for rectal cancer has already been discussed. Suffice it to say that imaging is especially critical in selecting patients for a local excision. The best candidates have either a T1N0 or a T2N0 lesion. For the T2 lesions, local excision alone is not sufficient as therapy alone, and either preoperative or postoperative adjuvant therapy should be added. The selection criteria for a local excision are summarized in Table 30-1.

Technique

Historically, there are three approaches to local excision of rectal cancer: transanal, transcoccygeal, and transsphincteric. The transsphincteric approach has been associated with fecal

TABLE 30-1. Properties of distal rectal adenocarcinoma amenable to local excision for curative intent[124]

Physical features
Tumors <4 cm in diameter
Tumor <40% of bowel circumference
Tumor within 10 cm of dentate line
Tumor freely mobile on digital rectal examination
ERUS
T1, T2 lesions
No regional lymph node involvement

incontinence secondary to sphincter dysfunction, and thus has fallen out of favor. Recently, a newer technique, TEM, has provided a minimally invasive option for local excision which also allows the operator to reach lesions that are located more proximally and would have required a transcoccygeal or transsphincteric approach in the past.

Transanal Excision

Local excision can be accomplished via a transanal approach for the majority of low rectal cancers. In our prospective study of 48 local excisions for rectal cancer, 33 were performed using a transanal approach.[86] Before local excision, all patients should receive a full mechanical and antibiotic bowel preparation. After induction of anesthesia, the patient is flipped over and placed in the prone-jackknife position, with the buttocks taped apart. A pudendal nerve block should then be administered, which aids in postoperative pain control and more importantly relaxes the sphincter complex. An anal retractor alone or in combination with a retractor with self-retaining hooks are then used to dilate the anus and expose the lesion. Once adequate visualization has been obtained, traction sutures are often placed 1–2 cm distal to the tumor, and the line of dissection is marked on the mucosa using electrocautery. This line of dissection should be approximately 1–2 cm from the border of the tumor circumferentially (Figure 30-8). If visualization is not initially adequate, serial traction sutures should be used to prolapse the lesion into the field of view. Next, the electrocautery is used to make a full-thickness incision along the previously marked mucosa (Figure 30-8B). Upon completion of this incision, the perirectal fat should be visible beneath the lesion to confirm a full-thickness excision. In anterior lesions, care must be taken not to injure the back wall of the vagina in females, or the prostate in males. The lesion is then excised leaving visible perirectal fat at the base of the lesion. The defect in the bowel wall is then closed transversely using interrupted 3-0 polyglycolic sutures.

The complications most closely associated with transanal excisions include urinary retention, urinary tract infections, delayed hemorrhage, infections of the perirectal and ischiorectal space, and fecal impactions. However, the overall incidence of these complications is quite low, and the mortality rate is 0% in most series.

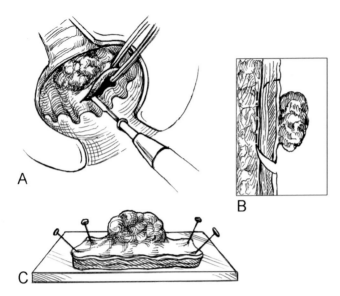

FIGURE 30-8. Transanal excision. **A** A transanal excision is performed by marking out a 1 cm or greater margin around the tumor. **B** A full-thickness excision is then performed to obtain adequate radial as well as lateral margins. **C** The specimen is then oriented accurately for the pathologist.

Transcoccygeal Excision

The transcoccygeal approach was used historically over the transanal approach for larger, more proximal lesions. It was originally popularized by Kraske who found it beneficial when operating on lesions within the middle or distal third of the rectum. This approach is especially useful for lesions on the posterior wall of the rectum, but can certainly be used for anterior or lateral lesions as well. In our series, the transcoccygeal approach was used where the distal margin was approximately 4.8 cm from the dentate line as compared with 3.0 cm for the transanal approach.[86]

All patients should undergo a full antibiotic and mechanical bowel preparation the day before surgery. The patient is again placed in the prone-jackknife position with the buttocks taped apart after the induction of general anesthesia. The tape will be released for closure to facilitate the approximation of the subcutaneous tissues and skin. Unlike the transanal approach, a pudendal block is not required, because the sphincters do not require relaxation. The patient is prepped and draped in a sterile manner with povidone-iodine solution, and an incision is made in the posterior midline adjacent to the sacrum and coccyx down to the upper border of the posterior aspect of the external sphincter. The coccyx, which along with the anal coccygeal ligament lies immediately deep to the skin and subcutaneous tissue, is removed to improve exposure. To do so, the anal coccygeal ligaments and other attachments are cauterized from each side and from the lower edge of the coccyx. The dissection then proceeds along the undersurface, anterior edge, of the coccyx until a cutting wire can pass through the sacral coccygeal joint. The coccyx is

then removed with occasional bleeding from an extension of the middle sacral artery, which is easily controlled with electrocautery. The levator ani muscles will now be visible at the base of the wound and should be separated in the midline, exposing a membrane that resides just outside of the perirectal fat. Division of this membrane allows for complete mobilization of the rectum within the intraperitoneal pelvis.

For posterior-based lesions, the distal margin of the tumor can be palpated via a rectal examination, and then the mesorectum and rectum are transected at a point 1–1.5 cm distal to the tumor (Figure 30-9). The excision is then completed with a 1-cm margin surrounding the lesion. For posterior lesions, the transcoccygeal approach allows for the removal of perirectal nodes that lie in the surrounding mesorectal tissue. For anterior lesions, a posterior proctotomy is made, and then the lesion is approached under direct vision, again excising the lesion down to the perirectal fat with a 1-cm margin (Figure 30-10). After removal, the specimen is reoriented for the pathologist and all the rectal incisions are closed in either a longitudinal or transverse manner to avoid narrowing of the rectum, using an absorbable suture. An air test should be performed, filling the operative field with sterile saline, and insufflating air in the rectum in order to check for air leaks in the suture line. Once these air leaks are controlled, the levator ani is reapproximated in the midline, and the anal coccygeal ligament is reattached to the sacrum. The operation is completed with closure of the skin and subcutaneous tissue.

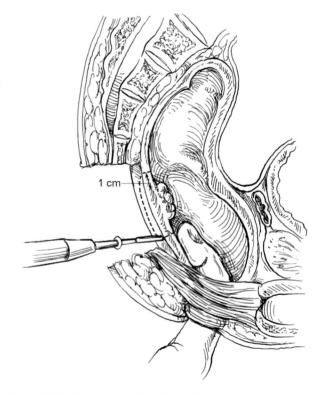

FIGURE 30-9. Transcoccygeal excision. For posterior lesions using a transcoccygeal or "Kraske" approach, one can palpate the lower border of the tumor to ensure an adequate distal margin.

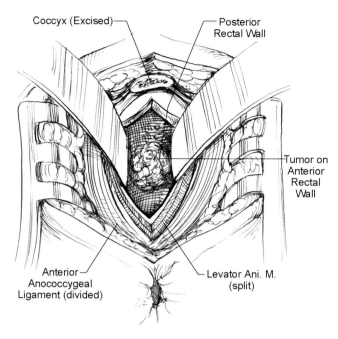

Coccyx (Excised)

Posterior
Rectal Wall

Tumor on
Anterior
Rectal
Wall

Anterior
Anococcygeal
Ligament (divided)

Levator Ani. M.
(split)

FIGURE 30-10. Transcoccygeal excision. Anterior lesions need to be approached by first making a posterior proctotomy and then excising the lesion through the rectum. The anterior and posterior walls of the rectum then need to be repaired, usually in a transverse manner in order to maintain the lumen diameter.

An unfortunate complication of this procedure is the development of a fecal fistula that extends from the rectum to the posterior midline incision. The incidence of this complication ranges from 5% to 20%,[86–88] and most heal after temporary diversion of the fecal stream via a loop ileostomy or colostomy. For this reason, the Kraske approach is used much less frequently than other methods for local treatment.

Transsphincteric Excision

The transsphincteric approach developed by York and Mason involves the complete division of the sphincters and the posterior wall of the rectum. The procedure starts similarly to the Kraske transcoccygeal approach, except the levator ani and the external sphincter muscles are divided in the midline. These muscles are carefully tagged so that they can be reapproximated exactly at the end of the procedure. Care must be taken to remain in the midline to avoid the nerve supply to the sphincters that lie in a posterolateral position bilaterally. Once the lesion is removed, the rectum, sphincters, and overlying musculature are closed in a careful stepwise manner. This procedure has an increased risk of incontinence secondary to sphincter dysfunction. Because the exposure provided from this approach is similar to that from the Kraske procedure, which carries less of a risk of incontinence, there are very few indications for this technique.

Transanal Endoscopic Microsurgery

TEM was first described in 1984 by Gerhard Buess of Tubingen, Germany.[89] The surgery is performed with the use of a special resectoscope which is 4 cm in diameter and available in lengths of both 12 and 20 cm. The scope is inserted with an obturator in place, which is then removed and replaced with an air-tight glass faceplate. The rectum is then manually insufflated, such as in rigid sigmoidoscopy, and the lesion is identified and centered in the field. The scope is then secured in position with the aid of a support arm that is attached to the operating table. The glass faceplate is then removed and replaced with a working adapter that contains four instrument ports and a fifth port for the stereoscope which is connected to a camera and projected onto a monitor. Carbon dioxide is then insufflated at low pressure (10–15 cm H_2O) to distend the rectum and allow for visualization of the lesion.

Once setup is complete, the operation proceeds in a manner similar to a transanal excision using a variety of special endoscopic instruments, which are introduced through the four ports in the working adapter. We begin with an injection of 1:100,000 solution of epinephrine in the submucosal plane around the lesion to aid with hemostasis. The margin of resection is then marked 1–1.5 cm circumferentially around the lesion using electrocautery. The lesion is then grasped and the excision proceeds along the previously marked line through the full thickness of the rectal wall and into the perirectal fat. The specimen is removed by temporarily removing the faceplate after complete excision. The defect is then closed using 3-0 long-lasting absorbable suture in a continuous or interrupted manner.

TEM allows for local excision of proximal rectal lesions that are not accessible via the transanal, transsphincteric, or transcoccygeal approaches. Despite favorable results of this relatively new technique, it has not gained widespread popularity secondary to the expense of the equipment, lack of familiarity with the equipment and setup, and complexity of the TEM operating system.

Outcomes: Retrospective Studies

The majority of the literature for local excision of rectal cancer comes from small retrospective reviews from single institutions. These studies are difficult to interpret because there is no uniform approach among the reviews. The length of follow-up varies from study to study, and many combine patients with tumors of different depth, positive margins, and different forms of local therapy including snare cautery and fulguration.

These retrospective reviews report a local recurrence rate of 5%–33% and survival rates of 57%–100%[90–94] (Table 30-2). These studies demonstrate that patients with superficial tumors and negative margins at the time of resection have low recurrence rates and a very good prognosis. Although these studies are not conclusive, they do suggest that local excision

TABLE 30-2. Series of local excision alone (retrospective series)

Author	No. of patients	Treatment arms	Follow-up	Recurrence local	Survival
Koscinski	58 (26 T1 and 32 T2)	47 TA, 6 TC, 5 TEM	Mean of 48 mo for Stage I and 59 mo for Stage II	T1, 5% T2, 28%	T1, 100% T2, 87.5%
Mellgren et al.[93]	261 (All T1 and T2)	108 LE via TA; 153 via APR	Mean of 52.8 mo	T1 estimated, 18% (LE), 0% (APR) T2 estimated, 47% (LE), 6% (APR)	T1, 72% (LE), 80% (APR) T2, 65% (LE), 81% (APR)
Horn	38 (17 T1, 14 T2, 7 requiring APR after LE)	3 endoscopic polypectomy, 35 TA, 5 salvage APR	Median of 50 mo	T1, 0% T2, 43%	T1, 100% T2, 82.6%
Gall et al.[121]	84 (54 T1, 19 T2, 11 T3) via LE; 383 APR	16 endoscopic polypectomy, 68 LE, 383 APR	Median of 77.5 mo	T1, 11% (LE), 0% (APR) T2, 22% (LE), 5% (APR)	T1, 74% ± 15% (LE), 100%–2% (APR) T2, 68% ± 24% (LE), 76% ± 11% (APR)
Morson et al.[82]	143 (115 T1, 20 T2, 7 T3)	143 LE; only 91 with negative margins		2/91 (2%) with negative margins 13/69 (19%) with positive margins	Corr. 5 y of 100% with negative margins Corr. 5 y of 83%–96% with positive margins
Whiteway	46 (13 T1, 18 T2, 15 T3)	46 TA and TSp; 27 for cure, 6 disseminated disease; 13 for high risk		Approximately 8 (17%)	Cancer specific survival of 87%

Source: From Ref. 124.
LE, local excision; TA, transanal excision; TC, transcoccygeal excision; TSp, transsphincteric excision.

may provide adequate oncologic control with considerably lower morbidity and mortality rates than APR for select distal rectal cancers.

Local Excision and Adjuvant Therapy

Local recurrence continues to be a major source of morbidity and mortality after both local excisions and radical resections for rectal cancer. The major risk factors for recurrence include the depth of invasion of the primary tumor, positive surgical margins, histologic grade of the tumor, and the presence of tumor in the regional lymph nodes. The addition of adjuvant or neoadjuvant radiation has been shown to decrease these local recurrence rates, and there is increasing evidence that chemoradiation may have a beneficial effect on survival. One of the major shortcomings of local excision is the inability to pathologically assess the regional lymph nodes. Microscopic disease can be present in the regional lymph nodes in up to 12% of T1 lesions, 22% of T2 lesions, and 58% of T3 and T4 lesions.[95,96] This microscopic disease may lead to local recurrence if left untreated. These findings have caused many observers to advocate the use of postoperative radiation after local excision in an attempt to eradicate any nodal disease, especially in more aggressive tumors with some of the risk factors previously mentioned. It also further emphasizes the need for preoperative ERUS or eMRI to identify patients with nodal disease who may be inappropriate for local excision.

Similar to the studies for local excision alone, many of the studies involving local excision combined with pre- or postoperative chemoradiation are small retrospective single-institution studies, and thus are difficult to interpret (Table 30-3). The patient population, radiation and chemotherapy protocols, and tumor characteristics are highly variable among these studies. The survival rates for these studies range from 33% to 100% depending on tumor stage and the use of adjuvant therapy. However, local recurrence rates are decreased when compared with local excision alone, ranging from 0% to 15% for T1 and T2 lesions, and 0% to 20% for T3 lesions.[76,91,94,97–99]

Prospective Studies

Unfortunately, there are very few prospective studies that use local excision for distal rectal adenocarcinoma with or without chemoradiotherapy (Table 30-4). We treated 48 patients with rectal adenocarcinoma via local excision, using postoperative chemoradiation for all T2 and T3 lesions. Over a mean follow-up period of 40.5 months, we found an overall survival of 93.8%, with recurrence rates by stage of 0% for T0 lesions, 9.5% for T1 lesions, 0% for T2 lesions, and 40% for T3 lesions. Of note, local recurrence was seen in three of five patients with lymphatic invasion and two of two patients with positive margins at the time of local excision.[86] From our results, we concluded that surgery alone was adequate for T1 lesions, whereas T2 lesions required a combination of surgery and chemoradiation for adequate results, provided that there were negative margins and no lymphatic involvement. If either of these characteristics were present, we recommended the addition of chemoradiation for T1 lesions, and radical resection for T2 lesions.

TABLE 30-3. Local excision plus XRT (retrospective series)

Author	No. of patients	Treatment arms	Follow-up	Local recurrence	Survival
Wong et al.[19]	25	21 TA, 4 endoscopic polypectomy or fulguration, all got 50 Gy XRT postop	Median 72 mo (minimum of 36 mo)	6/25 (24%)	Crude 5-y survival 96%
Mendenhall et al.[99]	67 (34 T1, 12 T2, 2 T3)	65 TA, 2 TC 48 received 45–60 Gy XRT postop	Median 65 mo (6–273 mo)	T1 = 11% T2–3 = 25%	T1 = 76% T2–3 = 77%
Bailey et al.[97]	63 (35 T1, 18 T2, 10 T3)	63 LE 34 XRT, 45–50 Gy	Median 44 mo (12–130)	4/53 (7.5%)	Crude 5-y survival 74.3%
Chakravarti et al.[91]	99 (58 T1, 41 T2)	52 LE alone	Median 51 mo (4–162 mo)	LE alone = 11% T1, 67% T2	Relapse-free 5-y survival
		47 LE plus 45–64.8 GY XRT (45 postop, 2 preop) 33 also had 5-FU		LE + CRT = 0% T1, 15% T2	LE alone = 80% T1, 33% T2 LE + CRT = 65% T1, 76% T2
Paty et al.[94]	125 (74 T1, 51 T2)	125 LE	Median 80.4 mo	T1 = 17%	10-y survival of 74% for T1 and 72% for T2
Willett et al. et al.[98]	56 (34 T1, 22 T2)	31 received 45–54 Gy and 15 of them got 5-FU 45 TA or TSp, 10 TC, 1 fulguration, 30 received 45 Gy postop XRT. Since 1986, received 5-FU	Median 48 mo	T2 = 26% Since 1985, 0/20 patients after chemoradiation	Actuarial 5-y recurrent-free survival of 72%

Source: From Ref. 124.

LE, local excision; TA, transanal excision; TC, transcoccygeal excision; TSp, transsphincteric excision; Gy, gray; CRT, chemoradiation therapy; XRT, radiation therapy.

Ota[100] published results on a study of 46 patients with a median follow-up time of 36 months. In this study, all patients received postoperative radiation, whereas T3 patients also received chemotherapy in addition to their radiation treatments. He reported a 6.5% local recurrence rate and a 3-year survival rate of 93%.

Steele et al. published a multicenter, prospective trial of local excision for rectal cancer in 110 patients.[81] All of these patients were thoroughly screened preoperatively to ensure that their tumors were within 10 cm of the dentate line, <4 cm in size, and involved <40% of the circumference of the bowel wall. Furthermore, all patients had to be N0M0, and statistical analyses were only performed on patients with negative margins at the time of resection. Patients were treated with postoperative chemoradiation only if they had T2 lesions. They published survival rates of 87% and 85% for T1 and T2

lesions, respectively, with an overall survival rate of 85%. They also found an overall disease-free survival rate of 78%, with 84% for T1 lesions, and 71% for T2 lesions. These data compare very favorably with APR, with a 5-year survival rate of 70% for Stage I disease. Unfortunately, the retrospective APR data are not separated into T1 and T2 lesions, making comparison difficult.

Transanal Endoscopic Microsurgery

Because TEM is still a relatively new technique, the data supporting its use are still being compiled. There are a few small, single-institution, retrospective, and prospective studies describing the use and outcomes of TEM for the excision of rectal cancer.[101–103] In general, these studies show survival and recurrence rates ranging from 83% to 100% and 0% to 27%,

TABLE 30-4. Local excision plus adjuvant therapy (prospective series)

Author	No. of patients	Treatment arms	Follow-up	Local recurrence	Survival
Ota[100]	46	LE Postop XRT (53 Gy) 5-FU for 7 T3's, 1 T2	Median 36 mo (18–73)	3/46 (6.5%) All T3's	Overall 3-y survival 93%
Bleday et al.[86]	48 (21 T1, 21 T2, 6 T3)	Postop XRT 54 Gy and 5-FU /500 mg/M² day 1–3, 28–30 for T2, T3 lesions	Mean 40.5 mo	4/48 (8%)	Overall 3-y survival 93.8%
Steele et al.[81]	110 (59 T1, 51 T2)	Postop XRT 54 Gy and 5-FU/ 500 mg/M² day 1–3, 29–31 for T2 lesions	Mean 48 mo	T1, 3/59 (5.1%) T2, 7/51 (13.7%)	Overall 6-y survival 85%

Source: From Ref. 124.

respectively. These rates are equivalent to those seen for transanal excision, but again comparison is difficult because of the differences in patient population, adjuvant therapy, and tumor characteristics (Table 30-5).

Recommendations

Patient selection is arguably the most important factor for obtaining comparable oncologic results with local excision or TEM versus APR in the treatment of low rectal cancers. All patients should receive a thorough history and physical including a digital rectal examination to assess the distance of the tumor from the anal verge, as well as its size and mobility. Ideally, tumors should be <4 cm in diameter and occupy <40% of the bowel circumference. Tumors within 5 cm from the dentate are amenable to resection via a transanal procedure, whereas more proximal tumors may require a TEM or transcoccygeal approach if an LAR is not feasible. Immobile tumors are not candidates for local excision because they are likely transmural. The overall health of the patient must be taken into account, because medically unfit patients are often good candidates for local excision. Even T2 and T3 lesions in these patients can be locally excised, accepting a higher rate of local recurrence for lower rates of morbidity and mortality. In this setting, these patients should receive adjuvant chemoradiotherapy and close follow-up.

After a thorough history and physical, all patients should undergo preoperative ERUS or eMRI to assess for transmural spread and regional lymphadenopathy. Tumors with evidence of nodal involvement should be considered advanced disease, and should be treated with a radical resection, either an APR or LAR with low pelvic anastomosis. T1 lesions have a very low probability of regional nodal involvement and are excellent candidates for local excision, whereas the opposite is true for T3 and T4 lesions, which should be treated via radical resection. The treatment of T2 lesions is somewhat controversial. Historically, better results have been seen with APR for T2 lesions; however, local excision with postoperative chemoradiation seems to be yielding similar results. If local excisions is offered to patients with T2 lesions, either preoperative or postoperative chemoradiation therapy should be part of the treatment plan.

CT scans of the abdomen and pelvis should be obtained in order to look for any signs of distant spread. PA and lateral views of the chest are necessary for similar reasons. In the presence of incurable distant metastases, there is a role for local excision for small T2 and T3 lesions, because these patients are likely to succumb to their distant disease before local recurrence causes any major problems. A full colonoscopy should also be performed preoperatively to assess for any synchronous polyps or carcinomas.

After this thorough preoperative evaluation has been completed, patients may then undergo local excision. Surgical margins should be 1 cm, although the key factor is a negative margin regardless of size. These excisions must be full thickness and include some perirectal fat. Local excisions are still considered total excisional biopsies, because final therapy awaits pathologic evaluation. After excision, these tumors should be evaluated for surgical margins, depth of invasion, histologic grade, and vascular or lymphatic invasion. Tumors with positive margins must be treated with additional therapy, either via reexcision, chemoradiation, or radical resection. Tumors are then categorized into low or high risk based on their level of differentiation and the presence or absence of vascular or lymphatic invasion. Patients with low-risk T1 lesions do not receive any additional therapy, whereas patients with high-risk T1 lesions and low-risk T2 lesions are given adjuvant chemoradiation. Patients with high-risk T2 and any T3 lesions should undergo radical resection (Table 30-6). Close follow-up is essential for all patients in order to detect local recurrence as early as possible.

Other Local Techniques

Small rectal cancers can be treated definitively using electrocoagulation or endocavitary radiation (ecRT). Electrocoagulation uses standard electric cautery to ablate the tumor, frequently with a specialized operating proctoscope. ecRT is

TABLE 30-6. Treatment recommendations after initial resection

T stage	Low risk*	High risk†
T1	No further treatment	Adjuvant chemoradiation
T2	Adjuvant chemoradiation	Radical resection
T3	Radical resection	Radical resection

*Low risk: well or moderately differentiated with no evidence of lymphatic or vascular invasion.
†High risk: poorly differentiated or lymphatic invasion or vascular invasion.

TABLE 30-5. Transanal endoscopic microsurgery

Author	No. of patients	Treatment arms	Follow-up	Local recurrence	Survival
Lezoche et al.[101]	35 (All T2)	All had preop 50 Gy XRT then TEM	Median 38 mo (24–96 mo)	1/35 (2.85%)	Probability of survival at 96 mo = 83%
Farmer et al.[102]	49 (36 Tis, 10 T1, 3 T2, 1 T3)	All TEM	Median 33 mo (20–48 mo)	2/49 (5.6%) 1 patient had a salvage APR	1 death from disseminated cancer. Survival = 97.9%
Azimuddin	21 (7 Tis, 9 T1, 5 T2)	All TEM	Mean 15 mo	0% for T0 and T1 20% for T2	100% for all grades
de Graaf et al.[103]	76 (32 Tis, 21 T1, 18 T2, 5 T3)	All TEM	Median 10 mo, mean 13.9 mo (1–52 mo)	Tis = 0%, T1 = 10%, T2 = 33%, and T3 = 0%	1 patient died yielding overall survival of 98.7%

a high-dose low-voltage technique applied to a smaller rectal cancer through a special proctoscope. Both techniques have the disadvantage of not providing an intact specimen for histologic analysis. Treatment results using each technique have not been evaluated in any prospective trial; however, recent retrospective reviews[104,105] conclude that these two techniques are good treatment options in carefully selected patients.

Survival after Rectal Cancer Excision

Overall 5-year survival rates for colorectal cancer have shown improvement over recent decades with the combination of better surgery and adjuvant therapy. Reports from 20 years previous have assured us that a sphincter-sparing surgical approach does not sacrifice survival in selected patients where an adequate margin can be achieved.[106–108] Overall, 5-year survival rates after major surgery for rectal cancer are as follows: Stage I, 85%–100%; Stage II, 60%–80%; and Stage III, 30%–50%.[57,66,106,109–115]

Local excision of cancers confined to the rectal wall without lymphatic or distant spread (T1 and T2N0) can achieve cure rates of 80%–100% as discussed previously; however, the results published in retrospective trials are extremely unreliable because many studies span decades, have no standard entrance criteria, and no standard adjuvant therapy policy. In some retrospective studies, local recurrence seemed high but overall survival was not different than a comparative group of patients who underwent radical resection.[93] Future emphasis on earlier diagnosis, accurate preoperative staging, and appropriate choice of resection procedure, combined with improved adjuvant therapy, should influence favorably overall survival using this conservative technique.

Laparoscopically Assisted Resections for Rectal Cancer

The application of laparoscopy for the treatment of intraabdominal malignancies including proctectomy for rectal cancer is now being performed. In these operations, part of the procedure is done using the laparoscope and completion of the procedure is in the traditional manner. In particular, exploration and mobilization of the colon and rectum can be done with the laparoscope and laparoscopic instruments. Ligation of the vascular pedicle is performed with laparoscopic clips, vascular stapling devices, or radiofrequency coagulation devices. The pelvic dissection can be performed and well visualized laparoscopically in many patients. Most often, however, the actual resection of the bowel and an anastomosis are still more easily performed in an extracorporeal manner.

The main questions about laparoscopically assisted proctectomy for colorectal cancer are whether it provides the same TME specimen as traditional open techniques, and whether there is any other unique biologic alteration in the laparoscopic procedure that leads to a change in survival or in recurrence patterns. Concerning the latter point, there have been several reports of unusual wound recurrences at trocar sites in patients undergoing laparoscopic-assisted colectomy. However, a randomized trial of open versus laparoscopically assisted colon resection found no statistically significant differences in survival.[116] In a recent article from the United Kingdom, laparoscopically assisted LAR for rectal cancer revealed an increased risk of a positive circumferential margin compared with open surgery.[117] Going forward, the use of laparoscopy will increase with rectal resection; however, its use will need to be monitored and studied to make sure that the standard principles of a TME are adhered to.

Synchronous Cancers

Synchronous cancers of the large intestine occur with an incidence of approximately 3.5%.[118] Also, synchronous polyps are common with a primary cancer. If one finds two cancers within the colon and rectum, then one must plan an approach to the surgical resection that depends on the location of the two lesions. Certainly, two resections and two primary anastomoses can be performed in large bowel surgery with a complication rate that is similar to that of just one anastomosis.[119] If a patient has a small rectal cancer that is amenable to local excision along with a synchronous cancer of the colon, one can consider a local excision of the rectal lesion followed by primary resection of the colon lesion. It is important, however, to realize that surveillance after local excision of a rectal cancer needs to be more aggressive in monitoring for local recurrence and metachronous cancers or precancers than after resection of single bowel cancer.

Extended Resection for Locally Advanced Colon or Rectal Cancer

Carcinoma of the colon and rectum will sometimes invade adjacent organs or the abdominal wall. When this occurs, it has been shown that extended resection of the cancer along with the tissue or organ that it has adhered to can lead to a 5-year survival rate of >50%, provided the surgical margins are tumor free.[120,121] Patients with inflammatory adhesions to contiguous organs have a slightly higher survival rate than patients with malignant infiltration, but the distinction between malignant and inflammatory contiguity often cannot be made until after en bloc resection. The organs that are usually involved with adhesions from colon or rectal cancer include the uterus, small bowel, urinary bladder, and abdominal wall. In general, approximately 5% of patients will present with locally advanced lesions.[121]

Surgical Treatment of Recurrent Colorectal Carcinoma

Recurrent colorectal cancer affects between 12% and 50% of patients with Dukes B or C (TT2N0 through T3NN1) disease. Although adjuvant treatment has some effect on survival, surgery remains the mainstay in treatment of recurrent disease. Most often, the intent of surgery for recurrent disease is not curative, but to improve survival or palliate symptoms.

There are three main patterns of recurrence after resection of a primary colorectal cancer. The most common site of recurrence is the liver. However, isolated recurrences can also be seen locoregionally or in the lung. Although 60%–70% of patients who die of colorectal cancer have liver metastasis, the liver is an isolated site of recurrence in <20% of patients. Of the latter group, only 5%–10% will be candidates for curative hepatic resection.[122]

Locoregional recurrence of rectal cancer has been decreasing over the past 2 decades. With the use of adjuvant therapy and the wider application of TME, local failure has been reported as low as 3%. However, when a patient develops a local recurrence, it is often not just a suture line recurrence but a regional recurrence. The workup of these patients requires extensive imaging to identify features of the tumor which would make it unresectable.

Wanebo et al.[123] demonstrated a 25% actuarial 5-year survival after abdominal sacral resection for recurrent colorectal cancer. They concluded that patients presenting after a long disease-free interval could benefit from such a large procedure. Noncurative surgery has only a small role in the treatment of symptomatic pelvic recurrence, particularly with sacral involvement. Newer approaches such as cryoablation of perineal recurrences may replace heroic procedures and may be useful in symptomatic relief of nonresectable pelvic recurrence.

Appendix: Practice Parameters for the Treatment of Rectal Carcinoma

Prepared by the American Society of Colon and Rectal Surgeons

Preoperative Evaluation

A patient with a newly diagnosed rectal cancer requires preoperative assessment to identify tumor stage and operative risk factors that may affect the choice of the surgical procedure.

Examination

Digital rectal examination and sigmoidoscopy allow for the assessment of tumor location, size, and fixation.

Synchronous colon malignancies or coexisting adenomatous polyps should be identified preoperatively, if possible. Colonoscopy is preferred over barium enema.

Imaging Studies

Identifying the extent of local, regional, or distant metastasis may be useful if the findings would modify the approach to treatment. ERUS may be preferred to assess rectal wall penetration, MRI to evaluate perirectal tissue involvement, and CT scan to identify hepatic or pulmonary metastasis.

Laboratory Studies

Laboratory studies should be obtained as indicated by the patient's general condition and anesthetic requirements. The measurement of baseline CEA is useful if postoperative monitoring is planned.

Treatment Considerations

Where possible, the patient should participate in the treatment selection. They should understand the risks and benefits of therapy including short-term and long-term outcome and treatment alternatives.

Abdominoperineal Resection

This procedure is generally indicated for lesions of the lower one-third of the rectum or for higher lesions where tumor characteristics and anatomic factors favor such resection. Where possible, preoperative colostomy counseling is recommended.

Sphincter-preserving Resection

These procedures are possible for the majority of patients with rectal carcinoma. The choice of the anastomotic technique should be left to the discretion of the surgeon.

Transanal Procedures

Such procedures may be performed for cure in highly selected patients with favorable tumor characteristics or for patients in need of palliative therapy. These procedures include local excision, electrocoagulation, endocavitary irradiation, and laser ablation.

Hartmann's Procedure

This procedure may be indicated for patients who present with obstructed or perforated carcinoma and for patients in whom colorectal anastomosis is clinically inadvisable.

Abdominal Transsacral Resection

The indication for this procedure has been largely supplemented by other sphincter-preserving resections. It provides adequate treatment for mid rectal cancers in the hands of surgeons experienced with this approach.

Adjacent Organ Resection

Contiguous organ resection should be considered in the absence of metastatic disease.

Palliative Surgical Procedures

Such procedures, which may include contiguous organ resection, may be indicated to alleviate or significantly reduce the patient's symptoms caused by primary or recurrent tumor.

Adjuvant Therapy

Adjuvant chemotherapy or radiation therapy, preoperatively or postoperatively, may be used in combination with surgical resection to potentially improve results for cure or for palliation.

Reprinted from Dis Colon Rectum 1993;36(11):989–1006. Copyright © 1993. All rights reserved. American Society of Colon and Rectal Surgeons.

References

1. Floyd CE, Stirling CT, Cohn I Jr. Cancer of the colon, rectum and anus: review of 1,687 cases. Ann Surg 1966;163(6):829–837.
2. Reilly JC, Rusin LC, Theuerkauf FJ Jr. Colonoscopy: its role in cancer of the colon and rectum. Dis Colon Rectum 1982;25(6):532–538.
3. Travieso CR Jr, Knoepp LF Jr, Hanley PH. Multiple adenocarcinomas of the colon and rectum. Dis Colon Rectum 1972;15(1):1–6.
4. Heald RJ, Bussey HJ. Clinical experiences at St. Mark's Hospital with multiple synchronous cancers of the colon and rectum. Dis Colon Rectum 1975;18(1):6–10.
5. Langevin JM, Nivatvongs S. The true incidence of synchronous cancer of the large bowel. A prospective study. Am J Surg 1984;147(3):330–333.
6. Brahme F, Ekelund GR, Norden JG, Wenckert A. Metachronous colorectal polyps: comparison of development of colorectal polyps and carcinomas in persons with and without histories of polyps. Dis Colon Rectum 1974;17(2):166–171.
7. Dixon AK, Fry IK, Morson BC, et al. Pre-operative computed tomography of carcinoma of the rectum. Br J Radiol 1981;54(644):655–659.
8. Grabbe E, Lierse W, Winkler R. The perirectal fascia: morphology and use in staging of rectal carcinoma. Radiology 1983;149(1):241–246.
9. Adalsteinsson B, Glimelius B, Graffman S, et al. Computed tomography in staging of rectal carcinoma. Acta Radiol Diagn (Stockh) 1985;26(1):45–55.
10. Freeny PC, Marks WM, Ryan JA, Bolen JW. Colorectal carcinoma evaluation with CT: preoperative staging and detection of postoperative recurrence. Radiology 1986;158(2):347–353.
11. Thompson WM, Halvorsen RA, Foster WL Jr, et al. Preoperative and postoperative CT staging of rectosigmoid carcinoma. AJR Am J Roentgenol 1986;146(4):703–710.
12. Kane R. The accuracy of CT, MRI, and ultrasound in the detection of hepatic metastatic disease from colon cancer. Abstract. Proceedings of the 76th Scientific Assembly and Annual Meeting of the Radiological Society of North America, Chicago, IL, 1990.
13. Beynon J, Foy DM, Roe AM, et al. Endoluminal ultrasound in the assessment of local invasion in rectal cancer. Br J Surg 1986;73(6):474–477.
14. Hildebrandt U, Feifel G. Preoperative staging of rectal cancer by intrarectal ultrasound. Dis Colon Rectum 1985;28(1):42–46.
15. Hildebrandt U, Feifel G, Schwarz HP, Scherr O. Endorectal ultrasound: instrumentation and clinical aspects. Int J Colorectal Dis 1986;1(4):203–207.
16. Rifkin MD, Wechsler RJ. A comparison of computed tomography and endorectal ultrasound in staging rectal cancer. Int J Colorectal Dis 1986;1(4):219–223.
17. Beynon J, Roe AM, Foy DM, et al. Preoperative staging of local invasion in rectal cancer using endoluminal ultrasound. J R Soc Med 1987;80(1):23–24.
18. Solomon MJ, McLeod RS. Endoluminal transrectal ultrasonography: accuracy, reliability, and validity. Dis Colon Rectum 1993;36(2):200–205.
19. Wong WD, Orrom WJ, Jensen L. Preoperative staging of rectal cancer with endorectal ultrasonography. Perspect Colon Rectal Surg 1990;3:315–334.
20. Beynon J. An evaluation of the role of rectal endosonography in rectal cancer. Ann R Coll Surg Engl 1989;71(2):131–139.
21. Hulsmans FJ, Tio TL, Fockens P, et al. Assessment of tumor infiltration depth in rectal cancer with transrectal sonography: caution is necessary. Radiology 1994;190(3):715–720.
22. Orrom WJ, Wong WD, Rothenberger DA, et al. Endorectal ultrasound in the preoperative staging of rectal tumors. A learning experience. Dis Colon Rectum 1990;33(8):654–659.
23. Ng A, Recht A, Busse PM. Sphincter preservation therapy for distal rectal cancer: a review. Cancer 1997;79:671.
24. Gualdi GF, Casciani E, Guadalaxara A, et al. Local staging of rectal cancer with transrectal ultrasound and endorectal magnetic resonance imaging: comparison with histologic findings. Dis Colon Rectum 2000;43(3):338–345.
25. Brown G, Richards CJ, Bourne MW, et al. Morphologic predictors of lymph node status in rectal cancer with use of high-spatial-resolution MR imaging with histopathologic comparison. Radiology 2003;227:371–377.
26. Kim NK, Kim MJ, Yun SH, et al. Comparative study of transrectal ultrasonography, pelvic computerized tomography, and magnetic resonance imaging in preoperative staging of rectal cancer. Dis Colon Rectum 1999;42(6):770–775.
27. Meyenberger C, Huch Boni RA, Bertschinger P, et al. Endoscopic ultrasound and endorectal magnetic resonance imaging: a prospective, comparative study for preoperative staging and follow-up of rectal cancer. Endoscopy 1995;27(7):469–479.
28. Blomqvist L, Machado M, Rubio C, et al. Rectal tumour staging: MR imaging using pelvic phased-array and endorectal coils vs endoscopic ultrasonography. Eur Radiol 2000;10(4):653–660.
29. Adjuvant therapy of colon cancer: results of a prospectively randomized trial. Gastrointestinal Tumor Study Group. N Engl J Med 1984;310(12):737–743.
30. Wallengren NO, Holtas S, Andren-Sandberg A, et al. Rectal carcinoma: double-contrast MR imaging for preoperative staging. Radiology 2000;215(1):108–114.

31. Urban M, Rosen HR, Holbling N, et al. MR imaging for the preoperative planning of sphincter-saving surgery for tumors of the lower third of the rectum: use of intravenous and endorectal contrast materials. Radiology 2000;214(2):503–508.

32. Beets-Tan RG, Beets GL, Vliegen RF, et al. Accuracy of magnetic resonance imaging in prediction of tumour-free resection margin in rectal cancer surgery. Lancet 2001;357(9255): 497–504.

33. Burton RC. Postoperative wound infection in colonic and rectal surgery. Br J Surg 1973;60(5):363–365.

34. Clarke JS, Condon RE, Bartlett JG, et al. Preoperative oral antibiotics reduce septic complications of colon operations: results of prospective, randomized, double-blind clinical study. Ann Surg 1977;186(3):251–259.

35. Solla JA, Rothenberger DA. Preoperative bowel preparation. A survey of colon and rectal surgeons. Dis Colon Rectum 1990;33(2):154–159.

36. Platell C, Hall J. What is the role of mechanical bowel preparation in patients undergoing colorectal surgery? Dis Colon Rectum 1998;41(7):875–882; discussion 882–883.

37. Bucher P, Mermillod B, Gervaz P, Morel P. Mechanical bowel preparation for elective colorectal surgery: a meta-analysis. Arch Surg 2004;139(12):1359–1364; discussion 1365.

38. Morotomi M, Guillem JG, Pocsidio J, et al. Effect of polyethylene glycol-electrolyte lavage solution on intestinal microflora. Appl Environ Microbiol 1989;55(4):1026–1028.

39. Nichols RL, Broido P, Condon RE, et al. Effect of preoperative neomycin-erythromycin intestinal preparation on the incidence of infectious complications following colon surgery. Ann Surg 1973;178(4):453–462.

40. Muto T, Bussey HJ, Morson BC. The evolution of cancer of the colon and rectum. Cancer 1975;36(6):2251–2270.

41. Morson BC. Factors influencing the prognosis of early cancer of the rectum. Proc R Soc Med 1966;59(7):607–608.

42. Morson B. President's address. The polyp-cancer sequence in the large bowel. Proc R Soc Med 1974;67(6):451–457.

43. Tierney RP, Ballantyne GH, Modlin IM. The adenoma to carcinoma sequence. Surg Gynecol Obstet 1990;171(1):81–94.

44. Dukes CE. Simple tumors of the large intestine and their relationship to cancer. Br J Surg 1925;13:720.

45. Helwig EB. The evolution of adenomas of the large intestine and their relationship to carcinoma. Surg Gynecol Obstet 1947;84:36–49.

46. Jass JR. Do all colorectal carcinomas arise in preexisting adenomas? World J Surg 1989;13(1):45–51.

47. Gabriel WB, Dukes CE, Bussey HJ. Lymphatic spread in cancer of the rectum. Br J Surg 1935;25:395–413.

48. Corman ML. Principles of surgical technique in the treatment of carcinoma of the large bowel. World J Surg 1991;15(5):592–596.

49. McArdle CS, Hole D. Impact of variability among surgeons on postoperative morbidity and mortality and ultimate survival. BMJ 1991;302(6791):1501–1505.

50. Hodgson DC, Zhang W, Zaslavsky AM, et al. Relation of hospital volume to colostomy rates and survival for patients with rectal cancer. J Natl Cancer Inst 2003;95(10):708–716.

51. Meyerhardt JA, Tepper JE, Niedzwiecki D, et al. Impact of hospital procedure volume on surgical operation and long-term outcomes in high-risk curatively resected rectal cancer: findings from the Intergroup 0114 Study. J Clin Oncol 2004;22(1): 166–174.

52. Heald RJ. The 'Holy Plane' of rectal surgery. J R Soc Med 1988;81(9):503–508.

53. Adam IJ, Mohamdee MO, Martin IG, et al. Role of circumferential margin involvement in the local recurrence of rectal cancer. Lancet 1994;344(8924):707–711.

54. Havenga K, DeRuiter MC, Enker WE, Welvaart K. Anatomical basis of autonomic nerve-preserving total mesorectal excision for rectal cancer. Br J Surg 1996;83(3):384–388.

55. Cawthorn SJ, Parums DV, Gibbs NM, et al. Extent of mesorectal spread and involvement of lateral resection margin as prognostic factors after surgery for rectal cancer. Lancet 1990;335(8697):1055–1059.

56. Enker WE, Thaler HT, Cranor ML, Polyak T. Total mesorectal excision in the operative treatment of carcinoma of the rectum. J Am Coll Surg 1995;181(4):335–346.

57. Krook JE, Moertel CG, Gunderson LL, et al. Effective surgical adjuvant therapy for high-risk rectal carcinoma. N Engl J Med 1991;324(11):709–715.

58. Heald RJ. Rectal cancer: anterior resection and local recurrence—a personal view. Perspect Colon Rectal Surg 1988;1(2):1–26.

59. Masui H, Ike H, Yamaguchi S, et al. Male sexual function after autonomic nerve-preserving operation for rectal cancer. Dis Colon Rectum 1996;39(10):1140–1145.

60. Kapiteijn E, Marijnen CA, Nagtegaal ID, et al. Preoperative radiotherapy combined with total mesorectal excision for resectable rectal cancer. N Engl J Med 2001;345(9):638–646.

61. Nagtegaal ID, van de Velde CJ, van der Worp E, et al. Macroscopic evaluation of rectal cancer resection specimen: clinical significance of the pathologist in quality control. J Clin Oncol 2002;20(7):1729–1734.

62. Grinnell RS. Distal intramural spread of carcinoma of the rectum and rectosigmoid. Surg Gynecol Obstet 1954;99(4): 421–430.

63. Black WA, Waugh JM. The intramural extension of carcinoma of the descending colon, sigmoid, and rectosigmoid: a pathologic study. Surg Gynecol Obstet 1948;87:457.

64. Quer EA, Dahlin DC, Mayo CW. Retrograde intramural spread of carcinoma of the rectum and rectosigmoid: a microscopic study. Surg Gynecol Obstet 1953;96(1):24–30.

65. Williams NS, Dixon MF, Johnston D. Reappraisal of the 5 centimetre rule of distal excision for carcinoma of the rectum: a study of distal intramural spread and of patients' survival. Br J Surg 1983;70(3):150–154.

66. Pollett WG, Nicholls RJ. The relationship between the extent of distal clearance and survival and local recurrence rates after curative anterior resection for carcinoma of the rectum. Ann Surg 1983;198(2):159–163.

67. Goligher JC, Dukes CE, Bussey HJ. Local recurrences after sphincter saving excisions for carcinoma of the rectum and rectosigmoid. Br J Surg 1951;39(155):199–211.

68. Dukes CE. The surgical pathology of rectal cancer. Proc R Soc Med 1943;37:131.

69. Wolmark N, Fisher B, Wieand HS. The prognostic value of the modifications of the Dukes' C class of colorectal cancer. An analysis of the NSABP clinical trials. Ann Surg 1986;203(2): 115–122.

70. Nelson H, Petrelli N, Carlin A, et al. Guidelines 2000 for colon and rectal cancer surgery. J Natl Cancer Inst 2001;93(8): 583–596.

71. Quirke P, Durdey P, Dixon MF, Williams NS. Local recurrence of rectal adenocarcinoma due to inadequate surgical resection. Histopathological study of lateral tumour spread and surgical excision. Lancet 1986;2(8514):996–999.

72. Miles WE. A method of performing abdomino-perineal excision for carcinoma of the rectum and of the terminal portion of the pelvic colon (1908). CA Cancer J Clin 1971;21(6):361–364.

73. Takahashi T, Ueno M, Azekura K, Ohta H. Lateral node dissection and total mesorectal excision for rectal cancer. Dis Colon Rectum 2000;43(10 suppl):S59–68.

74. Jones OM, Smeulders N, Wiseman O, Miller R. Lateral ligaments of the rectum: an anatomical study. Br J Surg 1999; 86(4):487–489.

75. Rothenberger DA, Wong WD. Abdominoperineal resection for adenocarcinoma of the low rectum. World J Surg 1992;16(3): 478–485.

76. Wong CS, Stern H, Cummings BJ. Local excision and postoperative radiation therapy for rectal carcinoma. Int J Radiat Oncol Biol Phys 1993;25(4):669–675.

77. Rosen L, Veidenheimer MC, Coller JA, Corman ML. Mortality, morbidity, and patterns of recurrence after abdominoperineal resection for cancer of the rectum. Dis Colon Rectum 1982;25(3):202–208.

78. Pollard CW, Nivatvongs S, Rojanasakul A, Ilstrup DM. Carcinoma of the rectum. Profiles of intraoperative and early postoperative complications. Dis Colon Rectum 1994;37(9): 866–874.

79. Christian CK, Kwaan MR, Betensky RA, et al. Risk factors for perineal wound complications following abdominoperineal resection. Dis Colon Rectum 2005;48(1):43–48.

80. Williams NS, Johnston D. The quality of life after rectal excision for low rectal cancer. Br J Surg 1983;70(8):460–462.

81. Steele GD Jr, Herndon JE, Bleday R, et al. Sphincter-sparing treatment for distal rectal adenocarcinoma. Ann Surg Oncol 1999;6(5):433–441.

82. Morson BC, Bussey HJ, Samoorian S. Policy of local excision for early cancer of the colorectum. Gut 1977;18(12):1045–1050.

83. Mason AY. President's address. Rectal cancer: the spectrum of selective surgery. Proc R Soc Med 1976;69(4):237–244.

84. Nicholls RJ, Mason AY, Morson BC, et al. The clinical staging of rectal cancer. Br J Surg 1982;69(7):404–409.

85. Rafaelsen SR, Kronborg O, Fenger C. Digital rectal examination and transrectal ultrasonography in staging of rectal cancer. A prospective, blind study. Acta Radiol 1994;35(3):300–304.

86. Bleday R, Breen E, Jessup JM, et al. Prospective evaluation of local excision for small rectal cancers. Dis Colon Rectum 1997;40(4):388–392.

87. Killingback M. Local excision of carcinoma of the rectum: indications. World J Surg 1992;16(3):437–446.

88. Christiansen J. Excision of mid-rectal lesions by the Kraske sacral approach. Br J Surg 1980;67(9):651–652.

89. Beuss G, Gunther M. Endoscopic operative procedures for the removal of rectal polyps. Coloproctology 1984;6:254.

90. Benson R, Wong CS, Cummings BJ, et al. Local excision and postoperative radiotherapy for distal rectal cancer. Int J Radiat Oncol Biol Phys 2001;50(5):1309–1316.

91. Chakravarti A, Compton CC, Shellito PC, et al. Long-term follow-up of patients with rectal cancer managed by local excision with and without adjuvant irradiation. Ann Surg 1999; 230(1):49–54.

92. Gonzalez QH, Heslin MJ, Shore G, et al. Results of long-term follow-up for transanal excision for rectal cancer. Am Surg 2003;69(8):675–678; discussion 678.

93. Mellgren A, Sirivongs P, Rothenberger DA, et al. Is local excision adequate therapy for early rectal cancer? Dis Colon Rectum 2000;43(8):1064–1071; discussion 1071–1074.

94. Paty PB, Nash GM, Baron P, et al. Long-term results of local excision for rectal cancer. Ann Surg 2002;236(4):522–529; discussion 529–530.

95. Brodsky JT, Richard GK, Cohen AM, Minsky BD. Variables correlated with the risk of lymph node metastasis in early rectal cancer. Cancer 1992;69(2):322–326.

96. Heimann TM, Oh C, Steinhagen RM, et al. Surgical treatment of tumors of the distal rectum with sphincter preservation. Ann Surg 1992;216(4):432–436; discussion 436–437.

97. Bailey HR, Huval WV, Max E, et al. Local excision of carcinoma of the rectum for cure. Surgery 1992;111(5):555–561.

98. Willett CG, Compton CC, Shellito PC, Efird JT. Selection factors for local excision or abdominoperineal resection of early stage rectal cancer. Cancer 1994;73(11):2716–2720.

99. Mendenhall WM, Morris CG, Rout WR, et al. Local excision and postoperative radiation therapy for rectal adenocarcinoma. Int J Cancer 2001;96 suppl:89–96.

100. Ota DM. M.D. Anderson Cancer Center experience with local excision and multimodality therapy for rectal cancer. Surg Oncol Clin North Am 1992;1(1):147–152.

101. Lezoche E, Guerrieri M, Paganini AM, Feliciotti F. Long-term results of patients with pT2 rectal cancer treated with radiotherapy and transanal endoscopic microsurgical excision. World J Surg 2002;26(9):1170–1174.

102. Farmer KC, Wale R, Winnett J, et al. Transanal endoscopic microsurgery: the first 50 cases. ANZ J Surg 2002;72(12): 854–856.

103. de Graaf EJ, Doornebosch PG, Stassen LP, et al. Transanal endoscopic microsurgery for rectal cancer. Eur J Cancer 2002;38(7):904–910.

104. Eisenstat TE, Oliver GC. Electrocoagulation for adenocarcinoma of the low rectum. World J Surg 1992;16(3):458–462.

105. Papillon J, Berard P. Endocavitary irradiation in the conservative treatment of adenocarcinoma of the low rectum. World J Surg 1992;16(3):451–457.

106. Slanetz CA Jr, Herter FP, Grinnell RS. Anterior resection versus abdominoperineal resection for cancer of the rectum and rectosigmoid. An analysis of 524 cases. Am J Surg 1972; 123(1):110–117.

107. McDermott F, Hughes E, Pihl E, et al. Long term results of restorative resection and total excision for carcinoma of the middle third of the rectum. Surg Gynecol Obstet 1982;154(6):833–837.

108. Jones PF, Thomson HJ. Long term results of a consistent policy of sphincter preservation in the treatment of carcinoma of the rectum. Br J Surg 1982;69(10):564–568.

109. Manson PN, Corman ML, Coller JA, Veidenheimer MC. Anterior resection for adenocarcinoma. Lahey Clinic experience from 1963 through 1969. Am J Surg 1976;131(4): 434–441.

110. Strauss RJ, Friedman M, Platt N, Wise L. Surgical treatment of rectal carcinoma: results of anterior resection vs. abdominoperineal resection at a community hospital. Dis Colon Rectum 1978;21(4):269–276.

111. Sauer R, Becker H, Hohenberger W, et al. Preoperative versus postoperative chemoradiotherapy for rectal cancer. N Engl J Med 2004;351(17):1731–1740.

112. Heberer G, Denecke H, Pratschke E, Teichmann R. Anterior and low anterior resection. World J Surg 1982;6(5):517–524.

113. Localio SA, Eng K, Coppa GF. Abdominosacral resection for midrectal cancer. A fifteen-year experience. Ann Surg 1983;198(3):320–324.

114. Wilson SM, Beahrs OH. The curative treatment of carcinoma of the sigmoid, rectosigmoid, and rectum. Ann Surg 1976;183(5):556–565.

115. Whittaker M, Goligher JC. The prognosis after surgical treatment for carcinoma of the rectum. Br J Surg 1976;63(5):384–388.

116. Clinical Outcomes of Surgical Therapy Study Group. A comparison of laparoscopically assisted and open colectomy for colon cancer. N Engl J Med 2004;350(20):2050–2059.

117. Guillou PJ, Quirke P, Thorpe H, et al. Short-term endpoints of conventional versus laparoscopic-assisted surgery in patients with colorectal cancer (MRC CLASICC trial): multicentre, randomised controlled trial. Lancet 2005;365(9472):1718–1726.

118. Heald RJ. Synchronous and metachronous carcinoma of the colon and rectum. Ann R Coll Surg Engl 1990;72(3):172–174.

119. Whelan RL, Wong WD, Goldberg SM, Rothenberger DA. Synchronous bowel anastomoses. Dis Colon Rectum 1989;32(5):365–368.

120. Curley SA, Carlson GW, Shumate CR, et al. Extended resection for locally advanced colorectal carcinoma. Am J Surg 1992;163(6):553–559.

121. Gall FP, Tonak J, Altendorf A. Multivisceral resections in colorectal cancer. Dis Colon Rectum 1987;30(5):337–341.

122. Steele G Jr, Ravikumar TS. Resection of hepatic metastases from colorectal cancer. Biologic perspective. Ann Surg 1989;210(2):127–138.

123. Wanebo HJ, Gaker DL, Whitehill R, et al. Pelvic recurrence of rectal cancer. Options for curative resection. Ann Surg 1987;205(5):482–495.

124. Greenberg J, Bleday R. Local excision of rectal cancer. Clin Colon Rectal Surg 2005;16(1):40–46.

31
Adjuvant Therapy for Colorectal Cancer

Judith L. Trudel and Lars A. Påhlman

Colon Cancer

The stage of disease at presentation remains the most important prognostic factor for colon cancer patients.[1] Stage I disease carries an excellent prognosis of more than 95% 5-year survival rate, and surgical treatment alone is considered sufficient; adjuvant treatment is not indicated. In contrast, adjuvant treatment has repeatedly been shown to improve survival for Stage III disease. The role of adjuvant treatment for Stage II (node-negative) disease remains controversial.

Adjuvant Chemotherapy for Node-positive Disease (Stage III)

Overall 5-year survival from curative surgery for Stage III colon cancer is 30%–60%.[1] Recurrences are often systemic, hence the need for systemic adjuvant treatment in these high-risk patients. Adjuvant chemotherapy improves survival by approximately 10%–15%.

5-Fluorouracil (5-FU)/leucovorin (LV)-based adjuvant chemotherapy for Stage III disease is the standard of care in the United States today.[2] Historically, single-agent chemotherapeutic agents such as thiotepa or fluoropyrimidines did not prove helpful as adjuvant treatment of colon cancer. Progressively, several combination trials of chemotherapy and immune modulators helped refine the recommendations made for adjuvant treatment. In 1988, the NSABP (National Surgical Adjuvant Breast and Bowel Project) CO-1 trial documented a significant 8% improvement in overall 5-year survival for Stage II and Stage III disease when adjuvant chemotherapy with MOF (semustine, vincristine, and 5-FU) was used.[3] In 1989, the NCCTG (North Central Cancer Treatment Group) published a three-arm randomized study of 401 Dukes' Stage B and C patients comparing surgical resection alone to levamisole and to 5-FU plus levamisole. 5-FU plus levamisole significantly decreased the recurrence rates and improved overall survival, particularly in Dukes' C patients.[4] The large Intergroup 0035 study

confirmed the efficacy of 5-FU plus levamisole in 971 patients with Dukes' Stage C cancer in 1990[5]; death rates were reduced by 33% ($P = .0007$), and recurrence rates by 40% ($P < .0001$). In 1990, the NIH (National Institutes of Health) published a consensus statement establishing 5-FU plus levamisole as the standard adjuvant therapy for Stage III colon cancer.[6] A recent European study has confirmed a significant reduction of 25% in the odds of cancer death in Stage III patients receiving adjuvant 5-FU and levamisole.[7]

While the usefulness of 5-FU/levamisole in Stage III disease was being confirmed, LV emerged as a beneficial agent for the treatment of metastatic disease. Its applicability to Stage II and Stage III disease was confirmed by the IMPACT (International Multicenter Pooled Analyses of Colon Cancer Trials) study of 1526 patients, published in 1995. In this study, 3-year disease-free survival increased from 62% to 71% ($P = .0001$) whereas overall survival increased from 78% to 83% ($P = .029$) in the 5-FU/LV group compared with surgical controls.[8] The NSAPB C-03 randomized trial of 1081 Stage II and Stage III patients comparing MOF to 5-FU/LV had documented a similar advantage of 5-FU/LV, with a 3-year disease-free survival increase from 64% to 73% ($P = .0004$) and an overall survival increase from 77% to 84% ($P = .003$) in the 5-FU/LV group compared with MOF.[9]

The relative merits of levamisole and LV as modulators of 5-FU-based adjuvant chemotherapy, and the optimal duration of treatment were investigated in several studies published between 1998 and 2000. The NCCTG/NCIC (National Cancer Institute of Canada)[10] study of 915 patients compared 6 months 5-FU/levamisole; 6 months 5-FU/LV/levamisole; 1 year 5-FU/levamisole; and 1 year 5-FU/LV/levamisole. Triple therapy for 6 months was as effective as 12 months; and 6-month triple therapy provided superior 5-year overall survival and disease-free survival compared with 5-FU/levamisole. The Intergroup trial 0089 of 3759 patients compared 1 year 5-FU/levamisole; 5-FU/high-dose LV for 32 weeks; and 5-FU/low-dose LV with or without levamisole for six cycles.[11] There were no differences between the four treatment arms with regard to 5-year disease-free and overall survival. The NSABP CO-4 study[12] and the QUASAR Collaborative Group study[13] have later confirmed the survival advantage provided by LV modulation over levamisole. Based on the results of these studies, the new standard for treatment was changed to 6 months of adjuvant chemotherapy with 5-FU/LV for Stage III, node-positive disease.

The newer chemotherapeutic agents currently under study or in use for treatment of metastatic disease (e.g., irinotecan, capecitabine, oxaliplatin) are undergoing evaluation for their usefulness in the adjuvant treatment of patients with Stage II and Stage III disease. Recent data from the multicenter international randomized MOSAIC trial have confirmed that the addition of oxaliplatin to 5-FU/LV (FOLFOX) further decreases the risk of recurrence in Stage II and Stage III disease by 23%, resulting in a significant improvement in 3-year disease-free survival.[14] Another important trial, the PETACC 3 trial, will soon report the results. In that trial 5-FU/leucovourin is compared with irinotecan to 5-FU/LV (FOLFIRI) in both Stage II and Stage III colon cancer.

Several tumor characteristics such as microsatellite instability and the expression of DNA synthesis-associated enzymes have recently been found to predict chemoresistance to 5-FU and irinotecan.[15,16] This is an area of research that is evolving rapidly, and will certainly change the recommendations for adjuvant treatment in both node-positive and node-negative disease.

Adjuvant Chemotherapy for Node-negative Disease (Stage II)

Whereas the efficacy and benefits of adjuvant chemotherapy for Stage III node-positive disease is unequivocally documented through numerous randomized trials, the role of adjuvant chemotherapy for Stage II node-negative disease is still controversial. The data from the early studies that prompted the NIH recommendation for adjuvant treatment in Stage III disease did not support a similar recommendation for Stage II disease.[4,5] Recent metaanalyses have yielded conflicting results. The IMPACT-B_2 (International Multicenter Pooled Analysis of B_2 Colon Cancer Trials) Group published a pooled analysis of five trials conducted from 1982 to 1989 and regrouping 1016 patients with Stage B_2 colon cancer.[17] Relapse rates, all-cause death rates, 5-year event-free survival and overall survival were similar in patients treated with adjuvant 5-FU/LV compared with controls. Increasing age and poor tumor differentiation were indicators of poor prognosis.[17] A SEER-Medicare cohort analysis of 3700 patients with resected Stage II colon cancer did not reveal any improvement in 5-year survival in patients having received adjuvant chemotherapy compared with controls (74% versus 72%).[18] In contrast, a pooled analysis of four NSABP trials (CO1, CO2, CO3, and CO4) with widely different treatment and control arms regrouping 1565 patients with Dukes' B disease (Stage II) and 2255 patients with Dukes' C disease (Stage III) concluded that patients with Dukes' B

disease (Stage II) should be offered adjuvant chemotherapy.[19] The authors calculated a 30% relative reduction in mortality for Stage II patients having received adjuvant chemotherapy. That metaanalysis has since been widely criticized for its methodologic flaws, and the controversy rages on. The likelihood of reaching a resolution on this subject is remote: to detect a significant survival benefit among Stage II colon cancer patients (who have an estimated 5-year survival of 80%), an adjuvant trial with a no-treatment control arm would require a sample size of 5000–8000 patients.[20] The recent data from the MOSAIC trial showing a significant improvement of 3-year disease-free survival and a 23% reduction of recurrence risk using a combination of 5-FU/LV/oxaliplatin (FOLFOX) in Stage II disease will undoubtedly spur renewed interest in this debate.[14] At this time, the use of adjuvant chemotherapy for Stage II node-negative disease remains an unanswered question, mainly because the prognosis for Stage II node-negative disease is good overall, and many patients would face unnecessary treatment. For the time being, patients with Stage II colon cancer at high risk for tumor recurrence might be considered for adjuvant treatment on an individual basis, or might be entered in a clinical trial.

Radiotherapy

Local recurrence of rectal cancer after surgery with curative intent has always been recognized as a significant clinical problem. Combined chemoradiotherapy has been shown to increase both local control and survival for patients with locally advanced and node-positive rectal cancer.[21] In contrast, although local failure and recurrence after surgery for colon cancer had been described, there long existed an unwritten consensus that treatment failures in colon cancer surgery were primarily systemic rather than local. Thus, no prospective, randomized study was devised to provide data on the role of external beam radiotherapy in preventing local recurrence or improving survival after colon surgery. The recognition that selected individuals with colon cancer were at a high risk for local recurrence eventually came from retrospective reviews of patterns of failure after surgery with curative intent. Two large retrospective reviews[22,23] helped define the risk factors for local recurrence after surgery for colon cancer. Locoregional failure was identified in 19%[22] to 46%[23] of patients overall; at least half of local recurrences were in the original tumor bed. Only 13% of the local recurrences were salvageable surgically.[22] The most important risk factors for local recurrence were: 1) pathologic staging, with local recurrence rates of 35% in modified Astler-Coller Stages B3, C2, or C3 versus 7% in Stages A, B1, and C1[2]; 2) primary tumor localization in a fixed, nonperitonealized segment of the colon, with the highest failure rates in the cecum, descending colon, hepatic or splenic flexures, and sigmoid colon[22,23]; 3) colon carcinoma complicated by perforation or obstruction, with a two- to three-fold increase in local recurrence for any given pathologic stage.[22]

Identification of individuals at high risk for local recurrence after curative surgery for colon cancer triggered a number of studies on the role of external beam radiotherapy in preventing local recurrence or improving survival after colon surgery. Several disparate single-institutional retrospective studies suggested an improvement in local failure and recurrence rates with adjuvant radiotherapy compared with historical controls.[25–26] Wide variations in radiation techniques and doses, concurrent use and choice of chemotherapy, and patient selection criteria make comparison among studies difficult. Overall, local control rates ranged from 60% to 88%, a significant improvement over controls treated by surgery alone. A single randomized prospective study initiated jointly by the NCCTG and RTOG, comparing chemotherapy alone with F-FU/levamisole versus combined chemotherapy/radiotherapy closed prematurely because of poor accrual; although no differences were observed in overall survival between treatment arms, the study lacked sufficient statistical power to draw valid conclusions.[27]

At this time, the precise role of adjuvant radiotherapy in the treatment of colon cancer remains undefined. There are no data to support a systematic recommendation for therapy or a well-recognized adjuvant regimen. The potential risks of adjuvant radiotherapy for colon cancer, particularly radiation damage to surrounding organs (e.g., small bowel) are significant. Treatment for individuals deemed at high risk for local recurrence after curative surgery for colon cancer should be individualized.

Immunotherapy, Tumor Vaccines, and Gene Therapy

The goal of cancer immunotherapy treatments is to stimulate the body's immune system in order to improve host defense mechanisms against growing tumors. Colorectal cancer immunotherapy strategies have evolved dramatically over the past 30 years. Nonspecific immune stimulation with bacterial cell products (e.g., BCG) and cytokines (e.g., interleukin-2) has recently been superseded by more specific immune stimulation targeted against colorectal tumor-expressed antigens. Whereas some tumor antigens are present in normal tissues but overexpressed in cancer, other tumor antigens are restricted to cancer tissues. Vaccines stimulate the immune system to recognize and act specifically against these tumor-expressed antigens, through either the humoral or cellular pathway.

More than 25 Phase I and Phase II studies have explored a variety of vaccines based on whole colorectal tumor cells, virus-modified tumor cells, gene-modified tumor cells, tumor antigen-derived peptides, tumor cell lysates, proteins or carbohydrates, monoclonal antibodies, plasmid or viral vectors encoding tumor antigens, and dendritic cell-based vaccines. Promising results were observed in some animal models and Phase I and II studies, prompting ongoing research efforts.

A few Phase III studies have also yielded promising results.[28] Three large studies have looked at the effect of immune stimulation with autologous irradiated tumor vaccine plus BCG in patients with colorectal cancer. Hoover et al.[29] randomized 98 patients with colon or rectal cancer to surgical resection alone or surgical resection followed by vaccination with autologous irradiated tumor plus BCG. There was no difference in disease-free or overall survival in the 80 eligible patients, but subset analysis showed a significant improvement in disease-free survival for colon cancer patients. The Eastern Cooperative Oncology Group (ECOG) randomized Stage II and Stage III colon cancer patients to either observation or vaccination with autologous irradiated tumor plus BCG. There was no survival difference between groups, but patients with a marked delayed cutaneous hypersensitivity showed a trend toward better disease-free and overall survival, suggesting that survival correlated with the patient's immune response to vaccination.[30] Vermoken et al.[31] randomized 254 patients operated for colon cancer to either observation or vaccination with autologous irradiated tumor plus BCG immediately after operation, followed by a vaccine booster 6 months after operation. The overall risk for recurrence was decreased by 44% in all vaccinated patients, with a 61% reduction in Stage II patients. Vaccination significantly increased recurrence-free survival, and there was a trend toward improved overall survival.[31] Because of its marginal efficacy, the complexity in the preparation of the vaccine, and the introduction of more effective chemotherapeutic agents, tumor cell-based immunotherapy is not frequently used in colon cancer patients.

Gene therapy is based on the concept of transferring genetic material into target cells, which would allow for correction of genetic defects in tumor suppressor genes, inactivation of oncogenes, or insertion of treatment-sensitizing genes (such as drug-converting enzymes) or "suicide genes" into the colorectal cells. Correction of p53 mutations, inactivation of k-ras gene product p21, and the delivery of prodrug converting enzymes are currently being studied. The long-term potential for clinical usefulness of these techniques remains to be defined.

Rectal Cancer

Although surgery remains the central treatment of rectal cancer, the overall approach to treatment has changed dramatically over the last three decades. Surgical technique has been refined to become more focused and precise, with specific attention given to a locally more aggressive and meticulous technique. The modern multimodal therapy approach individualizes rectal cancer care, thus offering the best and most appropriate treatment to every single patient. Local and distant staging guides the decision for adjuvant radiotherapy and/or chemoradiotherapy and for available surgical approaches, i.e., local excision or an abdominal procedure.

Many prospective trials have demonstrated the beneficial effect of preoperative and postoperative radiation therapy in patients with rectal cancer who had surgery with curative intent.

The clinical benefits of radiotherapy in the treatment of rectal cancer can be broadly divided under four categories: first, radiotherapy lowers local failure rates and improves survival in resectable rectal cancer; second, radiotherapy allows surgery in nonresectable rectal cancer; third, it facilitates sphincter-preserving procedures in low-lying rectal cancer; and finally, it may offer a totally curative approach without major surgery.

Radiotherapy can either be used alone or in combination with chemotherapy. The numerous combinations and variations in radiotherapy and chemotherapy regimens make the evaluation and comparison of different multimodal therapy pathways difficult. In this section, we will review the results of various adjuvant treatment modalities in rectal cancer focusing on areas of clinical benefit. We will not discuss the role of curative radiation alone.

Benefit No. 1: Radiotherapy Lowers the Local Failure Rates and Improves Survival in Resectable Rectal Cancer

According to three recently published metaanalyses, there is no doubt that neoadjuvant treatment is superior to adjuvant treatment with regard to reduction in local failure rates and cancer-specific survival.[32–34] The results of two of three other trials that specifically studied preoperative versus postoperative radiotherapy support the conclusions from the metaanalyses. The first report was the Uppsala trial in which short-course preoperative radiotherapy in all patients was compared with postoperative prolonged course only in patients with advanced cancers (Stages II and III).[35] The other two trials compared neoadjuvant chemoradiotherapy with adjuvant chemoradiotherapy with the same schedules and doses. The results from the NSABP R-03 trial, which closed prematurely because of poor accrual, showed that 44% of patients having undergone preoperative chemoradiation were disease free at 1 year, compared with 34% of patients who had received postoperative chemoradiation.[36] The German CAO/ARO/AIO trial has randomized patients with T3-4, N0, or any T,N1 rectal cancer to neoadjuvant chemoradiation followed by surgery and additional postoperative chemotherapy or postoperative chemoradiation.[37] In this study, surgery was performed according to the principles of sharp mesorectal excision. The rates of complete resection (R0) and sphincter-saving surgery were similar in both groups, but the 5-year cumulative rate of local relapse was 6% for patients assigned to preoperative chemoradiation and 13% for the postoperative chemoradiation group. Survival was similar in both treatment arms. Grade 3 or 4 toxicity occurred in 27% of patients in the preoperative chemoradiation group and 40% of patients in the postoperative chemoradiation group. The results of this last study suggest that preoperative chemoradiation is the preferred adjuvant treatment in patients with locally advanced rectal cancer.

Neoadjuvant Therapy: Radiation Alone Versus Chemoradiation

The potential advantages of neoadjuvant therapy include increased tumor radiosensitivity with decreased small bowel toxicity, decreased overall radiation-associated complications, and decreased risk of tumor seeding during surgery. The primary disadvantage of neoadjuvant therapy is the risk for overtreatment in patients with early-stage disease. New imaging modalities such as endorectal ultrasound[38] and magnetic resonance imaging[39] now allow for increasingly precise preoperative identification of patients with T2 and T3 tumors, thus minimizing the number of patients who would be overtreated by neoadjuvant therapy. Our ability to identify lymph node metastases preoperatively with any of these imaging modalities remains more limited.

A short course of preoperative radiation, 20–25 Gy given over 1 week is biologically equivalent to the traditional postoperative course of 45–55 Gy given over 5–6 weeks. It was long held that neoadjuvant radiation alone only improved local control but did not improve survival. In 1993, the randomized Swedish Rectal Cancer Trial (SRCT) demonstrated that a short course (25 Gy) of preoperative radiotherapy with surgery within the following week significantly reduced local recurrence from 27% to 12%, and improved 5-year survival rates from 48% to 58% when compared with surgery alone.[40] The main objection to all trials showing improvement in local recurrence and survival rates with radiotherapy, including the SRCT, was the high rate of local recurrence in the control arm that has been attributed to nonstandardized surgical technique.[32–34] Case series from specialized centers have reported lower local recurrence rates with surgery alone using meticulous surgical technique compared with patients treated with radiation and surgery in prospective trials when surgery was not standardized.[41–43] Several reports from different countries have confirmed that surgical skill is of utmost importance, thus opening for discussion the real role of radiotherapy when surgical technique is optimized.[44–47]

The role of preoperative radiation in patients with rectal cancer treated with optimal surgery was addressed in the Dutch Rectal Cancer Trial. All participating surgeons had adopted the technical "gold standard" of total mesorectal excision (TME) before entering patients. In this randomized, multicenter study of 1861 patients with rectal cancer, 2-year local recurrence rates were significantly improved from 8.2% to 2.4% when preoperative radiation was given before TME.[48] Five-year figures confirm a reduction in local recurrence rates from 11.4% after TME alone versus 5.6% for preoperative radiotherapy followed by TME but this does not translate into an improvement in 5-year survival rates (van de Velde, personal communication). Thus, it seems that neoadjuvant radiotherapy still has a place in the treatment of rectal cancer, even when surgical technique is optimized.

The advisability of adding chemotherapy to preoperative radiation (and therefore to use neoadjuvant combined chemoradiotherapy) is undergoing intense scrutiny. Additional 5-FU-based chemotherapy may theoretically act as a radiosensitizer at the high cost of increased hematologic and gastrointestinal toxicity. Neoadjuvant chemoradiotherapy is recommended for advanced disease (T4, N0-2), but there is no randomized phase III study comparing neoadjuvant radiotherapy versus neoadjuvant chemoradiotherapy in resectable rectal cancer (T2-3, N0-2). Only one study is currently underway to examine this issue. In the EORTC 22921 trial, patients with T3, T4 NX rectal cancer are randomized to one of four treatment arms: preoperative radiotherapy followed by surgery only; preoperative radiotherapy followed by surgery and postoperative adjuvant chemotherapy; neoadjuvant chemoradiation followed by surgery only; and neoadjuvant chemoradiation followed by surgery and additional adjuvant chemotherapy.[49] The trial was closed in 2003 after enrolling 1100 patients. A preliminary analysis of acute toxicity has demonstrated that at the dose recommended in the trial, the addition of chemotherapy during the radiation increased the proportion of patients developing grade 2 diarrhea from 17% to 34%. However, compliance with the adjuvant therapy and the proportion of patients undergoing surgery did not change. The oncologic results of this trial have not yet been published.

Postoperative Adjuvant Therapy: Radiation Alone Versus Chemoradiation

The advantage of reserving adjuvant treatment for the postoperative setting is the ability to restrict its use to patients who are at identified risk for failure, based on their histopathologic staging. In the German CAO/ARO/AIO trial, 18% of patients diagnosed with Stage II or III rectal cancer based on endorectal ultrasound had pathologic Stage I disease and were probably overtreated. The disadvantages include the higher incidence of radiation-related complications, particularly small bowel radiation injury and a higher number of patients unable to complete the entire course of therapy because of treatment side effects. Other reasons are the relative radioresistance of the hypoxic surgical bed and the risk for repopulation of tumor cells from surgery to the start of radiotherapy.

Postoperative adjuvant radiation therapy alone decreases local recurrence, although not to the same extent as neoadjuvant treatment, and does not improve survival.[50–52] Several early studies revealed that the addition of 5-FU-based chemotherapy to postoperative radiotherapy increased local control (Mayo Clinic/NCCTG 79-47-51[53]) and significantly improved survival by 10%–15% (Gastrointestinal Tumor Study Group[54] and Mayo/NCCTG[53]). Despite the fact that all those trials were heavily underpowered, these findings prompted the National Cancer Institute Consensus Conference of 1990 to recommend combined modality chemoradiotherapy as the standard postoperative adjuvant treatment for patients with Stage II and Stage III rectal cancer.[55] Although a recently published Norwegian trial confirmed[56] these findings, many countries, especially in Europe, did not follow those recommendations mainly because by then neoadjuvant radiotherapy had been proven to be more efficacious.

Benefit No. 2: Radiotherapy Allows Surgery in Nonresectable Rectal Cancer

The definition of a nonresectable rectal cancer is controversial. These tumors are clinically tethered or fixed but it is often difficult to predict whether fixation is the result of fibrotic adhesions or tumor infiltration of the pelvic sidewalls or adjacent organs.[57] Such tumors probably involve the fascia propria of the rectum, and a standard surgical resection following the principles of sharp mesorectal excision often results in tumor involvement of the circumferential resection margin. For the purpose of this section, we will define a nonresectable rectal cancer as a tumor that cannot be resected without a very high risk of local recurrence. Magnetic resonance imaging is particularly useful to determine the relationship of the tumor with the fascia propria of the rectum, and it may be the best imaging modality for the preoperative staging of patients with fixed tumors. Based on available data, patients with such locally advanced rectal cancer tumors benefit from preoperative radiotherapy with the aim of downsizing the tumor. Approximately 10%–15% of all patients with rectal cancer fall into this category; half of those patients have no metastases, indicating that there is potential for a curative procedure.[26] Based on tumor characteristics, surgery alone is unlikely to be curative and it is indicated to offer radiotherapy to those patients.

It must be emphasized that short-course radiotherapy is not an option in unresectable rectal cancer; a standard dose of 45–55 Gy over 5–6 weeks must always be given.

Radiotherapy is used to downsize tumors in this group of patients. After completion of standard-dose radiotherapy, a 6- to 8-week waiting period allows the tumor to shrink, increasing the possibility for a curative procedure.

The role of additional chemotherapy remains unclear in this context. There is very little solid evidence from randomized trials using chemoradiotherapy. One old trial (1969) reported positive results from chemoradiotherapy in locally unresectable rectal cancer.[58] Two other negative trials, published in the late 1980s, reported increased toxicity.[59,60] One underpowered Swedish trial (2001) showed improved local recurrence rate and overall survival in patients randomized to chemoradiotherapy versus radiotherapy alone followed by surgery.[61] Several phase II trials have reported a reduction in local recurrence rates and impressive data regarding survival[62,63]; problems with interpretation of case-mix and definition of "nonresectability" make the results of those trials difficult to interpret. The LARCS Nordic trial, which randomized patients with unresectable rectal cancer to receiving either 50 Gy preoperatively or 50 Gy and chemotherapy preoperatively just closed and will help to shed some light on this question.

At this time, there is no good evidence supporting the use of chemotherapy in addition to radiotherapy for unresectable rectal cancer. Despite the lack of data and scientific evidence, most radiotherapists and medical oncologists have more or less accepted the concept of using chemoradiotherapy for nonresectable rectal cancer patients. It is likely that the trend will continue, until ongoing trials answer that question. The newer chemotherapeutic agents currently in use or under study for treatment of locally advanced and metastatic colon cancer (e.g., irinotecan, capecitabine, and oxaliplatin) will doubtless be evaluated for their usefulness in neoadjuvant and adjuvant treatment of rectal cancer in the near future. Their efficacy and usefulness is unknown at this time.[64]

Benefit No. 3: Radiotherapy Facilitates Sphincter-preserving Procedures in Low-lying Rectal Cancer

Several series claim that preoperative radiotherapy (and preferably chemoradiotherapy) downsizes tumors to the extent that it is possible to increase the number of patients in whom the sphincters can be preserved.[65–69] There is even a report showing complete response to chemoradiotherapy in some patients with T4 tumors; some of these patients were not operated on and reportedly remain alive and well.[70] Caution must be exercised when reading these studies. First, rates of sphincter preservation do not tell the entire story; second, the main criticism of these studies is that modern therapies are compared with historical controls. The dramatic recent changes in surgical technique (TME, staplers) and the modern approach to rectal cancer treatment may partially explain the increased rate of sphincter preservation. We now accept a 5- to 10-mm distal margin as curative procedure if a stapled anastomosis is done.[71,72] Modern randomized trials must be done to verify the sturdiness of the conclusions. In the French R9001 trial, patients with T2 and T3 tumors received preoperative 39 Gy (13 × 3 Gy) and were randomized to immediate surgery or surgery 5 weeks after irradiation. Surgeons were asked before any treatment to evaluate the possibility to preserve the sphincters. Delaying surgery for 5 weeks after the end of radiation only slightly increased the rate of sphincter preservation.[73] This small trial indicates that there might be a downstaging and downsizing effect, which in turn might increase the rate of sphincter preservation. Of note, the overall recurrence rate in the trial was 9%, which is considered a high figure; more crucially, the local recurrence rate was 12% among the patients in whom the surgeon had originally planned an abdominoperineal excision but changed intraoperatively to a sphincter-preserving procedure because of the downsizing effect of radiotherapy.[73]

The German trial (CAO/ARO/AIO trial), in which patients were randomized to pre- or postoperative chemoradiotherapy, has shown a clear tendency to more favorable stage in patients having had preoperative treatment compared with postoperative chemoradiotherapy. In a subgroup analysis of patients determined by the surgeon before randomization to require an abdominoperineal resection, the proportion of sphincter preservation rate was 39% in the preoperative chemoradiation group and 18% in the postoperative chemoradiotherapy group.

In a recent Polish study, more than 300 patients were randomized to either short-course radiotherapy (25 Gy) with immediate surgery or long-course chemoradiotherapy and delayed surgery. T3 or resectable T4 tumors located within the reach of the examining finger, without evidence of sphincter involvement, and resectable with a 1-cm macroscopic distal margin were included in the study. Sphincter preservation and local recurrence rates were analyzed. Sphincter preservation rates were identical in both groups (61% in the short-course radiotherapy with immediate surgery versus 59% in the prolonged chemoradiotherapy course and delayed surgery).[74] This trial was conducted to determine whether chemoradiotherapy and delayed surgery had an impact on sphincter preservation. Accordingly, this is not a subset analysis of the data from the trial, indicating the strength of the results. At this time, there is no evidence that prolonged-course radiotherapy combined with chemotherapy with delayed surgery impacts sphincter preservation. It is possible that increasing the waiting time from end of radiotherapy to surgery will achieve further downsizing, which might improve sphincter preservation.

An important consequence of increased sphincter preservation is poor function. Poor quality of life may be the price to pay for intact sphincters: up to 20% of all patients who undergo a low anterior resection are incontinent of solid stool.[68] This contrasts with reports that patients with a stoma had a better quality of life compared with those with an anterior resection.[75] This must be considered when selecting surgical options for individual patients.

Adjuvant Chemotherapy Alone in Rectal Cancer

In contrast to colon cancer, chemotherapy alone as adjuvant treatment in rectal cancer remains questionable. In the early 1980s, underpowered United States radiotherapy trials concluded that chemotherapy improved survival compared with surgery alone. Two large randomized trials comprising more than 4000 patients have studied the value of chemotherapy versus surgery alone in colon and rectal cancer patients. Combination 5-FU/levamisole and 5-FU/LV were found to improve survival in patients with colon cancer, but showed no benefit in patients with rectal cancer.[76,77] These results underscore the difference in chemotherapy effectiveness for rectal cancer and colon cancer. The reasons for this are unclear:

different tumor profiles or lack of proper surgical technique at the time of these trials may partly explain the results. At this time, adjuvant chemotherapy alone is not acceptable in rectal cancer. However, postoperative chemotherapy is currently used to reduce the risk of distant relapse in patients with rectal cancer treated with pre- or postoperative chemoradiation and radical surgery.

References

1. Jemal A, Thomas A, Murray T, et al. Cancer statistics, 2002. CA Cancer J Clin 2002;52:23–47.
2. National Comprehensive Cancer Network. Clinical practice guidelines in oncology. JNCCN 2003;1:40–53.
3. Wolmark N, Fisher B, Rockette H, et al. Postoperative adjuvant chemotherapy or BCG for colon cancer: results from the NSABP protocol C-01. J Natl Cancer Inst 1988;80:30–36.
4. Laurie JA, Moertel CG, Fleming TR, et al. Surgical adjuvant therapy of large bowel carcinoma: an evaluation of levamisole and the combination of levamisole and fluorouracil. The North Central Cancer Treatment Group and the Mayo Clinic. J Clin Oncol 1989;7:1447–1456.
5. Moertel CG, Fleming TR, Macdonald JS, et al. Levamisole and 5-fluorouracil for adjuvant therapy of resected colon cancer. N Engl J Med 1990;322:352–358.
6. NIH Consensus Conference. Adjuvant therapy for patients with colon and rectal cancer. JAMA 1990;264:1444–1450.
7. Taal BG, Van Tinteren H, Zoetmulder FA, et al. Adjuvant 5-FU plus levamisole in colonic or rectal cancer: improved survival in stage II or III. Br J Cancer 2001;85:1437–1443.
8. International Multicentre Pooled Analysis of Colon Cancer Trials (IMPACT) investigators: efficacy of adjuvant fluorouracil and folinic acid in colon cancer. Lancet 1995;345:939–944.
9. Wolmark N, Rockette H, Fisher B, et al. The benefit of leucovorin-modulated fluorouracil as postoperative adjuvant therapy for primary colon cancer. Results form National Surgical Adjuvant Breast and Bowel Project protocol CO-3. J Clin Oncol 1993;11:1879–1887.
10. O'Connell MJ, Laurie JA, Kahn M, et al. Prospectively randomized trial of postoperative adjuvant chemotherapy in patients with high-risk colon cancer. J Clin Oncol 1998;16:295–300.
11. Haller DG, Catalano PJ, MacDonald JS, et al. Fluorouracil (FU), leucovorin (LV) and levamisole (LEV) adjuvant therapy for colon cancer: five-year final report of INT-0089 [abstract]. Proc Am Soc Clin Oncol 1998;17:256.
12. Wolmark N, Rockette H, Mamounas E, et al. Clinical trial to assess the relative efficacy of fluorouracil and leucovorin, fluorouracil and levamisole, and fluorouracil, leucovorin and levamisole in patients with Dukes' B and C carcinoma of the colon: results from National Surgical Adjuvant Breast and Bowel Project CO-4. J Clin Oncol 1999;17:3553–3559.
13. QUASAR Collaborative Group: comparison of fluorouracil with additional levamisole, higher dose leucovorin or both as adjuvant chemotherapy for colorectal cancer—a randomized trial. Lancet 2000;355:1588–1596.
14. Topham C, Boni C, Navarro M, et al. Multicenter international randomized study of oxaliplatin/5FU/LV (FOLFOX) in stage II and III colon cancer (MOSAIC trial): final results. Eur J Cancer 2003;1(suppl 5):S324–325. Abstr 1085.

15. Fallik D, Borrini F, Boige V, et al. Microsatellite instability is a predictive factor of the tumor response to irinotecan in patients with advanced colorectal cancer. Cancer Res 2003;15:5738–5744.
16. Barratt PL, Seymour MT, Stenning SP, et al. DNA markers predicting benefit from adjuvant fluorouracil in patients with colorectal cancer: a molecular study. Lancet 2002;360:1381–1391.
17. International Multicentre Pooled Analysis of B2 Colon Cancer Trials (IMPACT B2) investigators: efficacy of adjuvant fluorouracil and folinic acid in B2 colon cancer. J Clin Oncol 1999;17:1356–1363.
18. Schrag D, Gelfand S, Bach P, et al Adjuvant chemotherapy for stage II colon cancer: insight from a SEER-Medicare cohort [abstract]. Proc Am Soc Clin Oncol 2001;20:488.
19. Mamounas E, Wieand S, Wolmark N, et al. Comparative efficacy of adjuvant chemotherapy in patients with Dukes' B versus Dukes' C colon cancer: results from four National Surgical Adjuvant Breast and Bowel Projects adjuvant studies (CO-1, CO-2, CO-3 and CO-4). J Clin Oncol 1999;17:1349–1355.
20. Buyse M, Piedbois P. Should Dukes' B patients receive adjuvant therapy? A statistical perspective. Semin Oncol 2001;28 (suppl 1):20–24.
21. Krook JE, Moertel CG, Gunderson LL, et al. Effective surgical adjuvant therapy for high-risk rectal carcinoma. N Engl J Med 1991;324:709–715.
22. Willett CG, Tepper JE, Cohen A, et al. Local failure following curative resection of colonic adenocarcinoma. Int J Radiat Oncol Biol Phys 1984;10:645–651.
23. Gunderson LL, Sosin H, Levitt S. Extrapelvic colon-areas of failure in a reoperation series: implications for adjuvant therapy. Int J Radiat Oncol Biol Phys 1985;11:731–741.
24. Willett CG, Fung CY, Kaufman DS, et al. Postoperative radiation therapy for high-risk colon carcinoma. J Clin Oncol 1993;11:1112–1117.
25. Schild SE, Gunderson LL, Haddock MG, et al. The treatment of locally advanced colon cancer. Int J Radiat Oncol Biol Phys 1997;37:51–58.
26. Amos EH, Mendenhall WM, McCarty PJ, et al. Postoperative radiotherapy for locally advanced colon cancer. Ann Surg Oncol 1996;3:431–436.
27. Martenson J, Willett CG, Sargent D, et al. A phase III study of adjuvant radiation therapy (RT), 5-fluorouracil (5-FU), and levamisole (LEV) vs. 5-FU and LEV in selected patients with resected, high-risk colon cancer: initial results of INT 0130 [abstract]. Proc Am Soc Clin Oncol 1999;18:235.
28. Hanna MG Jr, Hoover HC Jr, Vermoken JB, et al. Adjuvant active specific immunotherapy of stage II and stage III colon cancer with autologous tumor cell vaccine: First randomized phase III trials show promise. Vaccine 2001;19:2576–2582.
29. Hoover HC Jr, Brandhorst JS, Peters LC, et al. Adjuvant active specific immunotherapy for human colorectal cancer: 6.5 year median follow-up of a phase III prospectively randomized trial. J Clin Oncol 1993;11:390–399.
30. Harris JE, Ryan L, Hoover HC Jr, et al. Adjuvant active specific immunotherapy for stage II and II colon cancer autologous tumor cell vaccine: Eastern Cooperative Oncology Group Study E5238. J Clin Oncol 2000;18:148–157.
31. Vermoken JB, Claessen AM, Van Tinteren H, et al. Active specific immunotherapy for stage II and stage III human colon cancer: a randomized trial. Lancet 1999;353:345–350.

32. Camma C, Giunta M, Fiorica F, et al. Preoperative radiotherapy for resectable rectal cancer: a meta-analysis. JAMA 2000;284:1008–1015.

33. Colorectal Cancer Collaborative Group. Adjuvant radiotherapy for rectal cancer: a systematic overview of 8,507 patients from 22 randomised trials. Lancet 2001;358:1291–304.

34. Glimelius B, Grönberg H, Järhult J, Wallgren A, Cavallin-Ståhl E. A systematic overview of radiation therapy in rectal cancer. Acta Oncol 2003;42:476–492.

35. Påhlman L, Glimelius B. Pre- or postoperative radiotherapy in rectal and rectosigmoid carcinoma: report from a randomized multicentre trial. Ann Surg 1990;211:187–195.

36. Roh MS, Petrilli N, Wieand H, et al. Phase III randomized trial of preoperative versus postoperative multimodality therapy in patients with carcinoma of the rectum (NSABP R-03) [abstract]. Proc Am Soc Clin Oncol 2001;20:123a.

37. Sauer R, Fietkau R, Wittekind C, et al. Adjuvant versus neoadjuvant radiochemotherapy for locally advanced rectal cancer. Strahlenther Onkol 2001;177:173–181.

38. Garcia-Aguilar J, Pollack J, Lee SH, et al. Accuracy of endorectal ultrasonography in preoperative staging of rectal tumors. Dis Colon Rectum 2002;45:10–15.

39. Beets-Tan RGH, Beets GL, Vliegen RFA, et al. Accuracy of magnetic resonance imaging in prediction of tumour-free resection margin in rectal cancer surgery. Lancet 2001;357:497–504.

40. Swedish Rectal Cancer Trial: initial report from a Swedish multicentre study examining the role of preoperative irradiation in the treatment of patients with resectable rectal carcinoma. Br J Surg 1993;80:1333–1336.

41. Heald RJ, Karanjia ND. Results of radical surgery for rectal cancer. World J Surg 1992;16:848–857.

42. Enker WE. Potency, cure, and local control in the operative treatment of rectal cancer. Arch Surg 1992;127:1396–1401.

43. Moriya Y, Hojo K, Sawada T, Koyama Y. Significance of lateral node dissection for advanced rectal carcinoma at or below the peritoneal reflection. Dis Colon Rectum 1989;32:307–315.

44. Wibe A, Rendedal PR, Svensson E, et al. Prognostic significance of the circumferential resection margin following total mesorectal excision for rectal cancer. Br J Surg 2002;89:327.

45. Dahlberg M, Glimelius B, Påhlman L. Changing strategy for rectal cancer is associated with improved outcome. Br J Surg 1999;86:379–84.

46. Martling AL, Holm T, et al. Effect of a surgical training programme on the outcome of rectal cancer in the County of Stockholm. Lancet 2000;356:93–96.

47. Swedish Rectal Cancer Register. Available at: http://www.SOS.se/mars/kvaflik.htm (Swe).

48. Kapiteijn E, Matijnen CA, Naggtegaal ID, et al. Preoperative radiotherapy combined with total mesorectal excision for resectable rectal cancer. N Engl J Med 2001;345:638–646.

49. Bosset JF, Pierat M, Van Glabbeke M. Preoperative radiochemotherapy versus preoperative radiotherapy with or without postoperative chemotherapy: progress report of the EORTC 22921 trial [abstract]. Radiother Oncol 2000;56:S52.

50. Fisher B, Wolmark N, Rockette H, et al. Postoperative adjuvant chemotherapy or radiation therapy for rectal cancer. Results from NSABP protocol R-01. J Natl Cancer Inst 1988;80:21–29.

51. Wolmark N, Weiand HS, Hyams DM, et al. Randomized trial of postoperative adjuvant chemotherapy with or without radiotherapy for carcinoma of the rectum: National Surgical Adjuvant Breast and Bowel Project protocol R-02. J Natl Cancer Inst 2000;92:388–396.

52. Willett CG, Tepper JE, Kaufman DS, et al. Adjuvant postoperative radiation therapy for rectal adenocarcinoma. Am J Clin Oncol 1992;15:371–375.

53. Krook JE, Moertel CG, Gunderson LL, et al. Effective surgical adjuvant therapy for high-risk rectal carcinoma. N Engl J Med 1991;324:709–715.

54. Gastrointestinal Tumor Study Group. Adjuvant therapy of colon cancer: results of a prospective randomized trial. N Engl J Med 1984;310:737–743.

55. National Institutes of Health Consensus Conference: adjuvant therapy for patients with colon and rectal cancer. JAMA 1990;264:1444–1450.

56. Tveit KM, Guldvog I, Hagen S, et al. Randomised controlled trial of postoperative radiotherapy and short-term time-scheduled 5-fluorouracil against surgery alone in the treatment of Dukes B and C rectal cancer. Br J Surg 1997;84:1130–1135.

57. Påhlman L, Enblad P, Glimelius B. Clinical characteristics and their relation to surgical curability in adenocarcinoma of the rectum and recto-sigmoid: a population-based study in 279 consecutive patients. Acta Chir Scand 1985;151:685–693.

58. Moertel CG, Childs DS, Reitemeier RJ, et al. Combined 5-fluorouracil and supervoltage radiation therapy of locally unresectable gastrointestinal carcinoma. Lancet 1969;2:865–867.

59. Overgaard M, Berthelsen K, Dahlmark M, et al. A randomized trial of radiotherapy alone or combined with 5-FU in the treatment of locally advanced colorectal carcinoma. ECCO 5, meeting abstract 1989:0-0626.

60. Wassif-Boulis S. The role of preoperative adjuvant therapy in management of borderline operability of rectal cancer. Clin Radiol 1982;33:353–358.

61. Frykholm GJ, Pahlman L, Glimelius B. Combined chemo and radiotherapy versus radiotherapy alone in the treatment of primary, non-resectable adenocarcinoma of the rectum. Int J Radiat Oncol Biol Phys 2001;50:433–440.

62. Janjan NA, Abbruzzese J, Pazdur R, et al. Prognostic implications of response to preoperative infusional chemoradiation in locally advanced rectal cancer. Radiother Oncol 1999;51:153–160.

63. Bouzourene H, Bosman FT, Seelentag W, Matter M, Coucke P. Importance of tumor regression assessment in predicting the outcome in patients with locally advanced rectal carcinoma who are treated with preoperative radiotherapy. Cancer 2002;94:1121–1130.

64. Glynne-Jones R, Sebag-Montefiore D. Chemoradiation schedules—what radiotherapy? Eur J Cancer 2002;38:258–269.

65. Valentini V, Coco C, Cellini N, et al. Preoperative chemoradiation with cisplatin and 5-fluorouracil for extraperitoneal T3 rectal cancer: acute toxicity tumor response, sphincter preservation. Int J Radiat Oncol Biol Phys 1999;45:1175–1184.

66. Grann A, Minsky BD, Cohen AM, et al. Preliminary results of preoperative 5-fluorouracil, low-dose leucovorin and concurrent radiation therapy for clinically respectable T3 rectal cancer. Dis Colon Rectum 1997;40:515–522.

67. Hyams DM, Mamounas EP, Petrelli N, et al. A clinical trial to evaluate the worth of preoperative multimodality therapy in patients with operable carcinoma of the rectum: a progress report of National Surgical Breast and Bowel Project Protocol R-03. Dis Colon Rectum 1997;40:131–139.

68. Rouanet P, Saint-Aubert B, Lemanski C, et al. Restorative and nonrestorative surgery for low rectal cancer after high-dose radiation. Dis Colon Rectum 2002;45:305–315.

69. Mohiuddin M, Regine WF, Marks GJ, Marks JW. High dose preoperative radiation and the challenge of sphincter-preservation surgery for rectal cancer of the distal 2 cm of the rectum. Int J Radiat Oncol Biol Phys 1998;40:569–574.

70. Habr-Gama A, de Souza PM, Ribeiro U, et al. Low rectal cancer: impact of radiation and chemotherapy on surgical treatment. Dis Colon Rectum 1998;41:1087–1096.

71. Moore HG, Riedel E, Minsky BD, et al. Adequacy of 1 cm distal margin after restorative rectal cancer resection with sharp mesorectal excision and preoperative combined-modality therapy. Ann Surg Oncol 2003;1:80–85.

72. Karnjia ND, Schache DJ, Nort WR, Heald RJ. 'Close shave' in anterior resection. Br J Surg 1990;63:673–677.

73. Francois Y, Nemoz CJ, Baulieux J, et al. Influence of the interval between preoperative radiation therapy and surgery on downstaging and on the rate of sphincter-sparing surgery for rectal cancer: the Lyon R90-01 randomized trial. J Clin Oncol 1999; 17:2396–2402.

74. Bujko K, Nowacki MP, Bebenek M, et al. Sphincter preservation following preoperative radiotherapy for rectal cancer: report of a randomised trial comparing short-term radiotherapy versus conventionally fractionated radiochemotherapy. Radiother Oncol 2004;72(1):15–24.

75. Frigell A, Ottander M, Stenbeck H, Påhlman L. Quality of life of patients treated with abdominoperineal resection or anterior resection for rectal carcinoma. Ann Chir Gynaecol 1990;79: 26–30.

76. Taal BG, Van Tinteren H, Zoetmulder FA, et al. Adjuvant 5-FU plus levamisole in colonic or rectal cancer: improved survival in stage II or III. Br J Cancer 2001;85:1437–1443.

77. Glimelius B, Cedermark B, Dahl O, et al. Adjuvant chemotherapy in colorectal cancer: joint analyses of randomised trials by the Nordic Gastrointestinal Tumour Adjuvant Therapy Group. Eur J Cancer, ECCO 12, abstract-book 2003;39(suppl 1):S318. Abstr 1066.

32
Colorectal Cancer Surveillance

Brett T. Gemlo and David A. Rothenberger

The majority of colorectal cancers are resected for cure, leaving many patients eligible for ongoing surveillance. The best schema for clinically useful and cost-effective follow-up is still controversial, but the goals are clear. Rational follow-up should detect treatable recurrent cancers, identify and remove metachronous polyps, and identify possible hereditary influences in development of a colorectal cancer. In theory, such follow-up will increase the survival of patients with cancer and improve their quality of life by successfully treating recurrences, preventing metachronous cancers of the colon or rectum, as well as preventing subsequent hereditary cancers from developing in the patient and/or their family members. How to accomplish this is still controversial, but it is clear that accurate risk stratification and patient selection are central to any program of surveillance. The intensity of surveillance should be proportional to the patient's risk of recurrence, and those patients unfit for further surgery because of age or comorbidity may be best served by colonoscopic follow-up only.

Types of Surveillance

Metachronous Colorectal Neoplasms

Those patients who have undergone successful treatment of a colorectal malignancy have an increased risk of developing subsequent polyps or cancers compared with the rate at which an age-matched control population would develop their first colorectal neoplasm. The period of risk for the development of metachronous disease seems to be lifelong and cumulative. The risk of developing metachronous polyps ranges between 30% and 56%, and the risk of a second cancer is 2%–8%.[1–3] Because these cancers arise from adenomatous polyps, periodic colonoscopy with polypectomy should prevent the development of subsequent cancers. The starting point and appropriate interval for surveillance colonoscopy in the population of patients undergoing follow-up for colorectal cancer are controversial and poorly studied. In the past, most clinicians advocated colonoscopic follow-up 1 year after surgery to visualize the anastomosis and look for missed synchronous lesions. Recently, the utility of early follow-up colonoscopy 1 year after surgery compared with delaying colonoscopy until 3 years after surgery has been questioned. The Standards Task Force of the American Society of Colon and Rectal Surgeons (ASCRS) has recommended colonoscopy surveillance to begin 3 years after surgery assuming preoperative or intraoperative clearance was done and was negative.[4] If preoperative or intraoperative clearance examination could not be done, postoperative colonoscopy within 6 months of surgery is recommended. If multiple synchronous polyps are identified, during the clearance examination, it may be reasonable to do the first surveillance examination at 1 year. Otherwise, posttreatment colonoscopy should be performed at 3-year intervals. Follow-up surveillance colonoscopy every 3 years can be continued for the duration of an individual's active life. It is also acceptable to extend follow-up colonoscopy to every 5 years after a negative colonoscopy at 3 years. Once the patient is older than age 80, further examinations may be of limited usefulness although exceptions can be made for individuals who are healthy and active despite their advanced age.

Recurrent Cancer

The term "recurrent cancer" is a misnomer because the cancer does not disappear and then return. It simply progresses in sites not clinically detectable at the time of the original surgery. Locoregional recurrences are more common in cases of rectal cancer, and may represent inadequate tumor clearance at the time of surgery. Distant disease, typically in the liver or lungs, usually does not cause symptoms until the situation is quite advanced. Options for the detection of asymptomatic recurrences include physical examination, carcinoembryonic antigen (CEA) monitoring, colonoscopy, chest X-ray, (CXR), and various scans. In this high technology era, careful attention to new symptoms such as abdominal pain, change in bowel habits, weight loss, or anorexia is often lacking, but such symptoms are the first sign of recurrence in many cases. When present, a meticulous physical examination is conducted. This should include a digital rectal and vaginal examination for patients with rectal cancer. CEA testing is most useful in cases in which the level was increased preoperatively but decreased to normal levels after resection. Even in cases in which the preoperative CEA level is normal, serial CEA testing is often the first indication a patient has recurrent disease. Although CEA testing is controversial, the Standards Practice Task Force of the ASCRS recently recommended that CEA testing should be used as a part of follow-up for patients with colorectal cancer. This may be justified if its use is restricted to those who would tolerate reoperation if a recurrence were identified. Endoscopic follow-up is of limited usefulness in looking for recurrences because only 2% of recurrences are visible at colonoscopy. This is especially true for colonic anastomoses where recurrence is rare as compared with rectal anastomoses where mucosal recurrences are more likely to develop. Rigid proctoscopy is an alternative and, some suggest, superior way to assess a rectal anastomosis for recurrence. Patients with rectal cancer, especially those treated with transanal excision, should undergo endorectal ultrasound surveillance (usually every 3 months for the first year). There are currently insufficient data to recommend for or against routine use of CXR to identify an asymptomatic pulmonary metastasis. Its use should be restricted to patients who would tolerate a pulmonary resection. Computerized tomography (CT) and magnetic resonance imaging (MRI) scanning are very sensitive ways to detect liver and lung metastases, but are not recommended as a routine screening procedure. Positron emission tomography (PET) scanning may become the most sensitive way to detect recurrences, but although it is becoming more widely available, data supporting its use are still lacking. Although PET scanning is limited in its usefulness in detecting recurrence, it has been helpful in identifying patients with recurrence who have too many areas of distant recurrence to warrant operative therapy to remove the local, liver, or lung recurrence detected initially. Patients with isolated metastatic disease (fewer than eight liver metastases or 1 or 2 lobe lung involvement) may be candidates for operative treatment (see Chapter 34). As chemotherapy improves, operative therapy to resect residual disease may be more important to extract a cure.

Hereditary Cancer

Heredity is thought to be a major factor in 10%–25% of colorectal cancers. Patients who developed their cancer before age 50 years or who have first-degree relatives who developed colorectal or associated cancers such as endometrial, ovarian, ureteral, or bladder cancer or who have multiple family members with varying cancers especially if diagnosed before 50 years of age may have a hereditary cancer. Some inherited syndromes predispose the individual not only to development

of young-age-of-onset colorectal cancer but also other organ cancers. Thus, in addition to informing family members of their risks and need for intensive surveillance, the patient's follow-up plan may need to incorporate surveillance of other potential sites of cancer. Sometimes, genetic counseling and testing is useful and prophylactic surgery may be considered as in the case of hereditary nonpolyposis colon cancer syndrome.

Risk of Recurrence/Pattern of Recurrence

The risk of recurrence is proportional to the stage of the original disease. Most Stage IV patients have undergone palliative treatment and are not candidates for surveillance unless they were treated by operative removal of metastatic disease. Patients with Stage I colon cancer treated by radical surgery have such a low chance of recurrent disease that routine surveillance may not be justified. However, Stage I rectal cancer patients treated by local therapy are at significant risk of local recurrence and may deserve close follow-up. Patients with Stage II or III disease would seem to benefit most from close surveillance. Other tumor or surgery related factors such as degree of differentiation, presence of lymph node metastases, iatrogenic perforation, and poor primary tumor clearance, influence the risk of recurrence, and could be used to more accurately predict an individual patient's risk of recurrence, and guide the development of a specific follow-up program. To date, there is no standardized formula for doing this but an experienced clinician can individualize follow-up based on the risk of recurrence, the patient's overall health status, the patient's willingness to undergo serial testing and the ability for the patient to undergo aggressive retreatment if recurrence is identified.

The patterns of recurrence reflect the location of the primary tumor.[5] Rectal cancers tend to recur locally in the pelvis, but this tendency has diminished recently with improved mesorectal clearance techniques and the use of neoadjuvant chemoradiation. All colorectal cancers metastasize hematogenously to the liver and lungs as well as to regional lymphatics, and these areas need to be evaluated when looking for recurrent disease.

It is well established that 60%–80% of recurrences occur within 2 years of surgery, and more than 90% of recurrences are found within 5 years. Therefore, follow-up protocols should be most intensive for the first 2 years, and then taper off in frequency of evaluations over the next 3 years. The exception to this timing of recurrence is the patient who has had pelvic radiation. In such cases, recurrence tends to occur later so intensive surveillance may need to extend to 5 or 6 years. Subsequent to that, the risk of recurrence is so low that colonoscopic surveillance for metachronous cancers is all that is warranted. The development of symptoms at any time during follow-up should prompt a thorough diagnostic work-up and specific treatment.

Surveillance Effectiveness

The utility of a surveillance program should be manifest in an improvement in survival or quality of life when compared with patients who have received little or no follow-up. Several variables confound our ability to evaluate the advantages derived from intensive efforts to detect recurrent cancer before it becomes evident clinically. The first is the lead time bias that results from detecting asymptomatic recurrences. Early detection of such a recurrence for which no effective treatment can be offered will still result in a measured prolongation of survival from the time of diagnosis of the recurrence when compared with those patients treated for symptomatic recurrences because they were identified earlier. Even if the treatment provided does impart some benefit, the bias between groups persists.

The identification of recurrent disease does not necessarily result in improved outcomes. Only about 10% of recurrences are resectable with curative intent and chemotherapy offers little chance of cure. Those patients who are fortunate to have a lesion amenable to surgery are often not suitable surgical candidates as a result of age or comorbidity, and should not be subjected to intense follow-up because any information obtained cannot be acted upon. There is a subset of patients with resectable disease, who may benefit from radical re-resection, with 5-year survivals of 25%–30% in most series. PET scanning can assist in identifying this small group of individuals.[6]

The results of intensive follow-up programs reported in the literature have been disappointing. A recent review summarized the results of the six randomized, prospective trials of high-intensity versus low-intensity follow-up after surgical resection with curative intent for colorectal cancer.[7–13] Recurrences were not more common in the closely monitored group, but they were found earlier and were more likely to result in reoperation with curative intent. Despite this, only two of the six studies demonstrated a statistically significant improvement in overall survival as a result of intensive surveillance.

Because of the concern that inadequate sample size was in part responsible for the negative results encountered in the above studies, three separate metaanalyses have been conducted on these data.[6,14,15] Although this resulted in a more clearly discerned reduction in death from recurrent cancer, the reduction in absolute risk was only 7%.

Cost of Surveillance

Offsetting the survival benefits of an intensive surveillance program are the costs associated with such testing. Given the large number of patients involved, cost implications for Medicare and private insurers are significant. The heterogeneity of follow-up regimens results in 5-year Medicare-allowed charges of $910 to $26,717 per patient.[16] One of the above metaanalyses evaluated the cost-associated intensive follow-up in terms of cost per year of life gained and found it to be $6096.[17] Beart's hypothetical cost analysis of a program to closely follow Stage II and III patients resulted in a cost of $6558 per patient salvaged by resection.[18] Although these costs are significant, they seem to be below the accepted threshold of $30,000 per year of life gained.

Quality of Life

Intensive surveillance may have a negative impact on quality of life secondary to the anxiety, inconvenience, and cost associated with the testing. Conversely, intensive testing may be reassuring to patients and improve their quality of life. Investigators in Denmark found that although patients subjected to closer follow-up expressed greater confidence in their examinations, the increment in quality of life was marginal and did not justify the expense of follow-up.[19] Stiggelbout et al.[20] also showed no differences in health-related quality of life when different intervals of follow-up were studied but they did show patients had a strong preference for follow-up. Additional data are needed to determine methods and settings for follow-up that maximize both survival and the quality of life.

Recommendations

Recommendations for surveillance of patients who have undergone curative resection of colorectal cancer are as follows.

Virtually all patients can undergo follow-up studies that are focused on excluding hereditary cancer and on prevention of synchronous cancer by every 3- to 5-year surveillance colonoscopies to remove metachronous polyps. If hereditary cancer is likely, work-up appropriately and/or consider referral to experts in hereditary cancers. In addition to counseling the patient about their own risks for other sites of cancer development, the clinician must attempt to educate the patient's family members about their risks and surveillance or treatment options.

The search for treatable recurrent disease is more selective. It is helpful to first determine whether the patient has a significant risk of recurrence. If so, determine whether the patient prefers an aggressive approach to follow-up testing and whether the patient could tolerate retreatment if recurrence is identified. If there is a minimal risk of recurrence and/or the patient refuses or is not a candidate for aggressive follow-up, no additional testing is done. It is comforting for patients to know that should recurrence develop, you are available and palliative treatment can be instituted. Patients should still undergo routine colonoscopic surveillance every 5 years to detect metachronous polyps or cancer.

If there is a significant risk of recurrence and the patient wants aggressive follow-up and would tolerate retreatment, follow-up will include the search for recurrent disease. Typically this includes: history, physical examination, and serial testing as noted below every 3–6 months for the first 3 years, and then every 6–12 months for an additional 2 years. If pelvic radiation was used for rectal cancer, the closer interval of follow-up may need to be extended to 5 or 6 years. Careful attention to new symptoms and physical finding should be made.

Complete colonoscopy before resection, followed by an examination 1–3 years after surgery and every 3–5 years thereafter for the duration of the patient's productive life.

Serial CEA testing every 3 months for the first postoperative year or two and every 6–12 months thereafter for patients who desire an aggressive follow-up protocol and would tolerate aggressive retreatment for locoregional disease or hepatic or pulmonary metastasis.

Serial CXR every 6–12 months for patients who desire an aggressive follow-up protocol and would tolerate pulmonary resection.

Serial proctoscopy and selective endorectal ultrasound for rectal cancer patients who desire an aggressive follow-up protocol and would tolerate aggressive radical pelvic surgery with or without additional radiation and chemotherapy.

Based on the available evidence, there is no role for the routine use of liver function tests, hemoglobin, CT scanning, MRI, or PET scanning in asymptomatic patients.[4,7]

Future studies may more clearly define the role of these and other surveillance modalities.

References

1. Chen F, Stuart M. Colonoscopic follow-up of colorectal carcinoma. Dis Colon Rectum 1994;37(6):568–572.
2. Evers BM, et al. Multiple adenocarcinomas of the colon and rectum. An analysis of incidences and current trends. Dis Colon Rectum, 1988;31(7):518–522.
3. Reilly JC, Rusin LC, Theuerkauf FJ Jr. Colonoscopy: its role in cancer of the colon and rectum. Dis Colon Rectum 1982;25(6): 532–538.
4. Anthony T, et al. Practice parameters for the surveillance and follow-up of patients with colon and rectal cancer. Dis Colon Rectum 2004;47(6):807–817.
5. Kjeldsen BJ, et al. The pattern of recurrent colorectal cancer in a prospective randomised study and the characteristics of diagnostic tests. Int J Colorectal Dis 1997;12(6):329–334.
6. Jeffery GM, Hickey BE, Hider P. Follow-up strategies for patients treated for non-metastatic colorectal cancer. Cochrane Database Syst Rev 2002(1):CD002200.
7. Pfister DG, Benson AB 3rd, Somerfield MR. Clinical practice. Surveillance strategies after curative treatment of colorectal cancer. N Engl J Med 2004;350(23):2375–2382.
8. Pietra N, et al. Role of follow-up in management of local recurrences of colorectal cancer: a prospective, randomized study. Dis Colon Rectum 1998;41(9):1127–1133.
9. Schoemaker D, et al. Yearly colonoscopy, liver CT, and chest radiography do not influence 5-year survival of colorectal cancer patients. Gastroenterology 1998;114(1):7–14.
10. Ohlsson B, et al. Follow-up after curative surgery for colorectal carcinoma. Randomized comparison with no follow-up. Dis Colon Rectum 1995;38(6):619–626.
11. Secco GB, et al. Efficacy and cost of risk-adapted follow-up in patients after colorectal cancer surgery: a prospective, randomized and controlled trial. Eur J Surg Oncol 2002;28(4):418–423.
12. Kjeldsen BJ, et al. A prospective randomized study of follow-up after radical surgery for colorectal cancer. Br J Surg 1997;84(5):666–669.
13. Makela JT, Laitinen SO, Kairaluoma MI. Five-year follow-up after radical surgery for colorectal cancer. Results of a prospective randomized trial. Arch Surg 1995;130(10):1062–1067.
14. Figueredo A, et al. Follow-up of patients with curatively resected colorectal cancer: a practice guideline. BMC Cancer 2003;3(1):26.
15. Renehan AG, et al. Impact on survival of intensive follow up after curative resection for colorectal cancer: systematic review and meta-analysis of randomised trials. BMJ 2002;324(7341):813.
16. Virgo KS, et al. Cost of patient follow-up after potentially curative colorectal cancer treatment. JAMA 1995;273(23):1837–1841.
17. Renehan AG, O'Dwyer ST, Whynes DK. Cost effectiveness analysis of intensive versus conventional follow up after curative resection for colorectal cancer. BMJ 2004;328(7431):81.
18. Beart RW Jr. Follow-up: does it work? Can we afford it? Surg Oncol Clin North Am 2000;9(4):827–834; discussion 835–837.
19. Kjeldsen BJ, et al. Influence of follow-up on health-related quality of life after radical surgery for colorectal cancer. Scand J Gastroenterol 1999;34(5):509–515.
20. Stiggelbout AM, et al. Follow-up of colorectal cancer patients: quality of life and attitudes towards follow-up. Br J Cancer 1997;75(6):914–920.

33
Management of Locally Advanced and Recurrent Rectal Cancer

Robert R. Cima and Heidi Nelson

Of patients with newly diagnosed colorectal cancer who will undergo surgery with curative intent as part of their treatment, approximately 5%–12% will have tumors that have spread beyond the anatomic landmarks of a standard resection and have invaded adjacent organs or structures.[1–3] The goal of surgery in such cases is a wide, en bloc resection of the tumor and any involved adjacent organ or structure. Of patients who undergo resection with curative intent and receive adjuvant therapy, between 7% to 33% develop isolated local or regional recurrences.[4,5] In up to 20% of these recurrences, resection can be curative.[4,6,7]

Although tumor biology must influence the rate and location of recurrence, no tumor-specific characteristics have been clearly associated with local recurrence. The most important factor that influences tumor recurrence is the stage of disease at presentation.[8] Others include obstruction or perforation at presentation, adjacent organ involvement, tumor aneuploidy, increased tumor grade, mucin production, or evidence of venous or perineural invasion. Over the last decade, the adequacy of surgical resection and the use of preoperative chemoradiation have been shown to influence the rate of pelvic recurrence.[9–12] Detailed discussion of these aspects of rectal cancer treatment is addressed elsewhere in the textbook. The focus of this chapter is to discuss the evaluation, operative management, and multimodality treatment of patients with locally advanced rectal cancer. Because the preoperative evaluation, operative approach, and often the perioperative oncologic therapy are similar for primary locally advanced and recurrent rectal cancer, they will be discussed together. The outcomes for the different approaches are evaluated later in the chapter.

Locally advanced primary rectal cancers include tumors that are T4 N1-2 MX at the time of initial presentation. They are often associated with a higher rate of metastatic disease at the time of diagnosis and have a poorer overall prognosis than earlier-stage disease.[8] T4 tumors are found to be fixed by physical examination or to be invading adjacent organs or structures by diagnostic imaging studies. For T4 tumors,

standard surgery alone offers a limited chance of significant local tumor control and/or long-term survival. In cases in which an extended en bloc resection cannot be performed to achieve complete resection, patient survival is dismal: after no treatment or after palliative surgery, mean survival time is less than 1 year.[13]

Multimodality therapy incorporating radiation, chemotherapy, and surgery should be used to achieve local tumor control and to prevent or control systemic tumor dissemination, thereby improving patient survival for patients with locally advanced primary or recurrent colorectal cancers. To achieve these goals, appropriate surgery is combined with external-beam radiation therapy (EBRT), and, under ideal circumstances, intraoperative radiation therapy (IORT) and adjuvant or neoadjuvant chemotherapy.

Patients with isolated hepatic or pulmonary metastasis from a rectal cancer are known to have reasonable survival after surgical treatment; however, survival with an isolated, untreated, locoregional, rectal cancer recurrence is quite poor.[14,15] Most of these patients develop disabling complications, including severe pain from bony or nervous tissue involvement, urinary obstruction, fecal obstruction or incontinence, or persistent bleeding. Nearly 90% of rectal cancer recurrences after surgery alone occur in the central or posterior pelvis, and 19% occur at the anastomosis.[16] Stage T4 primary tumors are significantly associated with relapse in the anterior pelvic region.[16] EBRT alone or combined with systemic chemotherapy may result in temporary improvement of symptoms, but the 5-year survival rate is less than 5%.[14,15] Surgical palliation without the addition of systemic chemotherapy and radiation therapy adds little to the overall survival. For these patients, length of survival is perhaps less important than quality of life.

A patient who presents with a locally advanced primary or recurrent rectal cancer must be thoroughly evaluated for the presence of extrapelvic disease. If extensive extrapelvic disease is found, the degree and scope of surgical resection should be changed from one of curative intent to palliation.

An exception may be considered in younger patients with no significant comorbidities in whom a single, isolated, hepatic metastasis is found that could be surgically resected. However, if a patient has multiple sites of spread or significant comorbidities, extensive surgery involving multiple structures is not warranted, as the chance for cure is quite small. Whether a patient is a candidate for surgery is influenced by a number of factors, including the patient's overall physical condition and comorbid diseases and the extent of spread and fixation of the tumor outside of the rectum.

Preoperative Evaluation and Patient Selection

Complete resection of a locally advanced primary or recurrent rectal cancer is a significant undertaking. Complete resection may be technically possible in some patients, but if their overall physical condition does not make them an appropriate candidate, surgical palliation combined with chemoradiation is the more prudent course of action. To be considered for a complete resection, the patient should be in generally good health. Any significant cardiac or respiratory conditions should be thoroughly evaluated and treated. Patients who are in poor health, or who will not be able to tolerate multimodality therapy combined with complete surgical resection, or have an ASA classification of IV–V are not considered acceptable surgical candidates. Nearly as important as their physical condition is consideration of the patient's motivation and emotional preparedness for undergoing this extensive treatment. They should be thoroughly informed about and accepting of the short-term and long-term risks associated with the surgery, as well as possible subsequent surgeries or interventions required for postoperative complications.

If the patient is deemed an acceptable candidate for surgery, the next step is evaluation for the extent of local spread and the possibility of extrapelvic spread. A detailed history should be obtained. Symptoms that may suggest metastatic disease, such as back or bone pain outside of the pelvis, new respiratory symptoms, or headaches need to be carefully examined. A thorough physical examination, with particular attention placed on the rectal and vaginal examination, needs to be performed and any fixation of the tumor to rigid pelvic structures needs to assessed. Complete endoscopic evaluation of the colon needs to be performed, if technically possible, to rule out the presence of a synchronous lesion. Endoluminal ultrasound of the rectum may be combined with this evaluation in cases of recurrent disease to determine if there is a discrete mass adjacent to the intestine that might be amenable to endoscopic biopsy. Imaging should be repeated before surgery is considered and compared with similar previous studies to give some reassurance that there has been no progression or spread of the disease that might change or preclude any surgical intervention. The abdomen and pelvis need to be evaluated with a double contrast (intravenous and oral) computed tomography (CT) scan to exclude extrapelvic spread and to assess the extent of possible resection. CT scans are generally reliable for identifying the extent of disease and adjacent organ involvement but are less discriminating for predicting local tumor resectability.[17] Any suspicious hepatic lesion should be examined with ultrasound. If the lesion is worrisome for metastatic disease, it should be biopsied. Questionable findings on the chest X-ray film should be further investigated. Any worrisome lesion that is technically accessible should be biopsied percutaneously.

Although the above tests are the standard evaluation for diagnosing recurrence and excluding extrapelvic spread of the tumor, other, more tumor-specific tests have been proposed as adjuncts. Magnetic resonance imaging (MRI) might be more accurate than conventional CT scanning for detecting recurrences in the pelvis or elsewhere in the abdomen because of better image resolution. However, similar to CT scans, MRIs provide only anatomic details and may not be any better at distinguishing tumor recurrence from scar in a postoperative field, particularly after pelvic irradiation. To overcome this limitation, a metabolic-based imaging modality such as positron emission tomography (PET) has been studied.[18–22] Colorectal cancer is known to rapidly metabolize fluorine-18 fluorodeoxyglucose (FDG), which therefore can be used as a metabolic label to detect tumor deposits, not only in the pelvis, but throughout the entire body. Numerous nonrandomized studies have shown that FDG-PET imaging for recurrent colorectal cancer has a significantly higher sensitivity and specificity than CT scanning. When CT scanning was compared with FDG-PET imaging in postoperative patients with colorectal locoregional recurrences, the sensitivity of FDG-PET was significantly higher than CT plus colonoscopy (90% versus 71%, respectively), although the specificities were similar (92% versus 85%, respectively).[23] FDG-PET imaging has been shown to maintain this high sensitivity and specificity, 84% and 88%, respectively, even in the setting of the previously irradiated and postoperative pelvis.[18] Thus, FDG-PET might be a useful tool in the postoperative patient in whom there is a suspicion of recurrence but equivocal CT findings, and in whom extensive reoperative surgery might be extremely high risk.

Even the combination of physical examination and radiographic studies may not be able to prove that there is a pelvic recurrence of a rectal cancer, especially if the patient has undergone a previous pelvic operation or pelvic irradiation. We generally accept three ways of differentiating postoperative changes from tumor. The first is to document a change in the lesion, such as increase in size over time; the second is invasion of the adjacent organs; the third is histologic evidence obtained from endoscopic, CT- or ultrasound-guided biopsies of the suspicious tissue. However, occasionally pelvic disease is suspected from an increasing carcinoembryonic antigen or development of symptoms without any definable anatomic change on examination. In such situations, histologic proof should be vigorously sought. Exploratory pelvic surgery should be strongly discouraged because it poses an extreme risk to the patient and makes future evaluation of the pelvis even more difficult.

Determining Resectability

Locally advanced primary or locoregional recurrences of rectal cancers can extend to involve any of the pelvic organs or rigid bony structures of the pelvis. Resectability is based on the anatomic location and what other structures are fixed to the lesion. Although there are other schemes for assessing resectability, we use the following one to classify our patients who are being considered for possible resection. The tumor is classified as F0 when it is not fixed to any pelvic organ or structure, FR when the tumor is fixed but resectable, and FNR when the tumor is fixed and not resectable. FR is further subdivided by noting the anatomic extent of the fixation (anterior, posterior, and lateral).[24] Identifying the anatomic extent provides a better appreciation of the scope of the required resection. For example, anterior fixed lesions may require a hysterectomy, vaginectomy, a partial or complete cystectomy, or prostatectomy, whereas lesions that are fixed posteriorly may require a sacrectomy (Figures 33-1 to 33-3).

Although we have found this classification scheme to be extremely useful, it does not reliably predict resectability before surgery because new findings may be discovered at operation. However, in our experience, some factors are clearly associated with an unresectable tumor (Table 33-1). Any circumferential tumor that extends to the pelvic sidewall is considered unresectable. Evidence of bilateral ureteral obstruction is a very worrisome finding. Unless there is focal infiltration of the bladder trigone causing bilateral ureteral obstruction, this finding usually indicates that a bulky tumor has invaded both lateral pelvic sidewalls. This means that the disease is present at the level of the pelvic inlet, making complete resection impossible. Finally, S1 and S2 nerve root involvement or evidence of invasion of the sacral bone at the level of S1 and S2 indicates an unresectable tumor. A sacrectomy proximal to S2 results in sacroiliac joint instability and although internal fixation is possible, it is not warranted for cases of locally recurrent rectal cancer. Pain from nerve root involvement with tumor occasionally needs to be differentiated from sciatic nerve compression. Nerve compression symptoms may completely resolve after pelvic irradiation and chemotherapy. However, persistent buttock and perineal pain usually resulting from tumor expansion and ingrowth is a more ominous symptom.

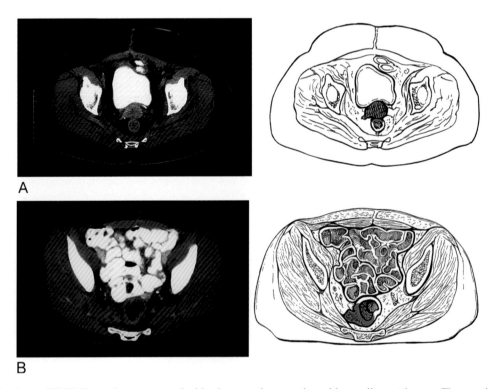

FIGURE 33-1. **A** A primary T3N0M0 rectal cancer treated with a low anterior resection without adjuvant therapy. The anterior recurrent tumor fixed at the base of the bladder was treated with preoperative chemoradiation and then resection with IORT. **B** After a primary low anterior resection for T2N0M0 rectal cancer without adjuvant therapy, this patient developed a lateral pelvic recurrence. After preoperative chemoradiation, the patient underwent an abdominal perineal resection with negative margins.

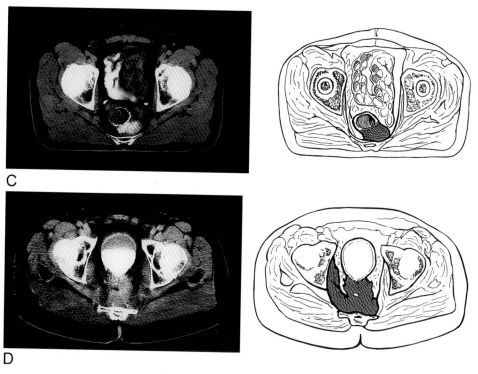

FIGURE 33-1. (*Continued*) **C** A recurrence after a T3N0M0 lesion treated with postoperative chemoradiation therapy was found to invade the sacrum. After additional EBRT and chemotherapy, IORT combined with an en bloc resection of the tumor and distal sacrum was performed with negative margins. **D** A massive recurrent cancer found in the pelvis after an abdominal perineal resection and postoperative chemoradiation. The tumor was fixed to vital pelvic structures and was deemed unresectable. (Reprinted from Nicholls RJ, Dozois RR, eds. Surgery of the Colon and Rectum. New York: Churchill Livingston © 1997 Elsevier Ltd., with permission from Elsevier.)

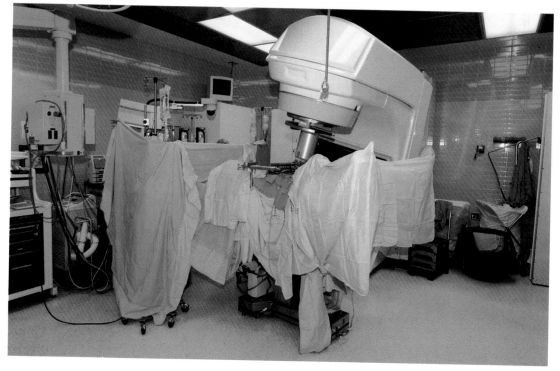

FIGURE 33-2. The IORT suite, showing the equipment, the position of the patient on the operating room table, and the linear accelerator.

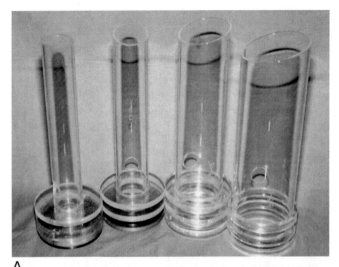

A

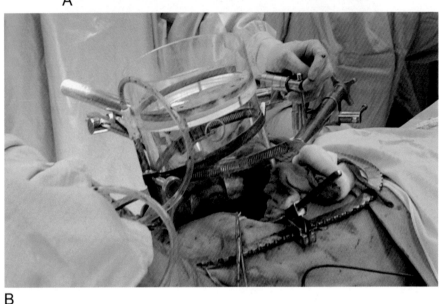

B

FIGURE 33-3. **A** The assortment of the lucite tubes used to direct the electron beam to a fixed site in the operative field in order to deliver the IORT. **B** Place of a large lucite tube to deliver the IORT into the pelvis. The tube is fixed in place by securing it to an external support apparatus attached to the operating table.

TABLE 33-1. Symptoms or findings suggestive of unresectability for cure

Sciatic pain
Bilateral ureteral obstruction
Multiple points of tumor fixation to the pelvic sidewall
Circumferential involvement of the pelvic sidewall
S1 or S2 bony or neural involvement
Extrapelvic disease

Multimodality Therapy for Advanced or Locally Recurrent Rectal Cancer

Surgery with curative intent is the mainstay of treatment for advanced or locally recurrent rectal cancer. However, surgery alone results in a high rate of local and distant failure.[13] To improve outcomes, surgery is combined with multimodality therapy, radiation, and chemotherapy. Radiotherapy is used to improve local control and systemic chemotherapy is used to treat possible disseminated disease.

Although EBRT may relieve symptoms and pain resulting from a large primary or recurrent rectal tumor, it alone does not offer a significant chance of cure.[25] However, when it is combined with sensitizing chemotherapy, the probability of achieving a resection with negative margins and the rate of local tumor control increases.[26–29] In the setting of a locally advanced or recurrent rectal cancer, centers have combined multimodality therapy with intraoperative radiotherapy—as electron beam radiation therapy, high-dose-rate brachytherapy, or traditional perioperative brachytherapy to further improve patient outcomes.[30–37] These forms of locally directed radiation reduce toxicity by limiting normal tissue exposure and deliver a high biologically equivalent dose to the localized area of the tumor.

In general, for patients who never received prior pelvic radiation therapy, a full course of EBRT (5040 cGy) is administered with concurrent 5-fluorouracil chemotherapy. Often, patients with recurrent rectal cancer have previously received a full course of pelvic EBRT. We treat such patients with an additional course of 2000 cGy of EBRT combined with additional 5-fluorouracil chemotherapy before repeating pelvic surgery. Therapeutic synergy between external beam and intraoperative radiation reaches its peak within 8 weeks of completion of external beam therapy. The disease is restaged clinically and radiographically 4 weeks after completion of the external beam and chemotherapy course. If there is no evidence of disease progression in the pelvis or extrapelvic metastasis, the patient is scheduled for surgery within the next 4 weeks.

Surgery

Before surgery, the magnitude of the operation and the possible complications are discussed in depth with the patient and family members. Very rarely in cases of locally advanced primary rectal cancers can the sphincter mechanism be preserved. In recurrent cancers, there is little role for an attempt at sphincter preservation. Therefore, the patient must be accepting of a permanent colostomy. In addition, the resection of adjacent structures or organs and the functional implications and reconstruction alternatives, such as an ileal conduit, need to be discussed.

Patients are admitted the night before surgery for mechanical and antibiotic bowel preparation, intravenous hydration, and instruction in preoperative incentive spirometry. At our institution, all cases of locally advanced or recurrent rectal cancers are scheduled in a dedicated IORT suite. This suite within the operating room complex houses the standard operating room equipment, a linear accelerator, and special anesthetic equipment that permits the anesthetized patient to be moved from operating to irradiating positions (Figure 33-2). In addition, remote controls are used to monitor the patient outside the suite while radiation is given. The patient is placed in the lithotomy position with both arms tucked and the legs supported in Allen stirrups. Special care is taken to ensure that the arms are well padded and in a neutral position to avoid any nerve injury. The calves are positioned and padded to avoid any pressure from directly resting on the stirrups because the lengthy operation may result in compartment syndrome and/or venous thrombosis.[38] Bilateral ureteral stents are inserted cystoscopically preoperatively.

A midline incision is usually made. Transverse abdominal incisions should be avoided because they compromise the placement of any stomas and may injure the inferior epigastric vessels, the primary blood supply of the rectus muscle.

Preservation of the rectus muscle is important in case a transpelvic rectus abdominis flap is required to reconstruct the pelvic floor. If the patient has had prior abdominal surgery, all adhesions need to be lysed. If any of the small bowel is adhered into the pelvis or in a region that might be indicative of tumor, a sample should be sent for intraoperative biopsy. If the bowel is involved with tumor, then that portion of the small bowel will need to be resected with the rectal tumor en bloc. Once all adhesions have been lysed, the entire abdomen needs to be thoroughly explored for evidence of extrapelvic tumor deposits. The liver, omentum, retroperitoneum, peritoneal lining, and the area of any prior surgical incision need to be carefully examined because they are frequently involved with recurrent disease. Any suspicious finding should be analyzed by frozen section. The presence of extrapelvic disease would be a contraindication to radical resection. Very rarely, exceptions may be made in a young patient who has limited pelvic and liver disease; in such cases, the pelvic recurrence and secondary liver tumor are resected simultaneously.

A self-retaining retractor is placed and the small bowel is packed into the upper abdomen to facilitate pelvic exposure. Because pelvic irradiation or prior pelvic surgery will have induced significant fibrosis in the tissues of the pelvis, we begin the dissection at the level of the aortic bifurcation. Starting at this level allows us to enter a virgin fascial plane, which aids in the posterior dissection to the level of the pelvic floor. Similarly, the ureters are identified before they enter the pelvis and are then mobilized along their length along the pelvic sidewall and into the bladder. Identifying the ureters all the way to their insertion into the bladder is important to ensure adequate length if an ileal conduit is required for urinary tract reconstruction.

For rectal cancer recurrences that are not fixed to any pelvic structure (F0), a completion abdominoperineal resection (APR) is required. The scope of the resection is similar to a standard APR but the pelvic fibrosis induced by any prior surgery will have distorted or eliminated the ideal, relatively bloodless plane between the mesorectum and sacral fascia. The distinction between fibrosis and tumor infiltration into adjacent tissue can be very difficult to discern at the time of the operation. If there is any question about the nature of the tissue, particularly when it occurs outside the realm of planned resection, for example, at the level of the sacral promontory or the lateral pelvic walls, a frozen section should be analyzed. If tumor cells are seen, a complete resection with negative margins is not feasible. As will be discussed later, it is in this setting that the use of IORT improves clinical outcomes.

When the tumor is fixed, either anteriorly or posteriorly, the scope of the operation is much larger than for the non-fixed lesion (F0). If the fixed tumor is considered resectable, we classify it as a FR (fixed, resectable) lesion. For anteriorly fixed tumors there are different operations that need to be considered, whereas for a primary or recurrent posteriorly fixed tumor that is fixed posteriorly, our operation of choice is an en bloc distal sacrectomy.

For the anteriorly fixed lesion, the choice of operation is influenced somewhat by the sex of the patient. In a woman, depending on the level and extent of the tumor, the resection may require only an en bloc excision of the posterior wall of the vagina, with immediate reconstruction. When the upper vagina or lower uterus is involved more extensively, en bloc hysterectomy and posterior vaginectomy would be necessary. A woman who has her uterus usually does not need a cystectomy. However, a man with an anteriorly fixed tumor usually needs a cystectomy or cystoprostatectomy. A partial cystectomy with a wide margin may be an option for an upper rectal lesion, but the functional results may be poor because of a decrease in bladder size and radiation-induced injury to the bladder. In such patients, an ileal conduit at the time of resection may be preferable to subjecting the patient to a second surgery.

Posteriorly fixed lesions require an en bloc distal sacrectomy. The proximal extent of the resection is to S2-3. A more proximal resection would require internal fixation of the sacroiliac joints to stabilize the pelvis. We consider a resection of this magnitude too extensive for primary or recurrent rectal cancer. Furthermore, when the resection is limited to the S2-3 level, it is generally possible to preserve one S3 root, which is usually sufficient to preserve bladder function. The sacrectomy proceeds through four distinct steps: 1) the anterior resection, 2) the posterior resection, 3) the use of IORT if required, and 4) the reconstruction of the pelvic tissue defect. The abdominal dissection is begun as described previously. The dissection in the posterior plane is performed to the level of proximal tumor extent along the sacrum. This permits reevaluation to ensure that the tumor does not extend above the S2-3 level. If it does, then the rectum is dissected free in the anterior and lateral planes, leaving the point of sacral fixation as the only point of attachment. A sacrectomy that needs to include a resection proximal to S3-4 requires bilateral ligation of the internal iliac arteries and veins. This is done to decrease blood loss during the sacrectomy. Once the rectum is completely freed anteriorly and laterally, all required abdominal wall stomas are created and an omental or rectus abdominis flap is mobilized and placed into the pelvis to be used for later reconstruction. The abdominal incision is closed and the patient is repositioned in the prone-jackknife position. A posterior midline incision from the region of the last lumbar vertebra to the coccyx is made. The gluteal muscles are dissected free of the sacrum and the proposed site of transection is identified. The important nervous structures to the lower pelvis and extremities, the pudendal and sciatic nerves, respectively, are identified and preserved. With the assistance of our orthopedic or neurosurgical colleagues, the sacrum is transected and the dural sac is closed. The defect is closed either over an omental flap or the mobilized rectus abdominis flap. Because the resulting tissue defect can be quite sizable, local muscle flaps may need to be mobilized in order to close the defect. Multiple closed suction drains should be used, because any pelvic fluid collection can easily become infected and lead to wound breakdown. The wound compli-

cations and breakdown in this heavily irradiated field are not uncommon and occur in as many as 65% of patients who undergo radical resection with concurrent IORT.[39] These postoperative wounds often require transfer of nonirradiated, well-vascularized tissue like muscle flaps to heal if that transfer was not done at the initial operation.

Use of IORT

In cases of close margins, known microscopically positive margins, or minimal gross unresectable disease in the pelvis or after the sacrectomy, our policy is to use intraoperative electron-beam radiation therapy (IORT). To give IORT, a lucite cylinder is positioned in the pelvis to target the at-risk area (Figure 33-3A,B). The patient is then positioned under the linear accelerator. Between 1000 to 2000 cGy is delivered, depending on the extent of margin involvement. A dose of 1000 cGy is recommended for minimal residual disease; 1500 cGy is given for gross residual disease less than 2 cm; and 2000 cGy is reserved for unresected or gross residual disease more than 2 cm. The IORT dose that can be given should take into account the total of any prior EBRT that has been administered.

Although we only have experience with EBRT, other institutions have used other ways of delivering intraoperative or prolonged local radiation therapy. At Memorial Sloan-Kettering, a combined-modality treatment protocol uses high-dose intraoperative brachytherapy (HDR-IORT).[30] The radiation is delivered via an array of catheters that are imbedded in a flexible rubber pad. This pad is then sutured to the area of concern and other normal tissue is packed away and protected. The catheters are connected to a high-dose-rate ^{192}Ir source. After the total dose is delivered, the pad is removed and the operation proceeds. Another approach is to use perioperative brachytherapy as a way to combine local delivery of radiation with extended surgery.[31–34] With this method, brachytherapy catheters are loosely secured to a mesh material that is then secured to the region of interest. The operation is completed and the ends of the catheters are brought out through a separate skin incision and secured to the skin. Then, usually between postoperative day 3 and 5, removable radioactive elements are placed into the brachytherapy catheters. Once the desired total dose is delivered, the catheters are removed at the bedside without the need for sedation or anesthesia. These techniques do not require a dedicated operating room with a linear accelerator to administer radiation regionally and may therefore expand where this type of surgery can be performed. One possible disadvantage with the use of the postoperative brachytherapy catheters is that it is difficult to protect normal tissue, particularly the small intestine, once the operation is complete. However, these alternative methods for delivering local radiation therapy, when combined with extended surgery and chemotherapy, seem to result in morbidity and survival outcomes that are comparable to our experience with intraoperative EBRT.

Results of Multimodality Treatment for Advanced Primary or Locally Recurrent Rectal Cancer

Disease recurrence and survival in patients with rectal cancer is highly dependent on the stage of disease and the mode of treatment. In recent reports, the combination of preoperative EBRT and total mesorectal excision surgery for resectable rectal cancer resulted in a recurrence-free rate of 94% for Stage II and 85% for Stage III tumors.[40] However, more locally advanced rectal cancers often have a higher recurrence rate.[41] Although the cause of death in these patients is usually attributable to systemic disease, a mortality rate of 16%–44% has been attributed to isolated local failure.[42,43] Also, advanced primary disease and recurrences in the pelvis are associated with significant pain, bleeding, and urinary or neurologic complications that often dominate the clinical picture and affect the patient's quality of life.[14] Traditionally, palliative pelvic radiation has been used, but it often only provides short-term palliation of symptoms or of local disease progression.[14,44] To better address the significant symptoms associated with advanced primary or recurrent rectal cancer and to perhaps improve survival, a number of institutions have used multimodality therapy, including preoperative chemoradiation, extensive surgery, and intraoperative-directed local radiation therapy.

For patients with advanced primary rectal cancer, studies have shown the benefit of combined preoperative chemoradiation followed by radical surgery. In a retrospective review of 60 patients with primary locally advanced rectal cancers,[45] 81% were able to undergo curative resection. Their overall 2-year survival was 91%, and their local regional recurrence rate was 7.5%. In another study, preoperative chemoradiation with extensive surgery improved overall survival and control of pelvic disease compared with preoperative radiation therapy alone.[35] In that study, the use of IORT improved local control in patients with microscopic residual disease or clinically fixed tumors. None of the patients treated with IORT developed local failure in the pelvis. Similar findings of improved local control and survival were reported in a series of patients with primary advanced rectal cancers who were given HDR-IORT.[36] These 22 patients with primary unresectable rectal cancer underwent multimodality therapy including preoperative chemotherapy, external beam irradiation, and extensive surgery with intraoperative brachytherapy, which led to actuarial 2-year local control of 81%. Local tumor control was 92% for patients who underwent resection with negative margins versus 38% for those with microscopic positive margins. The overall 2-year actuarial disease-free survival rates were 77% for patients with negative margins and 38% for patients with positive margins. In sum, series of patients with locally advanced primary rectal cancer who were treated with intraoperative radiation and surgery have shown an overall improvement in local control compared with historical controls.

Surgery alone has been used to treat recurrent rectal cancers. In the series by Garcia-Aguilar et al.[46] of 87 patients with recurrent rectal cancer, 64 patients underwent surgical exploration, and only 42 were able to undergo resection with curative intent. The estimated 5-year survival rate for patients who had curative-intent surgery was significantly better than that for patients who had only palliative or no surgery (35% versus 7%). In most series, recurrence and survival rates for patients with recurrent rectal cancer treated with surgery alone are less than those for patients with primary advanced rectal cancer, but are still better than historical data for patients treated with palliative therapies. In general, patients treated with multimodality therapy including IORT experience 3-year local control rates ranging from 25% to 78%, and long-term survival has been reported to be between 25% and 40%.[47–54]

The institution with the most experience using multimodality therapy including IORT for recurrent rectal cancer is the Mayo Clinic. Between 1981 and 1996, 394 patients were treated, 90 of whom had unresectable local or extrapelvic disease at the time of surgical exploration.[47] Although 304 patients underwent resection of the recurrent tumor, only 138 (45%) underwent a histologically confirmed curative resection. The 166 remaining patients had a palliative operation because of either gross (n = 139) or microscopic (n = 27) residual cancer in the pelvis. Nine percent of the patients who had surgery with curative intent underwent extended resections (i.e., sacrectomy, pelvic exenteration, cystectomy with ileal conduit) because of the advanced nature of the tumor. These patients were prospectively monitored to determine long-term survival and the factors influencing survival.

The 1-, 3-, and 5-year survival rates for the 304 patients were 84%, 43%, and 25%, respectively. The median survival time was 31 months. The 5-year survival rate was greater after curative (i.e., negative histologic margins) than after palliative surgery (37% versus 16%, $P < .001$). The presence of gross residual disease in patients who underwent nonpalliative resections resulted in decreased survival compared with those patients with microscopic residual disease. However, survival for patients who had extended resections was not significantly different than that for patients who had a limited resection (28% versus 21%, $P = 0.11$, respectively). Logistic regression analysis found several independent factors that contributed to the ability to perform a curative resection. On univariate analysis, initial surgery with end colostomy or painful recurrence were associated with having palliative surgery. On multivariate analysis, increasing number of tumor fixation sites was associated with a palliative resection. These factors also affected overall survival; patients with pain and more than one site of fixation had significantly lower survival rates. The best 5-year survival rates were in patients who had nonfixed tumors (41%) or asymptomatic recurrences (41%). Other institutions that have used a multimodality approach that included some form of intraoperative radiation have reported similar improvements in local recurrence and survival.[51–54]

Patients whose tumors can be resected with negative margins often have better outcomes. Because of this, some investigators have questioned the routine use of the intraoperative, locally directed radiation therapy.[55] Recently, Wiig and colleagues[56] reported a nonrandomized, prospective study evaluating the value of IORT in reoperative surgery for recurrent rectal cancer. The estimated overall 5-year survival was 30%. However, patients who had an R0 resection had a 60% survival compared with 25% and 0% for R1 and R2, respectively. The use of IORT did not improve survival or local recurrence when controlling for R-stage resection. However, other reports indicate that IORT improves local control and survival even in patients with R1 resections when compared with most control series of patients.[48] In addition, many series report that pelvic recurrences after multimodality therapy that included IORT occurred outside the intraoperative radiation field. In the most recent study to look specifically at the rate of local recurrence after the use of high-dose-rate brachytherapy, significantly more recurrences occurred outside of the IORT field than within the radiation field.[54] In that series, the time to pelvic recurrence was 16 months in patients who had a pelvic recurrence outside the radiation field, and 31 months in patients who had a pelvic recurrence within the radiation field; however, the difference was not statistically significantly ($P = .07$). To specifically address the benefit of adding IORT to the combined multimodality treatment of patients with advanced primary or recurrent rectal cancer would require a prospective, randomized trial. However, this would be a difficult undertaking given the relatively few institutions capable of delivering this complex therapy, the variations in different intraoperative radiation techniques, and the relatively limited number of patients for whom this therapy is appropriate. For now, most studies, although retrospective and often based on single institutions, suggest that combined multimodality therapy that includes IORT provides the best chance for cure for patients with locally advanced or recurrent rectal cancer.

Perioperatively related mortality was very low in patients who underwent this multimodality treatment (0.3%).[47] However, treatment-related morbidity was relatively high. In one series of 304 patients who underwent surgery with curative intent, 96 (32%) required prolonged hospitalizations, 78 (26%) of whom required readmissions and/or additional surgical procedures. The most frequent complications included pelvic abscesses (6.6%), bowel obstructions (5.3%), enteric fistulas (4.3%), and perineal wound complications (4.6%).[47] The complication rate was significantly higher in patients who underwent extended surgical resections and in patients who had recurrences fixed in more than two sites in the pelvis. These findings underscore the need for thorough preoperative patient selection to ensure that the patient is fit enough to tolerate the surgery and the potential complications, and that there is no evidence of disease outside of the region of resection.

Palliative Care for Advanced or Recurrent Rectal Cancer

Patients who present with locally advanced or recurrent rectal cancer must first be evaluated with the intent to cure. An equally important consideration is palliation of symptoms if a cure does not seem to be achievable. The local effect within the pelvis of an advanced or recurrent rectal cancer drives the need to address control of symptoms. These symptoms often include rectal bleeding, rectal obstruction, urinary obstruction caused by local invasion, and severe pain related to invasion of the pelvic sidewall or direct invasion of pelvic nerves. Over the past decade, the choice of palliative options has expanded and choice of option requires careful consideration of the presenting symptoms, possible future symptoms, extent of local and distant spread of the disease, and the overall physical condition of the patient.

Palliative interventions may be broadly classified as noninvasive, minimally invasive, and surgical. The primary noninvasive palliative option is radiotherapy. In patients who have never received pelvic radiation, a full course of external beam irradiation may be a very effective treatment for bleeding, pelvic pain, and near obstruction. The use of external beam radiotherapy may result in palliation of severe pelvic pain in 50%–90% of patients.[57,58] However, virtually all patients will experience progression of the tumor and recurrent symptoms before they die. Lingareddy and colleagues[44] have shown there is a significant use for palliative reirradiation in treating recurrent rectal cancers. In their study of 52 patients with recurrent rectal cancer, pelvic reirradiation resulted in complete palliation of bleeding, pain, and mass effect in 100%, 65%, and 24% of cases, respectively. The median initial radiation dose to the pelvis was 50 cGy; the median reirradiation dose was 30 cGy. Most patients had palliation of their symptoms until their deaths. Grade 3 and 4 toxicity were seen in 23% and 10% of patients, respectively. The 2-year overall actuarial survival was 25%.

Minimally invasive approaches to palliation usually involve mechanical means to reduce symptoms related to pelvic tumors. These include ureteral stents to alleviate urinary obstruction and expandable metal colonic wall stents or the use of lasers to relieve rectal obstruction. Self-expanding metal stents (SEMS) are useful for the nonsurgical management of rectal obstructions, bleeding, and malignant fistulas.[59] In a review of the literature, palliation with SEMS was achieved in 90% of patients.[60] In the largest series to report on SEMS for malignant rectal obstructions, stents could be deployed successfully in 36 of 37 patients with rectal obstructions,[61] and 28 had good long-term results with no need for subsequent intervention.[61]

Endoscopic lasers are an alternative to SEMS. The neodymium yttrium argon garnet (Nd:YAG) laser is the most frequently used. Endoscopic laser treatments remove the tissue intraluminally by coagulative necrosis or immediate tissue vaporization, depending on the amount of energy applied. Palliation of symptoms and marked improvement in quality of life is achieved after repeated laser sessions (usually 2–5) in 80%–90% of patients.[62,63] Unfortunately, laser therapy does not seem to be a durable treatment. Effective palliation decreases as a patient survives longer; successful palliation at 1 year was only 42%.[64]

There are no data on the use of palliative resections in patients with locally advanced or recurrent rectal cancer. However, a report from Memorial Sloan-Kettering has evaluated the role of palliative resection in 80 patients with Stage IV rectal cancer.[65] Twenty-four percent had clinical evidence of obstruction and 94% had either T3 or T4 lesions. None had received prior surgical or radiation therapy. They underwent radical resection of the primary lesion and surgical treatment of solitary hepatic metastasis, if present. There was one death, a 15% postoperative morbidity, and a 20% colostomy rate. The overall local recurrence rate was 6%, actuarial local control at 2 years was 94%, and median survival was 25 months. This study shows that in appropriately selected patients with Stage IV disease and complicated or advanced rectal cancer, surgical resection of the primary tumors can achieve very reasonable oncologic results and provide good palliation of symptoms related to the tumor.

Summary

For patients with advanced primary or recurrent rectal cancers, the only hope of cure requires a coordinated multidisciplinary approach to treatment. In general, EBRT, chemotherapy, extensive surgery, and the use of directed IORT seem to improve local control and survival. Surgery in these patients carries a higher morbidity rate than surgery for primary rectal cancer, but one that is acceptable in appropriately selected patients. Before proceeding with multimodality therapy, patients should be thoroughly evaluated for the presence of disseminated extrapelvic or metastatic disease, which would, in most instances, preclude a curative operation. Experience indicates that isolated anterior or posterior fixation of the tumor does not preclude a curative resection. In these cases, en bloc resection of involved organs or bony structures can result in resection with negative margins. However, tumors fixed to the lateral pelvic sidewall, fixed at multiple points, or fixed circumferentially are often unresectable or incurable. Available data from many institutions indicates that multimodality therapy for advanced primary or recurrent rectal cancer results in better local control and higher survival rates than palliative therapy.

References

1. Curly SA, Carlson GW, Shumate CR, et al. Extended resection for locally advanced colorectal carcinoma. Am J Surg 1992;163: 553–559.
2. Polk HC Jr. Extended resection for selected adenocarcinomas of the large bowel. Ann Surg 1972;175:892–899.
3. Bonfanti G, Bozzetti F, Doci R, et al. Results of extended surgery for cancer of the rectum and sigmoid. Br J Surg 1982;69: 305–307.
4. McDermott FT, Hughes ES, Pihl E, et al. Local recurrence after potentially curative resection for rectal cancer in a series of 1008 patients. Br J Surg 1985;72:34–37.
5. Wanebo HJ, Koness RJ, Vezeridas MP. Pelvic resection of recurrent rectal cancer. Ann Surg 1994;220;586–597.
6. Philipshen SJ, Heilweil M, Quan SHQ, et al. Patterns of pelvic recurrence following definitive resections of rectal cancer. Cancer 1984;53:1354–1362.
7. Rich T, Gunderson LL, Lew R, et al. Patterns of recurrence of rectal cancer after potentially curative surgery. Cancer 1983;52: 1317–1329.
8. Gunderson LJ, Sargent DJ, Tepper JE, et al. Impact of T and N substage on survival and disease relapse in adjuvant rectal cancer: a pooled analysis. Int J Radiat Oncol Biol Phys 2002;54: 386–396.
9. Heald RJ, Ryall RD. Recurrence and survival after total mesorectal excision for rectal cancer. Lancet 1986;1:1479–1482.
10. MacFarlane JK, Ryall RD, Heald RJ. Mesorectal excision for rectal cancer. Lancet 1993;341:457–460.
11. Swedish Rectal Cancer Trial. Improved survival with preoperative radiotherapy in respectable rectal cancer. N Engl J Med 1997;336:980–987.
12. Camma C, Giunta M, Fiorica F, et al. Preoperative radiotherapy for respectable rectal cancer: a meta-analysis. J Am Med Assoc 2000;284:1008–1015.
13. Kramer T, Share R, Kiel K, et al. Intraoperative radiation therapy of colorectal cancer. In: Abe M, ed. Intraoperative Radiation Therapy. New York: Pergamon Press; 1991:308–310.
14. Wong CS, Cummings BJ, Brierley JD, et al. Treatment of locally recurrent rectal carcinoma: results and prognostic factors. Int J Radiat Oncol Biol Phys 1998;40:427–435.
15. Knol HP, Hanssens PE, Rutten HJ, et al, Effects of radiation therapy alone or in combination with surgery and/or chemotherapy on tumor and symptom control of recurrent rectal cancer. Strahlenther Onkol 1997;173:43–49.
16. Hruby G, Barton M, Miles S, et al. Site of local recurrence after surgery, with or without chemotherapy, for rectal cancer: implications for radiotherapy field design. Int J Radiat Oncol Biol Phys 2003;55:138–143.
17. Farouk R, Nelson H, Radice E, et al. Accuracy of computed tomography in determining resectability for locally advanced primary or recurrent colorectal cancers. Am J Surg 1998;175: 283–287.
18. Moore HG, Akhurst T, Larson SM, et al. A case-controlled study of 18-fluorodeoxyglucose positron emission tomography in the detection of pelvic recurrence in previously irradiated rectal cancer patients. J Am Coll Surg 2003;197:22–28.
19. Ogunbiyi OA, Flanagan FL, Dehdashti F, et al. Detection of recurrent and metastatic colorectal cancer: comparison of positron emission tomography and computed tomography. Ann Surg Oncol 1997;4:613–620.
20. Miller E, Lerman H, Gutman M, et al. The clinical impact of camera-based positron emission tomography imaging in patients with recurrent colorectal cancer. Investig Radiol 2004; 39:8–12.

21. Valk PE, Abella-Columna E, Haseman MK, et al. Whole-body PET imaging with [^{18}F] fluorodeoxyglucose in management of recurrent colorectal cancer. Arch Surg 1999;134:503–511.

22. Arulampalam T, Costa D, Visvikis D, et al. The impact of FDG-PET on the management algorithm for recurrent colorectal cancer. Eur J Nucl Med 2001;28:1758–1765.

23. Whiteford MH, Whiteford HM, Yee LF, et al. Usefulness of FDG-PET scan in the assessment of suspected metastatic or recurrent adenocarcinoma of the colon and rectum. Dis Colon Rectum 2000;53:759–770.

24. Suzuki K, Dozois RR, Devine RM, et al. Curative reoperations for locally recurrent rectal cancer. Dis Colon Rectum 1996;39:730–736.

25. Guiney MJ, Smith JG, Worotniuk V, et al. Radiotherapy treatment for isolated loco-regional recurrence of rectosigmoid cancer following definitive surgery: Peter MacCallum Cancer Institute experience, 1981–1990. Int J Radiat Oncol Biol Phys 1997;38:1019–1025.

26. Aleksic M, Hennes N, Ulrich B. Surgical treatment of locally advanced rectal cancer. Options and strategies. Dig Surg 1998;15:342–346.

27. Rau B, Hohenberger P, Gellermann J, et al. T4 rectal carcinoma. Surgical and multimodal therapy. Chirug 2002;73:147–153.

28. Platell C, Cassidy B, Heywood J, et al. Use of adjuvant, preoperative chemo-radiotherapy in patients with locally advanced rectal cancer. ANZ J Surg 2002;72:639–642.

29. Gohl J, Merkel S, Rodel C, et al. Can neoadjuvant radiochemotherapy improve the results of multivisceral resections in the advanced rectal carcinoma (cT4a). Colorect Dis 2003;5:436–441.

30. Alektiar KM, Zelefsky MJ, Paty PB, et al. High-dose-rate intraoperative brachytherapy for recurrent colorectal cancer. Int J Radiat Oncol Biol Phys 2000;48:219–226.

31. Keuhne J, Kleisli T, Biernacki P, et al. Use of high-dose-rate brachytherapy in the management of locally recurrent rectal cancer. Dis Colon Rectum 2003;46:895–899.

32. Martinez-Monge R, Nag S, Martin EW. ^{125}Iodine brachytherapy for colorectal adenocarcinoma recurrent in the pelvis and para-ortics. Int J Radiat Oncol Biol Phys 1998;42:545–550.

33. Goes RN, Beart RW, Simons AJ, et al. Use of brachytherapy in management of locally recurrent rectal cancer. Dis Colon Rectum 1997;40:1177–1179.

34. Martinez-Monge R, Nag S, Martin EW. Three different intraoperative radiation modalities (electron beam, high-dose-rate brachytherapy, and iodine-125 brachytherapy) in the adjuvant treatment of patient with recurrent colorectal adenocarcinoma. Cancer 1999;86:236–247.

35. Weinstein GD, Rich TA, Shumate CR, et al. Preoperative infusional chemoradiation and surgery with or without an electron beam intraoperative boost for advanced primary rectal cancer. Int J Radiat Oncol Biol Phys 1995;32:197–204.

36. Harrison LB, Minsky BD, Enker WE, et al. High dose rate intraoperative radiation therapy (HDR-IORT) as part of the management strategy for locally advanced and recurrent rectal cancer. Int J Radiat Oncol Biol Phys 1998;42:325–330.

37. Willett CG, Shellito PC, Tepper JE, et al. Intraoperative electron beam radiation therapy for recurrent locally advanced rectal or rectosigmoid carcinoma. Cancer 1991;67:1504–1508.

38. Neagle CE, Schaffer JL, Heppenstall RB. Compartment syndrome complicating prolonged use of the lithotomy position. Surgery 1991;110:566–569.

39. Kim HK, Jessup JM, Beard CJ, et al. Locally advanced rectal carcinoma: pelvic control and morbidity following preoperative radiation therapy, resection and intraoperative radiation therapy. Int J Radiat Oncol Biol Phys 1997;38:777–783.

40. Kapiteijin E, Marijnen CAM, Nagtegaal ID, et al. Preoperative radiotherapy combined with total mesorectal excision for resectable rectal cancer. N Engl J Med 2001;345:638–646.

41. Tepper JE, O'Connell M, Niedzwiecki D, et al. Adjuvant therapy in rectal cancer: analysis of stage, sex, and local control—final report of intergroup 0114. J Clin Oncol 200220:1744–1750.

42. Lindel K, Willett CG, Shellito PC, et al. Intraoperative radiation therapy for locally advanced recurrent rectal or rectosigmoid cancer. Radiother Oncol 2001;58:83–87.

43. Hashiguchi Y, Sekine T, Sakamoto H, et al. Intraoperative irradiation after surgery for locally recurrent rectal cancer. Dis Colon Rectum 1999;42:886–893.

44. Lingareddy V, Ahmad NR, Mohiuddin M. Palliative reirradiation for recurrent rectal cancer. Int J Radiat Oncol Biol Phys 1997;38:785–790.

45. Platell C, Cassidy B, Heywood J, et al. Use of adjuvant, preoperative chemo-radiotherapy in patients with locally advanced rectal cancer. ANZ J Surg 2002;72:639–642.

46. Garcia-Aguilar J, Cromwell JW, Marra C, et al. Treatment of locally recurrent rectal cancer. Dis Colon Rectum 2001;44:1743–1748.

47. Hahnloser D, Nelson H, Gunderson LL, et al. Curative potential of multimodality therapy for locally recurrent rectal cancer. Ann Surg 2003;237:502–508.

48. Mannaerts G, Rutten HJT, Martijin H, et al. Comparison of intraoperative radiation therapy-containing multimodality treatment with historical treatment modalities for locally recurrent rectal cancer. Dis Colon Rectum 2001;44:1749–1758.

49. Mannaerts G, Martijin H, Crommelin MA, et al. Feasibility and first results of multimodality treatment, combining EBRT, extensive surgery, and IOERT in locally advanced primary rectal cancer. Int J Radiat Oncol Biol Phys 2000;47:425–433.

50. Haddock MG, Gunderson LL, Nelson H, et al. Intraoperative irradiation for locally recurrent colorectal cancer in previously irradiated patients. Int J Radiat Oncol Biol Phys 2001;49:1267–1274.

51. Calvo FA, Gomez-Espi M, Diaz-Gonzalez JA, et al. Intraoperative presacral electron boost following preoperative chemoradiation in $T_{3-4}N_x$ rectal cancer: initial local effects and clinical outcomes analysis. Radiother Oncol 2002;62:201–206.

52. Bussieres E, Gilly FN, Rouanet P, et al, Recurrences of rectal cancers: results of a multimodal approach with intraoperative radiation therapy. Int J Radiat Oncol Biol Phys 1996;34:49–56.

53. Shoup M, Guillem JG, Alektiar KM, et al. Predictors of survival in recurrent rectal cancer after resection and intraoperative radiotherapy. Dis Colon Rectum 2002;45:585–592.

54. Nuyttens JJ, Kolkman-Deurloo IK, Vermaas M, et al. High dose-rate intraoperative radiotherapy for close or positive margins in patients with locally advanced or recurrent rectal cancer. Int J Radiat Oncol Biol Phys 2004;58:106–112.

55. Wiig JN, Poulsen JP, Tveit KM, Olsen DR, Giercksky KE. Intraoperative irradiation (IORT) for primary advanced and recurrent rectal cancer: a need for randomised studies. Eur J Cancer 2000;36:868–874.

56. Wiig JN, Tveit KM, Poulsen JP, Olsen DR, Giercksky KE. Preoperative irradiation and surgery for recurrent rectal cancer.

Will intraoperative radiotherapy (IORT) be of additional benefit? A prospective study. Radiother Oncol 2002;62:207–213.

57. Allum WH, Mack P, Priestman TJ, et al. Radiotherapy for pain relief in locally recurrent colorectal cancer. Ann R Coll Surg Engl 1987;69:220–221.

58. Whiteley HW Jr, Stearns MW Jr, Leaming RH, et al. Palliative radiation therapy in patients with cancer of the colon and rectum. Cancer 1970;25:343–346.

59. Baron TH. Indications and results of endoscopic rectal stenting. J Gastrointest Surg 2004;8:266–269.

60. Khot UP, Lang AW, Murali K, et al. Systematic review of the efficacy and safety of colorectal stents. Br J Surg 2002;89: 1096–1102.

61. Spinelli P, Mancini A. Use of self-expanding metal stents for palliation of rectosigmoid cancer. Gastrointest Endosc 2001;53: 203–206.

62. Kimmey MB. Endoscopic methods (other than stents) for palliation of rectal carcinoma. J Gastrointest Surg 2004;8:270–273.

63. McGowan I, Barr H, Krasner N. Palliative laser therapy for inoperable rectal cancer: does it work? Cancer 1989;63:967–969.

64. Cutsem EV, Boonen A, Geboes K, et al. Risk factors which determine the long-term outcome of neodymium-YAG laser palliation of colorectal carcinoma. Int J Colorect Dis 1989;4:9–11.

65. Nash GM, Saltz LB, Kemeny NE, et al. Radical resection of rectal cancer primary tumor provides effective local therapy in patients with stage IV disease. Ann Surg Oncol 2002;9:954–960.

34
Colorectal Cancer: Metastatic (Palliation)

Michael D'Angelica, Kamran Idrees, Philip B. Paty, and Leslie H. Blumgart

Approximately 20% of patients with colorectal cancer present with established distant metastases.[1] In most cases, the metastases are detectable with noninvasive imaging, and patients can be assigned to AJCC (American Joint Committee on Cancer) Stage IV before any surgical intervention. Among these patients there is enormous heterogeneity with respect to sites of disease, extent of disease, symptoms, performance status, and comorbidities. The clinical spectrum at the time of diagnosis ranges from the asymptomatic patient with a single metastatic lesion to the rapidly deteriorating patient with colon obstruction and advanced, multiorgan metastases. It is therefore difficult to define rigid treatment algorithms that can be widely applied to all clinical settings.

Despite considerable progress in the treatment of advanced colorectal cancer, the vast majority of Stage IV patients are not curable by current treatment protocols. A recent analysis of data from the SEER (surveillance, epidemiology, and end results) population-based database estimates that the 5-year survival rate for Stage IV patients diagnosed between 1991 and 2000 was 8%.[2] However, despite a low overall cure rate, aggressive treatment is indicated for most patients to extend survival and enhance quality of life. Systemic chemotherapy, endoscopic treatments to palliate obstruction, surgical diversion, and surgical resection all have important roles in treatment of Stage IV patients. Treatment approaches must be individualized based on the extent and resectability of local and distant disease, the presence or absence of bowel obstruction, performance status, and comorbidities. For patients with good performance status and minimal symptoms from their primary cancers, standard treatment is systemic chemotherapy, which is well documented to increase survival and quality of life.[3,4] Surgical resection of the primary tumor and, when feasible, of the metastatic lesions can provide excellent palliation and can, in some cases, provide lasting cure.

In the past decade, there has been remarkable improvement in the efficacy of chemotherapy for colorectal cancer. First-line therapy with either FOLFOX or FOLFIRI now yields major responses in up to 50% of previously untreated patients, and achieves minor responses or stable disease in an additional 20% of patients.[5] Multiple, effective drug combinations are available as well, and second-line chemotherapy has become more effective and more likely to impact survival. Over the past 10 years, the median survival for patients with metastatic disease who are treated with chemotherapy has improved from 12–14 months to 21 months.[6] Although cure from chemotherapy alone remains extremely rare, effective chemotherapy combined with aggressive surgery may be increasing the overall cure rate. In this setting, the care of patients with advanced disease has become quite complex. The goal of this chapter is to provide a reference source for surgeons managing patients who present with Stage IV colorectal cancer.

Biology of Metastatic Disease

Metastasis is defined as the spread of malignant cells from a primary tumor to a distant organ. It is estimated that 90% of all cancer deaths are a result of metastasis.[7] The process of metastasis is a continuous and inefficient one that begins early in tumor formation and increases as tumors grow.[8] Metastatic foci themselves can go through the metastatic process and spread to other organs (i.e., metastases can metastasize).

Numerous clinical and laboratory studies have attempted to define the complex process of metastasis formation. It is a multistep process, and failure at any step results in failure of the overall process. The process relies on properties of the tumors cells, as well as the microenvironment of the primary and secondary sites.[9,10] A series of major events must occur (Figure 34-1).

The first step is tumorigenesis, which occurs after the initial malignant transformation. The tumor proliferates into a small mass of heterogenous cells that are of varying metastatic or malignant potential. These tumor cells undergo multiple and sequential genetic changes, characterized by the appearance of oncogenes and a decrease in tumor suppressor genes.

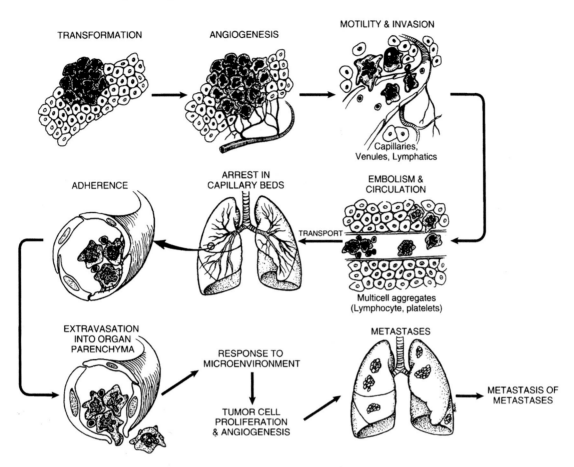

FIGURE 34-1. Schematic illustrating the multistep process involved in the development of metastasis. (Reprinted from DeVita VT Jr, Hellman S, Rosenberg SA. Cancer: Principles and Practice of Oncology. 6th ed. copyright 2001, with permission of Lippincott Williams & Wilkins.)

As the tumor grows beyond 1 mm in diameter and becomes relatively hypoxic, angiogenesis is initiated. The process of tumor angiogenesis is tightly regulated by pro- and anti-angiogenic factors secreted by both the tumor and its environment. As tumors successfully grow, suppressors of angiogenesis are inhibited and pro-angiogenic factors predominate, resulting in neovascularity and further growth of the tumor.[11] Some tumors may grow by utilizing other existing blood vessels in nearby tissues.

In the next step, some cells will develop an invasive phenotype. Most researchers believe that there is a selection process resulting in the clonal expansion of certain cell subpopulations with growth advantages and invasive properties. Whether this process represents a property of the whole tumor cell mass or true clonal selection of more invasive cell subpopulations is not known, and is a subject of intense research.[12] Malignant invasion is characterized by downregulation of cell adhesion, resulting in detachment of the cell from the primary tumor mass and the extracellular matrix. Stromal invasion is accomplished through interactions with the basement membrane, including adhesion, proteolysis, and migration, ultimately resulting in detachment and invasion through the basement membrane. This invasive phenotype

also enables these cells to enter thin-walled lymphatics and vasculature, allowing access to systemic circulation. The neovasculature from tumor-induced angiogenesis seems to be more susceptible to such invasion. This process of invasion is critically related to the expression (up-regulated or down-regulated) of adhesion molecules and factors influencing cell migration.[13,14]

Once inside the vascular system, cells or cell clumps (emboli) are circulated, and must survive hemodynamic filtering as well as immune surveillance. They must then arrest in a distant organ. This probably involves adhesion and/or trapping, based on size, within small capillary beds. There is likely a complex interaction between the malignant cell and the endothelium or exposed basement membrane, allowing cell arrest. Once arrested in a tissue bed, the cells extravasate into the tissue, enabling formation of a metastatic focus. There is debate as to whether proliferation occurs before or after actual extravasation into the tissue; some experimental models have shown that extravasation is not a prerequisite for growth in a secondary organ.[15] Paracrine growth factors, hormones, and the local tissue environment have critical roles in the ultimate outcome of extravasated cells. These metastatic cells can become dormant or proliferate; what determines this fate is not fully understood. Growth in the distant organ after deposition is a major limiting factor in the formation of metastasis, and some metastatic cells can remain dormant for years. Once deposited in the distant organ, the metastatic focus, if proliferating, must again go through tumorigenesis, angiogenesis, and evasion of the immune system.[16]

This complex multistep process of metastasis formation is related to multiple genetic changes among malignant cells. As the technology of measuring genetic changes improves, we are beginning to appreciate the changes that occur during this process. It seems that there are genes specific to tumorigenesis, invasion, angiogenesis, and other steps. Recently, a number of genes have been identified that suppress metastatic potential and, by their down-regulation, affect a cell's ability to metastasize without affecting tumorigenicity.[17] These discoveries provide a sense of the future challenge in elucidating the multiple, stepwise, and specific changes that regulate a cell's ability to metastasize. Advances in this field will have obvious and profound implications for the treatment of cancer.

Diagnosis/Staging

The clinical presentation of Stage IV patients is variable. Most present with symptoms referable to the primary tumor. However, symptoms from metastatic disease, asymptomatic metastatic lesions found on imaging studies, abnormalities in routine blood work, and cancers discovered on endoscopic screening procedures may also be the first signs of disease. Initial staging evaluation should include colonoscopy with biopsy, and imaging of the primary tumor, liver, and lungs. When feasible, endorectal ultrasound or magnetic resonance imaging (MRI) is recommended for rectal cancers to document the initial T and N stage. Spiral computed tomographic (CT) scanning of the chest/abdomen/pelvis is a highly accurate and efficient method of detecting metastases. Positron emission tomography (PET) scanning detects occult disease not seen on CT scan in 20% of Stage IV patients, and should be considered if such findings might affect patient management.[18]

Once the extent of disease workup is complete and distant metastases have been documented, the surgeon must make three important judgments. First is whether the patient is fit for aggressive treatment. Patients with poor performance status or serious cardiovascular, pulmonary, renal, neurologic, or gastrointestinal impairment may not tolerate chemotherapy or major surgery. Second is whether the primary tumor presents a clinically significant risk of bowel obstruction. Symptoms, radiographic findings, and endoscopic findings are important considerations. If the proximal colon is not dilated on radiographic studies and a colonoscope can traverse the tumor, it is generally safe to begin treatment with chemotherapy. The third determination is whether the patient's metastases can be surgically resected, and therefore treated with curative intent. If complete resection of all disease can be expected, then surgical intervention should assume a high priority.

Multidisciplinary Evaluation

Management of patients with advanced disease is often complex, and multidisciplinary evaluation can be helpful in determining initial therapy. The surgeon and medical oncologist should evaluate the patient in consultation with a radiologist and gastroenterologist. The goals, priorities, and expected course of treatment should be discussed. For rectal cancers that are bulky or symptomatic, the advice of a radiation oncologist is often helpful.

Palliative Management of the Primary Cancer—Stents, Laser

Approximately 8%–29% of patients with colorectal cancer initially present with symptoms of partial or complete bowel obstruction.[19] In a review of 713 obstructing carcinomas, 77% were left-sided and 23% were right-sided cases.[20] Furthermore, a majority of obstructing tumors are either Stage III or Stage IV.[21] Bowel obstruction is insidious in onset, with initial symptoms of mild discomfort and change in bowel habits. With disease progression, the symptoms can become worse, ranging from crampy abdominal pain, abdominal distension, nausea, abdominal tenderness, obstipation, and leukocytosis. Vomiting is a late symptom unless there is an associated small bowel obstruction. Without treatment, the process can progress to complete obstruction, ischemia, and perforation. The risk of cecal perforation is greatest in patients who have a competent ileocecal valve.

In the setting of metastatic cancer, the critical question is whether colon obstruction should be considered a contraindication for systemic chemotherapy or radiotherapy. The degree of symptoms, endoscopic findings, and radiographic findings are all relevant to this decision. When the cancer can be traversed with a colonoscope and there is no radiographic evidence for obstruction, many patients with partially obstructing cancers will tolerate aggressive chemotherapy. Patients must be instructed to monitor their symptoms closely, and to report any signs of worsening obstruction immediately. A liquid diet or pureed diet taken in small portions may help to reduce obstructive symptoms. For patients with advanced obstruction, nonresective palliative options include laser therapy, fulguration, colonic self-expanding metal stents, and creation of a diverting stoma.

Laser therapy has been used for palliation of obstructing rectal cancers for the past two decades.[22–24] In a large series of 272 patients who underwent palliative laser therapy for rectosigmoid cancers, the immediate success rate in treating obstructive symptoms was 85%.[25] Other studies have shown similar success rates, in the range of 80%–90%.[23,24] However, laser therapy is practical only for treating cancers of the distal colon and rectum, and is rarely used to treat proximal lesions. In addition, multiple therapy sessions are required to achieve lasting relief of symptoms. Serious complications such as bleeding, perforation, and severe pain have been reported in 5%–15% of patients, especially those undergoing multiple treatments.[22,24–26]

Surgical fulguration of rectal cancers is another method of opening the rectal lumen.[27,28] Fulguration, in combination with endoluminal debulking, can remove a large volume of tumor; however, unlike laser therapy, this procedure requires hospital admission and regional or general anesthesia.

Since their introduction in 1991, colonic stents have become an important method of palliation for obstruction in colorectal cancer patients, especially those with unresectable metastatic disease. These self-expanding metallic stents can potentially dilate the lumen to a near-normal diameter, providing quick relief of symptoms and, in some cases, allowing endoscopic assessment of the proximal colon. Stents can be placed in patients using minimal sedation, without need of prior endoscopic dilation and the concomitant increased risk of complications such as perforation or tumor fracture. Moreover, these stents can be placed across relatively long lesions by overlapping stents in a "stent-within-stent" manner.

In a retrospective series of 80 patients who underwent colonic stent placement for malignant large bowel obstruction, stents were successfully placed in 70 patients (87.5% overall technical success rate).[29] Satisfactory symptomatic relief and clinical decompression was achieved in 67 patients (83.7% overall clinical success rate). Two perforations occurred in this series, one of which resulted in death. Other complications included stent migration resulting in expulsion, reobstruction, and intractable tenesmus. Stenting of cancers in the mid and low rectum may result in debilitating urgency and incontinence.

A recent series of 52 patients with malignant obstruction secondary to either primary or recurrent disease, who underwent stent placement by colorectal surgeons, reported that 50 of 52 were successfully palliated.[30] One patient had a perforation, and in another patient obstruction was not relieved because of multiple sites of obstruction. The complication rate in this series was 25%; migration was the most common complication (15.4%), followed by reobstruction secondary to tumor ingrowth (3.8%), perforation, colovesical fistula, and severe tenesmus (2% each). Surgery was required in 17.3%, mostly because of complications or recurrent obstruction. Complications reported in the literature on colonic stents include stent malpositioning, migration, tumor ingrowth (through the stent interstices), tumor overgrowth (beyond the ends of a stent), perforation, stool impaction, bleeding, tenesmus, and postprocedure pain.

Laser therapy has also been used in certain situations, in conjunction with colonic stents, to recanalize and decompress large bowel. Overall, as more experience is gained, these endoscopic palliation therapies increasingly provide effective and durable palliation for patients with malignant obstruction.

Surgical Management of the Primary Cancer—Resection

The role of bowel resection in patients with unresectable metastases is controversial. It is important to recognize that there are no randomized data demonstrating a survival benefit for bowel resection in Stage IV patients. However, palliative resection of the primary tumor does provide durable local control, is generally well tolerated, and can benefit many Stage IV patients.[31] However, randomized trials of 5-fluorouracil (5-FU)-based chemotherapy versus best supportive care, conducted in the 1990s, have shown that Stage IV patients receiving systemic chemotherapy have increased length and quality of life.[3,4] Moreover, with modern multidrug regimens, the beneficial impact of chemotherapy continues to increase.[5,6] Thus, standard management for patients with unresectable metastatic colorectal cancer is systemic chemotherapy. The proper use of elective colon/rectal resection in nonobstructed patients is a source of continuing debate. Oncologists properly cite loss of performance status, risk of surgical complications, and delay in chemotherapy as major downsides to palliative resection. Surgeons, however, understand that elective operations have a far lower morbidity than emergency surgery and fear having to operate on patients who obstruct while receiving chemotherapy or who present with more advanced disease after multiple cycles of ineffective chemotherapy.

Four retrospective studies have evaluated nonoperative management of Stage IV colorectal cancer by comparing patients who did and did not undergo colorectal resection[32–35] (Table 34-1). The data come from the 1990s, when 5-FU-based chemotherapy was the standard systemic therapy. In all four studies, a strong majority of patients were treated by upfront bowel resection. Patients who were not initially resected were more likely to have rectal cancers, to have more extensive metastatic disease, and to be older. Operative mortality for the patients having upfront resection ranged from 1.6% to 9%. Patients who did not have initial bowel resection underwent a subsequent colorectal operation in 9.3%–32% of cases, although the indications for subsequent operation were often not specified. From these limited data, it is clear that upfront colon resection is frequently practiced, particularly for patients with colon primaries and with less extensive metastatic disease. However, it is not possible to assess the impact of colon resection on symptom control, tolerance to subsequent chemotherapy, quality of life, or survival.

A prospective study of 24 patients with unresectable Stage IV colorectal cancer and minimally symptomatic primary cancers treated by 5-FU-based chemotherapy was reported by Sarela and colleagues.[36] Eleven patients had metastases limited to the liver (six with greater than 50% replacement of the liver), 10 patients had lung metastases, and six patients had peritoneal metastases. In the follow-up period, four patients with sigmoid colon cancer developed bowel obstruction,

TABLE 34-1 Retrospective analysis of bowel resection for patients with unresectable Stage IV colorectal cancer

Study	Surgical group	N	Group features	Operative mortality (%)	Subsequent colon surgery (%)	Median survival (mo)
Vander bilt[34]	Resection	66	Proximal cancers	4.6	—	14.5
	No resection	23	Rectal cancers	—	9	16.6
MSKCC[33]	Resection	127	Proximal cancers, fewer metastases	1.6	—	16
		103	Rectal cancers, more metastases	—	29	9
Medicare[35]	Resection	6,469	Proximal cancers, younger age	9	—	10
	No resection	2,542	Rectal cancers	—	32	3
SEER[32]	Resection*	17,658	Proximal cancers, younger age	NR	—	Colon 11, rectum 16
	No resection	9,096	Rectal primary, older age	—	NR	Colon 2, rectum 6

*Resection group includes both initial and delayed bowel resection.
NR, not reported.

which was treated by operation in two cases and by endoluminal stenting in two cases. Three patients underwent right colectomy for abdominal pain with poor symptom relief. One patient underwent potentially curative resection after disease downstaging by chemotherapy. From this small study, it was concluded that a policy to defer resection of minimally symptomatic primary colorectal cancer is acceptable. However, it is noteworthy that 25% of the primary cancers (and 35% of the colon primaries) were ultimately resected.

Several retrospective studies have specifically examined the impact of rectal resection on patients with Stage IV rectal cancer.[37–40] The goals of radical surgery in this setting are to eliminate bleeding and obstruction, prevent local tumor progression, and prepare the patient for systemic chemotherapy. Moran et al.[37] reported that, among 95 patients undergoing rectal resection, local symptom control was excellent, and only one required subsequent reoperation for local recurrence. Longo et al.[38] reported that, among 103 patients, pelvic pain and sepsis were more common in the nonresected group (15%, 14%) than in the resected group (4%, 9%). Chu and colleagues[39] reported on 21 Stage IV patients treated by abdominoperineal resection. Perioperative morbidity (33%) and mortality (0%) were acceptable, and 20 of 21 patients had complete and durable resolution of local symptoms. Nash and colleagues[40] reported results for 80 patients treated by rectal resection without radiotherapy. There was only one perioperative death, and median hospital stay was 9 days. Only five patients developed local failure. Median survival was 25 months, with greatest survival seen in patients who received and responded to systemic chemotherapy. These studies document that surgical resection can achieve excellent palliation of local symptoms.

There are few published data evaluating the effectiveness of radiotherapy in palliative management of Stage IV rectal cancer. Crane et al.[41] reported on 55 patients who received chemoradiotherapy and 25 patients who received chemoradiotherapy followed by surgery. Both groups received systemic therapy (78% of patients). Pelvic symptom control was high (81%) in the chemoradiotherapy group, but not as high as in the chemoradiotherapy plus surgery group (91%).

There were limited data on the durability of symptom control over time.

To summarize the treatment options for Stage IV patients with unresectable metastases, treatment algorithms are shown for patients with Stage IV colon cancer (Figure 34-2) and Stage IV rectal cancer (Figure 34-3). The algorithms show multiple treatment options, reflecting the heterogeneity of disease presentation. The major variables to consider are location of the primary tumor, degree of colon/rectal obstruction, extent of metastatic disease, and fitness of the patient for surgery. For patents with nonobstructing primary tumors, upfront treatment with chemotherapy is favored because, in this era of increasingly effective chemotherapy, it is important that patients be given the full benefit of aggressive systemic therapy. However, it should be remembered that the goal of therapy is effective palliation, and surgical resection remains the most effective and durable local treatment option.

Liver Metastasis

Of the 150,000 new cases of primary colorectal cancer diagnosed in the United States each year, approximately 60% of these patients will develop liver metastases and about one-third will have disease limited to the liver.[1] Overall, it has been estimated that about 10% of all patients with colorectal liver metastases are candidates for potentially curative hepatic surgery.[42] Of those able to undergo complete hepatic resection, 25%–35% achieve long-term survival.[43] Therefore, only a small percentage of the overall number of patients with metastatic colorectal cancer are cured by liver surgery; this underlines the paramount importance of patient selection in determining optimal treatment. These statistics also highlight the fact that the majority of patients with liver metastases have unresectable disease, and require evaluation for chemotherapy or supportive care. It should be noted, however, that with improvements in chemotherapy, surgical technique, and ablative techniques, the number of patients eligible for hepatic surgery is on the rise.[44,45]

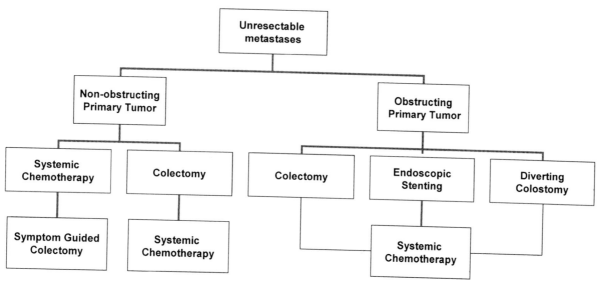

FIGURE 34-2. Treatment algorithms for patients with Stage IV colon cancer: use of palliative colon resection.

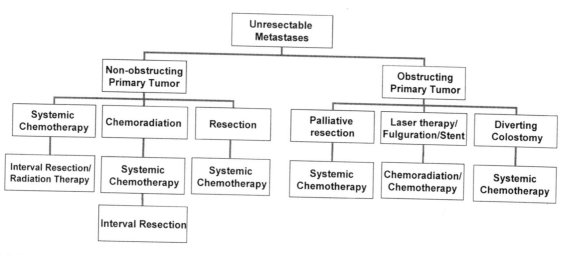

FIGURE 34-3. Treatment algorithms for patients with Stage IV rectal cancer: use of palliative rectal resection.

Natural History of Untreated Liver Metastases

To understand the impact of any therapy on outcome for patients with hepatic colorectal metastases, the natural history of untreated disease must be reviewed. This is especially relevant in understanding the impact of surgery for hepatic metastases, because there has never been a randomized trial comparing any therapy to surgery (nor is there ever likely to be). Before the 1980s, most hepatic metastases were left untreated. Several investigators have retrospectively studied untreated patients, documenting median survivals of 5–10 months; long-term survival was rarely seen.[46] The majority of these patients, however, had extensive disease, and most had their primary tumor in place, making comparison to modern surgical series irrelevant. Nonetheless, some investigators retrospectively identified patients with isolated, potentially resectable hepatic metastases who were left untreated. In these patients with limited metastases isolated to the liver, who would otherwise be potential candidates for surgery, 3-year survival was 14%–23% and 5-year survival was 2%–8%.[47,48] Whereas these studies were instrumental in demonstrating the relationship between bulk of disease and survival, they also clearly showed that, even in the best of circumstances, 5-year survival of patients with untreated liver metastases is distinctly uncommon.

Diagnosis and Patient Evaluation

In the patient who presents with liver metastases, the first consideration must be whether he or she is a potential surgical candidate, because resection remains the only potentially curative modality. A careful extent of disease workup should be initiated. First, a complete evaluation of the colon via colonoscopy should be performed within a year of presentation; this addresses the issue of synchronous and metachronous colonic neoplasms, as well as the issue of local recurrence (especially in rectal cancers). Complete cross-sectional imaging of the abdomen and pelvis with high-quality CT is also essential, to rule out extrahepatic disease. The additional advantage of routine chest CT is low compared with that of a plain chest X-ray, but should be considered in high-risk cases.[49] ^{18}F-FDG (Fluoro-deoxy-glucose) PET scanning is routinely performed because of early prospective data documenting its utility. The information obtained from PET scanning changes management decisions in patients with recurrent colorectal carcinoma 20%–50% of the time. The major strength of PET scanning seems to be the detection of occult extrahepatic disease.[18] Ongoing larger prospective studies will more clearly define the benefits of PET. A baseline serum carcinoembryonic antigen (CEA) level should also be drawn, as it is of prognostic value (see below), and serves as a baseline to follow after the conclusion of therapeutic interventions.

Once the issue of extrahepatic disease has been addressed, high-quality imaging of the liver is essential in determining bulk of disease and resectability. CT scans are the most common modality used to address liver disease and, with modern dynamic helical scanning techniques, this remains the mainstay of hepatic imaging. Routine CT scans can now evaluate the liver in combination with CT angiography or triphasic imaging of the parenchyma through various phases of intravenous contrast circulation. The most sensitive CT technique is CT portography, which is a CT scan performed after injection of contrast into the superior mesenteric artery. Because liver metastases derive their blood supply from the hepatic artery, when injected contrast enters the portal circulation, metastases appear like filling defects. Although this technique is considered the most sensitive method for evaluating the number of hepatic tumors, it often fails to define the anatomic relationships of tumor to hepatic vasculature, it requires an invasive procedure, and it is costly.[50,51] Additionally, with modern standard CT techniques, the marginal benefit is probably smaller than it once was.

Ultrasound and MRI are additional imaging techniques that can be useful in specific circumstances. Ultrasound is not an accurate method for addressing extrahepatic disease and, indeed, often cannot visualize the entire liver. However, in experienced hands, ultrasound is excellent at distinguishing neoplastic tumors from benign lesions such as cysts, focal nodular hyperplasia, or hemangiomata. Additionally, ultrasound can specifically evaluate the relationship of specific lesions to major vascular structures and the biliary tree. MRI is an excellent method for characterizing liver lesions. Particularly if there are multiple hepatic lesions, not all of which are suspected to be metastatic tumors, MRI can help distinguish malignant lesions from cysts, hemangiomata, and other benign lesions. MRI is also an excellent modality for evaluating relationships of tumor to the biliary tree (via magnetic resonance cholangiopancreatography—MRCP) and to hepatic vasculature. High-quality MRI and CT are probably equivalent for evaluating extent of liver disease, and as aids in surgical planning.[52] In any patient being considered for hepatic resection, a complete medical workup should be performed to assess the patient's fitness for undergoing a major abdominal operation. Any potential for liver dysfunction, such as alcohol abuse or chronic hepatitis, must be carefully evaluated. Pulmonary function should also be specifically evaluated, because patients undergoing major hepatectomy are at special risk for developing pulmonary complications, because of the upper abdominal transverse incision that is often necessary and the inevitable sympathetic pleural effusion. Likewise, any patient with a history of cardiac disease should be evaluated (as for any major abdominal surgery). We do not use chronologic age as a contraindication to hepatic surgery. We have previously reported that patients older than age 70 did as well as younger patients after hepatectomy.[53] This reflects careful patient selection and emphasizes the fact that physiologic age is more important than chronologic age.

Treatment Options

Chemotherapy

Until recently, chemotherapy was considered largely ineffective as treatment of unresectable metastatic colorectal cancer. However, with the development of irinotecan, oxaliplatin, hepatic arterial infusional chemotherapy with fluorodeoxyuridine (FUDR), and newer molecular-based therapies, there are now more effective chemotherapeutic options for these patients. For nearly 50 years, 5-FU was the only effective chemotherapeutic regimen for metastatic colorectal cancer. Despite many attempts to modify 5-FU with other agents, response rates generally ranged from 15% to 20%, and survival beyond 1 year was uncommon. The addition of leucovorin (5-FU/LV) and the use of infusional dosing techniques are associated with an increased response rate, and are frequently used despite no improvement in survival.[54]

Irinotecan (CPT-11) in conjunction with 5-FU/LV has been recently shown to be more effective than 5-FU/LV alone for treatment of metastatic colorectal cancer. Two randomized trials established the superiority of single-agent irinotecan over 5-FU/LV alone or best supportive care as second-line therapy.[55,56] Additionally, two randomized trials utilizing combined irinotecan/5-FU/LV as first-line chemotherapy have shown response rates of 40%, with modestly improved survival (median 15–17 months versus 12–14 months).[57,58] The addition of oxaliplatin has been particularly exciting because of the in vitro sensitivity seen in cisplatin-resistant cell lines, as well as its synergy with 5-FU.[58,59] In a trial comparing oxaliplatin/5-FU/LV (FOLFOX) to 5-FU/LV, response rates for FOLFOX were in excess of 50% (compared with 22% for 5-FU/LV). There was no difference in survival, but this is likely attributable to a 37% crossover from 5-FU/LV to FOLFOX during the trial.[60] Early analyses of comparisons of irinotecan/5-FU/LV to FOLFOX have so far shown FOLFOX to yield superior response rates.[61] Ongoing trials continue to define optimal timing, dosing, and sequence of various combination regimens. As these trials mature, and modern systemic chemotherapy regimens are refined, we are now seeing median survivals in excess of 20 months.[59,62]

Regional hepatic therapy via hepatic artery infusional (HAI) chemotherapy has been studied since the 1970s. This treatment takes advantage of the fact that hepatic metastases derive their blood supply from hepatic arterial branches.[63] Additionally, only a small proportion of systemically administered chemotherapy reaches the liver. The most frequently used agent for HAI is FUDR, which has a 90% hepatic extraction ratio. This permits maximal treatment of liver metastases and minimization of systemic side effects. However, HAI with FUDR limits treatment of occult extrahepatic disease. This can be addressed by giving additional systemic agents, or by using 5-FU via the hepatic artery with a higher "spillover" effect into the systemic circulation.

Early phase II trials of HAI FUDR or 5-FU for unresectable colorectal hepatic metastases demonstrated remarkable response rates ranging from 29% to 88%.[64-67] Subsequently, 10 randomized phase III trials comparing HAI chemotherapy to systemic chemotherapy have been completed (Table 34-2). From 1987 through 1990, five trials were done comparing HAI FUDR to intravenous FUDR or intravenous 5-FU/LV. All of these trials showed significantly increased response rates, but only trials comparing HAI chemotherapy to best supportive care showed improved survival. Most of these trials were underpowered and most allowed crossover, making conclusions about survival difficult. Two metaanalyses of the first seven trials have been performed on the assumption that each was underpowered, in an attempt to detect significant survival differences.[68,69] Both clearly confirmed the increased response rates, and both showed a modest survival benefit.

Since reporting of these seven trials, three more have been performed. The German Cooperative Group compared HAI FUDR to HAI 5-FU/LV to systemic 5-FU/LV. Response rates were significantly higher in patients receiving HAI chemotherapy (43% and 45% versus 20%), but there was no improvement in time to progression or overall survival. Similar to many of the previous trials, this study is difficult to interpret because only 70% of the HAI patients received the intended therapy and 51% of patients crossed over to other groups.[70] Another trial performed by the Medical Research

TABLE 34-2. Randomized trials comparing HAI to systemic chemotherapy for unresectable liver metastases

Study group	Year	Arms	n	Percentage receiving assigned treatment	Crossover allowed	Response rate (% CR + PR)	Median survival (mo)
MSKCC[161]	1987	HAI FUDR	48	94	Yes	50*	17
		IV FUDR	51	94		20	12
NCI[162]	1987	HAI FUDR	32	66	No	62*	17
		IV FUDR	32	92		17	12
NCOG[163]	1989	HAI FUDR	67	75	Yes	42*	17
		IV FUDR	76	86		10	16
City of Hope[164]	1990	HAI FUDR	31	100	Yes	55*	14
		IV 5-FU	10	100		20	12
NCCTG[165]	1990	HAI FUDR	39	85	No	48	13
		IV 5-FU/LV	35	100		12	11
French[166]	1992	HAI FUDR	81	87	No	44*	15*
		BSC or IV5-FU	82	50 got 5-FU		9	11
English[167]	1994	HAI FUDR	51	96	No	—	14
		BSC or IV5-FU	49	20 got 5-FU		—	8
German[70]	2000	HAI FUDR	54	69	Yes	43*	13
		HAI 5-FU/LV	57	70		45*	19
		IV 5-FU/LV	57	91		20	18
MRC/EORTC[71]	2003	HAI 5-FU/LV	95	66	No	22	15
		IV 5-FU/LV	126	87		19	15
CALGB[168]	2003	HAI FUDR	59	87	No	48*	23*
		IV 5-FU/LV	58	87		25	20

Source: Adapted from Cohen and Kemeny.[169]

Note: Response rate calculations are based on patients who received assigned treatment. Survival based on intent-to-treat calculation.

NCI, National Cancer Institute; NCOG, Northern California Oncology Group; NCCTG, North Central Cancer Treatment Group; MRC/EORTC, Medical Research Group/European Organization for Research and Treatment of Cancer; CR, complete response; PR, partial response.

*Statistically significant (P < .05)

Council and the European Organization for the Research and Treatment of Cancer compared HAI 5-FU/LV with systemic 5-FU/LV. This trial did not allow crossover, and showed similar response rates, time to progression, and overall survival. Again, only 66% of those patients assigned to HAI chemotherapy received the assigned therapy; additionally, HAI chemotherapy was with 5-FU rather than FUDR.[71] A Cancer and Leukemia Group B (CALGB) trial comparing HAI FUDR to systemic 5-FU/LV without crossover has recently been completed. Response rates were demonstrated to be significantly higher with HAI FUDR (48% versus 25%), as was overall survival (22.7 months versus 19.8 months).[72]

One of the major lessons learned from trials evaluating HAI chemotherapy was that, although control of hepatic disease was excellent, there was significant extrahepatic failure. Currently, with the explosion of new active systemic agents, a new paradigm has developed in the treatment of hepatic colorectal metastases. Many phase I and II trials are now evaluating combinations of HAI FUDR with systemically administered 5-FU/LV with irinotecan and/or oxaliplatin. Even in pretreated patients, impressive response rates in excess of 80% are being seen.[73] Although recent advances in cytotoxic chemotherapy for colorectal cancer over the last decade have been very exciting, the development of targeted molecular-based therapy provides even greater hope for more effective systemic treatments. Studies continue to focus on immune-based therapy including vaccines, monoclonal antibodies, and immunotoxins. Anti-angiogenic therapy with anti–vascular endothelial growth factor antibodies (bevacizumab) are also currently being evaluated. Inhibitors of the receptor for epidermal growth factor, a tyrosine kinase receptor, has also shown promising results, and drugs such as cetuximab (C225), ZD1839 (Iressa), and OSI774 (Tarceva) are actively being studied. Results of current clinical trials are anxiously awaited to see where these molecular-based targeted therapies will ultimately fit in among the armamentarium of systemic therapy for colorectal cancer.[62]

Resection

As described above, it is clear that patients with untreated hepatic colorectal metastases have poor survival. Although response rates to chemotherapeutic regimens are improving, the only therapy ever shown to be potentially curative for hepatic colorectal metastases is complete resection. When surgeons began attempting resections for metastatic colorectal cancer they were met with some skepticism.[74] The concept of treating what is generally acknowledged to be a "systemic" problem with "locoregional" therapy was certainly questionable. Additionally, liver resection performed in the 1970s and 1980s was associated with high morbidity and mortality, making its role in the treatment of advanced cancer suspect at that time.[75] Over the last 20 years, however, large series have demonstrated that liver surgery can now be practiced with acceptable safety, and that patients with isolated and resectable hepatic metastases have the potential for long-term survival.

In modern series, mortality rates for hepatectomy for metastatic colorectal cancer are uniformly 5% or less (Table 34-3). Nonetheless, morbidity for these operations remains substantial, and is usually reported between 20% and 50%. Fortunately, this morbidity does not generally translate into long hospital stays, intensive care unit stays, long-term disability, or early mortality. The most ominous complications, such as liver failure and significant hemorrhage, are now distinctly uncommon, thanks to better surgical technique and postoperative care. A recent review of more than 1800 liver resections (57% of a lobe or greater) over the last decade at our institution found that the median hospital stay was 8 days, morbidity was 45%, and mortality was 3%. Furthermore, of the 1245 hepatectomies performed for metastatic disease, mortality was 2.4%.[76]

Liver resection for metastatic colorectal cancer was performed sporadically in the 1970s, but was an unproven and suspect therapy. Dr. James Foster traveled to medical centers in the United States recording outcomes in patients undergoing

TABLE 34-3. Surgical series of hepatectomy for metastatic colorectal cancer with 100 or more patients

Author	No. of patients	Operative mortality (%)	1-y survival (%)	5-y survival (%)	10-y survival (%)	Median survival (mo)
Adson et al.[170]	141	2	82	25	—	24
Hughes et al.[171]	607	—	—	33	—	32
Schlag et al.[82]	122	4	85	30	—	28
Doci et al.[80]	100	5	—	30	—	33
Gayowski et al.[172]	204	0	91	32	—	40
Scheele et al.[173]	469	4	83	33	20	40
Fong et al.[174]	577	4	85	35	—	33
Jenkins et al.[175]	131	4	81	25	—	—
Rees et al.[176]	150	1	94	37	—	33
Jamison et al.[177]	280	4	84	27	20	42
Fong et al.[84]	1001	3	89	37	22	37
Minagawa et al.[178]	235	0	—	35	26	—
Figueras et al.[179]	235	4	87	36	—	46
Choti et al.[180]	226	1	—	40	26	40
Laurent et al.[181]	311	3	86	36	—	—

hepatectomy for colorectal metastases and, for the first time, documented 5-year survival rates of 25%.[77] Major institutional and multi-institutional reviews of patients undergoing hepatectomy for metastatic colorectal cancer have now clearly documented that, in well-selected patients, 5-year survival ranges from 25% to 40%, 10-year survival ranges from 20% to 26%, and median survivals range from 24 to 46 months (Table 34-4). These results obviously compare favorably to the results of no treatment (median survival 5–10 months) and to those of chemotherapy (median survival 10–14 months). Despite recent improvements in chemotherapy resulting in median survivals as high as 20 months (see above), complete resection still provides the best outcomes. True long-term cure from chemotherapy is extraordinarily rare, whereas at least half of the long-term survivors after liver resection are disease-free and presumably cured.[78] For these reasons, no trial has ever compared hepatectomy to no treatment or chemotherapy alone. Liver resection for resectable hepatic colorectal metastases is the treatment of choice.

Many studies of patients undergoing liver resection for isolated hepatic metastases have evaluated prognostic factors to help select those patients most likely to benefit from hepatectomy and, conversely, to identify those unlikely to benefit. The two most consistent negative prognostic factors are the presence of extrahepatic disease and the inability to resect all tumor; these two factors remain contraindications to hepatectomy. The exception to this rule is the patient with limited pulmonary metastases or colonic anastomotic recurrence, who may undergo combined resections with some success.[42] Although there are many inconsistencies in the major reported series, a list of other poor prognostic factors exist; these include lymph nodes involved by the primary colorectal tumor, synchronous presentation [or shorter disease-free interval (DFI)], larger number of tumors, bilobar involvement, CEA elevation greater than 200 ng/mL, and involved histologic margins.[79–83] Although it seems to be true that the stage of the primary tumor, the interval in which metastatic disease has developed, and the bulk of tumor in the liver (measured by size, number, and/or CEA level) can provide prognostic information on outcome after hepatectomy, none of these findings in and of themselves preclude the potential for long-term survival. We recently published a multivariate

analysis of 1001 patients who underwent potentially curative hepatectomy, and identified five factors as having the most influence on outcome.[84] These included size greater than 5 cm, DFI of less than 1 year, more than one tumor, lymph node-positive primary, and CEA greater than 200 ng/mL. Utilizing these five factors, we have developed a risk score predictive of recurrence after liver resection (Table 34-4).

Recurrence after hepatectomy for colorectal metastases is common, occurring in more than two-thirds of patients. In fact, long-term survival does not necessarily imply that there has been no recurrence. In a study of 96 actual 5-year survivors, nearly half had experienced a recurrence at some point and received further therapy.[78] In patients who do recur, the liver is the most common site of recurrence and is involved approximately 45% of the time. Most of these recurrences are isolated to the liver. Other common sites are lung, bone, and various intraabdominal sites.[85] Because many recurrences are isolated to the liver, repeat liver resection has been attempted by several surgeons with some success. Unfortunately, only 5%–10% of patients are candidates for a second liver resection, underscoring the importance of patient selection. Currently, at least 14 series reporting on more than 700 patients have documented that repeat hepatectomy for metastatic colorectal cancer is safe and effective in well-selected patients. Mortality is less than 5%, median survival from the time of the second liver resection ranges from 23 to 46 months, and 5-year survival ranges from 30% to 41%.[86] The factors most often associated with a poor outcome after repeat hepatectomy are size and number of tumors, as well as short DFI. Because of the potential for further effective therapeutic interventions after primary liver resection, patients eligible for such treatment should be followed with serial CEA and imaging studies to detect recurrences at an early and potentially treatable phase.

Because recurrence after hepatectomy for metastatic colorectal cancer is common, there is a sound rationale for use of adjuvant therapy. Indeed, adjuvant 5-FU-based systemic chemotherapy after liver resection was often given, but its use was not supported by prospective trials. A number of retrospective comparisons have been performed, but no definitive published data support the routine use of adjuvant postoperative 5-FU-based systemic chemotherapy. The effect of newer,

TABLE 34-4. Clinical risk score* and survival in 1001 patients undergoing liver resection for metastatic colorectal cancer

Score	1-y survival (%)	3-y survival (%)	5-y survival (%)	Median survival (mo)
0	93	72	60	74
1	91	66	44	51
2	89	60	40	47
3	86	42	20	33
4	70	38	25	20
5	71	27	14	22

Source: Adapted from Fong et al.[84]

*Each of the following five risk factors equals one point: node positive primary, DFI <12 mo, >1 tumor, size >5 cm, CEA >200 ng/mL. Score is total number of points in an individual patient.

more effective chemotherapeutic regimens on long-term survival after hepatectomy is not known, but is promising.

Because hepatic metastases derive their blood supply from the hepatic artery and the most common site of recurrence after hepatectomy is within the remnant liver, there is a strong argument for the use of HAI chemotherapy. Three randomized trials have addressed the efficacy of adjuvant HAI chemotherapy. In the German Cooperative multicenter study, HAI 5-FU/LV was compared with no treatment after hepatectomy. No significant differences in outcome were found; however, many patients in the HAI arm did not receive therapy, and 5-FU is not considered the optimal therapeutic for HAI chemotherapy.[87] In the recently published Intergroup study, adjuvant HAI FUDR combined with systemic 5-FU was compared with no treatment. A significant improvement in survival (46% versus 25% 4-year survival, $P = .04$) was demonstrated only when analyzed by actual treatment received. There was no significant difference in outcome when analyzed in an intent-to-treat manner.[88] The third trial, performed at Memorial Sloan-Kettering Cancer Center (MSKCC), compared systemic 5-FU/LV to systemic 5-FU/LV combined with HAI FUDR. Ninety-two percent of patients received therapy as assigned, and there was a significant improvement in 2-year survival (the primary endpoint) favoring the addition of HAI FUDR (86% versus 72%).[89]

Given the growing number of chemotherapeutic options for patients with metastatic colorectal cancer, there are many options for the patient who has had all of his or her liver metastases resected. Because HAI FUDR combined with systemic 5-FU/LV is the only therapy ever shown to improve survival in this setting, there is a strong argument for the use of this modality; however, the surgeon and medical oncologist need to have experience with pump implantation and management. With the advent of more effective systemic chemotherapy, such as irinotecan and oxaliplatin, as well as molecular targeted agents, new trials are needed to assess optimal adjuvant therapy.

Because the majority of patients with hepatic colorectal metastases are technically unresectable, the development of more effective chemotherapy has inspired many oncologists to use a "neoadjuvant" chemotherapy strategy in an attempt to render patients resectable. In a series from France, 701 patients with unresectable liver metastases received chronomodulated 5-FU/LV and oxaliplatin. Ninety-five (14%) of these patients became resectable, secondary to chemotherapeutic response, and underwent staged resection. The resections used techniques such as portal vein embolization and intraoperative ablation to extirpate all tumor, and achieved an actuarial 5-year survival rate of 35%.[44] Another study analyzed 23 previously treated patients with unresectable liver metastases. HAI FUDR was administered, and six patients (26%) were ultimately able to undergo an R0 resection.[45] These early studies suggest that patients with unresectable liver metastases should be treated aggressively with chemotherapy and reevaluated at intervals for the possibility of resection.

Although resection has become the gold standard for treatment of liver metastases, other methods of tumor destruction using thermal ablation techniques have also been developed. Cryotherapy has been used for decades, and utilizes probes to freeze tumors and surrounding normal hepatic parenchyma. Cryotherapy generally requires a laparotomy, and complications such as bleeding, liver cracking, and a cryoshock phenomena characterized by thrombocytopenia and disseminated intravascular coagulation can occur. More recently, radiofrequency ablation (RFA) probes have been developed that can heat liver tumors and a surrounding margin of tissue to create coagulation necrosis. RFA can be used percutaneously, laparoscopically, and at laparotomy under ultrasound, CT, or MRI guidance. Furthermore, RFA has low morbidity that generally ranges around 10% and is rarely serious. Although RFA can be used near blood vessels, because the heat-sink effect of blood flow protects the endothelium, major bile ducts can be seriously injured, limiting the use of RFA in central tumors situated near major bile ducts. Local recurrence after RFA is a significant problem, and seems to be strongly correlated with tumor size. Generally, recurrence is more common in tumors greater than 4 or 5 cm in diameter and in tumors abutting major blood vessels. With improvements in localization and monitoring of thermal application, however, these therapies are very promising alternatives to surgery. Perhaps the greatest application of ablative techniques will be in their use as additions to resection in patients with multiple bilobar tumors. Ongoing studies are currently evaluating these strategies.[90,91]

Lung Metastasis

It has been estimated that approximately 10% of patients with colorectal cancer will develop lung metastasis. Of these, only 10% will have metastases isolated to the lung; and of those patients with isolated lung metastases, only a small proportion (probably another 10%) will be considered candidates for pulmonary metastasectomy.[92] These estimates demonstrate that the majority of patients with metastatic colorectal cancer to the lung have advanced disease, and are thus treated with systemic chemotherapy or best supportive care. Few patients will be candidates for metastasectomy; this tiny proportion reflects extremely careful patient selection.

Data on the results of metastasectomy for colorectal lung metastases are inherently flawed because they have been retrospectively collected over long periods of time, and mostly reflect patient selection and tumor biology. There are no adequate control groups to compare survival; therefore, survival statistics are difficult to interpret. However, some patients who undergo pulmonary metastasectomy are cured, and long-term survival without complete resection is very rare, suggesting that patients do occasionally benefit.

Modern series of lung resection for metastatic colorectal cancer uniformly report operative mortalities of less than 2% (Table 34-5). Five-year survival rates range from 16% to 64%, but generally cluster around 30% to 40%. Most studies evaluate factors associated with outcome; however, given the limited number of cases, the statistical power of these studies to

TABLE 34-5. Outcome of patients undergoing pulmonary metastasectomy for colorectal cancer

Author	n	Operative mortality (%)	5-y survival (%)	Significant risk factors
Mori et al.[182]	35	—	38	None found
McCormack et al.[183]	144	0	44	Margin
McAfee et al.[93]	139	1	31	No. of lesions, CEA
Yano et al.[184]	27	—	41	No. of lesions
Saclarides et al.[185]	23	—	16	No. of lesions
van Halteren et al.[186]	38	—	43	DFI
Shirouzu et al.[187]	22	—	37	No. of lesions, size
Girard et al.[188]	86	1	24	CEA, margin
Okumura et al.[189]	159	2	41	No. of lesions, LN status
Zanella et al.[190]	22	0	62	None found
Zink et al.[191]	110	0	33	Size, CEA

Source: Adapted from Rizk and Downey.[96]
LN, lymph nodes.

detect significant factors is limited. Generally, the pathology of the primary tumor (grade, location, stage) has not been associated with outcome. The most frequently cited significant factors associated with adverse outcome are number and size of lung tumors, short DFI, increased CEA, and incomplete resection.

Although the majority of series evaluate disease limited to the lungs, several series have evaluated patients with both liver and lung metastases. Some authors advocate resection of synchronous limited extrapulmonary disease,[93] but the majority of studies that have analyzed synchronous liver and lung metastases report a uniformly poor outcome after combined resections. Long-term survival is very uncommon in this situation.[94,95] In the setting of isolated pulmonary recurrence after potentially curative partial hepatectomy, outcomes for pulmonary metastasectomy are more favorable and are similar to those for the initial hepatectomy.[94–96]

The surgical approach to patients who are potential candidates for pulmonary metastasectomy has been somewhat controversial. Based on older studies reported in the 1980s citing a 38% yield of contralateral thoracotomy in finding radiographically occult disease, routine bilateral thoracotomy had been advocated.[97] With modern-day CT, such an approach is not justified; indeed, the majority of surgeons perform pulmonary metastasectomy through a unilateral standard thoracotomy. The use of video-assisted thoracoscopic surgery (VATS) has increased in recent years, and is often used in metastasectomy when a minimal parenchymal resection is necessary. One problem with VATS is its inability to palpate the lung parenchyma; a prospective study evaluating confirmatory thoracotomy after VATS showed that 22% of lesions can be missed.[98] However, with improvements in radiology and VATS technique, a minimally invasive approach can be justified.

Peritoneal Metastasis

The peritoneal surface is involved in approximately 10%–15% of patients with colorectal cancer at time of initial presentation (synchronous metastases) and in 20%–50% of patients who develop recurrence (metachronous metastases).[99–102] As a site of colorectal cancer metastasis, the peritoneal surface ranks second only to the liver. Peritoneal metastasis occurs by direct implantation of cancer cells via one of four mechanisms: 1) spontaneous intraperitoneal (IP) seeding from a T4 colorectal cancer that has penetrated the serosal surface of the colon[103]; 2) extravasation of tumor cells at the time of colon perforation from an obstructing cancer; 3) iatrogenic tumor perforation through an area of serosal injury or enterotomy at the time of colon resection; 4) leakage of tumor cells from transected lymphatics or veins at the time of colon resection.[104] The risk of peritoneal metastasis is therefore highest in the setting of locally advanced cancers.

Peritoneal metastases are clinically important because of their frequent progression to malignant ascites and/or malignant bowel obstruction. In a French multicenter prospective study to assess the natural history of peritoneal carcinomatosis, 118 patients with T3 or T4 colorectal cancers were among the 370 study patients with nongynecologic malignancies.[105] Synchronous peritoneal carcinomatosis was found in 58.5% of the patients with colorectal cancer. The most frequent symptoms were ascites (29.7%) and bowel obstruction (19.5%).

Preoperative detection of peritoneal metastases is not reliable. Noninvasive imaging frequently misses small peritoneal lesions, even when these are widely disseminated. The sensitivity of CT scanning for lesions smaller than 5 mm is only 28%, as compared with 70% for lesions 2 cm or greater.[106] Thus, indirect signs such as bulky primary tumor, ascites, or bowel obstruction are important clues.

The extent of carcinomatosis is a major prognostic factor, and is best assessed by either laparoscopic or open exploration. Two different peritoneal carcinomatosis staging systems (Gilly's classification and Peritoneal Cancer Index of Sugarbaker) can be used to assess the extent of carcinomatosis.[107,108] These staging systems have both shown utility in determining the prognosis and treatment of patients with peritoneal carcinomatosis. By Gilly's classification, carcinomatosis is classified principally by the dimensions of the peritoneal tumor implants: Stage I, tumor nodules <5 mm in diameter localized in one part of the abdomen; Stage II, tumor nodules <5mm disseminated widely through the abdomen; Stage III, tumor nodules 5 mm to 2 cm in diameter; Stage IV, tumor nodules >2 cm. The Peritoneal Cancer Index scores the extent of carcinomatosis on the basis of tumor size and location within 13 regions of the abdomen and pelvis. The lesion with the largest size in each abdominopelvic region is scored on a scale of 0–3 (0, no tumor; 1, tumor up to 0.5 cm; 2, tumor up to 5.0 cm; 3, >5 cm or confluence). The total score of the Peritoneal Cancer Index can vary from 0 to 39. The Peritoneal Cancer Index is shown to correlate with survival. Median survival and 5-year survival after surgical debulking and IP chemotherapy were 48 months and 50% for peritoneal index <10, compared with 12 months and 0% for index >20.[109]

Standard management of patients known to have peritoneal metastases at initial presentation is systemic chemotherapy. Colon resection has an important role for patients with obstructing primary cancers, and also for patients with occult metastases that are first detected in the operating room. Historically, the median survival for patients with unresected peritoneal metastasis treated with 5-FU-based systemic chemotherapy was very poor (6–8 months).[102,105,110] However, patient survival is highly variable, depending on the extent of metastatic disease and response to chemotherapy.[111,112] Contemporary combination chemotherapy regimens have significantly greater efficacy, and can produce long periods of disease control in certain patients.[6]

In the past decade, a more aggressive treatment approach utilizing cytoreductive surgery and IP chemotherapy has been pioneered by Sugarbaker.[113] The goal of cytoreductive surgery is to remove all macroscopic disease with peritonectomy procedures and visceral resections. Perioperative IP chemotherapy is then used to destroy residual microscopic disease. IP delivery offers a pharmacokinetic advantage over standard intravenous delivery by producing high regional concentrations of drug while simultaneously minimizing systemic toxicities.[114,115] The most widely reported method of IP chemotherapy is intraoperative delivery of mitomycin in a hyperthermic (41C) circuit for 90 minutes.[116] An alternative approach is postoperative infusion of FUDR via an implanted IP catheter.[117]

Although few prospective trials have been completed for colorectal carcinomatosis, the available evidence suggests a survival benefit for cytoreductive surgery and IP chemotherapy. Phase II studies report 5-year survival rates ranging between 19% and 28%.[117,118] The most consistent and important prognostic factor in these studies is the ability to achieve complete resection of all gross disease. Five-year survival rates reported for patients with completely resected disease range from 27% to 54%.[117,119]

A phase III study conducted by the Netherlands Cancer Institute randomized 105 colorectal cancer patients with peritoneal carcinomatosis to either standard treatment (systemic 5-FU/LV with or without palliative colectomy) or experimental therapy (aggressive cytoreductive surgery, hyperthermic IP mitomycin, and systemic 5-FU/LV).[120] In the experimental arm, median operation time was 585 minutes, treatment toxicity was high, and treatment-related mortality was 8%. After a median follow-up of 22 months, median survival was 12.6 months in the standard therapy arm and 22.3 months in the experimental therapy arm. It is not known if the survival benefit observed in the experimental therapy arm is attributable to surgical debulking, IP chemotherapy, or both.

In summary, the standard therapy for patients with peritoneal metastases is systemic chemotherapy. However, there is evidence that aggressive surgical cytoreduction and IP chemotherapy will benefit patients with limited peritoneal tumor burden. Additional clinical trials are needed to define optimal use of this aggressive treatment approach.

Ovarian Metastasis

Approximately 7%–30% of ovarian neoplasms are metastatic cancers, the most common being colorectal and breast cancer.[121–124] In approximately 1%–7% of all women with primary colorectal cancer, ovarian metastases are discovered either at the time of colon surgery or during follow-up.[125–127] However, the risk of developing ovarian metastasis is substantially higher in woman with Stage IV disease, and approaches 90% in women with established peritoneal metastases. In addition, women with adenocarcinoma of the vermiform appendix have a very high risk of ovarian metastasis. Thus, in a woman with recent diagnosis of advanced colorectal cancer, any ovarian mass should be considered a metastasis from colorectal cancer until proven otherwise.

The pathogenesis of colorectal cancer ovarian metastasis is variable. Metastatic spread occurs primarily through the peritoneum, but can also occur via the blood stream, through lymphatic vessels, or by direct extension. Careful intraoperative assessment of the ovaries at the time of colon cancer surgery is essential. Synchronous metastases occur in 0%–8.6% of patients in various clinical studies,[128–132] whereas metachronous metastases develop in 1.4%–6.8% of colorectal cancer cases,[126,127,133,134] usually within 2 years after the primary resection.[129,135,136] Most often these metastatic lesions are large, and at least half of the cases have bilateral ovarian involvement.[136,137] Approximately 40% of these patients also have associated extraovarian pelvic metastasis.[136] Distinguishing a metastatic colorectal cancer from primary ovarian tumor is difficult by gross assessment alone, but a correct diagnosis can generally be determined through integration of clinicopathologic, immunohistochemical, and cytogenetic features. Most metastatic colorectal lesions are CK20+/CEA+/CK7− on staining, whereas primary ovarian neoplasms are CK20−/CEA−/CK7+.[138–141]

Clinical studies attempting to document the benefit of ovarian metastasectomy in patients with colorectal cancer are small and retrospective.[126,127,142,143] Although generally asymptomatic when first detected in the operating room or on

CT scan, ovarian metastases can compress or invade adjacent organs (ureter, bladder, bowel), rupture, and on rare occasions bleed. Survival of women with synchronous ovarian colorectal metastases is significantly worse than that of patients without such metastases.[126,144] In addition, ovarian metastases are frequently resistant to systemic chemotherapy even when other sites of metastatic disease are responding. Therefore, resection of synchronous ovarian metastases should be performed when encountered in the operating room. Bilateral oophorectomy and complete resection of gross disease is recommended. Reoperation for metachronous metastases should be considered in selected patients with good performance status and limited tumor burden elsewhere. The goal of metastasectomy is to prevent local tumor progression. Therefore, an aggressive surgical approach should be undertaken to achieve complete resection when possible, especially if disease is confined to the pelvis. The survival benefit of removing ovarian metastases has never been well documented. Complete metastasectomy is associated with significantly better outcome when compared with palliative debulking, especially in the setting of metastatic disease confined to the pelvis only. However, complete resection is only possible in 50% of these cases. For women with isolated ovarian metastases, median postresection survival is 18 months.[145] Women with other sites of disease have shorter survival, however, and 5-year survival after resection of established ovarian metastases is rare.[146,147] Although postresection chemotherapy with 5-FU was considered ineffective in studies done in the 1970s and 1980s, systemic chemotherapy should be strongly considered, particularly when residual disease is present. With the availability of stronger chemotherapeutic regimens containing oxaliplatin, irinotecan, and/or bevacizumab, better survival can be expected.[6,57,59,61]

The role of prophylactic oophorectomy in the absence of macroscopic disease is not well defined. Several clinical studies have failed to show a survival advantage, although the majority of evaluated patients were postmenopausal.[128,129,148,149] A randomized, prospective study comparing prophylactic oophorectomy versus no oophorectomy in Stage II or III colorectal cancer demonstrated an improvement in 5-year disease-free survival for the oophorectomy group (80%) compared with no oophorectomy (65%), but the benefit was not statistically significant ($P = .16$).[149] Some justification and benefits for prophylactic oophorectomy can be found in retrospective studies.[150–152] These studies have shown reduction in the incidence of ovarian carcinoma, resection of synchronous microscopic ovarian metastases, and prevention of metachronous ovarian metastases in the future. Based on the available data, it is reasonable to offer prophylactic oophorectomy to all postmenopausal patients. For premenopausal patients, only those with established peritoneal metastases, those with a clearly increased risk of developing ovarian carcinoma (strong family history, known carriers of breast cancer [BRCA] or hereditary nonpolyposis colorectal cancer [HNPCC] mutation), or those who have already completed their families should be considered for prophylactic oophorectomy.

Bone and Brain Metastases

Bone metastases from colorectal cancer reportedly occur in 7%–9% of cases, and most often present in the context of widespread metastatic disease.[153–155] Routine diagnostic bone imaging is not indicated in colorectal cancer patients, however, unless there are specific bone-related symptoms. There are no curative modalities, but palliation of pain, fractures, or spinal cord involvement are important issues for these patients. Symptomatic relief from bony metastases can usually be accomplished with radiation and medical therapy. However, pathologic fractures are best treated by operative internal fixation. The systemic issues related to bone metastases are serious and include debilitation, immobility, hypercalcemia, and thromboembolic disease.

Cerebral metastases from colorectal cancer are uncommon, occurring in 1%–4% of colorectal cancer cases.[156,157] Colorectal tumors account for approximately 3% of all metastatic brain tumors.[158] These are generally found in the context of widespread metastases to multiple organ sites, but on rare occasion can present as an isolated brain metastasis. There is no role for routine brain imaging at primary presentation or at presentation with metastases elsewhere, unless there are specific neurologic symptoms. Once brain metastases occur, symptoms are common; palliative therapies include steroids to decrease swelling and anticonvulsants to control seizures. Definitive therapy of colorectal brain metastases usually involves surgery, radiation, or a combination of the two. For isolated, single brain metastases, resection can result in survival beyond 1–2 years.[159,160]

References

1. Jemal A, Murray T, Ward E, et al. Cancer statistics, 2005. CA Cancer J Clin 2005;55(1):10–30.
2. O'Connell JB, Maggard MA, Ko CY. Colon cancer survival rates with the new American Joint Committee on Cancer sixth edition staging. J Natl Cancer Inst 2004;96(19):1420–1425.
3. Expectancy or primary chemotherapy in patients with advanced asymptomatic colorectal cancer: a randomized trial. Nordic Gastrointestinal Tumor Adjuvant Therapy Group. J Clin Oncol 1992;10(6):904–911.
4. Scheithauer W, Rosen H, Kornek GV, Sebesta C, Depisch D. Randomised comparison of combination chemotherapy plus supportive care with supportive care alone in patients with metastatic colorectal cancer. BMJ 1993;306(6880):752–755.
5. Tournigand C, Andre T, Achille E, et al. FOLFIRI followed by FOLFOX6 or the reverse sequence in advanced colorectal cancer: a randomized GERCOR study. J Clin Oncol 2004;22(2):229–237.
6. Hurwitz H, Fehrenbacher L, Novotny W, et al. Bevacizumab plus irinotecan, fluorouracil, and leucovorin for metastatic colorectal cancer. N Engl J Med 2004;350(23):2335–2342.

7. Hanahan D, Weinberg RA. The hallmarks of cancer. Cell 2000;100(1):57–70.

8. Fidler IJ. Critical determinants of metastasis. Semin Cancer Biol 2002;12(2):89–96.

9. Woodhouse EC, Chuaqui RF, Liotta LA. General mechanisms of metastasis. Cancer 1997;80(8 suppl):1529–1537.

10. Fidler IJ. Critical factors in the biology of human cancer metastasis: twenty-eighth G.H.A. Clowes memorial award lecture. Cancer Res 1990;50(19):6130–6138.

11. Folkman J. How is blood vessel growth regulated in normal and neoplastic tissue? G.H.A. Clowes memorial award lecture. Cancer Res 1986;46(2):467–473.

12. Hynes RO. Metastatic potential: generic predisposition of the primary tumor or rare, metastatic variants—or both? Cell 2003;113(7):821–823.

13. Bogenrieder T, Herlyn M. Axis of evil: molecular mechanisms of cancer metastasis. Oncogene 2003;22(42):6524–6536.

14. Chambers AF, Groom AC, MacDonald IC. Dissemination and growth of cancer cells in metastatic sites. Nat Rev Cancer 2002;2(8):563–572.

15. Al-Mehdi AB, Tozawa K, Fisher AB, Shientag L, Lee A, Muschel RJ. Intravascular origin of metastasis from the proliferation of endothelium-attached tumor cells: a new model for metastasis. Nat Med 2000;6(1):100–102.

16. Chambers AF, Naumov GN, Varghese HJ, Nadkarni KV, MacDonald IC, Groom AC. Critical steps in hematogenous metastasis: an overview. Surg Oncol Clin North Am 2001; 10(2):243–255, vii.

17. Shevde LA, Welch DR. Metastasis suppressor pathways: an evolving paradigm. Cancer Lett 2003;198(1):1–20.

18. Chin BB, Wahl RL. 18F-Fluoro-2-deoxyglucose positron emission tomography in the evaluation of gastrointestinal malignancies. Gut 2003;52(suppl 4):iv23–29.

19. Deans GT, Krukowski ZH, Irwin ST. Malignant obstruction of the left colon. Br J Surg 1994;81(9):1270–1276.

20. Phillips RK, Hittinger R, Fry JS, Fielding LP. Malignant large bowel obstruction. Br J Surg 1985;72(4):296–302.

21. Gandrup P, Lund L, Balslev I. Surgical treatment of acute malignant large bowel obstruction. Eur J Surg 1992;158(8):427–430.

22. Loizou LA, Grigg D, Boulos PB, Bown SG. Endoscopic Nd:YAG laser treatment of rectosigmoid cancer. Gut 1990; 31(7):812–816.

23. Daneker GW Jr, Carlson GW, Hohn DC, Lynch P, Roubein L, Levin B. Endoscopic laser recanalization is effective for prevention and treatment of obstruction in sigmoid and rectal cancer. Arch Surg 1991;126(11):1348–1352.

24. Mandava N, Petrelli N, Herrera L, Nava H. Laser palliation for colorectal carcinoma. Am J Surg 1991;162(3):212–214; discussion 215.

25. Brunetaud JM, Maunoury V, Cochelard D. Lasers in rectosigmoid tumors. Semin Surg Oncol 1995;11(4):319–327.

26. Gevers AM, Macken E, Hiele M, Rutgeerts P. Endoscopic laser therapy for palliation of patients with distal colorectal carcinoma: analysis of factors influencing long-term outcome. Gastrointest Endosc 2000;51(5):580–585.

27. Salvati EP, Rubin RJ, Eisenstat TE, Siemons GO, Mangione JS. Electrocoagulation of selected carcinoma of the rectum. Surg Gynecol Obstet 1988;166(5):393–396.

28. Eisenstat TE, Oliver GC. Electrocoagulation for adenocarcinoma of the low rectum. World J Surg 1992;16(3):458–462.

29. Camunez F, Echenagusia A, Simo G, Turegano F, Vazquez J, Barreiro-Meiro I. Malignant colorectal obstruction treated by means of self-expanding metallic stents: effectiveness before surgery and in palliation. Radiology 2000;216(2):492–497.

30. Law WL, Choi HK, Lee YM, Chu KW. Palliation for advanced malignant colorectal obstruction by self-expanding metallic stents: prospective evaluation of outcomes. Dis Colon Rectum 2004;47(1):39–43.

31. Rosen SA, Buell JF, Yoshida A, et al. Initial presentation with stage IV colorectal cancer: how aggressive should we be? Arch Surg 2000;135(5):530–534; discussion 534–535.

32. Cook AD, Single R, McCahill LE. Surgical resection of primary tumors in patients who present with stage IV colorectal cancer: an analysis of surveillance, epidemiology, and end results data, 1988 to 2000. Ann Surg Oncol 2005;12(8): 637–645.

33. Ruo L, Gougoutas C, Paty PB, Guillem JG, Cohen AM, Wong WD. Elective bowel resection for incurable stage IV colorectal cancer: prognostic variables for asymptomatic patients. J Am Coll Surg 2003;196(5):722–728.

34. Scoggins CR, Meszoely IM, Blanke CD, Beauchamp RD, Leach SD. Nonoperative management of primary colorectal cancer in patients with stage IV disease. Ann Surg Oncol 1999;6(7):651–657.

35. Temple LK, Hsieh L, Wong WD, Saltz L, Schrag D. Use of surgery among elderly patients with stage IV colorectal cancer. J Clin Oncol 2004;22(17):3475–3484.

36. Sarela AI, Guthrie JA, Seymour MT, Ride E, Guillou PJ, O'Riordain DS. Non-operative management of the primary tumour in patients with incurable stage IV colorectal cancer. Br J Surg 2001;88(10):1352–1356.

37. Moran MR, Rothenberger DA, Lahr CJ, Buls JG, Goldberg SM. Palliation for rectal cancer. Resection? Anastomosis? Arch Surg 1987;122(6):640–643.

38. Longo WE, Ballantyne GH, Bilchik AJ, Modlin IM. Advanced rectal cancer. What is the best palliation? Dis Colon Rectum 1988;31(11):842–847.

39. Chu QD, Davidson RS, Rodriguez-Bigas MA, Wirtzfeld DA, Petrelli NJ. Is abdominoperineal resection a good option for stage IV adenocarcinoma of the distal rectum? J Surg Oncol 2002;81(1):3–7.

40. Nash GM, Saltz LB, Kemeny NE, et al. Radical resection of rectal cancer primary tumor provides effective local therapy in patients with stage IV disease. Ann Surg Oncol 2002;9(10): 954–960.

41. Crane CH, Janjan NA, Abbruzzese JL, et al. Effective pelvic symptom control using initial chemoradiation without colostomy in metastatic rectal cancer. Int J Radiat Oncol Biol Phys 2001;49(1):107–116.

42. McCarter MD, Fong Y. Metastatic liver tumors. Semin Surg Oncol 2000;19(2):177–188.

43. Fong Y. Surgical therapy of hepatic colorectal metastasis. CA Cancer J Clin 1999;49(4):231–255.

44. Adam R, Avisar E, Ariche A, et al. Five-year survival following hepatic resection after neoadjuvant therapy for nonresectable colorectal. Ann Surg Oncol 2001;8(4):347–353.

45. Clavien PA, Selzner N, Morse M, Selzner M, Paulson E. Downstaging of hepatocellular carcinoma and liver metastases from colorectal cancer by selective intra-arterial chemotherapy. Surgery 2002;131(4):433–442.

46. Blumgart LH, Fong Y. Surgical options in the treatment of hepatic metastasis from colorectal cancer. Curr Probl Surg 1995;32(5):333–421.

47. Wagner JS, Adson MA, Van Heerden JA, Adson MH, Ilstrup DM. The natural history of hepatic metastases from colorectal cancer. A comparison with resective treatment. Ann Surg 1984;199(5):502–508.

48. Wood CB, Gillis CR, Blumgart LH. A retrospective study of the natural history of patients with liver metastases from colorectal cancer. Clin Oncol 1976;2(3):285–288.

49. Kronawitter U, Kemeny NE, Heelan R, Fata F, Fong Y. Evaluation of chest computed tomography in the staging of patients with potentially resectable liver metastases from colorectal carcinoma. Cancer 1999;86(2):229–235.

50. Kim HC, Kim TK, Sung KB, et al. CT during hepatic arteriography and portography: an illustrative review. Radiographics 2002;22(5):1041–1051.

51. Poyanli A, Sencer S. Computed tomography scan of the liver. Eur J Radiol 1999;32(1):15–20.

52. Hann LE, Winston CB, Brown KT, Akhurst T. Diagnostic imaging approaches and relationship to hepatobiliary cancer staging and therapy. Semin Surg Oncol 2000;19(2): 94–115.

53. Fong Y, Blumgart LH, Fortner JG, Brennan MF. Pancreatic or liver resection for malignancy is safe and effective for the elderly. Ann Surg 1995;222(4):426–434; discussion 434–437.

54. D'Angelica MI, Shoup MC, Nissan A. Randomized clinical trials in advanced and metastatic colorectal carcinoma. Surg Oncol Clin North Am 2002;11(1):173–191.

55. Rougier P, Van Cutsem E, Bajetta E, et al. Randomised trial of irinotecan versus fluorouracil by continuous infusion after fluorouracil failure in patients with metastatic colorectal cancer. Lancet 1998;352(9138):1407–1412.

56. Cunningham D, Pyrhonen S, James RD, et al. Randomised trial of irinotecan plus supportive care versus supportive care alone after fluorouracil failure for patients with metastatic colorectal cancer. Lancet 1998;352(9138):1413–1418.

57. Saltz LB, Cox JV, Blanke C, et al. Irinotecan plus fluorouracil and leucovorin for metastatic colorectal cancer. Irinotecan Study Group. N Engl J Med 2000;343(13):905–914.

58. Douillard JY, Cunningham D, Roth AD, et al. Irinotecan combined with fluorouracil compared with fluorouracil alone as first-line treatment for metastatic colorectal cancer: a multicentre randomised trial. Lancet 2000;355(9209):1041–1047.

59. Kuebler JP, de Gramont A. Recent experience with oxaliplatin or irinotecan combined with 5-fluorouracil and leucovorin in the treatment of colorectal cancer. Semin Oncol 2003;30 (4 suppl 15):40–46.

60. de Gramont A, Figer A, Seymour M, et al. Leucovorin and fluorouracil with or without oxaliplatin as first-line treatment in advanced colorectal cancer. J Clin Oncol 2000;18(16): 2938–2947.

61. Goldberg RM, Morton RF, Sargent DJ, et al. N9741: oxaliplatin (oxal) or CPT-11 + 5-fluorouracil (5FU)/leucovorin (LV) or oxal + CPT-11 in advanced colorectal cancer (CRC). Initial toxicity and response data from a GI Intergroup study. Proc Am Soc Clin Oncol 2002;21(128a):abstract 511.

62. O'Neil BH. Systemic therapy for colorectal cancer: focus on newer chemotherapy and novel agents. Semin Radiat Oncol 2003;13(4):441–453.

63. Ackerman NB, Lien WM, Kondi ES, Silverman NA. The blood supply of experimental liver metastases. I. The distribution of hepatic artery and portal vein blood to "small" and "large" tumors. Surgery 1969;66(6):1067–1072.

64. Oberfield RA, McCaffrey JA, Polio J, Clouse ME, Hamilton T. Prolonged and continuous percutaneous intra-arterial hepatic infusion chemotherapy in advanced metastatic liver adenocarcinoma from colorectal primary. Cancer 1979;44(2):414–423.

65. Weiss GR, Garnick MB, Osteen RT, et al. Long-term hepatic arterial infusion of 5-fluorodeoxyuridine for liver metastases using an implantable infusion pump. J Clin Oncol 1983;1(5):337–344.

66. Balch CM, Urist MM, Soong SJ, McGregor M. A prospective phase II clinical trial of continuous FUDR regional chemotherapy for colorectal metastases to the liver using a totally implantable drug infusion pump. Ann Surg 1983;198(5): 567–573.

67. Niederhuber JE, Ensminger W, Gyves J, Thrall J, Walker S, Cozzi E. Regional chemotherapy of colorectal cancer metastatic to the liver. Cancer 1984;53(6):1336–1343.

68. Harmantas A, Rotstein LE, Langer B. Regional versus systemic chemotherapy in the treatment of colorectal carcinoma metastatic to the liver. Is there a survival difference? Meta-analysis of the published literature. Cancer 1996;78(8):1639–1645.

69. Reappraisal of hepatic arterial infusion in the treatment of nonresectable liver metastases from colorectal cancer. Meta-Analysis Group in Cancer. J Natl Cancer Inst 1996;88(5):252–258.

70. Lorenz M, Muller HH. Randomized, multicenter trial of fluorouracil plus leucovorin administered either via hepatic arterial or intravenous infusion versus fluorodeoxyuridine administered via hepatic arterial infusion in patients with nonresectable liver metastases from colorectal carcinoma. J Clin Oncol 2000;18(2):243–254.

71. Kerr DJ, McArdle CS, Ledermann J, et al. Intrahepatic arterial versus intravenous fluorouracil and folinic acid for colorectal cancer liver metastases: a multicentre randomised trial. Lancet 2003;361(9355):368–373.

72. Kemeny N, Niedzwiecki D, Hollis DR. Hepatic arterial infusion (HAI) versus systemic therapy for hepatic metastases from colorectal cancer: a CALGB randomized trial of efficacy, quality of life (QOL), cost effectiveness, and molecular markers. Proc Am Soc Clin Oncol 2003;22(abstr 1010):252.

73. Leonard GD, Fong Y, Jarnagin W. Liver resection after hepatic arterial infusion (HAI) plus systemic oxaliplatin (Oxal) combinations in pretreated patients with extensive unresectable colorectal liver metastases. 2004 ASCO Annual Meeting Proceedings (Post-Meeting Edition). J Clin Oncol 2004; 22(14S):3542.

74. Silen W. Hepatic resection for metastases from colorectal carcinoma is of dubious value. Arch Surg 1989;124(9): 1021–1022.

75. Foster JH, Berman MM. Solid Liver Tumors. Philadelphia: Elsevier-Health Sciences Division; 1977.

76. Jarnagin WR, Gonen M, Fong Y, et al. Improvement in perioperative outcome after hepatic resection: analysis of 1,803 consecutive cases over the past decade. Ann Surg 2002;236(4): 397–406; discussion 406–407.

77. Foster JH. Survival after liver resection for secondary tumors. Am J Surg 1978;135(3):389–394.

78. D'Angelica M, Brennan MF, Fortner JG, Cohen AM, Blumgart LH, Fong Y. Ninety-six five-year survivors after liver resection

for metastatic colorectal cancer. J Am Coll Surg 1997;185(6): 554–559.

79. Scheele J, Stangl R, Altendorf-Hofmann A, Gall FP. Indicators of prognosis after hepatic resection for colorectal secondaries. Surgery 1991;110(1):13–29.

80. Doci R, Gennari L, Bignami P, Montalto F, Morabito A, Bozzetti F. One hundred patients with hepatic metastases from colorectal cancer treated by resection: analysis of prognostic determinants. Br J Surg 1991;78(7):797–801.

81. Rosen CB, Nagorney DM, Taswell HF, et al. Perioperative blood transfusion and determinants of survival after liver resection for metastatic colorectal carcinoma. Ann Surg 1992;216(4):493–504; discussion 504–505.

82. Schlag P, Hohenberger P, Herfarth C. Resection of liver metastases in colorectal cancer: competitive analysis of treatment results in synchronous versus metachronous metastases. Eur J Surg Oncol 1990;16(4):360–365.

83. Fortner JG, Silva JS, Golbey RB, Cox EB, Maclean BJ. Multivariate analysis of a personal series of 247 consecutive patients with liver metastases from colorectal cancer. I. Treatment by hepatic resection. Ann Surg 1984;199(3): 306–316.

84. Fong Y, Fortner J, Sun RL, Brennan MF, Blumgart LH. Clinical score for predicting recurrence after hepatic resection for metastatic colorectal cancer: analysis of 1001 consecutive cases. Ann Surg 1999;230(3):309–318; discussion 318–321.

85. Fong Y, Cohen AM, Fortner JG, et al. Liver resection for colorectal metastases. J Clin Oncol 1997;15(3):938–946.

86. Petrowsky H, Gonen M, Jarnagin W, et al. Second liver resections are safe and effective treatment for recurrent hepatic metastases from colorectal cancer: a bi-institutional analysis. Ann Surg 2002;235(6):863–871.

87. Lorenz M, Muller HH, Schramm H, et al. Randomized trial of surgery versus surgery followed by adjuvant hepatic arterial infusion with 5-fluorouracil and folinic acid for liver metastases of colorectal cancer. German Cooperative on Liver Metastases (Arbeitsgruppe Lebermetastasen). Ann Surg 1998;228(6):756–762.

88. Kemeny MM, Adak S, Gray B, et al. Combined-modality treatment for resectable metastatic colorectal carcinoma to the liver: surgical resection of hepatic metastases in combination with continuous infusion of chemotherapy—an intergroup study. J Clin Oncol 2002;20(6):1499–1505.

89. Kemeny N, Huang Y, Cohen AM, et al. Hepatic arterial infusion of chemotherapy after resection of hepatic metastases from colorectal cancer. N Engl J Med 1999;341(27):2039–2048.

90. Curley SA. Radiofrequency ablation of malignant liver tumors. Ann Surg Oncol 2003;10(4):338–347.

91. Nordlinger B, Rougier P. Nonsurgical methods for liver metastases including cryotherapy, radiofrequency ablation, and infusional treatment: what's new in 2001? Curr Opin Oncol 2002;14(4):420–423.

92. McCormack PM, Attiyeh FF. Resected pulmonary metastases from colorectal cancer. Dis Colon Rectum 1979;22(8): 553–556.

93. McAfee MK, Allen MS, Trastek VF, Ilstrup DM, Deschamps C, Pairolero PC. Colorectal lung metastases: results of surgical excision. Ann Thorac Surg 1992;53(5):780–785; discussion 785–786.

94. Nagakura S, Shirai Y, Yamato Y, Yokoyama N, Suda T, Hatakeyama K. Simultaneous detection of colorectal carcinoma liver and lung metastases does not warrant resection. J Am Coll Surg 2001;193(2):153–160.

95. Dematteo R, Minnard EA, Kemeny N. Outcome after resection of both liver and lung metastases in patients with colorectal cancer. Proc Am Soc Clin Oncol 1999. Abstr 958.

96. Rizk NP, Downey RJ. Resection of pulmonary metastases from colorectal cancer. Semin Thorac Cardiovasc Surg 2002;14(1): 29–34.

97. Roth JA, Pass HI, Wesley MN, White D, Putnam JB, Seipp C. Comparison of median sternotomy and thoracotomy for resection of pulmonary metastases in patients with adult soft-tissue sarcomas. Ann Thorac Surg 1986;42(2):134–138.

98. McCormack PM, Bains MS, Begg CB, et al. Role of video-assisted thoracic surgery in the treatment of pulmonary metastases: results of a prospective trial. Ann Thorac Surg 1996;62(1):213–216; discussion 216–217.

99. Sugarbaker PH, Cunliffe WJ, Belliveau J, et al. Rationale for integrating early postoperative intraperitoneal chemotherapy into the surgical treatment of gastrointestinal cancer. Semin Oncol 1989;16(4 suppl 6):83–97.

100. Dawson LE, Russell AH, Tong D, Wisbeck WM. Adenocarcinoma of the sigmoid colon: sites of initial dissemination and clinical patterns of recurrence following surgery alone. J Surg Oncol 1983;22(2):95–99.

101. Russell AH, Tong D, Dawson LE, et al. Adenocarcinoma of the retroperitoneal ascending and descending colon: sites of initial dissemination and clinical patterns of recurrence following surgery alone. Int J Radiat Oncol Biol Phys 1983; 9(3):361–365.

102. Chu DZ, Lang NP, Thompson C, Osteen PK, Westbrook KC. Peritoneal carcinomatosis in nongynecologic malignancy. A prospective study of prognostic factors. Cancer 1989;63(2): 364–367.

103. Willett CG, Tepper JE, Cohen AM, Orlow E, Welch CE. Failure patterns following curative resection of colonic carcinoma. Ann Surg 1984;200(6):685–690.

104. Hansen E, Wolff N, Knuechel R, Ruschoff J, Hofstaedter F, Taeger K. Tumor cells in blood shed from the surgical field. Arch Surg 1995;130(4):387–393.

105. Sadeghi B, Arvieux C, Glehen O, et al. Peritoneal carcinomatosis from non-gynecologic malignancies: results of the EVOCAPE 1 multicentric prospective study. Cancer 2000; 88(2):358–363.

106. Jacquet P, Jelinek JS, Steves MA, Sugarbaker PH. Evaluation of computed tomography in patients with peritoneal carcinomatosis. Cancer 1993;72(5):1631–1636.

107. Gilly FN, Beaujard A, Glehen O, et al. Peritonectomy combined with intraperitoneal chemohyperthermia in abdominal cancer with peritoneal carcinomatosis: phase I–II study. Anticancer Res 1999;19(3B):2317–2321.

108. Jacquet P, Sugarbaker PH. Clinical research methodologies in diagnosis and staging of patients with peritoneal carcinomatosis. Cancer Treat Res 1996;82:359–374.

109. Pestieau SR, Sugarbaker PH. Treatment of primary colon cancer with peritoneal carcinomatosis: comparison of concomitant vs. delayed management. Dis Colon Rectum 2000;43(10): 1341–1346; discussion 1347–1348.

110. Jayne DG, Fook S, Loi C, Seow-Choen F. Peritoneal carcinomatosis from colorectal cancer. Br J Surg 2002;89(12): 1545–1550.

111. Midgley R, Kerr D. Colorectal cancer. Lancet 1999;353(9150): 391–399.

112. Machover D. A comprehensive review of 5-fluorouracil and leucovorin in patients with metastatic colorectal carcinoma. Cancer 1997;80(7):1179–1187.

113. Sugarbaker PH. Colorectal carcinomatosis: a new oncologic frontier. Curr Opin Oncol 2005;17(4):397–399.

114. Speyer JL. The rationale behind intraperitoneal chemotherapy in gastrointestinal malignancies. Semin Oncol 1985; 12(3 suppl 4):23–28.

115. Sugarbaker PH, Graves T, DeBruijn EA, et al. Early postoperative intraperitoneal chemotherapy as an adjuvant therapy to surgery for peritoneal carcinomatosis from gastrointestinal cancer: pharmacological studies. Cancer Res 1990;50(18): 5790–5794.

116. Sugarbaker PH, Schellinx ME, Chang D, Koslowe P, von Meyerfeldt M. Peritoneal carcinomatosis from adenocarcinoma of the colon. World J Surg 1996;20(5):585–591; discussion 592.

117. Culliford ATT, Brooks AD, Sharma S, et al. Surgical debulking and intraperitoneal chemotherapy for established peritoneal metastases from colon and appendix cancer. Ann Surg Oncol 2001;8(10):787–795.

118. Verwaal VJ, van Ruth S, Witkamp A, Boot H, van Slooten G, Zoetmulder FA. Long-term survival of peritoneal carcinomatosis of colorectal origin. Ann Surg Oncol 2005;12(1):65–71.

119. Elias D, Blot F, El Otmany A, et al. Curative treatment of peritoneal carcinomatosis arising from colorectal cancer by complete resection and intraperitoneal chemotherapy. Cancer 2001;92(1):71–76.

120. Verwaal VJ, van Ruth S, de Bree E, et al. Randomized trial of cytoreduction and hyperthermic intraperitoneal chemotherapy versus systemic chemotherapy and palliative surgery in patients with peritoneal carcinomatosis of colorectal cancer. J Clin Oncol 2003;21(20):3737–3743.

121. Ulbright TM, Roth LM, Stehman FB. Secondary ovarian neoplasia. A clinicopathologic study of 35 cases. Cancer 1984; 53(5):1164–1174.

122. Webb MJ, Decker DG, Mussey E. Cancer metastatic to the ovary: factors influencing survival. Obstet Gynecol 1975; 45(4):391–396.

123. Israel SL, Helsel EV Jr, Hausman DH. The challenge of metastatic ovarian carcinoma. Am J Obstet Gynecol 1965; 93(8):1094–1101.

124. Demopoulos RI, Touger L, Dubin N. Secondary ovarian carcinoma: a clinical and pathological evaluation. Int J Gynecol Pathol 1987;6(2):166–175.

125. Barr SS, Valiente MA, Bacon HE. Rationale of bilateral oophorectomy concomitant with resection for carcinoma of the rectum and colon. Dis Colon Rectum 1962;5:450–452.

126. Blamey S, McDermott F, Pihl E, Price AB, Milne BJ, Hughes E. Ovarian involvement in adenocarcinoma of the colon and rectum. Surg Gynecol Obstet 1981;153(1):42–44.

127. Morrow M, Enker WE. Late ovarian metastases in carcinoma of the colon and rectum. Arch Surg 1984;119(12):1385–1388.

128. Cutait R, Lesser ML, Enker WE. Prophylactic oophorectomy in surgery for large-bowel cancer. Dis Colon Rectum 1983; 26(1):6–11.

129. Young-Fadok TM, Wolff BG, Nivatvongs S, Metzger PP, Ilstrup DM. Prophylactic oophorectomy in colorectal carcinoma: preliminary results of a randomized, prospective trial. Dis Colon Rectum 1998;41(3):277–283; discussion 283–285.

130. Burt CA. Carcinoma of the ovaries secondary to cancer of the colon and rectum. Dis Colon Rectum 1960;3:352–357.

131. Stearns MW Jr, Deddish MR. Five-year results of abdominopelvic lymph node dissection for carcinoma of the rectum. Dis Colon Rectum 1959;2(2):169–172.

132. Graffner HO, Alm PO, Oscarson JE. Prophylactic oophorectomy in colorectal carcinoma. Am J Surg 1983;146(2): 233–235.

133. Koves I, Vamosi-Nagy I, Besznyak I. Ovarian metastases of colorectal tumours. Eur J Surg Oncol 1993;19(6):633–635.

134. Harcourt KF, Dennis DL. Laparotomy for "ovarian tumors" in unsuspected carcinoma of the colon. Cancer 1968;21(6): 1244–1246.

135. Lindner V, Gasser B, Debbiche A, Tomb L, Vetter JM, Walter P. [Ovarian metastasis of colorectal adenocarcinomas. A clinico-pathological study of 41 cases.] Ann Pathol 1999;19(6): 492–498.

136. Rayson D, Bouttell E, Whiston F, Stitt L. Outcome after ovarian/adnexal metastectomy in metastatic colorectal carcinoma. J Surg Oncol 2000;75(3):186–192.

137. Abu-Rustum N, Barakat RR, Curtin JP. Ovarian and uterine disease in women with colorectal cancer. Obstet Gynecol 1997;89(1):85–87.

138. Loy TS, Calaluce RD, Keeney GL. Cytokeratin immunostaining in differentiating primary ovarian carcinoma from metastatic colonic adenocarcinoma. Mod Pathol 1996;9(11):1040–1044.

139. DeCostanzo DC, Elias JM, Chumas JC. Necrosis in 84 ovarian carcinomas: a morphologic study of primary versus metastatic colonic carcinoma with a selective immunohistochemical analysis of cytokeratin subtypes and carcinoembryonic antigen. Int J Gynecol Pathol 1997;16(3):245–249.

140. Wauters CC, Smedts F, Gerrits LG, Bosman FT, Ramaekers FC. Keratins 7 and 20 as diagnostic markers of carcinomas metastatic to the ovary. Hum Pathol 1995;26(8):852–855.

141. Dionigi A, Facco C, Tibiletti MG, Bernasconi B, Riva C, Capella C. Ovarian metastases from colorectal carcinoma. Clinicopathologic profile, immunophenotype, and karyotype analysis. Am J Clin Pathol 2000;114(1):111–122.

142. Blamey SL, McDermott FT, Pihl E, Hughes ES. Resected ovarian recurrence from colorectal adenocarcinoma: a study of 13 cases. Dis Colon Rectum 1981;24(4):272–275.

143. Herrera-Ornelas L, Mittelman A. Results of synchronous surgical removal of primary colorectal adenocarcinoma and ovarian metastases. Oncology 1984;41(2):96–100.

144. Huang PP, Weber TK, Mendoza C, Rodriguez-Bigas MA, Petrelli NJ. Long-term survival in patients with ovarian metastases from colorectal carcinoma. Ann Surg Oncol 1998;5(8): 695–698.

145. Wright JD, Powell MA, Mutch DG, et al. Synchronous ovarian metastases at the time of laparotomy for colon cancer. Gynecol Oncol 2004;92(3):851–855.

146. Miller BE, Pittman B, Wan JY, Fleming M. Colon cancer with metastasis to the ovary at time of initial diagnosis. Gynecol Oncol 1997;66(3):368–371.

147. MacKeigan JM, Ferguson JA. Prophylactic oophorectomy and colorectal cancer in premenopausal patients. Dis Colon Rectum 1979;22(6):401–405.

148. Ballantyne GH, Reigel MM, Wolff BG, Ilstrup DM. Oophorectomy and colon cancer. Impact on survival. Ann Surg 1985;202(2):209–214.

149. Sieleznef I, Salle E, Antoine K, Thirion X, Brunet C, Sastre B. Simultaneous bilateral oophorectomy does not improve prognosis of postmenopausal women undergoing colorectal resection for cancer. Dis Colon Rectum 1997;40(11):1299–1302.

150. Kontoravdis A, Kalogirou D, Antoniou G, Kontoravdis N, Karakitsos P, Zourlas PA. Prophylactic oophorectomy in ovarian cancer prevention. Int J Gynaecol Obstet 1996;54(3):257–262.

151. Sightler SE, Boike GM, Estape RE, Averette HE. Ovarian cancer in women with prior hysterectomy: a 14-year experience at the University of Miami. Obstet Gynecol 1991;78(4):681–684.

152. Rozario D, Brown I, Fung MF, Temple L. Is incidental prophylactic oophorectomy an acceptable means to reduce the incidence of ovarian cancer? Am J Surg 1997;173(6):495–498.

153. Barringer PL, Dockerty MB, Waugh JM, Bargen JA. Carcinoma of the large intestine: a new approach to the study of venous spread. Surg Gynecol Obstet 1954;98(1):62–72.

154. Besbeas S, Stearns MW Jr. Osseous metastases from carcinomas of the colon and rectum. Dis Colon Rectum 1978;21(4):266–268.

155. Buckley N, Peebles Brown DA. Metastatic tumors in the hand from adenocarcinoma of the colon. Dis Colon Rectum 1987;30(2):141–143.

156. Cascino TL, Leavengood JM, Kemeny N, Posner JB. Brain metastases from colon cancer. J Neurooncol 1983;1(3):203–209.

157. Rovirosa A, Bodi R, Vicente P, Alastuey I, Giralt J, Salvador L. [Cerebral metastases in adenocarcinoma of the colon.] Rev Esp Enferm Dig 1991;79(4):281–283.

158. Zimm S, Wampler GL, Stablein D, Hazra T, Young HF. Intracerebral metastases in solid-tumor patients: natural history and results of treatment. Cancer 1981;48(2):384–394.

159. Wronski M, Arbit E. Resection of brain metastases from colorectal carcinoma in 73 patients. Cancer 1999;85(8):1677–1685.

160. Ko FC, Liu JM, Chen WS, Chiang JK, Lin TC, Lin JK. Risk and patterns of brain metastases in colorectal cancer: 27-year experience. Dis Colon Rectum 1999;42(11):1467–1471.

161. Kemeny N, Daly J, Reichman B, Geller N, Botet J, Oderman P. Intrahepatic or systemic infusion of fluorodeoxyuridine in patients with liver metastases from colorectal carcinoma. A randomized trial. Ann Intern Med 1987;107(4):459–465.

162. Chang AE, Schneider PD, Sugarbaker PH, Simpson C, Culnane M, Steinberg SM. A prospective randomized trial of regional versus systemic continuous 5-fluorodeoxyuridine chemotherapy in the treatment of colorectal liver metastases. Ann Surg 1987;206(6):685–693.

163. Hohn DC, Stagg RJ, Friedman MA, et al. A randomized trial of continuous intravenous versus hepatic intraarterial floxuridine in patients with colorectal cancer metastatic to the liver: the Northern California Oncology Group trial. J Clin Oncol 1989;7(11):1646–1654.

164. Wagman LD, Kemeny MM, Leong L, et al. A prospective, randomized evaluation of the treatment of colorectal cancer metastatic to the liver. J Clin Oncol 1990;8(11):1885–1893.

165. Martin JK Jr, O'Connell MJ, Wieand HS, et al. Intra-arterial floxuridine vs systemic fluorouracil for hepatic metastases from colorectal cancer. A randomized trial. Arch Surg 1990;125(8):1022–1027.

166. Rougier P, Laplanche A, Huguier M, et al. Hepatic arterial infusion of floxuridine in patients with liver metastases from colorectal carcinoma: long-term results of a prospective randomized trial. J Clin Oncol 1992;10(7):1112–1118.

167. Allen-Mersh TG, Earlam S, Fordy C, Abrams K, Houghton J. Quality of life and survival with continuous hepatic-artery floxuridine infusion for colorectal liver metastases. Lancet 1994;344(8932):1255–1260.

168. Kemeny NND, Hollis DR, et al. Hepatic arterial infusion (HAI) versus systemic therapy for hepatic metastases from colorectal cancer: a CALGB randomized trial of efficacy, quality of life (QOL), cost effectiveness, and molecular markers. Proc Am Soc Clin Oncol 2003;22(abstr 1010):252.

169. Cohen AD, Kemeny NE. An update on hepatic arterial infusion chemotherapy for colorectal cancer. Oncologist 2003;8(6):553–566.

170. Adson MA, van Heerden JA, Adson MH, Wagner JS, Ilstrup DM. Resection of hepatic metastases from colorectal cancer. Arch Surg 1984;119(6):647–651.

171. Hughes KS, Simon R, Songhorabodi S, et al. Resection of the liver for colorectal carcinoma metastases: a multi-institutional study of patterns of recurrence. Surgery 1986;100(2):278–284.

172. Gayowski TJ, Iwatsuki S, Madariaga JR, et al. Experience in hepatic resection for metastatic colorectal cancer: analysis of clinical and pathologic risk factors. Surgery 1994;116(4):703–710; discussion 710–711.

173. Scheele J, Stang R, Altendorf-Hofmann A, Paul M. Resection of colorectal liver metastases. World J Surg 1995;19(1):59–71.

174. Fong Y, Blumgart LH, Cohen A, Fortner J, Brennan MF. Repeat hepatic resections for metastatic colorectal cancer. Ann Surg 1994;220(5):657–662.

175. Jenkins LT, Millikan KW, Bines SD, Staren ED, Doolas A. Hepatic resection for metastatic colorectal cancer. Am Surg 1997;63(7):605–610.

176. Rees M, Plant G, Bygrave S. Late results justify resection for multiple hepatic metastases from colorectal cancer. Br J Surg 1997;84(8):1136–1140.

177. Jamison RL, Donohue JH, Nagorney DM, Rosen CB, Harmsen WS, Ilstrup DM. Hepatic resection for metastatic colorectal cancer results in cure for some patients. Arch Surg 1997;132(5):505–510; discussion 511.

178. Minagawa M, Makuuchi M, Torzilli G, et al. Extension of the frontiers of surgical indications in the treatment of liver metastases from colorectal cancer: long-term results. Ann Surg 2000;231(4):487–499.

179. Figueras J, Valls C, Rafecas A, Fabregat J, Ramos E, Jaurrieta E. Resection rate and effect of postoperative chemotherapy on survival after surgery for colorectal liver metastases. Br J Surg 2001;88(7):980–985.

180. Choti MA, Sitzmann JV, Tiburi MF, et al. Trends in long-term survival following liver resection for hepatic colorectal metastases. Ann Surg 2002;235(6):759–766.

181. Laurent C, Sa Cunha A, Couderc P, Rullier E, Saric J. Influence of postoperative morbidity on long-term survival following liver resection for colorectal metastases. Br J Surg 2003;90(9):1131–1136.

182. Mori M, Tomoda H, Ishida T, et al. Surgical resection of pulmonary metastases from colorectal adenocarcinoma. Special reference to repeated pulmonary resections. Arch Surg 1991;126(10):1297–1301; discussion 1302.

183. McCormack PM, Burt ME, Bains MS, Martini N, Rusch VW, Ginsberg RJ. Lung resection for colorectal metastases. 10-year results. Arch Surg 1992;127(12):1403–1406.

184. Yano T, Hara N, Ichinose Y, Yokoyama H, Miura T, Ohta M. Results of pulmonary resection of metastatic colorectal cancer and its application. J Thorac Cardiovasc Surg 1993;106(5): 875–879.

185. Saclarides TJ, Krueger BL, Szeluga DJ, Warren WH, Faber LP, Economou SG. Thoracotomy for colon and rectal cancer metastases. Dis Colon Rectum 1993;36(5):425–429.

186. van Halteren HK, van Geel AN, Hart AA, Zoetmulder FA. Pulmonary resection for metastases of colorectal origin. Chest 1995;107(6):1526–1531.

187. Shirouzu K, Isomoto H, Hayashi A, Nagamatsu Y, Kakegawa T. Surgical treatment for patients with pulmonary metastases after resection of primary colorectal carcinoma. Cancer 1995;76(3): 393–398.

188. Girard P, Ducreux M, Baldeyrou P, et al. Surgery for lung metastases from colorectal cancer: analysis of prognostic factors. J Clin Oncol 1996;14(7):2047–2053.

189. Okumura S, Kondo H, Tsuboi M, et al. Pulmonary resection for metastatic colorectal cancer: experiences with 159 patients. J Thorac Cardiovasc Surg 1996;112(4):867–874.

190. Zanella A, Marchet A, Mainente P, Nitti D, Lise M. Resection of pulmonary metastases from colorectal carcinoma. Eur J Surg Oncol 1997;23(5):424–427.

191. Zink S, Kayser G, Gabius HJ, Kayser K. Survival, disease-free interval, and associated tumor features in patients with colon/rectal carcinomas and their resected intra-pulmonary metastases. Eur J Cardiothorac Surg 2001;19(6):908–913.

35
Anal Cancer

Mark Lane Welton and Madhulika G. Varma

This chapter, reviews the anatomy that defines anal and perianal squamous cell carcinomas (SCCs), discusses the cancers and precursor lesions that are most frequently found in these regions, and concludes with brief discussions of the less common malignancies of the anus and perineum.

New Anatomic Considerations

There are approximately 4200 new cases of anal cancer per year in the United States. This number may actually somewhat overestimate the true incidence because it is our impression that perianal or anal margin cancers are often classified as anal canal cancers because of proximity to the anus without actual involvement of the anal canal. As colorectal surgeons, the authors and editors are quite familiar with the landmarks that define the anal canal and anal margin. However, many caregivers involved in the diagnosis and treatment of this disease are less familiar with these landmarks in that their primary practices are internal medicine, gastroenterology, radiation oncology, medical oncology, dermatology, human immunodeficiency virus (HIV) medicine, etc. Many practitioners in these fields are not clear on the distinction between the dentate line and the anal verge and often lack the tools in their offices to visualize the anal landmarks. Given these limitations, we suggest a new terminology based on landmarks that all healthcare providers can easily visualize and understand. The new terminology is necessary because true anal canal lesions may have a more aggressive biology requiring chemoradiotherapy whereas lesions of the perianal skin may simply be treated with local excision. Thus, if the two classes of lesions are unwittingly grouped together, the response rates of anal cancer to chemoradiation therapy may be overstated.

The authors have proposed a new classification that may prove more useful to all caregivers who diagnose or treat patients with anal cancers. The classification system divides the region into three easily identifiable regions: intraanal, perianal, and skin (Figure 35-1).[1] **Intraanal** lesions are lesions that cannot be visualized at all, or are incompletely visualized, while gentle traction is placed on the buttocks. In contrast, **perianal** lesions are completely visible and fall within a 5-cm radius of the anal opening when gentle traction is placed on the buttocks (Figure 35-2). Finally, **skin** lesions fall outside of the 5-cm radius of the anal opening. A key component of this classification system is that all clinicians, including gastroenterologists, surgeons, nurse practitioners, and medical and radiation oncologists can perform this simple examination in their offices without the aide of an anoscope or a clear understanding of the anatomic landmarks (dentate line and anal verge) of the region.

Identification of a new zone, the transformation zone, is also proposed to help clinicians and pathologists understand how intraanal SCCs may be found 6, 8, or even 10 cm proximal to the dentate line in the anatomic rectum. The transition zone is a well-known region. It is an area 0 to 12 mm in length beginning at the dentate line where a "transitional urothelium-like" epithelium may be found in the rectal mucosa instead of the standard columnar mucosa of the rectum. A "transformation zone" is a common finding in the cervix. This transformation zone, which we would propose for the anorectum, is a region in which squamous metaplasia may be found overlying the normal columnar mucosa. This immature metaplastic tissue may extend up the rectum in a fluid and dynamic manner involving at times 10 cm or more of distal rectal mucosa. The "transformation zone" is an important region where metaplastic tissue susceptible to human papillomavirus (HPV) infection, in particular HPV 16, may be found.

Finally, the locations of all lesions within these zones should be clearly reported. Frequently, accurate reconstruction of the exact location of a lesion removed by a referring caregiver is not possible. This may lead to overtreatment of perianal and even skin lesions. In the distal rectum, it may still be necessary to refer to one established anatomic landmark, the dentate line (mucocutaneous junction), to accurately reflect how far proximally in the rectum a lesion was found. In contrast to the dentate line, the anal verge is poorly understood, poorly visualized, and often confused with anal margin, which represents a region, not an anatomic boundary.

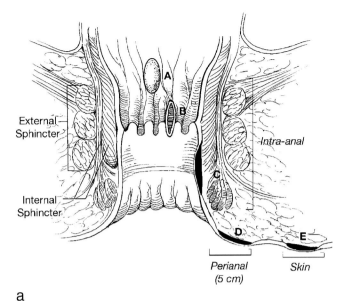

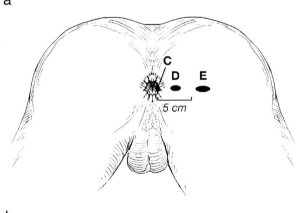

FIGURE 35-1. Classification system of anal cancers: a) coronal section. b) perianal view; A-C. intranal (anal canal) lesions, D. perianal (anal margin) lesions, E. skin lesions.

By adopting this new terminology, abandoning the use of some terms, and recording lesion locations clearly, we may begin to understand which lesions are amenable to local excision and which lesions require more radical intervention.

Terminology

The terminology used by pathologists when reporting premalignant lesions of the anus and perineum is often confusing to the treating clinicians. The terms SCC in situ (CIS), anal intraepithelial neoplasia (AIN), anal dysplasia, squamous intraepithelial lesion (SIL), and Bowen's disease may all be used to refer to the same histopathology. The training of the pathologist dictates the term chosen. AIN and anal dysplasia have both historically been broken into AIN I, II, and III and low-, moderate-, and high-grade dysplasia. However, as with other pathologic staging systems, the intra- and interobserver variability are too high with this many categories. Therefore,

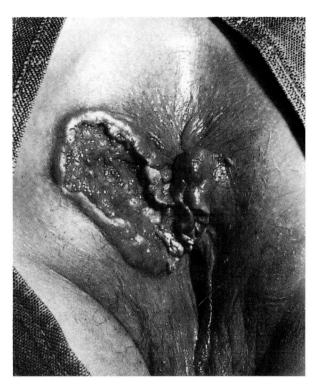

FIGURE 35-2. Perianal squamous cell carcinoma. (From Nivatvongs,[79] copyright © 1999. Reproduced by permission of Routledge/Taylor & Francis Group, LLC).

it has been suggested that when referring to intraanal, perianal, and skin lesions of the buttock that the tissue be classified as normal, low-grade squamous intraepithelial lesions (LSIL), high-grade squamous intraepithelial lesions (HSIL), or invasive cancer. Throughout the remainder of the chapter we will use this terminology and avoid CIS and Bowen's disease.

Lymphatic Drainage

Lymphatic drainage above the dentate line occurs via the superior rectal lymphatics to the inferior mesenteric lymph nodes and laterally to the internal iliac nodes. Below the dentate line, drainage is primarily to the inguinal nodes but may also involve the inferior or superior rectal lymph nodes.

Etiology and Pathogenesis of Anal Dysplasia and Anal SCC

The HPV is a necessary but not sufficient cause for the development of anal SCC (SCCA) and SILs.[2,3] HPV is a DNA papovavirus with an 8-kb genome and is the most common viral sexually transmitted infection.[4–6] Although most patients clear the virus with only 1% of the patients developing genital warts with low oncogenic potential (HPV serotypes 6 and

11),[7–9] an estimated 10%–46% of patients will develop sub-clinical infections that may harbor malignant potential (HPV serotypes 16, 18, 31, 33, 35).[10–13]

Transmission is not prevented by condoms because the virus pools at the base of the penis and scrotum thus abstinence is the only effective means of prevention. In women, the virus may pool and extend from the vagina to the anus. Anoreceptive intercourse may be associated with the development of intraanal disease but the presence of condylomata or dysplasia within the anus does not mandate that anoreceptive intercourse has occurred.[14]

In the rare patient who develops chronic infection, a variety of events must occur starting with the virus entering the basal and parabasal cells. This may occur through a disruption in the normal mucosal barrier that developed as a result of anoreceptive intercourse, other sexually transmitted diseases (ulcers from syphilis, gonorrhea), friable prolapsing hemorrhoidal tissues, or a firm bowel movement. As noted above, the squamous metaplastic tissue above the dentate line is a relatively "immature" incompletely developed squamous epithelium overlying the columnar epithelium and may not require trauma to disrupt an intact "barrier" making it particularly susceptible to HPV infection.[15] If high-risk viral DNA eludes immune surveillance and gains access to the nucleus of replicating cells (wound repair or metaplasia), the infection can become widespread and persistent lasting for decades resulting in an increased risk of cancer.

Cell-mediated immunity seems to be important to the cellular response prohibiting the virus from establishing a prolonged presence. This hypothesis is supported by the observation that cervical dysplasia patients with established high-risk lesions had a decreased ability to mount a T helper cell type 1 (Th1 IL-2) response in contrast to those patients with low-risk lesions.[16] Further support comes from the increased anal cancer rates observed in kidney transplant and HIV (+) patients, both populations with blunted cell-mediated responses.[17–22]

Oncogenic viruses lead to cellular proliferation in the latency phase by interfering with cell cycle control mechanisms.[15,23] Two "early region" viral genes, E6 and E7, inhibit cell cycle control resulting in increased proliferation. E7 binds directly to the retinoblastoma (Rb) tumor suppressor protein products p105, p107, and p130 related proteins leading to a complicated cascade of events involving E2F transcriptions factors, cyclin complexes, and other regulatory proteins allowing the cell to progress through G1 into S phase.[24] Cell cycle release by E7 allows for immortalization of the cells but is not sufficient for transformation of the infected cell. Accumulation of genetic errors seems necessary for transformation which is consistent with the clinical scenario of a longstanding low-grade infection preceding the development of malignancy.[25] The genetic errors may accumulate as a result of the E6 protein which binds to p53 with E6 associated protein (E6AP) leading to degradation of the complex through the ubiquitin pathway.[24,26] The unblocked

p53 protein is an important cell cycle regulating protein that leads to cell cycle arrest and apoptosis when genetic errors have accumulated, thus allowing for DNA repair and avoidance of replication of errors.

The E2 protein allows the HPV DNA to avoid intracellular detection by facilitating the attachment of the HPV DNA to the host chromatin. This also assures replication in a steady state with each cell division.[15,27–29] In uninfected epithelium, division occurs in the basal layers and maturation results in pyknotic condensed cells that slough from the tissue surface. In infected tissues, the viral DNA replication process is reactivated leading to the presence of specific proteins and viral particles that can be detected in the upper cell layers. In summary, through the combined effect of E7, E6, and E2, cells with genetic errors may proliferate, accumulate, and involve the entire thickness of the epithelium.[15] This may result in carcinogenesis.

As the infection with oncogenic viruses persists, the anal tissues may progress through low-grade to high-grade dysplasia and cancer. With this disease progression is an associated increased proliferation and angiogenesis, and decreased apoptosis.[30] In contrast to the mechanisms responsible for the increased proliferation and decreased apoptosis outlined in the above discussion, the mechanisms involved in increased angiogenesis are less well defined. However, in the cervix, angiogenic changes have long been recognized as an important and visible step in the progression of dysplasia to cancer. Colposcopy, a magnified view of the cervix, with the aid of acetic acid and Lugol's solution, allows for direct visualization of characteristic vascular patterns seen with LSIL and HSIL. Gynecologists are trained to recognize these vascular patterns and target their therapeutic destruction in the cervix accordingly. This therapeutic intervention, in combination with screening Pap smears, has led to the belief that cervical cancer is a largely preventable cancer.

Fortunately, the angiogenic changes associated with development of anal HSIL can also be visualized with the aid of acetic acid and Lugol's solution in the perianal skin, anus, and distal rectum through an operative microscope, colposcope, or loops in the office or operating room.[13] Targeted destruction is safe and may result in the same decrease in anal cancer incidence as was seen with cervical cancer when cervical Pap smears and targeted destruction was introduced for cervical disease.[31]

The cost effectiveness of such an anal cytology screening system to prevent anal cancer has been demonstrated using an economic model in both HIV-positive[32] and HIV-negative men who have sex with men (MSM).[33] These studies demonstrated that screening to identify patients with HSIL to be referred for treatment would be cost effective if performed annually for HIV-positive MSM and every 2–3 years for HIV-negative MSM.

Although the association of MSM and anal cancer is clear,[14,34,35] the association of HIV with the development and progression of anal cancer has been hard to separate from other confounding factors. Initial studies accumulating anal cancer rates from the pre-HAART (highly active antiretroviral therapy) era failed to show a correlation presumably because patients succumbed to complications of the HIV.[36,37] HPV is an indolent infection that leads to cancer in a minority of patients who generally suffer from a long-term infection. Thus, as might be expected, more recent studies reporting anal cancer rates in patients who are now surviving longer with effective HAART suggest an association with HIV and anal cancer.[17,18,38–40] The increase in anal cancer and dysplasia rates is seen in HIV-positive MSM, and HIV-positive heterosexual men and women who do not report anoreceptive intercourse.[17–19] Furthermore, HIV-positive patients are more likely to have HSIL, are more likely to progress from LSIL to HSIL over a 2–year time period, and both of these findings are increased in the patients with a lower CD4 count (<200 cells/mm).[38–40] Low CD4 counts are a surrogate measure for immunosuppression from the HIV infection and it is therefore suggested that HIV infection is associated with an increased risk of progression of anal disease.

Although the above articles suggest a permissive role for HIV in the development of anal cancer in HIV-positive men and women, a recent cancer registry report compared anal cancer rates from the pre-AIDS era to the post-AIDS era and found no correlation.[41] Nonetheless, data are accumulating that suggest that as men and women live longer in the HAART era, the indolent HPV infection will result in an increased risk for the development of anal cancer and this effect will be most significant in the most immunocompromised patients.

Epidemiology

The incidence of SCCA has been increasing in frequency over the last 30 years in the United States, Europe, and South America. This increase was noted to be quite pronounced in a recent 4–year review in which an increase from 3400 new cases for 1999 to 3900 new cases for 2002 was noted in the United States.[42,43] The California Cancer Registry found a statewide increase in anal cancers in non-Hispanic white men of approximately 2% per year between 1988 to 1999 with 1.0 case per 100,000 population in 1988 and 1.4 cases per population in 1999.[20] There was not a comparable increase for women over the same time period. Most alarming was the increase in the age-adjusted incidence for San Francisco white men aged 40–64 where the rates increased from 3.7 per 100,000 for 1973–1978, to 8.6 per 100,000 in 1984–1990 and ultimately to 20.6 per 100,000 in 1996–1999. This is the first report ever of anal cancer rates higher among men under age 40 compared with women of the same age group.[20] Previous reports have consistently shown a higher rate in women in all age groups.[44]

In Denmark during the years 1943–1987 there was a 1.5 fold increase in men and a 3-fold increase in women.[45] A significant decrease in the mean age of men diagnosed with SCCA from 68 to 63 years of age was also found. An even greater increase was found in city populations where a 3-fold increase in the incidence of anal cancers in Copenhagen and its suburbs was observed. A significant increase in incidence for the entire male population was still seen with the incidence observed between the years 1983–1987 representing an increase of 30%–40% of that seen in the 5-year span of 1943–1947. The rates in Copenhagen and surrounding areas were equal to the national level in 1943–1947 but in 1983–1987 the incidence in the city was 2.5-fold higher than that seen in the rest of the country. The average age of women patients with SCCA did not change but the incidence did increase 3-fold over the entire country with a significantly greater increase in Copenhagen when compared with the entire country. Men with anal cancer were significantly less likely to have been married when compared with men with colon cancer and stomach cancer. The same was not true of women with anal cancer. Similar findings were reported from Sweden where a dramatic increase in incidence of anal cancer was observed around 1960, with a greater change in women than men (2:1), and the steepest increase in the heavily populated cities.[44]

In another Copenhagen study, women with anal cancer were noted to have a higher risk of having had cervical neoplasia or cancer.[46] Risk factors for developing HSIL and anal cancer also included HIV seropositivity, low CD4 count, persistent infection with high-risk HPV genotypes (16, 18, 31, 33, 35), infection with multiple genotypes, cigarette smoking, anal receptive intercourse, and immunosuppression for organ allograft. Unlike cervical cancer, multiple partners was not a significant independent risk factor.[25,38,39,47–53]

Bowen's Disease

As mentioned above, the distinction between Bowen's disease and HSIL is unclear and seems to have more to do with the pathologist's training, cytopathology versus histopathology, than any biologic difference. Bowen's disease is both SCCA in situ and HSIL. The term Bowen's disease is applied to SCC in situ in both keratinizing and nonkeratinizing tissues. Thus, we believe the term is archaic and confusing, and should be abandoned in favor of HSIL. For purposes of this section of the chapter, we will use the term because it is in common usage.

Bowen's disease is frequently found as an incidental histologic finding after surgery for an unrelated problem, often hemorrhoids. The lesion is clinically unapparent but histologic assessment of the specimen reveals SCC in situ. Alternatively, patients may present with complaints of perianal burning, pruritus, or pain. Physical examination may reveal scaly, discrete, erythematous, or pigmented lesions.

The natural history of Bowen's disease is poorly defined. In the immunocompetent, fewer than 10% will progress to cancer.[54] However, in immunocompromised patients, the progression rate seems greater as evidenced by the higher rates of anal cancers observed in the HIV (+), and immunosuppressed transplant patients.[17-22] Because we are as yet unable to identify those patients that will progress, we favor treatment of Bowen's disease. An exception to this recommendation would be patients with advanced AIDS with poor performance statuses despite maximal medical therapy. This was a common problem in the early 1990s but since the advent of HAART, the vast majority of our AIDS patients are candidates for surgical intervention. The other exception might be the elderly patient with an asymptomatic lesion and a short life expectancy. Unlike perianal Paget's disease, there is no association with other visceral malignancies.[55]

The preferred treatment is fairly controversial but should be tailored to the given patient. The standard recommendation for the unsuspected lesion found after hemorrhoidectomy is to return the patient to the operating room for random biopsies taken at 1-cm intervals starting at the dentate line and around the anus in a clock-like manner. Frozen sections establish the presence of Bowen's disease and these areas are widely locally excised with 1-cm margins. Large defects are covered with flaps of gluteal and perianal skin. Bowen's recurrence rates in one series were as high as 23% despite this radical approach.[56] No cancers developed in this group, but complications including continence, stenoses, and sexual function, and HIV status were not reported. In another study of wide local excision, the authors noted a 63% persistence rate at 1 year and a 13% recurrence rate at 3 years. Eleven percent of the patients developed incontinence or stenosis.[57]

A less radical approach involves taking patients to the operating room and with the aide of an operating microscope, acetic acid, and Lugol's solution the lesions are visualized and targeted for electrocautery destruction. Similar to cervical disease, the Bowen's disease is visible because of its characteristic vascular pattern identifying the at-risk tissue for selective destruction.[13] This technique minimizes the morbidity of the procedure and saves the normal anal mucosa and perianal skin that would otherwise be sacrificed. Postoperative pain is significant as would be expected with any perianal procedure but in HIV (−) and otherwise immunocompetent patients there have been no recurrences and no progression to cancer. No patients developed incontinence or anal stenosis. In the HIV (+) patients, the recurrence rate is high but re-treatment is well tolerated and no cancers have developed in patients sent for surgical intervention.[31] Bowen's disease identified with the operative microscope and acetic acid may also simply be locally excised taking care to stay close to the lesion margin which is directly visualized with the operative microscope. The deep margin is kept equally close because wide local excision seems of limited benefit and increases morbidity. The resulting minimal defects heal in secondarily. High-risk patients, the immunocompromised, and patients practicing receptive anal intercourse, should be followed with Pap smears at yearly and three yearly intervals for the immunocompromised and immunocompetent, respectively.[32,33]

Other therapeutic modalities include topical 5-fluorouracil (5-FU) cream, imiquimod, photodynamic therapy, radiation therapy, laser therapy, and combinations of the above. The reports are generally small series with limited follow-up but there may be anecdotal success with each approach and the options may be kept in mind for challenging cases. Initial reports of the use of 5-FU cream were generally disappointing[58] but a recent report has suggested that Erbium:YAG laser pretreatment may improve the response of Bowen's disease.[59] Reports of the use of vidarabine and cidofovir support their consideration but the series are small with limited follow-up.[60,61] Imiquimod has been reported to be of benefit alone[62] and in combination with 5% 5-FU therapy in the immunosuppressed transplant and HIV (+) patient population.[63,64] Radiotherapy with a special skin patch or conventional external beam have also been reported.[65,66] Photodynamic therapy has been tried with success[67,68] and compared favorably to topical 5-FU in a randomized comparison.[69]

SCC of the Anal Margin

SCC arises from both the anal margin and the anal canal, although it is much less common in the former group. The distinction between the two locations has become more important as they are increasingly considered different entities with separate treatments and prognosis. Immunohistochemical studies of squamous cell tumors from the anal margin and anal canal demonstrate differences in expression of cadherin, cytokeratins, and p53 confirming that these tumors are of distinct histogenetic origin.[70] The anal margin is defined as the skin starting at the distal end of the anal canal to a 5-cm margin surrounding the anal verge.[71]

Clinical Characteristics

Tumors of the anal margin resemble SCC of other areas of skin and are therefore staged and often treated in a similar manner.[72] They have rolled, everted edges with central ulceration, and may have a palpable component in the subcutaneous tissues although the sphincter complex is not usually involved. Patients present in the seventh decade of life with equal incidence in men and women.[73,74] Presenting symptoms include a painful lump, bleeding, pruritus, tenesmus, discharge, or even fecal incontinence.[75] In general, anal margin tumors are characterized by a delay in diagnosis because of their location and indistinct features, and SCC is no exception. Patients have been noted to have symptoms anywhere from 0 to 144 months before diagnosis (median of 3 months),[76] and almost one-third are misdiagnosed at their first physician visit.[75] Patients were given erroneous diagnoses of hemorrhoids, anal fissures, fistulas, eczema, abscesses, or benign tumors. For anal margin tumors, however, there was no significant difference in survival between correctly diagnosed and misdiagnosed patients.[75]

TABLE 35-1. AJCC staging of SCC

	Anal margin	Anal canal
Primary tumor (T)		
Tx	Tumor cannot be assessed	Tumor cannot be assessed
T0	No evidence of primary tumor	No evidence of primary tumor
Tis	Carcinoma in situ	Carcinoma in situ
T1	Tumor ≤2 cm in greatest dimension	Tumor ≤2 cm in greatest dimension
T2	Tumor 2–5 cm in greatest dimension	Tumor 2–5 cm in greatest dimension
T3	Tumor ≥5 cm in greatest dimension	Tumor ≥5 cm in greatest dimension
T4	Tumor invades deep structures (muscle, bone, cartilage)	Tumor invades deep structures (vagina, urethra, bladder, but not sphincter)
Nodal status (N)		
Nx	Regional lymph nodes cannot be assessed	Regional lymph nodes cannot be assessed
N0	No regional lymph node metastasis	No regional lymph node metastasis
N1	Regional lymph node metastasis present	Perirectal lymph node metastasis present
N2		Unilateral internal iliac/inguinal lymph node metastasis present
N3		N1 and N2 and/or bilateral internal iliac and/or inguinal lymph node metastasis
Distant metastasis (M)		
Mx	Distant metastasis cannot be assessed	Distant metastasis cannot be assessed
M0	No distant metastasis	No distant metastasis
M1	Distant metastasis present	Distant metastasis present
Stage grouping (3b does not exist for anal margin)		
Stage 0	Tis	N0	M0	
Stage 1	T1	N0	M0	
Stage 2	T2,3	N0	M0	
Stage 3a	T1,2,3	N1	M0	or T4 N0 M0
Stage 3b	Any T	N2,3	M0	or T4 N1 M0
Stage 4	Any T	Any N	M1	

Staging

The staging of anal margin SCC is based on size of the tumor and lymph node involvement, both of which correlate with prognosis. Lymphatic drainage of the anal margin extends to the femoral and inguinal nodes and then to the external and common iliac nodes. Venous drainage occurs through the inferior rectal vein. Lymph node involvement is associated with the size and differentiation of the tumor.[76–78] In one study, the incidence of inguinal lymph node metastasis was noted to be 0% for tumors <2 cm, 23% for tumors 2–5 cm in size, and 67% in tumors >5 cm.[78] Distal visceral metastasis at presentation is rare but should be evaluated with a computed tomography (CT) scan of the abdomen and pelvis, to assess for liver metastases, as well as the presence of nodal disease. A chest X-ray can be performed to evaluate for lung metastasis. These tumors are generally slow growing and histologically are well differentiated with well-developed patterns of keratinization.[73,79] The American Joint Committee on Cancer (AJCC) staging system is described in Table 35-1.[71]

Treatment Options

Treatment of anal margin SCC traditionally consisted of surgical resection with wide local excision for smaller-sized tumors and abdominoperineal resection (APR) for larger, invasive tumors. However, it is well documented that wide local excision alone results in high locoregional recurrence rates (18%–63%) (Table 35-2)[73,80–84] and should be reserved for those lesions that can be excised with a 1-cm margin, are Tis or T1, and do not involve enough sphincter to compromise function.[74] A series of 27 patients with Tis and T1 lesions treated with wide local excision had a 100% 5-year survival[85] and in another study, all patients with small or superficial tumors locally excised had a survival of 100% whereas those with deep invasion did not survive 5 years.[83] Since it was introduced in the early 1970s, radiation therapy has become the mainstay of therapy for SCC of the anal canal and its application to tumors of the anal margin is increasing. In patients with T1 or early T2 lesions, local excision or radiation therapy provides similar local control rates (60%–100%),[78,86,87] but for less favorable lesions, chemoradiation is now used as the first-line therapy using a perineal field and inguinal fields, even without clinically detectable disease in the groin.[78,87] Pelvic lymph nodes are also treated for those patients with T3 and T4 tumors.[73,74,78,88] Local

TABLE 35-2. Results of local excision of anal margin tumors

Author	Year	N	Local recurrence (%)	Survival (%)
Beahrs and Wilson[85]	1976	27	0	100
Al-Jurf et al.[82]	1979	10	50	90
Schraut et al.[83]	1983	11	18	80
Greenall et al.[81]	1985	31	42	68
Jensen et al.[80]	1988	32	63	—
Pintor et al.[84]	1989	41	—	68

control rates for radiation therapy reported by T stage are as follows: T1, 50%–100%; T2, 60%–100%; T3, 37%–100%[78,86,87,89,90] (Table 35-3). In one study, the T3 lesions were separated into tumors 5–10 cm in size and those >10 cm with local control rates of 70% versus 40%, respectively.[89] Patients with persistent tumor can be treated with local excision or APR with a 50% salvage rate.[80,91] Those with recurrence after successful radiation can also be salvaged for cure.[92–95] The absolute 5-year survival rate for patients treated with local excision or APR ranges from 60% to 100% but is lower in patients with larger tumors.[81,82,96] Similarly, absolute 5-year survival in patients treated with radiation ranges from 52% to 90% with sphincter preservation in about 80%.[74] The use of chemoradiation specifically pertaining to SCC of the anal margin has not been well examined. However, one study did show an improvement in local control (64% versus 88%) with the addition of 5-FU and mitomycin to radiation.[89] In extrapolation of data from a randomized, multicenter study including early stage tumors, those of the anal margin and anal canal, it would be postulated that chemoradiation is superior.[93]

In summary, the choice of treatment is dependent on the stage of tumor, the anticipated functional result as a result of therapy, and the risk of complications. Although surgery may result in alteration of sphincter function, or a permanent colostomy, radiation therapy may also cause skin changes or proctitis that produces urgency, incontinence, or the need for diversion. For T1 and early T2 tumors, wide local excision may be less morbid and time consuming than radiation therapy and therefore a superior choice. However, if the excision will result in damage to the sphincters with impairment of fecal function, radiation provides similar local control and survival. T2 tumors should be treated with radiation therapy to the primary lesion and inguinal fields because of poor local control with excision and the significant risk of lymph node metastasis. This treatment modality is much less morbid than resection of the primary and bilateral lymph node dissection with similar control rates.[77] Those with T3, T4, or poorly differentiated tumors should receive radiation to the primary lesion and include inguinal and pelvic fields to treat regional nodes in these areas. APR should be reserved for those patients with persistent or recurrent disease after radiation therapy.[74,88]

TABLE 35-3. Radiation therapy for anal margin tumors by T stage

Author	Year	N	Local recurrence (%)			Cancer-specific 5-y survival (%)
			T1	T2	T3	
Cummings et al.[89]	1986	29	100	100	60	—
Cutuli et al.[90]	1988	21	50	71	37	72
Papillon and Chassard[78]	1992	54	100	84	50	80
Touboul et al.[87]	1995	17	100	60	100	86
Peiffert et al.[86]	1997	32	88	73	57	89

SCC of the Anal Canal

SCC incorporates all large-cell keratinizing, large-cell nonkeratinizing (transitional), and basaloid histologies. The terms epidermoid, cloacogenic, and mucoepidermoid carcinoma are all encompassed in the SCC group.[97] SCC of the anal canal is 5 times more common than SCC of the anal margin but its incidence is one-tenth that of rectal cancer. The incidence, epidemiology, and etiology have been described above.

Clinical Characteristics

The most common presenting symptom is bleeding, which occurs in >50% of patients with many complaining of anal pain. Other symptoms include palpable lump, pruritus, discharge, tenesmus, change in bowel habits, fecal incontinence, and rarely, inguinal lymphadenopathy.[75,98,99] A small number of patients will be asymptomatic. Unfortunately, most patients are diagnosed late, with up to 55% of patients being misdiagnosed at the time of presentation.[75] In another study of 172 patients with SCC, only 17 were diagnosed with tumors confined to the epithelium and subepithelial connective tissue.[100]

Evaluation

Physical examination should include a complete anorectal examination with external inspection of the anoderm, digital examination, anoscopy and proctoscopy, in addition to examination of inguinal areas. Careful notation should be made of the size, location, and mobility of the mass, associated perirectal lymphadenopathy, and in women, a pelvic examination should be performed to look for any associated lesions or invasion of tumor into the vagina. Complete examination and biopsy may require anesthesia for those patients with significant pain. Additional workup should include an endoanal/endorectal ultrasound to assess the depth of the tumor, presence of perirectal lymph nodes, and invasion of adjacent organs as an adjunct to the physical examination.[101–104] Ultrasound has been found to be superior to physical examination in assessing the involvement of internal and external anal sphincter muscle and perirectal lymph nodes. This has an impact on staging because physical examination often understages tumors. One study demonstrated that endorectal ultrasound T and N stage were significant predictors of relapse whereas the corresponding clinical staging was not.[103] Recently, a study of three-dimensional ultrasound has demonstrated improved accuracy in detecting perirectal lymph nodes and some suggestion of improved evaluation of tumor invasion.[105] Inguinal nodal involvement at the time of presentation can be difficult to determine. The sensitivity of radiologic imaging and clinical examination are poor.[106] Enlarged lymph nodes can be reactive to secondary inflammation in some cases and therefore should be biopsied with direct FNA (fine-needle aspiration) or ultrasound-guided FNA if detected by imaging. Excisional lymph node biopsy is rarely required but may be done if FNA is inconclusive. Studies of sentinel lymph node biopsy have demonstrated that the technique is safe and may result in more accurate staging[107] but the actual impact on initial and subsequent management remains unclear as long as inguinal fields are included during radiation therapy. CT scan or magnetic resonance imaging (MRI) of the abdomen and pelvis can add to locoregional staging as well as evaluating for liver metastasis. A chest X-ray is used as a screening tool for lung lesions and, if suspicious, a chest CT should be performed. Positron emission tomography (PET) scans are primarily useful for assessing persistent or residual disease after treatment. Colonoscopy can exclude any associated lesions proximal to the anal canal. Lastly, an HIV test should be performed for those at higher risk. HIV-positive patients with CD4 counts <200 need better monitoring of opportunistic infections, closer attention to toxic effects of chemoradiation with possible alterations in dosage, and management of antiretroviral therapy.[98,99,108,109]

Staging

The staging of anal canal SCC is based on the size of the tumor and lymph node metastasis. The TNM (tumor-node-metastasis) staging is listed in Table 35-1. The risk of nodal metastasis correlates with the size, depth of invasion, and the histologic grade of the tumor. In a series of 305 patients with SCC, lymph node metastasis was present in 16%. Nodal metastasis by T stage was as follows: T1 (0%), T2 (8.5%), T3 (29%), T4 (35%). Lymph node metastasis occurred in 47% of patients with T4 tumors >5 cm in size.[110] Inguinal metastases have been detected in 10%–30% of patients at the time of diagnosis[84,100,111,112] with an additional 5%–22% of patients developing clinically apparent lymph node metastases over time.[112] Nodal metastasis was almost double (58% versus 30%) in those tumors invading beyond the external sphincter compared with invasion of the internal sphincter.[113] Lymphatic drainage of the anal canal above the dentate line proceeds along the superior rectal vessels. At the dentate line, the drainage basin includes the internal pudendal, internal iliac, and obturator nodes. Below the dentate line, the lymphatic drainage is through the inguinal, femoral, and external iliac lymph nodes.[114] Mesenteric lymph nodes are more common in tumors of the proximal anal canal (50%) than the distal anal canal (14%).[98] An anatomic study of lymph node metastasis demonstrated that they most often occur above the peritoneal reflection and not in the perianal area. Additionally, almost half of the positive lymph nodes were <5 mm in size.[114] Distant visceral metastasis occurs in 10%–17% of patients at presentation and can be found in the liver, lung, bone, and subcutaneous tissues.[92,93] Subsequent metastasis is more common and was the cause of 40% of cancer-specific deaths in one series.[93]

Treatment

Surgery

The treatment of anal canal SCC was historically operative with APR being the standard of care. Unfortunately, local recurrence rates ranged from 27% to 47% and 5-year survival was 40%–70%.[83,84,97,98,100,106,115] The presence of pelvic lymph nodes decreased the 5-year survival to <20%.[99] Local excision was performed in those patients who could not tolerate an abdominal operation, refused a permanent colostomy, or had small, well-differentiated tumors. The recurrence rates and 5-year survival ranged from 20% to 80% and 45% to 85%, respectively.[79,80] However, in well-selected patients with early tumors, the 5-year survival was 100%.[83,84,100]

Radiation Therapy

Primary radiation therapy is quite effective in treating SCC because this tumor is extremely radiosensitive. It can be given as external beam radiation, brachytherapy, or in combination. Response is dose dependent with the best chance of tumor eradication occurring with at least 54 Gy of external beam radiation (Table 35-4).[116,117] However, this benefit is lost when radiation is administered in a split-course manner.[118,119] Local control and cure can be achieved in 70%–90% of selected patients with 60%–70% retaining sphincter function.[111,116] However, when tumors are larger than 5 cm or lymph nodes are involved, the cure rate decreases to 50%.[72,92,111,116] Better results with higher doses of radiation must be exchanged with increased radiation-induced complications when more than 40 Gy is administered. Serious late complications include anal necrosis, stenosis, and ulcerations, diarrhea, urgency, and fecal incontinence, cystitis, urethral stenosis, and small bowel obstruction. Significant impairment of fecal function caused by anal complications can lead to the placement of a colostomy. Most studies have found a dose-dependent effect on morbidity with the requirement of a colostomy in 6%–12% of patients.[95,111,120] However, a recent study examining risk factors predictive of requiring a colostomy for management of anal cancers found that tumor size was the only risk factor. Although radiation toxicities did occur, patients were not at an increased risk for requiring a stoma.[121] Brachytherapy used alone or in conjunction with external beam radiation is also effective with local control rates of 75%–79% and 5-year survival of 61%–65%, but 3%–6% of patients had serious complications that required surgery. The high rate of anal necrosis seen when both modalities are used has dampened

TABLE 35-4. Response to radiation based on dosage

| Author | Year | Local control (%) | |
		<54 Gy	>54 Gy
Hughes et al.[116]	1989	50	90
Constantinou et al.[117]	1997	61	77

TABLE 35-5. SCC of the anal canal: results of combination radiation and 5-FU plus mitomycin C

Author(s)	No. of patients	Dose (Gy)	Complete regression (%)	Follow-up (mo)	5-y survival (%)
Flam et al. (1987)[91]	30	41–50	87	9–76 →	—
Nigro (1987)[182]	104	30	93	24–132→	83
Habr-Gama et al. (1989)[183]	30	30–45	73	12–60 →	—
Sischy et al. (1989)[184]	79	40.8	90	20–55→	—
Cho et al. (1991)[185]	20	30	85	Av., 34	70
Cummings et al. (1991)[120]	69	50	85–93	>36	76
Lopez et al. (1991)[186]	33	30–56	88	Med., 48	79
Doci et al. (1992)[187]	56	36 + 18	87	2–45	81
Johnson et al. (1993)[188]	24	40.5–45	100	Med., 41	87
Tanum et al. (1993)[189]	86	50	T1*97 T2*80	46% >36	72
Beck and Karulf (1994)[190]	35	30–45	97	4–155	87
Smith et al. (1994)[191]	42	30	T1*90 T2*87	31 31	90 87

Source: Nivatvongs,[79] copyright © 1999. Reproduced by permission of Routledge/Taylor & Francis Group, LLC.

Comp., complete; med., median; av., average; →, survival at follow-up.

*Stage according to TNM classification.

the enthusiasm for this approach.[122,123] At this time, radiation therapy alone is not frequently used but may have a role in treating T1 tumors.[120,124]

Chemoradiation Therapy

The introduction of chemoradiation therapy by Nigro et al. in 1974 revolutionized the treatment of anal canal SCC by demonstrating equivalent local control and survival rates with preservation of sphincter function and thus avoidance of a colostomy.[125–127] Since that time, multiple studies have confirmed these results and now chemoradiation has become the standard therapy for SCC of the anal canal. Nigro et al. described using 30-Gy external beam radiation with 5-FU and mitomycin C, and demonstrated a complete pathologic response in 21 of 26 patients treated (81%). Since that time, various radiation doses (30–60 Gy) and chemotherapeutic regimens have been used with similar complete pathologic responses (45%–100%) and survival rates(70%–90%) (Table 35-5). As a result, operative treatment for anal canal SCC was largely abandoned and reserved for those patients with persistent or recurrent disease after chemoradiation. Although much controversy existed as to the benefit of chemoradiation therapy compared with primary radiation therapy, two randomized, controlled studies have been completed which demonstrate the superiority of chemoradiation therapy using

5-FU and mitomycin C to radiation alone.[92,93] Using 45 Gy with a boost for good response, both studies exhibited better local control rates with chemoradiation (Table 35-6) but no significant difference in survival. However, one study resulted in a higher complete response rate (80% versus 54%) and an improvement in colostomy-free survival (72% versus 47% at 3 years) which is significant.[92] Chemotherapy-related deaths occurred in 5.4% of patients in one series, and changes were made to the protocol which included a reduction of the dose for patients older than 70, bed-bound, frail, or with evidence of tumor-related sepsis.[93] The role of mitomycin C was also examined in a randomized trial which demonstrated better complete pathologic response rate (92% versus 85%), local control rate (84% versus 66%), colostomy-free survival rate (71% versus 59%), and disease-free survival (73% versus 51%) when mitomycin C was used in conjunction with 5-FU and radiation compared with 5-FU and radiation alone.[128] However, treatment toxicity was increased in the mitomycin C group (23% versus 7%) with a 4% chemotherapy-related mortality and overall survival was equivalent.

Although the use of mitomycin C has provided excellent results, cisplatin has gained favor because it is a radiation sensitizer, is less myelosuppressive than mitomycin C, and has been used for those patients who failed to respond to mitomycin C. In series of patients treated with 45–55Gy of radiation, 5-FU, and cisplatin, the reported rates of local control

TABLE 35-6. Results of two randomized trials examining radiation therapy alone and radiation therapy with chemotherapy for anal canal SCC

			Local control (%)			Overall survival (%)		
	N	Follow-up (y)	XRT	Chemo XRT	*P* value	XRT	Chemo XRT	*P* value
EORTC	110	5	50	68	.02	57	52	.17
UKCCCR	585	3	39	61	<.001	58	65	.25

(80%–83%), disease-free survival (77%–90%), and colostomy-free survival (71%–82%) were comparable to the best results obtained from mitomycin C regimens. Additionally, there were fewer severe toxicities reported.[129,130] A pilot study of the CALGB (Cancer and Leukemia Group B) using cisplatin demonstrated a complete response rate of 80%, colostomy-free survival of 56%, and overall survival of 78%. A randomized trial (RTOG 98-11) comparing cisplatin, 5-FU, 45 Gy to mitomycin C, 5-FU, 45 Gy is currently underway.[99,109]

Although the presence of inguinal metastasis at presentation indicates a worse prognosis, the overall 5-year survival is 48% (range, 30%–66%). Those with lymph nodes >2 cm in size, T3 or T4 tumors, or anal margin involvement had a worse survival (29%–32%).[112] For patients with obvious evidence of inguinal node metastasis, local control can be achieved in 90% of patients receiving chemoradiation compared with 65% receiving radiation alone. Surgical management with radical groin dissection can lead to significant complications and may be successful only 15% of the time.[106] The management of synchronous inguinal node metastasis is not standardized and different centers will use primary radiation therapy (45–65 Gy), chemoradiation, and selective lymph node dissection followed by radiation which has been reported to maintain disease-free intervals in up to 60% of patients.[73] For those with subclinical lymph nodes in the groin, chemoradiation is advocated with doses as low as 30–34 Gy. This minimizes toxicity but is effective in treating small-volume disease based on previous studies of small-sized tumors.[99] Whether or not inguinal fields should always be included when treating patients for anal canal SCC remains controversial.

Follow-up

No consensus has been reached on appropriate follow-up after treatment of SCC. It is generally agreed that early intervention for persistent disease and recurrent locoregional disease can lead to successful salvage therapy. Routine examination with digital rectal examination and proctoscopy every 2 months in the first year, every 3 months in the second year, and every 6 months thereafter has been recommended. Ultrasound examination has also become popular in detecting recurrence although the literature is mixed on its benefit.[103,131] CT scan or MRI performed after completion of chemoradiation may also be useful as a baseline for future comparison. MRI is useful for distinguishing surrounding tissues and detecting persistent or recurrent disease.

Treatment of Residual or Recurrent Disease

Persistent or recurrent disease localized to the pelvis after chemoradiation can be treated with salvage therapy. Patients need to be restaged with a CT of the chest, abdomen, and pelvis. MRI may be useful to assess resectability of pelvic

recurrence and PET scan may help to differentiate tumor from radiation-induced tissue changes or other undetectable metastases. APR can be performed for tumor localized to the pelvis with a 5-year survival of 24%–47%.[132–137] Those with positive margins, nodal disease at salvage, and persistent disease after chemoradiation have poorer outcomes.[137,138] Morbidity for APR in this setting is significant with an increased risk of perineal wound complications. This has prompted the use of plastic surgery reconstruction using rotational or advancement flaps to promote healing. The benefit of adjuvant chemotherapy after APR is currently unknown. Clinically evident inguinal disease after chemoradiation of the primary tumor can be treated with radical groin dissection if radiation has already been administered. Additional radiotherapy can be considered if maximal doses of radiation were not delivered. Radical groin dissection in selected patients can result in a 5-year survival of 55%.[139] Distant metastases have been found in 10%–17% of patients treated with chemoradiation,[92,93] and are usually treated with systemic chemotherapy such as cisplatin or 5-FU for palliation. If the metastases are isolated in the liver or lung and the primary disease is controlled, resection can be considered. The role of adjuvant maintenance chemotherapy is still under investigation in a Phase 3 randomized study in the United Kingdom.[109]

Uncommon Anal Canal Neoplasms

Adenocarcinoma

Anal canal adenocarcinomas are classified into three types. The first group may arise from the mucosa of the transitional zone in the upper canal and are indistinguishable from rectal adenocarcinoma. The second derives from the base of the anal glands which are lined with mucin-secreting columnar epithelium. The last can develop in the setting of a chronic anorectal fistula.[79] Adenocarcinomas account for 5%–19% of all anal cancers,[140–142] and have a more aggressive natural history than SCCs.[143]

The average age at presentation ranges from 59 to 71 years with equal gender distribution.[141,144] Patients may present with pain, induration, abscess/fistula, or a palpable mass. Other symptoms include bleeding, pruritus, seepage, prolapse, and weight loss.[79]

Because of the rarity and heterogeneity of this tumor, the role of surgery and chemoradiation has been difficult to assess, thus making definitive recommendations for treatment impossible. Many patients present with advanced local or metastatic disease making curative treatment challenging. The local disease may tend to be more advanced in those that arise in glands and fistulous tracts because these locations are outside the bowel wall and therefore the disease originates in a locally advanced location. Wide local excision may be feasible for those patients with a "rectal-type" tumor that is small, well differentiated, and does not invade the sphincter complex. All other tumors require APR. Chemoradiation alone has not been shown to be as effective for adenocarcinoma compared with SCC because of high local recurrence rates (54% versus 18%) and poor survival rates (64% versus 85%).[143] However, in another study analyzing treatments for anal canal adenocarcinoma including APR, surgery with radiation, and chemoradiation, similar locoregional recurrence rates (20%, 37%, 36%) and better overall survival was seen in the chemoradiation group (21%, 29%, 58%).[144] Other studies have suggested that a combined modality approach of surgery with chemoradiation does improve outcome with survival rates exceeding 60%.[140,141] Although no large series of patients has been treated in any uniform manner to substantiate the approach of chemoradiation therapy followed by surgery, the success of this approach for rectal adenocarcinoma would support its use.

Melanoma

Anorectal melanoma is characterized by unusual lesions that are often difficult to differentiate from benign pathology. For this reason, and its rarity, many patients present with advanced-stage disease. Although the anorectum is the most common site for primary melanoma of the gastrointestinal tract, it comprises only 0.5%–5% of all malignancies there. Fewer than 500 cases have been reported in the literature.[145] Patients are frequently female, Caucasian, and in their 60s. Isolated cases have been reported in African-American and Asian populations.[72,146,147]

Anorectal bleeding is the most common symptom described. However, anal pain, change in bowel habits, or tenesmus may also be reported. Weight loss and malaise may be indicative of advanced disease. A mass in the anal canal is the most frequent sign with a high likelihood of palpable inguinal lymph nodes. These tumors arise from the transitional epithelium of the anal canal, the anoderm, or the mucocutaneous junction. Although some lesions may seem to arise within the rectal mucosa, it is postulated that this is attributable to heterotopic epithelium within the rectum or mucosal spread from a primary foci within the anal canal.[146]

Most lesions are pigmented, with early lesions appearing polypoid and larger lesions having ulcerations, raised edges, or significant growth into the rectal vault. An early lesion may be indistinguishable from a thrombosed hemorrhoid and some cases have been incidentally diagnosed from a hemorrhoidectomy specimen. Approximately two-thirds of the lesions will be grossly pigmented or show histologic evidence of melanin.[148] Amelanotic lesions can be difficult to differentiate from undifferentiated SCC.

Surgical management of anorectal melanoma provides the only chance for cure. However, the choice of operation continues to be controversial because the prognosis is so poor. Up to 35% of patients present with metastatic disease,[149,150] and those patients with tumors >10 mm in thickness are not cured by any treatment.[150] Additionally, long-term survival rates,

which range from 0% to 29%,[145,148–152] do not seem to differ when wide local excision or APR is performed. However, some studies have shown fewer locoregional recurrences with a more radical operation,[148,149,153] thereby supporting the use of APR for earlier-stage tumors. In a recent study of anorectal melanomas stratified by tumor thickness, tumors >4 mm had inadequate local tumor control with wide local excision alone and APR was advocated.[150] Despite this, anorectal melanoma is largely a fatal disease and so the choice of treatment has little influence on the eventual outcome. Therefore, many authors advocate local excision to spare patients the morbidity of an APR and a colostomy. If the tumor is bulky and negative margins (1–2 cm) cannot be achieved, it involves the sphincter complex, or local resection will result in incontinence, then an APR is the recommended treatment option. If the patient already has signs of regional or systemic metastasis, radical excision should not be performed. The use of endoanal ultrasound and sentinel lymph node biopsies may further guide treatment for this disease.[145,151]

Adjuvant therapy for cutaneous melanoma has been studied extensively; however, the applicability of these data to anorectal melanoma remains uncertain. Many immunotherapeutic and chemotherapeutic agents such as dacarbazine, bacillus Calmette-Guerin, levamisole, and interferon-α have demonstrated no benefit.[151] Cytotoxic chemotherapy including cisplatin, vinblastine, and dacarbazine, combined with interleukin-2 or interferon-α2b has shown some improvement in survival; however, patients experienced significant treatment-related toxicity.[154] Radiation therapy has also been used to improve local and regional control, yet because of the small numbers of patients with anorectal melanoma, its efficacy is unknown. Because of its predilection for developing systemic metastasis, it is unclear whether efforts to achieve better local control are useful.

Gastrointestinal Stromal Tumors

Gastrointestinal stomal tumors (GISTs) of the anus are extremely uncommon with only 17 cases reported in the literature up to 2003.[155] GISTs are tumors of mesenchymal origin that are not derived from smooth muscle or Schwann cells. They are identified by immunohistochemical studies that stain positive for CD34 and CD117 antigens. It is important to differentiate them from true smooth muscle tumors, with which they were previously combined, as they have a different pathogenesis and biologic outcome. However, most series that have reported on leiomyomas and leiomyosarcomas in the past did not make this distinction, but in fact, reflect a large proportion of GISTs.[155,156] Because of the rarity of anal GISTs, they have only been studied with lesions of the rectum as a single entity.

Patients present in the fifth to seventh decade of life and are more often men. Most patients are asymptomatic but bleeding, anal pain, change in bowel habits, or urinary symptoms can occur. Pathologic factors implicated in aggressive tumors with metastatic potential are size >5 cm in diameter and high mitotic counts, pleomorphism, infiltration of muscularis propria, and coagulative necrosis. The presence of symptoms is also associated with a worse prognosis.

Treatment involves local excision for tumors <2 cm and APR for those with larger tumors or worse pathologic features.[155] In a study of anorectal stromal tumors, recurrence rates for local excision and radical resection were 60% and 0%, respectively.[157] The natural history of GISTs is indolent with a long latency period (>4 years) to recurrence or metastasis, which is usually by a hematogenous route.[156] The role of adjuvant therapy is still uncertain.

Small Cell Carcinoma/Neuroendocrine Tumors

Small cell or neuroendocrine tumors comprise less than 1% of all colorectal malignancies and are extremely rare in the anal canal. In a recent series of neuroendocrine carcinomas of the lower gastrointestinal tract, 16% were found in the anal canal.[158] Diagnosis involves identification of the classic histopathologic pattern. Hyperchromatic nuclei, pale nucleoli, high mitotic count, in addition to tumor growth in loose, non-cohesive sheets are seen, similar to small cell or oat cell carcinoma of the lung. Sixty-five to eighty percent of patients with extrapulmonary small cell tumors present with metastatic disease; therefore, it is important to stage them accurately. Those with disease limited to the anal canal are treated in a similar manner to those with adenocarcinoma, including chemoradiation and radical surgery. Those with disseminated disease may benefit from combination chemotherapy regimens used for small cell lung cancer such as cisplatin and etopside.[146,158]

Uncommon Anal Margin/Perianal Neoplasms

Basal Cell Carcinoma

The incidence of basal cell carcinomas (BCCs) of the anus, in comparison to sun-exposed areas of the body, is extremely low. It comprises about 0.1% of all BCCs diagnosed and fewer than 200 cases of BCC have been reported on the perianal and genital area.[159] BCCs of the anal margin account for only 0.2% of all anorectal cancers. The largest series of perianal BCCs thus far reported includes only 34 cases.[160]

The etiology of perianal BCC is likely different from BCC arising in sun-exposed skin. Although preexisting skin conditions such as basal cell nevus syndrome and xeroderma pigmentosum, immunodeficiency, and genetics may contribute to both types, radiation, chronic irritation or infection, history of trauma or burn have all been implicated in perianal lesions.[159,161] The majority of these carcinomas occur in men (60%–80%) and the average age at presentation is 65–75 years. Approximately one-third have a previous or concomitant history of BCC at other skin sites.[159,160,162]

The average size at presentation is <2 cm, although they can be as large as 10 cm and extend into the anal canal.[160] The clinical appearance can range from erythematous papules to nodules, plaques, and ulcers.[159] They tend to be mobile and superficial with little invasive or metastatic potential. Histologically they are similar to BCCs of other areas of the body and do not contain HPV.[159] It is extremely important to differentiate BCC from basaloid carcinoma histologically because these entities behave in a different manner.

It was previously thought that anorectal BCC was more aggressive than other cutaneous BCCs,[162] but it is likely that perianal BCC was not adequately differentiated from the more aggressive basaloid tumors thus suggesting a worse prognosis.

Treatment is wide local excision ensuring adequate margins which is possible in lesions <2 cm. Larger lesions may require excision with skin grafting or use of Mohs micrographic surgery to preserve uninvolved tissue. Recurrence rates for local excision range from 0% to 29%.[160,162] Cancer-specific survival in both series was 100% at 5 years. Recurrences can be treated with reexcision. Large lesions extending into the anal canal may be better treated with radiation or APR.

Paget's Disease

Paget's disease can be divided into two groups, mammary and extramammary. The former was identified on the nipple of the female breast with an underlying carcinoma by Sir James Paget in 1847.[163] The latter was described specifically in the perianal area by Darier and Couillaud in 1893[164] and comprises about 20% of the extramammary type.[146] Other sites of Paget's disease include the axilla, scrotum, penis, vulva, groin, thigh, and buttock where apocrine glands are found.

It is currently believed that Paget's cells represent an intraepithelial adenocarcinoma with a prolonged preinvasive phase that eventually develops into an adenocarcinoma of the underlying apocrine gland given enough time. The origin of these cells is not completely understood. One theory suggests that a pluripotent basal cell is the progenitor of the Paget's cell with the adenocarcinoma arising in the epidermis and extending into the dermis. The other theory supports the origin of Paget's cells from the apocrine glands that spreads into the overlying epidermis. The latter hypothesis may be more likely given the fact that the lesions tend to occur in areas of high-density apocrine glands.[73,146,165]

This is a rare condition with fewer than 200 cases reported in the literature to date.[166] Patients present in the seventh decade of life with equal distribution among men and women. The most common presenting symptom is intractable itching followed by bleeding, palpable mass, inguinal lymphadenopathy, weight loss, anal discharge and constipation. The median duration of symptoms is 3 years.[167,168] The lesions themselves often have an erythematous, eczematous appearance with well-demarcated borders mimicking a rash.

They may look ulcerated or plaque-like with oozing or scaling. A third of cases involve the entire anus.[169] These lesions are often misdiagnosed because of their similarity to other conditions. The differential includes Bowen's disease, Crohn's disease, condyloma acuminatum, hidradenitis suppurativa, pruritus ani, and SCC. Biopsy is essential to confirm the diagnosis.

Histologically, Paget's cells have large, round, eccentric, hyperchromic nuclei with pale-staining, vacuolated cytoplasm. The cytoplasm stains positive with periodic acid-Schiff stain because of the abundance of mucin and also stains positive for mucicarmine, cytokeratin 7, and Alcian blue, which stain mucoproteins, and differentiates it from Bowen's disease. Both mammary and extramammary Paget's disease have similar histologic features but mammary Paget's consistently presents with an associated invasive carcinoma, whereas in perianal Paget's disease, less than half (30%–44%) present with invasive adenocarcinoma.[165,169,170] However, the incidence of associated visceral malignancies in perianal Paget's disease is increased with various series reporting rates of 30%–50%. The most common sites include the gastrointestinal tract, anus, skin, prostate, neck, and nasopharynx.[165,169–171] There may also be synchronous lesions in the axillary or anogenital area in patients diagnosed with perianal disease, therefore a careful survey of other sites for malignancy and secondary disease is necessary.[146]

The treatment for perianal Paget's disease depends on the presence of invasion and other associated anorectal malignancies. For noninvasive lesions, wide local excision is the procedure of choice. In addition to resecting the lesion with grossly negative margins, it is important to map the extent of involvement of the lesion microscopically. This can be performed either by taking random biopsies 1 cm from the edge of the lesion in all four quadrants, including the dentate line, anal verge, and perineum[166,171] or by using toluidine blue and acetic acid to stain the Paget's cells, thereby directing the site for biopsy.[73] The use of intraoperative frozen sections ensures that any disease that extends beyond the gross lesion will be excised to reduce the chance of recurrence. Positive margins requiring reexcision are not uncommon when this technique is not used. In a recently reported series of 27 patients, 9 had positive margins and 12 required further surgery. Of the five patients who had mapping with 1-cm biopsies, none developed recurrence.[165] Another study reported positive margins in 53% of patients.[172] Preoperative mapping can also be performed using dermatologic punch biopsies. If the defect is small, the skin may be closed primarily. For larger lesions that require circumferential excision of the perianal skin, split-thickness skin grafts or sliding and rotational flaps may be required. Recurrence rates range from 37% to 100%.[165,170,173] Most recurrences were treated with wide reexcision with excellent results. For those who developed invasion, more radical surgery or adjuvant therapy was used.

Patients who have an invasive component or an associated anorectal malignancy should be considered for radical excision with APR. If positive inguinal lymph nodes are present, an inguinal lymphadenectomy should be added. Unfortunately, patients with invasive disease present with metastasis 25% of the time and all patients who die of this disease have an invasive component.[73,165] Too few cases of perianal Paget's disease exist to allow for a comparison of invasive and noninvasive groups. Disease-specific survival for all perianal Paget's disease at 5 years ranges from 54% to 70%[165,169–171] and at 10 years decreases to 39%–45%.[165,169]

The role of adjuvant chemoradiation therapy remains uncertain. It is currently used in some cases of invasive or aggressive recurrent disease. Concurrent anorectal malignancies may be another indication. Radiation has been associated with an increased rate of local complications when used for perianal Paget's disease[172] and is therefore reserved for patients who are not candidates for further surgical resection.[165]

Verrucous Carcinoma

The term verrucous carcinoma was initially coined in 1948 to describe a low-grade carcinoma of the oral mucosa that resembled viral warts. It has now been expanded to include those lesions described as giant condyloma acuminatum or Buschke–Lowenstein tumors. The latter was first described by Abraham Buschke in 1896 with respect to two invasive condylomata of the penis. Buschke and Lowenstein then further delineated these lesions of the anus in 1925.[174] These tumors were characterized by condylomatous features with growth to a large size, local invasion, and destruction of surrounding tissues and the absence of metastases. Although it is a well recognized entity, only 51 cases have been reported in the literature to date.[175] HPV is frequently detected.

These tumors are more frequently found in men with a 2.7:1 male to female ratio. The average age of patients is 45 years and is slowly decreasing. Patients usually present with complaint of an anal growth. Pain, perianal discharge/abscess, anorectal bleeding, pruritus, and a change in bowel habits may also occur.[175,176] The lesions themselves are generally slow growing with a soft, cauliflower-like appearance that can become nodular as it penetrates the underlying tissues. This direct expansion of the tumor causes erosion and even necrosis of the surrounding tissues thereby predisposing it to developing fistulas that drain purulent fluid. They usually arise from the perianal skin but can also present in the anal canal and distal rectum. At presentation they tend to be quite large measuring anywhere from 1.5 to 30 cm.[175] Regional lymphadenopathy may also occur secondary to infection.

The tumor, which is clinically difficult to distinguish from a malignancy, is histologically benign. Papillomatosis, acanthosis with hyperplasia of the prickle cell layer, variable hyperkeratosis, parakeratosis, and underlying inflammation are often found.[174] However, of all the cases of giant condyloma acuminatum reported, only 42% were histologically diagnosed as condyloma without any invasion. A malignant transformation was identified in 58% of the tumors; 8% had carcinoma in situ, and 50% had invasion that was termed verrucous carcinoma, SCC, or basaloid carcinoma.

The standard treatment for verrucous carcinoma is radical local excision. For those patients with extensive deep tissue involvement, multiple fistulas, or involvement of the anal sphincter, APR is indicated. Cure can be achieved only by radical excision. Neoadjuvant radiation therapy may be useful for those tumors with invasive carcinoma and to render a tumor resectable because of its large size; however, some controversy exists as to whether radiation promotes malignant transformation of the tumors. The most current studies do not support this concept, because the incidence of invasive lesions after radiation is extremely low.[176] It has been hypothesized that the high recurrence rates after radical excision may be attributable to spillage of residual tumor, which could potentially be prevented by reducing the tumor size with preoperative chemoradiation. Certainly, size and local extent of tumor invasion, not malignant histology, has the greatest impact on morbidity, recurrence, and mortality. Unfortunately, the rarity of this condition makes it difficult to study this issue prospectively.

HIV-related Anal Cancer

Kaposi's Sarcoma

Although Kaposi's sarcoma is the most common cutaneous malignancy in patients with AIDS,[177] the incidence of perianal lesions is quite small and decreasing with the increasingly effective antiretroviral therapy available today.[178] A study of 180 consecutive HIV-seropositive patients seen for anorectal symptoms revealed two perianal Kaposi's sarcomas. They were both small, round, purplish lesions that could easily have been mistaken for hemorrhoids. Both were treated with chemotherapy although radiation has been used for localized cutaneous lesions.[179]

Lymphoma

The incidence of non-Hodgkin's lymphoma (NHL) has been increasing in AIDS patients as treatment improves and life expectancy increases. NHL is the second most common AIDS-related neoplasm after Kaposi's sarcoma. Compared with lymphomas found in the general population, these tumors are characterized by B cells of a higher histologic grade that originates from extranodal tissue. They are also more aggressive, prone to dissemination, and resistant to treatment. Most lymphomas are found in the central nervous system and the gastrointestinal tract. However, anorectal lymphomas are extremely rare, comprising less than 1% of all anorectal neoplasms in the general population.[180] Although the anorectal area is devoid of lymphoid tissue, it is postulated that the exposure to chronic infections from anal receptive intercourse or an immunocompromised state may result in an "acquired" mucosa-associated lymphoid tissue.

The most common presenting symptoms are pain, pruritus, drainage, or a palpable mass. Some patients may have more constitutional symptoms such as fever, night sweats, or weight loss.[180] After appropriate staging, patients are treated with a standard regimen for NHL of chemotherapy and radiation therapy of the affected area.

There is no role for surgical treatment. Usual chemotherapeutic agents include cyclophosphamide, actinomycin, vincristine, and corticosteroids (CHOP). There are too few cases of anorectal lymphoma reported to discuss overall prognosis. However, younger patients without constitutional symptoms may fare better. Additionally, low CD4 counts and performance status may affect a patient's ability to endure aggressive therapy.[146] Isolated reports of immunocompetent patients with anorectal lymphoma have been reported with excellent response to treatment.[181]

References

1. Welton ML, Sharkey FE, Kahlenberg MS. The etiology and epidemiology of anal cancer. Surg Oncol Clin North Am 2004; 13:263–275.
2. Frisch M, Glimelius B, van den Brule AJ, et al. Sexually transmitted infection as a cause of anal cancer. N Engl J Med 1997;337:1350–1358.
3. Munoz N, Bosch FX, de Sanjose S, et al. Epidemiologic classification of human papillomavirus types associated with cervical cancer. N Engl J Med 2003;348:518–527.
4. Strickler HD, Schiffman MH. Is human papillomavirus an infectious cause of non-cervical anogenital tract cancers? BMJ 1997;315:620–621.
5. Koutsky L. Epidemiology of genital human papillomavirus infection. Am J Med 1997;102:3–8.
6. O'Mahony C, Law C, Gollnick HP, Marini M. New patient-applied therapy for anogenital warts is rated favourably by patients. Int J STD AIDS 2001;12:565–570.
7. Bauer HM, Ting Y, Greer CE, et al. Genital human papillomavirus infection in female university students as determined by a PCR-based method. JAMA 1991;265:472–477.
8. Pecoraro G, Morgan D, Defendi V. Differential effects of human papillomavirus type 6, 16, and 18 DNAs on immortalization and transformation of human cervical epithelial cells. Proc Natl Acad Sci USA 1989;86:563–567.
9. Woodworth CD, Doniger J, DiPaolo JA. Immortalization of human foreskin keratinocytes by various human papillomavirus DNAs corresponds to their association with cervical carcinoma. J Virol 1989;63:159–164.
10. van der Snoek EM, Niesters HG, Mulder PG, van Doornum GJ, Osterhaus AD, van der Meijden WI. Human papillomavirus infection in men who have sex with men participating in a Dutch gay-cohort study. Sex Transm Dis 2003;30: 639–644.
11. Palefsky JM, Gonzales J, Greenblatt RM, Ahn DK, Hollander H. Anal intraepithelial neoplasia and anal papillomavirus infection among homosexual males with group IV HIV disease. JAMA 1990;263:2911–2916.
12. Palefsky JM, Holly EA, Gonzales J, Berline J, Ahn DK, Greenspan JS. Detection of human papillomavirus DNA in

anal intraepithelial neoplasia and anal cancer. Cancer Res 1991;51:1014–1019.

13. Jay N, Berry JM, Hogeboom CJ, Holly EA, Darragh TM, Palefsky JM. Colposcopic appearance of anal squamous intraepithelial lesions: relationship to histopathology. Dis Colon Rectum 1997;40:919–928.

14. Holly EA, Whittemore AS, Aston DA, Ahn DK, Nickoloff BJ, Kristiansen JJ. Anal cancer incidence: genital warts, anal fissure or fistula, hemorrhoids, and smoking. J Natl Cancer Inst 1989;81:1726–1731.

15. Bosch FX, Lorincz A, Munoz N, Meijer CJ, Shah KV. The causal relation between human papillomavirus and cervical cancer. J Clin Pathol 2002;55:244–265.

16. Hildesheim A, Schiffman MH, Tsukui T, et al. Immune activation in cervical neoplasia: cross-sectional association between plasma soluble interleukin 2 receptor levels and disease. Cancer Epidemiol Biomarkers Prev 1997;6:807–813.

17. Palefsky JM, Holly EA, Ralston ML, Da Costa M, Greenblatt RM. Prevalence and risk factors for anal human papillomavirus infection in human immunodeficiency virus (HIV)-positive and high-risk HIV-negative women. J Infect Dis 2001;183:383–391.

18. Holly EA, Ralston ML, Darragh TM, Greenblatt RM, Jay N, Palefsky JM. Prevalence and risk factors for anal squamous intraepithelial lesions in women. J Natl Cancer Inst 2001;93:843–849.

19. Sobhani I, Vuagnat A, Walker F, et al. Prevalence of high-grade dysplasia and cancer in the anal canal in human papillomavirus-infected individuals. Gastroenterology 2001;120:857–866.

20. Cress RD, Holly EA. Incidence of anal cancer in California: increased incidence among men in San Francisco, 1973–1999. Prev Med 2003;36:555–560.

21. Penn I. Cancers of the anogenital region in renal transplant recipients. Analysis of 65 cases. Cancer 1986;58:611–616.

22. Penn I. Cancer in the immunosuppressed organ recipient. Transplant Proc 1991;23:1771–1772.

23. McGlennen RC. Human papillomavirus oncogenesis. Clin Lab Med 2000;20:383–406.

24. zur Hausen H. Immortalization of human cells and their malignant conversion by high risk human papillomavirus genotypes. Semin Cancer Biol 1999;9:405–411.

25. Martin F, Bower M. Anal intraepithelial neoplasia in HIV positive people. Sex Transm Infect 2001;77:327–331.

26. Werness BA, Levine AJ, Howley PM. Association of human papillomavirus types 16 and 18 E6 proteins with p53. Science 1990;248:76–79.

27. Chow LT, Broker TR. Papillomavirus DNA replication. Intervirology 1994;37:150–158.

28. Dollard SC, Wilson JL, Demeter LM, et al. Production of human papillomavirus and modulation of the infectious program in epithelial raft cultures. OFF. Genes Dev 1992;6:1131–1142.

29. Flores ER, Lambert PF. Evidence for a switch in the mode of human papillomavirus type 16 DNA replication during the viral life cycle. J Virol 1997;71:7167–7179.

30. Litle VR, Leavenworth JD, Darragh TM, et al. Angiogenesis, proliferation, and apoptosis in anal high-grade squamous intraepithelial lesions. Dis Colon Rectum 2000;43:346–352.

31. Chang GJ, Berry JM, Jay N, Palefsky JM, Welton ML. Surgical treatment of high-grade anal squamous intraepithelial lesions: a prospective study. Dis Colon Rectum 2002;45:453–458.

32. Goldie SJ, Kuntz KM, Weinstein MC, Freedberg KA, Welton ML, Palefsky JM. The clinical effectiveness and cost-effectiveness of screening for anal squamous intraepithelial lesions in homosexual and bisexual HIV-positive men. JAMA 1999; 281:1822–1829.

33. Goldie SJ, Kuntz KM, Weinstein MC, Freedberg KA, Palefsky JM. Cost-effectiveness of screening for anal squamous intraepithelial lesions and anal cancer in human immunodeficiency virus-negative homosexual and bisexual men. Am J Med 2000;108:634–641.

34. Daling JR, Weiss NS, Hislop TG, et al. Sexual practices, sexually transmitted diseases, and the incidence of anal cancer. N Engl J Med 1987;317:973–977.

35. Scholefield JH, Sonnex C, Talbot IC, et al. Anal and cervical intraepithelial neoplasia: possible parallel. Lancet 1989;2:765–769.

36. Rabkin CS, Yellin F. Cancer incidence in a population with a high prevalence of infection with human immunodeficiency virus type 1. J Natl Cancer Inst 1994;86:1711–1716.

37. Koblin BA, Hessol NA, Zauber AG, et al. Increased incidence of cancer among homosexual men, New York City and San Francisco, 1978–1990. Am J Epidemiol 1996;144:916–923.

38. Critchlow CW, Surawicz CM, Holmes KK, et al. Prospective study of high grade anal squamous intraepithelial neoplasia in a cohort of homosexual men: influence of HIV infection, immunosuppression and human papillomavirus infection. AIDS 1995;9:1255–1262.

39. Palefsky JM, Holly EA, Ralston ML, et al. Anal squamous intraepithelial lesions in HIV-positive and HIV-negative homosexual and bisexual men: prevalence and risk factors. J Acquir Immune Defic Syndr Hum Retrovirol 1998;17:320–326.

40. Palefsky JM, Holly EA, Hogeboom CJ, et al. Virologic, immunologic, and clinical parameters in the incidence and progression of anal squamous intraepithelial lesions in HIV-positive and HIV-negative homosexual men. J Acquir Immune Defic Syndr Hum Retrovirol 1998;17:314–319.

41. Frisch M, Biggar RJ, Goedert JJ. Human papillomavirus-associated cancers in patients with human immunodeficiency virus infection and acquired immunodeficiency syndrome. J Natl Cancer Inst 2000;92:1500–1510.

42. Greenlee RT, Murray T, Bolden S, Wingo PA. Cancer statistics, 2000. CA Cancer J Clin 2000;50:7–33.

43. Jemal A, Murray T, Samuels A, Ghafoor A, Ward E, Thun MJ. Cancer statistics, 2003. CA Cancer J Clin 2003;53:5–26.

44. Goldman S, Glimelius B, Nilsson B, Pahlman L. Incidence of anal epidermoid carcinoma in Sweden 1970–1984. Acta Chir Scand 1989;155:191–197.

45. Frisch M, Melbye M, Moller H. Trends in incidence of anal cancer in Denmark. BMJ 1993;306:419–422.

46. Melbye M, Sprogel P. Aetiological parallel between anal cancer and cervical cancer. Lancet 1991;338:657–659.

47. Holmes F, Borek D, Owen-Kummer M, et al. Anal cancer in women. Gastroenterology 1988;95:107–111.

48. Palefsky JM, Shiboski S, Moss A. Risk factors for anal human papillomavirus infection and anal cytologic abnormalities in HIV-positive and HIV-negative homosexual men. J Acquir Immune Defic Syndr 1994;7:599–606.

49. Caussy D, Goedert JJ, Palefsky J, et al. Interaction of human immunodeficiency and papilloma viruses: association with anal epithelial abnormality in homosexual men. Int J Cancer 1990;46:214–219.

50. Friedman HB, Saah AJ, Sherman ME, et al. Human papillo-mavirus, anal squamous intraepithelial lesions, and human immunodeficiency virus in a cohort of gay men. J Infect Dis 1998;178:45–52.

51. Palefsky JM, Holly EA, Ralston ML, Jay N, Berry JM, Darragh TM. High incidence of anal high-grade squamous intra-epithelial lesions among HIV-positive and HIV-negative homosexual and bisexual men. AIDS 1998;12:495–503.

52. Ogunbiyi OA, Scholefield JH, Raftery AT, et al. Prevalence of anal human papillomavirus infection and intraepithelial neoplasia in renal allograft recipients. Br J Surg 1994;81:365–367.

53. Daling JR, Sherman KJ, Hislop TG, et al. Cigarette smoking and the risk of anogenital cancer. Am J Epidemiol 1992;135:180–189.

54. Marfing TE, Abel ME, Gallagher DM. Perianal Bowen's disease and associated malignancies. Results of a survey. Dis Colon Rectum 1987;30:782–785.

55. Arbesman H, Ransohoff DF. Is Bowen's disease a predictor for the development of internal malignancy? A methodological critique of the literature. JAMA 1987;257:516–518.

56. Marchesa P, Fazio VW, Oliart S, Goldblum JR, Lavery IC. Perianal Bowen's disease: a clinicopathologic study of 47 patients. Dis Colon Rectum 1997;40:1286–1293.

57. Brown SR, Skinner P, Tidy J, Smith JH, Sharp F, Hosie KB. Outcome after surgical resection for high-grade anal intraep-ithelial neoplasia (Bowen's disease). Br J Surg 1999;86:1063–1066.

58. Bargman H, Hochman J. Topical treatment of Bowen's disease with 5-fluorouracil. J Cutan Med Surg 2003;7:101–105.

59. Wang KH, Fang JY, Hu CH, Lee WR. Erbium:YAG laser pre-treatment accelerates the response of Bowen's disease treated by topical 5-fluorouracil. Dermatol Surg 2004;30:441–445.

60. Snoeck R, Van Laethem Y, De Clercq E, De Maubeuge J, Clumeck N. Treatment of a bowenoid papulosis of the penis with local applications of cidofovir in a patient with acquired immunodeficiency syndrome. Arch Intern Med 2001;161:2382–2384.

61. Okamoto A, Woodworth CD, Yen K, et al. Combination ther-apy with podophyllin and vidarabine for human papillomavirus positive cervical intraepithelial neoplasia. Oncol Rep 1999;6:269–276.

62. Micali G, Nasca MR, Tedeschi A. Topical treatment of intraep-ithelial penile carcinoma with imiquimod. Clin Exp Dermatol 2003;28(suppl 1):4–6.

63. Smith KJ, Germain M, Skelton H. Squamous cell carcinoma in situ (Bowen's disease) in renal transplant patients treated with 5% imiquimod and 5% 5-fluorouracil therapy. Dermatol Surg 2001;27:561–564.

64. Pehoushek J, Smith KJ. Imiquimod and 5% fluorouracil ther-apy for anal and perianal squamous cell carcinoma in situ in an HIV-1-positive man. Arch Dermatol 2001;137:14–16.

65. Panizzon RG. Radiotherapy of skin tumors. Recent Results Cancer Res 2002;160:234–239.

66. Chung YL, Lee JD, Bang D, Lee JB, Park KB, Lee MG. Treatment of Bowen's disease with a specially designed radioactive skin patch. Eur J Nucl Med 2000;27:842–846.

67. Webber J, Fromm D. Photodynamic therapy for carcinoma in situ of the anus. Arch Surg 2004;139:259–261.

68. Varma S, Wilson H, Kurwa HA, et al. Bowen's disease, solar keratoses and superficial basal cell carcinomas treated by photodynamic therapy using a large-field incoherent light source. Br J Dermatol 2001;144:567–574.

69. Salim A, Leman JA, McColl JH, Chapman R, Morton CA. Randomized comparison of photodynamic therapy with topical 5-fluorouracil in Bowen's disease. Br J Dermatol 2003;148:539–543.

70. Behrendt GC, Hansmann ML. Carcinomas of the anal canal and anal margin differ in their expression of cadherin, cytoker-atins and p53. Virchows Arch 2001;439:782–786.

71. Anal Canal. AJCC Cancer Staging Manual, 6th ed. Greene FL, Page DL, Fleming ID, Fritz AG, Balch CM, Haller DG, Morrow M (eds). New York: Springer; 2002:125–130.

72. Gervasoni JE Jr, Wanebo HJ. Cancers of the anal canal and anal margin. Cancer Invest 2003;21:452–464.

73. Skibber J, Rodriguez-Bigas MA, Gordon PH. Surgical consid-erations in anal cancer. Surg Oncol Clin North Am 2004;13:321–338.

74. Newlin HE, Zlotecki RA, Morris CG, Hochwald SN, Riggs CE, Mendenhall WM. Squamous cell carcinoma of the anal margin. J Surg Oncol 2004;86:55–62; discussion 63.

75. Jensen SL, Hagen K, Shokouh-Amiri MH, Nielsen OV. Does an erroneous diagnosis of squamous-cell carcinoma of the anal canal and anal margin at first physician visit influence progno-sis? Dis Colon Rectum 1987;30:345–351.

76. Winburn GB. Anal carcinoma or "just hemorrhoids"? Am Surg 2001;67:1048–1058.

77. Mendenhall WM, Zlotecki RA, Vauthey JN, Copeland EM 3rd. Squamous cell carcinoma of the anal margin treated with radiotherapy. Surg Oncol 1996;5:29–35.

78. Papillon J, Chassard JL. Respective roles of radiotherapy and sur-gery in the management of epidermoid carcinoma of the anal mar-gin. Series of 57 patients. Dis Colon Rectum 1992;35:422–429.

79. Nivatvongs S. Perianal and anal canal neoplasms. In: Gordon PH, Nivatvongs S, eds. Principles and Practice of Surgery for the Colon, Rectum, and Anus. St. Louis: Quality Medical Publishing; 1999:448–471.

80. Jensen SL, Hagen K, Harling H, Shokouh-Amiri MH, Nielsen OV. Long-term prognosis after radical treatment for squamous-cell carcinoma of the anal canal and anal margin. Dis Colon Rectum 1988;31:273–278.

81. Greenall MJ, Quan SH, Stearns MW, Urmacher C, DeCosse JJ. Epidermoid cancer of the anal margin. Pathologic features, treatment, and clinical results. Am J Surg 1985;149:95–101.

82. Al-Jurf AS, Turnbull RP, Fazio VW. Local treatment of squa-mous cell carcinoma of the anus. Surg Gynecol Obstet 1979;148:576–578.

83. Schraut WH, Wang CH, Dawson PJ, Block GE. Depth of inva-sion, location, and size of cancer of the anus dictate operative treatment. Cancer 1983;51:1291–1296.

84. Pintor MP, Northover JM, Nicholls RJ. Squamous cell carci-noma of the anus at one hospital from 1948 to 1984. Br J Surg 1989;76:806–810.

85. Beahrs OH, Wilson SM. Carcinoma of the anus. Ann Surg 1976;184:422–428.

86. Peiffert D, Bey P, Pernot M, et al. Conservative treatment by irradiation of epidermoid carcinomas of the anal margin. Int J Radiat Oncol Biol Phys 1997;39:57–66.

87. Touboul E, Schlienger M, Buffat L, et al. Epidermoid carci-noma of the anal margin: 17 cases treated with curative-intent radiation therapy. Radiother Oncol 1995;34:195–202.

88. Mendenhall WM, Zlotecki RA, Vauthey JN, Copeland EM 3rd. Squamous cell carcinoma of the anal margin. Oncology (Williston Park) 1996;10:1843–1848; discussion 1848, 1853–1854.

89. Cummings BJ, Keane TJ, Hawkins NV, O'Sullivan B. Treatment of perianal carcinoma by radiation(RT) or radiation plus chemotherapy(RTCT). Int J Radiat Oncol Biol Phys 1986;12:170.

90. Cutuli B, Fenton J, Labib A, Bataini JP, Mathieu G. Anal margin carcinoma: 21 cases treated at the Institut Curie by exclusive conservative radiotherapy. Radiother Oncol 1988;11:1–6.

91. John MJ, Flam M, Lovalvo L, Mowry PA. Feasibility of nonsurgical definitive management of anal canal carcinoma. Int J Radiat Oncol Biol Phys 1987;13:299–303.

92. Bartelink H, Roelofsen F, Eschwege F, et al. Concomitant radiotherapy and chemotherapy is superior to radiotherapy alone in the treatment of locally advanced anal cancer: results of a phase III randomized trial of the European Organization for Research and Treatment of Cancer Radiotherapy and Gastrointestinal Cooperative Groups. J Clin Oncol 1997;15:2040–2049.

93. UKCCCR. Epidermoid anal cancer: results from the UKCCCR randomised trial of radiotherapy alone versus radiotherapy, 5-fluorouracil, and mitomycin. UKCCCR Anal Cancer Trial Working Party. UK Co-ordinating Committee on Cancer Research. Lancet 1996;348:1049–1054.

94. Roelofsen F, Bartelink H. Combined modality treatment of anal carcinoma. Oncologist 1998;3:413–418.

95. Allal AS, Mermillod B, Roth AD, Marti MC, Kurtz JM. Impact of clinical and therapeutic factors on major late complications after radiotherapy with or without concomitant chemotherapy for anal carcinoma. Int J Radiat Oncol Biol Phys 1997;39:1099–1105.

96. Bieri S, Allal AS, Kurtz JM. Sphincter-conserving treatment of carcinomas of the anal margin. Acta Oncol 2001;40:29–33.

97. Dougherty BG, Evans HL. Carcinoma of the anal canal: a study of 79 cases. Am J Clin Pathol 1985;83:159–164.

98. Rousseau DL Jr, Petrelli NJ, Kahlenberg MS. Overview of anal cancer for the surgeon. Surg Oncol Clin North Am 2004;13:249–262.

99. Clark MA, Hartley A, Geh JI. Cancer of the anal canal. Lancet Oncol 2004;5:149–157.

100. Boman BM, Moertel CG, O'Connell MJ, et al. Carcinoma of the anal canal. A clinical and pathologic study of 188 cases. Cancer 1984;54:114–125.

101. Roseau G, Palazzo L, Colardelle P, Chaussade S, Couturier D, Paolaggi JA. Endoscopic ultrasonography in the staging and follow-up of epidermoid carcinoma of the anal canal. Gastrointest Endosc 1994;40:447–450.

102. Drudi FM, Raffetto N, De Rubeis M, et al. TRUS staging and follow-up in patients with anal canal cancer. Radiol Med (Torino) 2003;106:329–337.

103. Giovannini M, Bardou VJ, Barclay R, et al. Anal carcinoma: prognostic value of endorectal ultrasound (ERUS). Results of a prospective multicenter study. Endoscopy 2001;33:231–236.

104. Goldman S, Glimelius B, Norming U, Pahlman L, Seligson U. Transanorectal ultrasonography in anal carcinoma. A prospective study of 21 patients. Acta Radiol 1988;29:337–341.

105. Christensen AF, Nielsen MB, Engelholm SA, Roed H, Svendsen LB, Christensen H. Three-dimensional anal endosonography may improve staging of anal cancer compared with two-dimensional endosonography. Dis Colon Rectum 2004;47:341–345.

106. Fuchshuber PR, Rodriguez-Bigas M, Weber T, Petrelli NJ. Anal canal and perianal epidermoid cancers. J Am Coll Surg 1997;185:494–505.

107. Perera D, Pathma-Nathan N, Rabbitt P, Hewett P, Rieger N. Sentinel node biopsy for squamous-cell carcinoma of the anus and anal margin. Dis Colon Rectum 2003;46:1027–1029; discussion 1030–1031.

108. Hoffman R, Welton ML, Klencke B, Weinberg V, Krieg R. The significance of pretreatment CD4 count on the outcome and treatment tolerance of HIV-positive patients with anal cancer. Int J Radiat Oncol Biol Phys 1999;44:127–131.

109. Eng C, Abbruzzese J, Minsky BD. Chemotherapy and radiation of anal canal cancer: the first approach. Surg Oncol Clin North Am 2004;13:309–320, viii.

110. Deniaud-Alexandre E, Touboul E, Tiret E, et al. Results of definitive irradiation in a series of 305 epidermoid carcinomas of the anal canal. Int J Radiat Oncol Biol Phys 2003;56:1259–1273.

111. Touboul E, Schlienger M, Buffat L, et al. Epidermoid carcinoma of the anal canal. Results of curative-intent radiation therapy in a series of 270 patients. Cancer 1994;73:1569–1579.

112. Gerard JP, Chapet O, Samiei F, et al. Management of inguinal lymph node metastases in patients with carcinoma of the anal canal: experience in a series of 270 patients treated in Lyon and review of the literature. Cancer 2001;92:77–84.

113. Cummings BJ. Treatment of primary epidermoid carcinoma of the anal canal. Int J Colorectal Dis 1987;2:107–112.

114. Wade DS, Herrera L, Castillo NB, Petrelli NJ. Metastases to the lymph nodes in epidermoid carcinoma of the anal canal studied by a clearing technique. Surg Gynecol Obstet 1989;169:238–242.

115. Ryan DP, Mayer RJ. Anal carcinoma: histology, staging, epidemiology, treatment. Curr Opin Oncol 2000;12:345–352.

116. Hughes LL, Rich TA, Delclos L, Ajani JA, Martin RG. Radiotherapy for anal cancer: experience from 1979–1987. Int J Radiat Oncol Biol Phys 1989;17:1153–1160.

117. Constantinou EC, Daly W, Fung CY, Willett CG, Kaufman DS, DeLaney TF. Time-dose considerations in the treatment of anal cancer. Int J Radiat Oncol Biol Phys 1997;39:651–657.

118. John M, Pajak T, Flam M, et al. Dose escalation in chemoradiation for anal cancer: preliminary results of RTOG 92-08. Cancer J Sci Am 1996;2:205.

119. Myerson RJ, Kong F, Birnbaum EH, et al. Radiation therapy for epidermoid carcinoma of the anal canal, clinical and treatment factors associated with outcome. Radiother Oncol 2001;61:15–22.

120. Cummings BJ, Keane TJ, O'Sullivan B, Wong CS, Catton CN. Epidermoid anal cancer: treatment by radiation alone or by radiation and 5-fluorouracil with and without mitomycin C. Int J Radiat Oncol Biol Phys 1991;21:1115–1125.

121. Nguyen WD, Mitchell KM, Beck DE. Risk factors associated with requiring a stoma for the management of anal cancer. Dis Colon Rectum 2004;47:843–846.

122. Ng Ying Kin NY, Pigneux J, Auvray H, Brunet R, Thomas L, Denepoux R. Our experience of conservative treatment of anal canal carcinoma combining external irradiation and interstitial implant: 32 cases treated between 1973 and 1982. Int J Radiat Oncol Biol Phys 1988;14:253–259.

123. Papillon J, Montbarbon JF. Epidermoid carcinoma of the anal canal. A series of 276 cases. Dis Colon Rectum 1987;30: 324–333.

124. Mitchell SE, Mendenhall WM, Zlotecki RA, Carroll RR. Squamous cell carcinoma of the anal canal. Int J Radiat Oncol Biol Phys 2001;49:1007–1013.

125. Nigro ND, Vaitkevicius VK, Considine B Jr. Combined therapy for cancer of the anal canal: a preliminary report. Dis Colon Rectum 1974;17:354–356.

126. Buroker TR, Nigro N, Bradley G, et al. Combined therapy for cancer of the anal canal: a follow-up report. Dis Colon Rectum 1977;20:677–678.

127. Nigro ND. An evaluation of combined therapy for squamous cell cancer of the anal canal. Dis Colon Rectum 1984;27:763–766.

128. Flam M, John M, Pajak TF, et al. Role of mitomycin in combination with fluorouracil and radiotherapy, and of salvage chemoradiation in the definitive nonsurgical treatment of epidermoid carcinoma of the anal canal: results of a phase III randomized intergroup study. J Clin Oncol 1996;14:2527–2539.

129. Hung A, Crane C, Delclos M, et al. Cisplatin-based combined modality therapy for anal carcinoma: a wider therapeutic index. Cancer 2003;97:1195–1202.

130. Gerard JP, Ayzac L, Hun D, et al. Treatment of anal canal carcinoma with high dose radiation therapy and concomitant fluorouracil-cisplatinum. Long-term results in 95 patients. Radiother Oncol 1998;46:249–256.

131. Lund JA, Sundstrom SH, Haaverstad R, Wibe A, Svinsaas M, Myrvold HE. Endoanal ultrasound is of little value in follow-up of anal carcinomas. Dis Colon Rectum 2004;47:839–842.

132. van der Wal BC, Cleffken BI, Gulec B, Kaufman HS, Choti MA. Results of salvage abdominoperineal resection for recurrent anal carcinoma following combined chemoradiation therapy. J Gastrointest Surg 2001;5:383–387.

133. Zelnick RS, Haas PA, Ajlouni M, Szilagyi E, Fox TA Jr. Results of abdominoperineal resections for failures after combination chemotherapy and radiation therapy for anal canal cancers. Dis Colon Rectum 1992;35:574–577; discussion 577–578.

134. Pocard M, Tiret E, Nugent K, Dehni N, Parc R. Results of salvage abdominoperineal resection for anal cancer after radiotherapy. Dis Colon Rectum 1998;41:1488–1493.

135. Ellenhorn JD, Enker WE, Quan SH. Salvage abdominoperineal resection following combined chemotherapy and radiotherapy for epidermoid carcinoma of the anus. Ann Surg Oncol 1994;1: 105–110.

136. Allal AS, Laurencet FM, Reymond MA, Kurtz JM, Marti MC. Effectiveness of surgical salvage therapy for patients with locally uncontrolled anal carcinoma after sphincter-conserving treatment. Cancer 1999;86:405–409.

137. Akbari RP, Paty PB, Guillem JG, et al. Oncologic outcomes of salvage surgery for epidermoid carcinoma of the anus initially managed with combined modality therapy. Dis Colon Rectum 2004;47:1136–1144.

138. Nilsson PJ, Svensson C, Goldman S, Glimelius B. Salvage abdominoperineal resection in anal epidermoid cancer. Br J Surg 2002;89:1425–1429.

139. Greenall MJ, Magill GB, Quan SH, DeCosse JJ. Recurrent epidermoid cancer of the anus. Cancer 1986;57:1437–1441.

140. Klas JV, Rothenberger DA, Wong WD, Madoff RD. Malignant tumors of the anal canal: the spectrum of disease, treatment, and outcomes. Cancer 1999;85:1686–1693.

141. Beal KP, Wong D, Guillem JG, et al. Primary adenocarcinoma of the anus treated with combined modality therapy. Dis Colon Rectum 2003;46:1320–1324.

142. Basik M, Rodriguez-Bigas MA, Penetrante R, Petrelli NJ. Prognosis and recurrence patterns of anal adenocarcinoma. Am J Surg 1995;169:233–237.

143. Papagikos M, Crane CH, Skibber J, et al. Chemoradiation for adenocarcinoma of the anus. Int J Radiat Oncol Biol Phys 2003;55:669–678.

144. Belkacemi Y, Berger C, Poortmans P, et al. Management of primary anal canal adenocarcinoma: a large retrospective study from the Rare Cancer Network. Int J Radiat Oncol Biol Phys 2003;56:1274–1283.

145. Malik A, Hull TL, Floruta C. What is the best surgical treatment for anorectal melanoma? Int J Colorectal Dis 2004;19: 121–123.

146. Billingsley KG, Stern LE, Lowy AM, Kahlenberg MS, Thomas CR Jr. Uncommon anal neoplasms. Surg Oncol Clin North Am 2004;13:375–388.

147. Chang AE, Karnell LH, Menck HR. The National Cancer Data Base report on cutaneous and noncutaneous melanoma: a summary of 84,836 cases from the past decade. The American College of Surgeons Commission on Cancer and the American Cancer Society. Cancer 1998;83:1664–1678.

148. Brady MS, Kavolius JP, Quan SH. Anorectal melanoma. A 64-year experience at Memorial Sloan-Kettering Cancer Center. Dis Colon Rectum 1995;38:146–151.

149. Thibault C, Sagar P, Nivatvongs S, Ilstrup DM, Wolff BG. Anorectal melanoma: an incurable disease? Dis Colon Rectum 1997;40:661–668.

150. Weyandt GH, Eggert AO, Houf M, Raulf F, Brocker EB, Becker JC. Anorectal melanoma: surgical management guidelines according to tumour thickness. Br J Cancer 2003;89: 2019–2022.

151. Bullard KM, Tuttle TM, Rothenberger DA, et al. Surgical therapy for anorectal melanoma. J Am Coll Surg 2003;196:206–211.

152. Moozar KL, Wong CS, Couture J. Anorectal malignant melanoma: treatment with surgery or radiation therapy, or both. Can J Surg 2003;46:345–349.

153. Roumen RM. Anorectal melanoma in The Netherlands: a report of 63 patients. Eur J Surg Oncol 1996;22:598–601.

154. Eton O, Legha SS, Bedikian AY, et al. Sequential biochemotherapy versus chemotherapy for metastatic melanoma: results from a phase III randomized trial. J Clin Oncol 2002; 20:2045–2052.

155. Tan GY, Chong CK, Eu KW, Tan PH. Gastrointestinal stromal tumor of the anus. Tech Coloproctol 2003;7:169–172.

156. Miettinen M, Furlong M, Sarlomo-Rikala M, Burke A, Sobin LH, Lasota J. Gastrointestinal stromal tumors, intramural leiomyomas, and leiomyosarcomas in the rectum and anus: a clinicopathologic, immunohistochemical, and molecular genetic study of 144 cases. Am J Surg Pathol 2001;25:1121–1133.

157. Walsh TH, Mann CV. Smooth muscle neoplasms of the rectum and anal canal. Br J Surg 1984;71:597–599.

158. Bernick PE, Klimstra DS, Shia J, et al. Neuroendocrine carcinomas of the colon and rectum. Dis Colon Rectum 2004;47: 163–169.

159. Gibson GE, Ahmed I. Perianal and genital basal cell carcinoma: a clinicopathologic review of 51 cases. J Am Acad Dermatol 2001;45:68–71.

160. Nielsen OV, Jensen SL. Basal cell carcinoma of the anus—a clinical study of 34 cases. Br J Surg 1981;68:856–857.

161. Espana A, Redondo P, Idoate MA, Serna MJ, Quintanilla E. Perianal basal cell carcinoma. Clin Exp Dermatol 1992;17: 360–362.

162. Paterson CA, Young-Fadok TM, Dozois RR. Basal cell carcinoma of the perianal region: 20-year experience. Dis Colon Rectum 1999;42:1200–1202.

163. Paget J. On disease of the mammary areola preceding cancer of the mammary gland. St. Barth Hosp Rep 1874;10:87–89.

164. Darier J, Couillaud P. Sur un cas de maladie de Pager de la region kerineo-anal er scrotale. Ann de Dermatole dr de Syph 1893;4:25–31.

165. McCarter MD, Quan SH, Busam K, Paty PP, Wong D, Guillem JG. Long-term outcome of perianal Paget's disease. Dis Colon Rectum 2003;46:612–616.

166. Beck D. Paget's disease and Bowen's disease of the anus. Semin Colon Rectal Surg 1995;6:143–149.

167. Berardi RS, Lee S, Chen HP. Perianal extramammary Paget's disease. Surg Gynecol Obstet 1988;167:359–366.

168. Tulchinsky H, Zmora O, Brazowski E, Goldman G, Rabau M. Extramammary Paget's disease of the perianal region. Colorectal Dis 2004;6:206–209.

169. Jensen SL, Sjolin KE, Shokouh-Amiri MH, Hagen K, Harling H. Paget's disease of the anal margin. Br J Surg 1988;75: 1089–1092.

170. Sarmiento JM, Wolff BG, Burgart LJ, Frizelle FA, Ilstrup DM. Paget's disease of the perianal region: an aggressive disease? Dis Colon Rectum 1997;40:1187–1194.

171. Beck DE, Fazio VW. Perianal Paget's disease. Dis Colon Rectum 1987;30:263–266.

172. Besa P, Rich TA, Delclos L, Edwards CL, Ota DM, Wharton JT. Extramammary Paget's disease of the perineal skin: role of radiotherapy. Int J Radiat Oncol Biol Phys 1992;24:73–78.

173. Marchesa P, Fazio VW, Oliart S, Goldblum JR, Lavery IC, Milsom JW. Long-term outcome of patients with perianal Paget's disease. Ann Surg Oncol 1997;4:475–480.

174. Grussendorf-Conen EI. Anogenital premalignant and malignant tumors (including Buschke-Lowenstein tumors). Clin Dermatol 1997;15:377–388.

175. Trombetta LJ, Place RJ. Giant condyloma acuminatum of the anorectum: trends in epidemiology and management—report of a case and review of the literature. Dis Colon Rectum 2001; 44:1878–1886.

176. Chu QD, Vezeridis MP, Libbey NP, Wanebo HJ. Giant condyloma acuminatum (Buschke-Lowenstein tumor) of the anorectal and perianal regions. Analysis of 42 cases. Dis Colon Rectum 1994;37:950–957.

177. Frisch M, Smith E, Grulich A, Johansen C. Cancer in a population-based cohort of men and women in registered homosexual partnerships. Am J Epidemiol 2003;157:966–972.

178. Gates AE, Kaplan LD. AIDS malignancies in the era of highly active antiretroviral therapy. Oncology (Huntingt) 2002;16: 441–451, 456, 459.

179. Yuhan R, Orsay C, DelPino A, et al. Anorectal disease in HIV-infected patients. Dis Colon Rectum 1998;41:1367–1370.

180. Place RJ, Huber PJ, Simmang CL. Anorectal lymphoma and AIDS: an outcome analysis. J Surg Oncol 2000;73:1–4; discussion 4–5.

181. Smith DL 2nd, Cataldo PA. Perianal lymphoma in a heterosexual and nonimmunocompromised patient: report of a case and review of the literature. Dis Colon Rectum 1999;42: 952–954.

182. Nigro ND. Multidisciplinary management of cancer of the anus. World J Surg 1987;11:446–451.

183. Habr-Gama A, da Silva e Sousa AH, Nadalin W, et al. Epidermoid carcinoma of the anal canal: results of treatment by combined chemotherapy and radiation therapy. Dis Col Rectum 1989;32:773–777.

184. Sischy B, Scotte Doggett RL, Krall JM, et al. Definitive irradiation and chemotherapy for radiosensitization in management of anal carcinoma: interim report on radiation therapy oncology group study no. 8314. J Nat Canc Inst 1989;81: 850–856.

185. Cho CC, Taylor CW III, Padmanabham A, et al. Squamous-cell carcinoma of the anal canal: Management with combined chemo-radiation therapy. Dis Colon Rectum 1991;34:675–678.

186. Lopez MJ, Myerson RJ, Shapiro SJ, Fleshman JW, Fry RD, Halverson JD, Kodner IJ, Monafo WW. Squamous cell carcinoma of the anal canal. Am J Surg 1991;162:580–584.

187. Doci R, Zucaki R, Bombelli L, Montalto F, Lomonica G. Combined chemoradiation therapy for anal cancer: a report of 56 cases. Ann Surg 1992;215:150–156.

188. Johnson D, Lipsett J, Leong L, Wagman LD, Terz JJ. Carcinoma of the anus treated with primary radiation therapy and chemotherapy. Surg Gynecol Obstet 1993;177: 329–334.

189. Tanum G, Tweit KM, Karlsen KO. Chemo-radiatiotherapy of anal carcinoma: Tumor response and acute toxicity. Oncology 1994;50:14–17.

190. Beck DE, Karulf RE. Combination therapy for epidermoid carcinoma of the anal canal. Dis Colon Rectum 1994;37: 1118–1125.

191. Smith DE, Shah KH, Rao AR, Frost DB, Latino F, Anderson PJ, Peddada AV, Kagan AR. Cancer of the anal canal: Treatment with chemotherapy and low dose radiation therapy. Radiology 1994;191:569–572.

36
Presacral Tumors

Eric J. Dozois, David J. Jacofsky, and Roger R. Dozois

The presacral or retrorectal space may be the site of a group of heterogeneous, and rare tumors that are often indolent and produce ill-defined symptoms. Because detection is often difficult and delayed, patients frequently present with tumors that have reached considerable size and involve multiple organ systems, complicating their treatment. The diagnosis and management of these tumors has evolved in recent years because of improved imaging modalities, a better understanding of tumor biology, adjuvant chemoradiation therapy, and a more aggressive surgical approach. Few surgeons have the opportunity to treat these complex lesions, and the care of these patients can be greatly optimized by an experienced, multidisciplinary team.

Anatomy and Neurophysiology

A thorough understanding of pelvic anatomy including soft tissue, neurologic, and osseous structures is essential in the evaluation and management of presacral tumors. The boundaries of the retrorectal region include the posterior wall of the rectum anteriorly and the sacrum posteriorly (Figure 36-1). This space extends superiorly to the peritoneal reflection and inferiorly to the rectosacral fascia and the supralevator space. Laterally, the area is bordered by the ureters, the iliac vessels, and the sacral nerve roots (Figure 36-2A). Several important vascular and neural structures are located in this area and injury to them may have important physiologic rectoanal sequelae, as well as neurologic and musculoskeletal consequences. If all sacral roots on one side of the sacrum are sacrificed, the patient will continue to have normal anorectal function. Likewise, if the upper three sacral nerve roots are left intact on either side of the sacrum, the patient's ability to defecate spontaneously and to control anorectal contents will remain essentially intact. If, however, both S-3 nerve roots are sacrificed, the external anal sphincter will no longer contract in response to gradual balloon dilation of the rectum and this will translate clinically into variable degrees of anorectal incontinence and difficult defecation.[1] If sacrectomy is to be performed, the surgeon must be familiar with the relationship between the thecal sac, sacral nerve roots, sciatic nerve, piriformis muscle, and sacrotuberous and sacrospinous ligaments (Figure 36-2B). From a structural standpoint, the majority of the sacrum can be resected. If more than half of the S-1 vertebral body remains intact, pelvic stability will be maintained. However, preoperative radiation to the sacrum may ultimately lead to stress fractures if only S-1 remains. As such, spinopelvic stability may be augmented with fusion in select patients. Knowledge of anatomy of the thigh and lower extremity is required in complex cases requiring muscle or soft tissue flaps. It is important to discuss with patients preoperatively the potential neuromuscular and visceral losses that may occur during the operation and how this will influence their function and quality of life.

Classification

General Considerations

Presacral lesions are rare. Reports from various large referral centers would indicate that their incidence may be as low as 1 in 40,000 hospital admissions (0.014%).[2] Spencer and Jackman[3] found precoccygeal cysts in only 3 of 20,851 proctologic examinations. Jao et al.[4] reported 120 patients over a 19-year period. Lesions found in the presacral space can be broadly classified as congenital or acquired, benign or malignant. Two-thirds of lesions are congenital and of these, two-thirds are benign and one-third are neoplastic. The presacral space has a complex embryologic development, and this potential space is composed primarily of connective tissue, nerves, fat, and blood vessels. Because this area contains totipotential cells that differentiate into three germ cell layers, a multitude of tumor types may be encountered. The classification first described by Uhlig and Johnson[5] has been used for many years by several authors and divides tumors into the broad categories: congenital, neurogenic, osseous, and miscellaneous. We have modified and updated this system to

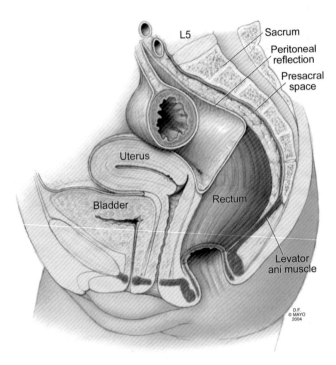

FIGURE 36-1. Relationship of pelvic structures to presacral space.

may have a morphologic appearance similar to that of the adult or fetal intestinal tract. The presence of glandular or transitional epithelium will differentiate this lesion from an epidermoid or dermoid cyst. Malignant transformation is rare.[7]

Teratomas are true neoplasms derived from totipotential cells and include all three germ layers. They may undergo malignant transformation to squamous cell carcinoma arising from the ectodermal tissue, or rhabdomyosarcoma arising from the mesenchymal cells. Anaplastic tumors are also seen in which the tissue of origin may not be distinguishable. Histologically, these tumors are referred to as either "mature" or "immature" reflecting the degree of cellular differentiation. Teratomas are more common in females and in the pediatric age group, and are often associated with other anomalies of the vertebrae, urinary tract, or anorectum.[8] In adults, malignant degeneration can occur in 40%–50%.[9] Incomplete

subcategorize tumors into malignant and benign entities, because this greatly impacts therapeutic approaches (Table 1).

Gross and Histologic Appearance

Epidermoid cysts result from closure defects of the ectodermal tube. They are histologically composed of stratified squamous cells, do not contain skin appendages, and are typically benign.

Dermoid cysts also arise from the ectoderm, but histologically they contain stratified squamous cells and skin appendages. These are also generally benign. Epidermoid and dermoid cysts tend to be well circumscribed and round and have a thin outer layer. Occasionally they communicate with the skin surface producing a characteristic postanal dimple. They are most common in females and the infection rate may be high because they are often misdiagnosed as a perirectal abscess and manipulated operatively.

Enterogenous cysts are lesions thought to originate from sequestration of the developing hindgut. Because they originate from endodermal tissue, they can be lined with squamous, cuboidal, or columnar epithelium. Transitional epithelium may also be found. These lesions tend to be multilobular with one dominant lesion and smaller satellite cysts. Similar to dermoid and epidermoid cysts, they can become infected and are more common in women. These are generally benign, but case reports have described malignant transformation within rectal duplications.[6]

Tailgut cysts, which are sometimes referred to as cystic hamartomas, are also multilocular cysts. These cysts are composed of squamous, columnar, or transitional epithelium that

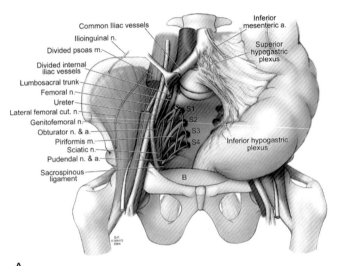

A

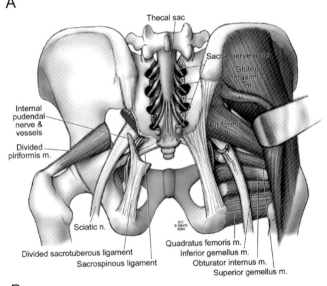

B

FIGURE 36-2. **A** Anterior view of pelvic anatomy. **B** Posterior view of pelvic anatomy with sacral elements removed.

TABLE 36-1. Classification of presacral tumors

Congenital
  Benign
    Developmental cysts (teratoma, epidermoid, dermoid, mucus-secreting)
    Duplication of rectum
    Anterior sacral meningocele
    Adrenal rest tumor
  Malignant
    Chordoma
    Teratocarcinoma
Neurogenic
  Benign
    Neurofibroma
    Neurilemoma (schwannoma)
    Ganglioneuroma
  Malignant
    Neuroblastoma
    Ganglioneuroblastoma
    Ependymoma
  Malignant peripheral nerve sheath tumors
(malignant schwannoma, neurofibrosarcoma, neurogenic sarcoma)
Osseous
  Benign
    Giant-cell tumor
    Osteoblastoma
    Aneurysmal bone cyst
  Malignant
    Osteogenic sarcoma
    Ewing's sarcoma
    Myeloma
    Chondrosarcoma
Miscellaneous
  Benign
    Lipoma
    Fibroma
    Leiomyoma
    Hemangioma
    Endothelioma
    Desmoid (locally aggressive)
  Malignant
Liposarcoma
Fibrosarcoma/malignant fibrous histiocytoma
    Leiomyosarcoma
    Hemangiopericytoma
    Metastatic carcinoma
  Other
    Ectopic kidney
    Hematoma
    Abscess

Source: Modified from Uhlig and Johnson.[5]

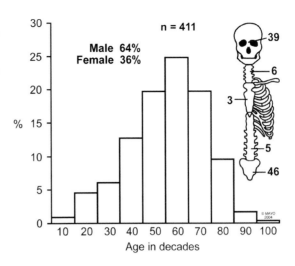

FIGURE 36-3. Distribution of chordomas. (Mayo Clinic orthopedic database.)

skull and for the sacrococcygeal region in the pelvis. More than half occur in the sacrum (Figure 36-3). They predominate in men and are rarely encountered in patients younger than 30 years of age. These tumors may be soft, gelatinous, or firm and may invade, distend, or destroy bone and soft tissue. The center of these tumors contains extracellular mucin. Hemorrhage and necrosis within tumors may lead to secondary calcification and pseudocapsule formation. Common symptoms include pelvic, buttock, and lower back pain aggravated by sitting and alleviated by standing or walking. Diagnosis is often delayed and these tumors may reach a considerable size.

Anterior sacral meningoceles are a result of a defect in the thecal sac and may be seen in combination with presacral cysts or lipomas. Typical symptoms include constipation, low back pain, and headache that is exacerbated by straining or coughing. It may be associated with other congenital anomalies such as spina bifida, tethered spinal cord, uterine and vaginal duplication, or urinary tract or anal malformations. Surgical management consists of ligation of the dural defect.

Neurogenic tumors include neurilemomas, ganglioneuromas, ganglioneuroblastomas, neurofibromas, neuroblastomas, ependymomas, and malignant peripheral nerve sheath tumors (neurofibrosarcoma, malignant schwannomas, neurogenic sarcomas). The most common malignant neurogenic lesion in the Mayo series was neurilemoma, which is more common in males and may occur at any age.[4] Neurogenic tumors tend to grow slowly and may reach considerable size. Differentiating between benign and malignant pathology preoperatively can be difficult, but is of paramount importance to guide operative approach.

Osseous tumors include chondrosarcoma, osteosarcoma, myeloma, and Ewing's sarcoma. These tumors arise from bone, cartilage, fibrous tissue, and marrow. Because of relatively rapid growth, these often reach considerable size. The lungs are a common sight of metastasis. All osseous tumors of the presacral space are associated with sacral destruction. Although

or intralesional resection increases the likelihood of malignant degeneration.[10] These also can become infected and be misdiagnosed as a perirectal abscess or fistula. Diagnosis is often delayed and these tumors may reach considerable size.

Sacrococcygeal chordoma is the most common malignancy in the presacral space. These tumors are believed to originate from the primitive notochord which embryologically extends from the base of the occiput to the caudal limit in the embryo. They can occur anywhere along the spinal column, but have a predilection for the pheno-occipital region at the base of the benign, giant cell tumors are locally destructive and can metastasize to the lungs ("benign metastasizing giant cell tumor").

Miscellaneous lesions in this region include metastatic deposits, inflammatory lesions related to Crohn's disease or diverticulitis, hematomas, and anomalous pelvic ectopic kidneys.

Overall, most presacral tumors occur in females and are cystic. Most solid tumors are chordomas and more often seen in males. Benign lesions are frequently asymptomatic and discovered incidentally during routine gynecologic examinations which may explain the greater incidence in females. By contrast, malignant tumors are more often symptomatic, but still frequently found late because of their vague symptomatology.

Diagnosis and Management

History and Physical Examination

Because of their indolent course, presacral tumors are often found incidentally at the time of periodic pelvic or rectal examination. Symptomatic patients typically complain of vague, longstanding pain in the perineum or low back. Pain may be aggravated by sitting and improved by standing or walking. In the Mayo Clinic series, pain was more common when the tumor was malignant as compared with benign (88% versus 39%).[4] Occasionally, patients complain of longstanding perineal discharge and their symptoms may be confused with anal fistula or pilonidal disease.[11] Several clues may alert the clinician to the presence of a retrorectal cystic lesion, including repeated operations for anal fistula, the inability of the examiner to uncover the primary source of infection at the level of the dentate line, a postanal dimple, or fullness and fixation of the precoccygeal area. All patients in the Mayo series with osseous tumors complained of low back pain, perineal pain, or both.[4] Some patients may give a history of referral to a psychiatrist because of a clinician's inability to ascertain the origin of the patient's chronic, ill-defined pain. Patients with larger tumors may complain of constipation and/or rectal and urinary incontinence, and sexual dysfunction because of the sacral nerve root involvement. Patients should be examined carefully, focusing on the perineum, rectal examination, and assessing for a postanal dimple. In the Mayo series, 97% of presacral tumors could be palpated on rectal examination.[4] Digital rectal examination will typically reveal the presence of an extrarectal mass displacing the rectum anteriorly with a smooth and intact overlying mucosa. Rectal examination is also critical in assessing the level of the uppermost portion of the lesion, degree and extent of fixation, and relationship to other pelvic organs such as the prostate. Rigid or flexible sigmoidoscopy can be used to assess the overlying mucosa and rule out transmural penetration of the tumor. A careful neurologic examination focusing on the sacral nerves and musculoskeletal reflexes is mandatory, and may also aid in the diagnosis of extensive local tumor invasion.

Diagnostic Tests

The presence of a presacral tumor can be confirmed with plain radiographs of the sacrum, or with more sophisticated imaging modalities such as computerized tomography (CT), magnetic resonance imaging (MRI), and endorectal ultrasound (ERUS). Simple anterior–posterior and lateral radiographs of the sacrum identify osseous expansion, destruction, and/or calcification of soft tissue masses, but are typically not helpful in rendering a specific diagnosis. A chordoma is the most common tumor causing these findings, but sarcomas or benign, locally aggressive tumors, such as giant cell tumor, neurilemoma, and aneurysmal bone cysts, may also cause extensive bony destruction. The characteristic "scimitar sign" denotes the presence of an anterior sacral meningocele, a diagnosis that can be confirmed with conventional myelography or MRI with gadolinium.[12]

In recent years, state of the art imaging such as CT, MRI, and positron emission tomography (PET) scan has dramatically changed the way in which these tumors should be evaluated. CT and MRI complement each other and are the most important radiographic studies in evaluating a patient with a presacral lesion. CT can determine whether a lesion is solid or cystic and whether adjacent structures such as the bladder, ureters, and rectum are involved (Figure 36-4A–C). CT is also the best study to evaluate cortical bone destruction. MRI is highly recommended because of its multiplanar capacity and improved soft tissue resolution that will be essential for planning specific lines of resection (Figure 36-5A,B). Sagittal views will assist in decision making in regard to need for and level of sacrectomy (Figure 36-5C). MRI is also more sensitive than CT in spinal imaging, showing associated cord anomalies such as a meningocele, nerve root, and foraminal encroachment by tumor, or thecal sac compression.[13] MRI is superior to CT in evaluating the extent of marrow involvement in bone. Angiogram and venogram can be added to the MRI (MR angiogram, venogram) to delineate vascular involvement and anatomy grossly distorted by tumor mass effect. This information is helpful to the vascular, plastic, and orthopedic surgeons for operative planning. Gadolinium-enhanced MRI imaging before, during, and/or after neoadjuvant therapy may also show the effectiveness of this treatment in terms of volume of tumor that appears vascularized and viable.

In patients with presacral cystic lesions thought to be the source of a chronically draining sinus, fistulogram may help clarify the diagnosis. ERUS has been used by some to characterize retrorectal tumors and their relationship to the muscularis propria of the rectum.[14]

Preoperative Biopsy

Historically, the role of preoperative biopsy of presacral tumors has been a controversial topic in the general surgical literature. Its necessity and how it is performed varies from author to author. In the past, some authors have considered any

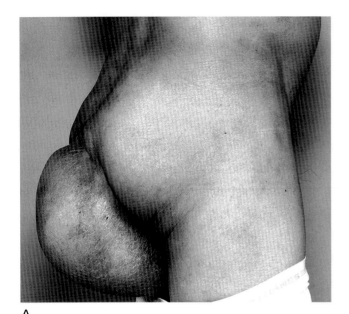

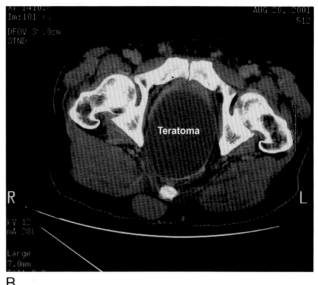

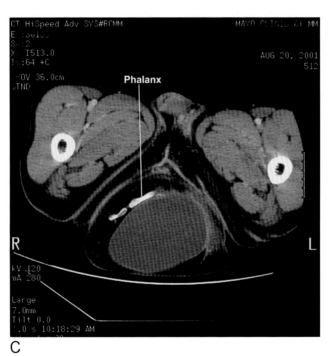

FIGURE 36-4. Massive cystic teratoma with sacral appendage **A**. CT image of teratoma, intrapelvic portion **B**, extrapelvic portion **C**, including fully developed phalanx.

presacral tumor deemed resectable a contraindication to pre-operative biopsy,[4,15–17] with only a minority stating that all solid tumors should be sampled preoperatively by biopsy.[18] This, in part, may have to do with the fact that the literature on this topic is sparse and outdated, especially when one considers the availability of modern imaging, better knowledge of tumor biology, and new opportunities for neoadjuvant therapy. Indeed, some patients will substantially benefit from preoperative chemotherapy and radiation, especially in osseous tumors such as Ewing's sarcoma, osteogenic sarcoma, and

neurofibrosarcoma. Likewise, very large tumors such as pelvic desmoids can be more easily removed after reducing their size with radiation. We consider preoperative tissue diagnosis essential to the management of solid and heterogenously cystic presacral tumors. For example, the surgical approach and necessary margins are dramatically different when faced with a neurofibroma as compared with a neurofibrosarcoma. When performed correctly, preoperative biopsy can only improve the overall management, not harm it. What is clear about preoperative biopsies of presacral tumors is that they should never be

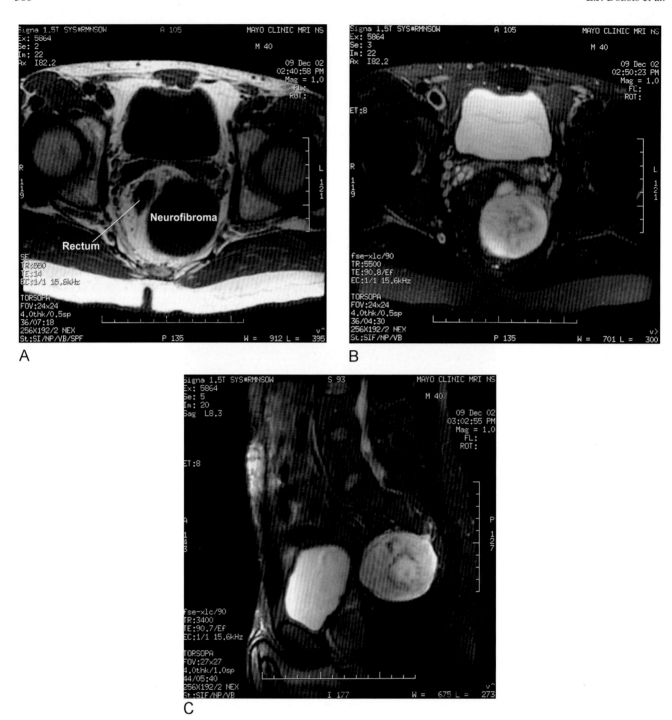

FIGURE 36-5. MRI of pelvic neurofibroma displacing the rectum anterior and lateral. **A** T1 weighted coronal image. **B** T2 weighted coronal image. **C** Sagittal view with tumor exiting the third sacral foramen.

performed transrectally or transvaginally. In the presence of a cystic lesion, such an approach is likely to result in infection rendering its future complete excision more difficult and increasing the likelihood of postoperative complications and recurrence. More importantly, inadvertent transrectal needling of a meningocele may lead to disastrous sequelae such as meningitis and even subsequent death. Moreover, because the

biopsy tract needs to be removed en bloc with the specimen, transrectal biopsy would mandate proctectomy in a patient whose rectum may otherwise have been spared.

There is rarely an indication to biopsy a purely cystic presacral lesion. From a technical standpoint, a presacral tumor biopsy should be done by a radiologist with experience in the evaluation and management of pelvic tumors. In planning the

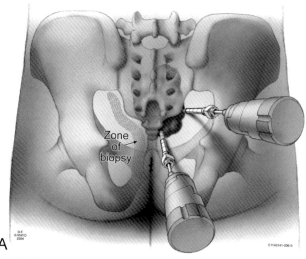

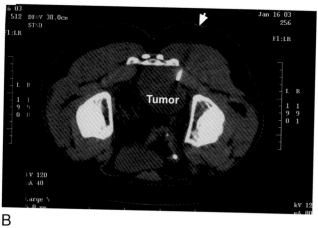

FIGURE 36-6. **A** Preoperative biopsy technique using CT guidance. **B** Parasacral approach to presacral neurogenic tumor.

approach for a biopsy, the surgeon should always consider the resection margins so that the needle tract can be removed en bloc with the specimen. The transperineal or parasacral approach is usually ideal and falls within the field of the pending surgical resection (Figure 36-6A,B). Transperitoneal, transretroperitoneal, transvaginal, and transrectal biopsy should be avoided. Biopsy tracts should never traverse neurovascular planes. Normal coagulation studies are required before biopsy, because hematoma formation and/or bleeding will potentially contaminate involved areas. PET–CT scan can be useful to guide biopsy needles into small focal areas of high tumor density.

Role of Preoperative Neoadjuvant Therapy

Modern protocols and the wide availability of neoadjuvant tumor irradiation and systemic chemotherapy has revolutionized the management of patients with complex malignancies. It is in large part because of these new treatment modalities before surgery that a preoperative diagnosis is of paramount

importance. Although some tumors, such as chondrosarcoma and chordoma, are poorly responsive to both chemotherapy and irradiation, there are a number of tumors seen in the presacral space whose rate of local recurrence can be markedly decreased with the addition of irradiation. Preoperative, as opposed to postoperative, irradiation can be extremely helpful in the face of large pelvic tumors. One of the significant advantages of preoperative irradiation is that it allows treatment to a smaller radiation field. Postoperative irradiation for a pelvic tumor would require irradiation of the entire surgical bed, previous tumor site, all contaminated surgical planes, and the sites of all skin incisions. This increased radiation exposure is associated with increased morbidity. Furthermore, should "spillage" occur during resection of a radiosensitive tumor, this contamination may be with previously irradiated necrotic, nonviable cells. A third, and perhaps most important, advantage of preoperative irradiation in sensitive tumors, is the fact that decreased tumor size is often observed. A decrease in tumor size in a pelvic tumor may allow the surgeon to spare vital structures that would have had to be sacrificed in order for wide margins to be achieved without prior radiation. Additionally, a smaller tumor often means a surgery of a lesser magnitude and therefore less risk for intraoperative complications.

Large tumors in the presacral space, especially sarcomas, are notorious for systemic metastasis. Neoadjuvant chemotherapy is the cornerstone of treatment for diagnoses such as Ewing's sarcoma and osteogenic sarcoma. A wide resection of a pelvic tumor of this type, which would cause a delay in systemic chemotherapy treatment, is not in the patient's best interest. Micrometastatic disease must be treated in patients with diagnoses such as these preoperatively, unless the tumor has caused an immediate complication that requires emergent surgery. Furthermore, one could argue that lymphoma or Ewing's sarcoma can be completely treated with chemoradiation, and that surgery may not be necessary at all.

As with extremity sarcomas, there are clearly some cases in which irradiation and chemotherapy are not required. Small, low-grade malignancies without metastatic disease that can be completely excised with a histologically negative wide margin may likely be observed without adjuvant treatment. This, however, implies that any subsequent recurrence would again be amenable to excision. If a recurrence would no longer be amenable to re-resection, then most oncologic surgeons would favor adjuvant treatment to minimize the risk of this recurrence. Most authorities advocate irradiation, either before or after resection, of nonextremity low-grade sarcomas with "marginal" or positive margins or for any patient with an intermediate or high-grade malignancy.

The efficacy of adjuvant chemotherapy for patients with nonextremity sarcomas has not been established firmly to date. One randomized trial examined the efficacy of adjuvant chemotherapy in patients with soft tissue sarcomas of the head and neck, breast and trunk, all of whom received postoperative radiotherapy.[19] Adjuvant chemotherapy consisted of doxorubicin, cyclophosphamide, and methotrexate, a regimen that admittedly is no longer commonly used for sarcoma management. However, the three-year actuarial disease-free survival rate in the chemotherapy group was 72% compared with 60% in the group without chemotherapy. These differences showed a trend, but were not statistically significant. However, one must understand that as improvements in local therapy continue, fewer patients will succumb to local recurrence and more patients will succumb to distant disease. It is in this setting that neoadjuvant chemotherapy may be of most benefit.

Surgical Treatment

Rationale for Aggressive Approach

The rationale for an aggressive surgical approach for presacral tumors is based on several arguments. The lesion may already be malignant or transform into a malignant state if left in place. In patients with teratomas, especially those in the pediatric age group, the risk of malignant transformation is considerable and continues to increase dramatically if removal is delayed or incomplete.[9] Untreated anterior sacral meningoceles may become infected and lead to meningitis, which is associated with high mortality.[20] Cystic lesions may become infected making their excision difficult and increasing the possibility of postoperative infection and future recurrence. A presacral mass in a young woman may cause dystocia at the time of delivery. Lastly, benign and malignant tumors left untreated may grow to considerable size, making surgical resection much more complicated.

Unfortunately, in the past, many surgeons have adopted a rather defeatist attitude toward sacrococcygeal chordomas and other tumors in this area based on a number of erroneous misconceptions. Chordomas are slow-growing tumors producing vague symptoms which leads to a delay in diagnosis for months or even years. Thus, patients may seek medical treatment late in the course of their disease and the presence of a large mass in this often unfamiliar and complex anatomic area makes some surgeons reluctant to consider aggressive surgical approach for fear of serious operative and postoperative complications. This same reluctance to operate may apply to other types of lesions as well. Moreover, chordomas have all too often been considered to have a benign clinical behavior characterized by slow local growth. We now know that these tumors will metastasize and that the longer the diagnosis is delayed, the greater risk of distant spread. Finally, and most importantly, tumors in this area have been treated inadequately in the past because of tumor violation, their large size and location, and fear of neurologic complication and/or musculoskeletal instability. Tumor violation can take place preoperatively when such tumors are biopsied transrectally, or intraoperatively when margins of resection are inadequate or tumor cells are spilled in an effort to be too conservative. When a surgeon is attempting to avoid injury to the rectal wall or important neurologic structures, they may inappropriately restrict excision and compromise oncologic outcome. For malignant lesions, wide margins and oncologic cure should be the primary goal of these procedures.

Role of Multidisciplinary Team

It is of great importance that an experienced team consisting of a colorectal surgeon, orthopedic oncologic surgeon, spine surgeon, urologist, plastic surgeon, vascular surgeon, musculoskeletal radiologist, medical oncologist, radiation oncologist, and specialized anesthesiologist evaluate and surgically treat tumors that are large and extend to or destroy the hemipelvis or the upper half of the sacrum. The importance of a multispecialty approach for presacral tumors was first described in 1953 by a Mayo Clinic team of surgeons. They found an improvement in outcome in this difficult to manage group of patients with the combined effort of multiple specialists.[21] This quote from their publication describes their convictions:

The surgical management of presacral and sacral tumors has been in general unsatisfactory. We feel that progress in treating these lesions may have been impeded rather than enhanced by the individual surgical specialists who came into contact with these lesions. Consequently, we have united our efforts in solving the problem and thereby utilizing the special assets of the three surgical specialties—neurologic, orthopedic and general surgery—in meeting this problem.

Surgical Approach

Careful surgical planning is important in deciding how to approach these tumors whether it be an anterior approach (abdominal), posterior approach (perineal), or a combined abdominoperineal approach. CT and MRI will help define the margins of resection and the relationship of the tumor to the sacral level (Figure 36-7). Small and low-lying lesions can be removed transperineally through a parasacral incision, whereas tumors extending above the S-3 level, especially if large, often require a combined anterior and posterior approach.

For large, malignant lesions requiring extended resection, a plastic surgeon has a significant role, because adequate soft tissue coverage can often be difficult. Most often, we use the transabdominal rectus abdominus myocutaneous (TRAM) flap, which fills dead space and can cover large cutaneous defects left by the resection. Healthy, well-vascularized tissue flaps, placed in the surgical bed, markedly decrease the incidence of wound-related complications.

Preoperative Considerations

Optimizing patients for surgery is of extreme importance in a majority of these cases. Adequate nutritional repletion with total parenteral nutrition or with a feeding tube, may be necessary in patients who present severely debilitated. In technically complex cases, when we expect a long operative time and significant debilitation postoperatively, we consider

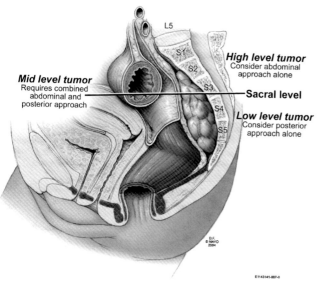

FIGURE 36-7. Relationship of tumor to sacral level and proposed approach.

placement of a temporary intravenacaval filter, because the risk of deep venous thrombosis and pulmonary embolus is high and postoperative anticoagulation may be contraindicated. Availability of blood products should be assessed. A multidisciplinary team meeting preoperatively, to review films and plan surgical strategy, avoids confusion during the day of surgery. An operating theater capable of managing massive transfusion requirements is mandatory, as is an anesthesiologist comfortable with the physiologic management needed during the procedure.

Posterior Approach

For low-lying tumors, the patient is placed in the prone jackknife position with the buttocks spread with tape (Figure 36-8A). An incision is made over the lower portion of the sacrum and coccyx down to the anus taking care to avoid damage to the external sphincter. Resection of the tumor may be facilitated by transection of the anococcygeal ligament and coccyx (Figure 36-8B). The lesion can then be dissected from the surrounding tissues including the rectal wall, in a plane between the retrorectal fat and the tumor mass itself. In the case of very small lesions, the surgeon may double-glove the left hand and, with the index finger in the anal canal and lower rectum, push the lesion outward, away from the depths of the wound (Figure 36-8C) facilitating dissection of the lesion off the wall of the rectum without injury. If necessary, the lower sacrum or coccyx or both can be excised en bloc with the lesion to facilitate excision.

Combined Abdominal and Perineal Approach

If the upper pole of the tumor extends clearly above the S-3 level, an anterior and posterior approach is usually indicated. Patients may be placed in the supine or lateral

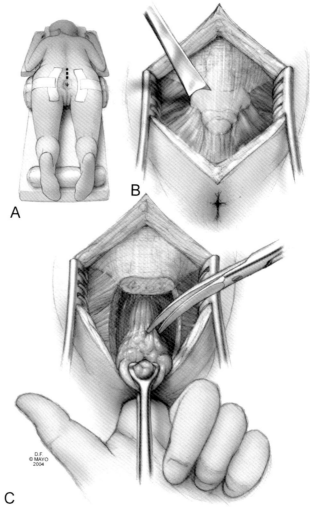

FIGURE 36-8. **A** Positioning for posterior approach. **B** Coccygectomy. **C** Index finger in anal canal to "push" tumor outward facilitating dissection.

position, depending on the surgeon's preference and previous experience. A variety of techniques and positioning to the abdominal perineal approach have been described.[22] If an anterior–posterior approach is necessary, the patient can be placed in a "sloppy-lateral" position to facilitate a simultaneous two-team approach (Figure 36-9A–C). We always recommend cystoscopy and bilateral ureteral stent placement before laparotomy. Through a midline incision, the abdomen should be carefully examined to rule out metastasis or other important pathology. After the lateral attachments to the sigmoid have been mobilized and the presacral space is entered just below the promontory, the posterior rectum can be dissected from the upper sacrum down to the upper extension of the tumor. The ureters are identified and protected. The rectum can then be mobilized laterally, and if necessary, anteriorly.

If a malignant tumor can be safely separated from the posterior wall of the rectum without compromising a wide

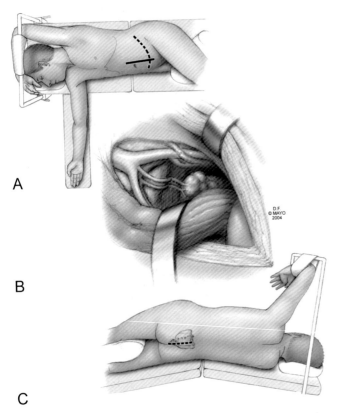

A

B

C

FIGURE 36-9. **A** Modified lateral position for anterior exposure via a midline (solid line) or ilioinguinal (dotted line) incision. **B** Anterior exposure of vessels and tumor. **C** Posterior approach to sacrum.

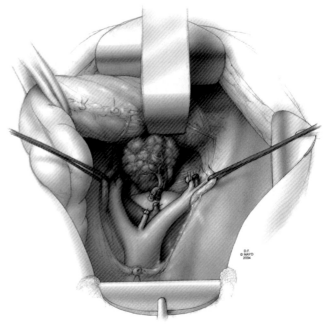

FIGURE 36-10. Ligation of middle sacral and internal iliac vessel.

margin, the lesion can be dissected in a plane between its capsule and the mesorectal fat to preserve the rectum. If the tumor is extremely large, markedly compressing and displacing the rectum, making dissection between the rectal vault and the tumor hazardous, one should remove the rectum en bloc with the tumor and the involved segments of the sacrum. It is mandatory in malignant cases that no structures attached to the specimen be separated with dissection and that they be removed en bloc with the primary tumor mass. In this situation, the upper rectum is transected with a stapler at the level of the promontory. Under these circumstances, it is imperative that the anterior wall of the rectum be completely freed from the seminal vesicles and prostate in men and the upper two-thirds of the vagina in women. The pelvic floor can then be reconstructed over the anal remnant and the sigmoid colostomy established in the left lower abdominal wall.

In the presence of very large tumors, blood loss during the procedure can be substantial. This may be minimized by ligating the middle and lateral sacral vessels and both internal iliac arteries and veins (Figure 36-10). When ligating the internal iliac artery, it is best to preserve the anterior division, which gives off the inferior gluteal artery, thereby reducing the risk of perineal necrosis. This is often performed in conjunction with permissive hypotension. A vascular surgeon can be helpful during this portion of the procedure especially in patients who have had prior irradiation or have distorted vascular anatomy. In a situation in which a large tissue defect is expected, one may elect to mobilize one rectus muscle (preferably the right if possible), on its vascular pedicle and place it in the presacral area for later use in the closure of the perineal wound when the patient is prone. In the anterior-posterior approach, when a flap will be used, a thick piece of silastic mesh is placed posterior to the vital structures and anterior to the bony structures to protect vital structures from injury during bony resection while in the prone or lateral position. After the abdominal incision is closed and the colostomy is matured, the anesthetized patient can then be moved from the supine to the prone position. The perineal approach is similar to that used for benign low-lying cystic or solid tumors, except that wider and more proximal dissection will be necessary. After an incision has been made over the sacrum and coccyx down to the anus, the anococcygeal ligament is transected and the levator muscles are retracted laterally. If the rectum is to be preserved, the tumor can be separated from the rectum by careful dissection of the plane between the rectum and the tumor. The orthopedic surgeon can then proceed with separation of gluteus maximus muscles on both sides, detachment of the sacrospinous and sacrotuberous ligaments, and division of the piriformis muscles bilaterally to protect the sciatic nerves (Figure 36-11A). A posterior laminectomy may be required to expose and ligate nerve roots to be sacrificed and/or the thecal sac (Figure 36-11B,C). In this manner the lesion can be removed en bloc with the lower sacrum and coccyx and involved sacral roots. If the surgeon previously

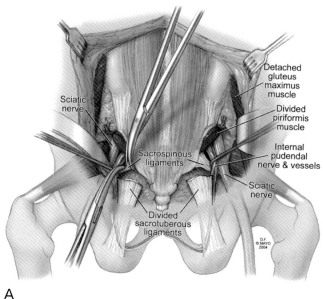

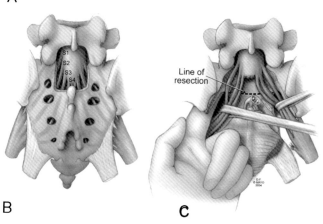

FIGURE 36-11. Posterior approach and exposure of sciatic nerves **A**, sacral nerve roots **B**, and ligation of thecal sac **C**.

elected to excise the rectum en bloc, it is preferable to remove the anus and anal canal with the rectal specimen. The wound is then closed in layers over suction silastic drain, or a TRAM flap is inserted and sewn into place by the plastic surgeon. More complex soft tissue procedures may be required if the tumor involves the posterior soft tissue elements.

Results of Treatment

Malignant Lesions

The results of surgical treatment of malignant presacral neoplasms and cysts depends on the natural behavior of the lesion and the adequacy of resection. In malignant cases, if wide margins are not achieved or if the tumor is violated, one can expect a high local recurrence rate and a poor overall outcome. In general, most malignant tumors reported in the literature have had a rather poor prognosis, but many such tumors had been incompletely resected or excised piecemeal, breaking oncologic principles. Kaiser et al.[23] found that local recurrence rate increased from 28% to 64% if the tumor was violated perioperatively.

In the literature, the prognosis for patients with chordomas has been variable, ranging from 15% to 76% at 10 years after surgical therapy. At the Mayo Clinic, the 5-year survival rate in 1976 was reported to be 75%; more recently we have found 5- and 10-year survivals of 80% and 50%, respectively [Chiu et al. An update of the Mayo Clinic experience 1980–1992 (unpublished data)].[4] Of 16 patients with chordomas that were completely resected, nine had no clinical or radiologic evidence of recurrence 4–14 years later. Isolated metastases to the lungs, ribs, spine, and long bones can sometimes be excised successfully and provide patients with symptomatic relief and a substantial prolongation of life. The 5-year survival for patients with malignant tumors other than chordomas was 17%. Only one patient with a neuroblastoma, one with a neurofibrosarcoma, and one with Ewing's sarcoma were alive without recurrence at 3, 5, and 7 years, respectively. However, these results likely were related to the lack of, or poor quality of, the adjuvant therapies available.

Cody et al.[24] reported their experience with malignant presacral tumors, 9 (38%) of which had chordomas. Excision of these tumors was described as "en bloc" or "in fragments." Forty-eight percent developed local recurrence; 60% of patients underwent open biopsy. For all treated patients, survival at 5, 10, 15, and 20 years was 69%, 50%, 37%, and 20%, respectively.

Lev-Chelouche et al.[15] reported on 21 patients with malignant presacral tumors, nine of which were chordomas. No patients underwent preoperative biopsy. Nearly all patients had a palpable lesion on rectal examination. Fifteen of 21 malignant lesions were completely excised. Most recurrences were seen in patients with incomplete resection and 50% of these died of disease.

Wang et al.[25] reported their series of 22 patients with malignant presacral tumors, five of which were chordomas and seven were leiomyosarcomas. Tumor size ranged from 1.5 to 40 cm. The average size of malignant tumors was 17 cm; 96% were palpable by rectal examination. CT was believed to be the best test to identify the lesions and define extent and degree of tumor invasion, but the diagnosis remained nonspecific. No patients underwent preoperative biopsy. Five patients had complete resection and 17 had incomplete resection. The overall 5-year survival rate for malignant tumors was 41%. No patients underwent preoperative adjuvant therapy. Postoperative chemotherapy and radiotherapy was used in selected patients with malignant tumors.

Bohm et al.[17] reported their series of 24 patients with congenital presacral tumors. They had four patients with chordomas and 20 with developmental cysts. All patients with chordoma

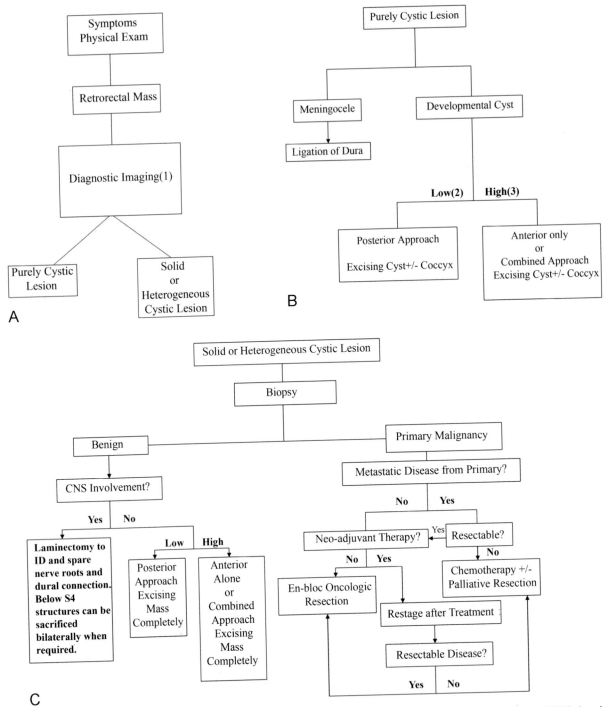

FIGURE 36-12. Proposed treatment algorithm. Notes: 1) conventional radiographs of pelvis, CT scan, MRI with gadolinium, ERUS, intralu-minal contrast studies of rectum, PET, myelogram; 2) lower than the third sacral vertebra; 3) higher than the third sacral vertebra.

underwent excision. Three of four chordoma patients had recurrence at 25, 32, and 55 months. Patients with recurrence presented with pain and neurologic disturbance. Complete local reexcision was done in the three patients with recurrence. Only 3 of 20 patients with developmental cysts developed recurrence, all of which underwent successful reexcision.

Congenital Cystic Lesions

In general, cystic lesions can be treated adequately by complete excision via a posterior approach. Large cystic lesions such as teratomas extending high into the pelvis can be excised via a combined abdominal–perineal approach. There continues to be some debate as to whether or not a coccygectomy needs to be done for all resections of congenital cystic lesions.[11] Some believe that the coccyx harbors totipotential cells that will lead to a high recurrence rate if not excised.[26] It should be remembered also that 10%–38% of patients with cystic lesions harbor a malignancy and that oncologic principles must be followed.[27]

In the Mayo series, 49 congenital cystic lesions were described including 15 epidermoid cysts, 16 mucus-secreting cysts, 15 teratomas, and 2 meningoceles.[4] Three teratocarcinomas were seen. Most lesions were in females with only three in males. Average size of cysts was 4–7 cm. Almost all cystic lesions were treated with a posterior approach. Of 66 patients with benign tumors, 10 had recurrence (four had giant cell tumors, six had congenital benign cysts), most of which were treated successfully with reexcision.

Lev-Chelouche et al.[15] reported 21 benign presacral lesions. Complete excision of benign lesions was possible in all cases with no recurrences during the 10-year follow-up.

Singer et al.[11] reported on seven patients with presacral cysts (six females, one male). All patients had previously been misdiagnosed and treated for pilonidal cysts, perirectal abscesses, fistula in ano, psychogenic disorder, proctalgia fugax, and posttraumatic or postpartum pain before the correct diagnosis was made. Patients underwent an average of 4.1 prior operative procedures. All patients were successfully treated with resection through a parasacrococcygeal approach after the correct diagnosis was made with CT fistulogram.

Algorithm

Based on the experience at our institution, we have established a decision-making algorithm to guide the management of presacral tumors (Figure 36-12).

Conclusion

Presacral tumors are rare, the differential diagnosis is extensive, and their discovery is notoriously difficult and late. A high index of suspicion is needed to identify these patients. Once a benign or malignant presacral lesion is discovered and histologically diagnosed, it should be treated, even if the patient is asymptomatic. CT and MRI imaging can help differentiate between benign and malignant, cystic and solid and accurately define extent of adjacent organ and bony involvement to guide operative planning. Completely cystic lesions, in general, do not require preoperative biopsy unless malignancy is suspected. All solid tumors and heterogenous cysts should be considered for biopsy to rule out malignancy, guide neoadjuvant therapy, and plan extent of resection. Biopsies should be done transperineally or parasacrally.

An aggressive approach, by an experienced, multidisciplinary team, that can achieve a tumor-free, en bloc resection, avoid tumor violation, restore spinopelvic stability, and minimize intraoperative and postoperative complications, should decrease the risk of local recurrence and improve survival.

References

1. Gunterberg B, Kewenter J, Petersen, et al. Anorectal function after major resection of the sacrum with bilateral or unilateral sacrifice of sacral nerves. Br J Surg 1976;63:546–554.
2. Whittaker LD, Pemberton JD. Tumors ventral to the sacrum. Ann Surg 1938;107:96–106.
3. Spencer RJ, Jackman RJ. Surgical management of precoccygeal cysts. Surg Gynecol Obstet 1962;115:449–452.
4. Jao SW, Beart RW Jr, Spencer RJ, et al. Retrorectal tumors. Mayo Clinic experience, 1960–1979. Dis Colon Rectum 1985; 28:644–652.
5. Uhlig BE, Johnson RL. Presacral tumors and cysts in adults. Dis Colon Rectum 1975;18:581–596.
6. Springall RG, Griffiths JD. Malignant change in rectal duplication. J R Soc Med 1990;83:185–187.
7. Caropreso PR, Wengert PA Jr, Milford HE. Tailgut cyst—a rare retrorectal tumor: report of a case and review. Dis Colon Rectum 1975;18:597–600.
8. Izant RJ Jr, Filston HC. Sacrococcygeal teratomas. Analysis of forty-three cases. Am J Surg 1975;130:617–621.
9. Waldhausen JA, Kilman JW, Vellios F. Sacrococcygeal teratomas. Surgery 1963;54:933–939.
10. Hickey RC, Martin RG. Sacrococcygeal teratomas. Ann NY Acad Sci 1964;114:951.
11. Singer MA, Cintron JR, Martz JE, et al. Retrorectal cyst: a rare tumor frequently misdiagnosed. J Am Coll Surg 2003;196: 880–886.
12. Lee KS, Gower DJ, McWhorter JM, Albertson DA. The role of MR imaging in the diagnosis and treatment of anterior sacral meningocele. Report of two cases. J Neurosurg 1988;69: 628–631.
13. Lee RA, Symmonds RE. Presacral tumors in the female: clinical presentation, surgical management, and results. Obstet Gynecol 1988;71:216–221.
14. Scullion DA, Zwirewich CV, McGregor G. Retrorectal cystic hamartoma: diagnosis using endorectal ultrasound. Clin Radiol 1999;54(5):338–339.
15. Lev-Chelouche D, Gutman M, Goldman G, et al. Presacral tumors: a practical classification and treatment of a unique and heterogeneous group of diseases. Surgery 2003;133:473–478.
16. Luken MG 3rd, Michelsen WJ, Whelan MA, et al. The diagnosis of sacral lesions. Surg Neurol 1981;15:377–383.
17. Bohm B, Milsom JW, Fazio VW, et al. Our approach to the management of congenital presacral tumors in adults. Int J Colorectal Dis 1993;8:134–138.
18. Eilbert FR. Expert commentary on retrorectal tumors: spectrum of disease, diagnosis and surgical management. Perp Col Rect Surg 1990;3:252–255.
19. Glenn J, Kinsella T, Glatstein E, et al. A randomized, prospective trial of adjuvant chemotherapy in adults with soft tissue sarcomas of the head and neck, breast, and trunk. Cancer 1985;55: 1206–1214.
20. Amacher AL, Drake CG, McLachlin AD. Anterior sacral meningocele. Surg Gynecol Obstet 1968;126:986–994.
21. MacCarty CS, Waugh JM, Coventry MB, et al. Surgical treatment of sacral and presacral tumors other than sacrococcygeal chordoma. J Neurosurg 1965;22:458–464.

22. Localio SA, Eng K, Ranson JHC. Abdominosacral approach for retrorectal tumors. Ann Surg 1980;191:555–560.

23. Kaiser TE, Pritchard DJ, Unni KK. Clinicopathologic study of sacrococcygeal chordoma. Cancer 1984;53:2574–2578.

24. Cody HS 3rd, Marcove RC, Quan SH. Malignant retrorectal tumors: 28 years' experience at Memorial Sloan-Kettering Cancer Center. Dis Colon Rectum 1981;24:501–506.

25. Wang JY, Hsu CH, Changchien CR, et al. Presacral tumor: a review of forty-five cases. Am Surg 1995;61:310–315.

26. Aktug T, Hakguder G, Sarioglu S, et al. Sacrococcygeal extraspinal ependymomas: the role of coccygectomy. J Pediatr Surg 2000;35:515–518.

27. Kang J-C, Kaiser AM, Tolazzi AR, et al. Presacral cysts: a risk for malignancy. Contemp Surg 2002;58:448–452.

514

37
Miscellaneous Neoplasms

Richard Devine and Marc Brand

Carcinoids

Carcinoid tumors originate from enterochromaffin cells, part of the diffuse endocrine system. Thus, they are considered to belong in the neuroendocrine group of tumors.[1] They are a confusing group of tumors with a wide range of behavior. Carcinoid tumors may be located in any of a number of locations within and outside the gastrointestinal (GI) tract, may be single or multiple, may produce a wide array of biochemical products, may produce symptoms from the biochemical products or the tumor itself, and exhibit varying degrees of biochemical and aggressive behavior relative to their location. This section will focus on carcinoid tumors of the small bowel, appendix, colon, and rectum.

History and Terminology[1,2]

The clinical and histologic recognition of carcinoid tumors was first described in 1888 by Lubarsch. He had noted two patients with multiple small tumors of the ileum at autopsy. The term carcinoid ("karzinoid") was first applied to these tumors in 1907 by Oberndorfer. The term implies that these tumors are similar to carcinoma, but behave somewhat differently. Specifically, carcinoid tumors are histologically similar to carcinoma, but have a more benign clinical course. Gossett and Masson described the argentaffin-reducing properties of appendiceal carcinoids in 1914, and the tumors became known as "argentaffinomas." The argentaffin reaction is characterized by reduction of silver salts to a black metallic silver stain.

The association between carcinoid tumors and serotonin production was first described by Lembeck in 1953. Around the same time, the first description of the carcinoid syndrome was published by Waldenstrom's group (1954). Within a few years, Sandler and Snow first recognized a variable nature of carcinoids. They described an "atypical" *gastric* carcinoid which only produced a serotonin *precursor* and had staining and flushing patterns different from "typical" carcinoids. The

staining pattern is described as "argyrophilic," implying that the reduction of silver salts to the black metallic silver stain occurs only in the presence of pretreatment with a reducing agent.

The amine precursor uptake and decarboxylation (APUD) abilities of these tumors were recognized by Pearse in 1969, and carcinoid tumors became known as "APUDomas." APUDomas, including carcinoid tumors, are now considered part of a group of tumors known as neuroendocrine tumors. Neuroendocrine tumors are derived from the diffuse neuroendocrine system. As such, carcinoid tumors share some characteristics with melanomas, pheochromocytomas, medullary carcinoma of thyroid, and pancreatic endocrine tumors.[3]

Pathology[3]

The light microscopic appearance of carcinoid tumors is rather bland. They are composed of monotonous sheets of small round cells. The cells themselves demonstrate uniform nuclei and cytoplasm. The ultrastructural appearance of carcinoid tumors demonstrates electron-dense neurosecretory granules which contain small clear vesicles. These neurosecretory granules correspond to the synaptic vesicles found in neurons.

The staining pattern of carcinoid tumors is related to the amines and peptides they produce as well as cytoplasmic proteins they contain. Silver staining was initially used to identify these tumors. Carcinoid tumors that are capable of taking up *and* reducing silver stains are described as "argentaffin positive," and this is attributed to the silver reducing ability of serotonin. Tumors that are only capable of silver uptake, and not silver reduction, may be demonstrated by addition of an external reducing agent. These tumors are described as "argyrophilic."

Silver staining has been supplanted by immunohistochemical stains for cytoplasmic proteins. Chromogranin, neuron-specific enolase, and synaptophysin are frequently used to identify a tumor as being a neuroendocrine tumor.

Carcinoid tumors have been described to grow in one of five histologic patterns. These histologic patterns have been

TABLE 37-1. Carcinoid tumor growth patterns

Sogo and Tazawa[4]	Martin and Potet[5]	Pattern	Description	Frequency	Prognosis
Type A	Type I	Insular	Solid nests with peripheral palisading	Most frequent pattern	Favorable
B	II	Trabecular	Ribbon-like anastomosing pattern	Second-most frequent pattern	Favorable
C	III	Glandular	Tubular, acinar, or rosette pattern	Least frequent pattern	Poor
D	IV	Undifferentiated	No recognizable pattern	Third-most frequent pattern	Poor
Mixed	Mixed	Any combination of the above	Any combination of the above	A + C most frequent mix	Most favorable
				A + B next most frequent	Favorable

designated as A-D[4] or I-IV,[5] with the fifth pattern in each system being a combination of several patterns. These growth patterns are described in Table 37-1.

Pathophysiology

Carcinoid tumors are known to produce at least 30 bioactive compounds.[2] These compounds may be amines (including serotonin and histamine), proteins (a wide variety of hormones and kinins), and prostaglandins. Serotonin, an amine, is the most well-known of these compounds.

Serotonin is derived from tryptophan, an essential amino acid. The production of serotonin is a two-step process: hydroxylation of tryptophan to 5-hydroxytryptophan (5-HTP), followed by decarboxylation of 5-HTP to 5-hydroxytryptamine (5-HT, or serotonin). Serotonin is then stored and transported in platelets. Metabolism of serotonin occurs in the liver (monoamine oxidase) and then the kidney (aldehyde dehydrogenase) to produce 5-hydroxy-indole-acetic acid (5-HIAA) which is excreted in the urine.

Normally, less than 1% of tryptophan is converted into serotonin. The remainder is used for synthesis of proteins, niacin (vitamin B_7), and nicotinamide (vitamin B_3). Protein malnutrition, hypoproteinemia, and pellagra (vitamin B_3 deficiency) may develop if large quantities of tryptophan are diverted to serotonin production by carcinoid tumors.

Classification

Numerous classification schemes have been devised to categorize carcinoid tumors. These have been based on several features including site of origin and histologic growth pattern. The prognosis of carcinoid tumors is somewhat related to these classifications.

Carcinoid tumors are grouped by their site of origin into foregut, midgut, and hindgut tumors. Foregut tumors originate in the thymus, respiratory tract, stomach, duodenum, pancreas, and ovaries. Midgut tumors originate in the jejunum, ileum, appendix, and proximal colon. Hindgut tumors originate in the distal colon or rectum. The histologic classification pattern has already been described (Table 37-1).

Several studies have reviewed the distribution of site of origin of carcinoid tumors. Godwin[6] reported the most frequent sites of origin as the appendix, ileum, rectum, and bronchus (38%, 23%, 13%, 11.5%, respectively) in a series of 4349 carcinoid tumors. In another large series, Modlin and Sandor[7] reported the most frequent sites of origin as the bronchus, ileum, rectum, and appendix (32.5%, 17.6%, 10%, 7.6%, respectively) in 5468 carcinoid tumors.

Clinical Presentation[3]

Carcinoid tumors may be found incidentally or may present as a result of the production of local or systemic symptoms. Local symptoms are related to the site of origin or site of metastasis, whereas systemic symptoms are related to production of bioactive compounds.

Local Symptoms

Small bowel carcinoids may produce local symptoms of periodic abdominal pain, small bowel obstruction (caused by intussusception or mesenteric fibrosis and small bowel kinking), intestinal ischemia, and GI hemorrhage. Appendiceal carcinoids are often found incidentally at the time of appendectomy. Rectal carcinoids are often found incidentally at the time of colorectal cancer screening examinations. The symptoms of rectal carcinoids, when present, are related to bleeding and change in bowel habits. Liver metastases may be the initial presentation, manifested by hepatomegaly and right upper quadrant pain.

Systemic Symptoms and the Carcinoid Syndrome[2]

Systemic symptoms produced by carcinoid tumors are referred to as the carcinoid syndrome. These consist of a combination of vasomotor symptoms (flushing and blood pressure changes), diarrhea, and bronchospasm. These symptoms are brought on by release of active tumor products into the circulation. The liver is capable of metabolizing and inactivating large quantities of tumor products. Therefore, the carcinoid syndrome occurs only in the presence of liver metastases (for GI carcinoids), or a primary carcinoid tumor located outside the portal venous system. Episodes of symptoms of the carcinoid syndrome may be precipitated by routine daily experiences such as emotional stress, heat, alcohol consumption, or straining at stool.

Flushing symptoms and hypotension are thought to be caused by a variety of bioactive tumor products. These include catecholamines, histamine, tachykinins, and kallikrein. Four different patterns of flushing have been described, and each is related to a specific site of origin. Type 1 flushing is a diffuse, erythematous rash, which may last up to 5 minutes, and is associated with the early stage of metastases from midgut carcinoid tumors. Type 2 flushing is a violaceous rash with telangiectasias, which may also last up to 5 minutes, and is associated with the later stages of metastases from midgut carcinoid tumors. Type 3 and 4 flushing is associated with bronchial and gastric carcinoid tumors, respectively.

The heart may be affected by carcinoid tumor products, particularly in those patients with midgut carcinoids and liver metastases. It is thought to be caused by the effects of serotonin on the heart. Specifically, serotonin has an effect on myofibroblasts resulting in fibroplasia, increased vascular tone, bronchoconstriction, and platelet aggregation. Together, these effects may cause pulmonary hypertension, tricuspid and pulmonary valve stenosis, and right ventricular hypertrophy and fibrosis. The left side of the heart is typically protected from the effects of carcinoid products by the lungs, which are capable of inactivating these substances.

Carcinoid crisis is a life-threatening condition. It may be brought on by anesthesia, embolization or manipulation of the tumor, administration of chemotherapy, or occur spontaneously. Life-threatening manifestations of the carcinoid crisis include profound flushing and hypotension, bronchoconstriction, arrhythmias, and hyperthermia. Other manifestations include diarrhea, confusion, and stupor. The crisis may be limited or avoided by pretreatment with somatostatin and histamine blockade (both H_1- and H_2-receptors) before treatments known to induce a crisis.

Diagnostic Studies

Biochemical Studies

Carcinoid tumors are often difficult to diagnose preoperatively, particularly those in the small bowel and appendix. In a study by Thompson and von Heerden,[8] less than 10% of 145 patients with GI carcinoids were accurately diagnosed before surgery, and all had carcinoid syndrome at presentation.

The diagnosis of carcinoid tumor before surgery relies on biopsy of an accessible lesion (in the foregut, hindgut, or liver), or the identification of biochemical products from the tumor. Although carcinoid tumors may produce many substances, the most widely used tests are related to serotonin. The most widely accepted test currently used to diagnose the presence of a carcinoid tumor is a 24-hour urine specimen analyzed for 5-HIAA (a serotonin metabolite). Urinary 5-HIAA excretion under normal circumstances is between 2–8 mg/24 hours. Excretion exceeding these levels has shown high sensitivity and specificity (73% and 100%,

TABLE 37-2. Dietary and medicinal intake affecting urinary 5-HIAA[70-72]

Foods rich in serotonin	Medicines affecting urine 5-HIAA
Bananas	Guaifenesin
Plantains	Acetaminophen
Pineapples	Salicylates
Plums	L-Dopa
Kiwi	
Walnuts	
Hickory nuts	
Pecans	
Avocados	
Tomatoes	

respectively) in diagnosing carcinoid syndrome.[9] It is important to avoid foods and medications that can produce a false-positive result by affecting urinary 5-HIAA levels. These are listed in Table 37-2.

Carcinoid tumors vary in their ability to produce serotonin. Midgut tumors typically produce high levels of serotonin and its metabolites. Foregut tumors typically lack the ability to convert (decarboxylate) 5-HTP (5-hydroxytryptophan) into 5-HT (serotonin), resulting in low urinary levels of 5-HIAA. However, the kidney may decarboxylate sufficient 5-HTP into 5-HT, thus increasing urinary serotonin levels. Hindgut carcinoids rarely produce 5-HTP or 5-HT, and urine and blood tests are typically negative. Platelet serotonin levels may be more sensitive than urine or blood tests. The results of three different tests in a series of 44 patients with carcinoid tumors is shown in Table 37-3.[10]

Imaging Studies

Localization of primary carcinoids in the GI tract is often difficult. Carcinoids in the foregut and hindgut are frequently diagnosed by endoscopy and biopsy.[11] However, ileal and appendiceal carcinoids are more common and less easily localized. These primary sites often remain unknown, despite small bowel contrast studies or computed tomographic (CT) scanning, until surgical exploration identifies the primary site.[12] If these studies are positive, it is usually the mesenteric kinking and fibrosis that is evident rather than the mass itself. Contrast studies may show small bowel obstruction, extrinsic filling defects, or kinking, angulation, and separation of small bowel loops.[11]

TABLE 37-3. Comparison of urine and platelet biochemical studies in carcinoid patients

	Number	Platelet 5-HT (%)	Urine 5-HIAA (%)	Urine Serotonin (%)
Foregut	14	50	29	55
Midgut	25	100	92	82
Hindgut	5	20	0	60

Multiple newer imaging techniques have been used in an attempt to identify both the primary tumor as well as metastases. These may be categorized as morphologic and functional imaging studies. Morphologic studies include ultrasound, CT, and magnetic resonance imaging (MRI). These studies may be useful, as they are in many types of cancers, in identifying distant metastases. In addition, CT scans may show a characteristic stellate soft-tissue stranding in the mesentery.[13] Functional studies are based on tumor uptake and scintigraphic imaging of various isotopes. The first of these was metaiodobenzylguanidine (MIBG),[14] but this has since been replaced by newer agents and techniques. The two scintigraphic imaging techniques currently in use are somatostatin receptor scintigraphy (SRS) and positron emission tomography (PET). Both techniques rely on differential uptake of the radiotracer by the tumor relative to normal tissue. SRS relies on somatostatin receptors on the cell surface, whereas PET relies on metabolic utilization of the localizing agent. A recent study by Hoegerle et al.[15] compared both morphologic and functional imaging modalities in localizing primary and metastatic carcinoid tumors in 17 patients. The results are summarized in Table 37-4, and suggest that the two approaches are complementary. ^{18}F-Dopa-PET imaging is more sensitive in localizing primary tumors and lymph node involvement, whereas CT or MRI is more sensitive in identifying distant disease.

Prognosis

The behavior and prognosis of carcinoid tumors are highly variable and are affected by multiple factors including tumor size, depth, presence and location of metastases, and primary tumor location.

TABLE 37-4. Morphologic and functional imaging in carcinoid tumors

| | PET | | | |
Tumor site	^{18}F-Dopa	[18]FDG	SRS	CT/MRI
Primary	7/8	2/8	4/8	2/8
Lymph nodes	41/47	14/47	27/47	29/47
Distant metastases	12/37	11/37	21/37	36/37

[18]FDG, ^{18}F-fluorodeoxyglucose; SRS, somatostatin receptor scintigraphy.

The TNM staging of carcinoid tumors is similar to that of GI adenocarcinomas. T-stage is related to depth of penetration, and nodal and metastatic staging are related to its absence or presence. Prognosis is affected by the TNM stage, as shown in Table 37-5. The effect of primary tumor location on prognosis (survival, likelihood of carcinoid syndrome, and additional tumors) is shown in Table 37-6.

Treatment

Tumor-directed Therapy[16,17]

The mainstay of treatment for carcinoid tumors is surgical resection. Difficulty arises in selecting the extent of surgery relative to the extent of disease, magnified by two considerations: 1) carcinoid tumors are often located in an area where "local excision" is an option (appendix, rectum), and 2) the benefit of debulking procedures. The surgical decision is based on the likelihood of residual primary disease, lymph node metastases, and the benefit of debulking the tumor burden to reduce the symptoms of the carcinoid syndrome. Guidelines for extent of surgical resection are summarized in Table 37-7.[16,17]

TABLE 37-5. TNM staging and survival of GI carcinoid tumors[73]

TNM stage		Definition	5-y survival (%)	Comment
T	1	Submucosa	82	Survival differences
	2	Muscularis propria		related to tumor
	3	Subserosa		depth in absence
	4	Perforated or invading neighboring structure	52	of metastases
N	0	Absent	95	Survival differences
	1	Present	83	related to presence and proximity of metastases
M	0	Absent	—	
	1	Present	38	

TABLE 37-6. Effect of primary carcinoid location on prognosis[16]

Primary carcinoid location	Overall 5-y survival (%)	Incidence of metastases (%)	Carcinoid syndrome	Multiplicity of carcinoid tumors (%)	Second primary cancer (%)
Appendix	99	<1 cm, 0 1–1.9 cm, 11 >2 cm, 30–60	Rare	4.2	13
Small bowel	Related to metastasis (see Table 37-4)	<1 cm, 20–30 1–2 cm, 80 LN 20 liver >2 cm, >80 LN 40–50 liver	Common	30–50	20–30
Colon	20–52	Frequent	Rare	Infrequent	25–40
Rectum	No mets–92 LN mets–44 Distant mets–7	<1 cm, 3 1–2 cm, 11 >2 cm, 74	Rare	0–3	7–32

LN, lymph node.

TABLE 37-7. Guidelines for extent of surgical resection

Primary tumor	Factor	Extent of resection
Appendix	<1 cm	Appendectomy
	1–1.9 cm	Individualize, appendectomy, or right hemicolectomy
	>2 cm	Right hemicolectomy
Small bowel	Locally limited disease	Resection of primary and metastatic tumors
	Extensive disease	Resection or bypass of primary tumor Debulking of metastases
Colon		Colectomy
Rectum	<1 cm	Local excision
	1–1.9 cm	Individualize, local excision, or proctectomy
	>2 cm	Proctectomy

Small bowel carcinoid tumors are frequently associated with lymph node metastases and structural abnormalities (intussusception, mesenteric fibrosis, and small bowel kinking). Lymph node metastases are common, even when the tumors are small. Lesions less than 1 cm in diameter have a 20%–30% incidence of lymph node involvement. Additionally, there are often multiple small bowel lesions. Therefore, surgical management involves formal resection and wide mesenteric excision of the associated region of lymph node drainage as well as thorough exploration for additional lesions.[16,17]

Appendiceal carcinoids typically behave differently than small bowel carcinoids. They are frequently found during appendectomy, are less likely to have lymph node metastases (0% for lesions less than 1 cm, 11% for lesions between 1 and 1.9 cm, and 30%–60% for lesions greater than 2 cm in diameter) and multicentric disease is rare. Therefore, appendectomy is adequate treatment for lesions less than 1 cm, whereas lesions greater than 2 cm are treated by formal resection (right hemicolectomy). Treatment for intermediate-size appendiceal carcinoids (1–1.9 cm) must be individualized, balancing the risk of a more extensive surgery against the risk of residual disease. Factors that suggest an increased likelihood of residual disease, and are thus used to indicate a formal right hemicolectomy, include lymphovascular invasion, involvement of the mesoappendix (by direct extension or in lymph nodes), or a positive surgical margin.[16,17]

Colonic carcinoid tumors generally behave in an aggressive manner and frequently have lymph node metastases and a poor prognosis. Therefore, they are treated with formal resection.[16,17]

Rectal carcinoid tumors are minimally aggressive lesions, and behave in a manner similar to appendiceal carcinoids. They have a similar rate of lymph node metastases and multiple lesions are uncommon. Surgical treatment also shows similarity in that local (transanal) excision is adequate for lesions less than 1 cm in diameter whereas formal proctectomy is advised for lesions larger than 2 cm in diameter. Treatment for intermediate-size rectal carcinoids (1–1.9 cm) must be individualized, balancing the risk of a more extensive

surgery against the risk of residual disease. Muscular invasion is the factor that suggests an increased likelihood of residual disease, and is thus used to indicate a formal proctectomy.[16,17]

Treatment of hepatic metastases is of significant benefit, especially when metastatic disease is confined to the liver.[18] Tumor debulking may be in the form of hepatic resection, ablative therapy (cryotherapy, radiofrequency ablation), radiolabeled octreotide, or hepatic artery embolization and chemoembolization. The expected 5-year survival rate for patients with carcinoid liver metastases is 20%. Death is often related to liver failure from local tumor progression or carcinoid heart disease. However, several studies have demonstrated a 5-year survival rate approximating 70% when these metastases are treated with a combination of the listed techniques. Similar survival rates have been achieved with the use of liver transplantation in a small number of patients.[19]

Systemic Therapy

Medical treatment for patients with carcinoid tumors has two purposes: palliation of systemic symptoms of the carcinoid syndrome, and treatment of metastases. The palliation of symptoms may use medications directed at specific symptoms, or medications causing a generalized reduction in hormone production. Specific agents that may help control symptoms of the carcinoid syndrome are listed in Table 37-8. Somatostatin analogs are helpful in controlling many of the symptoms of the carcinoid syndrome by reducing synthesis and systemic release of hormone products. Octreotide is a long-acting somatostatin analog with a half-life of 90 minutes. In doses of 400 μg/day, octreotide improved the major symptoms of flushing and diarrhea in more than 80% of patients.[3] Lanreotide is another somatostatin analog with a longer half-life than octreotide, and both agents are available in long-acting depot forms.

Chemotherapy has largely been ineffective in patients with metastatic carcinoid tumor.[20] Single agent regimens using 5-fluorouracil, streptozotocin, dacarbazine, dactinomycin, doxorubicin, etoposide, cisplatin, and carboplatin have had objective tumor response rates between 0%–30% in small series of patients. Similarly poor results have been found when combination chemotherapy has been used in the adjuvant

TABLE 37-8. Medical treatment of carcinoid syndrome symptoms[2,3]

Symptom	Drug category	Specific agents
Flushing	H$_2$-Blockade	Cimetidine, ranitidine, famotidine
	α$_1$-Blockade	Doxazosin, phenoxybenzamine
	Phenothiazine	Chlorpromazine
	Corticosteroid	Prednisone
Diarrhea	Serotonin blockade	Ketanserin, ondansetron, cyproheptadine, methysergide
	Opiate blockade	Codeine, loperamide
Bronchospasm	Phenothiazine	Chlorpromazine
	Bronchodilator	Salbutamol
	Corticosteroid	Prednisone

setting or to treat metastatic carcinoid tumor. Interferon has been used in the treatment of metastatic carcinoid tumors with some success. Patients have experienced an objective response rate near 50%, with a duration of 2.5 years. However, interferon therapy produces significant side effects of a flu-like syndrome, fatigue, and fever which may limit its use.

GI Stromal Tumors

In the past, most spindle cell sarcomas arising from the mesenchymal elements of the GI tract were considered smooth muscle neoplasms and were considered leiomyomas, leiomyosarcomas, and leiomyoblastomas. With advances in electron microscopy and immunohistochemistry, it was discovered that many of these tumors lacked structural or immunophenotypic features associated with smooth muscle differentiation and the more generic term "stromal tumor" was introduced.[21] Further advances in immunohistochemistry allowed pathologists to separate these tumors into those that are true smooth muscle tumors (leiomyomas) and those that are thought to arise from GI pacemaker cells (GI stromal tumors).

GI stromal cell tumors (GISTs) are mesenchymal tumors arising from the intestinal wall, omentum, or retroperitoneum that stain positive for the CD117 antigen, a marker for the KIT oncoprotein. Sixty to seventy percent of GISTs also stain positive for CD34, a hematopoietic progenitor cell antigen.[22] Leiomyomas are stain negative for KIT and CD34 and positive for desmin or smooth muscle actin.[23]

Because of structural and immunohistochemical similarities between GISTs and the interstitial cells of Cajal, it is thought GISTs arise from these cells or other pluripotential mesenchymal stem cells. The interstitial cells of Cajal are located in the muscle layer of the GI tract and form a complex network that regulates intestinal motility.

The stomach is the most common location of GISTs (45%–55%) with small bowel the next most common location (25%–35%). Only 10%–20% of GISTs are located in the colon and rectum. The gender distribution is close to equal in all locations.

GISTs occur throughout the colon but are most often located in the rectum. Miettinen et al.[23,24] retrieved all cases coded as leiomyomas, leiomyosarcomas, smooth muscle tumors, or stromal tumors at the Armed Forces Institute of Pathology and the University of Helsinki from 1970 to 1996 for rectal tumors and 1970 to 1998 for colon tumors. The most common location was the rectum and anus (80%). Older reports of colorectal leiomyosarcomas (the majority of which were probably GISTs) also show an increased incidence in the anorectal area with about 1/3 occurring in the colon and 2/3 in the anorectal area.[25]

The most common clinical presentation is hematochezia, abdominal or rectal pain, or a mass found incidentally on physical examination or endoscopically. As might be expected, how patients present is largely related to the size of the tumor.[26–28]

Complete surgical excision, if possible, continues to be the treatment of choice. Because GISTs rarely spread to the lymphatic system, removal of the regional lymph nodes is not necessary or recommended.[29] Wide margins are not necessary, but complete en bloc removal of the tumor and its pseudocapsule should be performed. Because of high local recurrence rates, enucleation of the tumor (leaving the pseudocapsule) or cutting across tumor should be avoided.

The use of imatinib mesylate (Gleevac in the United States, Glivec in Europe, Novartis Pharmaceuticals) has significantly impacted the treatment of GISTs. The KIT oncoprotein, detected in almost all GIST tumors by positive immunohistochemical staining for the CD117 antigen, is a transmembrane receptor tyrosine kinase encoded for by the C-kit protooncogene.[29,30] In GIST tumors, abnormal activation of the KIT oncoprotein results from a mutation in the C-kit gene. This abnormal activation results in unregulated cellular proliferation. Imatinib is a selective tyrosine kinase inhibitor and acts by blocking the abnormal activation of the KIT oncoprotein.

Demetri et al.[31] used imatinib in 147 patients with metastatic or unresectable GIST tumors. Fifty-four percent had a partial response with shrinkage of their tumors and 41% of the patients had stable disease. Van Oosterom et al.[32] found an objective response in 70% (25 of 36 patients) of patients with KIT-positive metastatic GIST tumors.

The use of imatinib as a postoperative adjuvant to surgery is currently being investigated and patients who have a resected primary GIST should be considered for entry into a clinical trial.[29] Patients who present with marginally resectable or unresectable tumors should be considered for a course of preoperative imatinib. Katz et al.[30] reported two cases of patients with unresectable GIST tumors treated with imatinib. In both cases there was a dramatic decrease in the size of the tumors and both patients eventually had surgical excision of their tumors.

The incidence of local recurrence or metastatic disease after complete surgical excision is high. About 50% of patients with potentially curative resection will develop a recurrence.[29] Of 40 patients with rectal tumors reported by Yeh et al.,[27] 48% developed a recurrence or metastasis. They also found local recurrences were higher in the group that had wide local excision compared with those who had a more radial resection, such as an abdominoperineal resection or anterior resection (55% versus 24%).

Leiomyomas

Leiomyomas of the colon and rectum are usually small (less than 1 cm) nodules arising from the smooth muscle of the muscularis mucosa. They are differentiated from GISTs by staining negative for CD117 (KIT) and positive for desmin and smooth muscle actin.[33] They are almost always found incidentally on endoscopy or in surgical resections done for other pathology. Of 88 cases reported by Miettinen et al.,[33] 29% were in the rectum and 49% in the sigmoid colon. The leiomyomas in this series were almost all removed by snare polypectomy. There were no recurrences. Walsh and Mann[34] also reported a series of 26 patients who had leiomyomas arising from the muscularis mucosa. Twenty-two tumors had some sort of local excision (12 by biopsy forceps). No recurrence was noted in any of these patients. Small incidental leiomyomas found on endoscopy are benign tumors that are adequately treated by snare polypectomy alone.

Squamous and Adenosquamous Carcinoma

Squamous and adenosquamous carcinomas of the colon are thought to be variants of the same tumor.[35] Squamous cell cancers have pure epithelial features without glandular elements; adenosquamous cancers have both epithelial and glandular features. A review of the National Cancer Institute's database found approximately one in 2000 cases of colorectal cancer was adenosquamous.[36] By 1999, only 59 cases of squamous cell carcinoma and 56 cases of adenosquamous cell cancer had been published. A review of the National Cancer Institute database added 145 cases of adenosquamous cancer in 1999.

To be considered a primary colon rectal tumor, these tumors should be located proximal to the distal rectum to exclude anal canal cancers that have extended proximally. Patients with a history of squamous cell cancer elsewhere are also excluded because of the possibility this may represent metastatic disease.

The mean age of patients in reported cases of pure squamous cell cancer is 58[37] and 66 for a large series of patients with adenosquamous cancer. The anatomic location seems to be similar to that of adenocarcinoma with most lesions found in the proximal and distal colon and few in the middle colon (transverse and descending).[36,37]

Patients tend to present with advanced disease. Cagie et al.[36] reviewed 145 patients with adenosquamous disease and found only 11% presented with node negative, superficially invasive cancer (Astler-Coller Stage A and B). Forty-four percent had tumors with full-thickness invasion or positive lymph nodes and 40% had distant metastasis. Those patients with T_1, or T_2, N0, M0 lesions appeared to have a prognosis similar to that of patients with adenocarcinoma. Patients with T_3 lesions, positive lymph nodes, or metastatic disease have a worse prognosis.[36] In a combined series of squamous and adenosquamous cancer, Frizelle et al.[35] reported a 5-year survival rate of 86% for patients with Stage II disease and only 24% for patients with Stage III.

The primary treatment of these tumors is surgical. Because, by definition, these tumors are located in the colon or proximal to mid rectum, a segmental resection with anastomosis should be feasible. In rectal tumors, preoperative adjuvant chemoradiation should be considered. This recommendation is based on improved control of local disease with preoperative adjuvant therapy in patients with adenocarcinoma and the good response to chemoradiation in patients with squamous cell cancer of the anus.[35] No recommendations based on data can be made concerning postoperative adjuvant chemotherapy in patients with these tumors. The prognosis, however, is so poor in patients with nodal disease that adjuvant chemotherapy seems a reasonable option. At the very least, these patients deserve to have a consultation with an oncologist.

Lymphomas

Most primary GI lymphomas are located in the stomach or small bowel; only 6%–12% of primary GI lymphomas occur in the colon. Primary colonic lymphomas represent less than 1% of large bowel malignancies.[38] Approximately 70% involve the cecum or ascending colon.[39,40] The most common presenting symptoms are abdominal pain, palpable abdominal mass, hematochezia or melena, and weight loss.[39,41]

Several authors use Dawson's criteria to establish a diagnosis of primary intestinal lymphoma as opposed to generalized lymphoma secondarily involving the GI tract. Dawson's criteria are: 1) absence of enlarged superficial lymph nodes when the patient is first seen; 2) no enlargement of mediastinal lymph nodes; 3) the total and differential white count are normal; 4) at laparotomy, only regional lymph nodes have metastatic disease; 5) the liver and spleen are unaffected.[42]

The majority of lymphomas in the colon and rectum are non-Hodgkin's lymphomas of B cell origin, diffuse large cell type. In a series of 32 patients reported by Myung et al.,[41] 22 were of diffuse large cell type and 27 of B cell origin. Other pathologic types that occur in the colon include low-grade lymphoma tissue (MALT lymphomas), mantle cell lymphoma, and T cell lymphoma.[38,43,44]

GI lymphoid tissue exists in intestinal mucosa, submucosa, and lamina propria. Low-grade B cell lymphomas arising from these specialized lymphoid tissues are referred to as MALT (mucosa-associated lymphoid tissue) tumors. MALT tumors are low-grade tumors with an indolent course and are usually located in the stomach, but cases of colonic involvement have been reported.[45–47] Currently, gastric MALT tumors are thought to arise in response to *Helicobacter pylori* infection and it has been shown that eradication of the *H. pylori* infection will lead to complete regression in the majority of cases.[48] MALT tumors in the colon are usually solitary lesions, but can also present as multiple polypoid lesions. In a series of 17 colonic MALT tumors reported by Yatabe et al.,[49] treatment consisted of endoscopic (three patients) or surgical excision (14 patients); three of the patients also had chemotherapy. There are two case reports of complete regression of a colonic MALT with either chemotherapy or treatment of a concomitant *H. pylori* infection.[47,50]

Multiple lymphomatous polyposis is a mantle cell lymphoma that involves the GI tract. Multiple lymphomatous polyps can involve the GI tract from the stomach to the rectum, but can also involve the colon alone. The most common presenting symptoms are weight loss, diarrhea, abdominal pain, rectal bleeding, and anemia. On endoscopic examination, it can be confused with familial adenomatous polyposis or nodular lymphoid hyperplasia. The treatment is chemotherapy.[51,52]

Treatment of localized, primary colonic lymphoma is primarily surgical excision.[40,45] Aviles et al.[45] followed surgical excision with adjuvant chemotherapy consisting of cyclophosphamide, doxorubicin, vincristine, prednisone, and bleomycin. In 40% of their cases, epirubicin was used in place of doxorubicin. In node negative patients, their event-free survival rate at 10 years was 80%. In two other series of more advanced lesions, the 5-year survival rate was only 33% and 39% in patients treated with both surgery and chemotherapy.[39,40]

Extramedullary Plasmacytoma

The most common type of plasma cell neoplasm is multiple myeloma. Of 1272 patients with a plasma cell neoplasm seen at M.D. Anderson Cancer Center, 94% had multiple myeloma and only 2% (22 patients) had an extramedullary plasmacytoma (EMP).[53] More than 75% of EMPs occur in the upper respiratory tract, and when they do occur in the GI tract, they are usually found in the stomach or small intestine.[53,54] Therefore, EMPs occurring in the colon are very rare and by 2004, only 22 have been reported in the English language.[55]

To be considered an EMP, metastatic multiple myeloma must be excluded by evaluating the urine for Bence-Jones protein, serum electrophoresis, and bone marrow biopsy. Pathologic diagnosis is established by histologic and immunohistochemical findings consistent with a localized collection of monoclonal plasma cells.[55,56]

Hashiguchi et al.[55] recently reviewed all the reported cases of colonic EMPs. Patient ages ranged from 15 to 90 with a mean of 52.3. The cecum (36.4%) and rectum (22.7%) were the most common sites involved. Treatment consisted of surgery alone in 18 cases (81.8%), radiotherapy in two cases (9%), and both surgery and radiotherapy in one case. In the 22 plasmacytoma cases report by the M.D. Anderson group, only two were in the colon. Radiation treatment alone was used in 18 of the 22 cases with good results. In seven of the 22 cases (32%), multiple myeloma developed after a median of 1.8 years, including one of the two colon cases.[56]

Melanoma

Primary melanomas of the GI tract are rare and the majority are located in either the anorectal area or the esophagus.[57] An electronic search of the medical literature from 1966 to 2004 found only four reports of primary colonic melanoma.[58,59]

Malignant melanoma will often metastasize to the GI tract, and autopsy studies have shown malignant melanoma is one of the most common metastatic lesions to involve the GI tract. Up to 60% of patients dying of melanoma will have metastasis to the GI tract.[60] It is unusual, however, for colonic metastasis to be diagnosed while the patient is alive.

In a recent Mayo Clinic review, 2965 patients were treated between 1960 and 2000 with metastatic melanoma. Only 24 patients (0.8%) had symptoms from metastatic melanoma to the colon. The mean age at diagnosis of metastatic disease was 60.4 and the average time between diagnosis of the primary and metastasis was 8.47 years. The presenting symptoms were bleeding (50%), pain (20%), obstruction (20%), and weight loss (17%). Eighteen of the 24 had segmental resection and the 1-year survival was 37%. The 5-year survival was 21%.[60]

Long-term survival from literature review of patients with isolated colonic metastasis was 58.7 months. Therefore, surgery for metastatic melanoma to the colon with either palliative or curative intent is indicated.

Colonic Complications of Leukemia

Colonic complications of leukemia may be broadly divided into two categories: complications caused by leukemic invasion of the bowel and complications caused by the profound immunocompromise, as a result of the disease and its treatment.

Leukemic infiltration of the colon is not common. In a paper by Hunter and Bjelland,[61] 13 of 142 leukemic patients had a significant GI complication and only one had evidence of colonic infiltration. In an autopsy study, 16 of 148 patients who died of leukemia had evidence of leukemia infiltrates in the colon.[62]

Endoscopic and radiologic findings are varied; a small localized ulceration,[63] diffuse polyposis,[64] a colitis-like appearance,[65] and plaque-like bowel thickening have all been described. The most common CT finding is a diffuse thickening of the bowel wall.[66]

Symptoms of leukemic infiltration are nonspecific, such as abdominal pain, bloating, diarrhea, and hematochezia.[67] The treatment consists of treating the underlying leukemia. Surgery is indicated only if complications arise.

Neutropenic enterocolitis is a serious life-threatening complication of the chemotherapeutic treatment of leukemias. Cartoni et al.[68] reported a 6% incidence of neutropenic colitis in 1450 consecutive patients treated for leukemia with a mortality rate of 15%. Hogan et al.[69] reported a 15% incidence of neutropenic colitis in a group of 78 patients treated for acute myelogenous leukemia. In the report by Hogan et al., the median onset of symptoms (fever, pain, diarrhea) was 10 days after the start of chemotherapy and all patients had absolute neutrophil counts of less than 0.5×10^9/L. CT and ultrasound findings consist of thickening of the bowel wall in the ileocecal region. Cartoni et al. showed that detection of bowel wall thickening on ultrasound was associated with a worst prognosis than if no thickening was detected (a 29% mortality versus 0% mortality).

Treatment consists of bowel rest, parenteral nutrition, and broad spectrum antibiotics. Surgery should be reserved for complications such as documented evidence of bowel perforation or massive bleeding.

References

1. Creutzfeldt W. Carcinoid tumors: development of our knowledge. World J Surg 1996;20:126–131.
2. Lips CJM, Lentjes EGWM, Hoppener JWM. The spectrum of carcinoid tumors and carcinoid syndrome. Ann Clin Biochem 2003;40:612–627.
3. Jensen RT, Doherty GM. Carcinoid tumors and the carcinoid syndrome. In: DeVita VT, Hellman S, Rosenberg SA, eds. Cancer: Principles and Practice of Oncology. 6th ed. Philadelphia: Lippincott Williams & Wilkins; 2001:1813–1832.
4. Soga J, Tazawa K. Pathologic analysis of carcinoids: histologic reevaluation of 62 cases. Cancer 1971;28:990–998.
5. Martin ED, Potet F. Pathology of endocrine tumors of the GI tract. Clin Gastroenterol 1974;3:511–532.
6. Godwin JD. Carcinoid tumors. An analysis of 2,837 cases. Cancer 1975;36:560.
7. Modlin IM, Sandor A. An analysis of 8305 cases of carcinoid tumors. Cancer 1997;79:813.
8. Thompson GB, von Heerden JA. Carcinoid tumors of the gastrointestinal tract. Presentation, management, and prognosis. Surgery 1998;98:1054.
9. Feldman JM. Carcinoid tumors and syndrome. Semin Oncol 1987;14:237.
10. Kema IP, deVries GE, Sloof MJH, Biesma B, Muskiet FAJ. Serotonin, catecholamines, histamine, and their metabolites in urine, platelets, and tumor tissue of patients with carcinoid tumors. Clin Chem 1994;40:86.
11. Thompson GB, van Heerden JA, Martin JK, et al. Carcinoid tumors of the gastrointestinal tract: presentation, management, and prognosis. Surgery 1985;98:1054.
12. Bancks NH, Goldstein HM, Dodd GD. The roentgenologic spectrum of small intestinal carcinoid tumors. Am J Roentgenol Radium Ther Nucl Med 1975;123:274–280.
13. Picus D, Glazer HS, Levitt RG, Husband JE. Computed tomography of abdominal carcinoid tumors. Am J Radiol 1984;143:581–584.
14. Fischer M, Kamanabroo D, Sonderkamp H, Proske T. Scintigraphic imaging of carcinoid tumors with I-131-metaiodobenzylguanidine. Lancet 1984;2:165.
15. Hoegerle S, Altehoefer C, Ghanem N, et al. Whole-body 18F-dopa PET for detection of gastrointestinal carcinoid tumors. Radiology 2001;220(2):373–380.
16. Memon MA, Nelson H. Gastrointestinal carcinoid tumors: current management strategies. Dis Colon Rectum 1997;40(9):1101–1118.
17. Stinner B, Kisker O, Zielke A, Rothmund M. Surgical management for carcinoid tumors of small bowel, appendix, colon, and rectum. World J Surg 1996;20:183–188.
18. Pasieka JL. Carcinoid syndrome symposium on treatment modalities for gastrointestinal carcinoid tumors. Can J Surg 2001;44(1):25–33.
19. Le Treut YP, Delpero JR, Dousset B, et al. Results of liver transplantation in the treatment of metastatic neuroendocrine tumors. A 31-case French multicentric report. Ann Surg 1997;225(4):355–364.
20. Kvols LK. Neoplasms of the diffuse endocrine system. In: Kufe DW, Pollock RE, Weichselbaum RR, et al., eds. Cancer Medicine. 6th ed. Hamilton, ON: BC Decker; 2003:1275.
21. Fletcher CDM, Berman JJ, Corless C. Diagnosis of gastrointestinal stromal tumors: a consensus approach. Hum Pathol 2002;33(5):459–465.
22. Davila RE, Faigel DO. GI stromal tumors. Gastrointest Endosc 2003;58:80–87.
23. Miettinen N, Sarlomo-Rikala M, Sobin LH, Lasota J. Gastrointestinal stromal tumors and leiomyosarcomas in the colon. A clinicopathologic, immunohistochemical, and molecular genetic study of 44 cases. Am J Surg Pathol 2000;24:1339–1352.
24. Miettinen M, Furlong M, Sarlomo-Rikala M, Burke A, Sobin LH, Lasota J. Gastrointestinal stromal tumors, intramural leiomyomas, and leiomyosarcomas in the rectum and anus. A clinicopathologic, immunohistochemical, and molecular genetic study of 144 cases. Am J Surg Pathol 2001;25:1121–1133.
25. Akwari OE, Dozois R, Weiland L, Beahrs OH. Leiomyosarcoma of the small and large bowel. Cancer 1978;42:1375–1384.
26. Haque S, Dean PJ. Stromal neoplasms of the rectum and anal canal. Hum Pathol 1992;23:762–768.
27. Yeh C, Chen H, Tang R, Tasi W, Lin P, Wang J. Surgical outcome after curative resection of rectal leiomyosarcoma. Dis Colon Rectum 2000;43:1517–1521.
28. Tworek JA, Goldblum JR, Weiss SW, Greenson JK, Appelman HD. Stromal tumors of the anorectum. A clinicopathologic study of 22 cases. Am J Surg Pathol 1999;23:946–954.
29. Eisenberg BL, Judson I. Surgery and imatinib in the management of GIST: emerging approaches to adjuvant and neoadjuvant therapy. Ann Surg Oncol 2004;11:465–475.
30. Katz D, Segal A, Alberton Y, et al. Neoadjuvant imatinib for unresectable gastrointestinal stromal tumor. Anticancer Drugs 2004;15:599–602.
31. Demetri GD, Von Mehren M, Blanke CD, et al. Efficacy and safety of imatinib mesylate in advanced gastrointestinal stromal tumors. N Engl J Med 2002;347:472–480.
32. Van Oosterom AT, Judson I, Verweij J, et al. Safety and efficacy of imatinib (STI571) in metastatic gastrointestinal stromal tumors: a phase 1 study. Lancet 2001;358:1421–1423.
33. Miettinen M, Sarlomo-Rikala M, Sobin LH. Mesenchymal tumors of muscularis mucosae of colon and rectum are benign leiomyomas that should be separated from gastrointestinal stromal tumors: a clinical pathologic and immunohistochemical study of eighty-eight cases. Mod Pathol 2001;14(10):950–956.
34. Walsh TH, Mann CV. Smooth muscle neoplasms of the rectum and anal canal. Br J Surg 1984;71:597–599.
35. Frizelle FA, Hobday KS, Batts KP, Nelson H. Adenosquamous and squamous carcinoma of the colon and upper rectum. A clinical and histopathologic study. Dis Colon Rectum 2001;44:341–346.
36. Cagie B, Nagy NW, Topham A, Rakinic J, Fry RD. Adenosquamous carcinoma of the colon, rectum, and anus: epidemiology, distribution, and survival characteristics. Dis Colon Rectum 1999;42:258–263.

37. Juturi JV, Francis B, Koontz PW, Wilkes JD. Squamous cell carcinoma of the colon responsive to combination chemotherapy: report of two cases and review of the literature. Dis Colon Rectum 1999;42:102–109.

38. Lee HJ, Han JK, Kim TK, et al. Primary colorectal lymphoma: spectrum of imaging findings with pathologic correlation. Eur Radiol 2002;12:2242–2249.

39. Zibhelboim J, Larson MV. Primary colonic lymphoma. Clinical presentation, histopathologic features, and outcome with combination chemotherapy. J Clin Gastroenterol 1994;18(4):291–297.

40. Fan CS, Changchien CR, Wang JY, et al. Primary colorectal lymphoma. Dis Colon Rectum 2000;43:1277–1282.

41. Myung SJ, Kwang RJ, Yan SK, et al. Clinicopathologic features of ileocolonic malignant lymphoma: analysis according to colonoscopic classification. Gastrointest Endosc 2003;57(3): 343–347.

42. Dawson IM, Cornes JS, Morson BC. Primary malignant lymphoid tumors of the intestinal tract. Br J Surg 1961;49:80–89.

43. Chim CS, Shek TWH, Chung LP, Liang R. Unusual abdominal tumors. Case 3. Multiple lymphomatous polyposis in lymphoma of the colon. J Clin Oncol 2003;21(5):953–955.

44. Isomoto H, Maeda T, Akashi T, et al. Multiple lymphomatous polyposis of the colon originating from T-cells: a case report. Dig Liver Dis 2004;36:218–221.

45. Aviles A, Neri N, Huwerta-Guzman J. Large bowel lymphoma: an analysis of prognostic factors and therapy in 53 patients. J Surg Oncol 2002;80:111–115.

46. Arima N, Tanimoto A, Hamada T, et al. MALT lymphoma arising in giant diverticulum of ascending colon. Am J Gastroenterol 2000;95:3673.

47. Avner HW, Beham-Schmid C, Lidner G, et al. Successful non-surgical treatment of primary mucosa-associated lymphoid tissue lymphoma of colon presenting with multiple polypoid lesions. Am J Gastroenterol 2000;95:2387.

48. Yoon SS, Coit DG, Portlock CS, Karpeh MS. The diminishing role of surgery in the treatment of gastric lymphoma. Ann Surg 2004;240:28–37.

49. Yatabe Y, Nakamura S, Nakamura T, et al: Multiple polypoid lesions of primary mucosa-associated lymphoid tissue lymphoma of colon. Histopathology 1998;32:116–125.

50. Raderer M, Pfeffel F, Pohl G, Mannhalter C, Valencak J, Chutt A. Regression of colonic low-grade B-cell lymphoma of the mucosa associated lymphoid tissue type after eradication of *Helicobacter pylori*. Gut 2000;46:133–135.

51. Isomoto H, Maeda T, Akashi T, et al. Multiple lymphomatous polyposis of the colon originating from T-cells: a case report. Dig Liver Dis 2004;36:218–221.

52. Lam KC, Yeo W, Lee J, Chow J, Mok TSK. Unusual abdominal tumors. Case 4. Multiple lymphomatous polyposis in mantle cell lymphoma. J Clin Oncol 2003;21:955–956.

53. Liebross RH, Hu CS, Cox JD, Weber D, Delusalle K, Alexanian R. Clinical course of solitary extramedullary plasmacytoma. Radiother Oncol 1999;52:245–249.

54. Lattuneddu A, Farneti F, Lucci E, et al. A case of primary extramedullary plasmacytoma of the colon. Int J Colorectal Dis 2004;19:289–291.

55. Hashiguchi K, Iwai A, Inoue T, et al. Extramedullary plasmacytoma of the rectum arising in ulcerative colitis: case report and review. Gastrointest Endosc 2004;59:304–307.

56. Mendenhall WN, Mendenhall CM, Mendenhall NP. Solitary plasmacytoma of bone and soft tissue. Am J Otolaryngol 2003;24:395–399.

57. Schuschter LM, Green R, Fraker D. Primary and metastatic diseases in malignant melanoma of the gastrointestinal tract. Curr Opin Oncol 2000;12:181–185.

58. Avital S, Romaguera RL, Sands L, Marchetti F, Hellinger MD. Primary malignant melanoma of the right colon. Am Surg 2004;70:649–651.

59. Sarah P, MaNiff JF, Madison MD, Wen-Jen Poo H, Bayar S, Sallem RR. Colonic melanoma, primary or regressed primary. J Clin Gastroenterol 2000;30:440–444.

60. Tessier DJ, McConnell EJ, Young-Fadok T, Wolff BG. Melanoma metastatic to the colon. Case series and review of the literature with outcome analysis. Dis Colon Rectum 2003;46: 441–447.

61. Hunter RB, Bjelland JC. Gastrointestinal complications of leukemia and its treatment. AJR Am J Roentgenol 1984;142: 513–518.

62. Prolla JC, Kisner JB. The gastrointestinal lesions and complication of the leukemias. Ann Intern Med 1964;61: 1084–1099.

63. Matsushita M, Hajiro K, Okazaki K, et al. A minute erosion representing leukemic infiltration of the colon. Endoscopy 1997;29:55–56.

64. Utsunomiya A, Hanada S, Terada A, et al. Adult T-cell leukemia with leukemic cell infiltration into the gastrointestinal tract. Cancer 1988;61:824–828.

65. Gos P, Rosito MA, Tarta C, et al. Leukemic rectosigmoiditis. Endoscopy 2000;32:520.

66. Khalil RM, Singer AA. CT appearance of direct leukemic invasion of the bowel. Abdom Imaging 1997;22:464–465.

67. Rabin MS, Bledin AG, Lewis D. Polypoid leukemic infiltration of the large bowel. AJR Am J Roentgenol 1978;131:723–724.

68. Cartoni C, Dragoni F, Micuzzi A, et al. Neutropenic enterocolitis in patients with acute leukemia: prognostic significance of bowel wall thickening detected by ultrasonography. J Clin Oncol 2001;19:756–761.

69. Hogan W, Letendre L, Litzow M, et al. Neutropenic colitis after treatment of acute myelogenous leukemia with idarubicin and cytosine arabinoside. Mayo Clin Proc 2002;77: 760–762.

70. Nutall KL, Pingree SS. The incidence of elevations in urine 5-hydroxyindoleacetic acid. Ann Clin Lab Sci 1998;28:167.

71. Feldman JM, Butler SS, Chapman BA. Interference with measurement of 3-methoxy-4-hydroxymadelic acid and 5-hydroxyindoleacetic by reducing metabolites. Clin Chem 1974;20:607.

72. Feldman J, Lee E. Serotonin content of foods: effect on urinary excretion of 5-hydroxyindoleacetic acid. Am J Clin Nutr 1985;42:639–643.

73. Neary P, Redmond PH, Houghton T, Watson GRK, Bouchier-Hayes D. Carcinoid disease: Review of the literature. Dis Colon Rectum 1997;40(3):349–362.

38
Hereditary Nonpolyposis Colon Cancer

Lawrence C. Rusin and Susan Galandiuk

Colorectal cancer affects 148,300 patients in the United States annually (72,600 males and 75,700 females) causing 56,600 deaths each year.[1] Those patients who have two or more first- and/or second-degree relatives with colorectal cancer have a potentially definable inheritable disorder. Approximately 5%–6% of colorectal cancers have a known germline genetic mutation. Hereditary nonpolyposis colon cancer (HPNCC) is one of the syndromes and accounts for 3% of newly diagnosed colorectal cancer cases.[2]

HNPCC is characterized by the early onset of colorectal cancer (mean age, 45 years), with multiple generations affected. These cancers tend to be proximal to the splenic flexure, poorly differentiated, and have an increased frequency of synchronous and metachronous cancers. There is also an excess of extracolonic cancers, including endometrial, ovarian, gastric, small bowel, hepatobiliary, and transitional cell carcinomas. Over a patient's lifetime, there is an 80% risk of cancer, with colon cancer being the most frequently diagnosed cancer.[3] The syndrome is characterized by an autosomal dominant mode of inheritance. Germline mutations in mismatch repair (MMR) genes, which normally repair mistakes in DNA replication, are responsible for HNPCC.

Historical Perspectives

Alfred Warthin, a pathologist at the University of Michigan, first described a family with inherited intestinal cancer in 1895. Detailed descriptions of this family (known as "Family G") as well as other families were published in 1913. Gastric cancer was the predominant cancer.[4] Nearly 50 years later, after spending time at the University of Michigan, Henry Lynch published the pedigrees of two large midwestern families ("Family N" from Nebraska and "Family M" from Michigan). In his article, he commented on the wide spectrum of cancers diagnosed and the probability of an inheritable gene. By the mid-1980s, after further studies, two patterns of disease presentation became apparent, so-called Lynch I (colorectal cancer only) and Lynch II (colorectal and other malignancies). Concurrent observations determined that there was

a paucity of colonic polyps in these patients, and that there was considerable overlap between Lynch I and II syndromes. The syndrome became known as HNPCC.[5]

To promote research collaborative studies, the International Collaborative Group on HNPCC met in Amsterdam in 1990.[6] A set of diagnostic guidelines was agreed on that would allow researchers to gather homogenous populations to be studied. Once HNPCC was well categorized, rapid progress was made elucidating the genetic defect as well as in diagnosis and treatment of the disease. Colorectal tumors were found to have multiple mismatched nucleotides. This unique genetic abnormality was termed replication error phenotype or RER+. Most of these mismatched bases were in areas of the gene called "microsatellites," so the term microsatellite instability (MSI) became prevalent.[7] Extensive research in yeast and *Escherichia coli* had identified a group of genes referred to as MMR genes. Using linkage studies, the first human homolog, MSH2, was identified in 1993 by Fishel.[8]

Genetics

What Are Microsatellites?

Microsatellites are short tandem repeating base sequences that are usually mononucleotide or dinucleotide base repeats. Most often, the repeats are found in the noncoding or intronic portion of the gene. However, microsatellites can occur anywhere within the gene. There are well over 200 polymorphic microsatellite loci identified.[9] The most common sequences are repeats of adenine or thymine or the dinucleotide repeats of cytosine/adenine (CA_n) or guanine/thymine (GT_n). When the number of repeats in a microsatellite sequence in a cancer cell is different from the surrounding normal tissue, this is termed "microsatellite instability."

Different Types of DNA Repair

There are several intracellular mechanisms that repair DNA damage and maintain genomic stability and fidelity. "Base excision repair" (BER) repairs mutations caused by reactive oxygen species related to aerobic metabolism. Oxidative DNA damage produces a stable 8oxo 7-8 dihydro-2′ deoxyguanosine (8 oxoG), which readily misrepairs with adenine residues resulting in G:C→T:A transversion mutations. "Nucleotide excision repair" (NER) repairs damage caused by exogenous agents such as mutagenic and carcinogenic chemicals as well as ultraviolet radiation. Several genes have been cloned XPA through XPG. MMR genes repair single base mismatches as well as insertion/deletion loops (IDL) of up to 10 nucleotides. MMR gene dysfunction is characterized by MSI and is responsible for HNPCC. The so-called mutator phenotype of HNPCC is characterized by an increased genome-wide mutation rate. This is in contradistinction to sporadic colon cancer or familial polyposis, which is characterized by loss of whole portions of chromosome alleles known as loss of heterozygosity (LOH).[10]

MMR Function in Single Cells

This MMR repair system has been well studied and elucidated in single cell organisms. There are three main components of this repair system, namely, MutS, MutL, and MutH.

MutS recognizes base mismatches and IDL. Acting as an adenosine triphosphatase (ATPase) homodimer, MutS attaches to the abnormal DNA, undergoes a conformational change, and translocates or slides along the DNA, allowing the formation of a large DNA loop. As the DNA is being shortened into the loop, the abnormal mismatches are included in the DNA loop. MutL, another ATPase, again acting as a homodimer, identifies the loop segment of DNA that includes the mismatch. The loop continues to enlarge, and a DNA-methylated (DAM) GATC base sequence is encountered. The new DNA strand is recognized because it is not methylated. At this point, MutH, an endonuclease, is activated and a nick in the DNA strand is made. This can occur on either the 3′ or 5′ side of the DNA strand. Bidirectional exonucleases excise the abnormal DNA strand and DNA polymerase resynthesizes a new strand.[11]

MMR Function in Humans

MMR genes have been found in every organism studied and are homologous with yeast and bacterial MMR genes. In humans, five MutS genes have been identified (*MSH2, MSH3, MSH4, MSH5, MSH6*) and four MutL genes (*MLH1, PMS1, PMS2, MLH3*). No MutH gene equivalent has been discovered. In humans, MutS and MutL presumably directly activate exonucleases without the need for a MutH gene.

Unlike single cell MMR genes that function as a homodimer, human MMR genes function as a heteroduplex (Figure 38-1). MSH2 acts as a "scout" and identifies the mismatches in the new DNA strand. It then complexes with MSH6 to form the MutSα complex that identifies single nucleotide misrepairs. Alternatively, MSH2 can complex with hMSH3 forming MutSβ complex that repairs IDL with up to 10 base pairs.

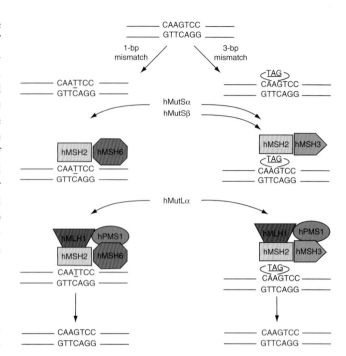

FIGURE 38-1. The DNA MMR system can correct either single base-pair mismatches or larger loops of mismatched DNA. hMSH2 serves as the "scout" that recognizes mismatched DNA. It forms a complex with either hMSH6 or hMSH3, depending on the number of mismatched nucleotides. A second heterodimeric complex (hMLH1/hPMSI) is then recruited to excise the mispaired nucleotides. hMUTSα = hMSH2/hMSH6; hMuTSβ = hMSH2/hMSH3; hMutLα = hMLH1/hPMS1. bp = base pair. (Reprinted with permission from Chung and Rustgi.[29])

These pathways are not mutually exclusive as MutSα can recognize 2–4 base IDL, but there is less affinity. Likewise, MutSβ can recognize single base pair insertions and deletions. Both MSH3 and MSH6 must be abnormal to have complete loss of hMSH2-dependent MMR.[12]

MLH1 and PMS2 bind to form a second heteroduplex that interacts with the MutS duplex, stimulating excision and resynthesis. The exact mechanism of action of the human MutL MMR genes is not known. The most frequently mutated genes in HNPCC are *MLH1* (33%) and *MLH2* (31%) and rarely *PMS2* or *PMS1*.[13] Of the mutations identified, 90% occurred in *MLH1* and *MSH2*.[14] Recently, a metaanalysis of index families fulfilling the Amsterdam criteria, worldwide, revealed that a mutation in *MLH1* is found in 25.5%–29.6% of families, and *MSH2* is found in 14.8%–21.6% of families. In general, the overall mutation discovery rate is less than 50%.[14]

MutS has two functions—mismatch recognition and ATPase activity. Both functions are essential for repair in 7 of 8 possible single-base mismatches. The C:C misrepair is not recognized, but fortunately occurs least frequently.[10] It is generally agreed that mismatched DNA stimulates ATP hydrolysis as part of the repair mechanism, but there is disagreement as to the role this has in MMR gene function. It is agreed that the MutS with adenosine 5′-diphosphate (ADP) has the highest affinity for the mismatch.

In the translocation model, ATP enables MutSα or β to move like a motor protein away from the mismatch. This allows formation of an α loop similar to that described in the *E. coli* model. When the MutS ADP is attracted to the MMR, it is converted to MutS ATP, which has reduced affinity for the mismatch and activates the binding sites for translocation along the newly synthesized DNA. This draws flanking DNA toward the mismatch, causing it to form into an α loop.[15]

The molecular switch theory proposes that this transposition from ADP to ATP in the MutS gene switches the repair complex on and off. MutS ADP has a high affinity for the misrepaired gene and then it binds to it. When this occurs, ADP is transformed to ATP and causes a conformational change in the MutS complex. A clamp is formed around the mismatched DNA. Several of these clamps surround the misrepair and signal either a repair process or induce apoptosis via a P53 independent pathway. When ATP is hydrolyzed to ADP, the clamp is switched off and is released from the DNA strand. The MutS complex is now recycled and can recognize a new mismatch. The ATP hydrolysis in this model turns the MMR switch off and on but is not intrinsically involved in the actual repair.[16]

The third theory is called "transactivation." MutS binds both ATP and the mismatch DNA simultaneously in order to activate MMR. The ATPase in this model functions as a proofreader and binds only to heteroduplex DNA. Once the mismatch and the ATP are bound, it is believed that a signal is produced to authorize DNA repair.[17]

Genes Implicated in HNPCC Carcinogenesis

When MMR genes are dysfunctional, the myriad genes that have microsatellites in their coding region can become inactivated, causing acceleration of tumorigenesis. Transforming growth factor beta Type II receptor gene (*TGFβRII*) has a 10 adenine-repeating tract in its coding area. *TGFβRII* was found to be mutated in 70%–90% of cancers with MSI.[18,19] *TGFβRII* acts as a tumor suppressor gene and is a strong inhibitor of epithelial growth. Insulin-like growth factor II receptor gene (*IGFRII*) binds insulin-like growth factor I, thus antagonizing its growth stimulating effects. IGFRII also activates TGFβI from its latent to active form. There is a long 8 repeat guanine tract in *IGFRII*. In 90% of tumors studied, either *TGFRII* or *IGFRII* was abnormal but not both. This suggests that the genes are part of the same tumorigenesis pathway.[20]

The *BAX* gene is another gene found to be mutated in up to 54% of MSI-H colorectal tumors.[19] It is involved in apoptosis and is a downstream gene often activated by the P53 gene. It is of note that MSI-H tumors have wild-type *P53*. In the coding region of the *BAX* gene, there is an 8 guanine repeating tract spanning codons 38–41 that is highly susceptible to frameshift mutations.[21] Other genes with microsatellites in the coding region are *MSH3*, *MSH6*, *TCF4*, *BLM* (19), *Capase-5*,[22] and the *PTEN* gene and *APC*.[23]

Because only 50% of HNPCC tumors have mutations in known MMR genes, a search for other unique gene pathways that could affect DNA repair is ongoing. *RAF* oncogenes are a family of genes that encode kinases and mediate cellular responses to growth signals. *BRAF* is a *RAF* gene that is common in MMR-deficient tumors and in colorectal tumors that have a normal *KRAS* gene. Both BRAF and KRAS mutations are found in all stages of colon cancer and in adenomas greater than 1 cm.[24] Another DNA repair gene is *MED1* that has endonuclease activity and could function as a MutH gene. It has four hypermutable tracts of adenine repeats. *MED1* alteration may contribute to progressive MSI as part of "mutators mutation" phenomena.[25]

Pathologic Features

There are unique pathologic features associated with the mutator phenotype of HNPCC. Cancers are often mucinous or poorly differentiated with signet ring cells.[26] Despite what appears to be unfavorable histology, the incidence of lymph nodes is 35% compared with 65% in sporadic colon cancer.[27] In 9% of patients, there is an extensive peritumoral lymphocytic infiltration that may be the result of an enhanced immunologic response (Figure 38-2A). Others have described a Crohn's-like lymphocytic reaction with the accumulation of both B and T lymphocytes around the tumor (Figure 38-2B).[28] Flow cytometry showed most HNPCC tumors to be diploid. Because HNPCC cancers have small unstable tracts, large chromosomes are not lost. This is in contradistinction to the frequent aneuploidy of sporadic colon cancer where tumorigenesis is related to the LOH.[29]

Clinical Features of HNPCC

Affected individuals in HNPCC have an increased risk of colon cancer and other extracolonic cancers as demonstrated in Table 38-1. Colon cancer is the most frequently diagnosed cancer in HNPCC (80%) and endometrial cancer is the most frequent extracolonic cancer (50%–60%).[29] Colorectal cancers in HNPCC are proximal to the splenic flexure (68% in HNPCC versus 49% of sporadic cancers), are more likely to have associated synchronous cancers (7% HNPCC versus 1% sporadic colon cancer), and will have increased metachronous cancers at 10 years (29% HNPCC versus 5% sporadic cancers).[30] Similarly, women with HNPCC-related endometrial cancer have a 75% risk of a second cancer during a 26-year follow-up. The median age of onset of colon cancer is 42 years and for endometrial cancer it is 49 years.[31]

Despite being termed hereditary nonpolyposis colon cancer, a polyp is still the precursor lesion for a colorectal cancer. The phenotype is not the extensive polyposis as seen in familial

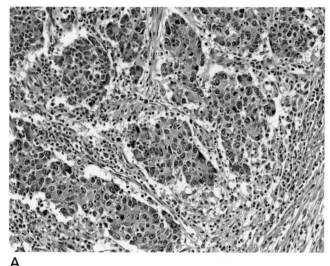

A

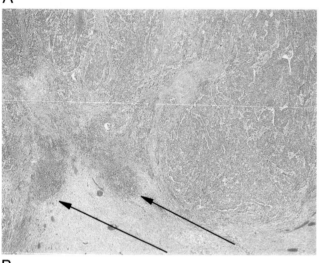

B

FIGURE 38-2. **A** Medullary carcinoma type pattern with peritumoral lymphocytic infiltrate. **B** MSI-H cancer with marked peritumoral lymphocytic infiltrate (Crohn's-like reaction), × 20 magnification. (Courtesy of Robert E. Petras, MD, National Director Gastrointestinal Pathology Services, Ameripath Inc., Oakwood Village, OH and Associate Professor of Pathology, Northeastern Ohio University College of Medicine).

adenomatous polyposis (FAP). In a Danish surveillance study, 70% of mutation carriers developed adenoma by age 60 as opposed to 37% in the control group. The adenomas in the mutation carrier group were larger and had a higher proportion of villous components and high-grade dysplasia. Adenomas were located in the proximal colon and 70% of the polyps had absent MMR genes on immunohistochemistry.[32] One cancer is prevented for every 2.8 polyps removed in HNPCC patients[33] compared with one cancer being removed for every 41–119 polypectomies in the general population.[34] It is estimated that malignant transformation occurs in 3 years in HNPCC as opposed to 10 years in sporadic colon cancer.

TABLE 38-1. Lifetime risks for cancer associated with the hereditary nonpolyposis colorectal cancer syndrome

Type of cancer	Persons with HNPCC	General population
Colorectal	80–82	5–6
Endometrial	50–60	2–3
Gastric	13	1
Ovarian	12	1–2
Small bowel	1–4	0.01
Bladder	4	1–3
Brain	4	0.6
Kidney, renal, pelvis	3	1
Biliary tract	2	0.6

Source: Reprinted with permission from Chung and Rustgi.[29]

In other studies, HNPCC polyps are found throughout the colon and not necessarily clustered near the proximal colon where the predominance of cancers are seen.[35]

Two other types of polyps—the flat adenoma and serrated adenoma—have been implicated as possible precursors of the HNPCC cancers. Flat adenomas are found proximally in up to 50% of HNPCC patients[36] (Figure 38-3A and B). Approximately 20% of flat adenomas will be MSI-H and will also have a mutation in the *TGFβRII* gene.[36] These polyps are difficult to detect during colonoscopy without dye spray techniques (e.g., methylene blue). Furthermore, flat adenomas with advanced histology (high-grade dysplasia or cancer) are significantly smaller (10.75 mm) than comparable polypoid lesions (20 mm).[37] It has been proposed that hyperplastic polyps, serrated adenomas, and serrated adenocarcinomas form a morphologic continuum. Carcinomas associated with serrated adenomas have a predilection for the cecum and the rectum and are often mucinous in nature. MSI is found in 37% of the cases.[38]

Genotype–Phenotype Relationships

There are very few studies that evaluate phenotype–genotype correlations. One study of 35 families found the *MSH2* mutation to be associated with a late age onset of rectal cancer and more extracolonic cancers than in the *MLH1* mutation-positive group.[39] Mutations in MSH2 were associated with an increased risk of rare extracolonic cancers in another study.[40] Amsterdam-positive families with known mutations were compared with Amsterdam-positive families without a known mutation. The subgroup without mutations had an increased risk of rectal cancer, fewer HNPCC-related cancers, a lower frequency of multiple colorectal cancers, and a later age of onset.[41]

The Muir-Torre syndrome is characterized by sebaceous adenomas, sebaceous carcinomas, and keratoacanthomas associated with multiple visceral tumors. Colorectal cancers are most frequently found (51%) and are often proximal to the splenic flexure (60%). Although only 25% of Muir-Torre patients develop a polyp, 90% of patients who develop polyps

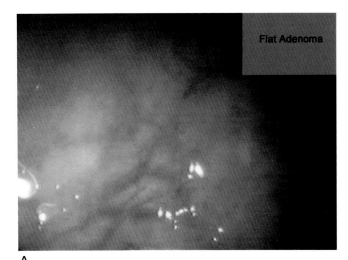

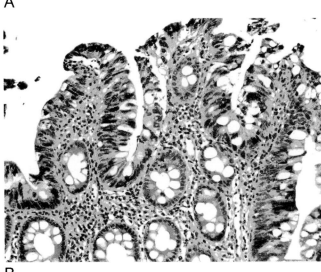

FIGURE 38-3. **A** Colonoscopic view of a flat adenoma in the cecum that could easily be overlooked. Such polyps are more easily seen using dye-spraying techniques. **B** Microscopic view of same polyp after endoscopic removal, showing severe dysplasia, ×100 magnification. (Courtesy of Dr. Robert E. Petras, MD, National Director Gastrointestinal Pathology Services, Ameripath Inc., Oakwood Village, OH and Associate Professor of Pathology, Northeastern Ohio University College of Medicine).

will develop colon cancer. The second most frequent tumors are genitourinary (24%).[42]

Germline mutations in *MLH1*[43] and *MSH2*[39] have been identified. As expected, many of the tumors exhibit MSI. The visceral tumors are often low grade, and prolonged survival in the presence of metastatic disease has been reported. The median age of diagnosis is 55 years and only 60% will have a positive family history.[42] Aggressive screening and surveillance for colorectal and genitourinary cancers as recommended for HNPCC are warranted.

MUTSα (a heterodimer of MSH6 and MSH2) senses and repairs single base mismatches. In a study of 91 familial non-HNPCC patients, six patients (7.0%) were found to have *MSH6* mutations but none were found in 58 HNPCC patients. These tumors were microsatellite low (MSI-L), had a median onset of 61 years, and did not fulfill classic Amsterdam criteria.[44] Other studies of 90 mutation-negative HNPCC families and HNPCC-like families found only one *MSH6* mutation.[45]

Despite this discrepancy, the International Collaborative Group has collected more than 30 potentially pathogenic *MSH6* mutations. Thirty-five percent of these mutations involve only one amino acid.[46] *MSH6* is the third most frequently affected gene in HNPCC. Because MutSβ (heterodimer of MSH2 and MLH1) can act redundantly to repair single base mismatches, and insertion–deletions of large dinucleotide sequences is intact, there are less frame shifts. This results in less loss of function in affected genes. A weaker phenotype occurs with slower tumorigenesis and cancers that are MSI-L.[45] *MSH6* knockout mice display an MSI-L phenotype and the majority of tumors in mice are endometrial or cutaneous with few intestinal cancers.[47]

Colorectal cancers are more frequently left-sided in *MSH6* carriers.[48] The risk of endometrial cancer is increased over *MSH2* or *MLH1* carriers (76% versus 30%) and colon cancer is decreased (32% versus 80%). The median age of onset is 55 years.[49] Therefore, a distinct phenotype has emerged, characterized by a clustering of endometrial cancer, a decreased frequency of colorectal cancer, later age of onset, and MSI-L cancers. Some *MSH6* cancers are MSI-H. Combined MSI testing and immunohistochemistry, as well as a distinct phenotype, are used to select families for *MSH6* mutation analysis.[49]

Diagnosis

The key to the diagnosis of HNPCC is a detailed family history and subsequent construction of a family pedigree. Amsterdam criteria (Table 38-2) were created to define clinical criteria to identify patients with a high probability of

TABLE 38-2. Amsterdam criteria

Amsterdam criteria
- At least three family members with colorectal cancer, one of whom is first-degree relative of the other two.
- At least two generations with colorectal cancer.
- At least one individual <50 y at diagnosis of colorectal cancer.

Amsterdam criteria II
- At least three family members with HNPCC-related cancer, one of whom is first-degree relative of the other two.
- At least two generations with HNPCC-related cancer.
- At least one individual <50 y at diagnosis of HNPCC-related cancer.

Modified Amsterdam criteria
- Two first-degree relatives with colorectal cancer involving two generations.
- At least one case diagnosed before 55 y *or*
- Two first-degree relatives with colorectal cancer and a third relative with endometrial cancer or another HNPCC-related cancer.

Source: Modified with permission from Chung and Rustgi.[29]

having an inheritable form of colon cancer not associated with diffuse polyposis. For day-to-day clinical purposes, the original definition was too restrictive because it did not account for the extracolonic malignancies associated with HNPCC, the decrease in the average family size, the late onset variants of HNPCC, and the problems with incomplete data recovery. Modifications of the Amsterdam criteria have occurred and are known as Amsterdam II and modified Amsterdam criteria (Table 38-2). A National Cancer Institute workshop on HNPCC was held in 1996. Out of this meeting, a broader, less-specific set of guidelines was introduced (Table 38-3).[50] These criteria, known as the Bethesda criteria, were formulated to increase sensitivity at the expense of specificity and focused on individual patients. Because MSI status is linked to HNPCC and the clinical criteria were broadened, MSI testing of this population can define a subpopulation for genetic testing.

It is important to remember that HNPCC is a clinical diagnosis and genetic testing cannot prove a family does *not* have HNPCC. Gene testing can potentially decrease the cost and morbidity of screening and surveillance, help with surgical decisions, stratify patients for chemoprevention, and help patients cope with job and family planning.

Table 38-4 compares the sensitivity and specificity of several of the clinical criteria for identifying a pathologic mutation. This table is derived from a cohort of 70 families. Only 18 families had a mutation found and six of these were inconclusive.[51]

Genetic Testing

Gene sequencing of *MSH2* and *MLH1* is now commercially available. This testing may not be covered by insurance companies and the cost is approximately $1750. Furthermore, interpretation of gene testing is complicated because mutations are spread diffusely throughout MSH2 and MLH1. Mutations themselves are a broad spectrum of truncating, frameshift, and missense mutations. A missense mutation results in the substitution of a single amino acid, and the effect on protein function may be negligible. This type of missense mutation is often reported as a mutation of unknown significance. Approximately 31% of *MLH1* mutations are this

TABLE 38-4. Direct mutation finding (n = 70)

Category	Sensitivity (%)	Specificity (%)
Amsterdam [n = 28]	61	67
Amsterdam II [n = 34]	78	61
Bethesda [n = 56]	94	25
Bethesda (1–3) [n = 44]	94	49

Source: Adapted and reproduced from Syngal et al.,[51] with permission from the BMJ Publishing Group.

type.[52] Missense mutations must meet strict criteria to be considered pathologic: Is the amino acid change conserved across species? What is the mutation population frequency? Does the mutation segregate with cancer in kindreds? Finally, does the alteration affect gene function? A data bank of known mutations is kept by the International Collaborative Group of HNPCC now known as InSiGHT.

Only half of well-characterized HNPCC families have a mutation identified. This suggests that there are other unknown MMR genes or that current techniques are lacking in sensitivity. Before genes are sequenced, they are amplified by polymerase chain reaction (PCR) and both alleles are sequenced simultaneously. A wild-type allele may mask a very short mutated allele. A technique called conversion has been used to detect these hidden mutations. Patient mononuclear cells are fused with a specially designed rodent cell line. One quarter of the hybrids contain a single copy of the human genes, thus the human gene is now haploid and can be analyzed and characterized.[53] In a series of 10 suspected HNPCC families, no mutations were found on initial gene sequencing, but a mutation was found in all 10 when the conversion technique was used.[54]

Once criteria to identify HNPCC families had been broadened, direct gene testing by sequencing was less effective (Table 38-4). Two techniques that are more cost effective—MSI testing and immunohistochemistry—are performed before gene sequencing if the strict Amsterdam criteria or the Bethesda 1–3 criteria are not fulfilled. MSI testing is done on tissue. An international workshop was held and five validated microsatellite markers were selected to ensure uniformity of diagnosis between different laboratories. These microsatellite loci include two polyadenine sequences (BAT25 and BAT26) and three dinucleotide repeat sequences (D2S123, D5S346, D17S250).[55] Microsatellite testing can be done on fresh tissue or paraffin blocks. A typical test for MSI is seen in Figure 38-4. If none of the markers are unstable, the tumor is called microsatellite stable (MSS). When only one marker is unstable, this is termed MSI low (MSI-L), and microsatellite high (MSI-H) will have two or more markers positive. When a tumor is MSI-H, then gene sequencing of *MSH2* or *MLH1* can be performed. The cost of MSI testing is $700.

Immunohistochemistry is a technique using antibodies to MSH2 and MLH1. This is a standard laboratory procedure (Figures 38-5 and 38-6) to identify which MMR gene is abnormal so that only one MMR gene needs to be sequenced.

TABLE 38-3. Modified Bethesda guidelines

Amsterdam criteria
- Patient with two HNPCC-related tumors.
- Patient with colorectal cancer with first-degree relative with HNPCC-related cancer; one of the cancers at <50 y or adenoma at <40 y.
- Patient with colorectal cancer or endometrial cancer at <50 y.
- Patient with right-sided, undifferentiated colorectal cancer at <50 y.
- Patient with signet ring colorectal cancer at <50 y.
- Patient with adenoma at <40 y.

Source: Modified from Rodriguez-Bigas et al.,[50] with permission from Oxford University Press.

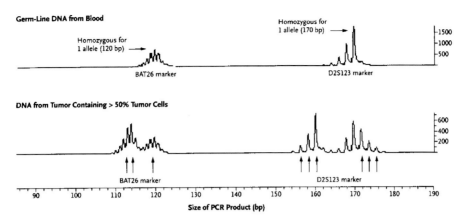

FIGURE 38-4. Detection of MSI with the use of fluorescent labeling of PCR products analyzed in an automatic sequencer. Two markers are analyzed in the same track: the mononucleotide repeat marker BAT26 is shown on the left, and the dinucleotide marker D2S123 is shown on the right. The upper tracking is from germline DNA from blood. The lower tracing is from DNA extracted from a histologic section of a tumor containing more than 50% tumor cells. For marker BAT26, germline DNA shows a single peak, indicating that the patient is homozygous for this marker (arrow). Tumor DNA shows, in addition to the normal allele (single arrow), a new allele (double arrows) that has lost approximately five nucleotides. This constitutes microsatellite stability. For marker D2S123, germline DNA is homozygous, whereas tumor DNA shows two new alleles (triple arrows), one with a loss of approximately 10 nucleotides (left) and one with a gain of two nucleotides (right). Thus, the tumor shows MSI with both markers. All peaks display "stutter"—that is, small amounts of material with a gain or a loss of one or a few nucleotides. This is a normal phenomenon. (Reprinted with permission from Lynch HT, De la Chapelle A. Hereditary colorectal cancer. N Engl J Med 2003;348:919–932. Copyright © 2003 Massachusetts Medicine Society. All rights reserved).

If immunohistochemistry reveals that one gene is absent, this is presumptive evidence that the patient probably has HNPCC. Recently, 28 families with a known *MSH2* or *MLH1* mutation were studied. The MSI panel identified all families as being MSI-H, but in five cases a mutant protein was expressed that could be detected by immunohistochemistry thereby producing a false test.[56]

A cost analysis has been performed on four different gene testing strategies: 1) gene sequencing for Amsterdam-positive individuals ("Amsterdam" strategy); 2) tumor MSI analysis of individuals who meet less stringent modified clinical criteria

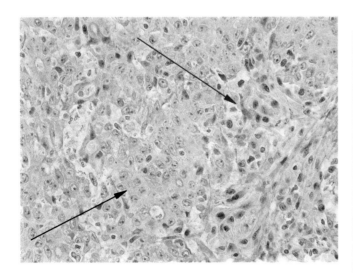

FIGURE 38-5. hMLH1 immunohistochemistry. Blue arrow indicates positive nuclear staining for the presence of hMLH1 protein within an inflammatory cell. Black arrow demonstrates the absence of protein within cancer cells, × 400 magnification. (Courtesy of Robert E. Petras, MD, National Director Gastrointestinal Pathology Services, Ameripath Inc., Oakwood Village, OH and Associate Professor of Pathology, Northeastern Ohio University College of Medicine).

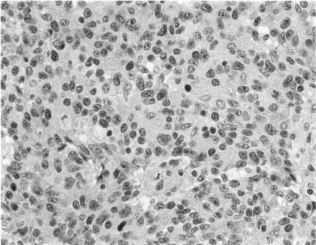

FIGURE 38-6. hMSH2 immunohistochemistry. Positive nuclear staining demonstrates the normal presence of hMSH2 protein, × 400 magnification. (Courtesy of Robert E. Petras, MD, National Director Gastrointestinal Pathology Services, Ameripath Inc., Oakwood Village, OH and Associate Professor of Pathology, Northeastern Ohio University College of Medicine).

and germline mutation of individuals with MSI-H tumors ("modified" strategy); 3) MSI testing of all colorectal cancers and germline analysis of individuals with MSI-H tumors ("test-all" strategy); and 4) germline mutation analysis of individuals who satisfy the Amsterdam criteria and tumor MSI analysis of the remaining individuals who meet less stringent criteria ("mixed" strategy). The least expensive strategy was the Amsterdam only strategy, but only 10% of mutations were identified. The modified and mixed strategies identified 60% and 75% of the mutations, respectively. These strategies were $400.00 less expensive than the test-all strategy in the model. Only seven mutations were missed by the mixed strategy per 1000 colorectal cancers. The cost for finding each of these seven extra mutations in the test-all strategy was $51,000 per mutation.[57] Currently, a mixed strategy seems most appropriate. MSI testing of all colorectal cancers may become standard in the future because of its potential relationship to increased survival and response to chemotherapy. This would make testing all colorectal cancers the best medical practice.

Before genetic testing in HNPCC is done, informed consent must be obtained. Testing should begin with an affected individual (an HNPCC cancer has been diagnosed). It is best to choose a proband with the earliest age of onset of cancer. For a patient who meets the Amsterdam II criteria or the first three Bethesda criteria, it is reasonable to proceed to germline testing. When the clinical risk is lower, MSI testing or immunohistochemistry should be performed first. If the tumor stains positive for MSH2 and MLH1 or is MSS or MSI-L, no further genetic testing is performed. However, if the tumor is MSI-H, or there is absent staining on immunohistochemistry for MLH1 or MSH2, then gene sequencing is performed. Note that only 50% of Amsterdam families have an MMR mutation on gene sequencing, and that HNPCC is a clinical diagnosis, *not* a genetic diagnosis. Further genetic testing can be performed in a research setting when mutations in *MSH2* and *MLH1* are not found. Conversion testing as previously described can be performed as well as testing for *hMSH6* (especially in MSI-L patients or when there are late onset HNPCC pedigrees).

Because of the high number of missense mutations in HNPCC, the gene-sequencing test may be reported as a mutation of unknown variance. This is a non-informative test. When the proband has a negative or a non-informative test, no further gene testing in the at-risk family members is possible. All family members require intensive surveillance. When the proband has a positive mutation, the family members that test positive are carriers of the abnormal gene and need extensive surveillance and/or prophylactic surgery. However, when the proband's test is positive and the at-risk family members are mutation negative, these family members are not carriers of an MMR gene. Their colon cancer risk is that of the general population. They should be screened accordingly. The cost of screening family members for a known mutation is $300.

There are also a number of ethical considerations regarding the ordering of genetic testing with respect to insurance discrimination. Currently, nearly all states have passed legislation prohibiting genetic discrimination in health insurance; however, only "asymptomatic" individuals are protected by such legislation.[58,59]

Registries

Once a diagnosis of HNPCC is suspected, a referral to a registry for inherited colorectal cancer or to a cancer center with a high-risk clinic is important. A registry has a database or list of families and their members who have a high frequency of colorectal cancer. Personnel at the registry consist of a coordinator, oftentimes a genetic counselor, and a physician director. The whole focus of the registry is patient care, education of patients, families, and referring physicians, and promotion of collaborative research. No single physician has the time to educate high-risk individuals about autosomal dominant inheritance and the cancer risk of inherited colorectal cancers; to gather factual medical data about widely dispersed family members and construct a pedigree; to give counsel about the risks and benefits of gene testing; to perform gene testing and carefully and confidentially explain the results; and finally to coordinate treatment and life-long surveillance. Registry personnel provide further support for myriad problems such as family stress, health insurance difficulties, and job discrimination. A local registry can be found by accessing the Collaborative Group of the Americas on Inherited Colorectal Cancer at http://www.cgaicc.com. To emphasize the need for expert counseling and care, a study of 177 patients undergoing genetic testing for FAP was performed. Of those patients, only 18% received pretest counseling, 16% gave a written consent, and a full 30% were given incorrect test interpretation.[60]

Surveillance

In 1997, a number of medical societies proposed uniform screening criteria for colorectal cancer, proposing separate criteria for average- and high-risk patient groups. Patients with HNPCC or a family history thereof constitute one of these high-risk groups. Because of the 80% lifetime risk of developing colorectal cancer, the American Cancer Society recommends colonoscopy every 2 years beginning at age 21, and annual colonoscopy recommended beginning at age 40.[61] Because cancers in HNPCC can occur at very young ages and develop within 2 years of a negative colonoscopy,[62] it is important to stress to patients that if they have symptoms, they should be checked regardless of their age and even if they have had a recent negative colonoscopy. Colonic neoplasia in individuals with HNPCC seems to develop more rapidly than in average-risk nonaffected individuals.[63] For this reason, many, including the authors, believe that colonoscopy in these individuals should be performed annually rather than every

2 years, even in young individuals. Adenomas in HNPCC patients occur earlier and are more likely to be villous.[64]

The value of screening colonoscopy in HNPCC was demonstrated by Jarvinen and colleagues[65] who studied a group of 252 individuals belonging to 22 HNPCC families. Of these, 137 participated in screening colonoscopy every 3 years, whereas the remainder refused such evaluation. Colorectal cancer developed in 8% of the screened family members, compared with 16% of those who refused screening. In those individuals who were known to have a DNA MMR gene mutation, the rate of colorectal cancer in those who underwent screening was 18% compared with 41% in those who did not undergo screening. All cancers that developed in the screened group were either Dukes' A or B lesions, with no attributable deaths, compared with more advanced lesions in the unscreened group and nine deaths attributed to cancer (8%). Jarvinen and colleagues demonstrated that colonoscopic screening at 3 yearly intervals in HNPCC family members not only reduced the risk of colorectal cancer by half but prevented deaths caused by colorectal cancer and reduced the mortality by two-thirds. Similarly, the study by Rekonen-Sinislao and associates[66] also demonstrated an earlier cancer stage at diagnosis and better 10-year survival in those individuals in whom colorectal cancer was detected during a colonoscopic screening examination compared with those in whom diagnosis was made based on symptoms.

Because of the high risk of endometrial cancer in women, annual transvaginal ultrasound to examine the endometrium, preferably with endometrial aspiration, is recommended beginning between ages 25 and 35 years because the increased risk for gynecologic cancer in these patients begins at age 25.[67,68] There are no data demonstrating the efficacy of this type of screening. One recent study has even shown such screening not to be effective.[69,70] It is important to note that, should a patient from an HNPCC family be diagnosed with endometrial cancer, they should undergo surveillance colonoscopy before hysterectomy in the event that colonic pathology is present and colonic resection is required at the same surgery.

Treatment

As with other colorectal conditions, there is not one operation that suits all patients. The majority of patients with a diagnosis of HNPCC, based on the finding of an existing colorectal cancer or an advanced adenoma, will be offered colectomy and ileorectal anastomosis (IRA). This is thought to be the operation of choice, which removes the "at risk" organ, reduces cancer risk, preserves anal sphincter function, and retains the reservoir capacity of the rectum. This operation eliminates the need for annual surveillance colonoscopy, because only rigid or fiberoptic examination of the rectum is required. The estimated risk of rectal cancer after colectomy

and IRA is, however, 12% at 12 years.[71] This operation is clearly not suited for those who will not be compliant with follow-up examinations. Colectomy and IRA may not be the ideal operation for the patient with impaired anal sphincter function because of either obstetric injury or age or for patients with decreased mobility. The operation also is not suited for patients with more than three bowel movements per day, because these individuals will frequently have significant diarrhea and poor functional results after colectomy. In some patients, a lesser resection may be in order as a result of any of these reasons. It is however *essential* that both the patient and physician recognize the need for ongoing annual colonoscopy, because the risk for a metachronous colon cancer in HNPCC is 45%.[72] *Conversely*, in the very young patient with a long projected life expectancy or in the patient who is not likely to be compliant with follow-up examinations, total colectomy with stapled ileal pouch anal anastomosis may be the preferred procedure, because it removes nearly all of the at-risk colorectal mucosa.

In cases of rectal cancer not involving the sphincters, either an anterior resection, coloanal anastomosis or colectomy and ileal pouch anal anastomosis can be considered. In the event that the latter option is chosen, preoperative endorectal ultrasound staging is desirable. In cases of a uT2 or uT3 or possible uN1 cancers, preoperative chemoradiation should be given whenever possible, because ileal pouches tolerate radiation poorly.

In women undergoing colectomy, strong consideration should be given to performing a hysterectomy and bilateral salpingo-oophorectomy in the patient who has completed childbearing, because of the increased risk of both endometrial and ovarian carcinoma.

There is controversy as to whether surgical treatment or continued surveillance should be offered to the asymptomatic patient who has a mutation identified by genetic testing, but an as yet "normal" colon. Several studies have examined this question using decision analysis methods; however, factors such as patient compliance must be taken into account.[73,74]

Prognosis

The survival rate in HNPCC patients with colorectal cancer is better than that of patients with sporadic colorectal cancer when matched for stage and age of onset.[75,76] There is some question of whether or not patients with Stage II or III microsatellite unstable colorectal cancers benefit from 5-fluorouracil-based adjuvant therapy. Whereas some studies report that patients with microsatellite unstable tumors do not benefit from such therapy, other studies suggest a benefit.[77,78] One possible explanation for the differences in such studies could be attributable to different underlying causes of this MSI (e.g., *MLH1* gene-promoter methylation in some patients with sporadic colorectal cancer). Although germline mutations are involved in HNPCC, other mechanisms such as somatic mutations and the loss of heterozygosity of mismatch-repair genes may be involved in microsatellite unstable tumors.[79]

Chemoprevention

Currently, there is much interest in chemoprevention. Whereas data exist regarding the efficacy of nonsteroidal antiinflammatory drugs (NSAIDs) in reducing the risk of colorectal cancer in the general population, such data are lacking for HNPCC.[80,81] Currently, NSAIDs and novelose undigested starch are being studied in HNPCC. The CAPP II trial is a controlled, randomized trial of colorectal polyp and cancer prevention using aspirin and resistant starch in carriers of HNPCC. It is a Phase II multicenter study with a multifactorial design, being performed at 33 centers. Patients are randomized to active agent or placebo, the active agents consisting of 600 mg of aspirin and 30 g of resistant starch for 2–4 years.[82] The accrual goal is 1000 HNPCC gene carriers. This study, which began in January 1999 and is projected to end in December 2006, is designed to detect differences in adenoma incidence.[69,82]

Calcium and vitamin D intake have been associated with a decreased risk of sporadic colorectal cancer.[83] Supplemental dietary calcium is thought to inhibit the proliferative effect of bile acids and fatty acids on the colonic mucosa by precipitating these luminal surfactants.[84] A trial of supplemental calcium in HNPCC families did not demonstrate a decrease in epithelial proliferation, although the sample size was small and the study was conducted before genetic testing was available.[69,85]

Conclusion

Our knowledge about HNPCC continues to grow. This disorder is associated with a germline mutation in one of several MMR genes. Genetic testing is currently available for mutations in genes *hMLH1* and *hMHS2*. Suspicion of this disorder in a given patient is raised by a family history of early age onset cancer, an increased number of first-degree relatives with colorectal cancer, or an HNPCC-related cancer. Endometrial cancer is the most common extracolonic cancer. Although there is debate regarding the frequency and beginning of screening, most clinicians believe that colonic examinations yearly or every 2 years should be performed beginning in patients in their early 20s. Prophylactic colectomy may be offered to known mutation carriers as well as members of at-risk families who develop advanced adenomas. Removal of all of the colon and IRA or colectomy and IPAA are the operations of choice, because they remove most "at-risk" colonic mucosa. In the event of the former, continued surveillance of the rectum is mandatory. With careful surveillance and management, colorectal cancer can be prevented in these patients and the mortality rate decreased. In those who develop colorectal carcinoma, the overall survival rate is more favorable than that of patients with sporadic colorectal cancer.

Appendix I: Practice Parameters for the Identification and Testing of Patients at Risk for Dominantly Inherited Colorectal Cancer

Prepared by The Standards Task Force, The American Society of Colon and Rectal Surgeons, The Collaborative Group of the Americas on Inherited Colorectal Cancer
–Take a family history. This is the first step in recognizing families possibly affected by inherited colorectal cancer.
–Document a suspicious pedigree; a family tree based on the recollection of family members is not solid enough evidence. Request medical records to confirm diagnosis.
–Identify criteria for genetic testing. FAP is easily recognized clinically when patients present with more than 100 colorectal adenomas. Fewer adenomas are needed for a diagnosis when a patient is part of an established kindred. The Amsterdam criteria are a way of clinically identifying families with hereditary nonpolyposis colorectal cancer, where an MMR gene mutation can be detected.
–Testing for MSI in tumors is a screen for families with hereditary nonpolyposis colorectal cancer where the clinical pattern of the disease is suggestive but not strong enough to fulfill Amsterdam criteria.
–Offer surveillance to families not meeting the above criteria for genetic testing. Families with more than two first-degree relatives affected with colorectal cancer, especially if one is affected at a young age (<45 years), need to be offered endoscopic surveillance even if genetic testing is not indicated.
–Adhere to all protocols for genetic testing. Institutional review board approval, informed consent, and pretest and posttest counseling are the key elements of genetic testing for inherited colorectal cancer.
Summary: It is hoped that these guidelines will assist in the recognition and management of patients affected by syndromes of inherited colorectal cancer.

Reprinted from Dis Colon Rectum 2001;44(10):1403–1412. Copyright © 2001. All rights reserved. American Society of Colon and Rectal Surgeons.

Appendix II: Practice Parameters for the Treatment of Patients with Dominantly Inherited Colorectal Cancer (FAP and Hereditary Nonpolyposis Colorectal Cancer)

Prepared by The Standards Task Force, The American Society of Colon and Rectal Surgeons
James Church, MD; Clifford Simmang, MD; on behalf of the Collaborative Group of the Americas on Inherited Colorectal Cancer and the Standards Committee of The American Society of Colon and Rectal Surgeons.

Section 1. Familial Adenomatous Polyposis

Guideline 1: Treatment Must Be Preceded by Thorough Counseling about the Nature of the Syndrome, Its Natural History, Its Extracolonic Manifestations, and the Need for Compliance with Recommendations for Management and Surveillance; Level of Evidence: III

Dominantly inherited colorectal cancer syndromes show a striking pattern of cancer in affected families. This is because of the high penetrance (penetrance = percent of patients with the mutation who have the disease) and often-severe expression (expression = clinical consequences of the mutation) of the mutations involved. FAP has a penetrance of close to 100%, colorectal cancer occurs at an average age of 39 years, and every affected patient is guaranteed at least one major abdominal surgery. Despite these calamitous prospects, families with FAP adapt well to their disease. Most patients are compliant with recommended treatments, take a keen interest in the syndrome, and have an active role in encouraging relatives to undergo screening. However, when a relative has a bad outcome, either because of severe disease or complications of treatment, family psychology may be affected. Noncompliance, denial, or a refusal to accept recommendations may ensue. The best way of avoiding both bad outcomes and an unfortunate response to them is to provide comprehensive, integrated counseling, support, and clinical services. These sorts of services are best provided through a department, registry, or center with personnel who have experience in managing patients and families with these syndromes.

Guideline 2: Prophylactic Colectomy or Proctocolectomy Is Routine. The Timing and Type of Surgery Depend on the Severity of the Polyposis Phenotype and to a Lesser Extent on the Genotype, Age, and Clinical and Social Circumstances of the Patient; Level of Evidence: III

The recommendation for prophylactic colectomy or proctocolectomy in FAP is based on the very high rates of colorectal cancer seen in patients who are not screened. In unscreened patients, the incidence of cancer is more than 60%. Appropriate screening and timely surgery can minimize this. The risk of cancer is not uniform, however, and is related to the severity of the colonic polyposis. Debinski and coworkers showed the rate of cancer for patients with >1000 colonic polyps was twice that of patients with <1000 colonic polyps. In its turn, the severity of the colorectal polyposis is often related to the site of the APC mutation in a family. The "hot spot" mutation at codon 1309 is in an area of the gene where mutations always cause severe disease. Mutations in codons 3 and 4 are classically associated with attenuated FAP whereas mutations in the part of codon 15 that is 3′ of codon 1450 are usually associated with mild colorectal disease. Mutations in exons 5–15E have a variable colorectal phenotype, where some family members have relatively mild disease and others severe. The important aspects of surgery to consider are its timing, its type, and the technical options to be used.

Timing of Surgery

Even in patients with severe disease, cancer is rare under the age of 20. At-risk family members start screening (either genetic or with flexible sigmoidoscopy) at around puberty. If there is a positive genotype or an adenoma is seen on sigmoidoscopy, colonoscopy is recommended. The risk of cancer of any individual patient can be estimated from the size and number of the adenomas seen on colonoscopy, and surgery planned accordingly. For patients with mild disease and low cancer risk, surgery can be done in mid-teen years (15–18 years). Where there is severe disease, or if the patient is symptomatic, surgery is done as soon as convenient after diagnosis.

Type of Surgery

There are three main surgical options: colectomy and IRA, proctocolectomy with ileostomy (TPC), and proctocolectomy with ileal pouch–anal anastomosis (IPAA). For any of these options, there are choices of technique. The IPAA can be stapled, leaving 1–2 cm of anal transitional epithelium and low rectal mucosa, or it can be hand-sewn after a complete anal mucosectomy. The operation can be done conventionally (i.e., open), laparoscopically, or laparoscopically assisted. The ileostomy may be a regular end stoma or one of the varieties of continent ileostomy (K or T).

Choice of Procedure

TPC is almost never done as a first operation except when a proctocolectomy is required and there is a contraindication to a pouch-anal anastomosis (e.g., a mesenteric desmoid tumor prevents the pouch from reaching the pelvic floor, a low rectal cancer invades the pelvic floor, or poor sphincters mean inability to control stool).

There is debate among authorities on which of the other two options should be preferred. Some recommend IPAA for all or almost all FAP patients, basing their recommendation on the risk of rectal cancer after IRA and equivalent quality of life after the two operations. Others have shown better functional outcomes after IRA and recommend it for patients with mild colorectal polyposis. However, the risk estimates of rectal cancer that are an overriding concern for the proponents of universal IPAA are based on data collected before restorative proctocolectomy was an option and may well be overestimates, especially when applied to patients with mild disease. The risk of rectal cancer after IRA is strongly related to the severity of colorectal polyposis at presentation, and IRA is a reasonable option in mildly affected patients (<20 rectal adenomas, <1000 colonic adenomas). Retrospective data show that such patients have a very low risk of rectal cancer and include all those with attenuated FAP.[30] Bowel function is usually good after IRA, the operation is simple, and complication rates are relatively low. Bowel function after a stapled IPAA is almost as good as with an IRA, and the anastomosis is usually safe enough to allow consideration of the option of avoiding a temporary ileostomy.

There is no argument that patients with severe rectal (>20 adenomas) or colonic (>1000 adenomas), or those with a severely dysplastic rectal adenoma, a cancer anywhere in the large bowel, or a large (>3 cm) rectal adenoma should have a primary IPAA. A stapled IPAA is associated with a risk of anal transitional neoplasia in 30% of patients, although if serious neoplasia occurs (high-grade dysplasia or carpeting of the mucosa), the transitional zone can usually be stripped transanally and the pouch advanced to the dentate line. Even mucosectomy and hand-sewn IPAA is associated with anal neoplasia, although at a lower rate. The disadvantage of anal mucosectomy is worse function and increased complication rates. Both IRA and IPAA require lifelong surveillance of the rectum or pouch, because both are at risk of developing adenomas.

Choice of Technique

Mobilization of the colon using minimally invasive techniques such as laparoscopy or a Pfannenstiel incision is ideal for performing colectomy in children, because it minimizes the trauma of the surgery and the pain of the incisions. Its cosmetic result is appealing and it allows an early return to full activities. Whether minimally invasive techniques lower the risk of postoperative intraabdominal desmoid tumors is unknown, but the concept is attractive. A preoperative erect abdominal X-ray will usually show the position of the flexures and indicate whether use of a Pfannenstiel incision for mobilizing the colon is feasible.

Guideline 3: Lifetime Follow-up of the Rectum (after IRA), Pouch (after IPAA), and Ileostomy (after TPC) Is Required; Increasing Neoplasia in the Rectum Is an Indication for Proctectomy; Level of Evidence: III

The combination of a germline APC mutation, stasis of stool, and glandular epithelium is potent at producing epithelial neoplasia. Adenomas and carcinomas have been described in the rectum, the ileostomy, and the ileal pouch itself, with the risk and severity of neoplasia increasing with time. The risk of severe neoplasia is mainly determined by the position of the mutation in the gene, as reflected by the severity of the polyposis. Severely affected patients have such a high risk of rectal cancer after IRA that subsequent proctectomy is almost routine and initial IPAA is to be preferred. Yearly endoscopic surveillance of the bowel after the index surgery for FAP is standard. Two-thirds of patients undergo spontaneous regression of rectal polyps after IRA, an effect that lasts 3–4 years. Subsequent surveillance will give a picture of the stability of the rectal mucosa. Small (<5 mm) adenomas can be watched, although random biopsies are done to exclude severe dysplasia. Increasing number and size of adenomas are indications for more frequent surveillance, and adenomas >5 mm should be removed cleanly with a snare. Repeated fulguration of rectal polyps over many years can cause dense scarring that makes cancers flat and hard to see, and rectal dissection during proctectomy can be very difficult. Chronic rectal scarring makes rectal biopsy difficult, because the forceps tend to "bounce off" the scarred mucosa. Furthermore, scarring leads to reduced rectal compliance, increased stool frequency, and a tendency to seepage and incontinence. Severe dysplasia, or villous adenomas >1 cm, are indications for proctectomy. Proctoscopy is best done with a video endoscope, because comfort is enhanced and the view is better. Excellent preparation and a good view are essential to pick up early cancers that can be flat and subtle.

Sulindac (Clinoril®; Merck & Co., Inc., West Point, PA), either by mouth or by suppository, is effective in making polyps disappear. Celecoxib reduces polyp load, as does the sulindac metabolite exisulind. However, cancers have been reported in cases where sulindac had been effective in minimizing rectal polyps in the rectum of FAP patients who had had IRA, and these anecdotal cases make the long-term use of chemoprevention for rectal polyposis suspect. If it is used in patients who cannot tolerate rectal polypectomy, or who are unwilling or unable to have a proctectomy, close surveillance (every 6 months) with random biopsies to look for severe dysplasia is needed.

There have been at least three recent reports describing adenomas in ileal pouches, with a frequency and severity that depend on time from the initial surgery. Two prospective studies have independently calculated the rate of pouch polyposis as 42% at 7 years. There have been anecdotal reports of large adenomas and more than 100 adenomas in an ileal pouch. In general, these have been treated successfully by oral sulindac, in a dose of 150–200 mg twice daily. The full impact of pouch polyposis will not be obvious until the cadre of FAP patients with ileal reservoirs reaches a mean follow-up of 20 years. This is the time to most ileostomy cancers, and to the highest rates of rectal cancers after IRA.

Guideline 4: Use of Chemoprevention as Primary Therapy for Colorectal Polyposis Is Not Proven and Is Not Recommended; Level of Evidence: I–II

Sulindac, celecoxib, and exisulind are nonsteroidal antiinflammatory drugs that have been shown to reduce the number and size of colorectal adenomas in patients with FAP. Although many studies are short-term, two show effectiveness of sulindac maintained over 4 years. These studies were in patients who had undergone colectomy and IRA. A recent randomized, placebo-controlled, double-blind study of sulindac in genotype-positive, phenotype-negative FAP patients failed to show any effect of sulindac on polyp progression. Furthermore, there have been case reports of cancers occurring in patients with sulindac-mediated ablation of polyps, and the only report of a permanent, complete resolution of rectal polyposis comes from Winde and coworkers who used sulindac suppositories. The effect on polyps is dependent on continued compliance, and there are significant side effects with each medication. These medications should not be used as an alternative to surgery, except in patients with pouch polyposis or in selected patients with rectal polyposis after IRA in whom surgery is risky or unwanted by the patient. In these groups of patients, close surveillance (proctoscopy or pouchoscopy every 6 months) is indicated.

Guideline 5: Treatment of Duodenal Adenomas Depends on Adenoma Size and the Presence of Severe Dysplasia. Small Tubular Adenomas with Mild Dysplasia Can Be Kept under Surveillance, but Adenomas with Severe Dysplasia Must Be Removed; Level of Evidence: II–III

The incidence of duodenal adenomas in FAP patients is in the range of 80%–90%. All FAP patients therefore undergo screening esophagogastroduodenoscopy starting at age 20 years. The risk of invasive cancer developing in a duodenal adenoma, or in the duodenal papilla, is considerably higher than that for the average population, but in absolute terms it is still low. The aim of endoscopy is not to eradicate all neoplasia but to make sure that there is no severe dysplasia. Studies of the natural history of duodenal neoplasia in FAP show that rapid progression of dysplasia is uncommon, occurring in only 11% of cases over a mean follow-up of 7 years. Prospective, randomized studies have shown that treatment with nonsteroidal antiinflammatory drugs is ineffective in treating duodenal adenomas, although a recent report indicates that celecoxib may have some effect. If they are not medically treated, low-risk adenomas (small, tubular, low-grade dysplasia) may be biopsied and left alone. High-risk adenomas (>1 cm, villous) are treated. Adenomas with confirmed high-grade dysplasia must be removed. As endoscopic or even transduodenal excision or destruction is ineffective in the long term; duodenectomy has to be considered for duodenal adenomas with high-grade dysplasia after the diagnosis has been confirmed on review by an experienced gastrointestinal pathologist.

Guideline 6: Duodenectomy or Pancreaticoduodenectomy Is Recommended for Patients with Persistent or Recurrent Severe Dysplasia in the Papilla or Duodenal Adenomas; Level of Evidence: III

A review of literature reporting treatment of advanced duodenal adenomas shows that recurrence is almost guaranteed unless the duodenum is removed. Transduodenal polypectomy or endoscopic polypectomy may be temporarily effective, but does not offer a permanent cure. The results of pancreas-preserving duodenectomy or pancreaticoduodenectomy for benign or early malignant disease are good, with low recurrence and acceptable morbidity. The outcome of surgery for established cancer is not good, with recurrence and death the usual outcome. Although the risk of duodenal/periampullary cancer is relatively low in patients with FAP, patients with persistent high-grade dysplasia in the duodenum or papilla are a high-risk group. Careful surveillance is needed, and conservative surgery or endoscopic therapy may be tried. If the severe dysplasia returns or persists, consideration must be given to duodenectomy.

Guideline 7: Surgery for Intraabdominal Desmoid Tumors Should Be Reserved for Small, Well-defined Tumors with a Clear Margin; Abdominal Wall Desmoid Tumors Should Be Excised Whenever Possible; Level of Evidence: III

Desmoid tumors are histologically benign overgrowths of fibroaponeurotic tissue occurring rarely in the general population but in 12%–17% of patients with FAP. In the general population, desmoids are usually found in limbs or limb girdles; in FAP, desmoids are usually (80%) intraabdominal and often (80%) present within 2–3 years of an abdominal surgery. Intraabdominal desmoid tumors usually involve the mesentery of the small bowel, where they are intimately involved with the mesenteric vessels. They tend to infiltrate diffusely, kink adjacent bowel loops, and may obstruct the ureters. Attempts at excision are often unsuccessful, involve removal of a variable length of small intestine, and are associated with a high morbidity and a high recurrence.

Intraabdominal desmoid tumors may affect prophylactic colorectal surgery by limiting the length of the small bowel mesentery. This will sometimes prevent an IPAA. The most common scenario in which this occurs is in patients with Gardner's variant of FAP who need proctectomy after a previous ileorectal anastomosis. Patients need to be warned about this possibility and the likelihood of ileostomy before undergoing the surgery. The second most common site for desmoids in FAP is in the abdominal wall. Abdominal wall desmoid tumors are easier to excise than intraabdominal tumors, recurrence rates are lower, and the morbidity associated with excision is less. They should be excised with a 1-cm margin. It is often necessary to use mesh to cover the defect in the abdominal wall.

Guideline 8: Intraabdominal Desmoid Tumors Involving the Small Bowel Mesentery Are Treated According to Their Rate of Growth and Their Presentation. Clinically Inert Tumors Should Be Treated with Sulindac or Not Treated at All. Slowly Growing or Mildly Symptomatic Tumors May Be Treated with Less Toxic Regimens Such as Sulindac and Tamoxifen or Vinblastine and Methotrexate. Rapidly Growing Tumors Need Aggressive Therapy with Either Very High-dose Tamoxifen or Antisarcoma-type Chemotherapy. Radiation Is an Option if Collateral Damage Is Not a Big Concern; Level of Evidence: III

Intraabdominal desmoid tumors vary in their clinical behavior from aggressive, relentless growth to indolent, asymptomatic coexistence. There is no single, predictably effective way of managing intraabdominal desmoids. Evidence suggests that sulindac is partially effective but that a response to this nonsteroidal antiinflammatory agent may not be noticeable for up to 2 years. The role of high-dose antiestrogens is uncertain, with one report describing good results in aggressive desmoids with tamoxifen in a dose of 120 mg/day. Toremifene, a more potent antiestrogen than tamoxifen, has some effect on desmoid tumors but seems to work better in non-FAP desmoids than FAP. A pilot study of the antifibrosis agent pirfenidone resulted in some modest responses. Most aggressive desmoids receive chemotherapy, and there are two regimens reported. The combination of vinblastine and methotrexate has low toxicity and produces some responses. Non-FAP desmoids seem more likely to respond to this combination, although no prospective studies have been done. Antisarcoma therapy such as doxorubicin and dacarbazine is much more toxic but seems to be more effective for rapidly growing intraabdominal desmoid tumors associated with FAP. Radiation is effective in destroying tumors but its effect on the small bowel can be disastrous, causing fistulas and necrosis.

Intraabdominal desmoids that are not growing may be treated by sulindac alone. If they are growing slowly or causing symptoms, it is reasonable to add tamoxifen in a dose range of 80–120 mg/day. The dose should be gradually increased to these levels over a few weeks. If the tumor continues to grow, chemotherapy is appropriate. Really rapid growth is an indication for antisarcoma therapy, whereas a slower growth rate means vinblastine/methotrexate can be tried. A recent report of successful intestinal transplantation after resection of abdominal desmoids reinforces the extent of the surgery needed to remove them, but also offers some hope for tumors that fail to respond to anything else.

Section II: HNPCC

Guideline 1: Treatment Must Be Preceded by Thorough Counseling about the Nature of the Syndrome, Its Natural History, Its Extracolonic Manifestations, and the Need for Compliance with All Recommendations for Management and Surveillance; Level of Evidence: III

Hereditary nonpolyposis colorectal cancer is a dominantly inherited syndrome attributed to an inactivating mutation in one of the human DNA MMR genes. The syndrome is more complex than FAP because more genes are involved, penetrance is less complete, and expression is more varied. Furthermore, the clinical criteria defining HNPCC are arbitrary and not particularly accurate, and the yield of testing for germline mutations is lower than for FAP. HNPCC has a penetrance of at least 80%, and colorectal cancer occurs at a mean age of 46 years. Affected patients usually have at least one surgery and are committed to lifelong surveillance of several organs. Careful counseling is necessary to allow patients and their families to understand the implications of these complexities.

Guideline 2: When Patients with HNPCC as Defined by Genotype or Compliance with Amsterdam I Criteria Are Diagnosed with More Than One Advanced Adenoma or a Colon Cancer, They Should Be Offered the Options of Prophylactic Total Colectomy and IRA or Hemicolectomy Plus Yearly Colonoscopy. The Choice of IRA Assumes the Anal Sphincter and Rectum Function Normally; Level of Evidence: III

When patients known to be affected with HNPCC are diagnosed with advanced neoplasia, they can be offered a choice of conventional partial colectomy with surveillance of the remaining large bowel or total colectomy with rectal surveillance. Surveillance involves colonoscopy or proctoscopy (after IRA) every 1–2 years for life. There is evidence that cancers can occur in HNPCC within 2 years of a negative colonoscopy, but that cancers found on screening examinations performed with a 3-year interval can be cured. The risk of metachronous cancer after conventional treatment of an index cancer is 45% in patients with HNPCC, high enough to make prophylactic colectomy a reasonable option. The downside of colectomy and IRA lies in its effect on bowel function and quality of life. In a study of patients having IRA for FAP, quality of life was maintained, although stool frequency increased. These patients were younger than typical HNPCC patients having surgery, but even older patients can do well after IRA provided their anal sphincters and rectums are normal. The outcome of partial colectomy and effective surveillance can be similar to that of colectomy and IRA in terms of minimizing metachronous cancers. Likely patient compliance, the anticipated quality and frequency of colonoscopy, and the relative costs and reimbursement of the two options therefore influence the choice. Even after IRA, the risk of rectal cancer is 12% in 12 years, so continuing surveillance of the rectum is mandatory.

HNPCC patients diagnosed by genotype with a normal colon are also candidates for prophylactic colectomy. If penetrance of the mutation in the family approaches 100%, this should be strongly considered. There have been two attempts to discern the relative benefits of surgery versus surveillance using decision analysis methods. Syngal and coworkers showed that prophylactic colectomy/proctocolectomy performed at the time of diagnosis led to a greater benefit in years of life expectancy gained than surveillance, but that this benefit decreased the longer surgery was delayed. Furthermore, if prophylactic surgery is performed at the time of diagnosis of a cancer, the gain in life expectancy is only 4 days for colectomy/IRA and 6 days for proctocolectomy. The advantage of surgery is further reduced if the gain in years is discounted. When the outcome of the analysis was quality-adjusted life years (QALYs), surveillance was the most effective strategy, with a gain of 14 QALYs compared with no surveillance, 3.2 QALYs compared with prophylactic proctocolectomy at diagnosis of HNPCC, and 0.3 QALYs compared with colectomy. A similar phenomenon was seen when comparing colectomy with proctocolectomy. Use of QALYs improved the relative value of the lesser operation. In the decision analysis published by Vasen and coworkers prophylactic colectomy at age 40 conferred an increase in life expectancy over surveillance of 8–18 months. In the same scenario, Syngal et al. calculated a benefit for surgery of 9.6 months. These analyses do not take costs into account, however, and they assume a level of compliance and quality of endoscopy that may not be realistic. In the absence of a randomized comparison of surveillance and surgery, both options must be explained to the patient and individual circumstances, such as comorbidity, gastrointestinal physiology, likely compliance, and ease of colonoscopy, taken into account.

Guideline 3: Patients with HNPCC Who Have a Rectal Cancer Should Be Offered the Options of Total Proctocolectomy and IPAA or Anterior Proctosigmoidectomy, Assuming that the Sphincters Can Be Saved; Level of Evidence: III

Rectal cancer is an uncommon index cancer in patients with HNPCC. Surgical options, assuming the sphincters can be saved, are restorative proctocolectomy (with IPAA) and anterior resection. There are substantial differences in bowel function after these two procedures, but the risk of metachronous colon cancer after a primary rectal cancer is not known. The decision to preserve the proximal colon and commit to a program of intensive surveillance is therefore based on likely compliance of the patient with surveillance and the likely impact of the surgery on quality of life.

Guideline 4: Female Patients with HNPCC and Uterine Cancer in Their Family May Be Offered Prophylactic Hysterectomy Once Their Family Is Complete or When Undergoing Surgery for Other Intraabdominal Conditions; Level of Evidence: III

The lifetime risk of uterine cancer in HNPCC is 42%, and although it is most common in families with hMSH6 mutations, it is also associated with hMSH2 and hMLH1 mutations. Screening for endometrial cancer in females with HNPCC has been shown in at least one study to be ineffective in detecting cancer, and so where uterine cancer is a feature in families, affected females should be offered prophylactic hysterectomy. Oophorectomy should be done at the same time, because the risk for ovarian cancer associated with HNPCC is high and in a multi-institution review of HNPCC-associated ovarian cancer, synchronous endometrial cancer was present in 21.5% of 80 patients.

Brown and coworkers have shown that an increased risk for gynecologic cancer begins by age 25 years. Although the mean age at gynecologic cancer in their series of 67 affected females (43 uterine, 24 ovarian) was 49.3 years, five gynecologic cancers were diagnosed before age 35. The timing of prophylactic hysterectomy and oophorectomy is therefore debatable. It is tempting to offer surveillance during the childbearing years and delay surgery until the patient has had a chance to have her family. Until more data are available, this is the best option. Surgery can be done at the time of another abdominal surgery, or as a separate operation once the patient's family is complete.

Levels of evidence

Level I: Evidence from properly conducted randomized, controlled trials.
Level II: Evidence from controlled trials without randomization, or cohort or case-control studies or multiple times series, dramatic uncontrolled experiments.
Level III: Descriptive case series or opinions of expert panels.

References

1. Jemal A, Thomas A, Murray T, et al. Cancer statistics, 2002. CA Cancer J Clin 2002;52:23–47.
2. Burt RW, Peterson GM. Familial colorectal cancer: diagnosis and management. In: Young GP, Roger P, Leven B, eds. Prevention and Early Detection of Colorectal Cancer. London: WB Saunders; 1996:171–194.
3. Aarnio M, Mecklin JP, Aaltonen LA, et al. Lifetime risk of different cancers in hereditary nonpolyposis colorectal cancer. Int J Cancer 1995;64:430–433.
4. Warthin A. Hereditary with reference to carcinoma. Arch Intern Med 1913:546–555.

5. Lynch HT, Shaw MW, Magnuson CW, et al. Hereditary factors in cancer. Study of two large midwestern kindreds. Arch Intern Med 1966;117:206–212.
6. Vasen HF, Mecklin JP, Lynch HT. The International Collaborative Group on Hereditary Non-Polyposis Colorectal Cancer (ICG-HNPCC). Dis Colon Rectum 1991;34:424–425.
7. Ionov Y, Punado MA, Malklosyan S, et al. Ubiquitous somatic mutations in simple repeated sequences reveal a new mechanism for colonic carcinogenesis. Nature 1993;363:558–561.
8. Fishel R, Lesco MK, Roa MR, et al. The human mutator gene homolog MSH2 and its association with hereditary nonpolyposis colon cancer. Cell 1993;75:1027–1038.
9. Gyapuy G, Morissette J, Vignal A, et al. The 1993–94 genethon genetic linkage map. Nat Genet 1994;7:246–339.
10. Charames GS, Bapat B. Genomic instability and cancer. Curr Mol Med 2003;3:589–596.
11. Jacob S, Praz F. DNA mismatch repair defects: role in carcinogenesis. Biochimie 2002;84:27–47.
12. Johnson R, Korovali G, Prakash L, et al. Requirement of the yeast MSH3 and MSH6 genes for MSH2 genomic stability. J Biol Chem 1996;271:7285–7288.
13. Liu B, Parsons R, Papadoupolos N, et al. Analysis of mismatch repair genes in hereditary nonpolyposis colorectal cancer patients. Nat Med 1996;2:169–174.
14. Mitchell J, Farrington S, Dunlop M, et al. Mismatch repair genes in MLHI and in MSH2 and colorectal cancer: a HUGE review. Am J Epidemiol 2002;156:885–902.
15. Allen D, Markhov AM, Grilley M, et al. MutS mediates heteroduplex loop formation by a translocation mechanism. EMBO J 1997;16:4467–4476.
16. Gardia S, Acharya S, Fishel R. The role of mismatched nucleotides in activating the hMSH2-hMSH6 molecular switch. J Biol Chem 2000;275:3922–3930.
17. Junrope M, Obmolova G, Rausch K, et al. Composite active site of an ABC ATPase: MutS uses ATP to verify mismatch recognition and authorize DNA repair. Mol Cell 2001;7:1–12.
18. Parsons R, Myeroff L, Liu B, et al. Microsatellite instability and mutations of the transforming growth factor β type II receptor gene in colorectal cancer. Cancer Res 1995;55:5548–5550.
19. Calin G, Gofa R, Tibiletti M, et al. Genetic progression in microsatellite instability high (MSI-H) colon cancers correlates with clinico-pathological parameters: a study of the TGFβRII, BAX, hMSH3, hMSH6, IGFIIR, and BLM genes. Int J Cancer 2000;89:230–235.
20. Souza R, Apple R, Yin J. Microsatellite instability in the insulin-like growth factor II receptor gene in gastrointestinal tumors. Nat Genet 1996;14:255–257.
21. Rumpino N, Yamumoto H, Ionov Y, et al. Somatic frameshifts mutation in the BAX gene in colon cancers of the microsatellite mutator phenotype. Science 1997;275:967–969.
22. Schwartz S, Yamanoto H, Navano M, et al. Frameshifts mutations at mononucleotide repeats in capase-5 and other target genes in endometrial and gastrointestinal cancer of the microsatellite mutator phenotype. Cancer Res 1999;59: 2995–3002.
23. Shin K, Park Y, Park J. PTEN gene mutation in colorectal cancers displaying microsatellite instability. Cancer Lett 2001;174: 189–194.
24. Rajagopalan H, Bardelli A, Lingauer C, et al. RAF/RAS oncogenes and mismatch repair status. Nature 2002;418:934.
25. Riccio A, Aaltonen L, Godwin AK, et al. The DNA repair gene MBD4 (MED 1) is mutated in human carcinomas with microsatellite instability. Nat Genet 1999;23:266–268.
26. Mecklin JP, Sipponen P, Jarvinen HJ, et al. Histopathology of colorectal carcinomas in cancer family syndrome. Dis Colon Rectum 1986;29:849–853.
27. Guillem JG, Pueg-LaCalle J Jr, Cellini C, et al. Varying features of early age-onset colon cancer. Dis Colon Rectum 1999;42: 36–42.
28. Jass JR. Pathology of hereditary nonpolyposis colorectal cancer. Ann NY Acad Sci 2000;910:62–73.
29. Chung D, Rustgi A. The hereditary nonpolyposis colorectal cancer syndrome: genetics and clinical implications. Ann Intern Med 2003;138:560–570.
30. Muller A, Fishel R. Mismatch repair and the hereditary nonpolyposis colorectal cancer syndrome. Cancer Invest 2002;20: 102–109.
31. Aarino M, Mecklin JP, Aaltonen LA, et al. Life-time risk of different cancers in HNPCC. Int J Cancer 1995;64:430–433.
32. DeJong A, Morreau H, Van Puijenbroek M, et al. The role of mismatch repair gene defects in the development of adenomas in patients with HNPCC. Gastroenterology 2004;126:42–48.
33. Jarvinen HJ, Mecklin JP, Sistonen P. Screening reduces colorectal cancer rate in families with hereditary nonpolyposis colon cancer. Gastroenterology 1995;108:1405–1411.
34. Winawer SJ, Zauber AG, Ho MN, et al. Prevention of colorectal cancer by colonoscopic polypectomy: The National Polyp Study Workgroup. N Engl J Med 1993;329:1977–1981.
35. Lanspa ST, Lynch HT, Smyrk TC, et al. Colorectal adenomas in the Lynch syndromes: results of a colonoscopy screening program. Gastroenterology 1990;98(5 pt 1):1117–1122.
36. Olschwang S, Slezak P, Roze M, et al. Somatically acquired genetic alterations in flat colorectal neoplasias. Int J Cancer 1998;77:366–369.
37. Saitoh Y, Waxman I, West AB, et al. Prevalence and distinctive biologic features of flat colorectal adenomas in a North American population. Gastroenterology 2001;120:1657–1665.
38. Makinen MJ, George SMC, Jemvall P, et al. Colorectal carcinoma associated with serrated adenoma-prevalence, histological features, and prognosis. J Pathol 2001;193:286–294.
39. Weber TK, Conlon W, Pitrelli NJ, et al. Genomic DNA-based h MSH2 and h MLH1 mutation screening in 35 eastern United States hereditary nonpolyposis colorectal cancer pedigrees. Cancer Res 1997;57:3798–3803.
40. Vasen HF, Winjen JT, Menko FH, et al. Cancer risk in families with hereditary nonpolyposis colorectal cancer diagnosed by mutation analysis. Gastroenterology 1996;110: 1020–1027.
41. Bisgaard ML, Jager AL, Myrhoj T, et al. Hereditary nonpolyposis colorectal cancer (HNPCC): phenotype-genotype correlation between patients with and without identified mutation. Hum Mutat 2002;20:20–27.
42. Schwartz RA, Torre DP. The Muir-Torre syndrome: 25 year retrospective. J Am Acad Dermatol 1995;33:90–104.
43. Kruse R, Lamerti C, Wang Y, et al. Is the mismatch repair deficient type of Muir-Torre syndrome confined to mutations in the MSH2 gene? Hum Genet 1996;98:747–750.
44. Kolodner RD, Tytell JD, Schmeits JL, et al. Germ-line MSH6 mutations in colorectal cancer families. Cancer Res 1999;59: 5068–5074.

45. Huang J, Kuismanen SA, Liu T, et al. MSH6 and MSH3 are rarely involved in genetic predisposition to nonpolypotic colon cancer. Cancer Res 2001;61:1619–1623.

46. Karrola R, Raevaara TE, Lonnqvist KE, et al. Functional analysis of MSH6 mutations linked to kindreds with putative HNPCC. Hum Mol Genet 2002;11:1303–1310.

47. de Wind N, Decker M, Claij N, et al. HNPCC-like cancer predisposition in mice thru loss of MSH3 and MSH6 mismatch repair protein function. Nat Genet 1999;23:359–362.

48. Berends MJW, Wu Y, Sijmons RH, et al. Molecular and clinical characteristics of MSH6 of 25 index cases. Am J Hum Genet 2002;70:26–37.

49. Wagner A, Hendricks Y, Meijers-Heyboer EJ, et al. MSH6 germline mutations; analysis of a large Dutch pedigree. J Med Genet 2001;58:318–322.

50. Rodriguez-Bigas M, Boland CR, Hamilton SR, et al. A National Cancer Institute Workshop on HNPCC: meeting highlights and Bethesda guidelines. J Natl Cancer Inst 1997;89:1758–1762.

51. Syngal S, Fox EA, Eng C, et al. Sensitivity and specificity of clinical criteria for HNPCC associated mutations in MSH2 and MSL1. J Med Genet 2000;37:641–645.

52. Peltomaki P, Vasen HF. Mutations predisposing to hereditary nonpolyposis colorectal cancer: database and results of a collaborative study. International Collaborative Group on HNPCC. Gastroenterology 1997;113:1146–1158.

53. Yan H, Kinzler KW, Vogelstein B. Genetic testing—present and future. Science 2000;289:1890–1892.

54. Yan H, Papadopolous N, Marra G, et al. Conversion of diploidy to haploid. Nature 2000;403:723–724.

55. Boland CR, Thibideau SN, Hamilton S, et al. A National Cancer Institute Workshop on microsatellite instability for cancer detection and familial predisposition: development of international criteria for the determination of microsatellite instability in colorectal cancer. Cancer Res 1998;58:5248–5257.

56. Wahlberg SS, Schmeits J, Thomas G, et al. Evaluation of microsatellite instability and immunohistochemistry for the prediction of germ-line MSH2 and MLH1 in hereditary nonpolyposis colon cancer families. Cancer Res 2002;62:3485–3492.

57. Reyes C, Allan BA, Tiederman JP, et al. Comparison for selective strategies for genetic testing of patients with hereditary nonpolyposis colorectal carcinoma. Cancer 2002;95:1848–1856.

58. Rothstein MA. Policy recommendations. In: Rothstein MA, ed. Genetics and Life Insurance. Medical Underwriting and Social Policy. Cambridge, MA: The MIT Press; 2004.

59. Rothstein MA. Genetic privacy and confidentiality: why they are so hard to protect. J Law Med Ethics 1998;26:198–204.

60. Giardello FM, Brensinger JD, Petersen GM, et al. The use and interpretation of commercial APC gene testing for familial adenomatous polyposis. N Engl J Med 1997;336:823–827.

61. Byers T, Levin B, Rothenberger D, et al. American Cancer Society guidelines for screening and surveillance for early detection of colorectal polyps and cancer: update 1997. CA Cancer J Clin 1997;47:154–160.

62. Vasen HF, Nagengast FM, Khan PM. Interval cancers in hereditary nonpolyposis colorectal cancer. Lancet 1995;345:1183–1184.

63. Lynch HT, Lynch J. Lynch syndrome: genetics, natural history, genetic counseling and prevention. J Clin Oncol 2000;18(21 suppl):19S–31S.

64. Jass JR, Stewart SM. Evolution of hereditary non-polyposis colorectal cancer. Gut 1992;33:783–786.

65. Jarvinen HJ, Aarnio M, Mustonen H, et al. Controlled 15-year trial on screening for colorectal cancer in families with hereditary nonpolyposis colorectal cancer. Gastroenterology 2000;118:829–834.

66. Rekonen-Sinislao L, Aarnio M, Pekka-Mecklin J, et al. Surveillance improves survival of colorectal cancer in patients with hereditary nonpolyposis colorectal cancer. Cancer Detect Prev 2000;24:137–142.

67. Burke W, Petersen G, Lynch P, et al. Recommendations for follow-up care of individuals with an inherited predisposition to cancer. I. Hereditary nonpolyposis colon cancer. JAMA 1997;227:915–919.

68. Brown GJ, St. John DJ, Macrae FA, et al. Cancer risk in young women at risk of hereditary nonpolyposis colorectal cancer: implications for gynecologic surveillance. Gynecol Oncol 2001;80:346–349.

69. Lynch P. If aggressive surveillance in hereditary nonpolyposis colorectal cancer is now state of the art, are there any challenges left? [Editorial] Gastroenterology 2000;118:969–971.

70. Dove-Edwin I, Boks D, Goff S, et al. The outcome of endometrial carcinoma surveillance by ultrasound scan in women at risk of hereditary nonpolyposis colorectal carcinoma and familial colorectal carcinoma. Cancer 2002;94:1708–1712.

71. Rodriguez-Bigas MA, Vasen HF, Pekka-Mecklin J, et al. Rectal cancer risk in hereditary nonpolyposis colorectal cancer after abdominal colectomy. International Collaborative Group on HNPCC. Ann Surg 1997;225:202–207.

72. Fitzsimmons RJ Jr, Lynch HT, Stanislav GV, et al. Recognition and treatment of patients with hereditary nonpolyposis colon cancer (Lynch syndromes I and II). Ann Surg 1987;206:289–294.

73. Syngal S, Weeks JC, Schrag D, et al. Benefits of colonoscopic surveillance and prophylactic colectomy in patients with hereditary nonpolyposis colorectal cancer. Ann Intern Med 1998;129:787–796.

74. Vasen HF, van Ballegooijen M, Buskens E, et al. A cost-effectiveness analysis of colorectal screening of hereditary nonpolyposis colorectal carcinoma gene carriers. Cancer 1998;82:1632–1637.

75. Watson P, Lin K, Rodriguez-Bigas MA, et al. Colorectal carcinoma survival among hereditary non-polyposis colorectal cancer family members. Cancer 1998;83:259–266.

76. Sankila R, Aaltonen LA, Jarvinen HA, et al. Better survival rates in patients with MLH1 associated hereditary nonpolyposis colorectal cancer. Gastroenterology 1996;110:682–687.

77. Ribic CM, Sargent DJ, Moore MJ, et al. Tumor microsatellite-instability status as a predictor of benefit from fluorouracil-based adjuvant chemotherapy for colon cancer. N Engl J Med 2003;349:247–257.

78. Elsaleh H, Joseph D, Grieu F, et al. Association of tumour site and sex with survival benefit from adjuvant chemotherapy in colorectal cancer. Lancet 2000;355:1745–1750.

79. Iacopetta B, Elsaleh H, Zeps N. Microsatellite instability in colon cancer [correspondence]. N Engl J Med 2003;349:1774–1776.

80. Giovannucci E, Rimm EB, Meir J, et al. Aspirin use and the risk for colorectal cancer and adenoma in male health professionals. Ann Intern Med 1994;121:241–246.

81. Thun MJ, Namboodiri MM, Calle EE, et al. Aspirin use and risk of fatal cancer. Cancer Res 1993;53:1322–1327.

82. Galandiuk S. Ongoing clinical trials. Dig Surg 2003;20:464–475.

83. Garland C, Shekelle RB, Barret-Connor E, et al. Dietary vitamin D and calcium and risk of colorectal cancer. A 19-year prospective study in men. Lancet 1985;1:307–309.

84. Lapré JA, De Vries HT, Koeman JH, et al. The antiproliferative effect of dietary calcium on colonic epithelium is mediated by luminal surfactants and dependent on the type of dietary fat. Cancer Res 1993;53:784–789.

85. Cats A, Kleibeuker JH, Van der Meer R, et al. Randomized, double-blinded, placebo-controlled intervention study with supplemental calcium in families with hereditary nonpolyposis colorectal cancer. J Natl Cancer Inst 1995;87:598–603.

39
Inflammatory Bowel Disease: Diagnosis and Evaluation

Walter A. Koltun

History

In 1932 Crohn, Ginzburg, and Oppenheimer[1] described 13 patients with "regional ileitis" included in a total of 52 cases of nonspecific granulomatous inflammation of the intestine. Before their publication, numerous others had reported various cases of what were in retrospect, probably Crohn's disease (CD), as early as 1813,[2] but it was their published description that established the formal classification of the disease syndrome and association with noncaseating granulomas. The surgeon involved in the care of the majority of the patients, Dr. A.A. Berg, did not want his name included in the article. Because of the variable clinical and anatomic manifestations of the illness, "Crohn's disease" has subsequently become as common a descriptor of this disease entity as the term "regional enteritis."

The difficulty in distinguishing the colonic form of CD and ulcerative colitis (UC) confused the diagnosis and treatment of these illnesses until their differences were clarified by classic publications by Brooke[3] in 1959 and Lockhart-Mummery and Morson[4] in 1960. These authors pointed out both the segmental and granulomatous features of the colitis in CD. In addition, Brooke contributed significantly to the treatment of these inflammatory illnesses by pioneering surgical techniques in the 1950s that created a more functional ileostomy, which until that time was a miserable and disabling consequence of colectomy.[5] Truelove et al.[6] in 1959 reported on a double-blind, controlled study demonstrating the value of high-dose cortisone as treatment for severe colitis. Other turning points in the management and treatment of CD include the demonstration of the therapeutic value of metronidazole,[7] 6-mercaptopurine,[8] and more recently, the tumor necrosis factor (TNF)-α antagonist, infliximab.[9]

The surgical management of UC has been a continuous evolution starting with colectomy/ileostomy,[10,11] supplanted by the continent Kock ileostomy,[12] and finally the definitive reconstruction procedure known as the ileal pouch–anal anastomosis (IPAA), first described by Parks and Nicholls[13] in 1978 and subsequently refined by Utsunomiya.[14] The IPAA is now the standard of care for the surgical correction of UC.

Epidemiology

The causes of UC and CD are unknown, and thus epidemiologic data have been collected over many years in the hopes of providing some clues to the etiologies of these illnesses. Much of these data must be viewed with caution, however. Variations in diagnostic criteria, definitions of disease, and biases resulting from surveys done in tertiary care specialty centers, make universal conclusions difficult. However, some general statements can be made using such data that relate to disease prevalence and associated risk factors (Table 39-1).

The prevalence of inflammatory bowel disease (IBD) varies greatly with region of the world studied. Prevalence is the product of incidence and disease duration. Because IBD symptoms tend to wax and wane in severity, prevalence may be underestimated in some studies. IBD is found most frequently in the more temperate climates of North America and Europe. Studies from those regions show prevalence rates much higher than those in Asia, South America, or Africa. Prevalence rates as high as 300–400 per 100,000 population are found in Minnesota (USA), Manitoba (Canada), and the United Kingdom. Conversely, prevalence rates of approximately 23/100,000 are found in Japan, 10/100,000 in Singapore, and 75–120/100,000 in Israel. The relative incidence of Crohn's versus UC is again, variable, with either being found greater than the other depending on geographic region studied.[15–19]

It is generally recognized that both CD and UC have been increasing in incidence to a remarkable degree over the past 20–30 years with two- to tenfold increases depending on population and region studied.[18,20] These dramatic increases suggest an environmental effect, because a genetic factor would probably not alter disease rates so rapidly.

CD usually occurs in the third decade of life, whereas chronic UC in the fourth decade. There may be a bimodal distribution of disease incidence with a second peak in the sixth or seventh decade, but this is unclear and may simply be attributable to difficulty in differentiating it from other colitides such as diverticulitis or ischemic colitis.[21]

TABLE 39-1. Epidemiologic and associated risk factors for IBD

Epidemiology
  Race/ethnicity
    Whites and blacks > Hispanic, Native American, Asian
    Jews > non-Jews
  Geography
    Northern climates > Southern
    Scandinavia, North America, Europe > Asia, Africa, South America,
      Japan, Spain
  Sex
    CD: F > M
    UC: M > F
  Age at greatest incidence
    CD: third decade
    UC: fourth decade
  Residence
    Urban > rural
    Indoor > outdoor

Risk factors
  Diet
    Sugar consumption, ↑ CD
    ETOH, ↓ UC
    Margarine, no association
    Coffee, no association
    Fiber, no association
    Food additives, no association
  Childhood diarrheal illness ↑ IBD
  Higher socioeconomic status ↑ IBD
  Oral contraceptive use ↑ IBD
  Cigarettes ↑ CD
        ↓ UC
  Appendectomy ↓ UC
  NSAIDs ↑ symptoms IBD

Although originally thought to be relatively rare in blacks, more recent case control studies in the United States suggest a similar incidence to whites, although Africa itself has a very low incidence of IBD.[17] There is great variability in the incidence of IBD in Jews around the world, but nonetheless seems to be consistently higher than that found in the non-Jewish population in most countries studied.[22] IBD is more common in urban, "indoor" populations of individuals of middle to upper socioeconomic status, suggesting the "hygiene" hypothesis that relates the lack of early exposure to environmental antigens to the later development of disease.[15,19,23]

There is very little evidence that a specific dietary factor causes IBD although increased sugar consumption is associated with CD and alcohol intake is inversely related to chronic UC.[24,25] Childhood diarrheal illness, oral contraceptive and nonsteroidal antiinflammatory (NSAIDs) use are measurable risk factors for IBD, with NSAIDs reported as precipitating relapse in patients with inactive disease.[26] Smoking has been clearly shown to worsen CD, with increased risk of developing the disease de novo and increased risk of recurrence after surgical resection.[27,28] Conversely, smoking is protective for chronic UC, as is prior appendectomy.[27]

There is clearly a genetic predisposition to IBD. It is probably stronger in CD than UC. If an individual has IBD, there

is a 10%–20% risk of having another family member with IBD. Twin studies have shown that the concordance rate for identical twins is much higher than that for dizygotic or paternal twins (approximately 50% versus 15%), stressing the role genes have in the disease. However, the fact that identical twins do not have a 100% concordance, reinforces the fact that there must also be a nongenetic component to the illness. In families who have multiple affected members, the age of onset is probably earlier and some studies suggest that the anatomic pattern, extent and severity of disease may be similar.[29–31] Genetic techniques of analysis, including linkage and transmission disequilibrium testing using both sporadic and family registries of IBD patients have identified seven areas of the human genome (on chromosomes 1, 5, 6, 12, 14, 16, 19) that are significantly relevant to disease susceptibility,[32] underscoring the complexity of the genetic predisposition to IBD. It seems that no one gene locus is responsible for disease, but that many gene products have a role in the illness. The strongest genetic linkage is with CD and mutations in a locus on chromosome 16 which has now been identified as being in the *NOD2/CARD15* gene.[33,34] This gene is involved in innate host defense against enteric bacteria and mutations in this gene are believed to be responsible for approximately 15%–30% of patients with CD. Its discovery represents a breakthrough in the conceptualization of disease pathogenesis in IBD. Overall, both the epidemiology and now the molecular genetic evidence furthers the concept that IBD is the consequence of environmental exposure to a causative agent in a genetically susceptible individual.

Signs and Symptoms

Gastrointestinal Symptoms

Crohn's Disease

CD can affect any portion of the gastrointestinal (GI) tract from the mouth to the anus. It is usually discontinuous, usually involving several areas of the bowel at once, with sections of normal intestine interposed. The inflammation of CD involves the entire bowel wall, from mucosa to serosa and even into adjacent structures. These features are responsible for its presenting symptomatology.

The most common complaints of any patient with CD are abdominal pain and diarrhea, being found in more than 75% of patients. Weight loss, fever, and bleeding are present in approximately 40%–60% of patients, whereas anal symptoms of abscess and/or fistula occur in 10%–20% of patients. Many classification systems for CD have been suggested but the anatomic one has direct practical relevance in explaining symptoms. CD is most frequently found in the ileocecal region, making up approximately 40% of patients. Abdominal pain usually correlates with disease in this region.[20] Colonic disease is found in approximately 30% of patients and most directly correlates with symptoms of diarrhea and bleeding.

The remaining 30% of patients have disease confined to the small bowel proximal to the terminal ileum and correlates with abdominal pain, bloating, and a sense of postprandial nausea especially if partial obstruction caused by inflammation or strictures occurs. Anal disease is typically associated with patients having the terminal ileal and colonic distributions of disease.

The more recently developed Vienna classification of CD segregates patients into three categories based on behavior: inflammatory (B1), stricturing (B2), and fistulizing (B3).[35] This classification attempts to characterize disease biology but is imperfect. Patients will frequently change categories as disease progresses, because inflammatory disease usually becomes stricturing or fistulizing disease. Louis et al.,[36] over a 10-year period, found that in 125 patients with CD, the B2 and B3 categories (stricturing and fistulizing) each increased from approximately 10% to approximately 30%–40% with a compensatory decrease in the inflammatory, B1category. Thus duration of disease has a critical role in defining the category in this classification system.

Clinical severity of symptoms is widely variable, because CD typically has a waxing and waning course characterized by periods of disease activity interspersed with periods of remission. At any one time, approximately 50% of CD patients will be in clinical remission. The majority of patients (60%–75%) will have alternating years of quiescence and disease activity. Approximately 10%–20% will have either a chronic, unremitting course or repetitive annual flaring of disease. Prolonged quiescence is found in approximately 10%–15% of patients. The only useful predictor of future disease activity is past clinical behavior.

Ulcerative Colitis

The inflammation of UC characteristically starts in the rectum and extends proximally. So-called backwash ileitis is the only possible area of the small bowel that can be affected in UC, or CD should be suspected. Clinical symptoms relate to the extent and location of disease. Thus, rectal disease results in increased stool frequency, hematochezia, and tenesmus. Diarrhea is a frequent symptom and with tenesmus can result in incontinence, especially at night. Despite severe rectal inflammation, constipation with a sense of incomplete evacuation can be a complaint in 20%–25% of patients, but blood and mucous are nearly always present. With more proximal involvement, abdominal complaints increase including left lower quadrant pain and pain associated with peristalsis or stool evacuation. With increasing severity and extent of disease, nausea, vomiting, and weight loss ensue. Weight loss is attributed both to the loss of serum proteins through the diseased mucosa and the reluctance of the patient to eat in order to avoid exacerbation of symptoms. The development of systemic signs of illness such as tachycardia, fever, and increasing fluid requirement bespeaks severe disease. High-dose steroids may disguise worsening abdominal complaints,

including peritonitis in such circumstances and should not divert the clinician from recognizing the gravity of the development of such symptoms and signs. So-called "toxic megacolon" is a moniker that should be discarded, because severe life-threatening colitis may occur without colonic dilatation and urgent surgical intervention should be based on the triad of toxicity defined by tachycardia, fever, and increased white blood cell count.

Extraintestinal Manifestations

Musculoskeletal

The most common non-GI complaints in IBD patients relate to the musculoskeletal system. Osteopenia and osteoporosis are very common, in part because of therapeutic steroid use, occurring in as many as 50% and 15% of IBD patients, respectively. Such bone density loss is now recognized as leading to significant comorbidity and complications in IBD patients. One study found a 40% increased risk of bone fractures in IBD patients.[37] The arthropathies associated with IBD are found in up to 30% of patients and are divided into two broad categories. Peripheral arthritis usually affects multiple small joints and has little relation to GI disease activity. Axial arthritis (ankylosing spondylitis) is associated with certain human leukocyte antigen subtypes (B27) and is found in approximately 5% of both CD and UC patients. Its severity usually parallels disease activity. Recently, anti-TNF therapies have been shown to be effective in both CD and the arthropathy of IBD.[38,39]

Cutaneous

Pyoderma gangrenosum and erythema nodosum occur in approximately 0.5%–5% of patients with IBD. These, as well as oral lesions such as aphthous stomatitis and pyostomatitis vegetans, are more frequently associated with CD than UC and usually parallel underlying GI disease activity. The new appearance of pyoderma gangrenosum around the ileostomy of an IBD patient after colectomy is unexplained but is a clear clinical phenomenon.[40] There is a reported increased rate of psoriasis and eczema in IBD patients that does not parallel disease activity. One-third to one-half of patients with pyoderma gangrenosum have IBD.[41]

Hepatobiliary

Primary sclerosing cholangitis (PSC) has a reported incidence of approximately 3% in both CD and UC patients. It may present independently of intestinal disease activity, and colectomy in UC patients does not affect progression of liver disease. The presence of PSC in the UC patient increases the risk for malignant disease in both the colon and hepatobiliary system.[42]

Several studies have suggested an increased incidence of gallstones in IBD, especially CD although this is disputed.

The mechanism is presumed to be attributable to an altered enterohepatic biliary circulation caused by ileal disease.[43]

Ophthalmologic

Iritis, uveitis, and episcleritis can affect 2%–8% of UC and CD patients and are generally unrelated to disease activity. Iritis and uveitis present as blurred vision, eye pain, and photophobia and require prompt treatment to avoid scarring and even blindness. Episcleritis is typically less threatening and is characterized by scleral injection, burning, and tearing.

Coagulopathy

There is an identified increased risk of deep venous thrombosis, mesenteric thrombosis, and pulmonary embolism in IBD patients that is not explained simply by increased hospitalization and surgery. Decreased protein S and antithrombin III levels attributed to mucosal loss and increased levels of acute phase reactants including factors V and VIII have been implicated. The mortality of postoperative mesenteric thrombosis in the IBD patient has been reported to be as high as 50%,[44] but probably occurs more frequently than previously recognized with an overall lower mortality and morbidity in its milder forms.[45,46] Anticoagulation and work-up for coagulation disorders are usually recommended.

Disease Severity Assessment

Crohn's Disease

The CD activity index (CDAI) is the most frequently used method for quantitating disease severity in CD. It was developed by Best et al.[47] using multiple regression analysis and includes a total of eight items that are measured, multiplied by respective weighting factors, and then summated to yield a score (Table 39-2). It is generally accepted that a total score less than 150 points is quiescent disease, whereas more than 450 is severe, active disease. Relapses are defined as a score increasing to more than 150 or an increase of 100 points over baseline. The CDAI is most frequently used in longitudinal clinical studies to evaluate the results of experimental interventions. It suffers from many deficiencies including its reliance on subjective complaints and that it is time consuming, requiring the patient to keep a diary for 7-day periods defining symptomatology. Some measured symptoms, such as diarrhea and belly pain, may reflect short gut caused by prior surgery or strictures that do not represent active, inflammatory disease.[47] Other indices have been developed in an attempt to address these criticisms. The Harvey Bradshaw index (or modified CDAI) and the Van Hees index, which relies entirely on nine objective factors such as erythrocyte sedimentation rate (ESR), albumin, temperature, and stool consistency are two such measurement tools, but they are infrequently used, even in protocol settings.[48]

The Vienna classification, discussed above, is an attempt to classify or categorize subsets of CD patients and is not used as a severity assessment tool.[35]

Ulcerative Colitis

The benchmark study evaluating the effect of cortisone on UC by Truelove et al.[6] in 1955 also described the still most often used clinical assessment tool for severity assessment in UC (Table 39-3). The simplicity and clinical relevancy of the factors in this index allow for its daily use as a clinical tool and also for clinical response in study protocols. Variations on its initial format have included the creation of a "moderate" category for patients displaying features intermediate in value between the mild and severe categories. This index also does not take into account variability in the anatomic extent or observed severity of disease within the colon. Modern clinical studies requiring disease assessment will thus often use a variation on the Truelove and Witts classification which will include additional criteria based on colonoscopic appearance and possibly pathologic severity as well.[49,50]

TABLE 39-2. The CDAI

Item	Data collected	Calculation	Weighing factor
No. of liquid stools	7-day diary	Sum of 7 days	2
Abdominal pain	0–3 scale, 7-day diary	Sum of score for each day	5
General well-being	0–4 scale, 7-day diary	Sum of score for each day	7
Symptoms*	At clinic visit	Sum (6 total possible)	20
Lomotil use	7-day diary	Yes = 1, No = 2	30
Abdominal mass	At clinic visit	None = 0, questionable = 2, definite = 5	10
Hematocrit (HCT)	At clinic visit	M (47 subtract patient's HCT) F (42 subtract patient's HCT)	6
Weight	At clinic visit	% below ideal weight	1

*Symptoms include presence or absence of each of arthritis/arthralgia, iritis/uveitis, erythema nodosum/pyoderma gangrenosum/aphthous stomatitis, anal fissure/fistula/abscess, other fistula, or temperature >100°F.

TABLE 39-3. Truelove and Witts UC activity index

	Mild	Severe
Bowel frequency/24 hours	<4	>6
Blood in stool	+	+++
Fever	Absent	>37.5
Pulse	<90	>90
Hgb	>75% nL	<75% nL
ESR	<30	>30

Evaluation

Radiology

The diagnosis of IBD depends on the triad of clinical presentation, radiologic work-up, and histopathology of tissue biopsy. Thus, radiologic studies are critical in the evaluation of the patient with suspected or confirmed IBD.

Plain X-rays

Conventional radiologic studies have a significant role in the work-up and management of IBD. Plain abdominal radiographs can show signs of obstruction, perforation (free air), and at times thickening of the bowel or loss of haustral markings. The initial presentation of any patient with belly pain and a known or suspected diagnosis of IBD will incorporate a plain and upright film looking for these signs. On the plain film, air can act as a contrast medium and can allow the identification of the more subtle findings of nodularity of the mucosa suggesting ulceration or pseudopolyp formation. Chronic colitis may result in an ahaustral, tube-like colon that can be seen with air contrast (see Figure 39-1). Fulminant or rapidly worsening colitis may result in toxic dilatation ("toxic megacolon") that mandates surgical intervention and the specific avoidance of colonoscopy or contrast enema studies that may result in perforation. Incidental discoveries of

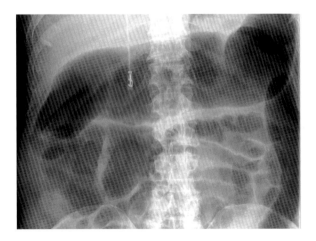

FIGURE 39-1. Plain radiograph of a patient with worsening symptoms of ulcerative colitis. Note the ahaustral left and transverse colon, signs of small bowel ileus and enlarged ("mega") transverse colon.

gallstones or renal calculi that occur with increased incidence in patients with IBD may also be made.

Contrast Radiologic Studies

Contrast studies will more frequently be used in the patient with CD than UC because of its predisposition for small bowel involvement. For the colitic patient, whether caused by CD or UC, colonoscopy is usually the preferred study, frequently obviating the need for barium enema. However, a double-contrast barium enema may still be used to discover or delineate extent of disease in the patient with GI symptoms, especially when caused by CD. Colonic contrast studies in the CD patient can show segmental disease, strictures, and fistulas. Reflux into the terminal ileum occurs in approximately 85% of patients and can reveal ileal disease more effectively than small bowel follow through because of less superposition of intestinal loops. When fistulas or near obstructing strictures are suspected, a water-soluble dye, such as Gastrografin is preferred. This minimizes the complications associated with possible extravasation of the dye if a fistula or intestinal perforation is present or subsequent impaction of barium if passed proximal to a stricture. Not infrequently in the patient with CD, an unsuspected rectal fistula tracking to a diseased terminal ileum is found on rectal contrast study (see Figure 39-3, below). Such a fistula can be easily missed on colonoscopy because it originates with the diseased terminal ileum and the rectum infrequently has other evidence of CD.

The difficulty of reaching the small bowel using fiberoptic instruments results in the common use of small bowel contrast studies to assess the degree of CD involvement of the small bowel. Small bowel series can effectively show areas of stricturing and upstream dilatation but may be difficult to perform or interpret because of slow intestinal transit from strictures, overlying loops of bowel, and pain associated with compression spot views (Figure 39-2). Enteroclysis is preferred over simple small bowel follow through, although its need for the placement of a naso-intestinal tube makes patient cooperation and satisfaction with this study much less. High-density barium must be used as the contrast agent, because water-soluble dyes rapidly dilute out in the small bowel, making detailed assessment of the intestinal mucosa difficult. After placement of the nasal tube beyond the pylorus, relatively small boluses of barium are injected that coat the walls of the intestine and then air is insufflated distending the bowel allowing detailed examination of the mucosa. Repetitive infusions of dye and air, with subsequent spot compression films, can result in remarkable detail being revealed but results are clearly dependent on operator expertise and patient cooperation.

GI contrast studies surpass computed tomography (CT) for detecting enteroenteric and enterocolic fistulas.[51] The discovery of an enteric fistula can be made when orally consumed contrast material is seen in a distal portion of bowel without illuminating intervening intestine, such as can occur with ileal disease fistulizing into the rectum. Sometimes the dye will

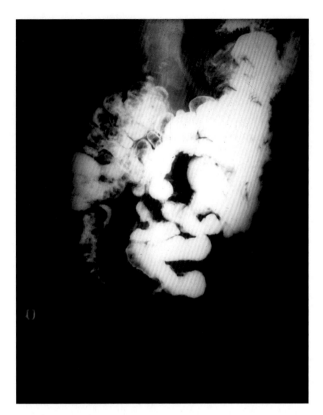

FIGURE 39-2. Small bowel follow through contrast study showing terminal ileal stricturing disease, with displacement of adjacent bowel loops caused by ileal thickening.

directly illuminate the fistula or involved organ, such as the bladder, as it tracks from the bowel, whether the contrast is given orally or rectally (Figure 39-3).

Sinography or fistula-gram can be used to delineate the path or origin of fistulous disease in CD patients, whether involving the abdominal wall or perineum. Such studies can

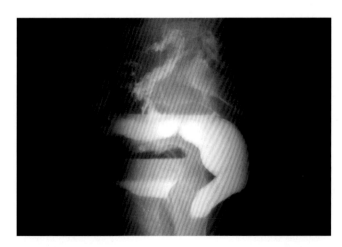

FIGURE 39-3. Colonic contrast study in CD patient showing complex fistulizing disease. Contrast is present in the proximal, diseased ileum and air and contrast in the bladder because of fistulizing disease.

also be done via the drainage catheter after percutaneous drainage of an abscess to document intestinal communication and, again, should be done with water-soluble contrast. Such anatomic localization assists in directing subsequent surgical care (especially when fistulous disease involving the urinary tree is found) and assessing response to therapy.

Retrograde studies through a stoma, especially an ileostomy, can provide very good evaluation for disease. The effectively foreshortened intestine allows better delineation of disease with less overlapping bowel loops and better double-contrast definition.

Computed Tomography

Abdominal and pelvic CT is probably the most frequently obtained study in the acute work-up of patients with IBD, especially CD. Such studies should be done with orally ingested low-density barium or iodinated contrast material that has been allowed to traverse the entire GI tract. Because of strictures or slow transit time, rectal administration of contrast will sometimes be necessary. CT scanning is especially useful for delineating enterovesical or colovesical fistulas and scans should be obtained before administering intravenous contrast, as contrast originating from the bowel will be seen in the bladder defining the fistula. Air within the bladder without prior instrumentation is also a very sensitive sign defining the presence of a fistula.

The great advantage of CT is its ability to look at the entire thickness of the intestine and its adjacent structures. Thus, thickened intestine, phlegmon, abscess, air in extraintestinal structures, and fistula formation are signs of CD that can be found on CT scan (Figure 39-4). Percutaneous drainage of abscess collections done under CT guidance can also be performed. Although less frequently performed for UC, CT findings that can be seen include increased perirectal and presacral fat, inhomogeneous areas of colonic thickening, target or "double halo" sign of the colon, and changes consistent with cancer development such as strictures or mass lesions.[51]

Magnetic Resonance Imaging

Magnetic resonance imaging (MRI) is playing an increasing role in the evaluation of IBD patients. Intestinal CD can be identified simply by thickened bowel loops on conventional MRI. MRI differs from CT, however, in that the intensity of T2-weighted signals from areas of disease correlate with severity of inflammation, especially after gadolinium administration. Such signal intensity in both the mesentery and bowel decreases with resolution of acute inflammation and may hold promise for monitoring the response of patients to medical therapy.[52,53]

MRI's value in defining perineal disease in the CD patient approaches, and may exceed, that achieved with examination under anesthesia.[52,53] Endorectal coil placement may improve

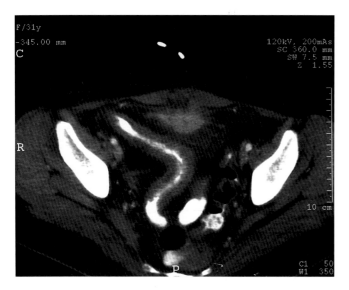

FIGURE 39-4. CT scan of CD patient with severe terminal ileal thickening and early abscess formation under anterior abdominal wall.

sensitivity but is infrequently necessary and sometimes impossible in the diseased anus. Intravenous injection of gadolinium highlights the fistula tract, and combined with MRI's ability to accurately define soft tissue anatomy, can result in remarkable delineation of disease.[54,55] MRI testing is expensive, however, and is probably unnecessary in the conventional perineal CD patient because an examination under anesthesia performed by a competent surgeon is usually as accurate and can also provide simultaneous treatment.[56] However, MRI is finding a role in reassessing the failed patient for unrecognized pathology and, more recently, in defining whether medical treatment with infliximab has truly healed a patient's fistulous disease. Several studies using gadolinium-enhanced MRI have shown that many fistulas that respond to exclusive medical management are, in fact, still present but quiescent.[57,58]

Ultrasound

The role of ultrasound in IBD is presently very limited. European centers are more familiar with its use for assessing the GI tract in IBD patients where it is sometimes used to longitudinally follow a patient's response to therapy. In the hands of an experienced operator, so-called transabdominal bowel sonography (TABS) can look for bowel wall thickening, fistula formation, and can even assess functional effects of strictures by observing bowel peristalsis and distention in the vicinity of such pathology.[59] This method of noninvasive intestinal evaluation has not gained wide popularity in the United States.

Intrarectal ultrasound can be used to document and map perianal fistula formation by injecting a solution of hydrogen peroxide into the external opening. The resulting bubbles are easily seen on ultrasound as they outline the path of the fistula tract. However, such uncomfortable and operator-dependent

techniques of fistula assessment have been largely replaced by MRI scanning (see above).

Nuclear Medicine

The injection of radionuclide-labeled white cells allows subsequent scintigraphic imaging of the abdominal organs and is increasingly being used as a technique to visualize actively inflamed bowel. Most techniques use indium[111] labeling of autologous leucocytes that are harvested from the patient, labeled, and then reinjected. Indium[111] has the advantage of a long half-life that allows scanning at 6, 12, and 24 hours with any visualized bowel activity as being abnormal. A fixed area of activity suggests an abscess. Newer techniques using technetium-99m–hexamethylpropyleneamine oxime (HMPAO) provide for better image quality because of their relatively selective labeling of granulocytes and also result in a lower radiation dose to the patient. Some studies using this tracer have shown very high sensitivity rates, but specificity is less because of its inability to differentiate between IBD and infectious causes of disease.[60] The advantage of such radionuclide scanning techniques relate mostly to their ability to differentiate between inflamed versus quiescent disease and their use will probably increase as newer labeling agents are devised.

Endoscopy

Colonoscopy has strongly influenced the diagnosis and evaluation of the patient with IBD. It is the study of choice for the patient with suspected UC because it can directly visualize the entire extent of the disease process. It is similarly relevant for CD when involving the colon, and can also be used to intubate and evaluate the terminal ileum. Most significantly, colonoscopy provides biopsies, which allows a tissue diagnosis to be made by the pathologist. There are numerous indications for colonoscopy in the IBD patient (Table 39-4) and it has a significant role in both medical and surgical treatment. The gross appearance of the colon as seen on colonoscopy can frequently differentiate between CD and UC (Table 39-5). Its use in the patient with severe disease is controversial. Although studies exist suggesting it can be safely done in the

TABLE 39-4. Indications for colonoscopy in IBD

• Diagnosis:	–Gross appearance
	–Tissue biopsy
• Disease extent	
• Disease complications:	–Fistulas
	–Stricture
	–Bleeding
• Preoperative "staging"	
• Monitor response to therapy	
• Stricture management:	–Biopsy
	–Dilatation
• Cancer surveillance	

TABLE 39-5. Gross (colonoscopic) features of colitis

	UC	CD
Early	Edema	Aphthous ulcers
	Confluent erythema	Patchy, asymmetric erythema
	Loss of vascular markings	Anal disease: Waxy skin tags Linear fissures
Intermediate	Granularity	Linear serpiginous ulcers
	Bleeding	Pseudopolyps
	Micropurulence	Anal disease: Fistulas Abscesses
Advanced/late	Ulcerations, transmural disease	Confluent ulcers
	Pseudopolyp formation	Deep "bear claw" ulcerations
	Purulence	Strictures
	Variable thinning/ thickening of colon	Mucosal bridging
	Mucosal bridging	

severely colitic patient, the risk of perforation caused by insufflation, biopsy, or mechanical bending of the scope is generally acknowledged as being high and thus colonoscopy is generally avoided in the acute setting. However, such severely ill patients still need endoscopic evaluation to rule out concurrent diseases such as pseudomembranous or cytomegalovirus-induced colitis. Rigid or flexible procto-scopic evaluation is thus recommended, with biopsies done in the lower rectum below the peritoneal reflection to minimize the risk of free perforation.

The flexible sigmoidoscope is conveniently used for the evaluation of the unsedated office patient, but is limited by its 65-cm length to visualizing the colon up to approximately the splenic flexure. This can often be adequate, however, and in the case of UC, definitive. In the patient with typical presenting symptoms of bloody diarrhea and tenesmus, a flexible sigmoidoscopy with biopsies and stool culture for pathogens and ova/parasites may complete the work-up and make the diagnosis.

There is an increasing experience with through-the-scope (TTS) pneumatic dilatation of colonic or ileocolonic strictures in CD. The technique incorporates repetitive insufflation of the TTS balloon for 15- to 60-second periods, with the larger balloons (25 mm) being associated with more patient pain and complications than the smaller ones (12 mm). In a prospective study of 55 patients, long-term success (mean follow-up of 34 months) with complete relief of obstructive symptoms was achieved in 62% of patients whereas 19 (38%) required operation and six (11%) suffered a perforation.[61]

Upper endoscopy or esophagogastroduodenoscopy (EGD) will infrequently be used in the management of CD because gastroduodenal CD occurs in less than 5% of patients. When CD does affect the stomach or duodenum, however, strictures are common and therapeutic dilatation and biopsies to evaluate for malignancy via EGD are necessary. More frequently,

EGD is useful in the evaluation of the differential diagnosis of upper abdominal pain or dysphagia in the IBD patient. Esophageal candidiasis brought on by immunosuppression, duodenal or gastric ulcerative disease caused by steroids or reflux disease from downstream partial obstruction all occur with increased frequency in the IBD patient and is well evaluated by EGD. So-called push enteroscopy using specially designed flexible scopes has been developed to improve access by the endoscopist to the jejunum, but its use is very limited. The preferred study for evaluation of small bowel CD is still small bowel contrast follow through or enteroclysis.

Wireless Capsule Endoscopy

Wireless capsule endoscopy (WCE) is a recent unique development for the visualization of the small bowel. An 11×26 mm capsule is swallowed that transmits two video images per second to a receiver worn on the belt. Over the 8-hour battery life of the device, more than 50,000 images are transmitted and stored which are subsequently evaluated at 25 frames per second by dedicated software and the human eye. Subtle small bowel lesions, usually out of the reach of the colonoscope or upper endoscope, can be appreciated. Its role in CD is still being clarified, but criteria for its use include the recommendation of prior colonoscopy and intubation of the terminal ileum. Many studies using WCE have found CD in this most common of regions that can be easily reached by a colonoscope obviating the need for the more expensive WCE. In addition, a small bowel contrast series is also necessary because the size of the capsule may cause it to impact at a stricture precipitating acute bowel obstruction requiring surgery. Other problems include its limited battery life in patients with slow transit, the inability to biopsy, and its imperfect localization of identified lesions. Nonetheless, this technology provides an added and potentially more sensitive tool in the diagnosis and management of patients with CD.[53,62,63]

Pathology

Ulcerative Colitis

UC begins in the rectum and extends proximally a variable distance with the worst disease being distal and the least disease being proximal. Disease may be limited to the rectum (ulcerative proctitis), extend to only the left colon, or completely to the cecum (pancolitis). The terminal ileum may be inflamed in continuity with the cecum (backwash ileitis). Disease is in continuity and segmental or "skip" disease does not occur, although so-called "rectal sparing" or some degree of patchiness can be seen in the actively treated patient, especially when enema therapy has been given. The gross appearance of the inflammatory process depends on the severity and duration of the disease (Table 39-5). In early disease, inflammation is restricted to the mucosa but in its severest, toxic form it can become transmural and indistinguishable grossly and histopathologically from CD, with deep ulcerations, pseudopolyp formation, and variable areas of thickened and thinned colonic wall.

The histopathologic features of UC are listed in Table 39-6. There are no pathognomonic features of UC and in its extreme form it can resemble CD. However, typical UC is associated with inflammation limited to the mucosa or lamina propria including relatively uniform crypt distortion and crypt abscesses. Goblet cell mucin depletion is common and the inflammatory infiltrate is usually neutrophilic, two features that distinguish it from CD where mucin depletion is uncommon and the inflammation is usually mononuclear. More severe UC leads to the entire loss of the crypt with deeper submucosal and transmural inflammation and ulceration. In the chronic, more quiescent phase, UC will have mucosal reconstitution but will still have crypt distortion, foreshortening, and branching. Inflammation will be variably reduced, even absent, but when present still relatively uniform in distribution. Dysplasia in longstanding UC is common but can only be interpreted in the setting of noninflamed bowel, because many of its features are common with inflammation, namely, crypt distortion, increased mitotic index, and nuclear atypia.

Crohn's Disease

The gross features of CD include its ability to affect any portion of the GI tract, its transmural inflammation, and its propensity to create fistulas and strictures, including in the perianal area. Skip lesions are common, resulting in multiple areas of bowel affected simultaneously with intervening segments of normal intestine. Diseased bowel may fistulize into adjacent bowel that is otherwise unaffected, a type of bystander injury that only requires surgical removal of the offending segment of intestine with primary repair of the fistula in the remaining, healthy bowel. Serositis is common in CD, as is fat wrapping or creeping fat, all nonspecific responses to the transmural inflammation seen. On the mucosal surface, the earliest changes are aphthous ulcers, which are tiny white pinpoint lesions representing mucosal ulcerations in the vicinity of enlarged lymphoid follicles. These are thought to then enlarge and coalesce into the larger, deeper, longitudinal serpiginous ulcers often found in CD. These will have a deep, fissuring appearance and will extend ever deeper into the bowel wall, infrequently perforating freely, but instead recruiting an inflammatory response from adjacent organs that tend to wall off the inflamed bowel and that can then lead to fistulization. Healing is associated with granulation tissue and stricture formation, features not usually found in UC.

Microscopically, the inflammatory infiltrate is frequently mononuclear and there is minimal goblet cell dropout in the mucosa. When crypt abscesses occur, they are nonuniform, affecting some crypts and not others. Vasculitis is sometimes seen (20%) and neuronal hyperplasia is common, both features that are rarely seen in UC. The classic noncaseating granuloma is found in 20%–60% of patient biopsies and is composed of epithelioid and giant cells of the Langhans type. Granulomas probably wax and wane in their presence and can also be found in adjacent tissues affected in continuity, such as bladder, lymph nodes, ovaries, and perianal squamous epithelial skin tags. Their significance is unclear, with some suggesting they indicate a less-aggressive form of CD.

Indeterminate Colitis

Approximately 10%–15% of colitis patients will have either clinical or pathologic features that do not allow a clear diagnosis of either CD or UC to be definitively made. This is often attributable to rapidly deteriorating, fulminant colitis, where even UC can have transmural or irregular mucosal involvement. Sometimes the gross anatomic appearance is complicated by incomplete response to various medications, especially when delivered transanally as enemas, which can lead to relative "rectal sparing" and therefore suggest CD over UC. Frequently, the correct diagnosis involves the judgment of an experienced clinician who considers not only the histopathology, but also the clinical characteristics of the patient, the history of disease progression, and even more subtle data such as serum antineutrophil cytoplasmic antibody (ANCA) and ASCA testing (see Serum Tests for IBD). More than half of such indeterminate cases can usually be resolved with such consideration of the entire clinical picture. This is especially important in the patient who is a candidate for pelvic pouch reconstruction, where the results of such surgery are significantly worse in the misdiagnosed Crohn's diseased patient.[64]

TABLE 39-6. Histology of IBD

	UC	CD
Early	Crypt distortion, branching	Patchy crypt distortion
	Goblet cell mucin depletion	Minimal goblet cell mucin depletion
	Vascular congestion (without inflammation)	Aphthoid ulcers
	Mucosal inflammation	
Intermediate	Uniform crypt abscesses	Focal crypt abscesses
	Loss of mucosa with retention of crypts	Vasculitis (20%)
	Lamina propria neutrophils	Noncaseating granulomas (20%–60%)
		Mononuclear cell infiltrate
Advanced/late	Crypt destruction	Transmural inflammation
	Neuronal hyperplasia uncommon	Neuronal hyperplasia common
	Deeper submucosa inflammation	Mucosal and submucosal thickening
	Pseudo polyp, mucosal bridging	Fibrosis and strictures
	Dysplasia common	Dysplasia uncommon

Serum Tests for IBD

Serum tests for IBD can be divided into several categories: acute phase reactants, nutritional parameters, and inflammatory markers. The prototypic acute phase reactant is the ESR, which is frequently used, especially in CD despite its imperfect correlation with disease activity. It is a necessary component to determine the CDAI (see section above). Some have suggested ESR correlates better with colitis, either CD or UC, than small bowel CD. This may be attributable to the fact that ESR may be normal in CD patients with noninflammatory disease who nonetheless may be very symptomatic because of the presence of "burned-out" fibrotic strictures.[65] Conversely, an acute abscess from a longstanding fistula in ano may increase the ESR without any evidence for flaring of intestinal disease. Similar difficulties have been encountered in correlating disease status with other acute phase reactants, such as C-reactive protein (CRP), orosomucoid (α-1-acid glycoprotein), α-1-antitypsin, and α-2-globulin.[66] The fecal excretion of α-1-antitrypsin when measured as a clearance ratio has some correlation to active intestinal disease but difficulty with collection methodology makes this test rarely used. Presently, ESR and CRP are the only two tests frequently used in the clinical arena.

Nutritional parameters are often used to assess the consequence of acute and subacute disease in IBD. Albumin, prealbumin, and iron studies (transferrin, serum iron) are reflective of the combined effects of decreased food intake (to minimize symptoms), compromised absorption (from inflammation or surgical shortening of the bowel), and increased losses (from loss of proteins and blood from mucosal ulceration). B12 is often decreased in CD patients with ileal disease or after surgical resection. Such nutritional tests are nonspecific, but extremely valuable in clinical decision making from either a surgical or medical perspective. Other relevant serum studies include liver function testing that may reveal subclinical PSC.

Research into the immune regulatory pathways that have a role in the inflammation seen in IBD has resulted in the identification of numerous chemokines that are altered in IBD.[48] Many of these, including interleukin (IL)-1, IL-2, IL-6, IL-8, TNF, CD45, soluble IL-2, and interferon-gamma have not been used beyond investigative protocols for a number of reasons. Frequently, serum levels of these cytokines do not correlate with the abnormal levels found in the tissues affected, thus obviating their use as serum tests. A possible exception may be the soluble IL-2 receptor (sIL-2r). Increased serum levels of sIL-2r seem to correlate with mucosal inflammatory activity. Levels decrease with response to therapy in parallel with the CDAI, and high levels have been predictive of clinical relapse.[67]

Perinuclear ANCA (pANCA) is an autoantibody found in the serum of approximately 50%–70% of UC patients but only 20%–30% of CD patients.[68] It does not correlate with disease activity, but is thought to indicate a more aggressive disease type, because of its association with patients who are relatively resistant to medical management and also with patients who frequently suffer pouchitis after ileal pouch anal anastomosis.[69,70] Another serum antibody, that to a common yeast, *Saccharomyces cerevisiae* (ASCA), has been shown to be present in 50%–70% of CD patients but only 10%–15% of UC patients. Thus, the measurement of both ANCA and ASCA is increasingly being used to try to differentiate between CD and UC when disease is limited to the colon and confusing features, such as rectal sparing, exist.

Although strictly speaking not a serum test, there has been the recent discovery of certain genetic mutations as being associated with CD. The presence of these mutations can be assayed using the DNA of leukocytes harvested by peripheral blood draw. Three mutations affecting the *NOD2/CARD15* gene on the short arm of chromosome 16 have been identified as being associated with CD.[33,34] The *NOD2/CARD15* gene codes for an intracellular protein that has high binding affinity for bacterial peptidoglycan and may have a role in innate immunoresponsiveness to enteric bacteria. Mutations in this gene are found in approximately10%–30% of CD patients versus 8%–15% of healthy controls. The relative risk of developing CD if mutations are carried in both copies of this gene is 10–40 times that of the general population. The presence of this mutation in a patient with CD is associated with ileal disease, earlier age of onset, and possibly fibrostenosing characteristics.[29,71] Mutations can be easily assayed by polymerase chain reaction techniques, and holds promise for possibly predicting responsiveness to medical or surgical therapies.

Evaluation of the Acute IBD Patient

The clinical and laboratory evaluation of the presenting IBD patient will depend on many factors. Obviously, a good history and physical examination will focus the clinical caregiver in one or another area that will then direct subsequent testing and care. Many of the testing regimens described previously in this chapter apply to a greater or lesser degree based on clinical circumstances. There is no one good test for IBD, so the clinical judgment, experience, and acumen of the physician is key in patient management. Nonetheless, there are some basic and fundamental testing regimens that should be at least considered, if not repetitively performed, whenever IBD is considered the possible diagnosis. A basic outline of evaluation of the acutely presenting IBD patient is found in Table 39-7. It is important to remember that the patient with a known diagnosis of IBD will frequently still require such a basic work-up whenever their disease flares. This is in part attributable to the recognition that these patients are at significant risk for the development of a superimposed secondary diagnosis not infrequently related to iatrogenic causes. These might include pseudomembranous or cytomegalovirus colitis, stress- or steroid-induced gastric ulceration, fungal sepsis, or neutropenia. In addition, a known IBD patient presenting with worsening symptoms may now have progression of disease or the development of a directly related complication, such as an intraabdominal abscess, bowel obstruction, toxic colitis, or

TABLE 39-7. Evaluation of the IBD Patient

	Test	Purpose
Serum labs	CBC	r/o anemia, leukocytosis
	Electrolytes, renal function	r/o electrolyte disturbance 2° diarrhea, dehydration
	ESR or CRP	↑ in systemic disease
	LFTs, albumin	r/o PSC, nutritional compromise
Stool studies	C. diff.	r/o infectious causes
	O & P	r/o infectious causes
	Pathogens	r/o infectious causes
X-rays	Plain abdominal X-rays	r/o free air, toxic colitis, stones, obstruction
	SBFT / enteroclysis	For small bowel disease
	Barium / Gastrografin enema	For fistulas, strictures, distribution of disease
	CT scan	For abscess, obstruction, fistulas, adjacent organ involvement
Endoscopy	Flexible / rigid scope	For biopsy to r/o CMV, granulomas, pseudomembranes
	Colonoscopy	For biopsy, visualize extent and severity of disease

LFTs: liver function tests
O & P: ova and parasites
C. Diff: Clostridium difficile toxin
SBFT: small bowel follow through
CMV: cytomegalovirus

colovesical fistula. Thus, the studies outlined in Table 39-7 should be regularly considered for the acutely presenting IBD patient, tempered by the good clinical judgment of the caring physician.

References

1. Crohn BB, Ginzburg L, Oppenheimer GD. Regional ileitis. Jour AMA 1932;99:1323–1329.
2. Combe C, Saunders W. A singular case of stricture and thickening of the ileum. Med Trans R Soc Med 1806;16–18.
3. Brooke BN. Granulomatous diseases of the intestine. Lancet 1959;II:745–749.
4. Lockhart-Mummery HE, Morson BC. Crohn's disease (regional enteritis) of the large intestine and its distinction from ulcerative colitis. Gut 1960;1:87–105.
5. Brooke BN. The management of an ileostomy including its complications. Dis Colon Rectum 1993;36:512–516.
6. Truelove SC, Witts LJ, Bourne WA, et al. Cortisone and corticotropin in ulcerative colitis. Br Med J 1959:387–394.
7. Sutherland L, Singleton J, Sesslons J. Double blind, placebo controlled trial of metronidazole in Crohn's disease. Gut 1991;32:1071–1075.
8. Korelitz BI. Immunosuppressive therapy of inflammatory bowel disease: a historical perspective. Gastroenterologist 1995;3(2):141–152.
9. Targan SR, Hanauer SB, van Deventer SJ, et al. A short-term study of chimeric monoclonal antibody cA2 to tumor necrosis factor alpha for Crohn's disease. Crohn's Disease cA2 Study Group. N Engl J Med 1997;337(15):1029–1035.
10. Dennis C. Ileostomy and colectomy in chronic ulcerative colitis. Surgery 1945;18:435–452.
11. Strauss AA, Strauss SF. Surgical treatment of ulcerative colitis. Surg Clin North Am 1944;24:211–224.
12. Kock NG. Intra-abdominal reservoir in patients with permanent ileostomy. Arch Surg 1969;99:223–231.
13. Parks AG, Nicholls RJ. Proctocolectomy without ileostomy for ulcerative colitis. Br Med J 1978;2:85–88.
14. Utsunomiya J. Restorative proctocolectomy for ileal reservoir. Int J Colorectal Dis 1986;1:2–19.
15. Ekbom A, Helmick C, Zack M, et al. The epidemiology of inflammatory bowel disease: a large, population-based study in Sweden. Gastroenterology 1991;100:350–358.
16. Yang SK, Hong WS, Min YI, et al. Incidence and prevalence of ulcerative colitis in the Songpa-Kangdong district, Seoul, Korea. J Gastroenterol Hepatol 2000;15:1037–1042.
17. Sonnenberg A, McCarty DJ, Jacobsen SJ. Geographic variation of inflammatory bowel disease within the United States. Gastroenterology 1991;100:143–149.
18. Loftus EV Jr, Schoenfeld P, Sandborn WJ. The epidemiology and natural history of Crohn's disease in population-based patient cohorts from North America: a systemic review. Aliment Pharmacol Ther 2002;16:51–60.
19. Blanchard JF, Bernstein CN, Wajda A, et al. Small-area variations and sociodemographic correlates for the incidence of Crohn's disease and ulcerative colitis. Am J Epidemiol 2001;154:328–335.
20. Munkholm P, Langholz E, Nielsen OH, et al. Incidence and prevalence of Crohn's disease in the country of Copenhagen 1962–87: a sixfold increase in incidence. Scand J Gastroenterol 1992;27:609–614.
21. Hellers G. Crohn's disease in Stockholm County 1955–1974. A study of epidemiology, results of surgical treatment and long term prognosis. Scand J Gastroenterol 1979;490(suppl):580.
22. Gilat T, Grossman A, Fireman Z, et al. Inflammatory bowel disease in Jews. Front Gastrointest Res 1986;11:135–140.
23. Sonnenberg A. Occupational distribution of inflammatory bowel disease among German employees. Gut 1990;31:1037–1040.
24. Reif S, Klein I, Lubin F, et al. Pre-illness dietary factors in inflammatory bowel disease. Gut 1997;40:754–760.
25. Boyko EJ, Perera DR, Koepsell TD, et al. Coffee and alcohol use and the risk of ulcerative colitis. Am J Gastroenterol 1989;84:530–534.
26. Tanner AR, Raghunath AS. Colonic inflammation and nonsteroidal anti-inflammatory drug administration. An assessment of the frequency of the problem. Digestion 1988;41:116–120.
27. Vessey M, Jewell D, Smith A, et al. Chronic inflammatory bowel disease, cigarette smoking, and use of oral contraceptives: findings in a large cohort study of women of childbearing age. Br Med J (Clin Res Ed) 1986;292:1101–1103.
28. Calkins BM. A meta-analysis of the role of smoking in inflammatory bowel disease. Dig Dis Sci 1989;34:1841–1854.
29. Ahmad T, Armuzzi A, Bunce M, et al. The molecular classification of the clinical manifestations of Crohn's disease. Gastroenterology 2002;122:854–866.
30. Satsangi J, Grootscholten C, Holt H, et al. Clinical patterns of familial inflammatory bowel disease. Gut 1996;38:738–741.
31. Bayless TM, Tokayer AZ, Polito JM II, et al. Crohn's disease: concordance for site and clinical type in affected family members—potential hereditary influences. Gastroenterology 1996;111:573–579.

32. Zhang WJ, Koltun WA. Genetic factors in the etiology and potential management of inflammatory bowel disease. Semin Colon Rectal Surg 2001;12(1):2–8.

33. Hugot JP, Chamaillard M, Zouali H, et al. Association of NOD2 leucine-rich repeat variants with susceptibility to Crohn's disease. Nature 2001;411:559–603.

34. Ogura Y, Bonen DK, Inohara N, et al. A frameshift mutation in NOD2 associated with susceptibility to Crohn's disease. Nature 2001;411:603–606.

35. Gasche C, Scholmerich J, Brynskov J, et al. A simple classification of Crohn's disease: report of the Working Party for the World Congresses of Gastroenterology Vienna 1998. Inflamm Bowel Dis 2000;6:8–15.

36. Louis E, Collard A, Oger AF, et al. Behaviour of Crohn's disease according to the Vienna classification: changing pattern over the course of the disease. Gut 2001;49:777–782.

37. Bernstein CN, Blanchard JF, Rawsthorne P, et al. The prevalence of extraintestinal diseases in inflammatory bowel disease: a population-based study. Am J Gastroenterol 2001;96:1116–1122.

38. Generini S, Giacomelli R, Fedi R, et al. Infliximab in spondyloarthropathy associated with Crohn's disease: an open study on the efficacy of inducing and maintaining remission of musculoskeletal and gut manifestations. Ann Rheum Dis 2004;63(12):1664–1669.

39. Nahar IK, Shojania K, Marra CA, et al. Infliximab treatment of rheumatoid arthritis and Crohn's disease. Ann Pharmacother 2003;37(9):1256–1265.

40. Sheldon DG, Sawchuk LL, Kozarek RA, et al. Twenty cases of peristomal pyoderma gangrenosum: diagnostic implications and management. Arch Surg 2000;135(5):564–568.

41. Powell FC, Schroeter AL, Su WPD, et al. Pyoderma gangrenosum: a review of 86 patients. Q J Med 1985;217:173–186.

42. Poritz LS, Koltun WA. Surgical management of ulcerative colitis in the presence of primary sclerosing cholangitis. Dis Colon Rectum 2003;46(2):173–178.

43. Cohen S. Liver disease and gallstones in regional enteritis. Gastroenterology 1971;60:237–245.

44. Talbot RW, Heppel J, Dozois RR, et al. Vascular complications of inflammatory bowel disease. Mayo Clin Proc 1986;61:140–145.

45. Fichera A, Cicchiello LA, Mendelson DS, et al. Superior mesenteric vein thrombosis after colectomy for inflammatory bowel disease: a not uncommon cause of postoperative acute abdominal pain. Dis Colon Rectum 2003;46(5):643–648.

46. Remzi RH, Fazio VW, Oncel M, et al. Portal vein thrombi after restorative proctocolectomy. Surgery 2002;132(4):655–661.

47. Best WR, Becktel JM, Singleton JW, et al. Development of a Crohn's disease activity index, national cooperative Crohn's disease study. Gastroenterology 1976;70:439–444.

48. Poritz LS, Koltun WA. Techniques of disease activity assessment in Crohn's disease. Semin Colon Rectal Surg 2001;12(1):16–21.

49. Powell-Tuck J, Day DW, Buckell NA, et al. Correlations between defined sigmoidoscopic appearances and other measures of disease activity in ulcerative colitis. Dig Dis Sci 1982;27:533–537.

50. Rutegard I, Ahsgren L, Stenling R, et al. A simple index for assessment of disease activity in patients with ulcerative colitis. Hepatogastroenterology 1990;37:110–112.

51. Carucci LR, Levine MS. Radiographic imaging of inflammatory bowel disease. Gastroenterol Clin North Am 2002;31(1):93–117.

52. Maccioni F, Viscido A, Broglia L, et al. Evaluation of Crohn's disease activity with magnetic resonance imaging. Abdom Imaging 2000;25:219–228.

53. Schreyer AG, Golder S, Seitz J, et al. New diagnostic avenues in inflammatory bowel diseases. Capsule endoscopy, magnetic resonance imaging and virtual enteroscopy. Dig Dis 2003;21(2):129–137.

54. Koelbel G, Schmiedl U, Majer MC, et al. Diagnosis of fistulae and sinus tracts in patients with Crohn disease: value of MR imaging. AJR Am J Roentgenol 1989;152:999–1003.

55. O'Donovan AN, Somers S, Farrow R, et al. MR imaging of anorectal Crohn disease: a pictorial essay. Radiographics 1997;17(1):101–107.

56. Borley NR, Mortensen NJ, Jewell DP. MRI scanning in perianal Crohn's disease: an important diagnostic adjunct. Inflamm Bowel Dis 1999;5(3):231–233.

57. Bell SJ, Halligan S, Windsor AC, et al. Response of fistulating Crohn's disease to infliximab treatment assessed by magnetic resonance imaging. Aliment Pharmacol Ther 2003;17(3):387–393.

58. Van Assche G, Vanbeckevoort D, Bielen D, et al. Magnetic resonance imaging of the effects of infliximab on perianal fistulizing Crohn's disease. Am J Gastroenterol 2003;98(2):332–339.

59. Gasche C, Moser G, Turetschek K, et al. Transabdominal bowel sonography for detection of intestinal complication in Crohn's disease. Gut 1999;44:112–117.

60. Arndt JW, Grootscholten MI, van Hogezand RA, et al. Inflammatory bowel disease activity assessment using technetium-99m-HMPAO leukocytes. Dig Dis Sci 1997;42:387–393.

61. Gevers AM, Couckuyt H, Coremans G, et al. Efficacy and safety of hydrostatic balloon dilation of ileocolonic Crohn's strictures: a prospective long-term analysis. Acta Gastroenterol Belg 1994;57:320–322.

62. Iddan G, Meron G, Glukhovsky A, et al. Wireless capsule endoscopy. Nature 2000;405:417.

63. Fireman Z, Mahajna E, Broide E, et al. Diagnosing small bowel Crohn's disease with wireless capsule endoscopy. Gut 2003;52:390–392.

64. Guindi M, Riddell RH. Indeterminate colitis. J Clin Pathol 2004;57:1233–1244.

65. Camilleri M, Proano M. Advances in the assessment of diseases activity in inflammatory bowel disease. Mayo Clin Proc 1989;64:800–807.

66. Brignola D, Lanfarnchi GA, Campieri M, et al. Importance of laboratory parameters in the evaluation of Crohn's disease activity. J Clin Gastroenterol 1986;8:245–248.

67. Louis E, Belaich J, Kemseke CV, et al. Soluble interleukin-2 receptor in Crohn's disease: assessment of disease activity and prediction of relapse. Dig Dis Sci 1995;40:1750–1756.

68. Cambridge G, Rampton DS, Stevens TR, et al. Anti-neutrophil antibodies in inflammatory bowel disease: prevalence and diagnostic role. Gut 1992;33:668–674.

69. Sandborn WJ, Landers CJ, Tremain WJ, et al. Association of antineutrophil cytoplasmic antibodies with resistance to treatment of left-sided ulcerative colitis: results of a pilot study. Mayo Clin Proc 1996;71:431–436.

70. Sanborn WJ, Landers CJ, Tremain WJ, et al. Antineutrophil cytoplasmic antibody correlates with chronic pouchitis after ileal pouch anal anastomosis. Am J Gastroenterol 1995;90:740–747.

71. Lesage S, Zouali H, Cezard JP, at al. CARD 15/NOD2 mutational analysis and genotype-phenotype correlation in 612 patients with inflammatory bowel disease. Am J Hum Genet 2002;70:845–857.

40
Medical Management of Inflammatory Bowel Disease

Stephen B. Hanauer, Wee-Chian Lim, and Miles Sparrow

Crohn's disease and ulcerative colitis (UC) are chronic inflammatory diseases of the gastrointestinal tract, collectively known as inflammatory bowel disease (IBD). IBD afflicts approximately 1.3 million Americans and seems to be increasing in frequency in many parts of the world,[1] producing chronic relapsing symptoms that are associated with increased morbidity and decreased quality of life. Although its etiopathogenesis is yet to be fully elucidated, it is thought to involve a complex interplay of genetic, environmental, microbial, and immune factors. Since the discovery of sulfasalazine's unanticipated efficacy in UC,[2] numerous agents have been added to the therapeutic "arsenal." Recent advances in our knowledge of the immunopathogenesis of IBD have also opened an exciting new door to biologic therapy. Pharmacotherapy remains the cornerstone of IBD management, with most patients requiring lifelong therapy because of the chronicity of the disease and its typical onset before 30 years of age.[3] Surgery is usually reserved for treating medically refractory disease or specific complications. With the exception of curative proctocolectomy in UC, neither medical nor surgical therapy can offer a cure for IBD. Therefore, the aims of therapy are to control symptoms, improve quality of life, and minimize short- and long-term complications of both the disease and its therapy.

An important principle in the medical therapy of IBD is that there are two phases to treatment: inducing symptomatic remission of active disease and maintaining this remission for the long term. Establishing the anatomic extent and clinical severity of disease is essential to guiding the therapeutic approach. Other important considerations include patient response to previous or current treatment, presence of complications, and side effects of the pharmacologic agents. Tailoring treatment according to the patient's unique needs and preferences has an important role in enhancing treatment adherence, which is crucial to an optimal long-term outcome. Therapeutic strategies continue to evolve with advancing knowledge, and this chapter details the current approach to medical treatment in IBD.

Medical Management of Crohn's Disease

Crohn's disease, a form of chronic idiopathic IBD, is manifested by focal, asymmetric, transmural, and, occasionally, granulomatous inflammation affecting any part of the gastrointestinal tract, from mouth to anus. The incidence in the United States and other Westernized countries is estimated at 5/100,000 with a prevalence of 50/100,000. Although any age group can be affected, diagnosis is usually made in the second and third decades of life.

This section will cover both the induction and maintenance phases of medical treatments for Crohn's disease, with therapeutic strategies organized according to disease severity. Special mention will be made of the role of infliximab, because this has now become standard therapy for management of moderate–severe and fistulizing Crohn's disease. Areas of particular interest to our surgical colleagues will then be discussed including medical management of perianal fistulae, indications for surgery, and medical strategies to reduce postoperative recurrence of Crohn's disease.

Induction Therapy for Crohn's Disease

Mild–Moderate Crohn's Disease

Patients with mild–moderate Crohn's disease are generally ambulatory and tolerate liquid and solid intake. These patients typically do not have severe abdominal tenderness, inflammatory masses, bowel obstruction, weight loss of >10%, and are not manifesting signs of systemic toxicity [e.g., fever (>37.5°C), tachycardia (>90/minute), anemia (<75%) of normal value, an increased erythrocyte sedimentation rate (ESR) (>30 mm/hour)].[4] Aminosalicylates and antibiotics are the mainstay of therapy for mild–moderate Crohn's disease, although the topically acting steroid, budesonide, is increasingly being used as a drug of choice for mild–moderate disease, with minimal side effects.

Sulfasalazine (Azulfidine®) was the first aminosalicylate trialed in the 1970s and 1980s. It was proven to be beneficial over placebo in the treatment of ileocolonic and colonic Crohn's disease when given in doses of 3–6 g daily, with 40%–50% of patients achieving clinical remission.[5] Sulfasalazine, is a compound consisting of sulfapyridine and 5-aminosalicylic acid (5-ASA, also known as mesalamine) attached by an azo bond that is cleaved into the active moiety, 5-ASA and its carrier molecule, sulfapyridine, by colonic bacterial azo-reductases and hence has minimal efficacy in Crohn's disease of the small bowel.[2] Its use is also limited by more side effects at higher doses secondary to the systemic absorption of sulfapyridine. Slow acetylators are more apt to develop intolerance, including headache, nausea, vomiting, and dyspepsia, whereas dose-independent hypersensitivity reactions include fever, rash, pneumonitis, hepatitis, pancreatitis, hemolytic anemia, bone marrow suppression, and reversible sperm abnormalities. Sulfasalazine also impairs folate absorption and patients receiving sulfasalazine should receive daily folic acid (1 mg/day) supplements.

Because of these limitations with sulfasalazine, newer formulations of 5-ASA or mesalamine were developed that minimized side effects and utilized varying drug delivery systems to deliver the active drug intact to the mucosa of the small bowel and colon. Delayed-release formulations of mesalamine include Eudragit-S coated mesalamine (Asacol®) that releases 5-ASA in the terminal ileum and cecum at pH 7, and Eudragit-L–coated mesalamine formulations (Salofalk®, Mesasal®, and Claversal®) that releases in the mid-ileum at pH 6. Pentasa® (a sustained-release formulation of mesalamine microgranules enclosed within a semipermeable membrane of ethylcellulose) is designed for controlled release throughout the small and large intestine, beginning in the duodenum. Newer azo-bonded formulations designed for release in the colon include the 5-ASA dimer, olsalazine (Dipentum®), and balsalazide (Colazal®), which is composed of 5-ASA molecules azo-bonded to 4-aminobenzoyl-β alanine. Mesalamine in doses of 3.2–4.0 g daily is well tolerated and has been successful in inducing remission in 40%–50% of patients with mild–moderate Crohn's disease. However, results of clinical trials have produced conflicting results, and there have been no adequately powered trials to date comparing mesalamine with sulfasalazine in Crohn's disease.[6] The use of rectal mesalamine, although frequently used for left-sided Crohn's disease, is not supported by evidence from clinical trials.

Antibiotics are an alternative first-line therapy in mild–moderate Crohn's disease, and seem to work better in patients with colonic rather than small bowel disease. Metronidazole, when compared with sulfasalazine in a crossover trial, had initial similar efficacy, although more patients who failed sulfasalazine therapy responded when "crossed over" to metronidazole than vice versa.[7] Side effects to metronidazole include a metallic taste, and most importantly peripheral neuropathy that can be irreversible, when administered long term in doses of >1 g/day.[8]

A more effective and possibly better-tolerated alternative to metronidazole is ciprofloxacin in doses of 1 g daily. Trials using this dose show it to be equally efficacious to mesalamine, 4 g/day, with approximately 50% of the patients entering clinical remission.[9] In uncontrolled trials, combinations of ciprofloxacin and metronidazole have yielded superior results to using either agent alone.[10,11]

Controlled-release oral budesonide is the only Food and Drug Administration (FDA)-approved agent for treating mild–moderate Crohn's disease involving the ileum or right colon. Budesonide is a more potent glucocorticoid than prednisolone, but has a hepatic first-pass metabolism of 90% such that only 10% reaches the systemic circulation; thus, steroid side effects are greatly minimized.[12] When administered for 8–12 weeks at a dose of 9 mg/day, budesonide led to a higher remission rate than mesalamine, 4 g/day (69% versus 45%), but when compared with conventional corticosteroids the results are conflicting.[13] In a recent metaanalysis of trials comparing budesonide to conventional corticosteroids, budesonide was slightly less effective than prednisone, but was associated with significantly fewer steroid side effects. For a subgroup of patients with ileocecal disease, however, budesonide induced remission in 65%–75% of patients.[12]

Regardless of the treatment strategy chosen, response to therapy should be evaluated after several weeks; 8–16 weeks of therapy may be needed for maximal benefits. Patients achieving remission should be considered for maintenance treatment; treatment failures should be offered an alternative first-line therapy or considered for treatment options offered to patients with moderate–severe Crohn's disease.

Moderate–Severe Crohn's Disease

Patients with moderate–severe Crohn's disease have either failed therapy for mild–moderate disease, or have significant systemic toxicity symptoms including fever, weight loss of >10%, abdominal pain and tenderness, nausea and vomiting without bowel obstruction, or significant anemia.[4] The treatment options for these patients include corticosteroids (prednisone or budesonide), infliximab, and at a relatively early stage, immunomodulator therapy with either thiopurines or methotrexate. Antibiotics may also be used for moderate–severe disease, but only for infectious complications such as abscesses, fistulae, or when used in conjunction with surgical drainage procedures. In patients for whom steroids are either ineffective or contraindicated, infusions of infliximab can provide an alternative therapy.

Corticosteroids are the mainstay of therapy in moderate–severe Crohn's disease and clinical trials with prednisone at doses of 40–60 mg daily for 8–12 weeks have achieved remission in 50%–70% of patients.[5] In clinical practice, prednisone is usually initiated at 40 mg daily and is continued at this dose until remission has been achieved—usually within 7–28 days. Subsequently, prednisone is tapered by 5–10 mg weekly until patients are on 20 mg, and then by 2.5–5 mg weekly from 20 mg until it is discontinued.[14]

Corticosteroids are neither safe nor effective as maintenance therapy[15] and therefore, once steroids are initiated, maintenance strategies must be simultaneously devised. In patients with moderately severe ileal or ileocolonic Crohn's disease, budesonide 9 mg daily is an effective first-line alternative to prednisone. Treatment failures are usually switched to a conventional corticosteroid.

More than 50% of patients with moderate–severe Crohn's disease who are initially treated with steroids will become steroid dependent or steroid resistant, and may require therapy with an immunomodulator. Patients who smoke and those with colonic disease are particularly at risk; adjunctive treatment strategies usually are needed.[16] No demonstrable benefit has been shown in these patients when combining 5-ASA therapy with steroid therapy.[17]

In recent years, steroid-dependent or refractory patients have been treated with the thiopurines—azathioprine (AZA) (2–2.5 mg/kg daily) or 6-mercaptopurine (6-MP) (1–1.5 mg/kg daily), although dose-response studies for these agents have not been performed.[18] Recently, genetic polymorphisms of thiopurine methyltransferase, the primary enzyme metabolizing 6-MP, have been identified that may allow clinicians to more accurately monitor and dose these medications according to measurements of the metabolites 6-thioguanine and 6-methylmercaptopurine.[19] Prospective studies to assess the value of this therapeutic monitoring have not been performed.[20] The use of thiopurines in moderate–severe active Crohn's disease is limited by their slow onset of action—3–4 months; however, their addition to steroid therapy has been shown to increase remission rates and to allow steroid-sparing.[18] Patients on thiopurines require regular complete blood counts to monitor for leukopenia; these should be performed every 1–2 weeks initially, and then every 3 months once doses are stabilized. Despite previous concerns, there is no increased risk of lymphoproliferative disorders with the thiopurines and they are considered safe during pregnancy.[21]

Parenteral methotrexate, in a dose of 25 mg weekly either subcutaneously or intramuscularly, is an alternative steroid-sparing agent for patients with moderate–severe Crohn's disease. Parenteral methotrexate has been shown to induce remissions and to be steroid sparing.[22] Nausea and asymptomatic mild increases of liver function tests are the most frequently encountered side effects; more serious side effects such as leukopenia and hypersensitivity pneumonitis are seen only rarely. Patients taking methotrexate should be counseled to avoid alcohol, and this drug is absolutely contraindicated in pregnancy.

Infliximab is a chimeric monoclonal antibody to tumor necrosis factor, and is indicated for the induction and maintenance of moderate–severe Crohn's disease patients who are not responding to corticosteroids and immunomodulators.[23] Infliximab is also effective at reducing the number of draining fistulae in patients with fistulizing Crohn's disease.[24]

Emerging indications for infliximab include maintenance therapy for luminal[25] and fistulizing disease,[26] steroid-sparing in steroid-dependent patients, early use in hospitalized patients when rapid amelioration of symptoms is desired, and to curtail some of the extraintestinal manifestations of Crohn's disease.[27]

Generally, infliximab is started at 5 mg/kg for both induction and maintenance therapy of moderate–severe Crohn's disease; some patients in the maintenance phase may require an increased dose of 10 mg/kg. A three-dose induction regimen of infliximab given at 0, 2, and 6 weeks has been found to be the optimal dosing strategy for several reasons.[28] First, a three-dose induction regimen is at least as good as, if not superior to, a single-dose induction regimen. Second, a three-dose induction regimen may be beneficial and allow patients to develop an immunologic tolerance to infliximab. As a result, this regimen may reduce the formation of antibodies to infliximab (previously known as human anti-chimeric antibodies—HACA), and reduce subsequent acute infusion reactions or delayed hypersensitivity reactions, both of which are at least in part related to these antibodies. In the United States, the FDA-approved recommended dose is 5 mg/kg given at 0, 2, and 6 weeks as an induction regimen. Reinfusion every 8 weeks is necessary to maintain response in most patients and is recommended to help reduce the formation of antibodies to infliximab.

Concurrent immunomodulator therapy with AZA, 6-MP, or methotrexate may also improve outcome by reducing the formation of antibodies to infliximab or reducing the incidence of acute infusion reactions or delayed hypersensitivity reactions; most evidence to support this hypothesis is only anecdotal. Given the risk of reactivation of latent tuberculosis, all patients should be screened for tuberculosis with tuberculin skin testing (and chest X-ray if skin testing is positive) before initiating therapy with infliximab.[27]

Severe–Fulminant Crohn's Disease

Patients with severe or fulminant Crohn's disease have ongoing symptoms despite oral steroids or infliximab given as an outpatient and present with high fever, cachexia, persistent vomiting, or may have evidence of an intestinal obstruction or an abscess. These patients almost always require hospital admission and resuscitation with intravenous fluids. Patients with clinical signs of a bowel obstruction or an abscess require an urgent surgical consultation, and intravenous antibiotics should be administered immediately, especially if sepsis is suspected. If sepsis can be excluded, then high-dose intravenous steroids should be started at doses equivalent to 40–60 mg of prednisone by either divided doses or continuous infusion. If patients do not respond to steroids within 5–7 days, alternative therapies such as infliximab, cyclosporine (CSA), or tacrolimus can be considered. Currently, there is no evidence base to support the use of these agents in this setting other than anecdotal experience.

Responders to parenteral steroids or CSA are then transitioned to an equivalent oral dose, whereas those failing medical treatments require surgery.[4]

Management of Perianal Crohn's Disease

Perianal complications of Crohn's disease include ischiorectal abscesses and perianal fistulae, and often require surgical intervention.[29] Abscesses require surgical drainage with or without the placement of setons, whereas fistulae should be treated at least initially with medical therapy including antibiotics, immunomodulators, or infliximab. Asymptomatic, nondraining fistulae can be safely observed without treatment once coexisting sepsis has been excluded. Initial medical treatment of abscesses should be with the antibiotics metronidazole or ciprofloxacin. Metronidazole in doses of 10–20 mg/kg is effective in reducing or stopping fistula drainage, although it seems that continuous therapy is needed to avoid recurrence, and side effects may be troublesome, especially peripheral neuropathy. In such cases, ciprofloxacin 500 mg per os twice a day is a reasonable alternative, or the two antibiotics can be given as combination therapy.[30,31]

The next line of treatment for perianal disease should be with an immunosuppressant agent such as AZA, 6-MP, CSA, or tacrolimus. Steroids have no role in perianal Crohn's disease. There are no long-term controlled trials assessing the thiopurines for perianal disease, although anecdotal success has been reported in some 40%–50% patients. Intravenous CSA is particularly potent; however, symptoms recur as soon as patients are begun on oral CSA.[32] Similarly, oral tacrolimus is effective, but is also associated with significant nephrotoxicity at effective doses.[33]

The role of infliximab in perianal Crohn's disease deserves special mention. In a placebo-controlled trial, patients who had previously not responded to antibiotics, steroids, or immunomodulators were given 5 mg/kg infliximab at 0, 2, and 6 weeks. Of these patients, 68% had a positive clinical response defined as a reduction by half the number of draining fistulae, and 55% had cessation of draining of all fistulae. The average duration of closure of fistulae was 12 weeks,[24] although maintenance therapy to prevent recurrent drainage or abscess has been demonstrated to be efficacious in the same manner as for luminal disease.[26] Patients receiving infliximab for perianal fistulae may benefit from temporary setons to ensure that recurrent abscess formation is prevented.

Maintenance Therapy for Crohn's Disease

Once remission has been achieved, the aim of therapy must now turn to maintaining this symptomatic improvement. Whereas corticosteroid therapy is successful in inducing remission in the majority of patients, it has no role as maintenance therapy in Crohn's disease, and carries the risk of steroid dependence.[15]

After a medically induced remission with corticosteroids, there is no evidence that aminosalicylates are effective in maintaining remission, unlike in UC.[17] In contrast, the thiopurines—AZA (2–2.5 mg/kg) and 6-MP (1–1.5 mg/kg)—have been proven to be steroid sparing and to maintain medically induced remission.[34] Although the optimal dose and duration of therapy are yet to be defined, maintenance benefits have been proven for up to 4 years of therapy.[35] For patients who have responded to 25 mg/week methotrexate as induction therapy, maintenance benefits using a lower dose of 15 mg/week have been demonstrated, with almost two-thirds of patients maintaining a steroid-free remission at 1 year.[36] Patients on either the thiopurines or methotrexate require regular monitoring of blood counts and liver enzymes[37]; hence, only reliably compliant patients should be chosen for these therapies. The evidence base for maintenance infliximab therapy is rapidly expanding. In a large, multicenter randomized, controlled trial involving 573 patients, those patients receiving 5 or 10 mg/kg infliximab every 8 weeks after a three-dose induction regimen at 0, 2, and 6 weeks were more likely to maintain a steroid-free remission at 30 and 54 weeks than those who did not receive maintenance infliximab therapy.[25]

Indications for Surgery in Crohn's Disease

Unlike UC, surgery for Crohn's disease is not curative, and yet is required in up to two-thirds of patients at some stage of their course to improve symptoms and quality of life. The most common indications for surgery are medically refractory disease, to avoid medication side-effects, or to treat complications of disease such as hemorrhage, perforation, obstruction, or abscess.[4] Although surgical resection is usually done, the disease predictably recurs at the anastomotic site, and stricturoplasty is a reasonable surgical alternative if previous small bowel resections place the patient at risk of short bowel syndrome. Any patient who fails to respond to 7–10 days of intensive inpatient management should be strongly considered for surgery. (See Chapter 42 for surgical management of Crohn's disease).

Postoperative Prophylaxis for Crohn's Disease

Postoperative disease recurrence at 1 year after first resection for Crohn's disease is seen endoscopically in 60%–80% of patients and clinically in 10%–20%, with smoking being the strongest predictive factor for recurrence.[38] Luminal factors also seem to be responsible for disease recurrence, as fecal diversion prevents recurrence, only for it to recur once continuity is reestablished.[39] Hence, there has been increasing interest in medical therapies given postoperatively to delay disease recurrence.[40] Most studies are small and short-term, and have given conflicting results. Aminosalicylates and metronidazole have both been proven to reduce postoperative recurrence in certain subgroups of patients, particularly those with isolated ileal disease. A metaanalysis of six trials evaluating mesalamine at various doses for this purpose showed that the risk reduction for endoscopic recurrence was 18% and for clinical recurrence was 10%, although no dose response was established.[41] Metronidazole (20 mg/kg) given for just 3 months from the time of ileal resection reduced clinical relapse versus placebo at 1 year from 25% to 4%, although many patients would have difficulty managing such high doses of the drug for longer periods.[2,42] Similarly, ornidazole administered for 12 months can also reduce endoscopic and clinical recurrences but, unfortunately, also is poorly tolerated by many patients. More recently, giving 6-MP 50 mg daily has been shown to be more effective than either mesalamine or placebo at reducing relapse; larger trials are needed to further validate these results.[43]

Thus, at present, there are no consistent recommendations regarding medical therapy after surgical resection for Crohn's disease. Many patients with longstanding strictures have a good postoperative prognosis, whereas patients with rapid progression of perforating complications and smokers have a worse prognosis. All patients should be advised to stop smoking. The choice of a specific postoperative recommendation requires some estimate of the patient's risk of recurrence as well as a thorough discussion with the patient regarding risks and benefits of medical therapy attempting to reduce the risk of clinical disease recurrence.

Medical Management of UC

In contrast to Crohn's disease, UC is characterized by diffuse mucosal inflammation that is limited to the colon. It invariably affects the rectum, and may extend proximally in a diffuse, continuous, circumferential pattern to involve part or all of the large intestine. The incidence is estimated at 2–14/100,000 person-years, affecting approximately 690,000 individuals in the United States, with a peak incidence in the third decade of life.[1]

This section will discuss the induction and maintenance phases of medical treatments for UC, with therapeutic strategies organized according to disease severity. Similar to Crohn's disease, the clinical goals for UC are to induce and maintain remission. The anatomic extent and clinical severity of disease help guide the therapeutic approach.

Induction Therapy for UC

Patients with UC typically present with bloody diarrhea, rectal urgency, and tenesmus. The primary goal of therapy is to induce clinical remission and promote mucosal healing.[14] Clinical remission is achieved when the inflammatory symptoms of diarrhea, bleeding, passage of mucopus, tenesmus, and urgency resolve, and with patients' renewed ability to distinguish gas from feces. In endoscopic remission, there is regeneration of an intact mucosa with a visible submucosal vascular pattern, without ulceration, significant friability, or granularity. Pseudopolyps, mucosal bridging, and areas of "atrophic mucosa" with distorted vasculature represent previous episodes of severe inflammation. Histologically, remission is characterized by the absence of neutrophils in the epithelial crypts, although it is not customary to perform biopsies to confirm histologic remission.[44]

Clinical remission usually precedes endoscopic healing, which usually precedes histologic remission. To successfully begin maintenance therapy, it is imperative to achieve clinical remission; failure to do so virtually guarantees a relapse, with the need to reinstitute intensive and sometimes more aggressive inductive treatment. It has also been demonstrated that failure to achieve endoscopic remission and the presence of residual polymorphonuclear leukocytes in the epithelial crypts are predictors of disease relapse.[45]

Therapies for inducing remission are based on the anatomic extent of disease and clinical severity. Proctitis and distal colitis refer to inflammation limited to below the splenic flexure, and thus amendable to the reach of topical and oral therapy. In extensive disease, the inflammation extends proximal to the splenic flexure and requires systemic medication. Supplementary topical therapy is often beneficial to treat prominent rectal symptoms of urgency or tenesmus. Disease severity is classified as mild, moderate, severe, or fulminant. Patients with mild disease have less than four stools daily, with or without blood, no systemic signs of toxicity, and a normal ESR. Moderate disease is characterized by features of both mild and severe disease. Severe disease is characterized by more than six bloody stools per day, abdominal tenderness with signs of systemic toxicity including fever (>37.5°C), tachycardia (>90/minute), anemia (<75% of normal value), and an increased ESR (>30 mm/hour). Fulminant colitis is manifested by more that 10 bloody stools per day, anemia requiring transfusion, signs of systemic toxicity, abdominal distension, and tenderness.[46] For patients with mild–moderate UC, oral and/or topical mesalamine is the mainstay of therapy, whereas topical corticosteroids may be useful in those with distal disease. Oral corticosteroids are reserved for those with moderate–severe disease and for those who did not respond to optimized doses of oral 5-ASA and topical therapies. Patients with severe colitis or those refractory to maximal oral and topical doses of corticosteroids and 5-ASA should be treated with intravenous corticosteroids. Failure to show significant improvement with intravenous corticosteroids is an indication for intravenous CSA, infliximab or a curative colectomy.

Mild–Moderate Proctitis

From a management standpoint, it is best to separate patients with proctitis from those with distal colitis. Although both are amendable to topical therapy, the choice of a topical pharmacologic agent is guided by the proximal extent of disease. Patients with proctitis have disease limited to the rectum, allowing effective topical therapy with suppositories. Mesalamine suppositories 1–1.5 g/day (Canasa®) either nightly or in divided doses are highly effective for proctitis up to 20 cm, and superior to oral 5-ASA therapy[47] and to topical corticosteroids. The proportion of patients achieving remission increases with the duration of treatment and is not dose dependent. Response is usually seen within 2–3 weeks, with higher response rates (63%–79%) at 4–6 weeks.[48] In patients not responding to rectal mesalamine alone, combination therapy with a topical corticosteroid (foam or enema) is better than either therapy alone.[49] Oral mesalamine may be given to those patients failing topical therapies or as an alternative for those who are unable to tolerate topical therapy, but higher dose regimens are usually required. Systemic corticosteroids are rarely required in patients with ulcerative proctitis and should only be reserved for patients with severe or refractory disease.

Mild–Moderate Distal Colitis

Topical 5-ASA is the treatment of choice for patients with distal colitis and achieves higher response rates than topical corticosteroids or oral 5-ASA therapy. Remission rates increase with the duration of therapy (63%–72% after 4 weeks) and are independent of dose; there are no apparent advantages of giving doses greater than 1 g/day.[48] Treatment is initiated with nightly mesalamine enema 4 g/60 mL (Rowasa®) administered at bedtime. Although topical 5-ASA is the most effective therapy for distal colitis, compliance may be difficult. Generally, mesalamine suppositories are easier to retain because of their smaller volume and more viscous state. Retention of mesalamine enemas is more difficult and may be associated with leakage and occasional abdominal discomfort. Mesalamine gel and foam formulations are easier to retain, but are not available in the United States. If enema retention is problematic for patients, loperamide (Imodium®) may be taken before enema administration to reduce rectal urgency and improve anal sphincter tone. Alternatively, initial therapy with mesalamine suppositories will allow for rapid improvement of rectal inflammation and improve ability to retain enemas. Smaller volume enemas (30 mL), that are easier to retain, may also be used to reach the upper rectum, reserving higher volume suspensions (60 mL) for more proximal spread up to the splenic flexure.

If a response is not seen within 2–4 weeks, an additional mesalamine enema or suppository may be added in the morning. Alternatively, combination therapy of mesalamine enemas at night and morning topical corticosteroids [e.g., hydrocortisone foam: 80 mg per application (Cortifoam®), or enema 100 mg/60 mL (Cortenema®)] may be considered, which is superior to either therapy alone.[50] The systemic bioavailability of rectally administered hydrocortisone approaches 80% because of low first-pass hepatic inactivation, and absorption tends to increase as colonic inflammation is reduced. Therefore, steroid-related side effects may begin to manifest after 2–4 weeks of treatment.

Newer formulations of corticosteroids, such as budesonide, are another therapeutic option to treat mild–moderate distal colitis. Their high first-pass hepatic metabolism markedly reduces systemic bioavailability, endogenous cortisol suppression,[51] and thus reduces the potential for steroid-induced side effects. A metaanalysis showed that budesonide enemas (2 mg/100 mL, Entocort® enema) are as effective and offer an alternative to conventional topical corticosteroids.[52] 5-ASA enemas have achieved higher clinical remission rates than budesonide enemas although both had similar endoscopic and histologic outcomes.[53] Because the budesonide enema formulation is not available in the United States, our approach is to add budesonide 2 mg tablet into the mesalamine suspensions for night-time administration. Similarly, a compounding pharmacist can produce a combination of 2 mg budesonide/500 mg mesalamine suppository for nightly or twice daily use in proctitis.

A small proportion of patients have mesalamine hypersensitivity. They may demonstrate worsening of rectal bleeding and urgency with rectal mesalamine, usually within 3–5 days of administration. In patients with mesalamine hypersensitivity, rectal mesalamine should be discontinued, which usually provides symptomatic relief within 72 hours. Treatment with topical corticosteroids is usually effective in achieving remission in this group of patients.

For patients with mild–moderate colitis who are not responding to topical mesalamine (with or without topical corticosteroid), oral mesalamine may be added as combination therapy and is superior to either oral or topical therapies alone.[54] For those who are unable to tolerate or refuse topical therapy, oral mesalamine is an effective alternative for inducing remission. However, it is not as efficacious as topical therapy because of "right-sided constipation" in patients with distal colitis, resulting in decreased 5-ASA delivery to the diseased left colon. Oral corticosteroids are reserved for patients failing the aforementioned therapy.

Mild–Moderate Extensive UC

When a patient has mild–moderate extensive UC, inflammation extends beyond the reach of topical therapy and oral pharmacologic therapy is required. Oral sulfasalazine or one of the newer 5-ASA formulations is the treatment of choice. In clinical trials, response rates with oral 5-ASA are similar for patients with distal and extensive colitis. Sulfasalazine achieves remission in 64%–80% of patients, at dosages of 2–6 g/day. There is a dose response for sulfasalazine, with larger doses achieving higher remission rates. Unfortunately, as many as 30%–40% patients are unable to tolerate higher therapeutic doses because of systemic absorption of the sulfapyridine conjugate. Patients on sulfasalazine should also receive daily folic acid (1 mg/day) supplementation because of inhibition of folate absorption.

As mentioned previously, the development of sulfa-free 5-ASA delivery forms have enabled clinicians to deliver larger amounts of the active moiety without the dose-limiting systemic toxicity. Effectiveness of these newer 5-ASA formulations to induce remission in mild–moderate extensive UC has been confirmed in a recent metaanalysis.[55] Clinical improvement or remission can be achieved in as many as 84% of patients with Asacol® (2.4–4.8 g/day), Salofalk®, Claversal®, Mesasal® (1.5–3 g/day), Pentasa® (2–4 g/day), olsalazine (1–3 g/day), and balsalazide (6.75 g/day). All of the newer 5-ASA formulations have similar pharmacokinetic profiles, are therapeutically equivalent[56] and have similar efficacy to sulfasalazine when equimolar doses are used (1 g sulfasalazine = 400 mg mesalamine = 1.125 g balsalazide) and a dose response is similarly observed. Patients who do not respond to the lower therapeutic dose range within a few weeks should receive doses at the upper end. Adding topical mesalamine or a topical steroid can be a useful adjunct and can help alleviate troublesome rectal symptoms.

The newer 5-ASA formulations are well tolerated and hypersensitivity reactions are rare. Cases of pneumonitis, pericarditis, pancreatitis, and idiosyncratic nephritis have been reported. About 80% of sulfasalazine-intolerant patients will tolerate mesalamine. Up to 30% of patients on olsalazine have worsening of diarrhea resulting from increased ileal secretion, and this dose-related phenomenon usually improves as the colitis heals. However, mesalamine can rarely cause hypersensitivity colitis, which is manifested by worsening diarrhea when 5-ASA therapy is initiated.

Patients with mild–moderate extensive UC not responding to optimal doses of oral mesalamine (with or without topical mesalamine) and those with more severe but nontoxic systemic symptoms will require the addition of oral corticosteroids. Prednisone at doses of 40–60 mg/day is usually initiated and is effective within 1–2 weeks. Oral prednisone demonstrates a dose-response effect between 20–60 mg; 60 mg is only modestly more effective than 40 mg at the expense of greater side effects.[57] Once remission has been achieved, the dose can be tapered by 5–10 mg every week until the patient is on 20 mg, and then tapered by 2.5–5 mg every week thereafter, while maintaining remission with 5-ASA therapy.

Severe UC

Patients with severe colitis that is refractory to maximal oral treatment with prednisone, 5-ASA, and topical medications should be hospitalized for further management. Initial patient evaluation should include blood tests for hematology, a metabolic panel, and total cholesterol level. An infectious process should be ruled out by stool analysis for ova, parasites, and *Clostridium difficile* toxin, fecal culture and sensitivity, and a rectal biopsy for cytomegalovirus.[58] Indiscriminate use of nonsteroidal antiinflammatory drugs (NSAIDs), anticholinergic agents, and antimotility (e.g., loperamide, diphenoxylate) should be avoided because of the potential of worsening colitis or inducing toxic megacolon.

The mainstay of treatment for severe colitis is parenteral corticosteroids in daily doses equivalent to 300 mg hydrocortisone or 48 mg methylprednisolone. There seems to be no added benefit to using higher daily doses of steroids. Rectal corticosteroids may be added as adjunctive therapy for those who are able to tolerate and retain enemas, although no controlled studies have confirmed any incremental benefit. There are no data concerning the efficacy of 5-ASA in severe colitis and these may be discontinued, particularly in patients who were recently started on this therapy.

In the original Oxford experience, patients were treated with bowel rest, IV steroids, antibiotics, and rectal steroids for 5–7 days, and then assessed for response. Bowel rest and total parenteral nutrition (TPN) alone have minimal benefit as primary therapy for acute severe UC.[59] Nutritional support should be provided for severely malnourished patients with the recognition that enteral nutrition has the benefit of fewer complications compared with TPN. If patients are nauseated or vomiting, parenteral nutrition may be required. The routine use of antibiotics has been shown to have no primary, therapeutic benefit in the treatment of severe UC; however, most experienced centers administer broad-spectrum antibiotics to patients with fulminant or anticipated transmural disease.[60,61]

Patients with signs of transmural and fulminant colitis (fever, leukocytosis, abdominal tenderness, "thumbprinting" on abdominal radiograph) who are at risk of toxic megacolon and perforation should be placed on bowel rest and started on broad-spectrum antibiotics. Abdominal radiograph should be done to assess for colonic dilation and to look for free air. Narcotics and anticholinergics, which may worsen colonic atony and dilation, must be avoided. Because the failure rate of medical therapy in hospitalized severe UC patients approaches 40%, they should also be followed closely by an experienced surgeon. Patients failing to respond to 7 days of intravenous corticosteroids are unlikely to benefit from prolonging this treatment and should either be considered for intravenous CSA or referred for surgery.[62]

Patients with toxic megacolon are managed as above. In addition, the gastrointestinal tract should be decompressed with the insertion of a nasogastric tube and a rectal tube. Other maneuvers, such as assisting the patient to roll from a supine to prone position every 2 hours and a knee-elbow position, may help redistribute gas to the distal colon and rectum, and aid in the expulsion of bowel gas. These patients should be monitored closely in the intensive care unit for any signs of deterioration. Serial abdominal radiographs are usually reviewed every 12 hours and electrolyte abnormalities, such as hypokalemia that may aggravate colonic dysmotility, are treated aggressively. Medical therapy may avoid the need for surgery in up to two-thirds of patient cases.[63] Failure to improve within 72 hours is an indication for surgery; any clinical, laboratory, or radiologic deterioration on medical therapy mandates an immediate colectomy.

Intravenous CSA is an effective "rescue" therapy for severe steroid-refractory UC and acts as a bridge to maintenance therapy with the slower-acting thiopurines, AZA or 6-MP.[64] Patients who are noncompliant, have a history of inadequately controlled seizures or active infection should not be treated with CSA. Hypocholesterolemia (serum cholesterol <120 mg/dL) and hypomagnesemia (serum magnesium <1.5 mg/dL) significantly increase the risk of seizures in patients treated with CSA. Whereas hypomagnesemia can be corrected promptly, cholesterol levels are far more difficult to correct, and should be checked early in potential candidates for intravenous CSA.

Before initiating therapy, the risks and benefits of CSA therapy should be reviewed in detail with the patient and an introductory meeting with the surgeons initiated. While continuing intravenous steroids, CSA is started as a continuous infusion of 2–4 mg/kg daily. A recent study confirmed the efficacy of low-dose CSA, which improves its toxicity profile.[65] CSA serum levels are obtained every 48 hours, with a target therapeutic level of 200–400 ng/mL [measured via high-performance liquid chromatography (HPLC)]. Daily inquiries should be made regarding symptoms of CSA toxicity such as paraesthesia, tremors, headache, and nausea. Blood pressure must be monitored and hypertension adequately controlled with a calcium channel blocker. Serum electrolytes are also monitored for CSA-induced nephrotoxicity, hyperkalemia, and hypomagnesemia, and careful attention given to any evidence of infection, especially at central venous catheter sites. Clinical improvement is generally seen within 4–5 days of initiating CSA treatment. Patients who have not demonstrated a significant improvement within 7 days of intravenous CSA therapy, or whose condition deteriorates during CSA therapy, are candidates for surgery.[66]

Most recently, infliximab has been used in patients with refractory[67] or steroid-resistant[68] UC. Two large trials, ACT I and ACT 2, have demonstrated efficacy of infliximab dosed at 5 mg/kg at 0, 2, 6 weeks and then every 8 weeks in moderate–severe UC (Sandborn and Rutgeerts, in press) and as a single dose for severe UC to prevent colectomy (Janerot, in press). The ultimate positioning of infliximab for UC remains to be determined.

Maintenance Therapy for UC

The second goal of therapy in UC is to sustain the symptomatic improvement of a clinical remission. Clinical remission is achieved when the following inflammatory symptoms resolve: diarrhea, bleeding, passage of mucopus, tenesmus, and urgency. Endoscopic remission implies maintenance of an intact mucosa without ulceration, friability, or granularity and histologic remission presumes the absence of neutrophils in the epithelial crypts. It has been demonstrated that up to 40% of symptom-free patients had an abnormal sigmoidoscopy and 90% had microscopic inflammatory activity.[69]

Aminosalicylates are the primary maintenance therapy to prevent relapse of remitted UC.[70] AZA and 6-MP are useful steroid-sparing agents for steroid-dependent patients and for maintaining remission in those patients not adequately sustained by 5-ASA alone.[57] Corticosteroids, methotrexate, and nicotine are ineffective maintenance agents. Prolonged

administration of CSA at a dosage of more than 5 mg/kg daily is not advisable because of the risk of nephrotoxicity and, hence, has no role as maintenance therapy.[71]

Patients experiencing their first episode of proctitis that has responded promptly to topical treatment may not need maintenance medication as long-term remission may persist. If relapse does occur, there is usually a rapid response to retreatment. Rarely, patients with a mild first episode of extensive colitis may opt to be followed without maintenance medication although the vast majority of patients will require therapy to prevent relapse.[57,71]

5-ASA–induced Remission of UC

Remission can be maintained with oral and/or topical 5-ASA formulations alone after induction therapy for mild–moderate UC. Once remission is attained, topical 5-ASA is the most effective maintenance therapy to prevent relapse of distal disease. Mesalamine suppositories (1–1.5 g/day) and enemas (1–4 g daily) are effective for patients with proctitis and distal colitis, respectively. A dose response is not seen above 1 g/daily in distal disease; however, the frequency of administration is of primary importance.[48] An attempt is usually made to reduce the frequency of topical therapy: initially every night,[36] then every other night, then every third night.[72] Most patients can continue on the lowest frequency of topical therapy that maintains remission and quality of life. The practice of alternate night dosing or every third night dosing does not substantially decrease remission maintenance rates.[48] Patients who flare after a period of quiescence maintained on mesalamine suppositories may have disease extension.[73] These patients will require repeat endoscopy and if extension of colitis is documented, oral therapy will be required.

Oral maintenance therapy for distal colitis is less effective than topical; however, most patients still prefer an oral aminosalicylate for its convenience, and transitioning to an oral maintenance regimen can be attempted. Patients requiring a combination of oral and topical 5-ASA to achieve remission often require combination 5-ASA therapy to maintain remission. An attempt to reduce and taper off rectal mesalamine may be made, but patients who require topical therapy to improve will usually require some regular administration of topical therapy to maintain remission. One study suggested that combination therapy with oral and intermittent rectal mesalamine (twice a week) is better than oral therapy alone.[74]

An oral aminosalicylate is the primary maintenance therapy for extensive colitis. A recent Cochrane review affirmed its efficacy as maintenance therapy in UC.[70] In contrast to topical 5-ASA, there is a dose-dependent efficacy in the maintenance effects of all oral 5-ASA. However, sulfasalazine is often limited by its dose-dependent adverse effects and although the optimal maintenance dose was determined to be 4 g/day, dose reduction to the lower 2 g/day is recommended to best balance sulfasalazine's efficacy and side effects.

There is currently no evidence to suggest that the newer 5-ASA formulations are more effective than sulfasalazine, but they have markedly lower incidence of adverse events, allowing a clinical response with an oral dose of up to 4.8 g/day without increasing toxicity. In the absence of an extensive evidence base for dosing mesalamine maintenance therapy, it has been our experience that the optimal maintenance dose is the same dose required to induce remission. We also administer oral therapy with aminosalicylates on a twice-daily schedule to improve compliance. Adherence to therapy is critical to an optimal long-term outcome, because patients who take less than 80% of the prescribed 5-ASA have a fivefold increase in the risk of relapse.[75] Risk factors for poor adherence include being single, being of the male gender, and use of multiple medications.[76]

Steroid-induced Remission in UC

Corticosteroids (oral or topical) are ineffective maintenance agents and should be tapered and weaned off once remission has been achieved. 5-ASA remains the primary maintenance therapy after a steroid-induced remission, but will usually require higher doses equivalent to 2.4–4.8 g of mesalamine daily. Approximately one-fifth of patients that were treated with corticosteroids are steroid-dependent at 1 year[77]; these patients typically experience a relapse of symptoms when corticosteroids are tapered below a threshold dose of 15–20 mg/day. Because chronic long-term use of corticosteroids is unacceptable, patients should be considered for long-term immunosuppressive drug therapy with the thiopurines or a curative colectomy. AZA at doses of 2–2.5 mg/kg and 6-MP at doses of 1–1.5 mg/kg daily are effective steroid-sparing[78–80] and maintenance agents[81,82] in up to two-thirds of patients. The thiopurines have a slow onset of action and, while allowing time for them to take effect, patients are typically maintained on corticosteroids that are gradually tapered in the subsequent 2–3 months.

CSA-induced Remission in UC

Steroid-refractory patients achieving remission with intravenous CSA are transitioned to oral CSA. The usual prescribed oral dose is twice the daily intravenous dose. In addition to oral prednisone 40–60 mg/day, AZA (2–2.5 mg/kg/day), or 6-MP (1–1.5 mg/kg/day) is initiated before discharge. Long-term outcome studies have demonstrated the importance of maintenance therapy with AZA or 6-MP that will allow more than half of severe, steroid-refractory UC patients to avoid surgery in the long term after a CSA-induced remission.[83,84] Because of the risk of opportunistic infection during the period of triple immunosuppressive therapy, *Pneumocystis carinii* prophylaxis with one double-strength trimethoprim-sulfamethoxazole tablet taken 3 times weekly is now standard therapy. Patients are followed up closely with the goal of maintaining CSA blood trough levels in the range of 150–300 ng/mL (HPLC). Corticosteroids are gradually tapered within the ensuing 3 months and once adequate time (usually 3 months) has been allowed for the effect of AZA or 6-MP to "kick in," CSA is tapered by reducing the dose by 50% for 2 weeks followed by complete withdrawal. A patient who relapses while on drug taper will usually be referred for surgery.

Refractory UC Disease

Some patients continue to have active inflammatory disease despite maximal medical therapy with 5-ASA and steroids, yet are not so acutely ill as to warrant hospitalization for intravenous steroids and/or CSA or surgery. Conditions contributing to refractoriness must be excluded: treatment nonadherence, concurrent use of NSAIDs, infection, and 5-ASA hypersensitivity. Concomitant irritable bowel syndrome (IBS) may masquerade as "refractory" disease; the absence of inflammatory symptoms (urgency, rectal bleeding, fever), the prominence of abdominal bloating and cramping, and a normal flexible sigmoidoscopy aid in the diagnosis of IBS. Uncontrolled series have demonstrated the value of AZA and 6-MP in achieving remission in these steroid refractory, chronically active UC patients.[80,82,85] It is anticipated that infliximab will become an alternative option for this subgroup of patients who do not tolerate or respond to AZA or 6-MP. Colectomy may be the final option in these patients.

Indications for Surgery in UC

Between 30%–40% of UC patients will eventually require surgery, with the majority of patients requiring surgery within 10 years of initial diagnosis. Emergent surgery is indicated when there is massive hemorrhage, toxic megacolon, perforation, and severe colitis that is unresponsive to medical therapy. Elective surgery is indicated for those with cancer or dysplasia, failure of or suffering from complications of medical therapy, and rarely to correct malnutrition and growth retardation in children, and to control debilitating extraintestinal manifestations. Chapter 41 discusses the surgical management of UC.

Conclusion

The medical therapy of IBD is a complex and challenging area that requires close collaboration between the patient, gastroenterologist, and surgeon. The concepts or therapeutic goals of first inducing and then maintaining remission are important to understand, and different agents are used to achieve these goals in both Crohn's disease and UC, albeit with considerable overlap. Corticosteroids are successful at inducing remission in both diseases, but they have no role as maintenance agents, and steroid-sparing agents such as AZA or 6-MP, or methotrexate in the case of Crohn's disease, should be added at the first sign of steroid-dependence. Infliximab is now well established in the therapeutic armamentarium for both the induction and maintenance of remission of luminal and fistulous Crohn's disease, although its role in UC is yet to be defined, and awaits the outcome of further clinical trials. CSA may be an effective "bridge" to induce remission in UC until therapeutic serum levels of AZA or 6-MP can be achieved, but is not used for maintaining remission. "Saving the colon at all costs" can no longer be advocated, because surgery provides a viable alternative to patients failing medical therapy or in those experiencing severe complications from either disease and can result in prompt symptomatic improvement in suitably chosen patients.

References

1. Loftus EV Jr, Sandborn WJ. Epidemiology of inflammatory bowel disease. Gastroenterol Clin North Am 2002;31(1):1–20.

2. Harrison J, Hanauer SB. Medical treatment of Crohn's disease. Gastroenterol Clin North Am 2002;31(1):167–184, x.

3. Hanauer SB, Present DH. The state of the art in the management of inflammatory bowel disease. Rev Gastroenterol Disord 2003;3(2):81–92.

4. Hanauer SB, Sandborn W. Management of Crohn's disease in adults. Am J Gastroenterol 2001;96(3):635–643.

5. Summers RW, Switz DM, Sessions JT Jr, et al. National Cooperative Crohn's Disease Study: results of drug treatment. Gastroenterology 1979;77(4 pt 2):847–869.

6. Prantera C, et al. Mesalamine in the treatment of mild to moderate active Crohn's ileitis: results of a randomized, multicenter trial. Gastroenterology 1999;116(3):521–526.

7. Ursing B, et al. A comparative study of metronidazole and sulfasalazine for active Crohn's disease: the Cooperative Crohn's Disease Study in Sweden. II. Result. Gastroenterology 1982; 83(3):550–562.

8. Rustscheff S, Hulten S. An unexpected and severe neurological disorder with permanent disability acquired during short course treatment with metronidazole. Scand J Infect Dis 2003;35(4): 279–280.

9. Colombel JF, et al. A controlled trial comparing ciprofloxacin with mesalazine for the treatment of active Crohn's disease. Groupe d'Etudes Therapeutiques des Affections Inflammatoires Digestives (GETAID). Am J Gastroenterol 1999;94(3):674–678.

10. Greenbloom SL, Steinhart AH, Greenberg GR. Combination ciprofloxacin and metronidazole for active Crohn's disease. Can J Gastroenterol 1998;12(1):53–56.

11. Prantera C, et al. Use of antibiotics in the treatment of active Crohn's disease: experience with metronidazole and ciprofloxacin. Ital J Gastroenterol Hepatol 1998;30(6):602–606.

12. Kane SV, et al. The effectiveness of budesonide therapy for Crohn's disease. Aliment Pharmacol Ther 2002;16(8):1509–1517.

13. Thomsen OO, et al. A comparison of budesonide and mesalamine for active Crohn's disease. International Budesonide-Mesalamine Study Group. N Engl J Med 1998;339(6):370–374.

14. Hanauer SB. Inflammatory bowel disease. N Engl J Med 1996;334(13):841–848.

15. Steinhart AH, et al. Corticosteroids for maintaining remission of Crohn's disease. Cochrane Database Syst Rev 2001(3):CD000301.

16. Munkholm P, et al. Frequency of glucocorticoid resistance and dependency in Crohn's disease. Gut 1994;35(3):360–362.

17. Modigliani R, et al. Mesalamine in Crohn's disease with steroid-induced remission: effect on steroid withdrawal and remission maintenance. Groupe d'Etudes Therapeutiques des Affections Inflammatoires Digestives. Gastroenterology 1996;110(3): 688–693.

18. Sandborn W, et al. Azathioprine or 6-mercaptopurine for inducing remission of Crohn's disease. Cochrane Database Syst Rev 2000:2.

19. Aberra F, Lichtenstein G. Review article: monitoring of immunomodulators in inflammatory bowel disease. Aliment Pharmacol Ther 2005;21(4):307–319.

20. Cuffari C, Hunt S, Bayless T. Utilisation of erythrocyte 6-thioguanine metabolite levels to optimise azathioprine therapy in patients with inflammatory bowel disease. Gut 2001;48(5): 642–646.

21. Connell WR, et al. Long-term neoplasia risk after azathioprine treatment in inflammatory bowel disease. Lancet 1994;343(8908):1249–1252.

22. Feagan BG, et al. Methotrexate for the treatment of Crohn's disease. The North American Crohn's Study Group Investigators. N Engl J Med 1995;332(5):292–297.

23. Targan SR, et al. A short-term study of chimeric monoclonal antibody cA2 to tumor necrosis factor alpha for Crohn's disease. Crohn's Disease cA2 Study Group. N Engl J Med 1997;337(15): 1029–1035.

24. Present DH, et al. Infliximab for the treatment of fistulas in patients with Crohn's disease. N Engl J Med 1999;340(18):1398–1405.

25. Hanauer SB, et al. Maintenance infliximab for Crohn's disease: the ACCENT I randomised trial. Lancet 2002;359(9317): 1541–1549.

26. Sands BE, et al. Infliximab maintenance therapy for fistulizing Crohn's disease. N Engl J Med 2004;350(9):876–885.

27. Sandborn WJ, Hanauer SB. Infliximab in the treatment of Crohn's disease: a user's guide for clinicians. Am J Gastroenterol 2002;97(12):2962–2972.

28. Rutgeerts P, Van Assche G, Vermeire S. Optimizing anti-TNF treatment in inflammatory bowel disease. Gastroenterology 2004;126(6):1593–1610.

29. Sandborn WJ, et al. AGA technical review on perianal Crohn's disease. Gastroenterology 2003;125(5):1508–1530.

30. Bernstein LH, et al. Healing of perineal Crohn's disease with metronidazole. Gastroenterology 1980;79(2):357–365.

31. Solomon M. Combination ciprofloxacin and metronidazole in severe perianal Crohn's disease. Clin Invest Med 1992; 15(suppl):A41.

32. Hanauer SB, Smith MB. Rapid closure of Crohn's disease fistulas with continuous intravenous cyclosporin A. Am J Gastroenterol 1993;88(5):646–649.

33. Sandborn WJ, et al. Tacrolimus for the treatment of fistulas in patients with Crohn's disease: a randomized, placebo-controlled trial. Gastroenterology 2003;125(2):380–388.

34. Pearson DC, et al. Azathioprine for maintaining remission of Crohn's disease. Cochrane Database Syst Rev 2000(2):CD000067.

35. Bouhnik Y, et al. Long-term follow-up of patients with Crohn's disease treated with azathioprine or 6-mercaptopurine. Lancet 1996;347(8996):215–219.

36. Feagan BG, et al. A comparison of methotrexate with placebo for the maintenance of remission in Crohn's disease. North American Crohn's Study Group Investigators. N Engl J Med 2000;342(22):1627–1632.

37. Cunliffe RN, Scott BB. Monitoring for drug side-effects in inflammatory bowel disease. Aliment Pharmacol Ther 2002; 16(4):647–662.

38. Cottone M, et al. Review article: prevention of postsurgical relapse and recurrence in Crohn's disease. Aliment Pharmacol Ther 2003;17(suppl 2):38–42.

39. Rutgeerts P, et al. Effect of faecal stream diversion on recurrence of Crohn's disease in the neoterminal ileum. Lancet 1991;338(8770):771–774.

40. Lewis JD, Schoenfeld P, Lichtenstein GR. An evidence-based approach to studies of the natural history of gastrointestinal diseases: recurrence of symptomatic Crohn's disease after surgery. Clin Gastroenterol Hepatol 2003;1(3):229–236.

41. Camma C. Mesalamine in the prevention of clinical and endoscopic postoperative recurrence of Crohn's disease: a meta-analysis. Dig Liver Dis 2002;34(suppl):A86.

42. Rutgeerts P, et al. Controlled trial of metronidazole treatment for prevention of Crohn's recurrence after ileal resection. Gastroenterology 1995;108(6):1617–1621.

43. Hanauer SB, et al. Postoperative maintenance of Crohn's disease remission with 6-mercaptopurine, mesalamine, or placebo: a 2-year trial. Gastroenterology 2004;127(3):723–729.

44. Hanauer SB. Therapeutic expectations: medical management of ulcerative colitis. In: Bayless T, Hanauer SB, eds. Advance Therapy of Inflammatory Bowel Disease. Hamilton, ON: B.C. Decker; 2001:111–113.

45. Riley SA, et al. Microscopic activity in ulcerative colitis: what does it mean? Gut 1991;32(2):174–178.

46. Truelove SC, Witts LJ. Cortisone in ulcerative colitis: final report on a therapeutic trial. Br Med J 1955(4947):1041–1048.

47. Gionchetti P, et al. Comparison of oral with rectal mesalazine in the treatment of ulcerative proctitis. Dis Colon Rectum 1998;41(1):93–97.

48. Cohen RD, et al. A meta-analysis and overview of the literature on treatment options for left-sided ulcerative colitis and ulcerative proctitis. Am J Gastroenterol 2000;95(5): 1263–1276.

49. Mulder CJ, et al. Beclomethasone dipropionate (3 mg) versus 5-aminosalicylic acid (2 g) versus the combination of both (3 mg/2 g) as retention enemas in active ulcerative proctitis. Eur J Gastroenterol Hepatol 1996;8(6):549–553.

50. Banerjee S, Peppercorn MA. Inflammatory bowel disease. Medical therapy of specific clinical presentations. Gastroenterol Clin North Am 2002;31(1):185–202, x.

51. Danielsson A, et al. Pharmacokinetics of budesonide enema in patients with distal ulcerative colitis or proctitis. Aliment Pharmacol Ther 1993;7(4):401–407.

52. Marshall JK, Irvine EJ. Rectal corticosteroids versus alternative treatments in ulcerative colitis: a meta-analysis. Gut 1997;40(6): 775–781.

53. Lemann M, et al. Comparison of budesonide and 5-aminosalicylic acid enemas in active distal ulcerative colitis. Aliment Pharmacol Ther 1995;9(5):557–562.

54. Safdi M, et al. A double-blind comparison of oral versus rectal mesalamine versus combination therapy in the treatment of distal ulcerative colitis. Am J Gastroenterol 1997;92(10): 1867–1871.

55. Sutherland L, MacDonald JK. Oral 5-aminosalicylic acid for induction of remission in ulcerative colitis. Cochrane Database Syst Rev 2003(3):CD000543.

56. Sandborn WJ. Rational selection of oral 5-aminosalicylate formulations and prodrugs for the treatment of ulcerative colitis. Am J Gastroenterol 2002;97(12):2939–2941.

57. Kornbluth A, Sachar DB. Ulcerative colitis practice guidelines in adults (update): American College of Gastroenterology, Practice Parameters Committee. Am J Gastroenterol 2004;99(7): 1371–1385.

58. Kumar S, et al. Severe ulcerative colitis: prospective study of parameters determining outcome. J Gastroenterol Hepatol 2004;19(11):1247–1252.

59. Keith J, Sitrin M. Nutritional/metabolic issues in the management of inflammatory bowel disease. In: Cohen RD, ed. Inflammatory Bowel Disease: Diagnosis and Therapeutics. Totowa, NJ: Humana Press; 2003:231–236.

60. Michetti P, Peppercorn MA. Use of antibiotics and other anti-infectious agents in ulcerative colitis. In: Bayless TM, Hanauer SB, eds. Advanced Therapy of Inflammatory Bowel Disease. Hamilton, ON: B.C. Decker; 2001:149–151.

61. Daperno M, et al. Review article: medical treatment of severe ulcerative colitis. Aliment Pharmacol Ther 2002;16(suppl 4): 7–12.

62. Gan SI, Beck PL. A new look at toxic megacolon: an update and review of incidence, etiology, pathogenesis, and management. Am J Gastroenterol 2003;98(11):2363–2371.

63. Present DH, et al. Medical decompression of toxic megacolon by "rolling." A new technique of decompression with favorable long-term follow-up. J Clin Gastroenterol 1988;10(5):485–490.

64. Loftus CG, Loftus EV Jr, Sandborn WJ. Cyclosporin for refractory ulcerative colitis. Gut 2003;52(2):172–173.

65. Van Assche G, et al. Randomized, double-blind comparison of 4 mg/kg versus 2 mg/kg intravenous cyclosporine in severe ulcerative colitis. Gastroenterology 2003;125(4):1025–1031.

66. Travis SP, et al. Predicting outcome in severe ulcerative colitis. Gut 1996;38(6):905–910.

67. Su C, et al. Efficacy of anti-tumor necrosis factor therapy in patients with ulcerative colitis. Am J Gastroenterol 2002;97(10): 2577–2584.

68. Probert CS, et al. Infliximab in moderately severe glucocorticoid resistant ulcerative colitis: a randomised controlled trial. Gut 2003;52(7):998–1002.

69. Rizzello F, et al. Review article: monitoring activity in ulcerative colitis. Aliment Pharmacol Ther 2002;16(suppl 4):3–6.

70. Sutherland L, et al. Oral 5-aminosalicylic acid for maintenance of remission in ulcerative colitis. Cochrane Database Syst Rev 2003;(3):CD000543.

71. Feagan BG. Maintenance therapy for inflammatory bowel disease. Am J Gastroenterol 2003;98(12 suppl):S6–S17.

72. Mantzaris GJ, et al. Intermittent therapy with high-dose 5-aminosalicylic acid enemas maintains remission in ulcerative proctitis and proctosigmoiditis. Dis Colon Rectum 1994;37(1): 58–62.

73. Ayres RC, et al. Progression of ulcerative proctosigmoiditis: incidence and factors influencing progression. Eur J Gastroenterol Hepatol 1996;8(6):555–558.

74. d'Albasio G, et al. Combined therapy with 5-aminosalicylic acid tablets and enemas for maintaining remission in ulcerative colitis: a randomized double-blind study. Am J Gastroenterol 1997; 92(7):1143–1147.

75. Kane S, et al. Medication nonadherence and the outcomes of patients with quiescent ulcerative colitis. Am J Med 2003; 114(1):39–43.

76. Kane SV, et al. Prevalence of nonadherence with maintenance mesalamine in quiescent ulcerative colitis. Am J Gastroenterol 2001;96(10):2929–2933.

77. Faubion WA Jr, et al. The natural history of corticosteroid therapy for inflammatory bowel disease: a population-based study. Gastroenterology 2001;121(2):255–260.

78. Rosenberg JL, et al. A controlled trial of azathioprine in the management of chronic ulcerative colitis. Gastroenterology 1975;69(1):96–99.

79. Kirk AP, Lennard-Jones JE. Controlled trial of azathioprine in chronic ulcerative colitis. Br Med J (Clin Res Ed) 1982;284(6325): 1291–1292.

80. Ardizzone S, et al. Azathioprine in steroid-resistant and steroid-dependent ulcerative colitis. J Clin Gastroenterol 1997;25(1): 330–333.

81. Hawthorne AB, et al. Randomised controlled trial of azathioprine withdrawal in ulcerative colitis. BMJ 1992;305(6844):20–22.

82. George J, et al. The long-term outcome of ulcerative colitis treated with 6-mercaptopurine. Am J Gastroenterol 1996;91(9): 1711–1714.

83. Chung PY, et al. Intravenous cyclosporin in ulcerative colitis: long-term follow-up of the university of Chicago experience [abstract]. Am J Gastroenterol 2003;98(9 suppl 1):S255.

84. Campbell S, Ghosh S. Combination immunomodulatory therapy with cyclosporine and azathioprine in corticosteroid-resistant severe ulcerative colitis: the Edinburgh experience of outcome. Dig Liver Dis 2003;35(8):546–551.

85. Adler DJ, Korelitz BI. The therapeutic efficacy of 6-mercaptopurine in refractory ulcerative colitis. Am J Gastroenterol 1990;85(6):717–722.

41
Surgical Management of Ulcerative Colitis

Phillip R. Fleshner and David J. Schoetz, Jr.

Ulcerative colitis (UC) is a diffuse inflammatory disease of the mucosal lining of the colon and rectum that manifests clinically as diarrhea, abdominal pain, fever, weight loss, and rectal bleeding. Because removal of the affected organ is curative, surgery has assumed a pivotal position in the management of these patients. Although removal of the entire colorectum and permanent ileostomy had been the standard operation for decades, increased experience with anal sphincter preservation has demonstrated the feasibility of performing surgical procedures that spare sphincter function while still removing all disease. This chapter considers the surgical alternatives, decision making, and techniques surrounding these procedures.

Indications for Surgery

The overall incidence of colectomy in a UC patient ranges from 23% to 45%.[1-3] This risk is higher in patients with pancolitis than in patients with left-sided disease.[1,2] Indications for colectomy include an acute flare unresponsive to medical measures, development of a life-threatening complication (e.g., toxic colitis, perforation, or hemorrhage), medical intractability, risk of malignancy, disabling extracolonic disease, and growth retardation in children. During an episode of acute colitis, the patient should be aggressively treated with intravenous steroids and bowel rest. The role of parenteral hyperalimentation in this situation is controversial. Encouraging results have been reported with the use of cyclosporine in acute colitis[4] yet long-term effectiveness of this particular treatment modality remains undefined. However, there is no reported increase in the incidence of perioperative complications after subtotal colectomy in patients treated before surgery with cyclosporine.[5,6]

Patients with life-threatening complications are generally easy to recognize and define. Nevertheless, these patients are frequently taking large doses of steroids and may appear deceptively well; consequently, appreciation of the severity of the disease and the timing of operation are of paramount importance. Medical intractability is the most common indication for operation and may seem difficult to define. In fact, there is probably no strict definition that a physician can uniformly apply. It is important to recognize that medical intractability is a problem the patient identifies in conjunction with the physician. Although a physician may believe that 12 months of steroids or other immunosuppressive management without complete resolution of symptoms is an adequate medical trial, the patient must be convinced that surgery is indicated. Only the patient can decide he or she feels fatigued, has missed much work or school, or is unable to do things he or she would like to do because of the systemic effects of active colitis and its treatment. If the surgeon waits until the patient has arrived at the conclusion that the disease is not satisfactorily controlled medically, the patient will graciously accept alternatives the surgeon has to offer. We believe this is a particularly important strategy for the surgeon to use if the patient is to be satisfied.

Patients with UC are also prone to the development of colorectal cancer. The risk of cancer is relatively low for the first 10 years after disease onset but then begins to increase at a rate of 1%–2% per year.[7] Thus, by the time the patients have had the disease for 20 years, the cumulative risk of colorectal cancer may be as high as 20%. The question of timing of surgery for cancer prophylaxis remains controversial. Certainly, with an established carcinoma, surgical treatment is mandatory. More controversial, however, is the management of patients with dysplasia. Most surgeons contend that during a surveillance biopsy program, identification of high-grade dysplasia by an experienced pathologist is an indication for colectomy. Patients with low-grade dysplasia should also be offered colectomy, although nonoperative management of these patients has been suggested by some because the natural history of low-grade dysplasia has not been well established.[8]

Elective colectomy may be indicated for some categories of severe extraintestinal manifestations of the disease. Persistent or recurrent monoarticular arthritis, uveitis, or iritis all respond favorably to colectomy. However, primary sclerosing cholangitis, ankylosing spondylitis, and sacroiliitis are not improved by colectomy. The response of pyoderma gangrenosum to colectomy is unpredictable.

Growth retardation is a common feature in children with UC. Contrary to popular belief, steroid therapy cannot be entirely blamed for delayed growth. Inadequate protein intake and excess loss in the colon are also contributory.[9] A rapid growth spurt is often observed after definitive surgery.

Emergency Versus Elective Procedures

Operative management of UC largely depends on whether the surgery is elective or emergent. Under elective conditions, the four available surgical options are: 1) total proctocolectomy and Brooke ileostomy, 2) total proctocolectomy and continent ileostomy, 3) abdominal colectomy with ileorectal anastomosis (IRA), and 4) ileal pouch–anal anastomosis (IPAA). Total proctocolectomy and Brooke ileostomy has been traditionally regarded as the optimal surgical approach and remains the operation with which alternative procedures should be compared. The technique has been well described and the immediate and late results are very satisfactory. Furthermore, patients avoid any risk for cancer, steroid medications are eliminated, and physician visits and reoperations are kept to a minimum. Although quality-of-life studies[10] have demonstrated excellent results, the loss of fecal continence and its attendant physical and psychologic sequelae continue to be significant drawbacks of the procedure. In addition, problems with nonhealing of the perineal wound, and the high incidence of small bowel obstruction and ileostomy revision, are not to be minimized.

Total proctocolectomy and continent ileostomy couples the benefit of complete large bowel excision with a reduction in some of the untoward aspects of an ileostomy, because no external appliance is needed and the stoma can be placed in a less conspicuous position on the abdominal wall. Continent ileostomy can be performed at anytime in UC patients having previously undergone total proctocolectomy and Brooke ileostomy if they find a standard ileostomy unsatisfactory. Because of increased surgical experience and improved surgical techniques, continent pouch morbidity has decreased since its initial clinical description. Most patients are ultimately happy with the results of the operation. Nonetheless, troublesome complications leading to incontinence continue to plague the postoperative course of a substantial number of patients.[11]

There are many attractive features of colectomy and IRA. The procedure avoids the perineal complications of total proctocolectomy, the risk of sexual dysfunction is minimal, is technically easy to perform, may provide perfect control of feces and flatus, and is well accepted by most patients. However, unlike the three other surgical options, ileorectostomy does not achieve total excision of colorectal mucosa. Many surgeons have not used this operation for UC, arguing that more than 25% of patients will require subsequent rectal

excision for persistent proctitis,[12,13] a small percentage of patients will develop cancer in the rectal remnant, and only half of the patients have satisfactory long-term functional results. Although we concur that this operation should not be advised in most UC patients, IRA does have a role in certain clinical situations. For example, an elderly patient with a long history of UC who develops a transverse colon cancer may be well served with an IRA in lieu of total proctocolectomy. Decisions must be made on an individualized basis, taking into account the compliance of the rectum and the integrity of the sphincter mechanism.

IPAA has the attractive features of complete excision of the colorectal mucosa, avoidance of a permanent intestinal stoma, continence via a normal route of defecation, and no prospect for a troublesome nonhealing perineal wound. Continence is usually preserved and the frequency of defecation is diminished with incorporation of a pelvic pouch into the operative procedure. Although the operation is associated with minimal mortality, the morbidity of this complex procedure is relatively high, and problems such as small bowel obstruction and pouchitis continue to be a cause for concern.

Under emergent conditions, surgical alternatives are limited. If the patient is septic, the diseased or perforated bowel should be removed. If the colon is bleeding, the colon should be removed. Traditionally, it has been taught that the rectum should also be removed. However, with the sphincter-saving alternatives that are currently available, careful preoperative proctoscopic evaluation to exclude a rectal etiology for the bleeding and a subsequent abdominal colectomy with end ileostomy can be safely performed. A subsequent procedure can then restore intestinal continuity. Similarly, with toxic colitis, it is seldom necessary to perform a proctectomy at the time of colectomy. In general, concerns over healing of the perineal wound in these frequently malnourished patients who are taking high-dose steroids should deter surgeons from doing proctectomy in the emergent setting. The authors have not found it necessary to use the blow-hole technique of Turnbull, but this is a philosophically acceptable approach in that it does not preclude subsequent continence-preserving alternatives. This technique is mainly of historical significance because most UC patients currently present for colectomy earlier and are not as nutritionally depleted as when this technique was frequently used.[14]

A few technical issues regarding subtotal colectomy in these patients must be stressed. Mesenteric dissection in the vicinity of the ileocecal valve should be flush with the colon to preserve ileal branches of the ileocolic artery and vein. These branches are necessary to facilitate subsequent construction of an ileal pouch. Distally, it is unnecessary to mobilize the rectum within the pelvis. In fact, dissection of the sigmoid to the sacral promontory, without violation of presacral planes, and a Hartmann procedure are recommended. This has shown to decrease the incidence of pelvic sepsis and facilitate subsequent pelvic surgery. The colon should be transected at the rectosigmoid junction and an intraperitoneal rectal stump created. Technically, closure of the rectal stump can be hazardous because the bowel is markedly inflamed and does not hold sutures or staples well. Bringing the distal site of transaction out as a mucous fistula, which can be either primarily matured or buried within the abdominal incision[15] or the subcutaneous tissue,[16] are alternative techniques to safely manage the very diseased rectal stump. A transanal rectal drain may prevent leakage from the diseased Hartmann pouch closure site.

There is a trend to avoid subjecting patients to multiple surgical procedures and to perform a definitive procedure at the time of emergent surgery. Although an IPAA can be successfully performed in patients undergoing surgery for emergent complications, the authors believe this generally is not a safe approach. These patients are usually on high doses of steroids and are nutritionally depleted. Patients with UC receiving high-dose steroids (more than 40 mg/day) have a significantly greater risk of developing pouch-related complications after colectomy than patients with UC receiving 1–40 mg/day and patients with UC who are not receiving corticosteroids.[8] From a practical standpoint, surgical options are limited in emergent situations. Salvage of the patient should be the primary concern. Abdominal colectomy is safe in these very ill, nutritionally depleted patients[5,15–18] and the procedure does not preclude any of the other surgical alternatives in the future. Additionally, the patient is able to live with an ileostomy and assess its impact on his or her life, thus allowing for an informed decision regarding subsequent continence-restoring surgery.

Brooke Ileostomy

The preoperative period should include effective patient education. A patient must be fully informed of the effects of an ileostomy on his or her quality of life. An ileostomy visitor, preferably age and sex matched and who has completely recovered from surgery, is invaluable during this period. Resistance to a permanent ileostomy can be tempered by stressing the beneficial aspects of this operation (e.g., curing the disease). It is also essential, when possible, to select the stoma site preoperatively with the help of an enterostomal therapist. As discussed in Chapter 44, the stoma should be placed in a flat area away from bony prominences, scars, and significant skin creases. Attention to these details will ensure a well-functioning ileostomy.

Operative Technique

A colectomy is performed in the standard manner with the patient in a modified lithotomy Trendelenburg position. The proctectomy phase of the procedure is remarkable for keeping the dissection close to the rectal wall, especially anteriorly in the area of Denonvilliers' fascia. Meticulous

dissection to minimize the risk of injury to pelvic autonomic nerves is essential. Perineal dissection should be performed in the intersphincteric plane. After the colorectum is removed, a Brooke ileostomy is constructed.[19] An appliance is then placed over the stoma. Bowel function is expected in 3–6 days.

In some situations, the end of the ileum does not reach far enough through the abdominal wall to allow primary maturation. In these situations, the mesentery is usually a limiting factor and selection of a more proximal site in the bowel may allow better mobilization. Alternatively, a loop-end ileostomy rather than an end ileostomy may reach more easily.

Postoperative Complications

A proctocolectomy with a Brooke ileostomy is a safe procedure with a predictable long-term outcome. It is, however, not entirely free of complications. Delayed healing of the perineal wound is not uncommon and can be quite problematic.[20] Failure of the wound to close should prompt investigation to exclude the presence of retained mucosa, foreign material, or Crohn's disease (CD). Sexual complications of proctocolectomy in men are much less common than in patients having a radical resection for cancer, yet permanent impotence or retrograde ejaculation can occur. Almost 30% of women complain of dyspareunia after this operation, presumably as a result of perineal scarring.[21] Intestinal obstruction is a troublesome complication that can be managed conservatively in most patients. Gentle irrigation of the stoma is an important therapeutic maneuver. Prolonged nonoperative treatment should not be pursued for fear of infarction. Although problems from the ileostomy have diminished markedly with the use of modern appliances and the Brooke modification, skin irritation, stomal stenosis, prolapse, and herniation remain significant causes of postoperative morbidity. Treatment of these problems can be as simple as reeducating a patient about the proper maintenance of the ileostomy. However, up to one-third of these patients ultimately require operative revision.[22] Despite the fact that these patients have undergone major abdominal surgery and have a permanent stoma, their quality of life as measured by validated questionnaires is very good and similar to that of the general population.[10] More than 90% of patients are happy with their current lifestyle. However, significant problems do remain. Almost 25% of patients are restricted in their social and recreation activities, and nearly 15% of patients who are knowledgeable of alternative procedures would consider conversion. In short, the Brooke ileostomy is generally well accepted, although a number of patients experience significant psychosocial and mechanical difficulties.

Current indications for the procedure include elderly patients, individuals with distal rectal cancer, patients with severely compromised anal function, and patients who choose this operation after appropriate education.

Continent Ileostomy

Physicians involved with patients requiring an ileostomy should be aware of the continent ileostomy. Although this procedure is less often performed today, it remains a viable alternative in patients who have discrete problems with an appliance. A continent ileostomy is usually reserved for patients who have failed Brooke ileostomy or those who are candidates for an IPAA but cannot have a pouch because of rectal cancer, perianal fistulas, poor anal sphincter function, or occupations that may preclude frequent visits to the toilet.

Preoperatively, a search for CD using barium examination of the stomach and small intestine is important. Suspicion of CD contraindicates construction of a continent ileostomy, because the risk of recurrent disease in the pouch is increased; this could necessitate resection of 45 cm of valuable small bowel and render the patient unable to maintain nutrition. Obesity and age over 40 years are associated with an increased risk of pouch dysfunction and represent relative contraindications to the continent ileostomy.[23]

The period before surgery must also include an open discussion with the patient, stressing that although continence is likely, major complications often occur. These setbacks generally must be corrected surgically, sometimes leading to pouch excision and creation of a standard Brooke ileostomy. The patient must comprehend that by learning to care for and intubate the reservoir, he or she has an important role in its functional outcome. Only highly motivated, emotionally stable individuals should consider this procedure.

Operative Technique

Patients undergoing combined total proctocolectomy/continent ileostomy have a proctocolectomy performed in the usual manner. Excision of a very short segment of terminal ileum and a diligent search for CD during the procedure are essential. In patients with a standard ileostomy undergoing conversion to continent ileostomy, the stoma is mobilized from the abdominal wall. Construction of the reservoir in these two patient groups is then performed in an identical manner.

The technique of constructing a continent ileostomy is conceptually difficult (Figure 41-1). Using the terminal 45–60 cm of the ileum, an aperistaltic reservoir is created by making an S-pouch or a folded two-limb pouch originally described by Kock et al.[23] In the classic technique, two 15-cm limbs of ileum are sutured together with continuous absorbable sutures to form a pouch. The antimesenteric border is incised and then folded over to form a reservoir. The ileum immediately distal to the reservoir is then scarified with electrocautery and 5 cm of adjacent mesentery is removed or thinned of fat and intussusception of this terminal 15 cm of ileum into the pouch is performed. The intussusception is secured with multiple nonabsorbable sutures and staples. The end of the ileum is then brought through the abdominal wall at the preoperatively identified site. Because

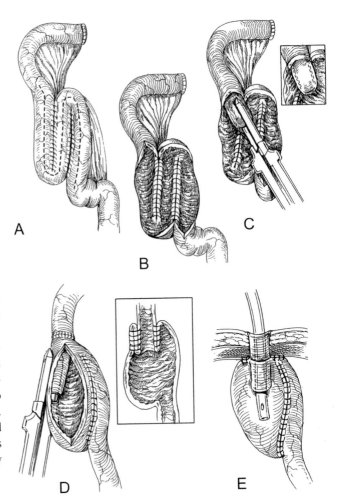

FIGURE 41-1. Continent ileostomy. **A** Three limbs of small bowel are measured and the bowel wall is sutured together. **B** After opening the bowel (see the dotted lines in A), the edges are sewn together to form a two-layered closure. **C** A valve is created by intussuscepting the efferent limb into the pouch and fixing it in place with a linear noncutting stapler. (Inset: staples in place on valve). **D** The valve is attached to the pouch sidewall with the linear noncutting stapler (a cross-section of the finished pouch is shown). **E** After closure of the last suture line, the pouch is attached to the abdominal wall and a catheter is inserted to keep the pouch decompressed during healing.

no external appliance is required, a continent ileostomy can be located lower on the abdominal wall for cosmetic reasons. The stoma is sutured flush with the skin and the pouch firmly anchored to the posterior rectus sheath. A wide plastic tube with large openings (i.e., Madina catheter; AStra Tech, Molndal, Sweden) is placed into the pouch to allow gravity drainage of the pouch in the early postoperative period. This tube is occluded for progressively longer periods beginning 10 days after surgery until it can be removed for 8 hours without distress. At this point, the pouch is significantly expanded, the tube is removed, and drainage is achieved by intubating the pouch three times a day.

Postoperative Complications

Postoperative complications that occur with sufficient frequency are nipple valve slippage, pouchitis, intestinal obstruction, and fistula. Nipple valve slippage[24,25] occurs because of the tendency of the intussuscepted segment to slide and extrude on its mesenteric aspect. Difficult pouch catheterization, chronic outflow tract obstruction, and incontinence ensue. Because of the frequency of this problem, many techniques other than simple surgical stapling have been described to stabilize the valve. Wrapping the valve with prosthetic materials does prevent valve slippage but also is accompanied by a potentially unacceptably high incidence of parastomal abscess and fistula formation.[11] Despite these technical modifications, nipple valve slippage remains the most common complication after continent ileostomy, occurring in almost 30% of patients.[11,24,25] Although nonoperative approaches have been attempted to correct this problem, surgical correction is virtually inevitable. Repair of the existing malfunctioning valve or creation of a new valve from the afferent ileal limb is performed.

Pouchitis is recognized in 25% of patients, making this the second most common postoperative complication after continent ileostomy.[11,23,24] Pouchitis refers to nonspecific inflammation that develops in the reservoir, and is thought to result from stasis and overgrowth of anaerobic bacteria. Patients present with a combination of increased ileostomy output, fever, weight loss, and stomal bleeding. The diagnosis is made by history and confirmed by pouch endoscopy. Pouchitis usually responds to a course of antibiotics and continuous pouch drainage.

Other complications include an incidence of intestinal obstruction after continent ileostomy of about 5%. Surgical intervention is mandatory when nonoperative therapy has been unsuccessful. The incidence of fistulas after creation of a continent ileostomy is approximately 10%. Fistulas usually originate in the pouch itself or at the base of the nipple valve. Pouch fistulas result from dehiscence of suture lines or, rarely, ileostomy tube erosion. These tracts may close with bowel rest, parenteral nutrition, and continuous pouch drainage. Fistulas from the base of the valve lead to incontinence, because ileal contents bypass the high-pressure zone of the nipple valve. These fistulas usually arise with tearing of the sutures anchoring the pouch to the anterior abdominal wall. Valve fistulas rarely heal without operation. At laparotomy, the valve is excised, the pouch rotated, and a new continent valve constructed from the afferent tract.

Patient satisfaction with a continent ileostomy is excellent.[26] Most patients note a marked improvement in their lifestyle, and almost all patients work and participate in social and recreational activities without restriction.[24] These observations are understandable in that 90% of patients eventually have total continence after one or more procedures. However, their enthusiasm is surprising considering that complications are quite frequent and often require major surgical intervention.[23,24] The often advertised Barnett modification of the Kock pouch (Figure 41-2) uses the afferent limb of small bowel to construct the nipple valve and wraps a portion of the residual efferent limb around the nipple valve.[27] This modification was designed to reduce the incidence of valve slippage and fistula formation. Another recently described variation[28] is the "T-pouch" in which a portion of ileum is folded into the side of the pouch rather than being intussuscepted (Figure 41-3). Theoretically, this eliminates valve slippage. Unfortunately, there are no controlled data to suggest that either of these modifications is any better than the standard procedure most centers are using.

Ileorectal Anastomosis

Before the advent of IPAA, abdominal colectomy with IRA was performed in UC patients who might otherwise have been offered a permanent ileostomy. Currently, IRA is mainly considered in patients with indeterminate colitis (IC), in

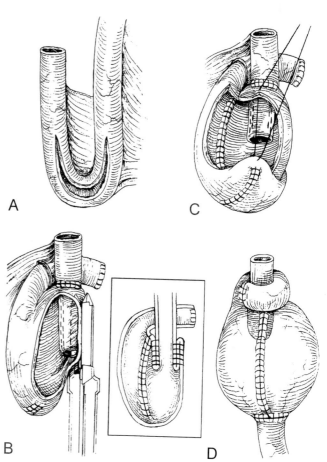

FIGURE 41-2. Barnett continent ileostomy reservoir (BCIR). **A** Two limbs of small intestine are sewn together and opened. **B** The afferent limb is intussuscepted to form a valve and the valve is stapled to the side of the reservoir. **C** The pouch is folded back and sutured closed. Insert shows cross-section of pouch. **D** Completed BCIR. The afferent limb of bowel has been divided and reattached to the apex of the pouch and the efferent limb is wrapped around the valve to form a collar.

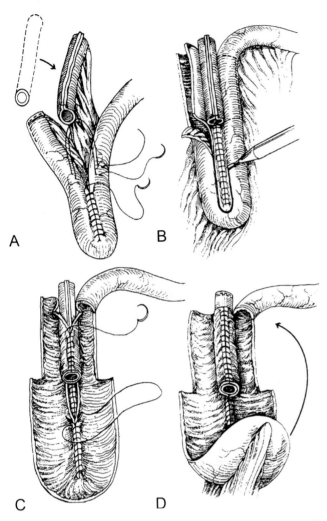

FIGURE 41-3. T-pouch. **A** Seromuscular sutures approximate the back wall of the pouch and fix the valve segment to the pouch through mesenteric windows. **B** The bowel is opened. **C** Edges of bowel are closed over the valve segment. **D** The reservoir is folded in half and closed.

high-risk or older patients who are not good candidates for IPAA, or if there is mild rectal disease in which rectal compliance remains adequate. The use of the operation may also be indicated in the teenager or young adult to rapidly regain good health, avoid a stoma, and return to school or work quickly. Functional results depend on the level of the anastomosis as well as the state of the rectum. Contraindications to IRA include a very diseased and noncompliant rectum, dysplasia or nonmetastatic cancer, perianal disease, and a severely compromised anal sphincter.

Postoperative Complications

IRA is a safe operation; mortality is low, particularly when it is performed as an elective procedure. The early morbidity of IRA is low, with the incidence of anastomotic leak being less than 10%, and major sepsis is very uncommon. Sexual

function is well preserved. The overall complication rate is much lower than that of an IPAA.[12] Although the frequency of defecation after IRA is variable, most patients pass between two and four semiliquid stools a day. Nocturnal defecation is quite common, but true incontinence is rare.[29]

The main concerns surrounding IRA for UC are the long-term issues regarding cancer risk in the retained rectum and the incidence of persistent rectal inflammation. The overall risk of cancer developing in the rectum after IRA approximates 6%, but this depends on the duration of follow-up.[30] Few of these cancers develop less than 10 years after operation, with most cancers appearing 15–20 years after operation. Cancer in the rectum after IRA produces few symptoms and early lesions are not always easily identified at sigmoidoscopy. Patients being offered IRA must realize the need for semiannual sigmoidoscopy with multiple biopsies to detect dysplasia, polyps, or invasive cancer. This recommendation is particularly important in young adults or children because these patients have the highest risk of developing cancer and are much more likely to be lost to follow-up.

The rectal stump may be the site of recurrent or persistent inflammation in 20%–45% of patients. Clinical features include severe diarrhea, tenesmus, bleeding, and urgency. Rectal excision is needed in those cases that do not respond to topical or systemic therapies. About one-quarter of patients require proctectomy after IRA for severe proctitis.[12,13] The only clinical factor that predicts a successful outcome is the degree of inflammation in the rectum preoperatively, minimal proctitis being associated with an excellent prognosis.[12] A great advantage of the IRA is that should a failure occur, other options remain. Conversion from an IRA to an IPAA may be required when there is a poor functional outcome because of poor rectal compliance, persistent and disabling proctitis, and with development of an upper rectal cancer. If conversion to IPAA is required, it can be performed safely, although poorer bowel function may be expected. However, quality of life is similar before and after conversion in these patients.[30]

Ileal Pouch–Anal Anastomosis

The most attractive of the continence-preserving alternatives is the IPAA, which consists of near total proctocolectomy, creation of an ileal reservoir, and preservation of the anal sphincter complex. The original operation as described by Sir Alan Parks included a complete stripping of the anal mucosa of the anal canal.[31] In an attempt to improve functional outcome, some surgeons[32,33] preserve the anal transition zone and perform a stapled anastomosis between the ileal pouch and the anal canal immediately cephalad to the dentate line ("double-stapled" technique). Both of these techniques remove the colorectum without creating a perianal wound, preserve innervation to the anus, bladder, and genitals, and retain the usual pathway for defecation. Preoperatively, the rectum should be evaluated sigmoidoscopically. Active rectal disease requires topical 5-aminosalicylic acid or steroid enemas to minimize rectal inflammation and facilitate mucosectomy. The anorectal sphincter mechanism must be intact to prevent leakage of watery ileal contents. Use of this procedure in patients with poor sphincter function or fecal incontinence must be carefully individualized. Preoperative evaluation also allows the surgeon to be certain that patients undergoing this operation are highly motivated and willing to cope with potential postoperative complications.

Operative Technique

After appropriate bowel preparation, the patient is brought to the operating room and placed in the modified lithotomy position. A midline incision is made and the abdomen explored to rule out evidence of CD. The colon is mobilized in the usual manner. A few technical points should be stressed. Omentectomy may be inappropriate, because there is a lower incidence of postoperative sepsis when the omentum is preserved.[34] Stapling of the distal ileum flush with the cecum is very important, as is preservation of the ileal branches of the ileocolic artery and vein. These vessels provide perfusion of the pouch after mesenteric division. The pelvic peritoneum is incised and rectal mobilization begun. Dissection is carried ventrally to the level of the prostate in men and the mid-portion of the vagina in women. Posteriorly, the dissection is carried past the end of the coccyx. Mobilization of the rectum should be flush with

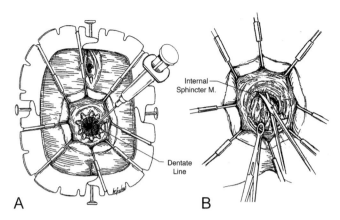

FIGURE 41-5. Mucosectomy. **A** A spinal needle is used to inject saline solution with epinephrine (1:200,000) into the submucosa from the dentate line to the levators. A circumferential incision through the mucosa is made at the dentate line. **B** A sleeve of mucosa is dissected free from the internal sphincter using sharp dissection.

fascia propria to minimize damage to nearby autonomic nerves traveling to urinary bladder and sexual organs.

Mucosal stripping is performed from a perineal approach. The use of a Lone Star™ retractor facilitates exposure and minimizes damage to the sphincter mechanism (Figure 41-4). A solution of dilute epinephrine is injected into the submucosal plane to facilitate mucosectomy and minimize bleeding (Figure 41-5). The excised mucosa and remaining proximal rectum are removed, leaving a short cuff of denuded rectal muscle distally for about 4 cm above the dentate line. Attention is then directed toward creation of the ileal reservoir. The terminal ileum is aligned in a J configuration and the pouch constructed with either a continuous absorbable suture or stapling device (Figures 41-6 to 41-9). Both limbs of the J are approximately 15–25 cm in length, the exact length guided by where the pouch reaches deepest into the pelvis. The prospective apex of the pouch must reach beyond the symphysis pubis to accomplish a tension-free ileoanal anastomosis. Selective division of mesenteric vessels to the apex of a proposed J-pouch will allow for more length (Figure 41-10). Superficial incision on the anterior and posterior aspects of the small bowel mesentery along the course of the superior mesenteric artery, and mobilization of the small bowel mesentery up to and anterior to the duodenum, are two additional important lengthening maneuvers. The pouch is then pulled into the pelvis and the anastomosis performed between the apex of the pouch and the dentate line, approximating full thickness of the pouch wall to the internal sphincter and anal mucosa (Figure 41-11). A proximal defunctioning loop ileostomy is created. One or two suction drains are placed in the presacral space and brought out through the left lower quadrant of the abdomen away from the ileostomy site.

In the double-stapled technique, the anorectum is divided by the abdominal operator approximately 2 cm above the dentate line using a right-angle linear stapler (Figure 41-12). After the pouch is created, the anvil of the mid-sized circular stapler

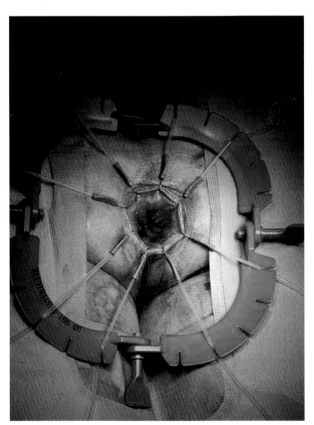

FIGURE 41-4. Lone Star™ retractor.

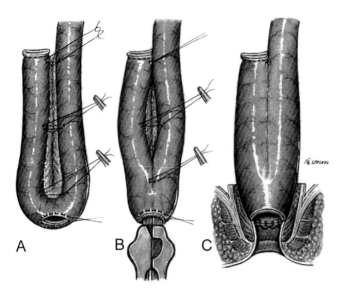

FIGURE 41-6. Ileal J-pouch creation. **A** The limbs of the ileum are oriented using stay sutures. **B** The common wall of the two limbs is then divided using a linear cutting stapler placed through an apical antimesenteric enterotomy. **C** The J-reservoir is then placed within the rectal muscular sleeve and sutured to the dentate line. (Reprinted from Veidenheimer MC. Mucosal proctectomy, ileal J-reservoir, and ileoanal anastomosis. In: Braasch JW, Sedgwick CE, Veidenheimer MC, Ellis FH Jr, eds. Atlas of Abdominal Surgery. Philadelphia: WB Saunders; copyright 1991, with permission from Elsevier).

device is tied in to the apex of the ileal pouch. Before proceeding with the anastomosis, integrity of the rectal staple line is tested using air insufflation. The stapler is placed transanally and the trocar advanced through the transverse staple line. The stapler is then closed as the abdominal surgeon ensures that no extraneous tissues are trapped within the stapling device.

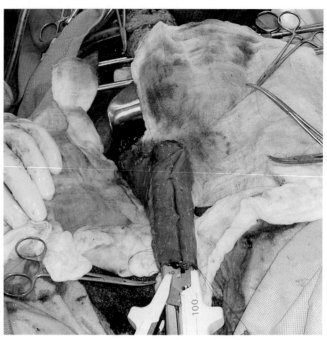

FIGURE 41-8. Ileal J-pouch. Intraoperative photograph showing application of the linear stapler through the apical enterotomy. Note how the stay sutures are helpful in advancing the bowel over the stapler.

Postoperative management is similar to that in patients who have had an ultra-low anterior resection or coloanal procedure protected by a loop ileostomy. Ileostomy output can be quite

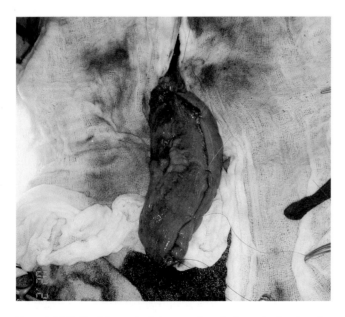

FIGURE 41-7. Ileal J-pouch. Intraoperative photograph showing the two limbs of the ileum properly oriented using stay sutures.

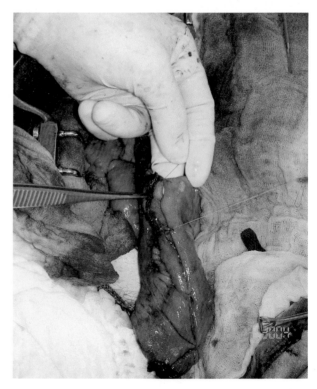

FIGURE 41-9. Ileal J-pouch. Intraoperative photograph showing the completed J-pouch.

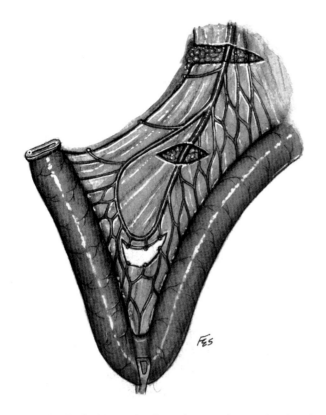

FIGURE 41-10. Ileal J-pouch. The peritoneum is scored to lengthen the mesentery. Selective division of mesenteric arcades is used to produce additional length (Reprinted from Veidenheimer MC. Mucosal proctectomy, ileal J-reservoir, and ileoanal anastomosis. In: Braasch JW, Sedgwick CE, Veidenheimer MC, Ellis FH Jr, eds. Atlas of Abdominal Surgery. Philadelphia: WB Saunders; copyright 1991, with permission from Elsevier).

high, because the stoma is more proximal than a traditional Brooke ileostomy. Patients should be encouraged to keep themselves well hydrated. In some instances, antidiarrheal medication is prescribed.

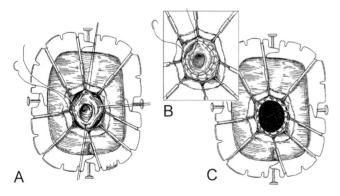

FIGURE 41-11. Hand-sewn ileoanal anastomosis. **A** After the pouch is gently pulled through the anal canal by the perineal surgeon, four sutures incorporating full thickness of the pouch and a generous bite of the internal sphincter are placed at right angles to anchor the efferent limb within the anal canal. **B** The anastomosis is completed by placing sutures between each anchoring suture. **C** The mucosally intact anastomosis is completed.

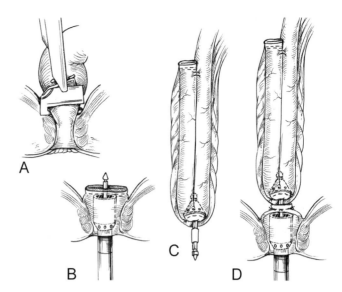

FIGURE 41-12. Double-stapled J-pouch anastomosis. **A** The anvil of a mid-sized circular stapler is tied into the apex of the J-pouch. **B** The anorectum is divided with a stapler within the levator muscles about 1–2 cm above the dentate line. Adjacent tissue such as the bladder or vagina must be excluded from incorporation in the staple line. The integrity of the staple line should be tested with air insufflation through an anoscope. **C** The perineal operator advances the mid-sized circular stapler against the anorectal transaction site and advances the trocar through the transverse staple line. **D** The anvil mechanism is positioned onto the rod of the circular stapler. Before completing the anastomosis, the abdominal operator must prevent extraneous tissue from being trapped into the stapling device.

Patients are usually discharged after 7–10 days in the hospital and return 6–8 weeks later to have the temporary ileostomy closed. Before closure, however, the pouch is thoroughly investigated. Digital rectal examination is used to assess anal sphincter tone and detect anastomotic strictures or defects. The pouch is examined endoscopically to ensure that the suture lines are healed, and a contrast study is performed to detect pouch leaks, fistulas, and sinus tracts. Only after confirmation that pouch abnormalities are not present is the ileostomy closed. Sphincter strengthening exercises should be encouraged in the period leading up to ileostomy closure, because they seem to improve functional results. In more than 90% of patients, the ileostomy can be closed through a peristomal incision. However, in the remainder, the midline abdominal incision must be reopened.

Postoperative Complications

Performing an ileoanal anastomosis is safe, with reported mortality rates ranging from 0% to 1%.[35] In distinct contrast to mortality, however, morbidity after IPAA remains considerable. Small bowel obstruction occurs in 20% of patients and results from adhesion formation to the large number of raw surfaces after colectomy and from kinking at the ileostomy site. Most of the obstructive episodes occur in the immediate period after either procedure. The most important factor predictive of small bowel obstruction is rotating the ileostomy 180 degrees (as some authors promote to reduce fecal spillage into the defunctionalized pouch).[36] Although an initial trial of nonoperative therapy is appropriate, surgical intervention may ultimately be required.

Although the incidence has steadily decreased with increasing surgical experience, pelvic sepsis still occurs in 5% of patients after IPAA. Pelvic sepsis may present in the immediate postoperative period or it may be delayed, manifesting as abscess formation (usually presacral) or a perineal fistula. The symptoms suggestive of early pelvic sepsis are fever, anal pain, tenesmus, and discharge of pus or secondary hemorrhage through the anus. Diagnosis is confirmed using computed tomography or magnetic resonance imaging which demonstrates the presence of an abscess or of edematous tissues. Because patients who develop sepsis in the early postoperative period have a higher likelihood of subsequent pouch failure,[37] an aggressive therapeutic approach should be adopted in these patients. Although most patients respond to intravenous antibiotics within 24–36 hours, patients with ongoing sepsis and an organized abscess should undergo early operative endoanal or imaging-guided percutaneous drainage. If drainage of the cavity is unsatisfactory, an attempt should be made to deroof the abscess and curette the cavity through the anus, creating a large communication between the abscess and the reservoir. Sometimes several local procedures are needed to eradicate sepsis. Rarely, an abdominal approach is needed.

The reported incidence of ileoanal anastomotic stricture has varied between 5% and 38%.[38–41] This difference depends in part on the definition of stricture used by different authors. For some, a stricture is a narrowing of the anastomosis that requires at least two dilations[39,40] whereas, for others, a stricture is narrowing associated with pouch-outlet obstruction and poor evacuation that requires repeated dilations. The etiology is usually anastomotic tension that also predisposes to infection from leakage. Full mobilization of the mesentery and avoidance of traction on the reservoir are key technical maneuvers to avoid stricture formation. Anchoring the pouch to surrounding tissues may prevent direct tension on the anastomosis itself. Avoidance of sepsis is paramount to a successful outcome. An apparent stricture may be noted when digital examination is performed for the first time after the operation. These asymptomatic, web-like strictures can be easily disrupted by gentle passage of the finger. More fibrotic strictures can usually be fractured digitally but occasionally the insertion of graded dilators under anesthesia is necessary. Operative management usually requires repeated dilatations yet reasonable function can be expected in more than 50% of patients.[39,40,42] Rarely, a transanal approach involving excision of the stricture and pouch advancement distally is necessary.[43,44]

Anastomotic separation is seen in approximately 10% of patients. If this complication is recognized during preileostomy closure contrast studies or as a defect on digital examination, ileostomy closure should be delayed until complete clinical and radiographic evidence of healing. Local drainage procedures for an associated abscess or a direct repair of the separation are sometimes necessary.[35] This aggressive approach will almost always be successful, allowing ileostomy closure.

The reported incidence of pouch-vaginal fistula ranges from 3% to 16%.[45–49] The patient complains of a vaginal discharge and clinical examination usually demonstrates the fistula. Occasionally, it is only detected by radiologic contrast enema (pouchogram). It is important to exclude a pouch-vaginal fistula by careful operative examination of the vagina as well as the anal canal before closing the defunctioning ileostomy. The fistula may present before ileostomy closure or after stoma closure.[46] The internal opening is usually located at the ileoanal anastomosis, but less often it may arise at the dentate line, perhaps as a form of cryptoglandular sepsis. Causative factors may include injury to the vagina or rectovaginal septum during the rectal dissection or anastomotic dehiscence with pelvic sepsis. The latter is probably the major predisposing factor because pelvic sepsis rates are significantly higher in patients with pouch-vaginal fistula than in those without.[50] CD has been reported to be more common in patients with pouch-vaginal fistula, yet is difficult to prove in the majority of cases. Management depends on the severity of symptoms. When these are minimal and acceptable to the patient, no action or the placement of a seton may be all that is necessary.[47] In those with a clinically significant degree of incontinence, a diverting ileostomy should be established if not already present. On defunctioning, sepsis is drained with or without placement of a seton suture and, once it has settled, repair is indicated. Simple defunctioning alone does not often lead to fistula closure.[51] Medical therapy is not indicated in managing these fistulas, although one recent series showed efficacy of infliximab.[52] Surgical options are divided into abdominal and local procedures. The former includes abdominal revision with advancement of the ileoanal anastomosis, and the latter fistulectomy with or without sphincter repair, endoanal advancement flap repair, and endovaginal or transvaginal repair. The height of the ileoanal anastomosis is the essential feature that influences the choice of operative approach. Pouch-vaginal fistula from an anastomosis at or above the anorectal junction should be approached abdominally with pouch dissection, repair of the vaginal defect, and creation of a new ileoanal anastomosis. Several authors have reported an approximately 80% success rate using this approach.[51,53,54] A fistula arising from an anastomosis within the anal canal should not be treated with an abdominal procedure because there is not sufficient distal anal canal length to be clear of the fistula. A local procedure is necessary in such circumstances and most surgeons have used either an endoanal ileal advancement flap procedure[45,46,48–50] or a transvaginal technique.[42,50,55] Although both approaches result in fistula closure in 50%–60% of cases, the transvaginal repair may have an advantage over the endoanal technique because it allows a direct approach to the fistula without the possibility of sphincter damage. Pouch-vaginal fistulas complicating CD are often difficult to treat, recurrence is common, and they frequently lead to pouch excision.[49–51]

The most frequent long-term complication after IPAA for UC is a nonspecific inflammation of the ileal pouch commonly known as pouchitis.[35,56–58] The presence of extraintestinal manifestations of UC before colectomy, especially primary sclerosing cholangitis, has been associated with the development of pouchitis.[56,59] Backwash ileitis does not predict the ultimate development of pouchitis. High-level expression of the serologic factor perinuclear antineutrophil cytoplasmic antibody before colectomy predicts the development of chronic pouchitis after IPAA.[60] The etiology of this nonspecific inflammation is unclear but, as with the continent ileostomy, may be attributable to an overgrowth of anaerobic bacteria. Presenting symptoms include abdominal cramps, fever, pelvic pain, and sudden increase in stool frequency. Treatment of pelvic reservoir pouchitis relies primarily on the use of antibiotics such as metronidazole and ciprofloxacin.[61,62] A mixture of probiotics can also be used in IPAA patients after resolution of the acute symptoms to prevent recurrence of pouchitis.[63] Although these regimens are almost always successful, occasionally steroid enemas or 5-aminosalicylates will be necessary. Patients with chronic pouchitis should be suspected of having CD. Uncommonly, an ileostomy with or without pouch excision is required for severe refractory pouchitis.

The number of bowel movements after successful ileoanal pouch procedures averages six per 24 hours. It should be pointed out that most patients are not particularly concerned with how often they defecate, because most can postpone defecation to accommodate social and recreational activities. Major incontinence is very unusual, although minor incontinence to mucus or stool, particularly at night, is observed in approximately 30% of patients. These patients are managed effectively with good perianal hygiene and the occasional use of a perineal pad. Although continence is clearly altered after pelvic pouch surgery, quality of life is extremely well preserved.[35,64] To obtain these results, however, approximately half of these patients regularly take a bulking agent or antidiarrheal medication to help regulate their bowels. Many patients also tend to eat less in the evening than at midday to minimize bowel movements when they are going out or while sleeping. Total failure, defined as removal of the pouch, occurs in only 5%–8% of cases and is usually caused by pelvic sepsis, undiagnosed CD, or an unacceptable functional outcome. Quality-of-life studies have disclosed that more than 95% of patients are satisfied with their pouch[35,65] and would not go back to an ileostomy.

Issues related to fertility, pregnancy, and the preferred method of delivery are of great importance in the female IPAA patient, many of whom are young and within their reproductive years. The ability of women desiring pregnancy to conceive after IPAA has been evaluated by several investigators. Most reports are characterized by small numbers of subjects attempting conception after surgery, and therefore do not permit any conclusions about fertility.[66–69] However, two larger studies have shown decreased postoperative fertility.[70–72] The severe decrease in postoperative fertility was attributed to probable tubal occlusion from adhesions, a phenomenon observed in another study.[67] However, physician recommendations against conception and patient concerns about having children affected with UC could not be discounted.[70] A second report from the same group on a different patient cohort found normal fecundity before UC diagnosis and from UC diagnosis to colectomy. However, fecundity decreased 80% after IPAA.[71] Placement of an anti-adhesion membrane around the fallopian tubes and ovaries during surgery may be useful in an attempt to reduce the incidence of these complications.

The optimal method of delivery remains controversial. Cesarean delivery decreases the risk of incontinence resulting from damage to the anal sphincters and yet is associated with complications inherent to abdominal surgery, including injury to the pelvic pouch and adhesion formation. Vaginal delivery may damage the pudendal nerve and the anal sphincter mechanism, but it reduces the problems associated with abdominal surgery and recovery is more rapid. Some short-term studies have shown the safety of vaginal delivery after IPAA.[73] However, vaginal delivery has been shown to cause occult sphincter damage[74] and injury to the innervation of the pelvic floor in normal females.[75] These factors could lead to an increased risk of fecal incontinence with age, which would be particularly devastating in a patient with a pelvic pouch.

Controversies

In approximately 10% of colitis patients, there are inadequate diagnostic criteria to make a definite distinction between UC and CD, especially in the setting of fulminant colitis.[76,77] These patients are labeled as having IC. Several major clinical concerns remain regarding performance of IPAA for IC, including a higher rate of perineal complications, development of CD, and eventual pouch loss.[78,79] Other investigators, however, have demonstrated acceptable outcomes of this procedure in IC.[80,81] Until the reasons underlying these discrepant data are uncovered, patients with IC should be counseled that undergoing IPAA may predispose them to a higher incidence of pouch-related complications. Although preoperative clinical factors that can predict those IC patients at risk for developing pouch complications or CD after IPAA have yet to be identified, a recent prospective study suggests that IC patients who express specific inflammatory bowel disease serologic markers before surgery have a significantly higher incidence of chronic pouchitis and CD after IPAA than IC patients who have a serologically negative profile.[82]

Another debated issue is whether IPAA should be offered to elderly patients. Two reasons to avoid these procedures in older patients relate to the higher incidence of anal sphincter dysfunction with increasing age and the morbidity of reoperations in these potentially medically more compromised patients. However, operations for rectal cancer with anastomosis to the anal sphincter are regularly performed in patients in their seventh and eighth decades, and thus many surgeons contend that an IPAA should also be made available. Many groups have demonstrated that IPAA in the elderly patient is safe and feasible.[83,84] It seems that chronologic age should not itself be used as an exclusion criterion. Pouch procedures are feasible in suitably motivated elderly individuals who understand the risks and problems of this procedure. Although bowel frequency remains constant in the first decade after the surgical procedure,[35,85,86] it is unclear what will occur as the patient continues to age. Perhaps the use of a double-stapled technique with preservation of the anal transition zone might improve function over time, but this remains unproven.

Another controversy relates to the use of the IPAA in UC patients who have an established colorectal cancer. The presence of distant metastatic disease is generally a contraindication to IPAA. These unfortunate patients should be managed with segmental colectomy or abdominal colectomy with IRA to facilitate early discharge and allow them to spend the rest of their lives relatively free of complications. Patients with middle and low rectal tumors, in accordance with basic principles of cancer surgery, may not be eligible for this procedure. Radiation therapy, if indicated, should be performed preoperatively; a pelvic pouch should not be subjected to radiation because of a high incidence of pouch loss. UC patients with cecal cancers represent another unique subgroup of patients. The sacrifice of a long segment of adjacent distal ileum with its mesenteric vessels may limit positioning of the reservoir into the pelvis. If a tension-free anastomosis cannot be ensured, a Brooke ileostomy may be necessary. Studies examining the use of the ileoanal pouch in patients with locally invasive cancers of the colon and upper rectum have been conflicting. In one series,[87] UC patients with a carcinoma had postoperative complications and functional results identical to UC patients without cancer. Metastatic disease developed in a small number of patients. In contrast, another study revealed that almost 20% of UC patients with cancer who had an IPAA died of metastatic disease.[88] Because both of these patients had T3 cancers at surgery, it is unclear that their course was adversely influenced by performing IPAA. This conservative management approach is also encouraged by surgeons at the Lahey Clinic,[89] where UC patients with a T3 cancer initially undergo an abdominal colectomy with ileostomy. An observation period of at least 12 months is recommended to ensure that no recurrent disease develops. Another reason to postpone IPAA in these patients is to allow adjuvant chemoradiation therapy to proceed unhindered without any added morbidity from a pouch–anal anastomosis and a relatively proximal ileostomy.

A number of innovations of the IPAA operation spurred by a desire to decrease complications and improve function have led to a series of technical controversies. Some authors believe that the entire rectal mucosa does not need to be removed. They favor leaving 1–2 cm of distal mucosa behind, transecting the rectum just above the puborectalis muscle and stapling the pouch to the rectal remnant. The potential advantages of the double-stapled approach include technical ease because it avoids a mucosectomy and the perineal phase of the operation, less tension on the anastomotic line, and improved functional results because sphincter injury is minimized and the anal transition zone with its abundant supply of sensory nerve endings is preserved.[90] However, surgeons who oppose this operative approach contend that residual diseased mucosa is at risk of malignancy. There have been nine reports of cancer developing after IPAA, eight in patients who underwent the procedure for dysplasia or colorectal cancer.[91–98] Two of these cases occurred in the preserved mucosa within the anal transition zone.[94,98] Although the origin of adenocarcinoma in these cases is a subject of debate, it is reasonably clear that a double-stapled technique should not be performed in the UC patient who is a high cancer risk (i.e., dysplasia or established cancer) at the time of IPAA. In addition, the potential for continuing colitis in this residual mucosa is another concern. Rauh and coworkers[99] have described a "short-strip pouchitis" that manifests as inflammation at the pouch anal anastomosis thought secondary to residual colitic mucosa. In an effort to resolve these issues, three prospective, randomized trials have demonstrated no significant differences in perioperative complications or functional results in those patients where a mucosectomy was done versus those patients where the distal rectal mucosa was preserved.[100–102] It is important that the surgeon performing an IPAA be familiar with both techniques in the event of failure or inability to use the stapler or when a hand-sewn anastomosis is contemplated but where anastomotic tension is excessive. It must be stressed that if a stapled technique is used, care should be taken to create an ileal pouch to anal anastomosis and not an ileal-to-rectum anastomosis.

Another technical controversial issue is the shape and size of the reservoir. Although the initial ileal reservoir created by Parks in the late 1970s was a triple-loop S pouch,[31] other pouch configurations have been described in an attempt to reduce pouch complications and improve functional outcome (Figure 41-13). Three other configurations that have been described are the double-loop J-pouch, the quadruple-loop W-pouch, and the lateral isoperistaltic H-pouch.[103–105] S-pouches were initially plagued with evacuation problems associated with a long (5-cm or more) exit conduit, frequently requiring pouch catheterization.[31] With shortening of the exit conduit to 2 cm or less, mandatory catheterization has been substantially reduced.[106] The long outlet tract formed in the H-pouch was also associated with pouch distention, stasis, and pouchitis.[107] The W-pouch has been favored by some surgeons[105] because its theoretically greater capacity may lead to fewer daily bowel movements. However, two randomized trials comparing the W- and J-pouch did not confirm this hypothesis.[108,109] In one study,[108] the median number of stools

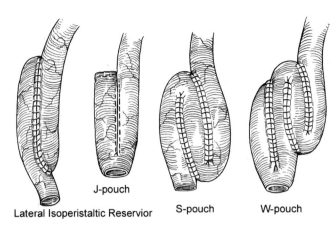

Lateral Isoperistaltic Reservior   J-pouch   S-pouch   W-pouch

FIGURE 41-13. Different ileal pouch configurations.

per day was the same in patients with a J- or W-pouch, and there was no difference in functional outcome between the two reservoirs in rates of incontinence, urgency, soiling, and the use of antidiarrheal agents. Johnston and coworkers[109] also demonstrated similar functional results between J- and W-pouches 1 year after surgery. At present, most centers perform a J-pouch because it is easier and faster to construct.[108,110] An S-pouch can provide additional length (2–4 cm) compared with the J-pouch and can be useful in minimizing anastomotic tension. However, the 2-cm exit conduit of the S-pouch may lengthen over time and obstructive defecation may develop.

A controversy that merits discussion relates to the routine use of a diverting loop ileostomy. Proponents of routine fecal diversion[111,112] contend that postoperative septic complications are minimized. Loop ileostomy also obviates the problem of immediate severe diarrhea through an edematous ileal pouch and a sphincter that has been damaged surgically by mucosectomy or double-stapling. However, many surgeons believe that the loop ileostomy is counterproductive.[113,114] Notwithstanding the additional operation and increased hospitalization associated with its closure, the morbidity of ileostomy closure is not insignificant, because small bowel obstruction and anastomosis leaks can occur. In addition, these ileostomies may be proximal in the small bowel and thus represent high-output stomas that can cause clinical dehydration. Some surgeons contend that omission of the ileostomy is safe when the anastomosis appears intact and under no tension, the procedure is not complicated by excessive bleeding or other technical difficulties, the terminal ileum is not affected by backwash ileitis, and the patients are not on high steroid doses before surgery. These criteria, however, have not been clearly studied in a prospective, randomized manner. It should be stressed that problems associated with the ileostomy or its closure such as dehydration, anastomotic leak, or bowel obstruction are easily managed with medical or surgical means. The development of a pouch-specific complication in those patients without an ileostomy is a particularly

morbid event requiring repeat laparotomy and fecal diversion in a septic patient. Clearly, more work is needed to further resolve the issue of whether an ileostomy should be routinely used in this procedure. It is clear that although associated with more skin irritation and stomal nursing care, a loop ileostomy is preferred over an end ileostomy for temporary fecal diversion after IPAA because of the ease of loop stoma closure.[115]

Many of the pelvic complications of the ileal pouch can be effectively managed by a perineal procedure. In some cases, however, these local procedures are not successful. The role of abdominal salvage surgery aimed at avoiding pouch excision or indefinite fecal diversion in patients with refractory pelvic sepsis, poor pouch function, or inflammation of retained rectal mucosa remains to be defined. Successful outcomes after salvage surgery have been reported in up to 90% of UC patients.[116–119] Others, however, have reported poorer results.[37,42] This great variability in success rates may be explained by variation in the severity of sepsis and its location in relation to the anastomosis.[37] The duration of follow-up is also an important factor, because failure after salvage continues steadily with time.[37,42] Various factors need to be considered when advising an abdominal salvage procedure, including feasibility of success, magnitude of operation, overall duration of treatment, and the patient's wishes. Counseling is essential and the patient must be given a realistic appraisal of the prospect of a successful outcome. The potential morbidity of removal of the reservoir resulting in a permanent ileostomy should also be discussed, including the possibility of a high-output ileostomy, pelvic nerve damage, and an unhealed perineal wound.

Conclusion

The approach to the UC patient requiring surgical intervention must begin with an open discussion concerning the pros and cons of each procedure. Surgeons should individualize treatment based on the patients' desires, fears, and expectations. In general, those patients desiring a minimum of complications without regard for continence should undergo total proctocolectomy with Brooke ileostomy. Those patients wishing to preserve fecal continence but also willing to accept a number of potential postoperative complications that in some cases may necessitate a stoma should consider an IPAA. The risk of complications and the unknown long-term effects of continence-preserving surgery require that patients be willing to undergo careful and regular follow-up. Patients not expected to comply with or take care of a continent ileostomy or IPAA should not be offered these procedures.

References

1. O'Keefe EA, Wright JP, Froggatt J, et al. Medium-term follow-up of ulcerative colitis in Cape Town. S Afr Med J 1989;76: 142–145.

2. Leijonmarck CE. Surgical treatment of ulcerative colitis in Stockholm county. Acta Chir Scand Suppl 1990;554:1–56.

3. Wexner SD, Rosen L, Lowry A, et al. Practice parameters for the treatment of mucosal ulcerative colitis. Dis Colon Rectum 1997;40:1277–1285.

4. Lichtiger S, Present DH, Kornbluth A, et al. Cyclosporine in severe ulcerative colitis refractory to steroid therapy. N Engl J Med 1994;330:1841–1845.

5. Fleshner PR, Michelassi F, Rubin M, et al. Morbidity of subtotal colectomy in patients with severe ulcerative colitis unresponsive to cyclosporin. Dis Colon Rectum 1995;38:1241–1245.

6. Hyde GM, Jewell DP, Kettlewell MGW, et al. Cyclosporin for severe ulcerative colitis does not increase the rate of perioperative complications. Dis Colon Rectum 2001;44:1436–1440.

7. Ransohoff DF. Colon cancer in ulcerative colitis. Gastroenterology 1988;91:1089–1094.

8. Lim CH, Dixon MF, Vail A, Forman D, Lynch DAF, Axon ATR. Ten year follow up of ulcerative colitis patients with and without low grade dysplasia. Gut 2003;52:1127–1132.

9. Motil KJ, Grand RJ, Davis-Kraft L, et al. Growth failure in children with inflammatory bowel disease: a prospective study. Gastroenterology 1993;105:681–691.

10. Camilleri-Brennan J, Steele RJ. Objective assessment of quality of life following panproctocolectomy and ileostomy for ulcerative colitis. Ann R Coll Surg 2001;83(5):321–324.

11. Fazio VW, Church JM. Complications and function of the continent ileostomy at the Cleveland Clinic. World J Surg 1988;12:148–154.

12. Leijonmarck CE, Lofberg R, Hellers G. Long-term results of ileorectal anastomosis in ulcerative colitis in Stockholm County. Dis Colon Rectum 1990;33:195–200.

13. Baker WNW, Glass RE, Richie JK, et al. Cancer of the rectum following colectomy and ileorectal anastomosis for ulcerative colitis. Br J Surg 1978;65:862–868.

14. Turnbull RB Jr, Hawk WA, Weakley FL. Surgical treatment of toxic megacolon. Ileostomy and colostomy to prepare patients for colectomy. Am J Surg 1971;122:325–331.

15. Ng RL, Davies AH, Grace RH, et al. Subcutaneous rectal stump closure after emergency subtotal colectomy. Br J Surg 1992;79:701–703.

16. Carter FM, McLeod RS, Cohen Z. Subtotal colectomy for ulcerative colitis: complications related to the rectal remnant. Dis Colon Rectum 1991;34:1005–1009.

17. Heuschen UA, Hinz U, Allemeyer EH, et al. Risk factors for ileoanal J pouch-related septic complications in ulcerative colitis and familial adenomatous polyposis. Ann Surg 2002; 235(2):207–216.

18. Alves A, Panis Y, Bouhnik Y, et al. Subtotal colectomy for severe acute colitis: a 20-year experience of a tertiary care center with an aggressive and early surgical policy. J Am Coll Surg 2003;197:379–385.

19. Brooke BN. The management of an ileostomy, including its complications. Lancet 1952;2:102–104.

20. Frizelle A, Pemberton JH. Removal of the anus during proctectomy. Br J Surg 1997;84:68–72.

21. Wickland M, Jansson I, Asztely M, et al. Gynaecological problems related to anatomical changes after conventional proctocolectomy and ileostomy. Int J Colorect Dis 1990;5: 49–52.

22. Carlsen E, Bergan A. Technical aspects and complications of end ileostomies. World J Surg 1995;19:632–636.

23. Kock NG, Darle N, Kewenter J, et al. Ileostomy. Curr Probl Surg 1977;14:1–52.

24. Litle VR, Barbour S, Schrock TR, Welton ML. The continent ileostomy: long-term durability and patient satisfaction. J Gastrointest Surg 1999;3:625–632.

25. Lepisto AH, Jarvinen HJ. Durability of Kock continent ileostomy. Dis Colon Rectum 2003;46(7):925–928.

26. Beck DE. Clinical aspects of continent ileostomies. Clin Colon Rectal Surg 2004;17:57–63.

27. Mullen P, Behrens D, Chalmers T, et al. Barnett continent intestinal reservoir. Multicenter experience with an alternative to the Brooke ileostomy. Dis Colon Rectum 1995;38(6):573–582.

28. Kaiser AM, Stein JP, Beart RW Jr. T-pouch: a new valve design for a continent ileostomy. Dis Colon Rectum 2002;45:411–415.

29. Newton CR, Baker WNW. Comparison of bowel function after ileorectal anastomosis for ulcerative colitis and colonic polyposis. Gut 1975;16:785–791.

30. Soravia C, O'Connor BI, Berk T, et al. Functional outcome of conversion of ileorectal anastomosis to ileal pouch-anal anastomosis in patients with familial adenomatous polyposis and ulcerative colitis. Dis Colon Rectum 1999;42:903–908.

31. Parks AG, Nicholls RJ. Proctocolectomy without ileostomy for ulcerative colitis. BMJ 1978;2:85–88.

32. Johnston D, Holdsworth PJ, Nasmyth DG, et al. Preservation of the entire anal canal in conservative proctocolectomy for ulcerative colitis: a pilot study comparing end-to-end ileo-anal anastomosis without mucosal resection with mucosal proctectomy and endo-anal anastomosis. Br J Surg 1987;74:940–944.

33. Wexner SD, James K, Jagelman DG. The double-stapled ileal reservoir and ileoanal anastomosis: a prospective review of sphincter function and clinical outcome. Dis Colon Rectum 1991;34:487–494.

34. Ambroze WL Jr, Wolff BG, Kelly KA, et al. Let sleeping dogs lie: role of the omentum in the ileal pouch-anal anastomosis procedure. Dis Colon Rectum 1991;34:563–565.

35. Michelassi F, Lee J, Rubin M, et al. Long-term functional results after ileal pouch anal restorative proctocolectomy for ulcerative colitis: a prospective observational study. Ann Surg 2003;238:433–441.

36. Marcello PW, Roberts PL, Schoetz DJ Jr, et al. Obstruction after ileal pouch-anal anastomosis: a preventable complication? Dis Colon Rectum 1994;37:1176–1177.

37. Heuschen UA, Allemeyer EH, Hinz U, et al. Outcome after septic complications in J pouch procedures. Br J Surg 2002;89: 194–200.

38. Marcello PW, Roberts PL, Schoëtz DJ Jr, et al. Long-term results of the ileoanal pouch procedure. Arch Surg 1993;128: 500–503.

39. Lewis WG, Kuzu A, Sagar PM, et al. Stricture at the pouch-anal anastomosis after restorative proctocolectomy. Dis Colon Rectum 1994;35:120–125.

40. Senapati A, Tibbs CJ, Ritchie JK, et al. Stenosis of the pouch anal anastomosis following restorative proctocolectomy. Int J Colorectal Dis 1996;11:57–59.

41. Prudhomme M, Dozois RR, Godlewski G, et al. Anal canal strictures after ileal pouch-anal anastomosis. Dis Colon Rectum 2003;46:20–23.

42. Galandiuk S, Scott NA, Dozois RR, et al. Ileal pouch–anal anastomosis. Reoperation for pouch-related complications. Ann Surg 1990;212:446–452.

43. Fazio VW, Tjandra JJ. Pouch advancement and neoileoanal anastomosis for anastomotic stricture and anovaginal fistula complicating restorative proctocolectomy. Br J Surg 1992; 79:694–696.

44. Fleshman J, McLeod RS, Cohen Z, Stern H. Improved results following use of an advancement technique in the treatment of ileoanal anastomotic complications. Int J Colorectal Dis 1988;3:161–165.

45. Wexner SD, Rothenberger DA, Jensen L, et al. Ileal pouch vaginal fistulas: incidence, etiology, and management. Dis Colon Rectum 1989;32:460–465.

46. Groom JS, Nicholls RJ, Hawley PR, et al. Pouch–vaginal fistula. Br J Surg 1993;80:936–940.

47. Keighley MR, Grobler SP. Fistula complicating restorative proctocolectomy. Br J Surg 1993;80:1065–1067.

48. Ozuner G, Hull T, Lee P, et al. What happens to a pelvic pouch when a fistula develops? Dis Colon Rectum 1997;40: 543–547.

49. Shah NS, Remzi F, Massmann A, et al. Management and treatment outcome of pouch-vaginal fistulas following restorative proctocolectomy. Dis Colon Rectum 2003;46:911–917.

50. Lee PY, Fazio VW, Church JM, et al. Vaginal fistula following restorative proctocolectomy. Dis Colon Rectum 1997;40: 752–759.

51. Paye F, Penna C, Chiche L, et al. Pouch-related fistula following restorative proctocolectomy. Br J Surg 1996;83:1574–1577.

52. Colombel JF, Ricart E, Loftus EV Jr, et al. Management of Crohn's disease of the ileoanal pouch with infliximab. Am J Gastroenterol 2003;98:2239–2244.

53. Cohen Z, Smith D, McLeod R. Reconstructive surgery for pelvic pouches. World J Surg 1998;22:342–346.

54. Zinicola R, Wilkinson KH, Nicholls RJ. Ileal pouch-vaginal fistula treated by abdominoanal advancement of the ileal pouch. Br J Surg 2003,90:1434–1435.

55. Burke D, van Laarhoven CJ, Herbst F, et al. Transvaginal repair of pouch–vaginal fistula. Br J Surg 2001;88:241–245.

56. Lohmuller JL, Pemberton JH, Dozois RR, et al. Pouchitis and extraintestinal manifestations of inflammatory bowel disease after ileal pouch-anal anastomosis. Ann Surg 1990;211: 622–627.

57. Fazio VW, Ziv Y, Church JM, et al. Ileal pouch-anal anastomoses complications and function in 1005 patients. Ann Surg 1995;222:120–127.

58. Meagher AP, Farouk R, Dozois RR, et al. Ileal J-pouch-anal anastomosis for chronic ulcerative colitis: complications and long-term outcome in 1310 patients. Br J Surg 1998;85: 800–803.

59. Sandborn W, LaRusso N, Schleck C, et al. Pouchitis after ileal pouch-anal anastomosis for ulcerative colitis occurs with increased frequency in patients with associated primary sclerosing cholangitis. Gut 1996;38:234–239.

60. Fleshner PR, Vasiliauskas EA, Kam LY, et al. High level perinuclear antineutrophil cytoplasmic antibody (pANCA) in ulcerative colitis patients before colectomy predicts the development of chronic pouchitis after ileal pouch-anal anastomosis. Gut 2001;49:671–677.

61. Madden MV, McIntyre AS, Nicholls RJ. Double-blind crossover trial of metronidazole versus placebo in chronic unremitting pouchitis. Dig Dis Sci 1994;39:1193–1196.

62. Shen B, Achkar JP, Lashner BA, et al. A randomized trial of ciprofloxacin and metronidazole in treating acute pouchitis. Inflamm Bowel Dis 2001;7:301–305.

63. Gionchetti P, Rizzello F, Helwig U, et al. Prophylaxis of pouchitis onset with probiotic therapy: a double-blind placebo-controlled trial. Gastroenterology 2003;124:1202–1209.

64. Holubar S, Hyman N. Continence alterations after ileal pouch-anal anastomosis do not diminish quality of life. Dis Colon Rectum 2003;46:1489–1491.

65. Köhler LW, Pemberton JH, Zinsmeister AR, et al. Quality of life after proctocolectomy. A comparison of Brooke ileostomy, Kock pouch, and ileal pouch-anal anastomosis. Gastroenterology 1991;101:679–684.

66. Counihan TC, Roberts PL, Schoetz DJ Jr, et al. Fertility and gynecologic function after ileal pouch-anal anastomosis. Dis Colon Rectum 1994;37:1126–1129.

67. Oresland T, Palmblad S, Ellstrom M, et al. Gynaecological and sexual function related to anatomical changes in the female pelvis after restorative proctocolectomy. Int J Colorectal Dis 1994;9:77–81.

68. Sjogren B, Poppen B. Sexual life in women after colectomy-proctomucosectomy with S-pouch. Acta Obstet Gynecol Scand 1995;74:51–55.

69. Tainen J, Matikainen M, Hiltunen KM, et al. Ileal J-pouch-anal anastomosis, sexual dysfunction, and fertility. Scand J Gastroenterol 1999;34:185–188.

70. Olsen KO, Joelsson M, Laurberg S, et al. Fertility after ileal pouch-anal anastomosis in women with ulcerative colitis. Br J Surg 1999;86:493–495.

71. Olsen KO, Juul S, Berndtsson I, et al. Ulcerative colitis: female fecundity before diagnosis, during disease, and after surgery compared with a population sample. Gastroenterology 2002; 122:15–19.

72. Johnson P, Richard C, Ravid A, et al. Female infertility after ileal pouch-anal anastomosis for ulcerative colitis. Dis Colon Rectum 2004;47(7):1119–1126.

73. Ravid A, Richard CS, Spencer LM, et al. Pregnancy, delivery, and pouch function after ileal pouch-anal anastomosis for ulcerative colitis. Dis Colon Rectum 2003;45:1283–1288.

74. Sultan AH, Kamm MA, Hudson CN, et al. Anal-sphincter disruption during vaginal delivery. N Engl J Med 1993;329:1905–1911.

75. Snooks SJ, Setchell M, Swash M, et al. Injury to innervation of pelvic floor sphincter musculature in childbirth. Lancet 1984;2:546–550.

76. Price AB. Overlap in the spectrum of non-specific inflammatory bowel disease—"colitis indeterminate." J Clin Pathol 1978;31:567–577.

77. Marcello PW, Schoetz DJ Jr, Roberts PL, et al. Evolutionary changes in the pathologic diagnosis after the ileoanal pouch procedure. Dis Colon Rectum 1997;40:263–269.

78. Koltun WA, Schoetz DJ Jr, Roberts PL, et al. Indeterminate colitis predisposes to perineal complications after ileal pouch-anal anastomosis. Dis Colon Rectum 1991;34:857–860.

79. Yu CS, Pemberton JH, Larson D. Ileal pouch-anal anastomosis in patients with indeterminate colitis. Long-term results. Dis Colon Rectum 2000;43:1487–1496.

80. Dayton MT, Larsen KR, Christiansen DD. Similar functional results and complications after ileal pouch-anal anastomosis in patients with indeterminate colitis vs ulcerative colitis. Arch Surg 2002;137:690–695.

81. Delaney CP, Remzi FH, Gramlich T, et al. Equivalent function, quality of life and pouch survival rates after ileal pouch-anal anastomosis for indeterminate and ulcerative colitis. Ann Surg 2002;236:43–49.

82. Hui T, Landers C, Vasiliauskas E, et al. Serologic responses in indeterminate colitis patients before ileal pouch-anal anastomosis may determine those at risk for persistent pouch inflammation. Gastroenterology 2003;124:A192.

83. Tan HT, Connolly AB, Morton D, et al. Results of restorative proctocolectomy in the elderly. Int J Colorectal Dis 1997;12:319–322.

84. Takao Y, Gilliland R, Nogueras JJ, et al. Is age relevant to functional outcome after restorative proctocolectomy for ulcerative colitis? Prospective assessment of 122 cases. Ann Surg 1998;227:187–194.

85. McIntyre PB, Pemberton JH, Wolff BG, et al. Comparing functional results one year and ten years after ileal pouch-anal anastomosis for chronic ulcerative colitis. Dis Colon Rectum 1994;37:303–307.

86. Bullard KM, Madoff RD, Gemlo BT. Is ileoanal pouch function stable with time? Dis Colon Rectum 2002;45:299–304.

87. Taylor BA, Wolff BG, Dozois RR. Ileal pouch-anal anastomosis for chronic ulcerative colitis and familial polyposis coli complicated by adenocarcinoma. Dis Colon Rectum 1988;31:358–362.

88. Stelzner M, Fonkalsrud EW. The endorectal ileal pullthrough procedure in patients with ulcerative colitis and familial polyposis with carcinoma. Surg Gynecol Obstet 1989;169:187–194.

89. Wiltz O, Hashmi HF, Schoetz DJ Jr, et al. Carcinoma and the ileal pouch-anal anastomosis. Dis Colon Rectum 1991;34:805–809.

90. Becker JM, Lamonte WS, Marie G, et al. Extent of smooth muscle resection during mucosectomy and ileal pouch anal anastomosis affects anorectal physiology and functional outcome. Dis Colon Rectum 1997;40:653–660.

91. Stern H, Walfisch S, Mullen B, et al. Cancer in an ileoanal reservoir: a new late complication? Gut 1990;31:473–475.

92. Puthu D, Rajan N, Rao R, et al. Carcinoma of the rectal pouch following restorative proctocolectomy: report of a case. Dis Colon Rectum 1992;35:257–260.

93. Rodriguez-Sanjuan JC, Polavieja MG, Naranjo A, et al. Adenocarcinoma in an ileal pouch for ulcerative colitis. Dis Colon Rectum 1995;38:779–780.

94. Sequens R. Cancer in the anal canal (transitional zone) after restorative proctocolectomy with stapled ileal pouch-anal anastomosis. Int J Colorectal Dis 1997;12:254–255.

95. Vieth M, Grunewald M, Niemeyer C, et al. Adenocarcinoma in an ileal pouch after prior proctocolectomy for carcinoma in a patient with ulcerative pancolitis. Virchows Arch 1998;433:281–284.

96. Iwama T, Kamikawa J, Higuchi T, et al. Development of invasive adenocarcinoma in a long-standing diverted ileal J-pouch for ulcerative colitis: report of a case. Dis Colon Rectum 2000;43:101–104.

97. Heuschen UA, Heuschen G, Autschbach F, et al. Adenocarcinoma in the ileal pouch: late risk of cancer after restorative proctocolectomy. Int J Colorectal Dis 2001;16:126–130.

98. Baratsis S, Hadjidimitriou F, Christodoulou M, et al. Adenocarcinoma in the anal canal following ileal pouch-anal anastomosis for ulcerative colitis using a double stapling technique. Dis Colon Rectum 2002;45:687–692.

99. Rauh SM, Schoetz DJ Jr, Roberts PL, et al. Pouchitis—is it a wastebasket diagnosis? Dis Colon Rectum 1991;34:685–689.

100. Seow-Choen A, Tsunoda A, Nicholls RJ. Prospective randomized trial comparing anal function after handsewn ileoanal anastomosis versus stapled ileoanal anastomosis without mucosectomy in restorative proctocolectomy. Br J Surg 1991;78:430–434.

101. Luukkonen P, Jarvinen H. Stapled versus hand sutured ileoanal anastomosis in restorative proctocolectomy: a prospective randomized trial. Arch Surg 1993;128:437–440.

102. Reilly WT, Pemberton JH, Wolff BG, et al. Randomized prospective trial comparing ileal pouch-anal anastomosis performed by excising the anal mucosa to ileal pouch-anal anastomosis. Ann Surg 1997;225:666–676.

103. Fonkalsrud EW. Total colectomy and endorectal ileal pullthrough with internal ileal reservoir for ulcerative colitis. Surg Gynecol Obstet 1980;150:1–8.

104. Utsunomiya J, Iwama T, Imago M, et al. Total colectomy, mucosal proctectomy and ileoanal anastomosis. Dis Colon Rectum 1980;23:459–466.

105. Nicholls RJ, Lubowski DZ. Restorative proctocolectomy: the four loop (W) reservoir. Br J Surg 1987;74:546–566.

106. Rothenberger DA, Buls JG, Nivatvongs S, et al. The Parks S ileal pouch and anal anastomosis after colectomy and mucosal proctectomy. Am J Surg 1985;149:390–394.

107. Stone MM, Lewin K, Fonkalsrud EW. Late obstruction of the lateral ileal reservoir after colectomy and endorectal ileal pullthrough procedures. Surg Gynecol Obstet 1986;162:411–417.

108. Keighley MRB, Yoshioka K, Kmiot W. Prospective randomized trial to compare the stapled double lumen pouch and the sutured quadruple pouch for restorative proctocolectomy. Br J Surg 1998;75:1008–1011.

109. Johnston D, Williamson MER, Lewis WG, et al. Prospective controlled trial of duplicated (J) versus quadrupled (W) pelvic ileal reservoirs in restorative proctocolectomy for ulcerative colitis. Gut 1996;39:242–247.

110. Fazio VW, Tjandra JJ, Lavery IC. Techniques of pouch construction. In: Nicholls RJ, ed. Restorative Proctocolectomy. Cambridge, MA: Blackwell Scientific; 1993;73–79.

111. Galandiuk S, Wolff BG, Dozois RR, et al. Ileal pouch-anal anastomosis without ileostomy. Dis Colon Rectum 1991;34:870–873.

112. Tjandra JJ, Fazio VW, Milsom JW, et al. Omission of temporary diversion in restorative proctocolectomy: is it safe? Dis Colon Rectum 1993;36:1007–1014.

113. Gorfine SR, Gelernt IM, Bauer JJ, Harris MT, Kreel I. Restorative proctocolectomy without diverting ileostomy. Dis Colon Rectum 1995;38:188–194.

114. Mowschenson PM, Critchlow JF, Peppercorn MA. Ileoanal pouch operation: long-term outcome with or without diverting ileostomy. Arch Surg 2000;135:463–465.

115. Fonkalsrud EW, Thakur A, Roof L. Comparison of loop versus end ileostomy for fecal diversion after restorative proctocolectomy for ulcerative colitis. J Am Coll Surg 2000;190:418–422.

116. Sagar PM, Dozois RR, Wolff BG, et al. Disconnection, pouch revision and reconnection of the ileal pouch–anal anastomosis. Br J Surg 1996;83:1401–1405.

117. Ogunbiyi OA, Korsgen S, Keighley MR. Pouch salvage. Long-term outcome. Dis Colon Rectum 1997;40:548–552.

118. Fazio VW, Wu JS, Lavery IC. Repeat ileal pouch–anal anastomosis to salvage septic complications of pelvic pouches: clinical outcome and quality of life assessment. Ann Surg 1998;228:588–597.

119. MacLean AR, O'Connor B, Parkes R, Cohen Z, McLeod RS. Reconstructive surgery for failed ileal pouch–anal anastomosis: a viable surgical option with acceptable results. Dis Colon Rectum 2002;45:880–886.

42
Surgery for Crohn's Disease

Scott A. Strong

Crohn's disease is a chronic, unremitting, incurable, inflammatory disorder that can affect the entire intestinal tract. Although the etiology remains uncertain, the distribution and behavior of the disease can be generally characterized. The presenting symptoms and signs, medical and operative options, and outcome likely depend on the disease genotype and phenotype. Specifically, the surgical procedures typically utilized in the operative management of Crohn's disease include nonresectional techniques such as internal bypass, fecal diversion, and strictureplasty as well as resectional procedures with or without concomitant anastomoses. The morbidity and risk for disease recurrence varies between the different procedures depending on myriad factors such as preoperative variables, site and behavior of disease, and postoperative influences.

Etiology and Incidence

The cause of Crohn's disease is unclear but recent investigations continue to provide insight into the etiology and pathogenesis of this inflammatory disorder that can affect any portion of the intestinal tract through a complex interplay between conditioning factors and effector mechanisms. The conditioning factors include genetic influences and triggering events that create a permissive host, whereas the effector mechanisms mediate tissue damage through dysregulation of the intestinal immune and nonimmune functions. Patients afflicted with symptomatic disease are likely genetically susceptible because abnormalities in seven loci on chromosomes 16q, 12, 6p, 14q, 5q, 19, and 1p have been identified in selected populations,[1] but there must be other factors at play because these variations have not been replicated in all populations and the proband concordance rate among monozygotic twins is only 50%–60%.[2,3] Initiating or triggering events such as environmental factors and microbial agents also probably contribute to disease susceptibility as evidenced by reports that describe the effects of tobacco usage[4–7] and fecal flora[8] on disease activity. In addition, abnormalities in immune

cellular function, nonimmune cell activity, protein expression, and cellular apoptosis hint as to the role of the dysregulated effector mechanisms in the pathogenesis of Crohn's disease.[9]

The prevalence of Crohn's disease in the United States is approximately seven cases per 100,000 persons, and the incidence has steadily increased over the past 5 decades.[10,11] Internationally, the prevalence is relatively high in northern Europe, significantly lower in southern Europe and Australia, and the lowest in South America, Asia, and upper Africa. This discrepancy in prevalence is likely multifactorial in nature, but it is recognized that the incidence and prevalence of Crohn's disease increases as a region becomes more urbanized.

The male-to-female ratio of the disease is 1.1–1.8:1 and the disease has a bimodal age distribution with the first peak occurring between the ages of 15–30 years and the second between 60–80 years; most persons experience the onset of disease symptoms before 30 years of age. The disorder is more common in whites than in blacks, Hispanics, or Asians, and a two- to fourfold increase in the prevalence has been found among the Jewish population in the United States, Europe, and South Africa compared with other ethnic groups.

Disease Classification

The original classification of Crohn's disease was described nearly three decades ago,[12] but inaccuracies associated with this and subsequent systems led to the most recent refinement, the Vienna Classification.[13] This scheme was generated by a World Congress of Gastroenterology Working Party that prospectively designed a simple phenotypic classification system based on objective and reproducible clinical variables that include age at diagnosis, anatomic location, and disease behavior. The age at diagnosis is stratified into patients <40 years and those ≥40 years. The anatomic location is classified as terminal ileum, colon, ileocolon, and upper gastrointestinal. Terminal ileal disease is defined as disease limited to the lower third of the small bowel with or without cecal involvement. Colon disease is any colonic involvement between the cecum and rectum without small bowel or upper gastrointestinal disease. Ileocolon disease is disease of the terminal ileum with colonic involvement noted between the cecum and rectum. And, upper gastrointestinal disease is defined as any disease location proximal to the terminal ileum regardless of involvement in other areas. The disease behavior is grouped as nonstricturing nonpenetrating (inflammatory), stricturing, and penetrating. Subsequent application of the Vienna Classification to clinical practice has demonstrated that the Crohn's disease phenotype markedly changes for a given patient over time[14–17] with 15% of patients experiencing a change in anatomic location and 80% of individuals with inflammatory disease ultimately demonstrating a stricturing or penetrating behavior. Moreover, the ability of experts to independently agree on disease phenotype using the Vienna Classification in controlled trials ranges from poor to fair.[18] It is unclear whether the varied classification systems fail because of the heterogeneity of the disease or inherent shortcomings of the classification schemes. Although these failings limit the utility of the Vienna Classification in clinical trials and disease management, recent advances in determining the genetic linkages associated with Crohn's disease will likely lead to a revised Crohn's disease classification system that combines genotype and phenotype characteristics.

Operative Indications

The indications for operative management of Crohn's disease include acute disease complications, chronic disease complications, and failed medical therapy. The acute complications are toxic colitis with or without associated megacolon, hemorrhage, and perforation, whereas the chronic disease complications include neoplasia, growth retardation, and extraintestinal manifestations. Failed medical therapy can take several forms including unresponsive disease, incomplete response, medication-related complications, and noncompliance with medication.

Toxic Colitis

Toxic colitis is a potentially fatal complication of Crohn's disease, particularly if accompanied by megacolon. Although several schemes exist to accurately identify toxic colitis, one reasonably simple system uses a definition that includes a disease flare accompanied by two of the following criteria: hypoalbuminemia (<3.0 g/dL), leukocytosis (>10.5 × 10^9 cells/L), tachycardia (>100 beats/minute), temperature increase (>38.6°C). Use of this relatively objective definition may aid in the diagnosis and care of these patients whose severe condition can be under-appreciated because of high dosages of steroids, immunomodulators, or biologic agents.

The initial management is directed at reversing physiologic deficits with intravenous hydration, correction of electrolyte imbalances, and blood product transfusions. Free perforation, increasing colonic dilatation, massive hemorrhage, peritonitis, and septic shock are indications for emergent operation after the patient has been adequately resuscitated. In the absence of these features, medical therapy is initiated with high dosages of intravenous corticosteroids, immunomodulators, and/or biologic agents.[19] Broad-spectrum antibiotics directed against intestinal flora are prescribed to minimize the risk of sepsis secondary to transmural inflammation or microperforation. Anticholinergics, antidiarrheals, and narcotics are avoided because they may worsen already impaired colonic motility or conceal ominous symptoms. Hyperalimentation may be started and the patient is closely observed with serial examinations and abdominal roentgenograms. Any worsening of the clinical course over the ensuing 24–72 hours mandates urgent laparotomy. If the patient improves minimally after 5–7 days of conventional therapy, the medical therapy should be altered or surgery should be advised. Experience with cyclosporine or infliximab in this setting is anecdotal, and should be weighed against operative therapy while understanding that surgery in this setting often relegates the patient to a life-long ileostomy.[20,21]

The principal operative options in patients with toxic colitis complicating Crohn's disease include subtotal colectomy with end ileostomy, total proctocolectomy with end ileostomy, and loop ileostomy with decompressive blowhole colostomy. Of these alternatives, subtotal colectomy with end ileostomy is the most widely practiced procedure. The most difficult aspect of the operation is managing the distal bowel stump. The distal limb may be closed with sutures or staples and then delivered to the anterior abdominal wall where it can lie without tension in the subcutaneous fat of the lower midline wound. Dehiscence of the closure during the postoperative period results in a mucous fistula instead of a pelvic abscess as witnessed when the closed stump is left within the peritoneal cavity. If the bowel wall is too friable to hold sutures or staples, a mucous fistula is primarily created. Rarely, instead of creating the fistula, the rectosigmoid stump must be exteriorized and wrapped in gauze to prevent retraction with a mucous fistula safely fashioned 7–10 days later.

The patient typically improves over the ensuing few days and can be typically discharged within a week of the operation. An ileoproctostomy can be recommended 6 months later in selected persons who demonstrate minimal mucosal inflammation, adequate rectal compliance, absence of significant anoperineal disease, and sufficient sphincter strength. Otherwise, the diseased rectum is left in place and the patient is counseled about the risk of neoplasia and the need for appropriate surveillance endoscopy.[22] In these individuals, proctectomy is usually recommended if disease-related symptoms prove to be too bothersome, neoplasia is identified, surveillance is limited because of stricturing, or laparotomy is warranted for other reasons. Disease-related symptoms are likely to occur in patients with prior anoperineal disease and proctectomy is often required within the first few postoperative years.[21,23]

Proctocolectomy with end ileostomy is rarely performed in the severely ill patient with toxic colitis because of the excessive rates of morbidity and mortality.[24–26] Proctectomy increases the difficulty of the procedure and risks pelvic bleeding as well as autonomic nerve damage. In rare instances of rectal perforation or profuse colorectal hemorrhage, or in the less severely ill patient who would not be a candidate for future ileoproctostomy, proctocolectomy may be a viable option. The surgeon must be cautioned, however, that the macroscopic and microscopic differentiation of ulcerative colitis from Crohn's proctocolitis is especially difficult in severe colitis, and primary proctocolectomy would nullify the future option of a restorative procedure in a patient with ulcerative colitis.

The need for loop ileostomy combined with decompression blowhole colostomy has virtually disappeared with improved medical recognition and more sophisticated management of toxic colitis. The operation is still useful in extremely ill patients or those in whom colectomy would be especially hazardous (e.g., contained perforation, high-lying splenic flexure, pregnancy). Contraindications to the procedure include colorectal hemorrhage, free perforation, and intraabdominal abscess. The operation is considered only a temporizing procedure, and a definitive operation is usually performed approximately 6 months later.

Hemorrhage

Crohn's disease may be responsible for life-threatening lower gastrointestinal hemorrhage and even exsanguination, but fortunately this is an infrequent complication.[27–30] More frequently, entities unrelated to disease involvement, including peptic ulcer disease and gastritis, may precipitate intestinal bleeding. Accordingly, gastric aspiration and possibly esophagogastroduodenoscopy are required to exclude sources of hemorrhage indirectly associated with Crohn's disease. The principal management of disease-related hemorrhage is determined by the severity and persistence of bleeding as well as the risk for recurrence. Localization of the bleeding site is essential regardless of the planned therapy. In a stable patient with colonic disease, endoscopic evaluation is preferred because this approach allows for disease assessment and therapeutic attempts at control of the identified bleeding site. However, indiscriminate usage of colonoscopy for bleeding colitis should be discouraged because this form of hemorrhage typically accompanies severe colitis, and colectomy with ileostomy is advised in this instance, regardless of the endoscopic findings.

A patient who requires ongoing resuscitation to maintain hemodynamic stability or in whom a small bowel source of active bleeding is suspected should undergo emergent mesenteric angiography to localize the source of hemorrhage and arrest ongoing bleeding through selective angiographic infusion of vasopressin or embolization. If the hemorrhage is localized but cannot be controlled by these interventional

modalities, the catheter is left in position and intraoperative angiography is performed to accurately identify the bleeding site and guide a limited bowel resection.[31] Otherwise, wide resection might be necessary to manage hemorrhage from a small ulcerated area within an extensive segment of affected bowel.

Laparotomy and resection with or without anastomosis are required if the patient's hemodynamic state cannot be sustained, bleeding persists despite 6 units of transfused blood, hemorrhage recurs, or another indication for surgery exists.

Perforation

Free perforation of the small bowel is also unusual and typically occurs at or just proximal to a strictured site.[32,33] The most appropriate treatment is resection of the involved bowel with immediate or delayed anastomosis. A nondiverted anastomosis should be avoided in the setting of delayed treatment, malnutrition, significant comorbidity, or severe sepsis. Resection with proximal ileostomy has an associated mortality rate of 4% compared with 41% with simple suture closure alone.[34] Perforation of the colon in patients with Crohn's disease is also rare and typically requires subtotal colectomy for optimal management because these cases often occur in the setting of severe colitis or steroid usage.[35]

Neoplasia

Overall, persons with Crohn's disease are at increased risk for developing cancer compared with the general population. In a population-based study from Canada,[36] these patients had an increased relative risk of developing carcinoma of the small intestine [17.4; 95% confidence interval (CI), 4.16–72.9] as well as malignancies of the liver and biliary tract (5.22; 95% CI, 0.96–28.5), and males were at a particular risk for lymphoma (3.63; 95% CI, 1.53–8.62). Their patients with Crohn's disease were also at increased risk for the development of colon cancer (2.64; 95% CI, 1.69–4.12) and the risk was similar to that seen in persons with ulcerative colitis (2.75; 95% CI, 1.91–3.97); the risk for rectal carcinoma, however, was similar to that demonstrated by a demographically matched cohort without inflammatory bowel disease.[36] Other population-based studies have supported the notion that Crohn's disease of the colon is associated with an increased risk of colorectal cancer,[37–39] whereas reports from some centers[40–42] have not noted the same association.

In a series of 22 patients with colorectal carcinoma complicating their Crohn's disease, 19 (86%) and 9 (41%) had adjacent or distant dysplasia, respectively, supporting a dysplasia-carcinoma sequence in Crohn's disease.[43] When a screening and surveillance program was adopted, dysplasia or cancer was detected in 16% of patients, and the probability of detecting dysplasia or cancer after a negative screening colonoscopy was 22% by the fourth surveillance examination. Accordingly, despite some controversy, many pundits[44,45] advocate that the endoscopic screening and surveillance protocols used for patients with ulcerative colitis should also be recommended for individuals with Crohn's disease of the large bowel. Specifically, a screening endoscopy should be performed 8–10 years after the onset of disease symptoms and four-quadrant random biopsies should be obtained every 10 cm along the length of the large bowel and directed biopsies should be procured from any strictures, lesions, or masses; subsequent surveillance endoscopy with similar biopsies should then be performed every 1–2 years. The finding of multifocal low-grade dysplasia, high-grade dysplasia, or invasive cancer would likely warrant review by a second experienced pathologist and confirmation would prompt a colectomy.

Growth Retardation

Abnormal linear growth secondary to delayed skeletal maturation is frequently encountered in children and adolescents with Crohn's disease. Specifically, more than half of children may have a subnormal height velocity and approximately one-quarter will have short stature.[46] Fortunately, surgical resection is often accompanied by growth response and associated psychologic benefit.

Extraintestinal Manifestations

Extraintestinal manifestations of Crohn's disease occur in nearly one-quarter of patients with Crohn's disease and can involve most organ systems.[47–49] Disorders of the skin, mouth, eye, and joints occur frequently with large bowel disease and their activity typically parallels the degree of intestinal inflammation. Operative management of the intestinal disease can provide beneficial control of the extraintestinal manifestation. Conversely, abnormalities affecting the hepatic, vascular, hematologic, pulmonary, cardiac, or neurologic systems behave independent of the intestinal disease. Other disorders such as nephrolithiasis and cholelithiasis are disease complications that likely arise from altered intestinal absorption.

Failed Medical Therapy

Antibiotics, probiotics, 5-aminosalicylate compounds, steroids, immunomodulators, and biologic agents all have a potential role in the management of Crohn's disease depending on the clinical presentation. Each medication within these therapeutic groups possesses appropriate dosing parameters, associated side effects, and an optimal time interval during which beneficial effects should appear. Before initiating treatment with any medication, the patient should be counseled about these features and objective criteria for disease response should be discussed and then sought after an established time interval. If the desired response is not achieved, prohibitive side effects arise, or noncompliance is problematic, the medication has failed and another medication should be trialed. When all appropriate medical therapy has failed, operative intervention is warranted. The continuation of ineffective medical management risks the development of further disease complications that may detrimentally impact surgical outcome.

Operative Considerations

Some fundamental observations that must be considered when operating for Crohn's disease are as follows:

- Crohn's disease is incurable
- Intestinal complications are the most common operative indication
- Operative options are influenced by myriad factors
- Asymptomatic disease should be ignored
- Nondiseased bowel can be involved by inflammatory adhesions or internal fistulas
- Mesenteric division can be difficult
- Resection margins should be conservative (2 cm)

Crohn's disease is a chronic inflammatory disorder that cannot be cured by medical therapy or operative intervention. Accordingly, treatment focuses on safely alleviating disease symptoms and restoring quality of life while attempting to maintain continuity of the intestinal tract. Of the various operative indications, intestinal complications including stricturing or penetrating disease that are unresponsive to medical therapy constitute the bulk of the indications, and the operative options depend on the multiple variables including patient age, anatomic location, disease behavior, symptoms, prior therapies, nutritional status, comorbid conditions, and associated sepsis. The patient's symptoms are especially important because the disease encountered at the time of surgery is often unanticipated despite preoperative evaluation.[50] In these instances, the findings must be compared with the presenting symptoms and signs, and any extensive disease that does not appear to be contributing to symptoms should be typically ignored. Exceptions to this axiom include the management of out-of-circuit bowel and short, uncomplicated small intestine strictures, which should be addressed in most patients.

Nondiseased bowel can be affected through inflammatory adhesions or internal fistulas. With adhesions, every attempt should be made to conserve the nondiseased bowel, although this can be especially difficult when managing enteroparietal or interloop abscesses. Most internal fistulas are best managed by wedge excision and primary closure of the fistula site in the secondarily affected small bowel. However, a short segmental resection with primary anastomosis may be required for fistulas targeting the rectosigmoid region because these often enter the bowel at the mesenteric margin and simple wedge excision may be vulnerable to breakdown of the suture line.

The mesentery of the diseased bowel is usually thickened because of fat deposition and enlarged mesenteric lymph nodes that straddle the ileocolic and sometimes superior mesenteric vessels. Attempts at simple division and ligation of the vessels may injure the remaining vascular pedicle leading to a rapidly spreading mesenteric hematoma that risks distal bowel ischemia. Instead, serial overlapping clamps applied to both sides of the intended transection line provide an ample margin or cuff on the mesenteric edge. Heavy, interlocking suture ligatures can then be used to under-run each pedicle caught within the clamps, eliminating concern for a spreading hematoma. Conservative (2 cm), macroscopically normal resection margins are associated with the same rate of operative morbidity and disease recurrence as extensive (12 cm), microscopically normal margins.[51] However, the luminal disease margin can be difficult to judge by inspecting the exterior of the bowel. Whereas inspection of the diseased bowel may reveal lymphadenopathy, creeping mesenteric fat, and corkscrewing of the serosal vessels, the nondiseased bowel may appear dilated with muscular hypertrophy and bowel wall edema. The key to discriminating between diseased and nondiseased bowel lies with palpation of the mesenteric margin of the bowel wall. A mesenteric ulcer will obscure the palpable transition from the mesentery to the bowel wall because of fat deposition between the terminal branches of the marginal vessels. If the surgeon's fingers passing from the mesentery onto the bowel can readily identify the edge of the bowel wall, the luminal mucosa will be macroscopically normal.

Operative Options

The surgical procedures performed for intestinal Crohn's disease can be divided into groups depending on whether resection of an intestinal segment is performed. The nonresectional procedures include internal bypass, fecal diversion, and strictureplasty, whereas the resectional procedures include resected bowel. Patients often undergo multiple procedures at the time of their single operation and these can be a combination of nonresectional as well as resectional procedures.

Internal Bypass

Internal bypass was the procedure of choice in the early days of surgery for Crohn's disease when mortality rates associated with resection were high because of lack of transfusion technology, antimicrobial medications, adequate anesthetic agents, and nutritional support services. However, with the advent of these modalities and recognition of complications such as recrudescent disease, mucoceles, and malignancy arising in diverted segments, this procedure was largely abandoned. However, bypass operations are still considered reasonable or desirable in specific circumstances. A complicated ileocecal phlegmon with dense attachment to the iliac vessels or retroperitoneum can be aptly managed by an exclusion bypass if the proximal end of the excluded ileal segment is exteriorized as a small mucus fistula and definitive resection is planned to occur in later months. Continuity bypass is sometimes the preferred method of managing symptomatic gastroduodenal Crohn's disease that is refractory to medical treatment where resection would entail extensive reconstruction of the upper intestinal tract or pancreaticobiliary system.

Fecal Diversion

Fecal diversion can be permanent or temporary. Many of the stomas created to permanently bypass unresected disease fail to control symptoms secondary to the out-of-circuit bowel, and resection is ultimately warranted. High complex fistulas and deep ulcerations are among the disease characteristics likely to mandate proctectomy with permanent ostomy for persistent disease symptoms despite fecal diversion.[52] Similarly, temporary diversion intended to heal distal disease or its sequelae is usually unsuccessful unless combined with a secondary procedure such as a rectal mucosal advancement flap that directly addresses the problem.[53] Even for free perforation of the small bowel, exteriorization of the proximal bowel alone is rarely the procedure of choice.

Strictureplasty

The incurable and pan-intestinal nature of Crohn's disease has led to a more conservative operative approach. For patients with multiple strictures of the small bowel, intestinal conservation may be maximally achieved by surgically widening the narrowed segment by performing a strictureplasty. This technique was initially described by Katariya et al.[54] for the successful treatment of tubercular small bowel strictures, and later used in strictures secondary to Crohn's disease.[55] The procedure safely relieves obstructive symptoms[56–58] with the operated patients demonstrating weight gain accompanied by improved food tolerance as well as discontinuation or reduction of steroid usage.[59] Moreover, patients undergoing strictureplasty alone are no more likely to require reoperation than those who undergo a concomitant resection,[60] and reoperation rates after first and second operations are also similar.[61]

The situations for which strictureplasty is considered are as follows:

- Diffuse involvement of the small bowel with multiple strictures
- Stricture(s) in a patient who has undergone previous major resection(s) of small bowel (>100 cm)
- Rapid recurrence of Crohn's disease manifested as obstruction
- Stricture in a patient with short bowel syndrome
- Nonphlegmonous fibrotic stricture

The contraindications to strictureplasty are as follows:

- Free or contained perforation of the small bowel
- Phlegmonous inflammation, internal fistula, or external fistula involving the affected site
- Multiple strictures within a short segment

- Stricture in close proximity to a site chosen for resection
- Hypoalbuminemia (<2.0 g/dL)

Multiple strictures in a patient with an albumin value <2.5 g/dL, preoperative weight loss, or advanced age may be regarded by some as a situation in which strictureplasty should be avoided because of concerns of sepsis, but a proximal diverting stoma with multiple strictureplasties should be considered in this instance.[57] Factors that do not seem to be associated with increased operative risk include perforative or phlegmonous disease remote from the strictureplasty site, steroid dosage, synchronous resection, number of strictureplasties, and length of stricture.

The length of the strictured segment dictates the type of strictureplasty technique used. Short (<10 cm) strictures are best managed by a Heineke-Mikulicz type of strictureplasty, whereas medium length (10–20 cm) strictures can be corrected by a Finney-type strictureplasty. Long (>20 cm) strictures are best managed by a side-to-side isoperistaltic strictureplasty.[62] Regardless the technique, the bowel is incised along its antimesenteric margin extending 1–2 cm beyond the diseased segment, which is identified by the presence of mesenteric ulceration. Biopsy of any suspicious mucosa is performed to exclude carcinoma[63–65] and closure is achieved using an absorbable suture in a one- or two-layer manner. The mesentery at each of the strictureplasty sites is then labeled with metallic clips to allow discrimination between the multiple sites in the unlikely event that postoperative hemorrhage occurs. Selective mesenteric angiography with intraarterial vasopressin infusion will control most bleeding episodes, but the radio-opaque metal clips will help avoid the need to open each of the strictureplasty sites to localize the bleeding site if reoperation is required.[66]

Many centers have used a Finney-type strictureplasty for recurrent terminal ileal disease with the anastomosis created between the terminal ileum and proximal colon.[67–70] Others have extrapolated this experience into patients undergoing their first operation for terminal ileal Crohn's disease.[71] A long ileocolostomy is constructed encompassing the entirety of the diseased bowel. Interestingly, subsequent endoscopic and imaging studies have revealed complete morphologic disease regression.[71]

Resection

The basic principles of resection should be followed whether an open or laparoscopic approach is used, and include mobilization of both diseased intestine as well as sufficient nondiseased bowel to facilitate the subsequent creation of a tension-free anastomosis or construction of an ostomy. Extensive mobilization may facilitate operations for terminal ileal disease complicated by fused ileal loops or a phlegmonous mass adherent to matted loops of small bowel, omentum, or retroperitoneal structures. Delivery of the ascending colon and terminal ileum into the wound or to the anterior abdominal wall enables separation of the involved intestinal loops and permits closer inspection to determine which segments require resection. Enteric fistulas often originate from diseased bowel that communicates with nondiseased intestine. Whereas the primary site usually requires resection, the secondarily affected bowel segments are typically treated by conservative wedge excision and simple closure of the resultant defect. The diseased bowel should be resected with conservative margins and the mesentery divided using the previously described methods. Removal of enlarged mesenteric lymph nodes is not a goal of resectional surgery because this practice risks vascular injury without reducing the likelihood of recurrent disease. The specimen should be opened after it has been delivered from the operative field to assure macroscopic disease-free resection margins.

A laparoscopic approach can be used for a variety of resectional procedures and is typically associated with longer procedure times, but shorter lengths of stay and briefer periods of recovery.[72–79] Although disease complicated by fistulas or phlegmons can prove challenging, experienced laparoscopic surgeons have been able to safely complete procedures in these instances without converting to a laparotomy.[80,81]

After the diseased bowel has been resected, the surgeon must decide whether to create an end stoma, an anastomosis, or a diverted anastomosis. In general, an end stoma is desirable in patients who are critically ill, demonstrate fecal peritonitis, or have coagulopathy. An anastomosis can be safely created in most other instances assuming a few general principles are respected that include the following:

- Adequate blood supply must be assured
- Tension or torsion are unacceptable
- Luminal size needs to be equivalent
- The mesenteric defect should be closed

A temporary diverting stoma should be considered to protect the anastomosis in instances of incompletely drained sepsis, excessive blood loss during a long operation, or severe hypoalbuminemia (<2.5 g/dL).

In operations for terminal ileal disease, the neoterminal ileum tends to be the usual site of disease recurrence. Accordingly, the optimal anastomotic configuration and preferred materials are subject to debate.[82–84] Some recent retrospective studies[85–88] and one prospective, randomized trial[89] suggest that larger side-to-side anastomoses are associated with a reduced risk for disease recurrence. Although many investigators have found no association between the materials used to create the anastomosis and morbidity rates,[86,87] at least three studies[85,90,91] have reported that a stapled anastomosis is safer than a hand-sewn anastomosis. Regardless, it is important to use a hand-sewn technique when the bowel wall is abnormally thickened because the stapling instruments are not designed to safely construct an anastomosis under these conditions.

Specific Anatomic Locations

Terminal Ileum

Terminal ileal disease is defined as disease limited to the lower third of the small bowel with or without cecal involvement. Approximately 20% of patients with Crohn's disease will express this phenotype, and usually present with symptoms suggestive of inflammation or obstruction. In the majority of cases, resection with construction of an ileal-ascending colon anastomosis is feasible and desirable. All nondiseased ascending colon should be preserved to provide the largest possible surface area for water absorption and to avoid a complex fistula involving retroperitoneal structures associated with recurrent disease involving an anastomosis that overlies the second portion of the duodenum. Alternatively, this is the situation in which some centers avoid bowel resection by creating a large Finney-type ileocolostomy.[71]

Terminal ileal disease with sparing of the ileocecal valve and cecum is ideally treated with resection and enteroenterostomy provided there is sufficient length (5–7 cm) of normal-appearing distal ileum after definitive ileal resection. Preservation of the ileocecal valve helps to minimize the risk of postoperative diarrhea. In many instances, a hand-sewn anastomosis is preferred because the distal segment may be too short to accommodate a stapled anastomosis.

Colon

Colon disease is any colonic involvement between the cecum and rectum without small bowel or upper gastrointestinal disease. Nearly 40% of patients have this disease distribution, and often complain of inflammatory disease symptoms including abdominal cramping, bloody diarrhea, and urgency.

Persons presenting with segmental disease are best treated with segmental resection to protect against dehydration and electrolyte imbalances associated with loss of the large intestine's physiologic role. In patients with disease limited to the ascending colon, the transverse colon is divided at the level of the middle colic vessels so that the mesenteric root naturally separates the anastomosis from the retroperitoneum, minimizing the risk for recurrent disease complicated by complex fistulas. Alternatively, a more proximal anastomosis may be wrapped with a pedicle of omentum, thereby preventing the anastomosis from lying in direct contact with the retroperitoneum. Disease involving the ascending and transverse colons is treated in a similar manner except an extended right colectomy is recommended because the mesentery of the ileum is more easily approximated to the mesentery of the sigmoid colon than the descending colon. Resection of the additional colonic segment avoids an internal hernia and does not adversely affect the functional outcome. Crohn's disease of the transverse, descending, and sigmoid colons presents a situation in which segmental resection and colocolic or colorectal anastomosis is most frequently used. Segmental

resection is particularly ideal for older individuals (>50 years) and patients with colitis who have previously undergone significant small bowel resection (>30 cm). In both instances, preservation of the ileocecal valve and colonic absorptive surface may protect against diarrhea and dramatically improve the functional outcome. Resection with coloproctostomy is used for these selected patients with left-sided disease, and a cecorectal anastomosis is constructed if the transverse colon is also involved. In younger patients and those without prior small bowel resection, the diseased segment and uninvolved proximal colon are resected and an ileosigmoid or ileorectal anastomosis is constructed.

Colonic strictureplasty has been described for short strictures and seems to be associated with a morbidity rate, risk for surgical recurrence, and postoperative quality of life comparable to that seen with resection.[92] However, given the 7% incidence of malignancy arising in a colonic stricture,[93] some surgeons argue that resection should be exclusively encouraged if all of the outcome measures are comparable.

Patients with extensive colonic involvement, relative rectal sparing, and adequate fecal continence without active anoperineal sepsis or compromised rectal compliance are candidates for colectomy with ileoproctostomy. Rectal compliance can be subjectively judged by distending the rectum during proctoscopy or objectively quantified with anorectal physiology testing; patients whose maximum tolerated rectal volume measures <150 mL will do poorly with an ileoproctostomy.[94] A rare patient presents with pan-colonic disease, significant upper rectal involvement, and sparing of the mid- and distal-rectum. Resection of all disease in this setting leaves an anastomosis only 6–8 cm above the anal verge, and is often associated with impaired function secondary to compromised compliance. Instead, an ileal J-pouch can be configured with 10-cm limbs and joined to the spared mid-rectum after subtotal proctocolectomy. Despite a likely increased disease recurrence compared with that seen with total proctocolectomy and ileostomy, the patient may enjoy several years without a stoma.

Patients with proctocolitis that warrants operative treatment usually require a total proctocolectomy with creation of an end ileostomy, especially those persons with colitis whose proctitis, sphincter dysfunction, or anoperineal sepsis is too severe for rectal preservation and ileoproctostomy. If proctectomy is required, the entirety of the rectum should be excised in a single or staged procedure because of the significant risk of cancer developing in the defunctioned rectal stump despite surveillance proctoscopy.[95] An unhealed perineal wound that persists 6–12 months after endoanal proctectomy should be evaluated to exclude concomitant pyoderma gangrenosum, perineal sinus, enteroperineal fistula, and malignancy. A simple shallow wound will usually respond to repeated wound debridements and diligent wound care with vacuum-assisted closure system and split-thickness skin grafts providing additional benefit. Wounds complicated by a perineal sinus or enteroperineal fistula require more extensive procedures that often include omental, muscle, or myocutaneous flaps.[96–98]

One center has chosen to offer patients with Crohn's disease isolated to the colon and rectum a total proctocolectomy with ileal pouch–anal anastomosis.[99] They have reported that the rates of Crohn's disease–related complications and pouch excision are 35% and 10%, respectively, after 10 years of follow-up. However, other reports suggest that 12%–29% and 45%–52% of patients with Crohn's disease subsequently require pouch excision 5 and 10 years after restorative proctocolectomy, respectively.[100–103] Consequently, a restorative proctocolectomy is usually avoided in the setting of recognized Crohn's disease, and is typically performed only as part of a controlled trial.

Ileocolon

Ileocolon disease is disease of the terminal ileum with colonic involvement noted distal to the cecum and proximal to the rectum. This disease phenotype occurs as often as terminal ileal disease, and the operative approach to these patients is similar to that already outlined for individuals with terminal ileal or colon disease. Specifically, the surgeon must conserve as much of the nondiseased colon as possible and avoid large mesenteric defects. This often requires the construction of two anastomoses, which does not seem to significantly increase operative morbidity.

Upper Gastrointestinal

Upper gastrointestinal disease is defined as any disease location proximal to the terminal ileum regardless of involvement in other areas, and represents the phenotype that is often the most difficult to manage because of its predilection for extensive disease and predominantly stricturing or penetrating behavior.

Small bowel disease proximal to the terminal ileum is often typified by several stenotic segments separated from one another by noninvolved bowel. These diseased segments range in length and can measure >50 cm. The prognosis for Crohn's disease diffusely involving the small bowel is significantly worse than that of localized disease.[104] The operative options in a symptomatic patient with diffuse jejunoileitis include internal intestinal bypass, strictureplasty, and resection. Intestinal bypass is reproved by most clinicians because of concerns about bacterial overgrowth and malignant degeneration. Resection risks immediate or future short bowel syndrome and is not generally recommended. An operation that consists of multiple strictureplasties is the procedure of choice using the previously discussed techniques to safely conserve small bowel and relieve symptoms secondary to luminal stenosis. The involved segments can be ignored only in the rare instance in which the diseased intestine appears to be inflamed without evidence of stricture or penetration.

Gastroduodenal Crohn's disease is relatively rare, and the most common presenting complaints are upper abdominal pain and symptoms of duodenal obstruction. Endoscopy will demonstrate macroscopic abnormalities in the majority of patients with the antrum most frequently involved.[105] Isolated gastric disease is exceedingly rare and any reports of successful treatment are purely anecdotal.[106] For duodenal disease, medical therapy is the mainstay of treatment for inflammatory and penetrating disease, whereas strictures present a different challenge.[107] Ulcer-like lesions are nonspecific, rarely cause stenosis, spontaneously regress, and are usually associated with other diseased sites. Contrarily, stenotic duodenal segments are typically unifocal and often respond poorly to medical management. Endoscopic balloon dilatation has been safely used to treat short duodenal strictures, and the procedure seems to be well tolerated while providing marked symptom relief.[108,109] In the past, the operative management of duodenal strictures was restricted to gastrojejunostomy with or without concomitant vagotomy.[110,111] Protagonists of truncal vagotomy cited the high risk for marginal ulceration whereas antagonists raised concerns about postoperative diarrhea. Recently, success with duodenal strictureplasty has been reported by several centers, and the technique seems to be the procedure of choice if the affected bowel is sufficiently supple and devoid of associated sepsis.[112–115]

Anoperineum

Crohn's disease will affect the anus or perineum in as many as 61%–80% of patients, and typically occurs with or following the onset of disease in other anatomic locations.[116] Involvement of this area can manifest itself as a fissure, skin tag or hemorrhoid, cavitating ulcer, abscess or fistula, anovaginal fistula, anorectal stricture, or carcinoma. These comprise the basis of the accurately descriptive and comprehensive Cardiff classification of anal Crohn's disease,[117] which has not been widely accepted by clinicians because it is perceived to be of minimal clinical relevance.[118,119] Whereas this classification system is solely based on the anatomic and pathologic features, scoring systems of disease activity have been proposed to complement this scheme. These include the Perianal Crohn's Disease Activity Index[120] and a newer system intended to evaluate and predict the outcome of operative management.[121]

The evaluation of anoperineal Crohn's disease should include a regional examination as well as investigations to determine the extent and activity of disease located elsewhere through varied imaging and endoscopic studies. The regional examination may be significantly enhanced by assessment with fistulography,[122,123] endoanal ultrasonography,[124–126] magnetic resonance imaging,[127–130] or examination under anesthesia. Comparative reports suggest that these modalities are associated with comparable accuracy,[131,132] and overall accuracy might be best enhanced by combining the results of any two modalities.[131]

The first priority of therapy is to drain any associated sepsis through the insertion of drainage catheters with or without placement of noncutting setons. The second priority focuses on stabilizing the infectious component using antibiotic therapy such as metronidazole or ciprofloxacin. In addition, attempts at medical management of the disease process are initiated with immunomodulators and biologic agents; 5-aminosalicylic acid compounds and steroids provide little benefit. The third priority is optimization of quality of life through continued medical therapy or operative intervention used individually or in combination. Asymptomatic fissures, skin tags, or hemorrhoids are best ignored because surgical treatment may escalate the disease to a point in which proctectomy is eventually required.[52,133,134] Cavitating ulcers may dramatically improve with operative debridement and intralesional steroid injection in combination with appropriately aggressive medical therapy.

Medical management typically includes antibiotics, immunomodulators, and biologic agents used individually or in combination. Metronidazole (20 mg/kg/day) prescribed for 6–8 weeks is associated with a 50%–56% healing rate, but nearly half of patients will experience disease exacerbation and paresthesias with dosage reduction.[135,136] Azathioprine (2–3 mg/kg/day) or 6-mercaptopurine (1.5 mg/kg/day) used alone heals 54% of fistulas compared with a 21% healing rate with placebo.[137] Three doses of infliximab (5 mg/kg) delivered at 0, 2, and 6 weeks can promote fistula closure in 55% of the patients, as compared with 13% of the patients treated with placebo, and the median length of time during which the fistula remains closed is 3 months.[138] However, ciprofloxacin (1000 mg/day) in combination with infliximab tends to be more effective than infliximab alone,[132,139] and re-treatment with infliximab every 8 weeks is more effective than placebo in maintaining fistula closure.[140,141] Lastly, concomitant immunosuppressive therapy with azathioprine, 6-mercaptopurine, or methotrexate may result in improved outcomes because of a reduction in the frequency of human antichimeric antibody formation, acute infusion reactions, and a reduced risk of delayed hypersensitivity-like reactions and formation of antinuclear antibodies.

The operative management of a perineal abscess or anoperineal fistula is predicated upon the patient's baseline continence, complexity of the fistula, amount of sphincter encompassed by the fistula, and severity of rectal involvement. In a review of 21 retrospective studies that focused on fistulotomy for a low-lying fistula, the postoperative incontinence rates ranged from 0% to 50%, and 6% to 60% ultimately required a stoma.[142] The initial healing rates in these studies ranged from 8% to 100%, with rates of 80%–100% in 13 of 21 studies, 60%–79% in five of 13 studies, and <60% in three of 21 studies. The clinical scenario best suited for fistulotomy is the continent patient with a simple, low-lying, posterior fistula without associated rectal disease. Fistulotomy for an anterior fistula in this setting, especially in a woman, may risk incontinence. If fistulotomy is likely to cause a disturbance in fecal continence in a patient with minimal rectal inflammation, a rectal mucosal advancement flap is recommended. The healing rates with this procedure range

from 50% to 80% in series containing at least 20 patients,[143–145] and a history of non-colon Crohn's disease is a predictor of failure.[144] Alternatively, a chronic indwelling noncutting seton can be used in this setting. These setons are more ideally suited for chronic drainage of a fistula complicated by rectal inflammation, with proctectomy required in 0%–33% of patients reported in series composed of at least 20 patients.[146–150] Fibrin sealant has also been used in these situations to obliterate the fistula tract, but success has been limited.[151–153] In some patients, the severity of rectal inflammation or extent of perineal sepsis mandates endoanal proctectomy and permanent fecal diversion.[116,142]

Anovaginal fistulas are more difficult to manage than anoperineal fistulas because they often originate from an anal ulcer and traverse a short distance through sometimes attenuated muscle. Fistulas that are not associated with an anal canal ulcer are usually managed with a rectal mucosal advancement flap if the rectal mucosa is noninflamed,[145,154] or an anocutaneous flap if the rectum is moderately diseased.[155] For women with an anovaginal fistula and anal canal ulceration or severe proctitis, proctectomy is often required.

Many clinicians are beginning to use medical therapy in combination with operative treatment. They are reporting that an examination under anesthesia before infliximab treatment accelerates healing[156] and infliximab treatment followed by definitive surgery has a beneficial additive effect in a multistep treatment regimen for the management of complex anal fistulas arising in patients with active proctitis.[157]

Strictures, which are typically situated at the top of the anorectal ring, should be ignored if asymptomatic or gently dilated if associated with complaints suggestive of outlet obstruction.[158,159] In selected patients with nondiseased rectums, a rectal sleeve advancement may be attempted.[160] Both squamous cell carcinoma and adenocarcinoma can complicate preexisting anoperineal Crohn's disease and persons with chronic involvement may require examinations under anesthesia with both directed and random biopsies of chronically indurated areas to exclude the possibility of malignant degeneration.[95,161–164] If a cancer is identified, the lymph node drainage basin should be closely examined and an oncologic resection planned with or without perioperative adjuvant therapy depending on the histology and stage of the tumor.

Special Circumstances

Enteroparietal Abscess

An enteroparietal abscess is likely best treated by initial external drainage using a computed tomography (CT)-guided catheter if the cavity is accessible or, otherwise, by surgical drainage. Conversely, some surgeons suggest that the abscess is best managed by laparotomy, resection, and occasional anastomosis.[165] Antagonists of this approach cite their concerns about short bowel syndrome after laparotomy because nondiseased bowel involved by the abscess often requires concomitant resection to manage the abscess.[166] Furthermore, successful CT-guided drainage procedures obviate the need for early as well as late operative intervention in nearly half of patients.[166] Patients with large, recurrent abscesses or fistulas after drainage are more likely to require subsequent laparotomy, but a fistula does not pose much operative difficulty if resection has been deferred for approximately 6 weeks.

Interloop Abscess

Interloop abscesses, which are considerably smaller than the enteroparietal form, are often occult or subtle in presentation and are usually identified only at the time of resection when separating loops of matted bowel.

Intramesenteric Abscess

Intramesenteric abscesses arise from penetrating disease eroding into the mesentery of the small bowel, colon, or rectum. In the small bowel, the abscess often dissects between the mesenteric leaves, extending sometimes to the origins of the superior mesenteric vessels. Resection of the bowel with a cuff of mesentery carries a particular risk for vascular injury or secondary hemorrhage. Instead, the abscess is identified by intraoperative needle aspiration, and the purulent fluid is drained back into the small bowel lumen by compression of the mesenteric leaves and needle aspiration. An exclusion bypass of the involved bowel is then performed by creating proximal and distal mucus fistulas, and constructing an enteroenterostomy above and below the diseased segment to restore bowel continuity. The excluded segment is then resected 6 months later. Intramesenteric abscesses of the sigmoid colon or rectum are best managed by external drainage combined with diverting end colostomy proximal to the site of disease. Resection with anastomosis to the normal rectum is performed 6 months later.

Retroperitoneal and Psoas Abscess

Abscesses arising in this anatomic location may be large and well-circumscribed or poorly localized with the infectious process extending deep to the psoas fascia in both caudad and cephalad directions. CT-guided drainage is usually first used followed by elective resection of the diseased segment. If a CT-guided approach fails, surgical drainage is warranted. A large, multilocular abscess is best treated by incising over the appropriate site, separating the oblique muscles, localizing the abscess by needle aspiration, incising the pyogenic membrane, and digitally disrupting any septations. A drainage catheter is inserted and continued until the cavity has collapsed after 4–6 weeks. If the abscess is initially identified at laparotomy, the diseased segment is mobilized, the involved bowel resected, and an anastomosis is usually constructed. The abscess is then unroofed and extraperitoneally drained,

and omentum is interposed between the bowel and the residual cavity. Sinography is completed immediately before catheter removal to assure collapse of the cavity. If the cavity persists, longer drainage is recommended.

Enterocutaneous Fistula

Enterocutaneous fistulas can develop before any surgical therapy, during the immediate postoperative period, or several weeks after an operation.[167] Early postoperative fistulas most likely represent breakdown of an anastomosis or an unrecognized enterotomy. Otherwise, they are the result of active penetrating disease. This latter presentation is best evaluated by imaging studies and endoscopy to determine the extent of disease and exclude possible septic foci that would require drainage. Medical therapy is then usually initiated with operative management warranted for significantly symptomatic fistulas that are unlikely to heal or fail to heal with medical treatment. Low-output fistulas that minimally soak a gauze dressing may be managed by nonoperative techniques, especially in patients with significant operative risk. If an operation is required, the fistulizing segment of bowel is typically diseased or situated proximal to an obstructed segment. Regardless, the fistulizing bowel and any other disease sites are addressed. Wedge excision or strictureplasty of the fistula site is not recommended because of the associated risk for postoperative leak and recurrent fistula.[168] However, strictureplasty may be performed in other diseased areas provided the previously mentioned guidelines are followed. In a patient with a complex fistula requiring a prolonged operation with extensive enterolysis, multiple anastomoses, enterotomy closures, or strictureplasties, a diverting stoma proximal to all procedure sites is often prudent to allow healing before restoration of the normal fecal flow. These persons often require home hyperalimentation for 3–6 months followed by stoma closure after preoperative imaging confirms complete healing of all suture lines and no areas of distal obstruction.

The management of a fistula developing during the early postoperative period depends on the timing of the presentation and other variables. If the operation was relatively straightforward and the fistula presents in the first 7–10 postoperative days, re-laparotomy, resection, or fistula repair, and probable proximal fecal diversion is warranted. Beyond that time interval or after a difficult operation, re-laparotomy may be associated with more harm than benefit because of formidable adhesions and the risk of iatrogenic bowel injury. An operation is indicated in these patients if they have evidence of sepsis or hemorrhage that cannot be managed by interventional radiology techniques or potentially life-threatening ischemic bowel. In addition, some individuals with fistulas that are particularly difficult to manage can be aided by a laparotomy whereby the upper abdomen is entered and a segment of jejunum proximal to the fistula site is brought out as a diverting stoma. These patients with postoperative fistulas treated nonoperatively will usually require home hyperalimentation, somatostatin, and possible gastric decompression until the fistula has healed.[169] If the fistula persists despite 6–12 months of management, operative intervention is planned after extensive evaluation of the fistula and intestinal tract.

Enteroenteric Fistulas

Enteroenteric fistulas are the most common type of internal fistula arising in people with Crohn's disease, and they have been reported to occur in 33% of patients whereas external fistulas affect 15% of people.[170] Isolated enteroenteric fistulas usually cause few symptoms unless obstructive or septic complications dominate the clinical presentation. However, nearly 40% of patients with internal fistulas initially managed by nonoperative methods will require surgery within 1 year, mainly because of disease intractability.[171] The principles of surgical management include resection of the fistula source, freshening of the defect in the adjacent bowel loop by wedge excision, and transverse closure of the defect. Primary bowel anastomosis can usually be safely performed after resection of the diseased segment is completed. However, certain clinical situations may pose particular difficulties.[172] If a phlegmonous reaction involving the rectosigmoid region is part of an ileosigmoid fistula, suture closure of the sigmoid defect may be vulnerable to breakdown. Instead, a limited sigmoid resection with primary anastomosis should be performed because the likelihood of anastomotic dehiscence is negligible.[173] In these cases, the sigmoid colon is diseased in nearly 40% of patients and the reoperative recurrence rate is significantly increased when preoperative endoscopy is omitted.[174]

Recurrence

Within a few decades of the first description of regional ileitis, the recurrent nature of the disease was recognized.[175] One year after an initial resection, 60%–80% of patients possess endoscopic recurrence, 10%–20% experience clinical relapse, and 5% demonstrate operative recurrence.[176] Physicians from many centers have tried to elucidate those factors responsible for its recurrent nature, but several of the parameters that initially were thought important in predicting disease recurrence have ultimately proved to be unrelated including age of disease onset,[177–185] gender,[177–185] anatomic location,[177–179,181,182,185] duration of preoperative symptoms,[180,183,186–188] previous resection,[189,190] operative indication,[178,179,185] and blood transfusion.[187,191,192] Although disease behavior may impact the likelihood of recurrence,[182] tobacco usage has been almost uniformly linked to recurrence. Specifically, smoking is an independent risk factor for symptomatic, endoscopic, and operative recurrence.[4–7]

The choice of operation might also impact the likelihood of recurrent disease, and various operative options may potentially affect the recurrence rate. Segmental colonic disease treated by limited resection with colocolonic or colorectal anastomosis for Crohn's disease of the large bowel has been described by a number of institutions over the past 3 decades[193–201] (Table 42-1). Although the majority of patients will experience symptomatic recurrence, more than 75% will maintain intestinal continuity for more than a decade after their initial resection with anastomosis. Despite the symptomatic recurrence rate, it is important to recall that segmental colonic resection delays the need for permanent ileostomy and partially conserves a portion of the large intestine's functional absorbing surface. Crohn's disease of the colon with relative rectal sparing can be adequately treated by colectomy with ileoproctostomy as described earlier. Longo and colleagues[202] reviewed the Cleveland Clinic's experience using this technique. The procedure was safely performed in 118 patients over a 26-year period. After an average 10 years of follow-up, 61% of patients maintained intestinal continuity with a functioning ileoproctostomy. The success of this operation is independent of patient age and duration of symptoms, but inversely linked, in part, to the presence of concomitant small bowel disease at the time of anastomosis. Many other authors have reported similar favorable findings.[197,199,200,202–207] (Table 42-2) One of the most common components of Crohn's disease that manifests itself after proctocolectomy is recurrence of disease in the ileostomy or remaining small bowel. Scammell and associates reported a 24% and 35% cumulative reoperative rate for recurrence at 5 and 10 years, respectively.[208] The majority of recurrences occurred within 25 cm of the stoma. Although the rates vary, these values largely agree with the experience of others.[199,206]

Various forms of medical therapy have been trialed to prevent the likelihood of recurrent Crohn's disease after operative management, but no clear prophylactic drug regime has emerged. First-line therapy generally consists of the 5-aminosalicylic acid compounds, which are only mildly protective and a recent metaanalysis of studies addressing this indication suggested that they were no better than placebo.[209] Second-line treatment includes immunomodulator medications that are potentially beneficial in postoperative patients with high risk for recurrence, endoscopic lesions noted in the neoterminal ileum, or disease-related symptoms.[210,211]

TABLE 42-1. Recurrence after segmental colonic resection

Author	No. of patients	Recurrence (%)	Follow-up (y)
de Dombal et al.[193]	42	37	15
Sanfey et al.[194]	13	8	7
Stern et al.[195]	5	20	5
Longo et al.[196]	18	62	5
Allan et al.[197]	36	66	15
Prabhakar et al.[198]	33	42	14
Bernell et al.[199]	134	49	10
Andersson et al.[200]	31	39	11
Martel et al.[201]	84	43	9

TABLE 42-2. Recurrence after total colectomy and ileoproctostomy

Author	No. of patients	Recurrence (%)	Follow-up (y)
Allan et al.[197]	63	53	15
Longo et al.[202]	131	65	10
Flint et al.[203]	37	41	6
Buchmann et al.[204]	105	30	8
Ambrose et al.[205]	63	48	10
Goligher[206]	47	49	15
Martel et al.[207]	39	41	10
Bernell et al.[199]	106	53	15
Andersson et al.[200]	26	46	9

Third-line therapy would likely include nitroimidazole antibiotics that prevent early endoscopic recurrence and postpone symptomatic relapse, but are not well tolerated.[212] Conventional corticosteroids, budesonide, and probiotics have been shown to ineffectively protect against postoperative disease recurrence, and the biologic agents have not been appropriately trialed.

Summary

Crohn's disease remains a chronic, incurable disorder that presents unique challenges to the surgeon. The proper care of these patients requires a thorough interview, examination, and evaluation because the presenting symptoms and signs can be quite subtle yet profoundly significant. Multiple factors must be considered to allow development of an appropriate treatment plan. Medical therapy often precedes or complements operative management, and although resection remains the principle operation of choice, the nonresectional techniques are often required to allow bowel conservation. The recurrent nature of the disease mandates that we continue to search for alterations in operative techniques and innovative medical therapies that reduce the need for repeat operations.

References

1. Brant SR, Shugart YY. Inflammatory bowel disease gene hunting by linkage analysis: rationale, methodology, and present status of the field. Inflamm Bowel Dis 2004;10:300–311.
2. Orholm M, Binder V, Sorensen TI, Rasmussen LP, Kyvik KO. Concordance of inflammatory bowel disease among Danish twins. Results of a nationwide study. Scand J Gastroenterol 2000;35:1075–1081.
3. Halfvarson J, Bodin L, Tysk C, Lindberg E, Jarnerot G. Inflammatory bowel disease in a Swedish twin cohort: a long-term follow-up of concordance and clinical characteristics. Gastroenterology 2003;124:1767–1773.
4. Cottone M, Rosselli M, Orlando A, et al. Smoking habits and recurrence in Crohn's disease. Gastroenterology 1994;106:643–648.
5. Timmer A, Sutherland LR, Martin F. Oral contraceptive use and smoking are risk factors for relapse in Crohn's disease. The Canadian Mesalamine for Remission of Crohn's Disease Study Group. Gastroenterology 1998;114:1143–1150.
6. Ryan WR, Allan RN, Yamamoto T, Keighley MR. Crohn's disease patients who quit smoking have a reduced risk of reoperation for recurrence. Am J Surg 2004;187:219–225.
7. Kane SV, Flicker M, Katz-Nelson F. Tobacco use is associated with accelerated clinical recurrence of Crohn's disease after surgically induced remission. J Clin Gastroenterol 2005;39:32–35.
8. Rutgeerts P, Goboes K, Peeters M, et al. Effect of fecal diversion on recurrence of Crohn's disease in the neoterminal ileum. Lancet 1991;338:771–774.
9. Gordon JN, Sabatino AD, Macdonald TT. The pathophysiologic rationale for biological therapies in inflammatory bowel disease. Curr Opin Gastroenterol 2005;21:431–437.
10. Binder V. Epidemiology of IBD during the twentieth century: an integrated view. Best Pract Res Clin Gastroenterol 2004;18:463–479.
11. Loftus EV Jr. Clinical epidemiology of inflammatory bowel disease: incidence, prevalence, and environmental influences. Gastroenterology 2004;126:1504–1517.
12. Farmer RG, Hawk WA, Turnbull RB. Clinical patterns in Crohn's disease: a statistical study of 615 cases. Gastroenterology 1975;68:627–635.
13. Gasche C, Scholmerich J, Brynskov J, et al. A simple classification of Crohn's disease: report of the Working Party for the World Congresses of Gastroenterology, Vienna 1998. Inflamm Bowel Dis 2000;6:8–15.
14. Louis E, Collard A, Oger AF, Degroote E, Aboul Nasr El Yafi FA, Belaiche J. Behaviour of Crohn's disease according to the Vienna classification: changing pattern over the course of the disease. Gut 2001;49:777–782.
15. Cosnes J, Cattan S, Blain A, et al. Long-term evolution of disease behavior of Crohn's disease. Inflamm Bowel Dis 2002;8:244–250.
16. Freeman HJ. Natural history and clinical behavior of Crohn's disease extending beyond two decades. J Clin Gastroenterol 2003;37:216–219.
17. Papi C, Festa V, Fagnani C, et al. Evolution of clinical behaviour in Crohn's disease: predictive factors of penetrating complications. Dig Liver Dis 2005;37:247–253.
18. Fedorak RN. Is it time to re-classify Crohn's disease? Best Pract Res Clin Gastroenterol 2004;18(suppl):99–106.
19. Santos JV, Baudet JA, Casellas FJ, Guarner LA, Vilaseca JM, Malagelada JR. Intravenous cyclosporine for steroid-refractory attacks of Crohn's disease. Short- and long-term results. J Clin Gastroenterol 1995;20:207–210.
20. Geoghegan JG, Carton E, O'Shea AM, et al. Crohn's colitis: the fate of the rectum. Int J Colorectal Dis 1998;13:256–259.
21. Yamamoto T, Keighley MR. Long-term outcome of total colectomy and ileostomy for Crohn disease. Scand J Gastroenterol 1999;34:280–286.
22. Lavery IC, Jagelman DG. Cancer in the excluded rectum following surgery for inflammatory bowel disease. Dis Colon Rectum 1982;25:522–524.
23. Guillem JG, Roberts PL, Murray JJ, Coller JA, Veidenheimer MC, Schoetz DJ Jr. Factors predictive of persistent or recurrent Crohn's disease in excluded rectal segments. Dis Colon Rectum 1992;35:768–772.

24. Scott HW, Sawyers JL, Gobbel WG Jr, Graves HA, Shull HW. Surgical management of toxic dilatation of the colon in ulcerative colitis. Ann Surg 1974;179:647–656.

25. Binder SC, Miller HH, Deterling RA Jr. Emergency and urgent operations for ulcerative colitis: the procedure of choice. Arch Surg 1975;110:284–289.

26. Koudahl G, Kristensen M. Toxic megacolon in ulcerative colitis. Scand J Gastroenterol 1975;10:417–421.

27. Cirocco WC, Reilly JC, Rusin LC. Life-threatening hemorrhage and exsanguination from Crohn's disease. Report of four cases. Dis Colon Rectum 1995;38:85–95.

28. Belaiche J, Louis E, D'Haens G, et al. Acute lower gastrointestinal bleeding in Crohn's disease: characteristics of a unique series of 34 patients. Belgian IBD Research Group. Am J Gastroenterol 1999;94:2177–2181.

29. Korzenik JR. Massive lower gastrointestinal hemorrhage in Crohn's disease. Curr Treat Options Gastroenterol 2000;3:211–216.

30. Kostka R, Lukas M. Massive, life-threatening bleeding in Crohn's disease. Acta Chir Belg 2005;105:168–174.

31. Fazio VW, Zelas P, Weakley FL. Intraoperative angiography and the localization of bleeding from the small intestine. Surg Gynecol Obstet 1980;151:637–640.

32. Freeman HJ. Spontaneous free perforation of the small intestine in Crohn's disease. Can J Gastroenterol 2002;16:23–27.

33. Werbin N, Haddad R, Greenberg R, Karin E, Skornick Y. Free perforation in Crohn's disease. Isr Med Assoc J 2003;5:175–177.

34. Greenstein AJ, Sachar DB, Mann D, Lachman P, Heimann T, Aufses AH Jr. Spontaneous free perforation and perforated abscess in 30 patients with Crohn's disease. Ann Surg 1987;205:72–76.

35. Bundred NJ, Dixon JM, Lumsden AB, Gilmour HM, Davies GC. Free perforation in Crohn's colitis. A ten-year review. Dis Colon Rectum 1985;28:35–37.

36. Bernstein CN, Blanchard JF, Kliewer E, Wajda A. Cancer risk in patients with inflammatory bowel disease: a population-based study. Cancer 2001;91:854–862.

37. Ekbom A, Helmick C, Zack M, Adami HO. Increased risk of large-bowel cancer in Crohn's disease with colonic involvement. Lancet 1990;336:357–359.

38. Munkholm P, Langholz E, Davidsen M, Binder V. Intestinal cancer risk and mortality in patients with Crohn's disease. Gastroenterology 1993;105:1716–1723.

39. Gillen CD, Walmsley RS, Prior P, Andrews HA, Allan RN. Ulcerative colitis and Crohn's disease: a comparison of the colorectal cancer risk in extensive colitis. Gut 1994;35:1590–1592.

40. Fireman Z, Grossman A, Lilos P, et al. Intestinal cancer in patients with Crohn's disease. A population study in central Israel. Scand J Gastroenterol 1989;24:346–350.

41. Persson PG, Karlen P, Bernell O, et al. Crohn's disease and cancer: a population-based cohort study. Gastroenterology 1994;107:1675–1679.

42. Jess T, Winther KV, Munkholm P, Langholz E, Binder V. Intestinal and extra-intestinal cancer in Crohn's disease: follow-up of a population-based cohort in Copenhagen County, Denmark. Aliment Pharmacol Ther 2004;19:287–293.

43. Sigel JE, Petras RE, Lashner BA, Fazio VW, Goldblum JR. Intestinal adenocarcinoma in Crohn's disease: a report of 30 cases with a focus on coexisting dysplasia. Am J Surg Pathol 1999;23:651–655.

44. Friedman S, Rubin PH, Bodian C, Goldstein E, Harpaz N, Present DH. Screening and surveillance colonoscopy in chronic Crohn's colitis. Gastroenterology 2001;120:820–826.

45. Winawer S, Fletcher R, Rex D, et al. for the U.S. Multisociety Task Force on Colorectal Cancer. Colorectal cancer screening and surveillance: clinical guidelines and rationale—update based on new evidence. Gastroenterology 2003;124:544–560.

46. Savage MO, Beattie RM, Camacho-Hubner C, Walker-Smith JA, Sanderson IR. Growth in Crohn's disease. Acta Paediatr Suppl 1999;88:89–92.

47. Rankin GB, Watts HD, Melnyk CS, Kelley ML Jr. National Cooperative Crohn's Disease Study: extraintestinal manifestations and perianal complications. Gastroenterology 1979;77:914–920.

48. Veloso FT, Carvalho J, Magro F. Immune-related systemic manifestations of inflammatory bowel disease. A prospective study of 792 patients. Clin Gastroenterol 1996;23:29–34.

49. Bernstein CN, Blanchard JF, Rawsthorne P, Yu N. The prevalence of extraintestinal diseases in inflammatory bowel disease: a population-based study. Am J Gastroenterol 2001;96:1116–1122.

50. Otterson MF, Lundeen SJ, Spinelli KS, et al. Radiographic underestimation of small bowel stricturing Crohn's disease: a comparison with surgical findings. Surgery 2004;136:854–860.

51. Fazio VW, Marchetti F, Church J, et al. Effect of resection margins on the recurrence of Crohn's disease in the small bowel. A randomized controlled trial. Ann Surg 1996;224:563–573.

52. Yamamoto T, Allan RN, Keighley MR. Effect of fecal diversion alone on perianal Crohn's disease. World J Surg 2000;24:1258–1262.

53. van Dongen LM, Lubbers EJC. Perianal fistulas in patients with Crohn's disease. Arch Surg 1986;121:1187–1190.

54. Katariya RN, Sood S, Rao PG, Rao PL. Stricture-plasty for tubercular strictures of the gastro-intestinal tract. Br J Surg 1977;64:496–498.

55. Lee ECG, Papaioannou N. Minimal surgery for chronic obstruction in patients with extensive or universal Crohn's disease. Ann R Coll Surg Engl 1982;64:229–233.

56. Tichansky D, Cagir B, Yoo E, Marcus SM, Fry RD. Strictureplasty for Crohn's disease: meta-analysis. Dis Colon Rectum 2000;43:911–919.

57. Dietz DW, Laureti S, Strong SA, et al. Safety and longterm efficacy of strictureplasty in 314 patients with obstructing small bowel Crohn's disease. J Am Coll Surg 2001;192:330–337.

58. Roy P, Kumar D. Strictureplasty. Br J Surg 2004;91:1428–1437.

59. Yamamoto T, Allan RN, Keighley MR. Long-term outcome of surgical management for diffuse jejunoileal Crohn's disease. Surgery 2001;129:96–102.

60. Ozuner G, Fazio VW, Lavery I, Milsom J, Strong S. Reoperative rates for Crohn's disease following strictureplasty. Dis Colon Rectum 1996;39:1199–1203.

61. Stebbing JF, Jewell DP, Kettlewell MG, Mortensen NJ. Recurrence and reoperation after strictureplasty for obstructive Crohn's disease: long-term results. Br J Surg 1995;82:1471–1474.

62. Michelassi F. Side-to-side isoperistaltic strictureplasty for multiple Crohn's strictures. Dis Colon Rectum 1996;39:345–349.

63. Marchetti F, Fazio VW, Ozuner G. Adenocarcinoma arising from a strictureplasty site in Crohn's disease. Report of a case. Dis Colon Rectum 1996;39:1315–1321.

64. Jaskowiak NT, Michelassi F. Adenocarcinoma at a strictureplasty site in Crohn's disease: report of a case. Dis Colon Rectum 2001;44:284–287.

65. Partridge SK, Hodin RA. Small bowel adenocarcinoma at a strictureplasty site in a patient with Crohn's disease: report of a case. Dis Colon Rectum 2004;47:778–781.

66. Ozuner G, Fazio VW. Management of gastrointestinal hemorrhage after strictureplasty for Crohn's disease. Dis Colon Rectum 1995;38:297–300.

67. Tjandra JJ, Fazio VW. Strictureplasty for ileocolic anastomotic strictures in Crohn's disease. Dis Colon Rectum 1993;36:1099–1103.

68. Yamamoto T, Keighley MR. Long-term results of strictureplasty for ileocolonic anastomotic recurrence in Crohn's disease. J Gastrointest Surg 1999;3:555–560.

69. Tonelli F, Ficari F. Strictureplasty in Crohn's disease: surgical option. Dis Colon Rectum 2000;43:920–926.

70. Futami K, Arima S. Role of strictureplasty in surgical treatment of Crohn's disease. J Gastroenterol 2005;40(suppl 16):35–39.

71. Poggioli G, Stocchi L, Laureti S, et al. Conservative surgical management of terminal ileitis: side-to-side enterocolic anastomosis. Dis Colon Rectum 1997;40:234–237.

72. Kishi D, Nezu R, Ito T, et al. Laparoscopic-assisted surgery for Crohn's disease: reduced surgical stress following ileocolectomy. Surg Today 2000;30:219–222.

73. Milsom JW, Hammerhofer KA, Bohm B, Marcello P, Elson P, Fazio VW. Prospective, randomized trial comparing laparoscopic vs. conventional surgery for refractory ileocolic Crohn's disease. Dis Colon Rectum 2001;44:1–8.

74. Msika S, Iannelli A, Deroide G, et al. Can laparoscopy reduce hospital stay in the treatment of Crohn's disease? Dis Colon Rectum 2001;44:1661–1666.

75. Tabet J, Hong D, Kim CW, Wong J, Goodacre R, Anvari M. Laparoscopic versus open bowel resection for Crohn's disease. Can J Gastroenterol 2001;15:237–242.

76. Duepree HJ, Senagore AJ, Delaney CP, Brady KM, Fazio VW. Advantages of laparoscopic resection for ileocecal Crohn's disease. Dis Colon Rectum 2002;45:605–610.

77. Benoist S, Panis Y, Beaufour A, Bouhnik Y, Matuchansky C, Valleur P. Laparoscopic ileocecal resection in Crohn's disease: a case-matched comparison with open resection. Surg Endosc 2003;17:814–818.

78. Bergamaschi R, Pessaux P, Arnaud JP. Comparison of conventional and laparoscopic ileocolic resection for Crohn's disease. Dis Colon Rectum 2003;46:1129–1133.

79. Huilgol RL, Wright CM, Solomon MJ. Laparoscopic versus open ileocolic resection for Crohn's disease. J Laparoendosc Adv Surg Tech A 2004;14:61–65.

80. Wu JS, Birnbaum EH, Kodner IJ, Fry RD, Read TE, Fleshman JW. Laparoscopic-assisted ileocolic resections in patients with Crohn's disease: are abscesses, phlegmons, or recurrent disease contraindications? Surgery 1997;122:682–686.

81. Watanabe M, Hasegawa H, Yamamoto S, Hibi T, Kitajima M. Successful application of laparoscopic surgery to the treatment of Crohn's disease with fistulas. Dis Colon Rectum 2002;45:1057–1061.

82. Cameron JL, Hamilton SR, Coleman J, Sitzmann JV, Bayless TM. Patterns of ileal recurrence in Crohn's disease. A prospective randomized study. Ann Surg 1992;215:546–551.

83. Scott NA, Sue-Ling HM, Hughes LE. Anastomotic configuration does not affect recurrence of Crohn's disease after ileocolonic resection. Int J Colorectal Dis 1995;10:67–69.

84. Kusunoki M, Ikeuchi H, Yanagi H, Shoji Y, Yamamura T. A comparison of stapled and hand-sewn anastomoses in Crohn's disease. Dig Surg 1998;15:679–682.

85. Hashemi M, Novell JR, Lewis AA. Side-to-side stapled anastomosis may delay recurrence in Crohn's disease. Dis Colon Rectum 1998;41:1293–1296.

86. Munoz-Juarez M, Yamamoto T, Wolff BG, Keighley MR. Wide-lumen stapled anastomosis vs. conventional end-to-end anastomosis in the treatment of Crohn's disease. Dis Colon Rectum 2001;44:20–25.

87. Tersigni R, Alessandroni L, Barreca M, Piovanello P, Prantera C. Does stapled functional end-to-end anastomosis affect recurrence of Crohn's disease after ileocolonic resection? Hepatogastroenterology 2003;50:1422–1425.

88. Scarpa M, Angriman I, Barollo M, et al. Role of stapled and hand-sewn anastomoses in recurrence of Crohn's disease. Hepatogastroenterology 2004;51:1053–1057.

89. Ikeuchi H, Kusunoki M, Yamamura T. Long-term results of stapled and hand-sewn anastomoses in patients with Crohn's disease. Dig Surg 2000;17:493–496.

90. Yamamoto T, Bain IM, Mylonakis E, Allan RN, Keighley MR. Stapled functional end-to-end anastomosis versus sutured end-to-end anastomosis after ileocolonic resection in Crohn disease. Scand J Gastroenterol 1999;34:708–713.

91. Resegotti A, Astegiano M, Farina EC, et al. Side-to-side stapled anastomosis strongly reduces anastomotic leak rates in Crohn's disease surgery. Dis Colon Rectum 2005;48:464–468.

92. Broering DC, Eisenberger CF, Koch A, et al. Strictureplasty for large bowel stenosis in Crohn's disease: quality of life after surgical therapy. Int J Colorectal Dis 2001;16:81–87.

93. Yamazaki Y, Ribeiro MB, Sachar DB, Aufses AH, Greenstein AJ. Malignant strictures in Crohn's disease. Am J Gastroenterol 1991;86:882–885.

94. Keighley MRB, Buchmann P, Lee JR. Assessment of anorectal function in selection of patients for ileo-rectal anastomosis in Crohn's colitis. Gut 1982;23:102–107.

95. Cirincione E, Gorfine SR, Bauer JJ. Is Hartmann's procedure safe in Crohn's disease? Report of three cases. Dis Colon Rectum 2000;43:544–547.

96. Rius J, Nessim A, Nogueras JJ, Wexner SD. Gracilis transposition in complicated perianal fistula and unhealed perineal wounds in Crohn's disease. Eur J Surg 2000;166:218–222.

97. Hurst RD, Gottlieb LJ, Crucitti P, Melis M, Rubin M, Michelassi F. Primary closure of complicated perineal wounds with myocutaneous and fasciocutaneous flaps after proctectomy for Crohn's disease. Surgery 2001;130:767–772.

98. Yamamoto T, Mylonakis E, Keighley MR. Omentoplasty for persistent perineal sinus after proctectomy for Crohn's disease. Am J Surg 2001;181:265–267.

99. Regimbeau JM, Panis Y, Pocard M, et al. Long-term results of ileal pouch-anal anastomosis for colorectal Crohn's disease. Dis Colon Rectum 2001;44:769–778.

100. Sagar PM, Dozois RR, Wolff BG. Long-term results of ileal pouch-anal anastomosis in patients with Crohn's disease. Dis Colon Rectum 1996;39:893–898.

101. Mylonakis E, Allan RN, Keighley MR. How does pouch construction for a final diagnosis of Crohn's disease compare with ileoproctostomy for established Crohn's proctocolitis? Dis Colon Rectum 2001;44:1137–1142.

102. Braveman JM, Schoetz DJ Jr, Marcello PW, et al. The fate of the ileal pouch in patients developing Crohn's disease. Dis Colon Rectum 2004;47:1613–1619.

103. Hartley JE, Fazio VW, Remzi FH, et al. Analysis of the outcome of ileal pouch-anal anastomosis in patients with Crohn's disease. Dis Colon Rectum 2004;47:1808–1815.

104. Cooke WT, Swan CH. Diffuse jejunoileitis of Crohn's disease. Quart J Med 1974;72:583–601.

105. Nugent FW, Roy MA. Duodenal Crohn's disease: an analysis of 89 cases. Am J Gastroenterol 1989;84:249–254.

106. Cary ER, Tremaine WJ, Banks PM, Nagorney DM. Case report: isolated Crohn's disease of the stomach. Mayo Clin Proc 1989;64:776–779.

107. Poggioli G, Stocchi L, Laureti S, et al. Duodenal involvement of Crohn's disease: three different clinicopathologic patterns. Dis Colon Rectum 1997;40:179–183.

108. Kelly SM, Hunter JO. Endoscopic balloon dilatation of duodenal strictures in Crohn's disease. Postgrad Med J 1995;71:623–624.

109. Kimura H, Sugita A, Nishiyama K, Shimada H. Treatment of duodenal Crohn's disease with stenosis: case report of 6 cases. Nippon Shokakibyo Gakkai Zasshi 2000;9:697–702.

110. Ross TM, Fazio VW, Farmer RG. Long-term results of surgical treatment for Crohn's disease of the duodenum. Ann Surg 1983;197:399–406.

111. Murray JJ, Schoetz DJ Jr, Nugent FW, Coller JA, Veidenheimer MC. Surgical management of Crohn's disease involving the duodenum. Am J Surg 1984;147:58–65.

112. Eisenberger CF, Izbicki JR, Broering DC, et al. Strictureplasty with a pedunculated jejunal patch in Crohn's disease of the duodenum. Am J Gastroenterol 1998;93:267–269.

113. Worsey MJ, Hull T, Ryland L, Fazio V. Strictureplasty is an effective option in the operative management of duodenal Crohn's disease. Dis Colon Rectum 1999;42:596–600.

114. Yamamoto T, Bain IM, Connolly AB, Allan RN, Keighley MR. Outcome of strictureplasty for duodenal Crohn's disease. Br J Surg 1999;86:259–262.

115. Takesue Y, Yokoyama T, Akagi S, et al. Strictureplasty for short duodenal stenosis in Crohn's disease. J Gastroenterol 2000;35:929–932.

116. Singh B, McC Mortensen NJ, Jewell DP, George B. Perianal Crohn's disease. Br J Surg 2004;91:801–814.

117. Hughes LE. Clinical classification of perianal Crohn's disease. Dis Colon Rectum 1992;35:928–932.

118. Alexander-Williams J, Hellers G, Hughes LE, Minervini S, Speranza V. Classification of perianal Crohn's disease. Gastroenterol Int 1992;5:216–220.

119. Francois Y, Vignal J, Descos L. Outcome of perianal fistulae in Crohn's disease—value of Hughes' pathogenic classification. Int J Colorectal Dis 1993;8:39–41.

120. Irvine EJ. Usual therapy improves perianal Crohn's disease as measured by a new disease activity index. McMaster IBD Study Group. J Clin Gastroenterol 1995;20:27–32.

121. Pikarsky AJ, Gervaz P, Wexner SD. Perianal Crohn disease: a new scoring system to evaluate and predict outcome of surgical intervention. Arch Surg 2002;137:774–777.

122. Kuijpers HC, Schulpen T. Fistulography for fistula-in-ano. Is it useful? Dis Colon Rectum 1985;28:103–104.

123. Weisman RI, Orsay CP, Pearl RK, Abcarian H. The role of fistulography in fistula-in-ano. Report of five cases. Dis Colon Rectum 1991;34:181–184.

124. Cho DY. Endosonographic criteria for an internal opening of fistula-in-ano. Dis Colon Rectum 1999;42:515–518.

125. Yee LF, Birnbaum EH, Read TE, Kodner IJ, Fleshman JW. Use of endoanal ultrasound in patients with rectovaginal fistulas. Dis Colon Rectum 1999;42:1057–1064.

126. Ratto C, Gentile E, Merico M, et al. How can the assessment of fistula-in-ano be improved? Dis Colon Rectum 2000;43:1375–1382.

127. Haggett PJ, Moore NR, Shearman JD, Travis SP, Jewell DP, Mortensen NJ. Pelvic and perineal complications of Crohn's disease: assessment using magnetic resonance imaging. Gut 1995;36:407–410.

128. deSouza NM, Gilderdale DJ, Coutts GA, Puni R, Steiner RE. MRI of fistula-in-ano: a comparison of endoanal coil with external phased array coil techniques. J Comput Assist Tomogr 1998;22:357–363.

129. Borley NR, Mortensen NJ, Jewell DP. MRI scanning in perianal Crohn's disease: an important diagnostic adjunct. Inflamm Bowel Dis 1999;5:231–233.

130. Orsoni P, Barthet M, Portier F, Panuel M, Desjeux A, Grimaud JC. Prospective comparison of endosonography, magnetic resonance imaging and surgical findings in anorectal fistula and abscess complicating Crohn's disease. Br J Surg 1999;86:360–364.

131. Schwartz DA, Wiersema MJ, Dudiak KM, et al. A comparison of endoscopic ultrasound, magnetic resonance imaging, and exam under anesthesia for evaluation of Crohn's perianal fistulas. Gastroenterology 2001;121:1064–1072.

132. West RL, Dwarkasing S, Felt-Bersma RJ, et al. Hydrogen peroxide-enhanced three-dimensional endoanal ultrasonography and endoanal magnetic resonance imaging in evaluating perianal fistulas: agreement and patient preference. Eur J Gastroenterol Hepatol 2004;16:1319–1324.

133. Jeffery PJ, Parks AG, Ritchie JK. Treatment of hemorrhoids in patients with inflammatory bowel disease. Lancet 1977;1:1084–1085.

134. Morrison JG, Gathright JB Jr, Ray JE, Ferrari BT, Hicks TC, Timmcke AE. Surgical management of anorectal fistulas in Crohn's disease. Dis Colon Rectum 1989;32:492–496.

135. Bernstein LH, Frank MS, Brandt LJ, Boley SJ. Healing of perineal Crohn's disease with metronidazole. Gastroenterology 1980;79:357–365.

136. Jakobovits J, Schuster MM. Metronidazole therapy for Crohn's disease and associated fistulae. Am J Gastroenterol 1984;79:533–540.

137. Pearson DC, May GR, Fick GH, Sutherland LR. Azathioprine and 6-mercaptopurine in Crohn disease. A meta-analysis. Ann Intern Med 1995;123:132–142.

138. Present DH, Rutgeerts P, Targan S, et al. Infliximab for the treatment of fistulas in patients with Crohn's disease. N Engl J Med 1999;340(18):1398–1405.

139. West RL, van der Woude CJ, Hansen BE, et al. Clinical and endosonographic effect of ciprofloxacin on the treatment of

perianal fistulae in Crohn's disease with infliximab: a double-blind placebo-controlled study. Aliment Pharmacol Ther 2004;20:1329–1336.

140. Hanauer SB, Feagan BG, Lichtenstein GR, et al., ACCENT I Study Group. Maintenance infliximab for Crohn's disease: the ACCENT I randomised trial. Lancet 2002;359:1541–1549.

141. Sands BE, Anderson FH, Bernstein CN, et al. Infliximab maintenance therapy for fistulizing Crohn's disease. N Engl J Med 2004;350:876–885.

142. Sandborn WJ, Fazio VW, Feagan BG, Hanauer SB; American Gastroenterological Association Clinical Practice Committee. AGA technical review on perianal Crohn's disease. Gastroenterology 2003;125:1508–1530.

143. Makowiec F, Jehle EC, Becker HD, Starlinger M. Clinical course after transanal advancement flap repair of perianal fistula in patients with Crohn's disease. Br J Surg 1995;82: 603–606.

144. Joo JS, Weiss EG, Nogueras JJ, Wexner SD. Endorectal advancement flap in perianal Crohn's disease. Am Surg 1998;64:147–150.

145. Sonoda T, Hull T, Piedmonte MR, Fazio VW. Outcomes of primary repair of anorectal and rectovaginal fistulas using the endorectal advancement flap. Dis Colon Rectum 2002;45:1622–1628.

146. Williams JG, MacLeod CA, Rothenberger DA, Goldberg SM. Seton treatment of high anal fistulae. Br J Surg 1991;78: 1159–1161.

147. Pearl RK, Andrews JR, Orsay CP, et al. Role of the seton in the management of anorectal fistulas. Dis Colon Rectum 1993;36:573–577.

148. Scott HJ, Northover JM. Evaluation of surgery for perianal Crohn's fistulas. Dis Colon Rectum 1996;39:1039–1043.

149. Sangwan YP, Schoetz DJ Jr, Murray JJ, Roberts PL, Coller JA. Perianal Crohn's disease. Results of local surgical treatment. Dis Colon Rectum 1996;39:529–535.

150. Faucheron JL, Saint-Marc O, Guibert L, Parc R. Long-term seton drainage for high anal fistulas in Crohn's disease—a sphincter-saving operation? Dis Colon Rectum 1996;39:208–211.

151. Lindsey I, Smilgin-Humphreys MM, Cunningham C, Mortensen NJ, George BD. A randomized, controlled trial of fibrin glue vs. conventional treatment for anal fistula. Dis Colon Rectum 2002;45:1608–1615.

152. Zmora O, Mizrahi N, Rotholtz N, et al. Fibrin glue sealing in the treatment of perineal fistulas. Dis Colon Rectum 2003;46: 584–589.

153. Loungnarath R, Dietz DW, Mutch MG, Birnbaum EH, Kodner IJ, Fleshman JW. Fibrin glue treatment of complex anal fistulas has low success rate. Dis Colon Rectum 2004;47:432–436.

154. Kodner IJ, Mazor A, Shemesh EI, Fry RD, Fleshman JW, Birnbaum EH. Endorectal advancement flap repair of rectovaginal and other complicated anorectal fistulas. Surgery 1993;114:682–689.

155. Hesterberg R, Schmidt WU, Muller F, Roher HD. Treatment of anovaginal fistulas with an anocutaneous flap in patients with Crohn's disease. Int J Colorectal Dis 1993;8:51–54.

156. Regueiro M, Mardini H. Treatment of perianal fistulizing Crohn's disease with infliximab alone or as an adjunct for exam under anesthesia with seton placement. Inflamm Bowel Dis 2003;9:98–103.

157. van der Hagen SJ, Baeten CG, Soeters PB, Russel MG, Beets-Tan RG, van Gemert WG. Anti-TNF-alpha (infliximab) used as induction treatment in case of active proctitis in a multistep strategy followed by definitive surgery of complex anal fistulas in Crohn's disease: a preliminary report. Dis Colon Rectum 2005;48:758–767.

158. Alexander-Williams J, Allan A, Morel P, Hawker PC, Dykes PW, O'Connor H. The therapeutic dilatation of enteric strictures due to Crohn's disease. Ann R Coll Surg Engl 1986;68:95–97.

159. Linares L, Moreira LF, Andrews H, Allan RN, Alexander-Williams J, Keighley MR. Natural history and treatment of anorectal strictures complicating Crohn's disease. Br J Surg 1988;75:653–655.

160. Marchesa P, Hull TL, Fazio VW. Advancement sleeve flaps for treatment of severe perianal Crohn's disease. Br J Surg 1998;85:1695–1698.

161. Slater G, Greenstein A, Aufses AH Jr. Anal carcinoma in patients with Crohn's disease. Ann Surg 1984;199:348–350.

162. Somerville KW, Langman MJ, Da Cruz DJ, Balfour TW, Sully L. Malignant transformation of anal skin tags in Crohn's disease. Gut 1984;25:1124–1125.

163. Connell WR, Sheffield JP, Kamm MA, Ritchie JK, Hawley PR, Lennard-Jones JE. Lower gastrointestinal malignancy in Crohn's disease. Gut 1994;35:347–352.

164. Ky A, Sohn N, Weinstein MA, Korelitz BI. Carcinoma arising in anorectal fistulas of Crohn's disease. Dis Colon Rectum 1998;41:992–996.

165. Ayuk P, Williams N, Scott N, Nicholson D, Irving M. Management of intra-abdominal abscesses in Crohn's disease. Ann R Coll Surg Engl 1996;78:5–10.

166. Sahai A, Belair M, Gianfelice D, Cote S, Gratton J, Lahaie R. Percutaneous drainage of intra-abdominal abscesses in Crohn's disease: short and long-term outcome. Am J Gastroenterol 1997;92:275–278.

167. Poritz LS, Gagliano GA, McLeod RS, MacRae H, Cohen Z. Surgical management of entero and colocutaneous fistulae in Crohn's disease: 17 years' experience. Int J Colorectal Dis 2004;19:481–485.

168. Lynch AC, Delaney CP, Senagore AJ, Connor JT, Remzi FH, Fazio VW. Clinical outcome and factors predictive of recurrence after enterocutaneous fistula surgery. Ann Surg 2004;240:825–831.

169. Hesse U, Ysebaert D, de Hemptinne B. Role of somatostatin-14 and its analogues in the management of gastrointestinal fistulae: clinical data. Gut 2001;49(suppl 4):iv11–21.

170. Greenstein AJ. The surgery of Crohn's disease. Surg Clin North Am 1987;67:573–596.

171. Broe PJ, Bayless TM, Cameron JL. Crohn's disease: are enteroenteral fistulas an addiction for surgery? Surgery 1982;91:249–253.

172. Young-Fadok TM, Wolff BG, Meagher A, Benn PL, Dozois RR. Surgical management of ileosigmoid fistulas in Crohn's disease. Dis Colon Rectum 1997;40:558–561.

173. Fazio VW, Wilk PJ, Turnbull RB Jr, Jagelman DG. Ileosigmoidal fistula complicating Crohn's disease. Dis Colon Rectum 1997;20:381–386.

174. Saint-Marc O, Vaillant J-C, Frileux P, Balladur P, Tiret E, Parc R. Surgical management of ileosigmoid fistulas in Crohn's disease: role of preoperative colonoscopy. Dis Colon Rectum 1995;38:1084–1087.

175. Crohn BB, Ginzburg L, Oppenheimer GD. Regional ileitis. JAMA 1932;99:214–220.

176. Froehlich F, Juillerat P, Felley C, et al. Treatment of postoperative Crohn's disease. Digestion 2005;71:49–53.

177. Michelassi F, Balestracci T, Chappell R, Block GE. Primary and recurrent Crohn's disease. Experience with 1379 patients. Ann Surg 1991;214:230–238.

178. Heimann TM, Greenstein AJ, Lewis B, Kaufman D, Heimann DM, Aufses AH Jr. Prediction of early symptomatic recurrence after intestinal resection in Crohn's disease. Ann Surg 1993; 218:294–298.

179. Cottone M, Orlando A, Viscido A, Calabrese E, Camma C, Casa A. Review article: prevention of postsurgical relapse and recurrence in Crohn's disease. Aliment Pharmacol Ther 2003;17(suppl 2):38–42.

180. Silvis R, Steup WH, Brand A, et al. Protective effect of blood transfusion on postoperative recurrence of Crohn's disease in parous women. Transfusion 1994;34:242–247.

181. Holzheimer RG, Molloy RG, Wittmann DH. Postoperative complications predict recurrence of Crohn's disease. Eur J Surg 1995;161:129–135.

182. Aeberhard P, Berchtold W, Riedtmann HJ, Stadelmann G. Surgical recurrence of perforating and nonperforating Crohn's disease. A study of 101 surgically treated patients. Dis Colon Rectum 1996;39:80–87.

183. Caprilli R, Corrao G, Taddei G, Tonelli F, Torchio P, Viscido A. Prognostic factors for postoperative recurrence of Crohn's disease. Gruppo Italiano per lo Studio del Colon e del Retto (GISC). Dis Colon Rectum 1996;39:335–341.

184. Raab Y, Bergstrom R, Ejerblad S, Graf W, Pahlman L. Factors influencing recurrence in Crohn's disease. An analysis of a consecutive series of 353 patients treated with primary surgery. Dis Colon Rectum 1996;39:918–925.

185. Anseline PF, Wlodarczyk J, Murugasu R. Presence of granulomas is associated with recurrence after surgery for Crohn's disease: experience of a surgical unit. Br J Surg 1997;84: 78–82.

186. Griffiths AM, Wesson DE, Shandling B, Corey M, Sherman PM. Factors influencing recurrence of Crohn's disease in childhood. Gut 1991;32:491–495.

187. Steup WH, Brand A, Weterman IT, Zwinderman KH, Lamers CB, Gooszen HG. The effect of perioperative blood transfusion on recurrence after primary operation for Crohn's disease. Scand J Gastroenterol 1991;188:81–86.

188. Wettergren A, Christiansen J. Risk of recurrence and reoperation after resection for ileocolic Crohn's disease. Scand J Gastroenterol 1991;26:1319–1322.

189. Nordgren SR, Fasth SB, Oresland TO, Hulten LA. Long-term follow-up in Crohn's disease. Mortality, morbidity, and functional status. Scand J Gastroenterol 1994;29:1122–1128.

190. Kim NK, Senagore AJ, Luchtefeld MA, et al. Long-term outcome after ileocecal resection for Crohn's disease. Am Surg 1997;63:627–633.

191. Scott AD, Ritchie JK, Phillips RK. Blood transfusion and recurrent Crohn's disease. Br J Surg 1991;78:455–458.

192. Hollaar GL, Gooszen HG, Post S, Williams JG, Sutherland LR. Perioperative blood transfusion does not prevent recurrence in Crohn's disease. A pooled analysis. J Clin Gastroenterol 1995;21:134–138.

193. de Dombal FT, Burton I, Goligher JC. Recurrence of Crohn's disease after primary excisional surgery. Gut 1971;12: 519–527.

194. Sanfey H, Bayless TM, Corman JL. Crohn's disease of the colon. Is there a role for limited resection? Am J Surg 1984;147: 38–42.

195. Stern HS, Goldberg SM, Rothenberger DA, et al. Segmental versus total colectomy for large bowel Crohn's disease. World J Surg 1984;8:118–122.

196. Longo WE, Ballantyne GH, Cahow E. Treatment of Crohn's colitis. Segmental or total colectomy? Arch Surg 1988;123:588–590.

197. Allan A, Andrews MB, Hilton CJ, Keighley MRB, Allan RN, Alexander-Williams J. Segmental colonic resection is an appropriate operation for short skip lesions due to Crohn's disease in the colon. World J Surg 1989;13:611–616.

198. Prabhakar LP, Laramee C, Nelson H, Dozois RR. Avoiding a stoma: role for segmental or abdominal colectomy in Crohn's colitis. Dis Colon Rectum 1997;40:71–78.

199. Bernell O, Lapidus A, Hellers G. Recurrence after colectomy in Crohn's colitis. Dis Colon Rectum 2001;44:647–654.

200. Andersson P, Olaison G, Hallbook O, Sjodahl R. Segmental resection or subtotal colectomy in Crohn's colitis? Dis Colon Rectum 2002;45:47–53.

201. Martel P, Betton PO, Gallot D, Malafosse M. Crohn's colitis: experience with segmental resections: results in a series of 84 patients. J Am Coll Surg 2002;194(4):448–453.

202. Longo WE, Oakley JR, Lavery IC, Church JM, Fazio VW. Outcome of ileorectal anastomosis for Crohn's colitis. Dis Colon Rectum 1992;35:1066–1071.

203. Flint G, Strauss R, Platt N, Wise L. Ileorectal anastomosis in patients with Crohn's disease of the colon. Gut 1977;18:236–239.

204. Buchmann P, Weterman IT, Keighley MR, Pena SA, Allan RN, Alexander-Williams J. The prognosis of ileorectal anastomosis in Crohn's disease. Br J Surg 1981;68:7–10.

205. Ambrose NS, Keighley MRB, Alexander-Williams J, Allan RN. Clinical impact of colectomy and ileo-rectal anastomosis in the management of Crohn's disease. Gut 1984;25:223–227.

206. Goligher JC. Surgical treatment of Crohn's disease affecting mainly or entirely the large bowel. World J Surg 1988;12: 186–190.

207. Martel P, Betton PO, Gallot D, Sezeur A, Malafosse M. Surgical treatment of Crohn's disease of the large intestine: do rectal complications influence the results of ileorectal anastomosis? Ann Chir 2000;125(6):547–551.

208. Scammell BE, Andrews H, Allan RN, Alexander-Williams J, Keighley MRB. Results of proctocolectomy for Crohn's disease. Br J Surg 1987;74:671–674.

209. Rutgeerts P. Strategies in the prevention of post-operative recurrence in Crohn's disease. Best Pract Res Clin Gastroenterol 2003;17:63–73.

210. Ardizzone S, Maconi G, Sampietro GM, et al. Azathioprine and mesalamine for prevention of relapse after conservative surgery for Crohn's disease. Gastroenterology 2004;127:730–740.

211. Hanauer SB, Korelitz BI, Rutgeerts P, et al. Postoperative maintenance of Crohn's disease remission with 6-mercaptopurine, mesalamine, or placebo: a 2-year trial. Gastroenterology 2004;127:723–729.

212. Rutgeerts P, Hiele M, Geboes K, et al. Controlled trial of metronidazole treatment for prevention of Crohn's recurrence after ileal resection. Gastroenterology 1995;108:1617–1621.

43
Less-common Benign Disorders of the Colon and Rectum

Walter E. Longo and Gregory C. Oliver

There are a variety of benign disorders of the colon and rectum that are uncommon but may be troublesome to diagnose and manage because of their obscurity and at times chronicity. The etiologies of these less-common disorders include bacterial, viral, parasitic, collagen vascular, ischemic, radiation related, and those involving immunocompromised states. It is often common that when the physician entertains these entities, that they never forget the encounter because of its misleading presentation and uncertain treatment. This chapter will describe the myriad of less-common disorders of the colon and rectum that one may encounter in clinical practice with emphasis on diagnosis, differential diagnosis, treatment, and long-term outcome.

Ischemic Colitis

Vascular disorders of the midgut and hindgut are extremely morbid conditions. This is because these diseases often afflict elderly individuals with various coexisting morbidities and limited physiologic reserve. This is compounded by the fact that these disorders are often diagnosed late, only after full-thickness intestinal injury has occurred, with perforation or gangrene. Major postoperative complications remain excessive and both early and late mortality rates continue to be significant. Ischemic colitis is the most common form of ischemic injury to the gastrointestinal (GI) tract.

It is paramount that the surgeon involved in the care of ischemia and hemorrhage of the colon and rectum has a thorough understanding of the anatomy of the large bowel. The superior mesenteric artery (SMA) and its branches, the inferior mesenteric artery (IMA) and its branches, as well as contributions of the iliac and pudendal arteries to the rectum contribute to the arterial supply of the large bowel. The ileocolic artery (ICA) arises from the right side of the terminal portion of the SMA and provides blood flow to the terminal ileum, appendix, cecum, and ascending colon. The right colic artery (RCA), which may originate from the ICA or the SMA, provides the predominant blood supply to the ascending

colon. It may be absent in up to 20% of patients. The middle colic artery is the first artery originating from the right side of the SMA, and its branches participate in the blood supply of the ascending colon, transverse colon, and the splenic flexure. The IMA arises from the abdominal aorta and gives rise to left colic and numerous sigmoidal branches, and finally terminates as the superior rectal artery. The superior rectal artery is the principal blood supply to the rectum. The remainder of the blood supply to the rectum comes from the middle and inferior rectal arteries, which are contributions from the internal iliac and internal pudendal arteries. There is variable and often unpredictable collateral blood supply to the colon and rectum. The collaterals between the SMA and IMA are the most important clinically and are the marginal artery of Drummond and the arc of Riolan. The venous drainage of the colon and rectum is more anatomically consistent. The venous blood flow from the colon and upper and middle rectum is via the SMV and inferior mesenteric vein to the portal system, whereas that of the lower rectum and anal canal is via the internal iliac veins.

Ischemic injury to the colon is now recognized to manifest distinct clinical subtypes, ranging in severity from transient segmental colopathy to fulminant gangrenous colitis.[1] The incidence of colonic ischemia in the general population remains unknown. Classically, colonic ischemia is described in elderly patients and those who have significant comorbidities. However, case reports reflect the heterogeneity of this disease. Etiologies including shock, autoimmune disease, coagulopathies, long-distance running, illicit drug use, and medication-induced colonic ischemia have been reported, in patients both young and old. Colonic ischemia remains a disease of variable clinical presentation and outcome.[2]

Ischemic colitis is often recognized as a specific entity characterized by sudden abdominal pain and diarrhea. A spectrum of disease exists, ranging from transient mucosal injury that spontaneously resolves to transmural disease with full-thickness gangrene. An intermediate form also exists in which, after resolution of symptoms, stricture formation occurs. An increased awareness and suspicion that ischemic colitis is present should initiate prompt diagnostic endoscopy. Unexplained abdominal symptomatology or unexplained clinical deterioration with abdominal symptoms should prompt the clinician to exclude the colon as the source of the problem. Unfortunately, routine laboratory and radiologic investigations often fail to identify colonic ischemia. Colonoscopy is responsible for the increasing awareness of colon ischemia and remains the procedure of choice to document its presence or absence and identify or exclude other colonic pathology.[3]

Two distinct forms of ischemic colitis have been repeatedly described throughout the last 40 years.[4] The spontaneous, usually self-limiting form of ischemic colitis contrasts drastically with the often catastrophic, more fulminant form. Despite the widely divergent outcomes, the initial presentations of the two forms may be identical and are not predictive of the patient's clinical course. Ischemic colitis is generally viewed as a nonocclusive form of intestinal ischemia. Although in some cases a specific anatomic abnormality may be identified, as in ligation of the IMA during repair of abdominal aortic aneurysms, the precipitating episode often resolves by the time of presentation. Diagnosis is dependent on a high index of suspicion for the disease. Correct interpretation of the symptoms, signs, and laboratory values associated with colonic ischemia must be followed by prompt diagnostic imaging, endoscopy, and/or operative exploration, depending on the severity of disease.[5]

Clinical risk factors are important to consider when evaluating a patient for ischemic colitis. Cardiovascular disease and hypertension are common, prevalent, preexisting medical conditions among our group of patients, and many of these patients are taking vasoactive medications, which may have limited the flow to the ischemic segments or have blunted the colon's ability to compensate for low blood flow.[6] Additionally, many have renal failure. The association between morbidity and mortality from ischemic colitis and patients with chronic renal failure has been described.[7] Certainly, one must have a low threshold for complete endoscopic evaluation of the entire colon in these patients when symptoms of an unexplained GI illness are present. Nevertheless, colonoscopy should be avoided in patients with peritoneal signs.

Nongangrenous ischemic colitis should be managed conservatively, because resolution is often self-limiting. Even strictures can be managed without operation because obstruction is rarely complete and endoscopy can differentiate benign from malignant strictures. Adequate hydration initially is important to maintain tissue perfusion. Systemic antibiotic therapy is given with monitoring of white blood cell count and hematocrit. There is no role for systemic anticoagulation. Abdominal pain, acidosis, and clinical deterioration all suggest impending infarction. Conservative therapy has no role once infarction develops and the prognosis is related to the time the diagnosis is made and the colon is resected. At surgery, all ischemic colon needs to be resected. Primary anastomosis should be avoided. Survival is almost uniformly inversely correlated with the

presence of infarction as well as the presence of coexisting morbidities. A recent series demonstrated that pain-associated ischemic colitis has a worse prognosis than melena-associated ischemic colitis.[8] Colonic ischemia affecting younger people is being recognized more frequently where identifiable causes include collagen vascular disease, hematologic disorders, long-distance running, and cocaine abuse.[9]

Total colonic ischemia remains a highly lethal condition. Risk factors for total colonic ischemia seem to be patients who have had profound blood loss after major abdominal surgery or patients with disease entities characterized by fluid shifts such as renal failure on hemodialysis. Regardless, prompt recognition and resection can be lifesaving in severe cases.[10] Ischemic proctosigmoiditis remains a rare entity, thought to be attributable to the abundant collateral blood supply located within the pelvis and perineum.[11] When this entity occurs, often an identifiable precipitating factor is identified. Conservative management is usually effective and proctectomy rarely required.

Collagen Vascular–associated Colitis

The collagen vascular diseases represent a collection of conditions that are believed to be the result of pathologic alterations in the immune system. They may occur in any organ and may be associated with GI manifestations.[12] Often these entities affect the blood supply to the colon and rectum and may produce ischemic changes and a colitis. Deposition of immune complexes in blood vessel walls resulting in either ischemia or thrombosis is the most widely accepted pathogenic mechanism. These entities include polyarteritis nodosa (PAN), cryoglobulinemia, Henoch-Schönlein purpura, Behçet's syndrome, systemic lupus erythematosus (SLE), scleroderma, and polymyositis.

Polyarteritis Nodosa

PAN is a systemic necrotizing vasculitis of small- and medium-sized arteries often with visceral involvement. Lesions are segmental and tend to involve bifurcations and branches of arteries. In the United States, the incidence is about 3–5 per 100,000 population per year. Men are affected more frequently than women and the age of onset is 40–60 years. Patients typically present with nonspecific signs and symptoms such as fever, weakness, headache, abdominal pain, weight loss, and malaise. PAN affects multiple systems including renal, musculoskeletal, nervous, GI, integument, cardiac, and genitourinary. The GI tract involvement is similarly nonspecific and presenting signs and symptoms include abdominal pain, nausea, and vomiting, bleeding, bowel infarction, and perforation, as well as cholecystitis, or hepatic/pancreatic infarction. PAN carries a high mortality rate when untreated. Nearly half of patients die within the first 3 months of onset. When immunosuppressive agents are combined with corticosteroids, the 5-year survival rate may increase to greater than 80%.

GI involvement of PAN is often a poor prognostic factor. Patients often have an abnormal visceral arteriogram with both saccular and fusiform aneurysms of the mesenteric vessels. Abdominal symptoms are often manifested as pain where organ damage caused by ischemia and hemorrhage may occur. GI hemorrhage, bowel perforation, and bowel infarction are often the underlying pathology. Some patients may present with a chronic wasting syndrome in which mesenteric angiography may establish the diagnosis. The Churg-Strauss syndrome (CSS) is a variant of PAN in which GI involvement caused by eosinophilic infiltration causes abdominal pain, bloody stool, and diarrhea. Surgical intervention is required for acute surgical conditions as a consequence of PAN or CSS. Bowel resection with avoidance of an intestinal anastomosis should be performed. A discussion with the family should include the poor prognosis with GI involvement.[13]

Cryoglobulinemia

Cryoglobulins are immunoglobulins that undergo reversible precipitation at low temperatures. Cryoglobulinemia may be associated with a particular disease such as autoimmune disease, lymphoproliferative disorder, infectious diseases, or it may be idiopathic form termed essential cryoglobulinemia. This disease is thought to be related to immune-complex disease with intravascular cryoglobulin deposits, reduced level of complement and complement fragments that act as chemotactic mediators of inflammation. Cryoglobulinemia may complicate chronic hepatitis infection, and many immune diseases including inflammatory bowel disease. The GI manifestations are rare and may result in ischemia or infarction secondary to a mesenteric vasculitis.[14]

Henoch-Schönlein Purpura

Henoch-Schönlein purpura is a distinct systemic vasculitis characterized by the tissue deposition of immunoglobulin A containing immune complexes. The clinical symptoms include abdominal manifestations, arthralgias or arthritis, palpable purpura, glomerulonephritis, and colicky abdominal pain. Although the disease is frequently seen in children, adults of any age may be affected. Abdominal symptoms are usually the result of vasculitis in which symptoms include abdominal pain, nausea, and vomiting, and GI bleeding may occur in up to 40% of patients. Intramural hematomas, intussusception, infarction, and perforation of the gut may be a sequelae of this disease.[15,16]

Behçet's Syndrome

Behçet's syndrome is a chronic relapsing inflammatory, multisystem disorder characterized by widespread vasculitis of large and small arterial and venous vessels. It is most prevalent around the Mediterranean and Japan. When it appears, it affects young men and runs an aggressive course. In Europe and North America, it mainly affects women. The etiology of the disease is unknown, but most authors believe it arises from a genetic predisposition with a triggering event such as streptococcal infection that leads to alteration in immune function.[17] The GI tract is affected in 15%–65% of cases, and when involved carries a poor prognosis.[18] Mesenteric ischemia and infarction are a result of large vessel disease and ulceration is a sequelae of small vessel disease involving the mucosa. The ileocecal region is the most frequently involved segment. Diarrhea, abdominal pain, colitis, pancreatitis, bleeding, and ulceration from the mouth to the anus are features of GI involvement.[19] It may also present with a mass in the ileocecal region and often mimics inflammatory bowel disease. Behçet's disease and inflammatory bowel disease share many of the extraintestinal manifestations involving the eye, mouth, liver, and joints. Behçet's disease behaves similarly to Crohn's disease with anorectal ulceration and rectovaginal fistula. It is often difficult to distinguish between Behçet's disease and inflammatory bowel disease, because of the similarity in extraintestinal symptoms, such as oral ulceration, erythema nodosum, uveitis, and arthritis. Histologically, the intestinal ulcers of patients with Behçet's disease are indistinguishable from those of patients with ulcerative colitis; however, the finding of the granuloma formation that is characteristic of Crohn's disease can be used to rule out Behçet's disease.

Endoscopic and radiographic evaluation of the small and large bowel will reveal deep ulcers, pseudopolyps, and mucositis. Surgery is often encouraged early in treatment before fatal complications occur. Wide surgical margins are preferred and intestinal anastomoses discouraged because anastomotic leaks, reperforation, and fistulization are common.[20] When these GI manifestations of Behçet's disease occur, the prognosis is poor.

Systemic Lupus Erythematosus

SLE is a chronic multisystem inflammatory disease that can affect any and every organ system of the body, and follows a relapsing and remitting form. It is an autoimmune disorder involving microvascular inflammation and the generation of autoantibodies. Although the specific cause of SLE is unknown, multiple factors are associated (genetic, hormonal, environmental) with this disease. Disturbances within the immune system result in the formation of immune complexes in the microvasculature leading to complement activation and inflammation. Antinuclear antibodies are present in the serum of virtually all patients with SLE and antibodies to native DNA are highly specific for the diagnosis of SLE.

GI symptoms are common in patients with active SLE. Nausea and dyspepsia are frequent complications. Abdominal pain may be related directly to active lupus. One of the most devastating complications of lupus is GI vasculitis and carries a 50% mortality rate.[21] Common sequelae include ulceration, hemorrhage, perforation, and infarction.[22,23] The diagnosis of small or large bowel vasculitis is frequently difficult to make because arteriography rarely demonstrates small vessel disease and computed tomography (CT), endoscopy, and small bowel series may also be unrevealing. The diagnosis is often made from surgical specimens after an acute surgical emergency. Medical treatment of abdominal lupus vasculitis often involves corticosteroids and cyclophosphamide.

Scleroderma

Scleroderma is a multisystem, multistage disorder of small arteries, microvessels, and connective tissue. The disease occurs in all races but affects women three to four times more often than men. Initial symptoms occur in the 20s to 40s. Systemic manifestations may include skin involvement, Raynaud's disease, polyarthritis, and lung, heart, kidney, and thyroid problems. In the GI tract, the disease may affect the esophagus, stomach, or small or large bowel. The GI symptoms may precede the diagnosis by several years, and are often the most difficult to treat. Overproduction of collagen, increased humoral immunity, and abnormal cellular immune function all contribute to the development of scleroderma in other organs. More importantly, the changes seen in the blood vessels in scleroderma have a role in the development of the clinical manifestations of the disease. The esophagus is the GI organ that is most frequently involved and more than 50% of patients diagnosed with scleroderma have esophageal manifestations. In the small bowel and the stomach, chronic intestinal pseudoobstruction, bacterial overgrowth, and malnutrition are the main consequences. These patients often require prokinetic agents which can be used to enhance gut motility. Antibiotic therapy is the treatment for bacterial overgrowth. Somatostatin is used when severe diarrhea develops which occasionally is seen in scleroderma.[24–26]

Scleroderma may also affect the large bowel and colonic motility. Clinically, patients may have severe constipation and may have fecal impaction, rectal prolapse, megacolon, and diverticula. GI bleeding arising from the colon has been reported to result from diverticulosis, stercoral ulcerations, and telangiectasias. Anorectal dysfunction frequently occurs with scleroderma and is similar to that of the esophageal dysmotility. These patients often have decreased internal anal sphincter pressures, a decreased or absent anorectal inhibitory reflex, and reduced rectal compliance. The treatment of constipation may prove difficult, and after conventional treatment fails, daily balanced electrolyte solutions containing polyethylene glycol may be required. Prokinetics are often tried, but results are disappointing. For fecal incontinence, efforts in controlling diarrhea are worthwhile. Antidiarrheals, however, may precipitate pseudoobstruction. Biofeedback may be considered. Finally, malnutrition may be a serious consequence of this disease and appropriate measures should be instituted.[27]

Polymyositis

Polymyositis is an inflammatory muscle disease of unknown etiology. It is characterized by weakness, high levels of striated muscle enzymes, and electromyographic or biopsy evidence of an inflammatory myopathy. This all is a result of immune-mediated muscle inflammation and vascular damage. The immune system is primed to act against previously unrecognized muscle antigens. It is a disease of adults and common among blacks. Symmetric proximal muscle pain and weakness, dysphagia, arthralgias, joint pain, and, when accompanied by a rash over the face, chest and hands, it is referred to as dermatomyositis. Serum creatine kinase is the most sensitive and specific laboratory study with levels 5–50 times that of normal. The erythrocyte sedimentation rate is usually increased, myoglobinuria may be present, and positive rheumatoid factor and antinuclear antibody may be found. Treatment includes systemic steroids and immunosuppressive agents. GI symptoms include impaired deglutition, impaired gastric emptying, bloating, constipation, and GI hemorrhage. Pneumatosis intestinalis, colonic dilatation, and diverticulosis may be seen. Certain subgroups of polymyositis-dermatomyositis may have an increased prevalence of malignancy. Overall, the 5-year mortality rate is 20%.[28]

Microscopic Colitis

Microscopic colitis is current terminology encompassing two subtypes: lymphocytic colitis and collagenous colitis. From a clinical perspective, disease manifestations and treatment are alike. These entities are separated by their histologic features. The clinical syndrome of watery diarrhea in the setting of normal radiologic studies of the GI tract and with a normal endoscopic mucosal appearance was problematic to many clinicians. Many patients were lumped into the rubric of irritable bowel syndrome for lack of any better understanding.

In 1976, Lindstrom[29] published the first article describing the association of colonic collagenous deposition and a watery diarrhea syndrome. Four years later, Read and colleagues[30] published the first article referring to microscopic colitis. In 1982, Kingham and associates[31] described six patients who presented with watery diarrhea and normal appearing colons by barium enema study and colonoscopy. However, random colonic biopsies revealed lymphocytic infiltrates in the colonic epithelium. Treating these six patients with antiinflammatory medications resolved their symptoms thus demonstrating the relationship between the infiltrate and the syndrome.

Pardi[32] estimates that microscopic colitis accounts for about 10% of cases of chronic diarrhea referred to major centers for study. Of this 10%, about half represent lymphocytic colitis and half collagenous colitis. Collagenous colitis occurs more often in women (studies exceed 80%) whereas there seems to be no gender differential in lymphocytic colitis.

Both entities principally afflict patients over the age of 60 but cases have been demonstrated in all age groups including pediatrics. Bo-Linn and associates[33] were able to demonstrate that watery diarrhea was secondary to marked depression of colonic absorption. This decreased function led to the associated findings of hypokalemia and, in severe cases, a protein-losing enteropathy. Crampy abdominal pain and weight loss are the major clinical complaints from patients. Stool frequency ranges from 3 to 20 per day. Despite this, dehydration is unusual as are fever, vomiting, and GI bleeding.

Clinical evaluation demands that when the patient comes to endoscopy, biopsies be obtained. Lymphocytic colitis tends to occur uniformly throughout the colon and rectum but collagenous colitis is often patchy, therefore requiring frequent colon biopsies at intervals throughout.[34] The histologic criteria for lymphocytic colitis requires more than 10 lymphocytes per 100 epithelial cells in the colon (Figure 43-1). Normal colons will have less than five lymphocytes per 100 cells. Additionally, a mixed mononuclear infiltrate is present in the lamina propria. The excess deposition of collagen in collagenous colitis occurs in the subepithelial layer of the bowel (Figure 43-2). It is interesting to note that it is not the thickness of the collagen layer that correlates with the severity of the diarrhea, but instead the degree of inflammatory infiltrate.[35] The terminal ileum may be affected by either type of microscopic colitis. Villous atrophy[36] and intraepithelial lymphocytosis[37] may be found on ileal biopsy. Ileal wall changes suggest that perhaps a small bowel luminal constituent is responsible for the inflammatory colonic changes. Studies demonstrating a high prevalence of arthritis (82%) and autoantibodies (50%) suggest the possibility of an autoimmune disorder.[38] Higher than expected prevalence of sprue-like HLA genes in microscopic colitis patients suggests an immunologic basis for the inflammatory changes.[39] Furthermore, diversion of the ileal content via a stoma led to morphologic resolution of colonic inflammatory changes on tissue microscopy. Closing the

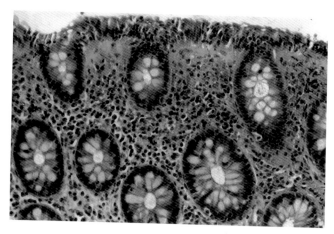

FIGURE 43-2. Collagenous colitis. H & E stain; magnification × 540. (© 2004 Frederick C. Skvara, MD).

stoma led to recurrent microscopic colitis.[40] Another factor related to possible pathogenesis of the colonic inflammatory process is bile acid malabsorption (BAM). One report found BAM present in 60% of those studied with lymphocytic colitis versus 27% in collagenous colitis.[41] Of note, 75% of patients with functional diarrhea demonstrated BAM. It therefore suggests that abnormalities of bile metabolism may be concomitant conditions but not causally related to the colonic inflammatory condition.

Recently, a report[42] linked the onset of microscopic colitis to a formulary change in which lansoprazole was substituted for omeprazole. Development of a watery diarrhea syndrome resulted in biopsy proven diagnosis, which resolved on discontinuation of the medication. This finding suggests that medication-induced colonic changes do occur and should be sought after in the evaluation of patients with microscopic colitis.

Treatment options are empiric and are directed at symptom management, management of the inflammatory process, and the potential role of disordered immunoregulation in the pathogenesis of this disease. Because there are multiple medications that impact the above targeted areas, it is recommended that therapy begin with the least toxic regimens. Initially, dietary modifications can be tried, eliminating caffeine, dairy, alcohol, and artificial sweeteners. Nonsteroidal antiinflammatory drugs (NSAIDs) should be discontinued. Loperamide and diphenoxylate/atropine are generally effective at symptom resolution. Bismuth subsalicylate has been demonstrated over an 8-week course to be safe and efficacious in disease management when dosed at 524 mg four times daily.[43] Cholestyramine induced remission in 19 of 22 patients[41] whereas mesalamine produced some response (range of 47%–50%). Steroids were more effective (70%–82% response). Immunomodulator therapy with azathioprine, 6-mercaptopurine, and others has been tried for steroid failures or those requiring chronic steroid maintenance with some success (89%).[44] Surgical options include ileostomy for diversion

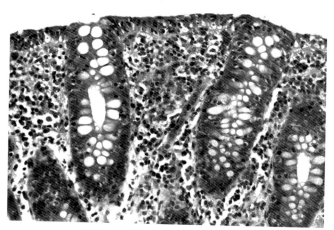

FIGURE 43-1. Lymphocytic colitis. Hematoxylin and eosin (H & E) stain; magnification × 540. (© 2004 Frederick C. Skvara, MD).

or colectomy, with or without restoration of continence. Surgery, as a treatment option, requires failure or intolerance to the medical options available and symptoms severe enough to warrant such aggressive intervention.

Eosinophilic Colitis

This rare condition is characterized by eosinophilic infiltration of the involved tissues and increased eosinophil counts in peripheral blood.[45] Eosinophilic colitis is usually encountered in the gastric antrum and proximal small bowel. Symptoms include abdominal pain, nausea, vomiting, and weight loss. When the mucosa is involved, bleeding, diarrhea and protein-losing enteropathy may be noted. Differential diagnosis includes tuberculosis, Crohn's disease, parasite infestations, allergic enteropathies, and collagen vascular disorders. Colonoscopic biopsies should differentiate eosinophilic colitis from these other grossly similar appearing conditions.[46] Therapy for symptomatic patients consists of steroids. Spontaneous remissions have been documented. Surgery has a role for management of complications, such as intussusception, obstruction, or hemorrhage and in cases in which diagnostic dilemmas require more tissue.[47]

Fungal Colitis

Fungal colitides do occur but are thankfully unusual in an immunologically normal patient. Clinical settings in which this diagnosis must be considered include human immunodeficiency virus (HIV) infections, immunocompromised states such as splenectomy, chronic liver disease, and steroid therapy as well as in chronically ill patients being treated with broad-spectrum antibiotics. The major pathogens in this category include *Candida* spp., *Histoplasma capsulatum*, and *Cryptococcus neoformans*. Outside the United States, other fungi may predominate such as is seen with *Penicillium marneffei* in Southeast Asia.[48]

Candida colitis is the more common of these entities found predominantly in patients in the intensive care unit. Usually, the infection is systemic involving septicemia, the pulmonary tract, the urinary tract, and the GI tract. Colonic involvement may be diffuse and thus results in diarrhea, fever, and abdominal pain. Perforation may occur with resultant peritonitis or fistulization. Stool cultures or endoscopic biopsies are diagnostic when typical spores, yeast, or pseudomycelia are demonstrated. Medical treatment is first-line therapy in the absence of peritonitis. This consists of oral nystatin 500,000–1,000,000 units four times daily or in sicker patients, ketoconazole 200–400 mg daily. Alternatively, amphotericin B 0.3–0.6 mg/kg can be administered intravenously.[49] Surgical intervention may be required in the face of free perforation or clinical findings of peritonitis. Despite aggressive surgical intervention, mortality is very high because of the severity of the associated conditions.

Histoplasmosis

H. capsulatum is found endemically throughout the Midwestern United States. Although principally a pathogen of the reticuloendothelial system, it can cause systemic infection in the immunocompromised host. Pulmonic disease is most common but ileocolitis does occur. A granulomatous process causing bleeding, ulceration, stricture formation, and perforation has been described.[50] Endoscopic examination can be confusing because the lesions may appear to resemble adenocarcinoma. Skip areas, pseudopolyps, ulcerations, and plaque-like lesions may be present but biopsies will reveal intracellular budding yeasts within the mucosa when this organism is present. Serologic tests and fungal cultures may also confirm the diagnosis. Although perforation is rare, emergent surgery with resection of the grossly affected tissue and proximal diversion may be necessary. Amphotericin B intravenously administered is indicated in severe cases whereas ketoconazole has been used effectively in patients less severely ill. Histoplasma colitis has been reported in otherwise healthy patients but the previously described assessment should demonstrate the responsible pathogen when present.[51]

Cryptococcus

Cryptococcosis usually affects the central nervous system. *C. neoformans* is acquired via inhalation of soil contaminated with this encapsulated yeast. Isolated GI infection is rare but does occur in immunocompromised patients. Colitis with perforation can occur spontaneously or after endoscopic biopsy and so surgical intervention to manage life-threatening complications may be necessary.[52] A high index of suspicion must be maintained when patients present with symptoms of colitis and a concomitant history of immune suppressive therapy or infection with HIV. Early medical therapy provides the best means of avoiding surgery in these very ill patients. Diagnosis is confirmed by biopsy of infected mucosa demonstrating encapsulated budding yeasts or via culture of stool. Ketoconazole is effective in less severely ill patients but amphotericin B is standard therapy in severely ill or immunocompromised patients.

Bacterial Colitis

Because bacterial pathogens can produce clinical syndromes, which may mimic other conditions in which surgery is more likely a therapeutic consideration, colorectal surgeons must have a basic understanding of the organisms that cause enterocolitis as well as diagnostic and therapeutic options (see Table 43-1). Bacterial pathogens cause disease within the GI tract in several ways: mucosal adherence leading to secretory diarrhea, toxin production, and mucosal invasion.[52] The very young and the elderly are at greater risk of serious sequelae as are immunocompromised hosts. The majority of infections worldwide occur in developing countries where water

TABLE 43-1. Clinical pathologic characteristics of bacterial colitis

Sign	Organisms capable of producing syndrome
Watery diarrhea	E. coli
	Salmonella
	Shigella
Dysentery	E. coli
	Salmonella
	Shigella
	Yersinia
	Campylobacter
Enteric fever or syndrome	Salmonella spp.
	Yersinia
	Campylobacter

contamination, poor food preservation techniques, and fecal contamination of food supplies is more likely. Each of the major bacterial pathogens is reviewed as to the clinical syndromes, complications, diagnosis, and treatment when necessary. For the most part, watery diarrhea syndrome requires supportive measures such as fluid and electrolyte replacement. Dysenteric syndromes characterized by bloody diarrhea, fever, and abdominal pain generally necessitate identification of the organism so that appropriate antibiotic therapy can be initiated (see Table 43-2). The goals of treatment are to decrease the period of bacterial shedding in the stools and to improve the patient's clinical condition, thus lessening the likelihood of invasive complications of infection.[53]

Escherichia coli

Based on the mechanism by which they cause diarrhea, four classes of E. coli are described. Enteropathic E. coli is primarily a problem causing outbreaks of severe diarrhea in nurseries. Diarrhea is caused by the bacteria adhering to the mucosa of the enterocytes and the production of a cytotoxin causing mucosal damage. Infection is primarily within the small bowel. The clinical syndrome may consist of watery diarrhea, vomiting, and fever. The process is generally self-limiting and so therapy is supportive. Trimethoprim-sulfamethoxazole (TMP/SMX) is effective and is recommended in complicated cases.

Enterotoxigenic E. coli is ubiquitous in developing nations and is the major organism causing traveler's diarrhea. Thirty to fifty percent of travelers from industrialized nations spending 3 weeks or more in developing nations will experience this infection.[52] The toxin produced does not damage the mucosa but causes a secretory diarrhea. Infection is self-limiting but may cause cramping and low-grade fevers. Treatment is supportive. For travelers wishing to avoid becoming ill with this pathogen, prophylaxis with bismuth subsalicylate, 2 tablets four times daily during periods of exposure is helpful. Unfortunately, salicylate intoxication is a concern in children and thus not recommended in this group.[53]

Enteroinvasive E. coli produces a syndrome much like Shigella. Mucosal invasion of enterocytes by this strain produces the illness but is usually self-limited. Treatment is supportive unless dysentery develops. Should this occur, TMP/SMX is indicated.

Enterohemorrhagic E. coli can cause serious dysenteric problems related to production of a cytotoxin. It has occurred in the United States in outbreaks associated with undercooked hamburger meat. Cramps, low-grade fever, and watery diarrhea progress to a more severe bloody diarrhea. Treatment remains supportive because no effective antimicrobial therapy is known. The clinical presentation may mimic inflammatory bowel disease or ischemic colitis. A hemolytic uremic syndrome or thrombocytopenia may complicate the recovery phase, especially in patients at either age extreme.[54]

Shigella

Although there are four species of Shigella known to cause clinical gastroenteritis, in the United States, S. sonnei predominates and S. flexneri is second most common. Shigella is

TABLE 43-2. Antibiotic therapy for bacterial colitis (adults)

Pathogen	Illness	Treatment
E. coli	Traveler's diarrhea	TMP/SMX 1 double strength tab b.i.d. × 3–5 d or ciprofloxacin 500 mg p.o. b.i.d. × 3–5 d
Salmonella	Bacteremia, sepsis, immuno-compromised host, dysentery	Ceftriaxone 1 g IV or IM q 12 h × 2 wk or cefoperazone 30 mg/kg q 12 h × 2 wk or chloramphenicol IV 75 mg/kg/d in 4 divided doses × 2 wk or ciprofloxacin 500 mg IV or p.o. q 12 h × 2 wk or ampicillin 100 mg/kg/d IV or IM q 6 h × 14 d
Shigella	Dysentery	TMP/SMX double-strength tablets (DS), one b.i.d. p.o. × 5 d or norfloxacin 400 mg tablets p.o. b.i.d. × 5 d or ciprofloxacin 500 mg p.o. b.i.d. × 5 d
Yersinia	Sepsis, severe abdominal pain with mesenteric adenitis	Gentamicin 7.5 mg/kg/d administered IV q 8 h for 7–10 d or TMP/SMX DS b.i.d. for 5 d or chloramphenicol IV 75 mg/kg/d given q 6 h for 7–10 d
Campylobacter	Dysentery or sepsis	Ciprofloxacin 500 mg p.o. t.i.d. × 5 d or azithromycin 500 mg q d × 3 d or gentamicin or chloramphenicol as for Yersinia, if severe
Tuberculosis	Enterocolitis	Isoniazid 300 mg p.o. q d and rifampin 600 mg p.o. q d for 4–6 mo
Aeromonas	Dysentery, enteric fever syndrome, immunocompromised patient	TMP/SMX DS p.o. b.i.d. × 7–10 d or doxycycline 100 mg p.o. b.i.d. or chloramphenicol IV 75 mg/kg/d given q 6 h for 7–10 d
Brucellosis	Colitis	Doxycycline 100 mg p.o. b.i.d. for 3–6 wk and streptomycin 1 g IM q 12–24 h for 14 d
Actinomycosis	Abdominal pain, mass, fever	Penicillin G 12–18 million units/d given q 4–6 h for 2–6 wk

b.i.d., twice a day; p.o., per os; q, every; IV, intravenously.

the prototypical pathogen causing a dysenteric syndrome based on the ability of this gram-negative rod to produce toxins permitting epithelial cell penetration and destruction. Malnourished and immunocompromised hosts are most at risk for the debilitating complications of infection.[55,56] Onset of infection follows fecal-oral transmission of a small number of inocula. Sexual transmission does occur but most cases originate from overcrowded housing and daycare facilities.[57] Watery diarrhea, fever, fatigue, and malaise herald the onset of colitis. Gross bleeding and mucous denotes dysentery and requires the more virulent properties usually associated with *S. dysenteriae* and least likely with *S. sonnei* as found in the United States.[58] Bowel obstruction and toxic megacolon are most frequently seen in *S. dysenteriae* infections in underdeveloped nations. Although stool volume is low, making dehydration unusual, the colonic inflammatory process leads to spasm and tenesmus (10–100 bowel movements per day). Diagnosis is best made by stool cultures for enteric pathogens. Endoscopic examination reveals a friable, edematous, erythematous mucosa with focal ulcerations and bleeding. The most often affected area is the rectosigmoid but the more severe the infection, the more proximal the changes progress. As to treatment, because infections with *S. sonnei* in the United States tend not to cause the dysenteric syndrome, supportive care is generally all that is necessary. Avoidance of antimotility agents is critical because their use exacerbates symptoms and predisposes to toxic megacolon. In the immunocompromised host or with the development of dysentery, TMP/SMX, ciprofloxacin, and ampicillin are usually effective at shortening the duration and severity of illness. Emergence of resistance to antibiotics is significant and so local knowledge of susceptibility patterns is important. Treatment should continue until stool cultures convert to no growth of the organism.

Salmonella

A gram-negative bacilli, *Salmonella* causes predominantly two clinical conditions. The first is typhoid fever caused by *S. typhi* and *S. paratyphi*, endemic in third world countries. The organism is ingested and is susceptible to destruction by normal gastric acidity, pancreatic enzymes, and enteric secretions.[52] Where these barriers to infection are altered either by postsurgical changes or acid-blocking medications, infection is more likely. Incubation periods range from 5 to 21 days with the onset of remitting fevers, headache, abdominal pains, and diarrhea. Hyperplasia of the reticuloendothelial systems can cause marked swelling in the ileocecal area. Hemorrhage, obstruction, and perforation may occur requiring emergent surgical intervention with resection and proximal diversion necessary.[59] The second and by far more common condition in the United States is non-typhoidal salmonellosis. *S. enteritidis* is usually responsible for causing a self-limited gastroenteritis in the warmer months of the year. Contaminated food products lead to nausea, vomiting, and abdominal pain. Most patients experience watery diarrhea but dysenteric symptoms may develop, especially in the immunocompromised host.[56,58] Infection is primarily small bowel but can progress to a colitis. Stool cultures, rectal swabs, or colonoscopic biopsies will assist in diagnosis. For severe infections in patients who are immune suppressed, have foreign body implants, hemolytic anemia, or pregnant, antibiotic therapy with ampicillin or TMP/SMX should be given as first-line therapy. In the majority of affected patients in the United States, supportive care will suffice.[58]

Campylobacter

This gram-negative rod is the most frequently identified cause of acute diarrheal illness in United States and industrialized nations. *C. jejuni* is the most common. Outbreaks generally occur during warm weather and are most frequently traced to poor handling or preparation of chicken products.[58] The organism can produce a spectrum of disease from watery diarrhea to dysentery depending on the strain's ability to produce enterotoxin, cytotoxin, or to cause mucosal invasion.[55,56] The terminal ileum and cecum are most frequently involved. Rarely, when the organism elaborates mucosal invasive properties, mesenteric lymphadenopathy may simulate appendicitis or produce an enteric fever-like syndrome. Most cases present with fever, abdominal pain, diarrhea, nausea, and malaise. Symptoms are generally self-limited resolving within 1 week but may linger up to 3 weeks. Immunocompromised patients are at greater risk for severe complications.[58]

Endoscopic findings range from segmental colonic ulcerations to a diffuse colitis. Disease limited to the ileocecal region may mimic Crohn's disease. Diagnosis requires stool cultures because clinically the disease mimics *Salmonella* and *Shigella*. Treatment with erythromycin or ciprofloxacin should be reserved for severely ill patients or any of those affected having an immunocompromised state, i.e., HIV, the very young, or the very old. Otherwise, treatment is supportive. Surgical intervention may be necessary to rule out appendicitis, or less frequently, to treat complications such as megacolon, hemorrhage, or perforation.[59]

Yersinia

Yersinia is a gram-negative coccobacillus capable of producing gastroenteritis commonly in Europe and North America. *Y. enterocolitica* and *Y. pseudotuberculosis* are most frequently associated with clinical disease, the latter being the more severe. Poor food handling and contaminated water are usually associated with outbreaks in the United States.[26] Of significant import to surgeons is that 40% of cases present in a manner very similar to acute appendicitis.[57–59] The organism invades Peyer's patches causing swelling in the terminal ileum, enlarged mesenteric nodes, localized pain, and watery diarrhea. At surgery, the appendix will appear normal. In severe cases, polyarthritis, erythema nodosum, and Reiter's syndrome may suggest the possibility of Crohn's ileocolitis. Colonoscopic evaluation may demonstrate erythema, aphthous ulcerations, and swelling of lymphoid tissue. Specific fecal culture techniques enhance identification, and serology is available, but both are time consuming.[56] Treatment of uncomplicated cases with antibiotics has not demonstrated clinical improvement except in the immunocompromised host or in the more complicated infection, i.e., enteric-like fever or mesenteric adenitis. In these more serious conditions, tetracycline, ciprofloxacin, TMP/SMX, or aminoglycoside are effective.[56,57,59]

Tuberculosis

Within the United States, tuberculosis occurs primarily in immunosuppressed populations (especially associated with HIV), among immigrants from underdeveloped nations, among the urban poor, and impoverished Native Americans.[58] Tuberculous enterocolitis is generally contracted via consumption of unpasteurized milk or from swallowing sputum infected from pulmonary tuberculosis. *Mycobacterium tuberculosis* and *M. bovis* predominate in the United States. Distal small bowel and cecal infections are noted and present with abdominal pain, weight loss, and fever. From exposure to illness, clinical illness can be delayed for up to a year.[59] Ulcers of varying depth, fistulas, and stenosis may result from the infectious process. Physical findings include generalized wasting and up to 50% of patients have a palpable mass in the right lower quadrant. Barium enema and/or CT may suggest the diagnosis but features can mimic inflammatory disease or malignancy. Tuberculous pericolonic adenitis may produce extrinsic compression and can lead to partial or complete obstruction. Tuberculous peritonitis can present as a surgical emergency mimicking acute appendicitis. Colonoscopic biopsy or fine-needle aspiration have permitted detection of acid-fast bacilli or caseating granulomas without the delay of awaiting culture reports. Diagnostic laparoscopy demonstrated tuberculous peritonitis with 95% accuracy in one series.[59] Stool cultures for viable tuberculosis organisms rarely demonstrate growth but is more likely in active cases of pulmonary tuberculosis. Serology tests have been developed and demonstrate sensitivity for intestinal tuberculosis of more than 80%.[58]

Treatment is usually medical with multi-drug regimens. Isoniazid and rifampin are first-line treatment but pyrazinamide and streptomycin or ethambutol may be added until sensitivity in the immunocompromised host can be established.[58] In more established cases, obstruction of the bowel secondary to sclerosing lesions or fistulous disease may require surgical intervention. It is still recommended that a medical trial be attempted because many patients will

improve and resolve without surgery.[59] Rectal tuberculosis, although rare, can cause stricturing. Most cases improve with anti-tuberculous drugs.

Neisseria gonorrhea

As a cause of proctitis, oroanal spread or anal-receptive sexual practices account for the majority of infections in the United States. Although heterosexual transmission is noted, the problem is more widespread in the homosexual population. Sexually transmitted diseases (STDs) are frequently encountered as co-infections with other STDs such as HIV, syphilis, and chlamydia. Gonococcal proctitis generally does not produce many symptoms or signs. Perianal itch, irritation, discharge, or tenesmus may be noted but are not generally troublesome. Physical examination may reveal a brownish purulent discharge, erythema, or fissuring of the mucosa. A mucopurulent discharge is the most common finding (71% in one study).[59] Cultures require a stool-free cotton swab of the rectal discharge which must be promptly plated on Thayer Martin media. A positive smear for gram-negative diplococci should be followed up with appropriate cultures. Treatment is best with a single dose of ceftriaxone intramuscularly. Alternatively, a single dose of oral cefixime, ciprofloxacin, or ofloxacin is effective.[58] Cure rates approach 97%.

Syphilis

Treponema pallidum infection of the anorectum is primarily a disease of anal-receptive males and females. Symptoms are usually minimal and frequently, when present, may be attributed to trauma from the sexual behavior or from mixed co-infections with other STDs. Chancres do occur but may be mistaken for idiopathic anal ulcers, cryptitis, or fissure disease.[58] Mucous, bleeding, and tenesmus may occur. In long-standing infections, a mass may be noted. Endoscopy may demonstrate ulcers but the mass may appear to represent carcinoma. Biopsies, of course, will fail to demonstrate tumor cells.[59] Darkfield examination of the discharge reveals *T. pallidum* organisms that are quite motile. Immunofluorescent stains are highly sensitive to detect this organism. Once diagnosed, parenteral penicillin G provides effective therapy. Missed primary infections may result in secondary- and tertiary-stage disease with the attendant long-term sequelae. Condyloma lata in the perianal area is evidence of secondary syphilis.

Aeromonas

Colitis caused by *Aeromonas* species seems primarily related to host immunity, i.e., HIV status, immunocompromised adults, children under the age of two, and in generally debilitated patients. Most infections in the United States are secondary to drinking untreated water. Watery stools, dysentery, vomiting, fever, and cramps are common to most enterocolitises making the diagnosis more obscure. Adults tend to have a more protracted, less severe diarrheal illness whereas children are more prone to an acute, fulminating illness. The latter are more likely to be complicated by hemolytic uremic syndrome, sepsis, and peritonitis.[58] In septic patients, mortality as high as 75% has been reported. *Aeromonas* colitis or severe associated illness should be treated with antibiotics. Quinolones are effective as are TMP/SMX, tetracycline, and chloramphenicol. Some antibiotic resistance has been emerging and so sensitivity testing should be performed. Endoscopic findings are nonspecific showing erythema (patchy or continuous), superficial ulcerations, exudates, and friable mucosa. Fortunately, in most patients, infections are mild and self-limited requiring no treatment.

Brucellosis

Brucellosis melitensis is a bacterium that may contaminate unpasteurized goat milk or cheese predominantly in underdeveloped nations. Rare in the United States, it can produce a nonspecific colitis. Cultures of the exudate will reveal the organism. Endoscopic examination reveals inflammatory changes of a protean nature.[58] Serologic tests contribute to early diagnosis and treatment can begin based on this alone. Single-agent therapy has an unacceptably high relapse rate so that currently, doxycycline 100 mg orally twice daily for 3–6 weeks and streptomycin 1 g intramuscularly (IM) every 12–24 hours for 14 days is preferred. Alternatively, TMP/SMX with streptomycin or rifampin is effective.

Actinomycosis

Actinomyces israelii is an anaerobic gram-positive bacterium normally found in the mouth, lungs, and GI tract of humans. Infection can be oro-cervical, pulmonary, or ileocolic. Fever, vomiting, weight loss, and diarrhea occur at the onset of the ileocolic infection. As the infection progresses, abdominal pain associated with palpable masses may develop. The lesions may fistulize to the abdominal wall where the characteristic sulfur granules within the discharge may be noted. Unfortunately, the enterocolic mass often suggests an obstructing neoplasm and so this diagnosis is usually made postoperatively. Obstruction may precipitate the need for surgical intervention. Although the ileocolic area is most often involved, mass lesions and stricturing lesions may occur anywhere else in the colon or rectum. Radiographs are typically nonspecific and seem to support the more common diagnosis of neoplasm. Pus or fistula drainage generally will demonstrate the classic microscopic appearance of *A. israelii* on Gram's stain.[59] Treatment of ileocolic actinomycosis is

resection. Concomitant treatment with high-dose penicillin G, 12–18 million units/day for 2–6 weeks is recommended. Oral penicillin, tetracycline, or erythromycin are usually continued for several weeks after any apparent cure.[59]

Miscellaneous Colitis

There are a number of unusual and rare causes of colitis that one may encounter. These may be diversion colitis, neutropenic enterocolitis, disinfectant colitis, corrosive colitis, colitis as a result of NSAIDs, and that related to toxic epidermal necrolysis (TEN) (Stevens-Johnson syndrome).

Diversion Colitis

Diversion colitis is a term used to describe the clinical entity of nonspecific inflammation of excluded colonic and rectal mucosa. Its importance lies in the difficulty to differentiate it from other colorectal inflammatory states when endoscopically evaluating the excluded segment of bowel. The etiology of diversion colitis is thought to be a deficiency of short-chain fatty acids which are the nutrients to the colonic mucosa.[60] This is supported by the fact that daily instillation of short-chain fatty acids results in improved endoscopic appearance of the diverted segment. Often this entity is asymptomatic, but when symptoms occur, rectal bleeding is the prominent symptom. Other symptoms include tenesmus, mucous discharge, and abdominal pain. Endoscopy may reveal mucous plugs, contact irritation, erythema, and ulcerations. Asymptomatic disease requires no pharmacologic treatment. Patients whom diversion is permanent and are symptomatic, twice daily irrigation of short-chain fatty acids is recommended for 2–4 weeks. Other treatments include 5-aminosalicylic acid (5-ASA) enemas and steroid enemas. Periodic examination of the diverted segment for neoplasia is warranted. Diversion colitis completely resolves once intestinal continuity is reestablished.[60–63]

Neutropenic Enterocolitis

Neutropenic enterocolitis is a potentially fatal condition that is now a commonly recognized complication of chemotherapy for neoplastic disease. However, this disease has been seen in patients who have undergone transplantation, and aplastic anemia. The exact pathogenesis remains challenging because other abdominal diseases mimic its presentation. The process has a predilection for the terminal ileum and cecum, but any segment of the bowel can be involved. Common presenting symptoms are abdominal pain, fever, diarrhea, abdominal distention, nausea, vomiting, and diarrhea with or without blood. A tip-off is coexisting neutropenia in the appropriate patient population. CT seems to be the most accurate method of diagnosis which reveals a thickened and inflamed terminal ileum and cecum. The management of these patients remains challenging. Bowel rest, intravenous fluids, broad spectrum of antibiotics with parenteral nutrition are the cornerstones of treatment. As the leukopenia resolves, often the patient improves. Surgery is reserved for perforation or peritonitis, or if lack of systematic improvement occurs despite conservative measures after a defined time period. Outcome can be unpredictable; however, coexisting morbidities often overwhelm the septic insult.[64–66]

Disinfectant Colitis

Commercially available endoscope disinfecting solutions readily cause colonic damage if allowed to contact the mucosa. These endoscopic cleaning solutions, often either hydrogen peroxide or glutaraldehyde, may produce a controversial lesion referred to as pseudolipomatosis. Furthermore, endoscopists may note the appearance of plaque-like lesions that resemble pseudomembranes upon withdrawal of the scope in an area that was previously noted to be normal in appearance. Clinically, in patients suspected of having developed disinfectant colitis, 24–48 hours after the procedure, abdominal cramping, bloody diarrhea, fever, and leukocytosis may develop. This entity remains self-limited although no long-term outcome is currently available. Efforts to prevent this include diligent rinsing and forced air drying. Automatic disinfecting machines should be routinely serviced and volume adjustments in the rinse cycle maintained.[67]

Corrosive Colitis

Glutaraldehyde and formalin are two potential corrosives used in a wide spectrum of medical care that may be responsible for corrosive colitis. A 2% solution of glutaraldehyde is widely used as a disinfectant because of its broad spectrum of action against acid and alcohol-resistant bacilli, hydrophilic viruses, and spores. Formalin enemas have been shown to improve the endoscopic and clinical features of patients with radiation proctitis. As with disinfectant colitis, these patients develop a self-limiting spectrum of symptoms such as abdominal pain, mucous diarrhea, and rectal bleeding within 48 hours of exposure to the corrosive agent. As always, other mechanisms that may mimic this condition need to be excluded. Treatment remains supportive with intravenous fluids as needed.[68–70]

NSAID and Salicylate-induced Colitis

The capacity of NSAIDs and salicylates to produce adverse side effects in the gastroduodenal mucosa is well known. In addition, NSAIDs may produce colonic mucosal injury. These drugs are also associated with the reactivation of quiescent inflammatory bowel disease, colonic stricture formation, and perforation and hemorrhage. Presenting symptoms are often diarrhea, rectal bleeding, and abdominal pain, along with a history of NSAID usage. Endoscopic findings range from patchy erythema and granularity to severe extensive mucosal ulcers. Often the clinical and endoscopic features are indistinguishable from idiopathic colitis. Treatment involves discontinuing NSAID and salicylate use as well as administering 5-ASA and steroid medications. At times, inpatient therapy is required. Relapse is not uncommon and chronic colitis may require surgery.[71]

Toxic Epidermal Necrolysis

TEN, also known as Stevens-Johnson syndrome, is a severe mucocutaneous exfoliative disease with an uncertain pathogenesis and a high mortality rate. The primary manifestation is the appearance of an erythematous confluent eruption that rapidly evolves into exfoliation of the skin at the dermal–epidermal junction, resulting in large sheets of necrotic dermis. This process seems to be immune-complex mediated and represents an idiosyncratic reaction to a drug or chemical agent. Sepsis, GI hemorrhage, leukopenia, fluid and electrolyte imbalance, and renal insufficiency are the major complications that contribute to the high mortality rate. Diffuse ulceration anywhere within the mucosal surface of the GI tract may occur. The colonoscopic appearance may resemble severe ulcerative or pseudomembranous colitis; however, biopsies show extensive necrosis and lymphocytic infiltration without crypt abscesses or neutrophils. The mucosal sloughing of the bowel may result in melena or intestinal perforation.[72]

Viral Colitis

Viral colitis is still relatively rare, however it is being seen with increasing frequency in this country. Etiologies include cytomegalovirus (CMV), herpes simplex virus, and viral colitides as a result of HIV or acquired immunodeficiency syndrome (AIDS). Although viral colitis is primarily a disease of immunocompromised patients, CMV colitis has been reported in immunocompetent individuals.

CMV Colitis

CMV is the most common viral cause of diarrhea and a frequent cause of diarrhea in patients with multiple negative stool test results. It is an affliction that typically occurs late in the course of HIV infection when CD4 counts plummet. Infection is most common in the colon, but concomitant disease may occur in the proximal gut. The clinical manifestations of CMV colitis vary greatly or one may be asymptomatic. Symptoms of these infections include fever, weight loss, abdominal pain, and diarrhea with or without blood. Patients may complain of fever and weight loss without diarrhea. As the disease progresses, frank ulceration, toxic megacolon, and perforation may occur. Anorectal herpes simplex virus infections may be concurrent with colitis; local problems include lymphadenopathy, tenesmus, severe pain, urinary retention, and lumbosacral dysesthesia. The diagnosis of CMV colitis may be challenging, and one often relies on endoscopic examination. Findings on endoscopy include patchy erythema, with or without ulcerations ranging from small to shallow that may be wide and deep. Because these processes are diffuse, biopsies should be obtained from multiple sites to facilitate diagnosis. Histopathologic examination of biopsy tissue will reveal the characteristic changes of these infections. The inclusions may be very atypical in appearance or few in number. They may also be present in tissue that macroscopically appears normal. Viral cultures can also be obtained on biopsy material. In the end, the diagnosis rests primarily on demonstrating viral cytopathic effect in tissue specimens.[73–75]

Treatment includes supportive care and antiviral agents. Agents of choice for CMV are 9-(1,3 dihydroxy-2-propoxymethyl) guanine (DHPG, ganciclovir) and phosphonoformate (Foscarnet) and for herpes simplex virus, acyclovir. Surgical therapy is required for complications such as bleeding and perforation. Because of the nature of the disease and the immunocompromised state of the patient, subtotal colectomy with ileostomy is advised. Mortality is high and often attributed to sepsis as a result of underlying opportunistic infection.[76,77]

Herpes Simplex Colitis

Herpes simplex virus, when involved in the GI tract, usually manifests itself as a proctitis. This remains a disease frequently afflicting homosexual males as well as those with AIDS. It usually presents with anorectal pain, discharge, tenesmus, and rectal bleeding as well as difficulty urinating, and sacral paresthesias. The diagnosis is established by history, sigmoidoscopic demonstration of an acute proctitis, and isolation of the virus by culture. A variety of immunoassays currently exist to aid in diagnosis. Oral acyclovir has been demonstrated to be effective in alleviating symptoms. Intestinal perforation associated with intestinal herpes simplex virus infection in an immunocompromised patient has been reported. Relapses are common, especially in sexually active homosexuals.[78–80]

Parasitic Colitis

Amebiasis

Amebiasis is the second leading cause of death from human parasitic disease worldwide. The causative protozoan parasite, *Entameba histolytica*, is a potent pathogen. Infection usually begins with the ingestion of cysts in food or water that have been contaminated by human species. *E. histolytica* trophozoites invade the intestinal mucosa causing amebic colitis. In some cases, amebas breach the mucosal barrier and travel through the portal circulation causing amebic

abscesses. Many individuals with *E. histolytica* infection have no symptoms and can clear their infection without any signs of disease. Symptomatic patients present with bloody diarrhea and abdominal pain and tenderness. The onset is often gradual with patients reporting several weeks of symptoms. The diarrhea may be profuse without blood; also, rectal bleeding without diarrhea may be an uncommon presentation. Fever is unusual and weight loss and anorexia may be present. Occasionally, individuals develop fulminant amebic colitis with widespread abdominal pain, fever, and peritonitis. Amebomas, which are localized inflammatory annular masses, may develop in the cecum or ascending colon, and can cause obstructive symptoms and mimic carcinoma. The diagnosis rests on the demonstration of *E. histolytica* in the stool or colonic mucosa of patients with diarrhea. Currently there are commercially available enzyme-linked immunoabsorbent assays (ELISA) that identify *E. histolytica*. The cornerstone of treatment for amebiasis is nitroimidazole derivatives such as metronidazole. Amebic colitis is treated by metronidazole followed by a luminal agent such as paromomycin, iodoquinol, or diloxanide to eradicate colonization. Although fulminant colitis is managed initially conservatively, perforation requires colectomy.[81,82]

Balantidiasis

Balantidium coli is the largest and least common protozoal pathogen of humans and is the only ciliate that produces important human disease. It is most frequently found in tropical and subtropical regions. Communities that are in close association with pigs have an increased prevalence of disease because of the high rate of carriage of this organism by these animals. *B. coli* infection is spread to humans by ingestion of cysts spread by contaminated water and food. The trophozoite invades the distal ileal and colonic mucosa and produces intense mucosal inflammation and ulceration. In the symptomatic patient, diarrhea with blood and mucus is accompanied by nausea, abdominal discomfort, and weight loss. If allowed to progress, it can develop into fatal fulminant colitis with peritonitis and colonic perforation. The diagnosis is made by identification of trophozoites excreted in the stool or from the margin of ulcers seen in the rectum. The most frequently used treatment is tetracycline 500 mg four times daily for 10 days.[83,84]

Cryptosporidiosis

Cryptosporidium colonizes both the small and large intestine and is commonly found in developing countries. It is now closely associated with immunocompromised patients, particularly associated with AIDS. This organism is able to reproduce both sexually and asexually; however, the oocyst is the infective form of the parasite. The organism may be transmitted by a variety of routes, including fecal-oral, hand to mouth, contaminated foods and water, and by pets. A wide range of clinical features exist from totally asymptomatic carriers to severe life-threatening disease. Clinically, patients develop voluminous watery diarrhea with fever and abdominal discomfort. In immunocompromised individuals, the disease is more severe and can be fatal. The diagnosis is made by identification of oocysts on fecal smears or in large intestinal mucosal biopsies. Treatment remains challenging and spiramycin and paromomycin have been moderately effective.[85]

Giardiasis

Giardiasis is a disease caused by the protozoan *Giardia lamblia*. It is a worldwide condition with the vast majority of patients being asymptomatic. It is common in hikers and bikers who drink from mountain lakes, adults who care for children who are in diapers, and there is an increased incidence in male homosexuals. Infection results from ingestion of the cyst and produces diarrhea, the most common complaint in the symptomatic patient. Malabsorption may also be manifested. The diagnosis is made by identification of trophozoites in the stool or by a *Giardia* ELISA. A negative stool examination does not exclude the diagnosis. The drug of choice for the treatment of *Giardia* is metronidazole or other nitroimidazole compounds that are better tolerated.[86–88]

Trypanosomiasis

Trypanosoma cruzi is the organism responsible for Chagas' disease or trypanosomiasis. It occurs primarily in Central America and is spread to humans by the bite of the bloodsucking vector Reduviid bug which carries the parasite. The local irritation from the bite results in scratching and subsequent inoculation of the organism into the circulation. Trypomastigotes convert to amastigotes and enter the bloodstream to infect and destroy muscle and nerve cells leading to motility disorders of the intestinal tract and congestive heart failure. Clinically, esophageal and colorectal symptoms develop with the latter manifesting as severe constipation with abdominal pain and distention. The diagnosis is made on linking clinical symptoms with a patient living in an endemic area. Medical treatment with nifurtimox and benzinidazole are effective in the acute phase by reducing parasitemia. Once the chronic form develops and tissue damage occurs, surgery is offered. Indications for surgery are megacolon, severe constipation, and chronic fecal impaction. Although various operations have been proposed, either the Duhamel retrorectal abdominotransanal pull through, or if the lower rectum is not involved, extended left hemicolectomy with colorectal anastomosis, may be used. Results have continued to be very favorable for an improved quality of life with low morbidity and mortality.[89–91]

Ascariasis

Ascariasis is caused by the large round worm *Ascaris lumbricoides*. It is endemic in tropical and subtropical areas and it is estimated that more than one-fifth of the world's population is affected. Infection occurs from ingestion of the eggs in contaminated food or water. After migrating from the small intestine into the portal venous system, they pass through the liver into the lungs where they are coughed up and swallowed. Intestinal ascariasis produces crampy abdominal pain, but with a large worm load, intestinal obstruction can occur. The diagnosis is made by finding eggs in the stool. Small bowel series may demonstrate worms in the distal ileum. A variety of drugs including pyrantel pamoate, mebendazole, and levamisole have been recommended. Surgery is required for unremitting intestinal obstruction, and if perforation has not occurred, manipulation of the worms through the ileocecal valve will prevent migration of worms through an intestinal anastomosis.[92,93]

Schistosomiasis

Five species of schistosome are known to produce disease in human intestine. Human infection occurs after penetration of the skin or mucous membranes by cercariae, the infective form of the parasite which is liberated into fresh water by the intermediate snail host. After 1–2 days in the subcutaneous tissue, the cercariae migrate through the venous system and lodge in the liver as mature adult worms. After producing fertilized eggs, miracidia develop within these eggs and eventually migrate into the intestinal lumen and thus the stool. *S. japonicum* preferentially invades the superior mesenteric veins thus involving the small intestine and the ascending colon, *S. mansoni* usually invades the inferior mesenteric veins penetrating the descending colon, and *S. hematobium* invades the bladder, pelvic organs, and rectum. Symptoms are referable either to the skin or the viscus involved with the disease. If migration through the bowel occurs, patients will develop severe lower abdominal pain, rectal bleeding, diarrhea, and passage of mucous. The diagnosis is made by the identification of the ova in fresh stool specimens. Rectal biopsy may also reveal the presence of eggs in the mucosa or submucosa. Treatment depends on which species is involved. Patients with longstanding schistosomal colitis are at risk for carcinoma, but this applies primarily to *S. japonicum*. Cirrhosis with portal hypertension may produce massive hemorrhage from varices requiring portal decompression.[94,95]

Strongyloidiasis

Strongyloides stercoralis is one of the major nematodes that infects humans. It is a soil-dwelling organism endemic to the rural southeastern United States and Appalachia that infects the upper small intestine of humans and rarely the colon. The infective (filariform) larvae in the soil penetrate the human skin, migrate through the circulation to the lungs and break out of the respiratory tree, and are then swallowed. In the upper small intestine, these larvae molt to become adult females which burrow into the submucosa and release eggs into the intestinal lumen. Sometimes these larvae may penetrate the colonic mucosa producing a colitis. Patients present with diarrhea, weight loss, and a microcytic anemia. The diagnosis can be made by stool aspirates during colonoscopy demonstrating *S. stercoralis* larvae on wet mount examination. Treatment is with oral thiabendazole 25 mg/kg by mouth twice daily for 3 months.[96–98]

Trichuriasis

Trichuris trichiura (whipworm) is found worldwide in both developed and developing countries. Human infection begins after ingestion of ova. Larvae are released into the small intestine and most frequently the cecum and the terminal ileum are colonized. In symptomatic individuals, diarrhea with blood and mucous occurs often associated with abdominal pain and tenesmus. Chronic infection can result in iron deficiency. Stool examination for the barrel-shaped eggs of *T. trichiura* confirms the diagnosis. Mebendazole is the treatment of choice in a dose of 100 mg twice daily for 3 days.[99–101]

Anisakiasis

Anisakiasis is a disease caused by human infection by the *Anisakis* larvae, a murine nematode found in raw or undercooked fish. With the increased popularity of eating sushi and raw fish in the United States, infection with *Anisakis* is expected to increase. These larvae are usually found in herring, mackerel, salmon, cod, halibut, rockfish, sardine, and squid. Most human infections have been reported from Japan and The Netherlands and involve the stomach. Invasion of the gastric or intestinal wall 1–5 days after eating raw fish may be characterized by the abrupt onset of abdominal pain, nausea and/or vomiting, diarrhea, or an ileus. For transient anisakiasis, supportive measures and reassurance are all that is needed. If the larvae have invaded the intestine or the stomach wall, diagnosis and cure occur with endoscopic or surgical removal if evidence of obstruction or perforation are found.[102–104]

Tapeworm

A number of adult tapeworms parasitize the intestinal tract of humans. Infection is acquired through the ingestion of the infected flesh of the intermediate host that is raw or inadequately cooked. The diagnosis of tapeworms is made by finding the ova in the feces. *Diphyllobothrium latum* is the fish tapeworm that results from the ingestion of raw fish. The worm produces vitamin B_{12} deficiency and fatigue. *Taenia solium* is the pork tapeworm acquired by eating inadequately cooked pork. Cysticercosis occurs when humans ingest the egg of *T. solium* and may present with a variety of neurologic symptoms. *T. saginata* are the organisms responsible for beef tapeworm. This beef tapeworm is found throughout the world and can achieve many meters in length. The clinical symptoms of all tapeworms are variable and include abdominal dis-

comfort, nausea, vomiting, cutaneous sensitivity, headache, and malaise. Many infections are asymptomatic. Treatment of all tapeworms is with either niclosamide or praziquantel.[105,106]

AIDS Diarrhea

AIDS can result in life-threatening opportunistic infections of the GI tract, of which many present with diarrhea. The etiology of diarrhea in the HIV-positive patient is multifactorial. There are various colitides, distinct ulcerative infections, and a number of malignancies that may occur. HIV infection can affect the entire GI tract and the hepatobiliary system. A number of reviews have emphasized diarrhea, weight loss, swallowing disturbances, and abdominal pain as the major gastroenterologic disorders in AIDS. GI manifestations range in severity from the inconvenience and discomfort of oral and perianal infections through to life-threatening diarrhea caused by intestinal cryptosporidiosis. In the evaluation of the HIV patient with diarrhea, one must be aware that there remains a wide range of infectious pathogens: viral (CMV, herpes simplex), bacterial (*M. avium–intracellulare*) and parasitic (*Cryptosporidium, Isopora belli*).[107,108]

The most important goal of evaluating diarrhea in HIV infection is to identify a treatable cause with the minimal amount of diagnostic testing. Evaluation of patients with diarrhea includes three stool samples and colonoscopy with biopsy. Rectal biopsy alone may miss proximal viral disease. Certain opportunistic pathogens such as *Giardia* or *Isopora* may reside in the foregut or midgut and require upper endoscopy for diagnosis. The diagnostic value of radiographic contrast studies in evaluating diarrhea is very low. A comprehensive investigation will reveal an etiologic agent in 90% of patients. If stool evaluation and flexible endoscopy are nondiagnostic, there is some rationale for a limited trial of empiric antibiotics. This approach should be undertaken in the appropriate clinical context. Treatment of pathogen-negative diarrhea consists of volume resuscitation and somatostatin analogs.[109–112]

The differential diagnosis of diarrhea in AIDS includes protozoa, viruses, bacteria, fungi, gut neoplasms, and pancreatic insufficiency. In all patients, at least three stool specimens for fecal leukocytes, ova and parasites, acid fast bacteria, *Clostridium difficile* toxin, bacteria and fat stain should be obtained. Specific therapies depending on the result of diagnostic testing should be implemented. Symptomatic therapy as well as empiric therapy when diagnostic testing is nonrevealing is often undertaken. Surgery is reserved for acute abdominal emergencies and in of itself carries a substantial mortality.

HIV Colitis

Diarrhea is the most frequent and often most morbid GI manifestations of HIV and AIDS. However, the role of HIV as a diarrheal pathogen remains controversial. Several investigators have identified HIV within the gut tissue in up to 40% of patients with AIDS. Despite the ability of HIV virus to infect colon cell lines, its ability to produce an HIV colitis remains controversial.

Radiation-induced Bowel Injury

The advent of radiation as a mainstay of treatment for gynecologic and urologic malignancies has produced an extensive literature on the topic of subsequent complications related to the effects of ionizing radiation on the GI tract. As advances in radiation oncology progressed, our understanding of the long-term aftereffects were slow to develop because of the time lag encountered between administration of treatment and the presentation of the chronic sequela of radiation therapy (RT). Changes in radiation protocols, methods of delivery, and the addition of chemotherapeutic regimens concomitant with administration of radiotherapy continue to evolve. So too will the long-term chronic complications. These developments render older literature on the subject mostly of historic interest. However, several critical principles have been learned and are meaningful in our understanding and treatment of radiation-induced GI complications.

Radiation injury to the bowel is biphasic; there is an acute injury demonstrable during administration of RT and a delayed, chronic injury that may be encountered months to years after completion of treatment.[113,114] Both total radiation dose and rate of administration of that dose are important factors in the incidence of bowel complications. Early work established radiation dose tolerance levels of the various organs. Between 1%–5% of patients receiving 4500 cGy are expected to experience radiation-induced complications over a 5-year period. The complication rate increases to 25%–50% when 6500 cGy are administered. The rectum tolerates 5500 cGy but at 8000 cGy, 25%–50% of patients will experience chronic complications.[115] Higher doses administered over shorter times result in more acute injury.[116] However, the absence of symptomatic acute-phase injury does not correlate with diminished chronic sequela.[117]

Risk factors within the population being treated with RT have been reported and they principally relate to factors that compound the effects of ionizing radiation or increase the likelihood that higher doses of radiation will be delivered to the bowel.[118] Examples of the former include conditions predisposing to intestinal ischemia, i.e., cigarette smoking, hypertension, diabetes mellitus, vasculitides, or arteriosclerotic processes. Examples of the latter include processes that fix the intestine within the field of radiation maximizing exposure, i.e., previous abdominopelvic surgery causing adhesions and inflammatory intraabdominal processes causing immobility of the bowel. For this reason, the terminal ileum is most frequently injured by RT because of fixation within the pelvis secondary to adhesions. In the absence of adhesions, the rectum and rectosigmoid are most frequently

injured because of their normal fixation anatomically within the pelvis. Currently, the most common indications for RT in the United States is cervical cancer, endometrial cancer, prostate cancer, and anorectal malignancies. Techniques to minimize tissue-volume exposure to administered RT include multiplanar delivery systems, patient positioning and blocking to remove other organs from the target area, and filling the bladder to displace other tissues from the pelvis.[118]

The acute effects of radiation on the intestines occurs during the administration of RT. It generally takes several weeks for the injury to become manifest. Concomitant administration of chemotherapy, especially common in the presurgical phase of treatment with rectal cancer, increases the tissue's susceptibility to the therapeutic properties of RT. Likewise, acute-phase radiation toxicity/enteritis is more likely to be noted. The acute injury is primarily mucosal with disruption of the rapidly dividing and growing cells at the base of the crypts. This leads to flattening of the villi and resultant diminution of absorptive and resorptive functions of the affected intestine. Mucositis, cramps, and diarrhea are the typical problems noted. Antimotility agents and, where applicable, antiinflammatory agents generally ameliorate symptoms. Sucralfate, mesalamine, or hydrocortisone enemas have been reported to be efficacious in the acute injury setting.[119] Low-residue or elemental diets together with glutamine supplementation improve the condition. Cessation of radiation or, at least, delaying the ongoing course generally permits most patients to resolve the acute toxicity. For the most part, preoperative radiation permits excision of the targeted tissues, excepting the distal portion of the rectum or anus being used when anastomosis (sphincter preservation) is possible. Nonirradiated proximal bowel is essential in maintaining acceptably low anastomotic leak rates when reconstruction is performed. When coloanal anastomosis is constructed in an irradiated field, many experienced surgeons elect to divert the fecal stream proximally to permit distal healing before restoration of continence, thus minimizing the deleterious effect of pelvic sepsis and anastomotic leakage.[118]

Chronic radiation injury is characterized by progressive, obliterative arteritis, as well as submucosal and transmural fibrosis (Figure 43-3). The endothelial thickening results in arterial and arteriolar thrombosis leading to ischemia. Submucosal collagen deposition leads to impaired tissue oxygenation, especially in the face of obliterative arterial disease (Figures 43-4 and 43-5). These pathologic changes cause the long-term problems associated with radiation such as obstruction, perforation, fistulization, and hemorrhage.[115–117] Evaluation of complications may necessitate GI contrast studies with barium, CT, magnetic resonance imaging, endoscopy, and fistulography. Detailed assessment is mandatory when surgical intervention is considered to optimize operative planning and to have adequate specialized help intraoperatively if the need exists.

Treatments for the complications of chronic radiation enteritis are directed toward symptom relief. Bleeding from

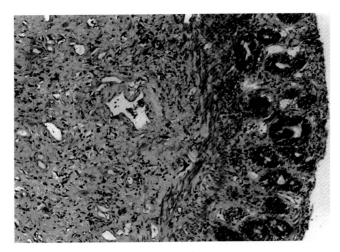

FIGURE 43-3. Radiation colitis demonstrating submucosal fibrosis/telangiectasia. H & E stain; magnification × 215. (© 2004 Frederick C. Skvara, MD).

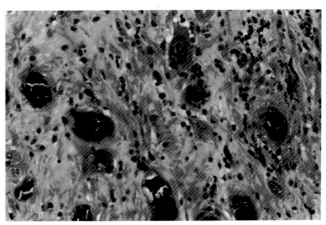

FIGURE 43-5. Radiation colitis prominence of fibroblasts. H & E stain; magnification × 540. (© 2004 Frederick C. Skvara, MD).

ischemic mucosa with telangiectatic vessels can be managed in one of several ways. Nd:YAG[119] and argon lasers have proven effective in ablating bleeding vascular lesions within reach of an endoscope. Argon is preferred because its energy is specifically absorbed by hemoglobin and so minimizes tissue damage to the already ischemic bowel.

A recent Cochrane Review comparing nonsurgical options for managing chronic radiation proctitis found sucralfate together with metronidazole effective in a small number of patients. The authors call for a multicenter placebo-based trial to reliably evaluate the outcomes of the various treatment regimens.[120]

Some clinical success has occurred with the administration of estrogen-progesterone therapy on a chronic basis. Transfusion needs and frequency of hospitalization have decreased in patients with bleeding secondary to chronic

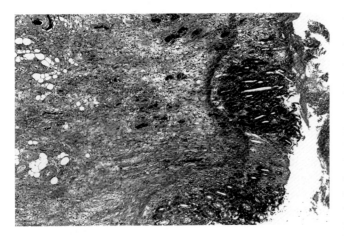

FIGURE 43-4. Radiation colitis demonstrating submucosal fibrosis/telangiectasia/mucosal atrophy. H & E stain; magnification × 86. (© 2004 Frederick C. Skvara, MD).

radiation enteritis.[121] Where bleeding occurs within the rectum, it is usually associated with radiation treatment of the cervix or prostate. Topical application of 4% formalin to these distal bleeding injuries has proven successful whether done in the office setting or the operating room, depending on the time entailed and amount of tissue needing treatment.[122,123] More recently, GI bleeding secondary to chronic radiation injury has been shown to respond well to hyperbaric oxygen therapy. The protocol frequently used treats the whole body for 60 minutes at 2 atmospheres of 100% O_2 for 30 days. Prostaglandin E_1 can be coadministered for its vasodilatory properties. A small number of patients have been thus treated with complete resolution of bleeding and mucosal healing.[124]

Fistulizing complications are best managed as conservatively as possible. When the severity of symptoms warrants consideration of surgery, the type of surgery will depend on how proximal in the GI tract the problem is and the organ to which the fistula connects. At laparotomy, as little adhesiolysis as possible should be performed because the already ischemic bowel tends to perforate (micro or macro) frequently necessitating more surgery. When possible, fistulizing tissue is best resected back to normal-appearing margins. When the amount of bowel is too excessive to permit resection, proximal diversion or bypass can be considered. Bypass is frequently avoided because diseased tissue is left behind, blind-loops create more symptoms, and bypass anastomosis still leaks at higher than normal rates. Enteric fistulas involving the genitourinary tract can be handled in the same manner with resection generally preferred where feasible. Frequently, within the pelvis, fecal diversion proximally proves safe and effective palliation in an otherwise high-risk situation. In the case of radiation-induced intestinal stenosis or obstruction, the same surgical considerations and options apply. Where feasible, resection and anastomosis of normal-appearing bowel are preferred. In the event of radiation-induced ischemic necrosis of the bowel, resection of necrotic tissue with diversion may be lifesaving. The most important determinant of operative morbidity and mortality was the location of the radiation injury itself.[125] Small bowel radiation injury in one series had a 38% mortality whereas colonic injury had a 15% mortality rate.

When long segments of small bowel have chronic radiation enteritis, malabsorptive problems arise. Because the malabsorption is secondary to tissue ischemia and subsequent fibrosis, treatment or resection will not restore this function. Patients with this chronic complication therefore require parenteral nutrition to sustain life and are subject to the metabolic complications of long-term parenteral alimentation. When the terminal ileum is affected by radiation, chronic diarrhea and electrolyte imbalance may occur because of failure to resorb bile salts. Symptomatic treatment with cholestyramine may alleviate these problems by binding the bile salts, and should be considered. Likewise, antimotility agents slow transit and so may allow the injured bowel more time to process intestinal contents and minimize the symptoms of chronic radiation enterocolitis.

Unless the clinical presentation of radiation injury to the bowel is emergent, a careful clinical assessment of the patient is vitally important to identify comorbid conditions. Patient nutrition, hydration, and sepsis need to be addressed and corrected wherever possible. Radiologic and endoscopic assessments need to be completed before finalizing a treatment plan. Therapeutic interventions should be considered beginning with the least invasive means first. Chronic radiation injury cannot be reversed because of the secondary ischemic changes. Therefore, goals for treatment should optimize quality of life while minimizing the morbidity and mortality of therapeutic intervention.[126]

C. difficile Colitis

C. difficile infection, an important source of colitis particularly in hospitalized patients, presents from either an asymptomatic infection to severe pseudomembranous colitis with bowel perforation and death. The majority of cases are seen after antibiotic usage. The remaining cases include patients receiving chemotherapy, patients with inflammatory bowel disease, and those with a variety of other medical problems. Almost all antibiotics have been associated with C. difficile infection. The most frequently implicated classes of drugs are the cephalosporins, ampicillin/amoxicillin, and clindamycin. Neither the antibiotic dosage nor the length of administration has been found to correlate with the development of C. difficile infection. The majority of infections occur 5–7 days into the course of antibiotics, but it may present weeks after cessation of the antimicrobials.[127]

Diarrhea is the most common symptom and is found in 90%–95% of cases. Patients with mild disease may present with diarrhea alone, or associated with a low-grade fever and abdominal pain. These patients may also have mild abdominal tenderness and an otherwise unremarkable abdominal examination. A small percentage of patients develop fulminant colitis with high fever and severe abdominal pain. Diarrhea may be absent in patients with severe disease and progress to toxic megacolon. Hypotension, oliguria, and other manifestations of septic shock may also be found in these severely ill patients.[128]

The laboratory diagnosis of C. difficile depends on the detection of the C. difficile toxins in the patient's stool. The most reliable laboratory tests for documenting C. difficile infection are the stool cytotoxin assay and stool cultures. However, stool cultures do not distinguish between carriers and those with acute infection. ELISA is a most popular test for C. difficile toxin in clinical laboratories. The ELISA tests have the advantage of being technically easier to perform and the results are available sooner; however, they are less sensitive than tissue culture. Patients suspected of having C. difficile infection can be evaluated endoscopically. The mucosal findings vary with the severity of the disease. In those with mild or moderate disease, endoscopy most often reveals normal mucosa or nonspecific inflammatory changes. In the great majority of those with severe disease, examination demonstrates the classic pseudomembranes which are round, punctate yellow or whitish lesions (Figure 43-6). Although the finding of pseudomembranes suggests the diagnosis of pseudomembranous colitis, biopsy of these lesions is recommended to definitively establish the diagnosis.[129]

When C. difficile infection occurs in patients receiving antibiotics, the offending antibiotic should be immediately discontinued if possible. In patients with mild disease, no other specific treatment is necessary. Most physicians will begin empiric antimicrobial therapy if there is a strong clinical evidence of colitis. Three orally administered antimicrobials have been shown to be effective against C. difficile infection: vancomycin, metronidazole, and bacitracin. Vancomycin used to be the drug of choice. In most patients, a significant improvement will occur within 2–5 days of

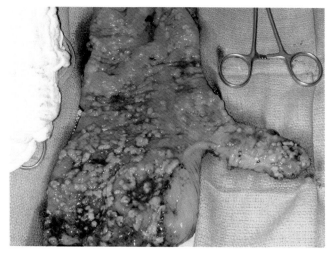

FIGURE 43-6. C. difficile colitis with classic pseudomembranes.

treatment. Vancomycin is costly and distasteful. Metronidazole is generally well tolerated and is much less expensive than vancomycin. Metronidazole, unlike vancomycin, is absorbed rapidly from the GI tract and consequently fecal concentrations are low. Despite this, metronidazole has been shown to be highly effective and is given in a dosage of 250 mg orally four times a day for 10 days. Bacitracin, when rarely used, has been shown to be as effective a treatment as vancomycin when 20,000–25,000 units were given four times a day for 7 days.[130]

In patients unable to take antimicrobials orally, intravenous metronidazole seems to be the most effective. Adequate fecal concentrations of metronidazole have been documented in patients with severe colitis after intravenous administration of this antimicrobial. Anion exchange resins have also been used successfully to treat *C. difficile* infection. Cholestyramine and colestipol, each given orally for 10 days, are thought to bind the *C. difficile* toxin in the lumen, thereby limiting the damage caused by the toxins. These agents have not proved to be as reliable as antimicrobials, and therefore it is recommended that they not be used as sole treatment except in cases of mild infection. It is also important that these resins are not given concomitantly with antibiotics because they have been shown to bind to antimicrobials in the intestinal lumen.[131]

Despite adequate medical therapy, surgical intervention may be required. Surgery may be necessary for patients in whom a perforation is suspected or those with toxic megacolon. When surgery is necessary, subtotal colectomy with ileostomy or fecal diversion via end ileostomy and mucous fistula are the most frequently performed procedures. Recurrence of *C. difficile* infection is not uncommon. Most suggest a second and longer course of antimicrobials for patients who have a symptomatic relapse. Some recommend a course of cholestyramine or colestipol after the antimicrobials. Recurrent infection is as responsive to antimicrobial treatment as are primary infections. Unfortunately, up to one-third of patients who relapse once will have further recurrences. Any patient with an unexplained abdominal illness who, in the last 2 weeks, has either been in the hospital or has received antibiotics should be suspected of *C. difficile* infection, even in the absence of diarrhea.[132] A recent review has established evidenced-based guidelines regarding antibiotic treatment for *C. difficile*–associated diarrhea in adults.[133] Surgery for fulminant colitis still commands a poor prognosis.[134]

References

1. Boley SJ, Schwartz S, Losl J, Sternhill V. Reversible vascular occlusion of the colon. Surg Gynecol Obstet 1973;116:52–60.
2. Ghandi S, Hansom MM, Vernava AM, et al. Ischemic colitis. Dis Colon Rectum 1996;39:88–100.
3. Longo WE, Gusberg RJ, Ballantyne GH. Ischemic colitis: patterns and prognosis. Dis Colon Rectum 1992;35:726.
4. Kaminski DL, Keltner RM, Willman VL. Ischemic colitis. Arch Surg 1973;106:558–563.
5. Arnott ID, Ghosh S, Ferguson A. The spectrum of ischemic colitis. Eur J Gastroenterol Hepatol 1999;11:295–303.
6. Guttmorson NL, Burbrick MP. Mortality from ischemic colitis. Dis Colon Rectum 1989;32:469–472.
7. Newman LA, Mittman N, Hunt Z, Alfonso AE. Survival among chronic renal failure patients requiring major abdominal surgery. J Am Coll Surg 1999;188:310–314.
8. Scharff J, Longo WE, Vartanian SM, et al. Ischemic colitis. Spectrum of disease and outcome. Surgery 2003;134:624–629.
9. Preventza OA, Lazarides K, Sawyer MD. Ischemic colitis in young adults: a single institution experience. J Gastrointest Surg 2001;5:328–332.
10. Longo WE, Ward D, Vernava AM, et al. Outcome of patients with total colonic ischemia. Dis Colon Rectum 1997;40:1448–1454.
11. Bharucha AE, Tremaine WJ, Johnson CD, Batta KP. Ischemic proctosigmoiditis. Am J Gastroenterol 1996;91:2305–2309.
12. Hostein J, Fournet J. Gastrointestinal manifestations of collagen diseases. Dig Dis 1986;4:240–252.
13. Guillevin L, Lhote F, Gayraud M, et al. Prognostic factors in polyarteritis nodosa and Churg-Strauss syndrome. A prospective study in 342 patients. Medicine 1996;75:17.
14. Baxter R, Nino-Marcia M, Bloom RJ, Kosek J. Gastrointestinal manifestations of essential mixed cryoglobulinemia. Gastrointest Radiol 1988;13:160–162.
15. Martinez-Frontonilla LA, Haase GM, Ernster JL, et al. Surgical complications in Henoch-Schonlein purpura. J Pediatr Surg 1984;19:434.
16. Cappel MS, Gupta AM. Colonic lesions associated with Henoch-Schonlein purpura. Am J Gastroenterol 1990;85:1186.
17. Kyle SM, Yeong ML, Isbister WH, Clark SP. Bechet's colitis: a differential diagnosis in inflammations of the large intestine. Aust NZ J Surg 1991;61:547–550.
18. Griffin JW, Harrison HB, Tedesco FJ, Mills LR. Behcet's disease with multiple sites of gastrointestinal involvement. South Med J 1982;75:1405–1408.
19. Iwama T, Utzunomiya J. Anal complications in Behcet's syndrome. Jpn J Surg 1977;7:114.
20. Matsumoto T, Uekusa T, Fukuda Y. Vasculo-Behcet's disease: a pathologic study of eight cases. Hum Pathol 1991;22:45–51.
21. Zizic TM, Classen JN, Stevens MB. Acute abdominal complications of systemic lupus erythematosus and polyarteritis nodosa. Am J Med 1982;73:525–531.
22. Zizic TM, Shulman LE, Stevens MB. Colonic perforations in systemic lupus erythematosus. Medicine 1975;54:411.
23. Papa MZ, Shiloni E, McDonald HD. Total colon necrosis: a catastrophic complication of systemic lupus erythmatosus. Dis Colon Rectum 1986;29:576–578.
24. Rose S, Young MA, Reynolds JC. Gastrointestinal manifestations of scleroderma. Gastroenterol Clin North Am 1998;27:563–594.
25. Abu-Shakra M, Guillemin F, Lee P. Gastrointestinal manifestations of systemic sclerosis. Semin Arthritis Rheum 1994;24:29–39.
26. Akesson A, Akesson B, Gustafson T, et al. Gastrointestinal function in patients with systemic sclerosis. Clin Rheumatol 1985;4:411.
27. Leighton JA, Valdovinos MA, Pemberton JA. Anorectal dysfunction and rectal prolapse in systemic sclerosis. Dis Colon Rectum 1993;36:182.

28. Chugh S, Dilawari JB, Sawhney IM, et al. Polymyositis associated with ulcerative colitis. Gut 1993;34:567–569.

29. Lindstrom CG. "Collagenous colitis" with watery diarrhea—a new entity? Pathol Eur 1976;11:87–89.

30. Read NW, Krejs GJ, Read MG, et al. Chronic diarrhea of unknown origin. Gastroenterology 1980;76:264–271.

31. Kingham JG, Levison DA, Ball JA, et al. Microscopic colitis: a cause of chronic watery diarrhea. Br Med J (Clin Res Ed) 1982; 285:1601–1604.

32. Pardi DS. Microscopic colitis. Mayo Clin Proc 2003;78: 614–617.

33. Bo-Linn GW, Vendrell DD, Lee E, et al. An evaluation of the significance of microscopic colitis in patients with chronic diarrhea. J Clin Invest 1985;75:1559–1569.

34. Pardi DS, Smyrk TC, Tremaine WJ, et al. Microscopic colitis: a review. Am J Gastroenterol 2002;97:794–802.

35. Lee E, Schilles LR, Vendrell D, et al. Subepithelial collagen table thickness in colon specimens from patients with microscopic colitis and collagenous colitis. Gastroenterology 1992; 103:1790–1796.

36. Marteau P, Lavergne-Slove A, Lemann M, et al. Primary ileal villous atrophy is often associated with microscopic colitis. Gut 1997;41:561–564.

37. Sapp H, Ithamukkala S, Brien TP, et al. The terminal ileum is affected in patients with lymphocytic or collagenous colitis. Am J Surg Pathol 2002;26:1484–1492.

38. Giardiello FM, Lazenby AJ, Bayless TM, et al. Lymphocytic (microscopic) colitis. Clinicopathologic study of 18 patients and comparison to collagenous colitis. Dig Dis Sci 1989;34: 1730–1738.

39. Fine KD, Do K, Schulte K, et al. High prevalence of celiac sprue-like HLA-DQ genes and enteropathy in patients with microscopic colitis syndrome. Am J Gastroenterol 2000;95:1974–1982.

40. Veress B, Lofberg R, Bergman L. Microscopic colitis syndrome. Gut 1995;36:880–886.

41. Fernandez-Banares F, Esteve M, Salas A, et al. Bile acid malabsorption in microscopic colitis and in previously unexplained functional chronic diarrhea. Dig Dis Sci 2001;46:2231–2238.

42. Thompson RD, Lestina LS, Benson SP, et al. Lansoprazole-associated microscopic colitis: a case series. Am J Gastroenterol 2002;97:2908–2913.

43. Fine KD, Lee EL. Efficacy of open-label bismuth subsalicylate for the treatment of microscopic colitis. Gastroenterology 1998;115:29–36.

44. Pardi DS, Loftus EV, Tremaine WJ, et al. Treatment of refractory microscopic colitis with azathioprine and 6-mercaptopruine. Gastroenterology 2001;120:1483–1484.

45. Schulze K, Mitros FA. Eosinophilic gastroenteritis involving the ileocecal area. Dis Colon Rectum 1979;22:47–50.

46. Partyka EK, Sanowski RA, Kozarek RA. Colonoscopic features of eosinophilic gastroenteritis. Dis Colon Rectum 1980;23:353–356.

47. Naylor TR, Pollet JE. Eosinophilic colitis. Dis Colon Rectum 1985;28:615–618.

48. Leung R, Sung JY, Chow J, et al. Unusual cause of fever and diarrhea in a patient with AIDS. *Penicillium marneffei* infection. Dig Dis Sci 1996;41:1212–1215.

49. Corman ML. Miscellaneous colitides. In: Corman ML, ed. Colon and Rectal Surgery. 4th ed. Philadelphia: Lippincott-Raven; 1998:1369–1370.

50. Clarkson WK, Bonacini M, Peterson I. Colitis due to *Histoplasma capsulatum* in the acquired immunodeficiency syndrome. Am J Gastroenterol 1991;86:913–916.

51. Lee SH, Barnes WG, Hodges GR, et al. Perforated granulomatous colitis caused by *Histoplasma capsulatum*. Dis Colon Rectum 1985;28:171–176.

52. Daly JS, Porter KA, Chong FK, et al. Disseminated, nonmeningeal gastrointestinal infection in an HIV-negative patient. Am J Gastroenterol 1990;85:1421–1424.

53. Arduino RC, DePont HL. Enteritis, enterocolitis and infectious diarrhea syndromes. In: Armstrong D, Cohen J, eds. Infectious Diseases. London: Mosby; 1999:2-35.1–2-35.10.

54. Sawyer MK, Gehlbach SH. Bacterial diseases of the colon. Prim Care 1998;15:125–145.

55. Ina K, Kusugami K, Ohta M. Bacterial hemorrhagic enterocolitis. J Gastroenterol 2003;38:111–120.

56. Goldsweig CD, Pacheco PA. Infectious colitis excluding *E. coli* O 157:H7 and *C. difficile*. Gastroenterol Clin North Am 2001;30:709–733.

57. Corman MC. Miscellaneous colitides. In: Corman MC, ed. Colon and Rectal Surgery. 4th ed. Philadelphia: Lippincott-Raven; 1998:1367–1368.

58. Niyogi SK. Shigellosis. J Microbiol 2005;43:133–143.

59. Beers MH, Berkow R, eds. Infectious disease. In: The Merck Manual. 17th ed. White House Station: Merck Research Laboratories; 1999:1147–1209.

60. Murray FE, O'Brien M, Birkett DH, et al. Diversion colitis: pathologic findings in a resected sigmoid colon and rectum. Gastroenterology 1987;93:1404.

61. Roediger WEW. The starved colon—diminished mucosal nutrition, diminished absorption and colitis. Dis Colon Rectum 1990;33:858.

62. Orsay CP, Kim DO, Pearl RK, et al. Diversion colitis in patients scheduled for colostomy closure. Dis Colon Rectum 1993;36:366.

63. Guillemot F, Colombel JF, Neut C, et al. Treatment of diversion colitis by short chain fatty acids. Prospective double blind study. Dis Colon rectum 1991;34:861.

64. Bavaro MF. Neutropenic enterocolitis. Curr Gastroenterol Rep 2002;4:297–301.

65. Moir CR, Scudamore CH, Benny WB. Typhlitis: selective surgical management. Am J Surg 1986;151:563.

66. Kiedan RD, Fanning J, Gatenby RA, et al. Recurrent typhlitis. A disease resulting from aggressive chemotherapy. Dis Colon rectum 1989;32:206.

67. Ryan CK, Potter GD. Disinfectant colitis: rinse as well as you wash. J Clin Gastroenterol 1995;21:6.

68. Stein BL, Lamoureux E, Miller M, et al. Glutaraldehyde-induced colitis. Can J Surg 2001;44:113–116.

69. Gan SI, Price IM. Waiting list induced proctitis: the hydrogen peroxide enema. Can J Gastroenteol 2003;17:727–729.

70. Cappell MS, Simon T. Fulminant acute colitis following a self administered hydrofluoric acid enema. Am J Gastroenterol 1993;88:122.

71. Gleeson MH, Davis AJM. Non-steroidal anti-inflammatory drugs, aspirin and newly diagnosed colitis: a case controlled study. Aliment Pharmacol Ther 2003;17:817–825.

72. Carter FM, Mitchell CK. Toxic epidermal necrolysis: an unusual cause of colonic perforation. Dis Colon Rectum 1993;36:773.

73. Bobak DA. Gastrointestinal infections caused by cytomegalovirus. Curr Infect Dis Rep 2003;5:101–107.

74. Dieterich DT, Rahmin M. Cytomegalovirus in AIDS: presentation in 44 patients and a review of the literature. J Acquir Immune Defic Syndr 1991;4:S29–35.

75. Wexner SD, Smithy WB, Trillo C, et al. Emergency colectomy for cytomegalovirus ileocolitis in patients with acquired immune deficiency syndrome. Dis Colon Rectum 1988;31:755.

76. Wilson SE, Robinson G, Williams RA, et al. Acquired immune deficiency syndrome (AIDS): indications for abdominal surgery, pathology and outcome. Ann Surg 1989;210:428.

77. Wastell C, Corless Keeling N. Surgery and human immunodeficiency virus-1 infection. Am J Surg 1996;172:89.

78. Colemont LJ, Pen JH, Pelckmans PA, et al. Herpes simplex virus Type I colitis: an unusual cause of diarrhea. Am J Gastroenterol 1990;85:1182–1185.

79. Wasselle JA, Sedgwick JH, Dawson PJ, et al. Intestinal herpes simplex infection presenting with intestinal perforation. Am J Gastroenterol 1992;87:1475.

80. Pollok RC. Viruses causing diarrhea in AIDS. Novartis Found Symp 2001;238:276–283.

81. Stanley SL. Amoebiasis. Lancet 2003;361:1025–1034.

82. Monga NK, Sood S, Kaushik SP, et al. Amebic peritonitis. Am J Gastroenterol 1976;66:366–373.

83. Knight R. Giardiasis, isosporiasis, and balantidiasis. Clin Gastroenterol 1978;7:31.

84. Castro J, Vasquez-Iglesias JL, Arnal-Monreal F. Dysentery caused by *Balantidium coli*. Endoscopy 1983;15:272.

85. Weber R, Bryan RT, Scwartz DA, et al. Human microsporidial infections. Clin Microbiol Rev 1994;7:426.

86. Wolfe MS. Giardiasis. Clin Microbiol Rev 1992;5:93.

87. Tanowitz HB, Weiss LM, Wittner M. Diagnosis and treatment of protozoan diarrheas. Am J Gastroenterol 1988;83:339.

88. Gunasekaran TS, Hassall E. Giardiasis diagnosed at colonoscopy with ileoscopy. Am J Gastroenterol 1996;91: 1011–1013.

89. Teixeira FV, Netinho JG. Surgical treatment of chagasic megacolon: Duhamel-Haddad procedure is a good option. Dis Colon Rectum 2002;10:1387–1392.

90. de Oliveira RB, Troncon LE, Dantas RO, Menghelli UG. Gastrointestinal manifestations of Chaga's disease. Am J Gastroenterol 1998;93:884–889.

91. Garcia SB, Aranha AL, Garcia FR, et al. A retrospective study of histopathologic findings in 894 cases of megacolon: what is the relationship between megacolon and colonic cancer? Rev Inst Med Trop Sao Paulo 2003;45:91–93.

92. Akgun Y. Intestinal obstruction caused by *Ascaris lumbricoides*. Dis Colon Rectum 1996;39:1159–1163.

93. Wasadikar PP, Kulkarni AB. Intestinal obstruction due to *Ascariasis*. Br J Surg 1997;84:410–412.

94. El-Garem AA. Schistosomiasis. Digestion 1998;59:589–605.

95. Sanguino J. Schistosomiasis of the colon and rectum. Hepatogastroenterology 1994;41:86.

96. Al Samman M, Haque S, Long J. Strongyloidiasis colitis: a case report and review of the literature. J Clin Gastroenterol 1999;28:77–80.

97. Weight SC, Barrie WW. Colonic *Strongyloides stercoralis* infection masquerading as ulcerative colitis. J R Coll Surg Edinb 1997;42:202–203.

98. Neva FA. Biology and immunology of human strongyloidiasis. J Infect Dis 1986;153:379–406.

99. Kaur G, Raj SM, Naing NN. Trichuriasis: localized inflammatory responses in the colon. Southeast Asian J Trop Med Public Health 2002;33:224–228.

100. Joo JH, Ryu KH, Lee YH, et al. Colonoscopic diagnosis of whipworm infection. Hepatogastroenterology 1998;45: 2105–2109.

101. Chandra B, Long JD. Diagnosis of *Trichuris trichiura* (whipworm) by colonoscopic extraction. J Clin Gastroenterol 1998;27:152–153.

102. Schuster R, Petrini J, Choi R. Anisakiasis of the colon presenting as bowel obstruction. Am Surg 2003;9:350–352.

103. Minamoto T, Sawaguchi K, Ogino T, Mai M. Anisakiasis of the colon: report of two cases with emphasis on the diagnostic and therapeutic value of colonoscopy. Endoscopy 1991; 23(1):50–52.

104. Shirahama M, Koga T, Uchida S, et al. Colonic anisakiasis simulating carcinoma of the colon. AJR Am J Roentgenol 1990;155:895.

105. Demiriz M, Gunhan O, Celasun B, et al. Colonic perforation caused by taeniasis. Trop Geogr Med 1995;47:180–182.

106. Fabijanic D, Giunio L, Ivani N, et al. Ultrasonographic appearance of colon taeniasis. J Ultrasound Med 2001;20:275–277.

107. Edwards P, Wodak A, Cooper DA, et al. The gastrointestinal manifestations of AIDS. Aust NZ J Med 1990;20:141–148.

108. Yeguez JF, Martinez SA, Sands DR, et al. Colorectal malignancies in HIV-positive patients. Am Surg 2003;69:981–987.

109. Fu CS, Conteas CN, LaRiviere MJ. Successful treatment of idiopathic colitis and proctitis using thalidomide in persons infected with human immunodeficiency. AIDS Patient Care STDS 1998;12:903–906.

110. Fine KD, Seidel RH, Do K. The prevalence, anatomic distribution, and diagnosis of colonic causes of chronic diarrhea. Gastrointest Endosc 2000;52:589–590.

111. Bonacini M, Skodras G, Quiason S, Kragel P. Prevalence of enteric pathogens in HIV-related diarrhea in the Midwest. AIDS Patient Care STDS 1999;13:179–184.

112. Monkemuller KE, Wilcox CM. Diagnosis and treatment of colonic disease in AIDS. Gastrointest Endosc Clin North Am 1998;8:889–911.

113. Palmer JA, Bush RS. Radiation injuries to the bowel associated with the treatment of carcinoma of the cervix. Surgery 1976; 80:458–464.

114. Bosch A, Frias Z. Complications after radiation therapy for cervical carcinoma. Acta Radiol Ther Phys Biol 1977;16: 53–62.

115. Novak JM, Collins JT, Donowitz M, et al. Effects of radiation on the human gastrointestinal tract. J Clin Gastroenterol 1979; 1:9–39.

116. Leupin N, Curschmann J, Kransbuhler H, et al. Acute radiation colitis in patients treated with short-term preoperative radiotherapy for rectal cancer. Am J Surg Pathol 2002;26: 498–504.

117. Nussbaum ML, Campana TJ, Weese JL. Radiation-induced intestinal injury. Clin Plast Surg 1993;20:573–580.

118. Corman ML. Vascular diseases. In: Corman ML, ed. Colon and Rectal Surgery. 4th ed. Philadelphia: Lippincott-Raven; 1998: 1058–1066.

119. Goldstein F, Khoury J, Thornton JJ. Treatment of chronic radiation enteritis and colitis with salicylazosulfapyridine and systemic corticosteroids. A pilot study. Am J Gastroenterol 1976; 65:201–208.

120. Denton A, Forbes A, Andreyev J, et al. Non-surgical interventions for late radiation proctitis in patients who have received radical radiotherapy to the pelvis. Cochrane Database Syst Rev 2002;(1):CD003455.

121. Alexander TJ, Dwyer RM. Endoscopic Nd:YAG laser treatment of severe radiation injury of the lower gastrointestinal tract: long-term follow-up. Gatrointest Endosc 1988;34:407–411

122. Parikh S, Hughes C, Salvati EP, et al. Treatment of hemorrhagic radiation proctitis with 4 percent formalin. Dis Colon Rectum 2003;46:596–600.

123. Luna-Perez P, Rodriguez-Ramirez SE. Formalin installation for refractory radiation-induced hemorrhagic proctitis. J Surg Oncol 2002;80:41–44.

124. Wurzer H, Schafhalter-Zoppoth I, Brandstatter G, et al. Hormonal therapy in chronic radiation colitis. Am J Gastroenterol 1998;93:2536–2538.

125. Miura M, Sasagawa I, Kubota Y, et al. Effective hyperbaric oxygenation with prostaglandin E_1 for radiation cystitis and colitis after pelvic radiotherapy. Int Urol Nephrol 1996;28:643–647.

126. Russell JC, Welsh JP. Operative management of radiation injuries of the intestinal tract. Am J Surg 1979;137:433–442.

127. Hurley BW, Nguyen CC. The spectrum of pseudomembranous enterocolitis and antibiotic-associated diarrhea. Arch Int Med 2002;162:2177–2184.

128. Surawicz CM, McFarland LV. Pseudomembranous colitis: causes and cures. Digestion 1999;60:91–100.

129. Kelly CP, Pothoularis C, LaMont JT. Clostridium difficile colitis. N Engl J Med 1994;330:257–261.

130. Mylonakis E, Ryan ET, Calderwood SB. Clostridium difficile-associated diarrhea. Arch Intern Med 2001;161:525–533.

131. Klinger PJ, Metzger PP, Seelig MH, Pettit PDM, Knudsen JM, Alvarez S. Clostridium difficile infection: risk factors, medical and surgical management. Dig Dis 2000;18:147–150.

132. Mazuki JE, Longo WE. Clostridium difficile colitis. Probl Gen Surg 2002;19:121–132.

133. Bricker E, Garg R, Nelson R, Loza A, Novak T, Hansen J. Antibiotic treatment for Clostridium difficile-associated diarrhea in adults. Cochrane Database Syst Rev 2005:CD004610.

134. Longo WE, Mazuski JE, Virgo KS, Lee P, Bahadursingh AN, Johnson FE. Outcome after colectomy for Clostridium difficile colitis. Dis Colon Rectum 2004;47:1620–1626.

44
Intestinal Stomas

Bruce A. Orkin and Peter A. Cataldo

Surgery involving ostomies is a major component of the general and colorectal surgeon's armamentarium. Proper creation, management, and closure of ostomies is critical both for the treatment of specific disorders as well as for the peace of mind of the patient.

An ostomy is a surgically created opening between a hollow organ and the body surface or between any two hollow organs. The word *ostomy* comes from the Latin word *ostium*, meaning mouth or opening. The suffix *–tomy* implies an intervention, either by surgery or injury. The word *stoma* comes from the Greek word for mouth and is used interchangeably with ostomy. An ostomy is further named by the organ involved. An ileostomy is an opening from the ileum to the skin, a colostomy is from the colon, a gastrostomy is from the stomach, and so forth. When two organs are joined, the descriptive term incorporates both. For instance, an anastomosis between the small bowel and colon might be called an *ileocolostomy*, between colon and the rectum, a *colorectostomy* or *coloproctostomy*. A loop ostomy is formed by bringing an intact loop of bowel through the skin and then dividing the antimesenteric side and maturing it so that there are two open lumens, the proximal and the distal.

Although ostomies used to be performed primarily for the permanent management of fecal output, the majority of ostomies today are created as a temporary measure, either as an end ostomy in the acute setting with later planned takedown and anastomosis, or as a proximal loop diversion to protect a low pelvic or risky anastomosis. It is estimated that 750,000 Americans are living with an ostomy and that 75,000 new stomas are created each year.

In this chapter we will be discussing ostomies brought to the surface of the body, focusing primarily on ileostomies and colostomies.

Indications for an Ostomy

There are many indications for stoma creation. The details of each will be discussed in the relevant chapters in this book. In general, however, an ostomy is created when an anastomosis is not possible for technical reasons or risk of failure, when

there is nothing distally to attach to such as after an abdominoperineal resection of the rectum, or for proximal diversion (Table 44-1).

Ostomies may be *temporary* or *permanent*. Temporary stomas divert the fecal stream away from an area of concern such as a high-risk anastomosis, located in a radiated field, low in the rectum, or after an injury. Permanent ostomies are required when the anorectum has been removed (abdominoperineal resection) in cancer or Crohn's disease. A permanent ostomy may also be an option in patients with severe fecal incontinence or complications of trauma or radiation such as a rectourethral fistula.

Creation of an ostomy is a traumatic event for most patients, both physically and mentally. Whenever possible, a detailed discussion of the proposed procedure, consequences, and alternatives should be undertaken. A trained enterostomal therapy nurse (ET) or wound ostomy care nurse (WOCN) should meet with the patient both before and after the surgery. When available, a *United Ostomy Association Visitor* should be called to meet with the patient, either before (if the surgery is elective) or after the surgery.

Stoma Physiology

The physiologic changes that occur in patients with ostomies are primarily related to the loss of continence and reduced colonic absorptive surface area. These affect fluid and electrolyte balance and lifestyle but generally have little effect on nutrition. However, once more than 50 cm of terminal ileum has been removed or taken out of continuity, nutritional consequences are likely.

Output

Ostomy output is directly related to the location of the opening in the bowel. Distal left or sigmoid colostomies normally produce formed stools that are of similar consisting to that of the anorectum. The more proximal the colostomy, the less surface area is available for water and electrolyte absorption and so the

TABLE 44-1. Indications for an ostomy

- Cancer
- Diverticular disease
- Inflammatory bowel disease—ulcerative colitis, Crohn's disease
- Radiation enteritis
- Complex perirectal, rectovaginal, or rectourethral fistulas
- Trauma
- Obstruction
- Perforation
- Motility and functional disorders including idiopathic megarectum and megacolon
- Infections—necrotizing fasciitis, Fournier's gangrene
- Congenital disorders—imperforate anus, Hirschsprung's disease, necrotizing enterocolitis, intestinal atresias

more liquid the stools. Right-sided colostomies not only produce a high volume but also have the additional disadvantage of a malodorous output because of the effects of colonic bacteria.

Initially after creation the output from an ileostomy tends to be fairly watery and green or bilious in color. Within a few days to a week of resumption of a regular diet, the material becomes thicker and more yellow-brown, although a greenish tinge often remains. The typical consistency is of watery porridge or applesauce. It is affected by diet, fluid intake, medications, and ongoing problems such as Crohn's disease or adhesions. If a substantial amount of small bowel has been removed, the output is looser and the patient is more prone to dehydration. It is not uncommon for some food to come through in a recognizable state. Foods notable for this include corn, other vegetables, and nuts. Some pills may also not be broken down in the small bowel, decreasing the bioavailability of these medications. Most ileostomates notice little odor from the output; however, certain foods, such as eggs and fish, may produce an offensive smell.[1]

Volume

In the healthy control subject, about 1000–2000 mL of fluid passes through the ileocecal valve daily. This is reduced by 80%–90% to 100–200 mL in normal stool as it passes through the colon. Unless the patient has diarrhea, left-sided colostomy output is similar to the feces that would be passed transanally, and there is little loss of total body fluid or sodium.[2]

Although postoperative ileostomy output may be high, it settles down to a regular volume seen. "Ileostomy dysfunction," although a general sounding term, refers to increased ileostomy output attributed to partial obstruction caused by inflammation and stenosis. This term was coined in the era of secondary maturation (i.e. before eversion of the exposed ileum became widely practiced during ileostomy construction). Historically, high outputs were anticipated for weeks after creation of an ileostomy but this was found to be caused by inflammation of the exposed small bowel serosa (serositis). Once primary maturation was adopted, this problem essentially disappeared.[3,4]

Postoperative colostomy output is also often liquid, but it rapidly becomes formed with the resumption of a normal diet and the return of ordered motility. The average output of an established ileostomy (in contrast to a newly created ileostomy) is about 200–700 mL with a median of about 500 mL per day. Total bowel rest results in a decrease in output by at least half and may be as low as 50–100 mL per day.[2]

The volume of ileostomy output varies fairly widely among patients but only mildly from day to day in a single individual. Although the average output is about 500 mL per day, a healthy, functioning ileostomy may produce up to 1000–1500 mL in a day especially in the early postoperative period. Outputs above this level usually cause dehydration.[5–9] Large amounts of fluid intake usually do not alter the output volume very much because most of it is absorbed and excreted through the kidneys.[7]

Ileostomates may generally eat a regular diet without restrictions. Decreased fluid intake slows the output and thickens it, whereas fatty food and large amounts of liquid increase transit and the fluidity of the effluent.[1] Prunes and cabbage may also increase the output.[7] Ileostomy effluent is generally weakly acidic at a pH of about 6.3.[2] When the terminal ileum has been resected but colon remains, more of the bile salts will enter the colon, which may result in a secretory diarrhea. This may be ameliorated by the use of oral bile binding agents such as cholestyramine (Questran).

Transit

An ileostomy discharges frequently and output is not eliminated by the timing of meals or rest. Yet, in most patients, the output increases with meals and certain foods. Surgical resection of the anus and rectum and/or colon effects the function of the proximal gastrointestinal tract and the integration of hormonal and neuroenteric activity. These interactions are complex and not well understood in health, much less in postoperative patients. Although the data are limited, it seems that small bowel transit times decrease after ileostomy, possibly related to mucosal hypertrophy and adaptation. The specific mechanisms are not known. Gastric emptying has been a subject of several studies but the results are conflicting. Soper et al.[10] found that gastric emptying is not altered in ileostomy patients. Yet, small bowel transit is longer than in control subjects (348 versus 243 minutes). In a more recent study, Robertson and Mathers[11] found that gastric emptying of liquids is not altered but emptying of solids is slowed.

Ileostomy output and dehydration may be decreased by prolonging the transit time to allow for more absorption. Codeine, loperimide, and Lomotil have all been shown to have this effect.[12,13]

Fluid and Electrolyte Balance

The average ileostomy puts out about 500 mL of water and 60 mmoles of sodium per day. This is 2–3 times higher than found in normal fecal output.[2] Consequently, the ileostomate must compensate by increasing intake or conserving other losses.

Urinary volume is relatively decreased in patients with ileostomies by as much as 40%, whereas renal sodium losses may be decreased by 55%.[14,15] Yet, despite the efforts of the kidneys to maintain balance, total body water and sodium reductions may be a chronic condition in ileostomy patients.[16–18]

The chronic dehydration and loss of fluid and electrolytes make ileostomy patients prone to dehydration. Rehydration is best accomplished with fairly large amounts of normal saline.[2] There is an inverse relationship between absorption of nutrients and electrolytes and transit time.[19]

Flora

The normal terminal ileum harbors few organisms in the healthy individual. After creation of an ileostomy, the distal ileum is rapidly colonized with a variety of bacteria. The microflora of an individual is fairly stable over time whereas there is great variability among individuals.[20] Staphylococci, streptococci, and fungi are increased whereas *Bacteroides fragilis* is rarely found in ileostomy effluent. The major variations in the flora of effluent from ileostomies, transverse colostomies, and feces per anum are in the relative numbers of anaerobes with log differences increasing from proximal to distal.[21,22]

Nutrition

The colon has little role in the maintenance of normal nutrition, working primarily to absorb fluid and to store feces so that the frequency of bowel evacuation may be limited. Thus, removal of the colon alone has little effect on nutrition. Patients who require a total proctocolectomy for disease such as ulcerative colitis or Crohn's disease are often malnourished because of their underlying problem. Postoperatively, they are able to gain weight and return to a much better level of nitrogen balance and general nutrition.

Loss of more than a few feet of the terminal ileum may result in loss of bile acids and poor absorption of fat and fat-soluble vitamins.[7,23] Specifically, vitamin B_{12}, necessary for normal hemoglobin synthesis, may not be adequately absorbed in patients with terminal ileal loss or significant Crohn's disease. This results in pernicious or macrocytic anemia, and these patients may require monthly administration of vitamin B_{12} (intramuscular or nasal). Absorption may also be impeded by distal ileal bacterial overgrowth.[24–26] Kidney stones may be a consequence of chronic dehydration and acid urine. Adding sodium bicarbonate to the diet as well as increasing fluid intake may help to prevent uric acid stone formation.[27–29]

Preoperative Considerations

Access, Adherence, Activity, Attire

Preoperative patient preparation is essential and patients should be counseled and marked. In many institutions this is done by an enterostomal therapist.

Factors to consider in relation to stoma placement include: occupation, clothing styles (including belt line), flexibility and range of motion, abdominal wall contour when sitting and standing, and physical limitations or disabilities.[30] Other factors include prior abdominal incisions, bony prominences, and abdominal girth. Although in most elective settings, the stoma therapist will provide preoperative marking, it is imperative for any abdominal surgeon to have this skill as well because at times a stoma therapist may not be available.

Siting through the umbilicus is a reasonable alternative when there is no other good location. Raza et al.[31] believed that this was a good option based on their series of 101 patients; only four needed revision and there were no parastomal hernias or prolapse. Fitzgerald et al.[32] noted that after closure in infants and children, the scar resembles a normal umbilicus and is cosmetically superior to that of an ostomy placed elsewhere.

Nevertheless, standard ostomy sites lie to either side of the midline overlying the rectus muscle and are the preferred location for stoma placement (Figure 44-1). In the supine position, a site is marked 5 cm away from prior incisions, bony prominences, the umbilicus, and the patient's belt line. This is usually located just lateral and inferior or in some cases superior to the umbilicus.

With the patient sitting and standing, the site is checked to ensure skin folds or crevices do not interfere with appliance fitting. In obese individuals, the stoma must not be hidden below a large abdominal pannus or stoma care will be very difficult. In this circumstance, a supraumbilical stoma is often more functional. Once proper placement is ascertained, the spot is marked with indelible ink. In complex cases, a stoma appliance can be fixed to the proposed site and worn for 24 hours to test placement.

End Ostomies

Most left colon colostomies are placed in the left lower quadrant of the abdominal wall, exiting through the rectus sheath. Most distal ileostomies are placed in the right lower quadrant. Occasionally, a higher or more lateral site may be chosen depending on body habitus, other scars, clothing, mesentery and bowel length, and surgical considerations. As noted, preoperative marking is essential, whenever possible, to select the best place for a stoma. The site is marked with indelible ink or scratched with a needle before preparation so the mark is not lost.

After the abdominal portion of the procedure is completed, the bowel and mesentery are again assessed for stoma construction with attention to length and viability. An adequate length of bowel should be mobilized to allow the intestine to come through the abdominal wall so it may protrude appropriately without undue tension. The blood supply to the end of the ostomy should be maintained to avoid ischemia. Similarly, the fascial and skin openings need to be large enough to avoid occluding the mesenteric vessels and the

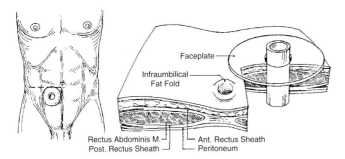

FIGURE 44-1. Stomal placement. The site is selected to bring the stoma through the rectus abdominis muscle. (From Beck DE. Intestinal stomas. In: Beck D, ed. Handbook of Colorectal Surgery. 2nd ed. Copyright 2003 by Taylor & Francis Group LLC (B). Reproduced with permission of Taylor & Francis Group LLC (B) in the format Textbook via Copyright Clearance Center).

lumen. It is usually fairly easy to bring out enough small intestine. Occasionally, if there is extensive inflammation, bowel wall thickening, or a very wide abdominal wall in the obese, it may be difficult. It may be more difficult to obtain a good length of colon, especially if the mesentery is thick or short. Mobilization of the proximal colon, especially around the splenic flexure, is often necessary. Ligation of some of the distal vascular arcades may also be necessary but should be done with great care to assure good distal perfusion. Although usually not necessary, the very end of the bowel may be stripped of mesentery for 1–3 cm and it will generally survive on submucosal perfusion. The surgeon should not hesitate to make a large fascial incision because a late hernia is preferable to early ischemic necrosis or retraction.

Although there are many variations in the details of ostomy creation, the principles are universal. The following describes the authors' technique. A Kocher clamp is applied to the fascial edge of the incision and a second is placed on the subcuticular layer. The surgeon holds a folded, wet gauze pad in the left hand beneath the abdominal wall through the incision, using the Kocher clamps to line up the abdominal wall layers. The abdominal wall is tented up with the left hand by pushing firmly on the abdominal wall from within. A 3- to 4-cm-diameter circular skin incision is made at the marked site using a #15 blade (Figure 44-2). With electrocautery, the skin disk is excised, leaving all of the subcutaneous fat. This allows the stoma to sit up rather than pull down as is more likely if the fat is removed. The assistant retracts the incision and the fat laterally and medially with a pair of Richardson or Army-Navy retractors. The subcutaneous fat is divided with the electrocautery vertically, progressively replacing the retractors deeper until the anterior fascia is encountered (Figure 44-2B). The fascia is divided vertically. Although some surgeons use a cruciate or plus-sign fascial incision ("+"), a vertical fascial incision is recommended because more fascia will remain intact between the ostomy site and the midline wound. The rectus muscle is split in the direction of its fibers and held apart with a large Kelly clamp. The retractors are

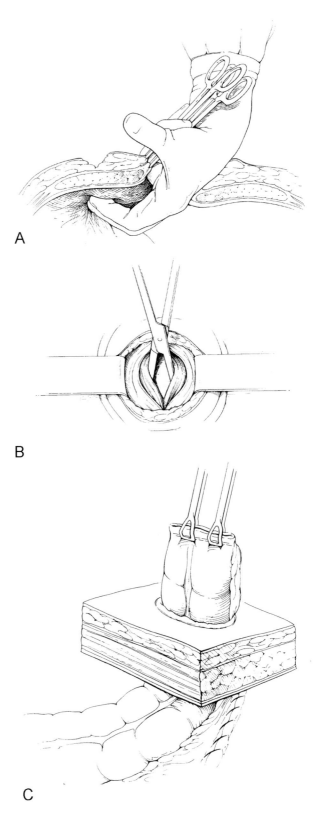

FIGURE 44-2. Colostomy creation. **A** Circular skin disk is removed. **B** Fascia is divided. **C** End of colon is brought through fascia and skin opening. (From Beck DE. End sigmoid colostomy. In: MacKeigan JM, Cataldo PA. eds. Intestinal Stomas. Principles, Techniques, and Management. Copyright 1993 by Taylor & Francis Group LLC (B). Reproduced with permission of Taylor & Francis Group LLC (B) in the format Textbook via Copyright Clearance Center).

repositioned to separate the muscles, exposing the posterior fascia. The posterior fascia and peritoneum are then incised with the electrocautery onto the wet lap pad. A large Kelly clamp is passed through the aperture and the pad is removed. The internal orifice may be viewed by lifting up on the Kocher clamps and levering the Kelly clamp up through the wound. The posterior opening may be enlarged as needed by incising the peritoneum and posterior fascia vertically, avoiding bringing the incision toward the midline wound. The opening is assessed and dilated by passing a finger, a thumb, and then two fingers. Any additional fascial widening needed is performed to allow easy passage of the bowel. A finger or clamp is kept in the opening at all times to avoid losing the tract, especially through the muscle plane. The end of the bowel to be used as the stoma is grasped with one or two large Babcock clamps placed through the aperture. This limb is then gently fed through the channel from within, rather than dragging it through with the Babcock clamps (Figure 44-2). This must be done carefully to avoid tearing the mesentery. If the fascial opening is too tight it should be further opened. The ileum should protrude 3–5 cm whereas the colon may protrude 1–2 cm. A bowel clamp such as a Glassman is placed across the protruding bowel to keep it at the correct level while the abdominal procedure is completed and the abdominal incision is closed. This clamp should not occlude the mesentery. It has been the authors' practice to place four interrupted 3-0 absorbable sutures from bowel seromuscular layer to the peritoneum and posterior fascia. We do not attempt to close the lateral gutter between the limb and abdominal wall.

Maturation

The maturation technique of an ileostomy or a colostomy differs because of the nature of the effluent and the size of the lumen. A matured ileostomy should protrude 1–3 cm after eversion to create a spigot or faucet effect. This directs the liquid output into the appliance and decreases the problem of ileal contents irritating the skin and getting underneath the faceplate. Because of the more formed nature of the stool, colostomies may be flatter, although a small amount of protrusion is beneficial for appliance placement and adherence. In general, the stoma is *matured primarily* by everting the end and sewing it to the skin edge as the last phase of the operation. An appliance is placed along with the dressings so that the effluent will be collected and the stoma will function normally as soon as the ileus resolves. The abdominal incision is closed and a wet towel is placed over the wound. After a long operation, there is a tendency to rush through this phase; however, it is critical to the success of the operation and the rehabilitation of the patient to spend the necessary time to create a well-formed stoma. The end of the bowel limb is excised removing the staple line or the straight clamp. The lumen is cleansed with Betadine-soaked gauze as needed.

End Ileostomy Maturation

Four sutures of a 3-0 absorbable material are placed to evert the ileum. These sutures are placed equidistant around the protruding bowel at the top, bottom, left, and right. The suture is first placed through the seromuscular and mucosa edge. A small but solid bite of the subcuticular edge of the skin opening is taken. The suture should not go through the surface of the skin because of the possibility of implantation of mucosa cells into the skin and resultant weeping patches and severe peristomal irritation. The third bite is taken through the seromuscular layer of the ileal wall at the level of the skin (Figure 44-3C2). Each of the four sutures is placed and tagged. The four tags are then grasped and the stoma is everted by gently pulling on the sutures while simultaneously pushing up on the seromuscular layer in between, half way down from the cut edge of the bowel to the skin with the back end of a forceps. This maneuver allows the ileum to evert and intussuscept. The four sutures are then tied down. One to two additional simple buried sutures are placed in between the everting ones to further approximately the mucosal–cutaneous junction. The midline wound is covered by a thin strip of nonadherent gauze and then the stoma appliance is placed. The opening in the faceplate should be cut to 5 mm

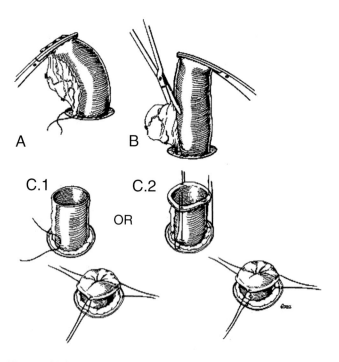

FIGURE 44-3. Ileostomy maturation. **A** Ligation. **B** Trimming of the ileal mesentery. **C.1** Serosa is attached to Scarpa's fascia and the mucosal edge sutured to dermis. **C.2** Triangular stitch from ileal end to serosa to dermis; tying sutures inverts the ileum to the skin. (From Beck DE. Intestinal stomas. In: Beck D, ed. Handbook of Colorectal Surgery. 2nd ed. Copyright 2003 by Taylor & Francis Group LLC (B). Reproduced with permission of Taylor & Francis Group LLC (B) in the format Textbook via Copyright Clearance Center).

larger than the diameter of the stoma to allow for swelling. The collection bag is oriented so that it hangs to the patient's side for the first few days while recumbent. Once the patient is ambulating well, it is rotated so that it hangs down toward the feet. Additional dressings are applied.

End Colostomy Maturation

Although a left-sided colostomy may be flush to the skin, slight eversion is preferred to improve appliance adherence and because weight gain may result in retraction. The procedure is similar to ileostomy maturation as outlined above. However, the stoma is trimmed so that only 1–2 cm protrudes. The four quadrant sutures do not need to include the third bite through the seromuscular layer at skin level unless this is needed to hold the stoma up. Because the stoma diameter is larger, two to three buried sutures may be placed in between each of the quadrant sutures.

Controversies

Several controversies exist about the creation of a stoma. Traditionally, absorbable sutures have been placed transabdominally from the seromuscular layer of the bowel to the posterior fascia and peritoneum to help fix the limb in place and reduce the incidence of parastomal hernias and prolapse or retraction. This has been questioned recently. It is still the authors' practice to place four interrupted 3-0 absorbable sutures from seromuscular layer of the bowel limb to the peritoneum and posterior fascia.

Other issues under discussion include whether an adhesion barrier should be placed around the limb as it exits the abdominal cavity because this may decrease the formation of adhesions and the incidence of small bowel obstruction. Some surgeons have adopted this practice. Perhaps even more controversial is whether a mesh patch should be placed prophylactically around the stoma to decrease the high incidence of parastomal hernias. Use of mesh around a stoma has always been viewed with skepticism because of the risk of infection and the subsequent need to remove the mesh. Yet, there are no data on the incidence of this problem.

Most stomas are primarily matured, however secondary maturation may be preferred when the bowel is too thickened and inflamed to evert, when it is too friable or weak to hold sutures, or when the patient is unstable and the additional time is not warranted. In cases of toxic colitis, megacolon, or distal obstruction, the bowel may be so distended and friable that it will not hold sutures. When operating for peritonitis, the colon or small bowel may be markedly thickened and inflamed. In these situations, the bowel may simply be exteriorized as a straight end and, in the manner of Jones, wrapped in a long length of moist gauze to hold it on the abdominal wall. The stoma may then be secondarily matured with the time interval determined by the appearance of the bowel and the condition of the patient. Usually, this is in the range of 2–7 days.

Hebert[33] described the *loop-end ostomy* for difficult-to-mature stomas in obese patients with a thick abdominal wall and a thickened or shortened mesentery. The bowel to be used as the stoma is divided with a linear stapler. The proximal end is brought through the abdominal wall aperture. The antimesenteric side is opened as the ostomy and the staple line is left along the side of the tract. A portion of the staple line may be excised as part of the maturation as needed (Figure 44-4).

Lateral Mesenteric Closure

A number of authors have advocated closing the lateral sulcus when constructing a colostomy or fixing the ileal mesentery to the falciform ligament when creating an ileostomy. This is done in an attempt to reduce the incidence of volvulus around the stomal limb and obstruction. Theoretically, a form of volvulus may occur because the bowel is fixed anteriorly at the abdominal wall and posteriorly by the mesentery. Yet, in clinical practice, this problem rarely occurs. In this author's experience with several hundred stomas, stomal volvulus has been a problem in only one patient. Yet, some surgeons cling to this religiously whereas others doubt its usefulness.

John Goligher of Leeds, England took this notion to its extreme by advocating creation of an *extraperitoneal colostomy* (Figure 44-5).[34] C.P. Sames described a similar technique.[35] The colon was extensively mobilized and tunneled

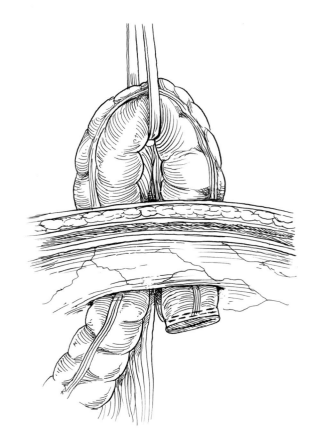

FIGURE 44-4. Loop-end colostomy.

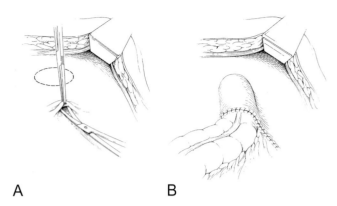

A   B

FIGURE 44-5. Extraperitoneal colostomy. **A** Peritoneum is opened, and an extraperitoneal tunnel is created with blunt dissection. **B** Colon is brought through the tunnel, and mesenteric defect is closed. (From Beck DE. End sigmoid colostomy. In: MacKeigan JM, Cataldo PA, eds. Intestinal Stomas. Principles, Techniques, and Management. Copyright 1993 by Taylor & Francis Group LLC (B). Reproduced with permission of Taylor & Francis Group LLC (B) in the format Textbook via Copyright Clearance Center).

from posterior to anterior beneath the peritoneum and then through the abdominal wall.

Mucous Fistula

The term mucous fistula refers to the distal end of the divided bowel that has been brought through the skin and matured as a stoma. Typically, when the bowel is completely transected, with or without resection of a segment, the proximal end may be made into an end stoma, e.g., ileostomy or colostomy. This is the functioning stoma through which the bowel contents empty. The other, or distal, end may be closed as in a Hartmann's procedure or may be brought to the surface and matured. This is referred to as a mucous fistula because it is an opening that occasionally produces mucous. A mucous fistula may be placed in a number of locations. Classically, this end of the bowel was brought out through the lower end of the vertical abdominal incision, but it may also be placed in its own site away from the wound and the primary ostomy, or it may even be brought up adjacent to the end ostomy and only opened a small amount as in the end-loop colostomy of Prasad et al.[36] (Figure 44-6).

The advantage of a mucous fistula is primarily that the distal portion of the bowel may be decompressed though this opening. This is important when an obstruction remains in the distal bowel such as an unresectable tumor. Closure of the distal end might result in a closed loop which, when filled with mucous, secretions, and bacteria, could rupture and result in peritonitis. A mucous fistula may also be used to access the distal bowel for purposes of observation, irrigation for washout, or for therapy. It is also a simple matter to find the distal limb when operating to close the ostomy. The obvious disadvantage of a mucous fistula is the second stoma site on

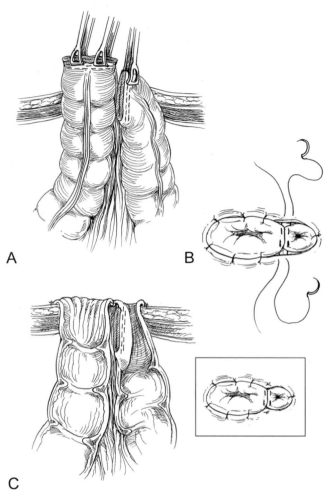

A   B

C

FIGURE 44-6. End-loop colostomy (Prasad). **A** The entire divided edge of the proximal limb and the antimesenteric corner of the distal limb are gently drawn through the opening in the abdominal wall. After the abdomen has been closed, the staple line of the proximal limb is excised completely and only the antimesenteric corner of the distal staple line is removed. **B** The proximal limb is matured flush with the skin by suturing the deep dermal skin to full-thickness colon with absorbable sutures. Transition sutures may be placed to help mature the mucous fistula, which has the appearance of a "ministoma." **C** Sagittal view of the completed end-loop colostomy. Note the portion of the distal staple line in the subcutaneous tissue.

the patient's abdominal wall. Although a mucous fistula does not produce a large amount of material, small amounts of mucous do emanate from time to time.

Diverting Stomas

Indications

Whether a colostomy or ileostomy, diverting stomas are nearly always created for a single purpose: to prevent fecal content from reaching a distal segment of the large bowel, either because of fear of leak (distal or difficult anastomosis) or to treat a leak (trauma, perforation, or anastomotic disruption). Once this principle is understood, the indications for and selection of an appropriate diverting stoma becomes straightforward.

Table 44-2 lists the common current indications for diverting ileostomies, colostomies, and end-loop stomas. These include protection of distal anastomoses, predominately ileal pouch-anal or coloanal anastomoses, complicated diverticulitis, treatment of anastomotic leaks and pelvic sepsis, large bowel obstruction, trauma, and fecal incontinence.

The end-loop stoma (including end-loop ileostomy, end-loop colostomy, end-loop ileocolostomy) as described by Prasad et al.[36] has created another option for fecal diversion which now allows the creation of a diverting stoma with remote intestinal segments (in association with colonic resection).

These three options exist for diverting stomas and the choice between these options will affect not only short-term complications, but the complexity of subsequent surgery and the quality of life (QOL) of the ostomate as well.

When deciding which stoma to create, the surgeon must thoughtfully consider the following principles:

1. Will the stoma achieve its primary purpose? Will it protect the anastomosis or treat the anastomotic leak?
2. Can a stoma be safely created? Can that segment of bowel reach an appropriate site on the abdominal wall and be matured successfully?
3. How will life with this stoma be, particularly if subsequent stoma takedown does not take place?
4. Will stoma choice affect subsequent stoma takedown? Loop stomas and end-loop stomas avoid the necessity of laparotomy for takedown versus the Hartmann procedure.
5. Will stoma choice limit future reconstructive options? Sigmoid colostomy may make a subsequent coloanal anastomosis more difficult versus loop ileostomy.

In both urgent and elective situations, these factors should be considered before initiating the surgical procedure. The patient can then be marked for potential stoma sites and counseled appropriately before surgery begins.

Although loop ostomies are usually meant to be temporary, a significant number are never closed. Because the patient must live with the loop stoma for at least several months, and sometimes for the remainder of his or her life, careful attention to ostomy construction remains very important.[37,38]

Another controversy exists regarding the distance between the diverting stoma and the distal area "to be protected." This pertains particularly to urgent operations without bowel preparation when treating an anastomotic leak or colonic perforation. Concerns exist that the column of stool between the stoma and the leak will continue to contaminate the peritoneal cavity preventing adequate treatment of intraabdominal sepsis. These concerns began in the early days of stoma creation when transverse loop colostomy and drainage were the preferred treatment for perforated diverticulitis. They continue today when a loop ileostomy is used in conjunction with drainage to treat an anastomotic leak or to protect a left-sided colonic anastomosis in emergency surgery without preoperative bowel preparation.

Loop Ileostomy Versus Transverse Loop Colostomy

When treating pelvic infection from a colonic source or particularly when choosing elective diversion for protection of low pelvic anastomosis, transverse loop colostomy and loop ileostomy are the major options. In nearly all situations, loop ileostomy is the superior choice. Transverse loop colostomy, except in rare circumstances, should be a procedure of historic significance only.[39]

Loop ileostomies are easy to construct, allow for better stoma placement, and are tolerated much better by ostomates. The effluent from both stomas is similar in volume and consistency. Therefore, colostomies offer no protection from fluid and electrolyte disturbances or skin irritation. In addition, loop ileostomies are easier and safer to "takedown" when restoring intestinal continuity.

In addition, loop transverse colostomies have a much larger lumen, rarely stay everted, often prolapse or retract, are usually placed in the epigastrium (a very inconvenient location), and are quite malodorous.

In a randomized, prospective trial by Williams et al.,[40] transverse loop colostomy was compared with loop ileostomy for elective protection of distal anastomoses. All ileostomies and colostomies objectively completely diverted the fecal stream. Nearly all complications were twice as common with transverse colostomies when compared with ileostomies (Table 44-3). Infection at the time of creation and at takedown, odor, leakage, and skin problems were all significantly higher in patients with transverse colostomies. In addition, multiple visits to the stoma therapist were needed in 58% of colostomy patients versus 18% of ileostomy patients. Others have expressed similar opinions and noted similar results.[41,42] Hernia formation at the ostomy closure site was much more common with transverse colostomies.[43,44]

Considering the available data, loop ileostomy should be the procedure of choice for proximal diversion of left-sided

TABLE 44-2. Indications for diverting stomas

- Protection of distal anastomosis
- Treatment of anastomotic leak
- Large bowel obstruction
- Trauma
- Diverticular disease
- Cryptoglandular sepsis
- Radiation complications
- Fecal incontinence
- Fulminant colitis

TABLE 44-3. Comparison of complications in a randomized trial of transverse loop colostomy and loop ileostomy[40]

	Transverse colostomy (%)	Loop ileostomy (%)
Prolapse	10	5
Skin problems	50	26
Leakage	31	18
Odor	53	6
Infection at takedown	30	0

anastomoses. The ileostomy is smaller, may be located in the right lower quadrant rather than the right upper quadrant as for a loop transverse colostomy, is less odorous, and easier to pouch and manage. Closure of the ileostomy is also an easier operation with fewer complications.[45]

Loop Colostomy

A loop colostomy can be created with any segment of the colon that can be mobilized to reach the abdominal wall. Only two sites, however, are generally used, the transverse colon and the left colon (sigmoid or descending). Because the transverse loop colostomy is rarely used today, construction of the left-sided loop colostomy will be described (Figure 44-7). If necessary, a transverse loop can be created in a similar manner using an appropriate segment of colon and matured in the right or left upper quadrant.

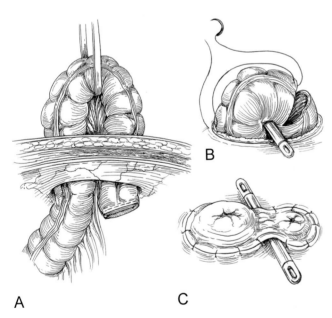

A   C

FIGURE 44-7. Loop-end colostomy. **A** A tape or rubber drain is passed through a small hole in the mesentery of the segment of colon to be exteriorized. **B** A plastic rod is placed through the mesenteric opening to support the loop on the skin and is sutured in place. The loop is opened transversely for about two-thirds of its circumference toward the distal end. The longer portion of the colon is everted with interrupted absorbable sutures. **C** Completed loop colostomy.

Loop Sigmoid Colostomy—Technique

The sigmoid and left colon are mobilized along the white line of Toldt as for a standard left colon resection, and an appropriate segment of colon is selected for stoma creation. In general, the most distal colonic segment available should be chosen. The bowel should be mobilized until the selected segment easily reaches the abdominal wall.

The peritoneum covering the mesentery adjacent to the bowel wall medially and laterally is then scored with electrocautery. A hemostat is passed immediately adjacent to the colon wall. Palpating the junction of the bowel wall and the mesentery with the index finger and thumb on the nondominant hand to guide the hemostat helps identify the correct site and avoids injury to the bowel wall. A Penrose drain or an umbilical tape is pulled through to encircle the bowel and identify the stoma site. A colored seromuscular suture is then used to mark the distal limb to prevent maturation of the incorrect end. The premarked stoma site, usually in the left lower quadrant, is excised. A disk approximately the size of a quarter is usually sufficient, but may need to be enlarged depending on the size of the colon. Smaller is better because it is easier to enlarge than decrease the size of the trephine. Small Richardson retractors expose the anterior rectus sheath. Counter pressure, applied from under the abdominal wall with the nondominant hand of the surgeon holding a wet gauze, facilitates this dissection.

The anterior rectus sheath is opened vertically for 3–4 cm. A small transverse extension may be made laterally in the midpoint. Medial extension should be avoided because this minimizes the fascial distance between the stoma site and the midline incision and may increase the risk of hernia. A curved instrument is used to bluntly spread the rectus abdominus in the direction of its fibers. The retractors are repositioned to spread the muscle, exposing the posterior rectus sheath. This is divided with the cautery onto the nondominant hand in the peritoneal cavity. The opening is enlarged to accept two fingers to the proximal interphalangeal joint.

The colon is passed, more by pushing than pulling, from the abdomen through the stoma site. Care is taken to avoid twisting the loop. The distal segment is oriented inferiorly and confirmed by the location of the colored suture. At times, a bar is placed beneath the loop to lie on the skin on either side of the opening for support. This is generally removed after 5–6 days. Once the colonic loop has traversed the abdominal wall without tension or evidence of ischemia, the abdomen is closed in standard manner and the incision is covered with a wet, sterile towel. There is no need to fix the colonic mesentery to the lateral peritoneal gutter because this maneuver has not been shown to decrease small bowel obstruction. Similarly, there is no need to fix the colonic wall to the fascia opening at the stomal site because this has not decreased the risks of parastomal hernia or stomal prolapse.

The colon is opened transversely just above the site where the distal-most portion meets the abdominal wall. Eighty percent of the colonic wall is transected. The distal end is matured primarily without eversion to the inferior one-third of the stoma trephine. The proximal end can be matured with or without slight eversion. If eversion is desired, classic tripartite sutures are passed from the dermis to the seromuscular layer 2–3 cm from the terminal end, and then full thickness to the terminal portion of the proximal stoma. After three everting sutures are placed, they are all tied, effectively everting the proximal or functional end of the stoma. Maturation is completed by adding sutures between the dermis and the cut end of the bowel as necessary to ensure mucocutaneous approximation. With this technique, the functional limb should occupy 75% of the circumference of the stoma trephine, with distal limb occupying the remainder. A support rod is generally unnecessary, but can be used if there is some tension on the stoma and retraction is a concern.

After surgery, a two-piece appliance with a clear collection bag is fit into place, and left undisturbed for 3–4 days. This allows for easy inspection of, and access to, the new stoma. Diet is advanced as intestinal activity resumes. Vascularity and patency of the stoma can be inspected by removing the stoma bag and, if necessary, peristomal evaluation can be performed by removing the appliance faceplate.

Loop Ileostomy

A loop ileostomy is created using the most distal ileal segment available that reaches the abdominal stoma site without creating tension on the stoma or distal anastomosis (especially when diverting an ileal pouch–anal anastomosis). Usually, this is 10–15 cm proximal to the ileocecal valve. Mobilization of the cecum and attachments of the terminal ileum to the retroperitoneum is occasionally required.

After selecting the appropriate ileal segment, a hemostat is passed under the bowel using the fingers of the nondominant hand to identify the mesenteric edge of the bowel and to protect it from injury. A Penrose drain or umbilical tape is pulled through this defect and clamped with a hemostat. A colored seromuscular suture is used to mark the distal portion to prevent maturation of the wrong stomal limb.

After identification and preparation of the ileal segment, the abdominal wall opening is created. A disk of skin, at the premarked stoma site, slightly smaller than a quarter, is excised. A defect through the abdominal musculature is created similar to that for a loop colostomy. The ileal segment is passed through the abdominal wall without twisting, ensuring that the previously placed suture, marking the distal end, is oriented caudally. The limb may be supported by a plastic rod, if the surgeon chooses.

After closing the abdominal incision in standard manner and protecting the wound with a sterile towel, the ileum is prepared for stoma creation. Two Allis clamps grasp the bowel at the junction between its distal-most portion and the abdominal skin. Electrocautery is then used to transect 80% of circumference of the bowel wall. The distal, or nonfunctional, end is

matured without eversion with three sutures between dermis and the full thickness of the terminal bowel. One suture is placed on the antimesenteric border of the distal end, whereas the other two are placed at the junction between the distal and proximal limbs. When passing sutures through the skin, only the inferior 25% of the stoma site circumference is used, leaving the remainder for the functional end. The proximal limb must be matured with eversion to prevent complications associated with caustic ileal effluent. *Tripartite bites* containing dermis, seromuscular layer of the bowel wall 2–3 cm proximal to the transected end, and full-thickness bowel wall at the transected end are then taken. Three sutures are placed on the antimesenteric border, and at the junction of the proximal and distal limbs of the stoma. After all three everting sutures are placed, they are tied sequentially and the proximal or functional end is everted. A single suture is placed between each of the prior sutures (only containing terminal bowel and dermis) to complete stoma maturation. A clear two-piece appliance is fixed to the stoma site in the operating room. This allows for visual inspection of the stoma in the postoperative period.

End-loop Stomas

End-loop stomas, as originally described by Unti et al.[46] consist of end-loop ileostomy, end-loop colostomy, and end-loop ileocolostomy. They offer the advantages of providing a well-everted, easily managed stoma in which laparotomy is not required for takedown and providing complete diversion of stool and decompression of the distal end. In addition, end-loop stomas may be created with remote intestinal segments (in association with bowel resection).

The technique for creation of all three is similar with the exception that two bowel segments must be approximated when creating an ileocolostomy. Creation of an ileocolostomy will be used to illustrate the technique. After right colon resection, the mesenteric defect is closed approximating the terminal ileum and the proximal transverse colon. A standard stoma trephine is created at the preselected stoma site (usually in the right upper or lower quadrant) as illustrated in the previous sections. The entire circumference of the terminal ileum and only the antimesenteric border of the previously stapled transverse colon are brought through the stoma site.

The abdominal incision is then closed. The antimesenteric corner of the transverse colon staple line is cut off with Mayo scissors. It is then matured to the stoma site dermis with three sutures without eversion. After this, the terminal ileal staple line is cut off completely. The ileum is everted as for standard end ileostomy. A single, full-thickness suture between the everted terminal ileum and the antimesenteric corner of the transverse colon completes the maturation.

As previously mentioned, this technique with minimal modification can be used to create an end-loop ileostomy or an end-loop colostomy. This technique produces upright stomas that are nearly indistinguishable from traditional end stomas to the ostomate. They are easy to pouch, requiring no support rod, and therefore are rarely associated with skin problems. Most importantly, laparotomy is not required for subsequent takedown. Because both the proximal and distal segments are located at one stoma site, a peristomal approach can nearly always be used to restore intestinal continuity. Complications will be discussed in the next chapter, but there are no complications unique to end-loop stomas, not seen in traditional loop stomas.

Turnbull Blowhole Procedure

As early as 1953, decompressive transverse colostomy was recommended for patients with toxic colitis.[47] Turnbull and Weakley[48,49] described a technique of intestinal decompression to be used in patients with toxic megacolon whose colon was so dilated and tissue-paper thin that any attempt to perform an acute resection was likely to result in massive peritoneal contamination and possible death. This procedure was used as a bridge to a more definitive resection after the patient had recovered from their acute illness.

Turnbull Blowhole Technique

A short, left paramedian incision is made to find a loop of distal ileum proximal to any terminal ileal disease. A small, lower midline incision can be substituted which may be incorporated into an incision used for a subsequent operation. The terminal ileum is exteriorized via a right lower quadrant incision and suspended over a bar. A 5-cm epigastric or right upper quadrant incision is made over the area of maximal transverse colon dilation for the "blowhole." The operative incision is closed. The ileostomy is primarily matured as a loop. The "blowhole" colostomy is matured in two layers (Figure 44-8). The seromuscular layer of the bowel wall is fixed to the fascia with several running sutures, leaving several centimeters of serosa exposed in the middle. The lumen is entered and the full thickness of the bowel wall is gently sutured to the skin with simple interrupted sutures. No attempt is made to evert this stoma because the tissue is likely to tear. Appliances are placed over both stomas.

Over the years, remarkable results have been reported in patients who are critically ill with a high expected mortality.[50,51] Remzi et al.[52] from the Cleveland Clinic reported their recent results, noting that even in Turnbull's own institution the procedure was now rarely performed. They described 17 patients over 18 years of age who underwent this procedure for inflammatory bowel disease, *Clostridium difficile* colitis, adult Hirschsprung's disease, and palliation for malignant bowel obstruction with metastases. Two of the patients with inflammatory bowel disease were pregnant. All four patients with metastatic carcinoma died of their disease. Twelve of the remaining 13 patients have been reconstructed, all with good results.

Obviously, the indications for this procedure have decreased over the past few decades because of better medical

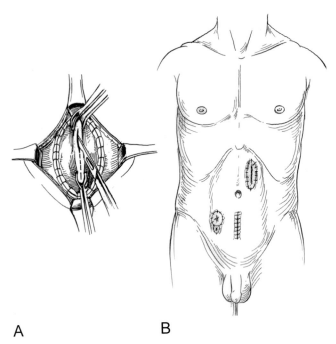

A   B

FIGURE 44-8. Blowhole colostomy and loop ileostomy "Turnbull procedure." **A** Through an incision made over the dilated transverse colon, the colon wall is sutured to the peritoneum to prevent intraabdominal contamination. The colon is opened and the edges of the opened bowel are sutured to the skin. **B** A loop ileostomy is created in the right lower quadrant usually through a lower midline incision.

management of inflammatory bowel disease, earlier referral for definitive surgery, and better critical care. Yet, the blowhole procedure is still a reasonable alternative in critically ill patients with toxic megacolon and large bowel obstruction and should remain a part of the colorectal surgeon's armamentarium.

Loop Ostomy Closure

Closure of a loop ostomy is generally a fairly straightforward procedure. Greater than 95% may be performed locally at the site of the stoma without having to reopen the midline or main abdominal incision. Occasionally, additional procedures may be necessary at the time of stomal closure such as repair of a parastomal hernia or even lysis of adhesions for an acute or chronic small bowel obstruction.

Closure of an end stoma is a much more extensive procedure than loop closure because the ends are separated and an intraabdominal approach is usually necessary. Closure of a Hartmann's procedure, especially if the distal end is in the pelvis, can be just as difficult as any resective procedure. Thus, this procedure should be performed with the same precautions, preparation, and concern as any colon resection.

The time interval between creation of the ostomy and closure will vary depending on the initiating disorder and the condition of the patient. It is best to wait until any inflammatory process has had adequate time to settle and for adhesions to soften. The patient should also be in as good condition as possible. Most temporary ostomies are closed in 2–3 months. A 6-week interval is the usual minimal period because adhesions tend to be severe before this. Periods of only 1–2 weeks or up to many years are occasionally used. Long time periods may be associated with disuse colitis or proctitis because the bowel normally obtains some of its nutrients such as glutamine from the passing contents. Irrigation with a solution of short-chain fatty acids may ameliorate this problem when symptomatic until continuity is reestablished. Atrophy and stenosis of the distal segment may rarely occur.

Loop Ileostomy Closure Technique

The only preparation necessary is a liquid diet the day before surgery and nothing after bedtime. Intravenous antibiotics are administered with the induction of anesthesia. A proctoscopic examination of the rectal anastomosis or the ileal pouch may be performed first with the patient in the lithotomy position. The patient is placed in the supine position. Some surgeons place a pursestring suture to close the ostomy lumen. The abdomen is prepped with Betadine solution and the patient is draped. A circumferential incision is made around the stoma at the mucocutaneous junction. If the skin is to be closed primarily, then the incision is extended as an ellipse laterally and medially for 1–2 cm. The edge of the stoma is grasped with straight hemostats at each of the four quadrants. These are used to hold the stoma up and retract it. Initially, Senn retractors are used to provide countertraction on the edges of the wound. These are replaced by small Richardson retractors as the wound becomes deeper. Using fine scissors and cautery, the dissection is carried down onto the antimesenteric surface of each limb, usually superior and inferior. Because the small bowel does not have fat appendages, the antimesenteric surface is smooth and unencumbered. It may be readily followed down to the anterior fascia on each side. The dissection is continued around, identifying the mesentery as it bulges out from under the loop, usually medially and laterally. The circumferential dissection of the subcutaneous portion of the loop is completed, exposing the anterior fascia all around. The serosa is freed from the fascia and rectus muscle using sharp dissection. There may be areas of tenacious adhesions and so care must be taken to avoid serosal tears and enterotomies. A finger may be inserted through a freed area and swept around the limb within the peritoneum to loose filmy adhesions and to identify areas of adherence. Additional intraabdominal adhesions may be released as needed to allow the loop to be exteriorized and to free 1–2 cm of the posterior fascia all around for later closure. If the fascial opening is very tight, it may be released by incising the rectus fascia superiorly or inferiorly for several centimeters and splitting the rectus muscle. This adds little risk but may provide significant visibility and may ease the dissection. The limb is carefully examined for serosal tears or enterotomies and these are repaired.

Continuity may be reestablished by either a sewn end-to-end anastomosis or by a stapled side-to-side anastomosis. If a sewn anastomosis is to be made, the opening in the loop must be cleared of adhesions and the mucocutaneous junction must be excised. Adhesions between the two limbs are divided so that the loop may be laid out in a straight line. The everted stoma is released and the eversion reduced. The attached skin and mucocutaneous junction are excised, leaving healthy, clean bowel edges. The opening usually encompasses about two-thirds of the cross-section of the bowel. The anastomosis is made with a single layer of inverting 3-0 suture using either absorbable material such as polyethylene glycol (Vicryl) or permanent material such as silk. The anastomosis is performed in two halves that are suspended between seromuscular, inverting stay sutures. These are placed just outside of the opening on either end and bridge the middle of the defect. The interrupted sutures are then placed sequentially from one side to the middle and then from the other side, inverting the mucosal edge. If the stoma must be excised, a standard end-to-end anastomosis may be made.

Currently, the anastomosis is usually made with a stapler in a side-to-side manner. This has proved to be reliable and faster, and bowel function may return sooner because it is typically a larger diameter anastomosis. After the limb has been mobilized, the skin is excised. The open end of the loop is held up with Babcock clamps. Throughout the procedure, the limbs are held vertically to reduce the risk of soilage. The two arms of the GIA stapler are placed into each of the two limbs of the loop. They are brought together with locking of the staples so that the mesentery is as lateral as possible and the staple line goes through the mid portion of the antimesenteric surface of the bowel. When locking the stapler, it is helpful to place two fingers between the bowel wall and the mesentery and to spread them, separating the mesenteric sides. The GIA stapler is fired and removed. The corners of the staple line are grasped with Allis clamps and pulled apart. Several Allis or Babcock clamps are placed in between to approximate the open edges of the bowel. This end is then stapled shut with a 60-mm linear stapler (TA-60). This creates a triangulated anastomosis that is wide and large. A crotch stitch is placed to complete the anastomosis. The limb is placed back into the abdominal cavity. The fascia is closed in a single layer with large, absorbable sutures. The skin may be closed with staples or subcuticular sutures or left open to heal secondarily.

Loop Colostomy Closure Technique

A loop colostomy may be closed in essentially the same manner as that of a loop ileostomy. Preparation usually includes both a mechanical washout and antibiotics. The dissection creates a larger wound and care must be taken to avoid cutting across fat epiploicae and diverticula. Because the lumen of the loop colostomy is larger than an ileostomy, a two-layered closure is often used. The mucosa is run with an absorbable suture and inverting, seromuscular (Lembert) sutures are placed using silk. A side-to-side stapled anastomosis is also safe and frequently used.

Closure of the Hartmann's Procedure

A Hartmann's procedure is used when a primary anastomosis is not feasible or safe as in the case of significant trauma, colonic obstruction, acute diverticulitis and toxic colitis, or megacolon. Typically, a variable amount of colon has been excised, a colostomy has been created, and the upper rectum has been closed. The entire colon may have been removed as in the case of toxic colitis, leaving an ileostomy and the closed rectum. In any case, the goal is to take down the stoma and reestablish continuity with either a colorectal or ileorectal anastomosis. Although this may be performed using hand-sewn techniques, the double-stapled method is now most often used. The advantages of an end-to-end stapled anastomosis are nowhere more clear than with this procedure.[53] At times, the procedure may be performed using a laparoscopic approach if adhesions are not too extensive.

A bowel preparation including both a mechanical washout and antibiotics is performed to cleanse the proximal colon. Enemas may be used to clear the rectum of mucous plugs and debris. If the proximal end is an ileostomy, then a clear liquid diet the day before surgery with nothing after bedtime is all that is necessary. The distal remaining bowel is cleansed at the beginning of the procedure using a sigmoidoscope and irrigating solution such as Betadine diluted 50% with saline. Some prefer to use a balloon catheter and enema procedure. The abdomen is prepped and draped. The abdominal cavity is entered through the old incision or laparoscopically. Adhesions are lysed as necessary and the rectal pouch is identified. Usually, little mobilization is needed if a stapled anastomosis is planned. The uterus or vagina or other tissues may need to be freed from the closed end. The ostomy is taken down from the abdominal wall. The end is trimmed, removing the skin and mucocutaneous junction. A standard double-stapled colorectal or ileorectal anastomosis is made with an appropriately sized stapler. A 29- or 33-mm stapler is usually used for a colorectal anastomosis, whereas a 25- or 29-mm stapler will usually fit into an ileorectal anastomosis. The anastomosis is tested with air or fluid and the donuts are examined for defects.

Results of Stoma Closure

Loop ostomy closure is still a significant operation with associated mortality and morbidity. There are actually quite a few studies that address these issues.[54–59] Fortunately, the risk of perioperative death is quite low at 0%–2%. Most of these deaths are attributable to nonsurgical conditions such as cardiac disease or pulmonary embolism. The rare, related death is attributable to sepsis from an anastomotic leak.

Overall complication rates of 15%–30% are consistently reported, although there are a few studies that report a wide range from 2.4% to 57%. These differences are probably related to the nature of the complications (attributed to the stoma closure or not) and the type of follow-up. There are no consistent differences between patients who had an elective or emergent ostomy.[54–65] In individual series, complication rates seem to decrease when subsequent time periods are analyzed, yet many reports from major institutions show similar rates from the 1970s through today.[66]

The most common complications of loop ostomy closure are wound infection (9%–34%), bowel obstruction (0%–10%), fecal fistula (0%–5%), and leak (0%–3%). Anastomotic strictures (0%–1%) and intraperitoneal abscess (0%–1%) after closure are fairly rare. Long-term consequences such as incisional hernias and small bowel obstructions are not uncommon with rates increasing over time from 2% to 10% or more for both.[54–56,60,61,67–69]

Risk factors that increase the complication rates of ostomy closure include diabetes, advanced age, type of ostomy being closed (end loop), increased operative time, and higher blood loss.[61] The most significant factors in several studies were steroid dependence and hypoalbuminemia.[64] A combination of factors, such as a high score, diabetes, and renal, cardiac, or pulmonary disease also portend a more difficult course.[59]

The surgical technique used for loop closure has been examined. Simple sutured closure of the anterior wall of the loop colostomy may have a lower complication rate than resection and anastomosis but there is no consensus on this.[62,70,71] Stapled and sewn anastomosis methods are of equal efficacy for colostomy closure.[63,72] The technique of loop ileostomy closure has been studied in several recent reports. Phang et al.[73] from the University of Minnesota reviewed a large series of ileostomy closures in which three techniques were used: simple sutured closure of the enterotomy, resection with hand-sewn anastomosis, and stapled anastomosis. Their overall complication rate was 24% which included wound infections (14%), small bowel obstructions (5%), and anastomotic leaks (3%). There was one death (0.3%) attributed to a cardiac event. The only difference was in the obstruction rate which was highest in patients who underwent resection with sutured anastomosis (12%) and lowest with simple enterotomy suture (2.3%). In a randomized trial, Hull et al.[74] from the Cleveland Clinic found that stapled and hand-sewn closures were equivalent in terms of complications, resumption of intestinal function, and length of stay. The only difference was that the stapled procedure was slightly faster. Others have also found these two techniques to be equivalent.[70]

The timing of ostomy closure has been a hotly debated topic for years. Some believe that early closure, even during the original hospital stay, will reduce costs and speed recovery. Others believe that early closure will abrogate the benefits of the diversion and result in higher complication rates. A careful review of the literature found 11 studies with specific data supporting delayed closure, usually for 3 months, and only two that found no difference between early and late closure.[55,60,63,71,75,76] Most surgeons recommend a 2- to 3-month interval.

It is generally believed today that loop ileostomies have a lower complication rate than loop colostomies. Closure of these stomas may also differ in morbidity although the support for this is limited.[40,70,77]

Closure of a Hartmann's procedure is a major operation with all of the risks of any resection and anastomosis in a reoperative setting. In this setting, most authors have also found that delaying the closure for 3 months is beneficial.[76,78–80] Recently, several small reports of successful laparoscopic closures of Hartmann's procedures have appeared.[81–84] This seems to be a reasonable approach; however, there should be a low threshold for conversion to an open procedure.

Minimally Invasive Stomas

Minimally invasive stomas can be created through three different approaches: 1) trephine stomas (those created with all exposure through the stoma site itself), 2) endoscopically assisted stoma creation, and 3) laparoscopically assisted stoma creation. Each offers its specific advantages and disadvantages as do traditional techniques for stoma creation. None of these techniques change the indications for, or proper siting of, a stoma. These less-invasive techniques should be used only when stoma creation is indicated and a properly sited stoma can be safely created.

Trephine Stomas

Trephine stomas originated with the very beginnings of stoma surgery.[85] Before the advent of general anesthesia, aseptic technique, and transabdominal surgery, stomas were created through either flank or iliac incisions which doubled as the stoma site after completion of the procedure.[86]

Currently, trephine stomas are rarely performed because of advances in surgical technique. Difficulty with exposure leads to two significant problems: 1) identifying the proper intestinal segment, and 2) discerning the proximal limb from the distal limb of the stoma. This can lead to a stoma that is distal to a site of a large bowel obstruction or maturation of the distal stomal segment resulting in iatrogenic bowel obstruction.[92] For these reasons, endoscopic and laparoscopic assistance have been added to trephine stoma creation.

Endoscopically Assisted Colostomy

Trephine stoma creation with endoscopic assistance is reserved for left-sided colostomies. Proximal to the left colon, its utility is severely limited by colonic distention secondary to passage of the endoscope. Endoscopic assistance is frequently used for sigmoid colostomy creation without bowel resection. Common indications include fecal incontinence, perianal sepsis, sacral decubiti in spinal cord–injured patients, and creation of covering stomas in association with complex anal surgery. Patients who have multiple abdominal operations, have had prior left-sided colon resection, or who are obese are poor candidates for this approach.

Endoscopically Assisted Colostomy Technique

Patients are prepared as for standard left-sided colostomy creation. An effective mechanical bowel preparation is essential to allow passage of the endoscope. A preselected stoma site is marked preoperatively by the enterostomal therapist, preferably in the left lower quadrant. The patient is placed in modified lithotomy position with legs in low stirrups, but the "foot" position of the operating table is left in its customary up position. The abdomen is prepped and draped in routine manner. The flexible sigmoidoscope (or colonoscope) is passed transanally into the sigmoid colon by the surgeon. The assistant identifies the endoscopic light transilluminating the left lower quadrant. The endoscope is then manipulated until the light approaches the premarked stoma site (Figure 44-9). The endoscope is left in place, resting on the "foot portion" of the operating room table. The surgeon then scrubs in. A circular disk of skin is removed from the premarked stoma site. The abdominal wall is traversed in standard manner and the colon identified by palpating the endoscope. The endoscope is

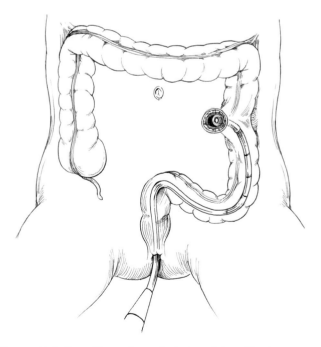

FIGURE 44-9. Sigmoidoscopic manipulation of sigmoid colon to premarked stoma site on abdominal wall.

withdrawn several centimeters and the sigmoid colon delivered through the stoma site, with care taken not to lose orientation of the proximal and distal ends. The sigmoid colon is then transected with a linear stapler as for standard end-loop stoma. To confirm orientation, the antimesenteric border of the distal staple line is transected. Air is insufflated via the endoscope and saline is drizzled over the distal stomal limb. Correct orientation is confirmed by air bubbles emanating from the distal colotomy. The distal antimesenteric border is matured without eversion and the proximal, functional end is matured in the standard manner. Insufflated air is once again confirmed to be originating from the distal limb to ensure correct orientation. The endoscope is withdrawn and the procedure terminated. Patients generally may resume a regular diet on the following day.

The limiting factors for the use of this technique include sigmoid length and fixation, abdominal wall obesity, prior surgery and adhesions, and the ability to pass the endoscopy through any strictures. As for all minimally invasive operations, the patient should be prepared for conversion to a laparoscopic or open approach.

Laparoscopic-assisted Stomas

End and loop colostomies as well as end-loop ileostomies can be created with laparoscopic assistance. Laparoscopy does not change the indications for stoma construction. Additionally, the techniques for stoma maturation are identical to those for open stomas. Initial reports of successful laparoscopic ostomy creation began to appear in 1991 through 1994.[87–89] Many more have been published since.

Laparoscopic Ileostomy

In many cases of laparoscopic-assisted ileostomy, laparoscopy is only necessary to facilitate the proper selection and identification of an appropriate ileal segment as well as ensure maturation of the proximal limb.

Laparoscopic Ileostomy Technique

A laparoscope is inserted through an umbilical port. A second port is inserted through the preoperatively marked stoma site. The terminal ileum is identified and its mobility assessed (Figure 44-10). If the ileum is free from attachments, a segment 10–15 cm proximal to the ileocecal valve is located and held with an atraumatic locking grasper through the stoma site port. Correct orientation of the proximal and distal limbs is confirmed, and the grasper is held firmly by the assistant. The ostomy site is enlarged to a standard stoma size by excising a disk of skin and dividing the fat and fascia vertically. The rectus muscle is split vertically and the posterior fascia and peritoneum are opened. The ileum is gently pulled through the opening, making sure that the site is wide enough to avoid injury to the bowel. This may be facilitated by using

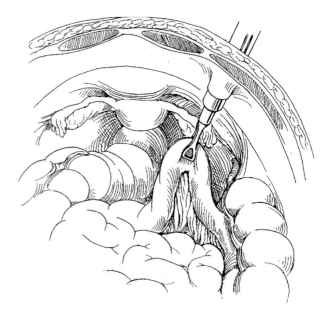

FIGURE 44-10. Laparoscopic ileostomy. Bowel is manipulated to the stomal opening using the laparoscopic Babcock grasper. (From Beck DE. Minimally invasive surgery. In: Beck D, ed. Handbook of Colorectal Surgery. 2nd ed. Copyright 2003 by Taylor & Francis Group LLC (B). Reproduced with permission of Taylor & Francis Group LLC (B) in the format Textbook via Copyright Clearance Center).

a large Babcock clamp and rocking the loop back and forth to see which side is most mobile. Pneumoperitoneum is reestablished with the ileum preventing release of carbon dioxide through the stoma site. Proper orientation is ensured, and then the pneumoperitoneum is released and the stoma is primarily matured.

If the terminal ileum is fixed to the right gutter or the right iliac fossa, mobilization will be required. In this situation, an additional trocar is placed in the left lower quadrant and retroperitoneal attachments and adhesions to the terminal ileum and cecum are freed as necessary to ensure construction of a tension-free stoma. During this dissection, the right-sided grasper is used to reflect the terminal end and cecum toward the upper abdomen to improve visualization, create traction, and facilitate safe dissection. The use of laparoscopy facilitates terminal ileal identification and allows for mobilization of ileal attachments. Numerous articles have attested to its safety and efficiency.[89,90]

Laparoscopic Sigmoid Colostomy

As in laparoscopic-assisted ileostomy, if the sigmoid colon is redundant and has minimal retroperitoneal attachments, then proper identification and orientation of the sigmoid colon are all that are required. This technique mirrors that described for laparoscopic-assisted ileostomy. If, however, the sigmoid colon is short and relatively fixed, then additional laparoscopic dissection will be required.

Laparoscopic Sigmoid Colostomy Technique

The patient is placed in the supine position. A rolled towel may be placed underneath the left hip. Both arms are carefully secured at the side and tucked. After prepping and draping, the patient is rotated to the right and placed in moderately steep Trendelenburg position. This facilitates exposure by allowing the small bowel to "fall out" of the left lower quadrant. The abdominal is entered through an umbilical or right rectus port and another port is placed through the premarked stoma site in the left lower quadrant. A 5-mm port is placed in the right lower quadrant and, if necessary, an additional port may be placed in the suprapubic region to facilitate retraction and dissection. The sigmoid colon is identified, grasped, and retracted medially. The sigmoid colon is mobilized from lateral to medial and from the rectosigmoid junction to the mid descending colon. Great care must be taken to protect the retroperitoneal structures including the ureter and gonadal bundle. While the assistant retracts the sigmoid colon medially, the surgeon gently separates the mesentery from the retroperitoneum by pushing the retroperitoneal structures posteriorly and laterally. Once the correct plane is entered, this dissection proceeds fairly easily. If the correct plane is not found, then tearing of the small gonadal and periureteric vessels often occurs. The extent of mobilization necessary varies and so the laxity of the sigmoid mesentery is assessed at regular intervals during the dissection to determine when there is adequate length to complete the exteriorization of the loop. Once the colon is mobilized, an appropriate segment is grasped and pulled up to the abdominal wall at the premarked stoma site. Proper orientation is ensured by carefully noting the proximal and distal limbs and the absence of twists.

The loop is held in place with correct orientation by the assistant with an atraumatic locking grasper placed through the stoma site trocar. The left lower quadrant trocar site is enlarged to a standard stoma size by excising a disk of skin and dividing the fat and fascia vertically. The rectus muscle is split vertically and the posterior fascia and peritoneum are opened. The colon is gently pulled through the opening, making sure that the site is wide enough to avoid injury to the bowel. This may be facilitated by using a large Babcock clamp and rocking the loop back and forth to see which side is most mobile. Pneumoperitoneum is reestablished and proper orientation is ensured. The pneumoperitoneum is released and the stoma is matured as a loop, end loop, or end stoma in routine manner as desired.

Patients resume intestinal activity and diet very quickly, often eating the evening of, or the day after, surgery. Discharge from the hospital is possible as soon as stoma teaching is complete. Multiple studies have attested to the safety and advantages of laparoscopic-assisted colostomy creation.[87,88,90,91,93–105]

Conclusion

Minimally invasively created ileostomies and colostomies are generally safe and well tolerated. They avoid the need for a major laparotomy and patients resume regular diet and activities fairly quickly in most cases. They have been shown to be safe and are now often the procedure of choice when a diverting ostomy is needed and no other abdominal procedure is necessary.

Technical Tips for Difficult Stomas

The creation of a stoma is, in reality, the creation of an anastomosis between the intestine and skin. All principles that apply to formation of anastomoses equally apply to stoma construction. Stomas should be well vascularized, approximated without tension, formed from healthy bowel, and constructed with attention to technical detail. In addition, the stoma should be placed properly, through a trephine of correct size, and created from an intestinal segment appropriate to accomplish the stoma's purpose whether temporary or permanent.

Often this is a simple, straightforward task. However, in emergency situations or in individuals with multiple prior abdominal incisions and operations, an obese abdominal wall, or short thick mesentery creation of a well-perfused, tension-free, properly placed stoma can present a significant challenge. As mentioned, preoperative planning is essential. In a patient with a challenging abdominal wall as a result of obesity or multiple incisions, preoperative marking (often with two alternative sites) may significantly ease stoma creation. For example, a supraumbilical site in the obese abdomen will decrease the thickness of the abdominal wall that must be traversed, therefore improving perfusion and decreasing tension (Table 44-4). A left-sided colostomy is often more difficult to construct than an ileostomy. However, in very obese individuals with significant mesenteric shortening, even an ileostomy can be challenging.

Generally, a supraumbilical stoma site is best for a colostomy because there is less of an abdominal wall pannus and greater colonic mobility. The peritoneal attachments of the left colon are mobilized completely, leaving the colon connected only by its midline blood supply. If this standard mobilization fails to create a tension-free stoma then the following steps, generally in ascending order, will nearly always lead to an acceptable left-sided colostomy (Figure 44-11): 1) the splenic flexure should be completely mobilized; 2) medial peritoneal attachments at the base of the colon mesentery should be transected; 3) the inferior

TABLE 44-4. Technical points for creation of an emergent ostomy

- Gentle handling of the friable bowel and mesentery
- Mobilize as much as necessary to reduce the risk of tension, tearing, and ischemia
- Large fascial opening to accommodate thick bowel and mesentery
- Site the stoma more superiorly than usual to avoid postoperative management problems
- Consider secondary maturation if eversion might be difficult or too time consuming

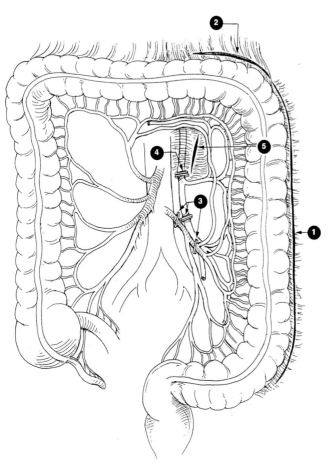

FIGURE 44-11. Operative measures to obtain left colon length. 1) Division of lateral colonic attachments; 2) division of the splenic flexure; 3) division of the inferior mesenteric artery at its aortic take-off and the inferior mesenteric vein; 4) second division of the inferior mesenteric vein at the inferior border of the pancreas; 5) incision of the splenic flexure mesentery. (From Rafferty JF. Obtaining adequate bowel length for colorectal anastomosis. Clin Colon Rectal Surg 2001;14:25–31, permission pending).

mesenteric artery can be transected proximal to the left colonic arterial takeoff to decrease tethering by the colonic blood supply; 4) "windows" should be created in the peritoneum overlying the colonic mesentery just below the stoma to create mesenteric lengthening.

Thickened mesentery associated with the terminal portion of the left colon can be trimmed, leaving only 1 cm (containing the marginal artery) attached to the colon wall. An oversized stoma trephine will decrease tension and venous compression, therefore improving vascularity to the stoma. These maneuvers will usually lead to a well-perfused, left-sided colostomy without tension. In the rare circumstance that, despite these maneuvers, this is not possible, a loop-end or "pseudo-loop" colostomy can be created. Following all previously prescribed maneuvers, the distal or terminal end of the left colon is stapled closed and left in the peritoneal cavity. Through an oversized stoma trephine, the antimesenteric border of the colon several

centimeters proximal to its closed end is brought through the abdominal wall guided by a Penrose drain. The antimesenteric border only is matured primarily to the abdominal wall without eversion (Figure 44-12). This is similar to the "blowhole" colostomy as described by Turnbull many years ago. This leads to a less than ideal, but functional stoma, which will allow recovery in an emergency setting. The stoma can be revised or reversed at a later date at an appropriate period.

Rarely, the bowel to be exteriorized is so edematous, rigid, and friable that sutures will not hold and will only tear and further compromise the bowel. At these times, the Jones technique is of particular usefulness. This is primarily used for end stomas and mucous fistulas. The stoma is brought out through a general fascia opening to avoid tearing and ischemia. At least 5 cm of bowel should sit above the skin. This spout is simply wrapped in a long roll of cotton gauze (Kerlix) which is kept moist. The stoma may be matured in 5–7 days or more at which time the edema will have decreased and the limb will have adhered to the fascia.

Finally, when creating a difficult stoma or if perfusion is a concern, it is occasionally best to create and mature the stoma before closure of the abdominal wall. This will facilitate any maneuvers necessary to create a functional, well-perfused stoma. At times, the barrier of a closed abdominal incision will lead the surgeon to accept a less than adequate result wanting to avoid reopening the abdomen. Technical points are summarized in Table 44-4.

Appliances Systems

In recent years, the quality and variety of ostomy appliances have increased markedly, and so there is now an appliance for almost every situation. Appliances are available for colostomies, ileostomies and urostomies. Most are disposable and available in one- or two-piece systems (Figure 44-13). The basic appliance has an adhesive faceplate with a central

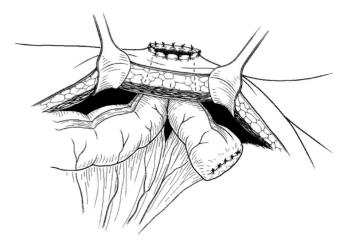

FIGURE 44-12. Trephine loop-end ostomy in patient with obese abdominal wall. (From Cataldo PA. Technique tips for the difficult stoma. Clin Colon Rectal Surg 2002;15:183–190, permission pending).

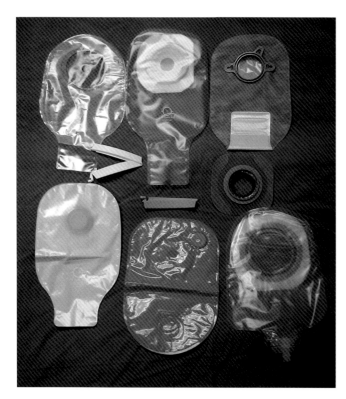

FIGURE 44-13. Ostomy appliances (picture).

opening and a collection piece or "bag." Most of the two-piece systems are connected by a Tupperware-style plastic ring. The central opening is sized to fit the stoma with a small 2- to 3-mm margin so that it is not too tight and does not erode into the mucosa. The ET/WOCN can assist patients and physicians in product selection.

There are many accessories that may be used with different pouching systems. Belts are available to lend additional support and security, especially during vigorous physical activity. Stoma Protectors may be used to minimize risk of stoma trauma at work or with contact sports. There are many pastes and creams and barrier inserts that may be used in patients with irregular peristomal surfaces or other local problems. Deodorant tablets may be taken orally or placed in the pouch. This is usually not necessary because current pouches are impervious to odor. Spray deodorants may be used in the room in which the appliance is changed. There are also a large variety of undergarments available, ranging from girdles and panties with built-in support panels to underwear with layered pockets to keep the plastic pouch from irritating the skin to sexy lingerie.

Ostomy Management

The most common problems encountered in the care of ostomy patients are attributed to stoma location and construction. Ostomy appliances should be changed when the stoma is least likely to function, usually before meals in the morning.

Left-sided colostomy patients are candidates to learn the process of colostomy irrigation. Colostomy irrigation is essentially a method of performing an enema through the colostomy to stimulate evacuation and avoid further drainage for a time. The goal of irrigation is not to actually wash the colon out but to stimulate motility and evacuation. This allows more freedom of activity for the patient with little worry of bowel action. Many ostomates may be trained to irrigation once every 1–3 days and a significant number are fairly dry in between.

Outcome and QOL

Long-term survival is primarily related to the underlying disease process, and many patients with a permanent ostomy live a long life. The overall well being of a patient is difficult to describe. Several measures of *Quality of Life* (QOL) have been developed that attempt to quantify specific areas or *domains* including physical well being and functional status, psychologic function, social interaction, somatic sensation, and sexual function.[106,107]

Recent studies have shown that patients with a well-constructed and managed ostomy often enjoy a very good QOL, and that a stoma may actually be preferable to a poorly functioning anorectum with incontinence, pruritus, odor. In addition, colostomy patients seem to function better than ileostomy patients. This is probably attributable to the less-frequent and more-formed output of the colostomy.[108] Of all ostomy patients, those with a colostomy who irrigate regularly have the best results in terms of confidence and participation in activities.[109] QOL improves markedly after surgery in all patients with inflammatory bowel disease and seems to improve over time in most patients.[110] Patients undergoing colostomy for cancer continue to worry about the risk of cancer recurrence and are less concerned about the consequences of the stoma.[108,111–113] "Lifestyle" is altered in between 40% and 80% of patients, especially those with ileostomies. Severe restrictions may be present in up to 10% of patients and mild to moderate restrictions in 30%–50%.[109,114]

Several studies have highlighted the importance of preoperative and postoperative counseling by an ET/WOCN. All patients improved their QOL after stomatherapy and this intervention seems to be most important during the first 3–6 months after surgery.[109,110]

Although most patients with major spinal cord injuries develop regular bowel habits with the standard management programs, some develop chronic bowel dysfunction with constipation, impaction, and incontinence. Colostomy has been performed in some of these patients as a last resort. Evaluation of these patients reveals that the large majority have a significant improvement in their QOL scores, that hospitalizations for bowel dysfunction may be reduced by 70%, and most wished they had undergone the procedure sooner. The colostomy resulted in simplified bowel care routine, less time spent on bowel management, and increased independence.[115,116]

Conclusions

Although permanent ostomies are becoming less common, they are still occasionally necessary. Temporary ostomies including loop ileostomies and colostomies, divided ostomies, and Hartmann procedures are still used quite often. The construction, care, and closure of stomas are major areas of concern for the general and colorectal surgeon. Patients are more aware of this aspect of their surgery than almost anything else. Thus, attention to this aspect of surgical care is critical. Appropriate preoperative preparation and postoperative support are necessary for all patients undergoing ostomy surgery. Early referrals to an ET/WOCN and the United Ostomy Association are very helpful.

References

1. Gazzard BG, Saunders B, Dawson AM. Diets and stoma function. Br J Surg 1978;65(9):642–644.
2. Hill GL. Physiology of conventional ileostomy. In: Dozois RR, ed. Alternatives to Conventional Ileostomy. Chicago: Yearbook Medical Publishers; 1985:31–35.
3. Brooke BN. The management of an ileostomy including its complications. Lancet 1952;2:102–104.
4. Turnbull RB Jr. Intestinal stomas. Surg Clin North Am 1958; 38:1361.
5. Crawford N, Broooke BN. Ileostomy chemistry. Lancet 1957;1:864–867.
6. Smiddy FG, Gregory SD, Smith IB, et al. Faecal loss of fluid, electrolytes and nitrogen in colitis before and after ileostomy. Lancet 1960;1:14–19.
7. Kramer P, Kearney MM, Ingelfinger FJ. The effect of specific foods and water loading on the ileal excreta of ileostomized human subjects. Gastroenterology 1962;42:535–546.
8. Kanaghinis T, Lubran M, Coghill NF. The composition of ileostomy fluid. Gut 1963;4:322.
9. Hill GL, Millward SF, King RFGJ. Normal ileostomy output: close relation to body size. Br Med J 1979;2:831–832.
10. Soper NJ, Orkin BA, Kelly KA, et al. Gastrointestinal transit after proctocolectomy with ileal pouch-anal anastomosis or ileostomy. J Surg Res 1989;46:300.
11. Robertson MD, Mathers JC. Gastric emptying rate of solids is reduced in a group of ileostomy patients. Dig Dis Sci 2000;45(7):1285–1292.
12. Newton CR. Effect of codeine phosphate, Lomotil and Isogel on ileostomy function. Gut 1978;19:377–383.
13. King RFGJ, Norton T, Hill GL. A double-blind cross-over study or the effect of loperimide hydrochloride and codeine phosphate on ileostomy output. Aust NZ J Surg 1982;52(2):121–124.
14. Gallagher ND, Harrison DD, Skyring AP. Fluid and electrolyte disturbances in patients with long established ileostomies. Gut 1962;3:219–223.
15. Bambach CP, Robertson WG, Peacock M, et al. Effect of intestinal surgery on the risk of urinary stone formation. Gut 1981;22:257–263.
16. Clarke AM, Chirnside A, Hill GL, et al. Chronic dehydration and salt depletion in patients with established ileostomies. Lancet 1967;2:740–743.
17. Hill GL, Goligher JC, Smith AH, et al. Long term changes in total body water, total exchangeable sodium and total body potassium before and after ileostomy. Br J Surg 1975;62:524–527.
18. Cooper JC, Laughland A, Gunning EJ, Burkinshaw L, Williams NS. Body composition in ileostomy patients with and without ileal resection. Gut 1986;27(6):680–685.
19. Holgate AM, Read NW. Relationship between small bowel transit time and absorption of a solid meal: influence of metoclopramide, magnesium sulfate, and lactulose. Dig Dis Sci 1983;28:812.
20. Vince A, O'Grady F, Dawson AM. The development of ileostomy flora. J Infect Dis 1971;128:638–641.
21. Finegold SM, Sutter VL, Boyle JD, Shimada K. The normal flora of ileostomy and transverse colostomy effluents. J Infect Dis 1970;122(5):376–381.
22. Gorbach SL, Nahas L, Wenstein L. Studies of intestinal microflora. IV. The microflora of ileostomy effluent: a unique microbial ecology. Gastroenterology 1967;53:874–880.
23. Percy-Robb IW, Jalan KN, McManus JP, et al. Effect of ileal resection on the bile salt metabolism in patients with ileostomy following proctocolectomy. Clin Sci 1971;41:371–382.
24. Gorbach SL, Tabaqchali S. Bacteria, bile and the small bowel. Gut 1969;10:963–972.
25. Hulten L, Kewenter J, Persson E, et al. Vitamin B12 absorption in ileostomy patients after operation for ulcerative colitis. Scand J Gastroenterol 1970;5:113–115.
26. Dotevall G, Kock NG. Absorption studies in regional enteritis. Scand J Gastroenterol 1968;3:293–298.
27. Modlin M. Urinary calculi and ulcerative colitis. Br Med J 1972;3(821):292.
28. Fukushima T, Sugita A, Masuzawa S, Yamazaki Y, Takemura H, Tsuchiya S. Prevention of uric acid stone formation by sodium bicarbonate in an ileostomy patient: a case report. Jpn J Surg 1988;18:465–468.
29. Christl SU, Scheppach W. Metabolic consequences of total colectomy. Scand J Gastroenterol Suppl 1997;222:20–24.
30. Bass EM, Del Pino A, Tan A, Pearl RK, Orsay CP, Abcarian H. Does preoperative stoma marking and education by the enterostomal therapist affect outcome? Dis Colon Rectum 1997;40: 440–442.
31. Raza SD, Portin BA, Bernhoft WH. Umbilical colostomy: a better intestinal stoma. Dis Colon Rectum 1977;20(3):223–230.
32. Fitzgerald PG, Lau GY, Cameron GS. Use of the umbilical site for temporary ostomy: review of 47 cases. J Pediatr Surg 1989;24(10):973.
33. Hebert JC. A simple method for preventing retraction of an end colostomy. Dis Colon Rectum 1988;31(4):328–329.
34. Goligher JC. Extraperitoneal colostomy or ileostomy. Br J Surg 1958;46(196):97–103.
35. Sames CP. Extraperitoneal colostomy. Lancet 1958;1(7020): 567–568.
36. Prasad ML, Pearl RK, Abcarian H. End-loop colostomy. Surg Gynecol Obstet 1984;158(4):380–382.
37. Winkler MJ, Volpe PA. Loop transverse colostomy. The case against. Dis Colon Rectum 1982;25(4):321–326.
38. Rutegard J, Dahlgren S. Transverse colostomy or loop ileostomy as diverting stoma in colorectal surgery. Acta Chir Scand 1987;153(3):229–232.
39. Boman-Sandelin K, Fenyo G. Construction and closure of loop transverse colostomy. Dis Colon Rectum 1985;28:772–774.

40. Williams NS, Nasmyth DG, Jones D, Smith AH. De-functioning stomas: a prospective controlled trial comparing loop ileostomy with loop transverse colostomy. Br J Surg 1986;73(7): 566–570.

41. Kockerling F, Parth R, Meissner M, Hohenberger W. Ileostomy–cecal fistula–colostomy—which is the most suitable fecal diversion method with reference to technique, function, complications and reversal? Zentralbl Chir 1997;122(1):34–38.

42. Arumugam PJ, Beynon J, Morgan AR, Carr ND. Randomized clinical trial comparing loop ileostomy and loop transverse colostomy for faecal diversion following total mesorectal excision. Br J Surg 2002;89(6):704–708.

43. Gooszen AW, Geelkerken RH, Hermans J, Lagaay MB, Gooszen HG. Quality of life with a temporary stoma: ileostomy vs. colostomy. Dis Colon Rectum 2000;43(5):650–655.

44. Edwards DP, Leppington-Clarke A, Sexton R, Heald RJ, Moran BJ. Stoma-related complications are more frequent after transverse colostomy than loop ileostomy: a prospective randomized clinical trial. Br J Surg 2001;88(3):360–363.

45. Hulten L. Enterostomies—technical aspects. Scand J Gastroenterol Suppl 1988;149:125–135.

46. Unti JA, Abcarian H, Pearl RK, et al. Rodless end-loop stomas. Seven-year experience. Dis Colon Rectum 1991;34(11): 999–1004.

47. Campbell FB, Campbell JG. Transverse colostomy for ulcerative colitis. J Int Coll Surg 1953;19(4):489–493.

48. Weakley FL, Turnbull RB Jr. Exclusion and decompression for toxic dilatation of the colon in ulcerative colitis. Proc R Soc Med 1970;63(suppl):73–75.

49. Turnbull RB Jr, Hawk WA, Weakley FL. Surgical treatment of toxic megacolon. Ileostomy and colostomy to prepare patients for colectomy. Am J Surg 1971;122(3):325–331.

50. Blansfield HN. The Turnbull procedure in the treatment of toxic megacolon. Conn Med 1973;37(12):609–611.

51. Shipp JD. Surgery for toxic megacolon: experience with the Turnbull-Weakley technique. Dis Colon Rectum 1974;17(3): 342–346.

52. Remzi FH, Oncel M, Hull TL, Strong SA, Lavery IC, Fazio VW. Current indications for blow-hole colostomy-ileostomy procedure. A single center experience. Int J Colorectal Dis 2003;18(4):361–364.

53. O'Connor TJ, Gaskin TA, Isobe JH. Reestablishing continuity after the Hartmann operation: use of the EEA stapling device. South Med J 1983;76(1):90.

54. Yajko RD, Norton LW, Bloemendal L, Eiseman B. Morbidity of colostomy closure. Am J Surg 1976;132(3):304–306.

55. Wheeler MH, Barker J. Closure of colostomy—a safe procedure? Dis Colon Rectum 1977;20(1):29–32.

56. Chapius P, Killingback M. Colostomy closure: technique and morbidity. Aust NZ J Surg 1979;49(3):363–368.

57. Samhouri F, Grodsinsky C. The morbidity and mortality of colostomy closure. Dis Colon Rectum 1979;22(5):312–314.

58. Khoury DA, Beck DE, Opelka FG, Hicks TC, Timmcke AE, Gathright JB Jr. Colostomy closure. Ochsner Clinic experience. Dis Colon Rectum 1996;39(6):605–609.

59. Ghorra SG, Rzeczycki TP, Natarajan R, Pricolo VE. Colostomy closure: impact of preoperative risk factors on morbidity. Am Surg 1999;65(3):266–269.

60. Mirelman D, Corman ML, Veidenheimer MC, Coller JA. Colostomies—indications and contraindications: Lahey Clinic experience, 1963–1974. Dis Colon Rectum 1978;21(3): 172–176.

61. Garber HI, Morris DM, Eisenstat TE, Coker DD, Annous MO. Colostomy closure. Morbidity reduction employing a semi-standardized protocol. Factors influencing the morbidity of colostomy closure. Dis Colon Rectum 1982;25(5):464–470.

62. Salley RK, Bucher RM, Rodning CB. Colostomy closure. Morbidity reduction employing a semi-standardized protocol. Dis Colon Rectum 1983;26(5):319–322.

63. Pittman DM, Smith LE. Complications of colostomy closure. Dis Colon Rectum 1985;28(11):836–843.

64. Mileski WJ, Rege RV, Joehl RJ, Nahrwold DL. Rates of morbidity and mortality after closure of loop and end colostomy. Surg Gynecol Obstet 1990;171(1):17–21.

65. Berne JD, Velmahos GC, Chan LS, Asensio JA, Demetriades D. The high morbidity of colostomy closure after trauma: further support for the primary repair of colon injuries. Surgery 1998;123(2):157–164.

66. Riesener KP, Lehnen W, Hofer M, Kasperk R, Braun JC, Schumpelick V. Morbidity of ileostomy and colostomy closure: impact of surgical technique and perioperative treatment. World J Surg 1997;21(1):103–108.

67. Garnjobst W, Leaverton GH, Sullivan ES. Safety of colostomy closure. Am J Surg 1978;136(1):85–89.

68. Henry MM, Everett WG. Loop colostomy closure. Br J Surg 1979;66(4):275–277.

69. Browning GG, Parks AG. A method and the results of loop colostomy. Dis Colon Rectum 1983;26(4):223–226.

70. Kohler A, Athanasiadis S, Nafe M. Postoperative results of colostomy and ileostomy closure. A retrospective analysis of three different closure techniques in 182 patients. Chirurg 1994;65(6):529–532.

71. Freund HR, Raniel J, Muggia-Sulam M. Factors affecting the morbidity of colostomy closure: a retrospective study. Dis Colon Rectum 1982;25(7):712–715.

72. Hasegawa H, Radley S, Morton DG, Keighley MR. Stapled versus sutured closure of loop ileostomy: a randomized controlled trial. Ann Surg 2000;231(2):202–204.

73. Phang PT, Hain JM, Perez-Ramirez JJ, Madoff RD, Gemlo BT. Techniques and complications of ileostomy takedown. Am J Surg 1999;177(6):463–466.

74. Hull TL, Kobe I, Fazio VW. Comparison of handsewn with stapled loop ileostomy closures. Dis Colon Rectum 1996;39(10): 1086–1089.

75. Aston CM, Everett WG. Comparison of early and late closure of transverse loop colostomies. Ann R Coll Surg Engl 1984;66(5): 331–333.

76. Khan AL, Ah-See AK, Crofts TJ, Heys SD, Eremin O. Reversal of Hartmann's colostomy. J R Coll Surg Edinb 1994;39(4): 239–242.

77. Edwards DP, Chisholm EM, Donaldson DR. Closure of transverse loop colostomy and loop ileostomy. Ann R Coll Surg Engl 1998;80(1):33–35.

78. Mosdell DM, Doberneck RC. Morbidity and mortality of ostomy closure. Am J Surg 1991;162(6):633–636; discussion 636–637.

79. Roe AM, Prabhu S, Ali A, Brown C, Brodribb AJ. Reversal of Hartmann's procedure: timing and operative technique. Br J Surg 1991;78(10):1167–1170.

80. Keck JO, Collopy BT, Ryan PJ, Fink R, Mackay JR, Woods RJ. Reversal of Hartmann's procedure: effect of timing and

technique on ease and safety. Dis Colon Rectum 1994;37(3):243–248.

81. Anderson CA, Fowler DL, White S, Wintz N. Laparoscopic colostomy closure. Surg Laparosc Endosc 1993;3(1):69–72.

82. Costantino GN, Mukalian GG. Laparoscopic reversal of Hartmann procedure. J Laparoendosc Surg 1994;4(6):429–433.

83. Vernava AM 3rd, Liebscher G, Longo WE. Laparoscopic restoration of intestinal continuity after Hartmann procedure. Surg Laparosc Endosc 1995;5(2):129–132.

84. MacPherson SC, Hansell DT, Porteous C. Laparoscopic-assisted reversal of Hartmann's procedure: a simplified technique and audit of twelve cases. J Laparoendosc Surg 1996;6(5):305–310.

85. Dinnick T. The origins and evolution of colostomy. Br J Surg 1934;22:142–153.

86. Biography-obituary, Jean Zulema Amussat. Bull Acad Med 1855–1856, Paris, p 21.

87. Lange V, Meyer G, Schardey HM, Schildberg FW. Laparoscopic creation of a loop colostomy. J Laparoendosc Surg 1991;1(5):307–312.

88. Romero CA, James KM, Cooperstone LM, Mishrick AS, Ger R. Laparoscopic sigmoid colostomy for perianal Crohn's disease. Surg Laparosc Endosc 1992;2(2):148–151.

89. Khoo RE, Montrey J, Cohen MM. Laparoscopic loop ileostomy for temporary fecal diversion. Dis Colon Rectum 1993;36(10):966–968.

90. Ludwig KA, Milsom JW, Garcia-Ruiz A, Fazio VW. Laparoscopic techniques for fecal diversion. Dis Colon Rectum 1996;39:285–288.

91. Oliveira L, Reissman P, Nogueras J, Wexner SD. Laparoscopic creation of stomas. Surg Endosc 1997;11:19–23.

92. Stephenson ER, Ilahi O, Koltun W. Stoma creation through the stoma site: a rapid safe technique. Dis Colon Rectum 1997;40:112–115.

93. Boike GM, Lurain JR. Laparoscopic descending colostomy in three patients with cervical carcinoma. Gynecol Oncol 1994;54(3):381–384.

94. Fuhrman GM, Ota DM. Laparoscopic intestinal stomas. Dis Colon Rectum 1994;37(5):444–449.

95. Hashizume M, Haraguchi Y, Ikeda Y, Kajiyama K, Fujie T, Sugimachi K. Laparoscopy-assisted colostomy. Surg Laparosc Endosc 1994;4(1):70–72.

96. Hunger T, Widmer MK, Rittmann WW. Laparoscopically assisted formation of end stage and loop ileostomies and colostomies. Helv Chir Acta 1994;60(6):965–967.

97. Jess P, Christiansen J. Laparoscopic loop ileostomy for fecal diversion. Dis Colon Rectum 1994;37(7):721–722.

98. Almqvist PM, Bohe M, Montgomery A. Laparoscopic creation of loop ileostomy and sigmoid colostomy. Eur J Surg 1995;161(12):907–909.

99. Khoo RE, Cohen MM. Laparoscopic ileostomy and colostomy. Ann Surg 1995;221(2):207–208.

100. Weiss UL, Jehle E, Becker HD, Buess GF, Starlinger M. Laparoscopic ileostomy. Br J Surg 1995;82(12):1648.

101. Hollyoak MA, Lumley J, Stitz RW. Laparoscopic stoma formation for faecal diversion. Br J Surg 1998;85(2):226–228.

102. Young CJ, Eyers AA, Solomon MJ. Defunctioning of the anorectum: historical controlled study of laparoscopic vs. open procedures. Dis Colon Rectum 1998;41(2):190–194.

103. Marusch F, Koch A, Kube R, Gastinger I. Laparoscopic creation of stomas–an ideal single indication in minimally invasive surgery. Chirurg 1999;70(7):785–788.

104. Decanini-Teran C, Belmonte-Montes C, Cabello-Pasini R. Laparoscopically created stomas. Rev Gastroenterol Mex 2000;65(4):163–165.

105. Swain BT, Ellis CN Jr. Laparoscopy-assisted loop ileostomy: an acceptable option for temporary fecal diversion after anorectal surgery. Dis Colon Rectum 2002;45(5):705–707.

106. McLeod RS, Lavery IC, Leatherman JR, et al. Factors affecting quality of life with a conventional ileostomy. World J Surg 1986;10:474.

107. Schupper H, Clinch J, Powell V. Definitions and conceptual issues. In: Spilker B, ed. Quality of Life Assessments in Clinical Trials. New York: Raven Press; 1990:11–24.

108. Baumel H, Fabre JM, Manderscheid JC, Domergue J, Visset J. Medicosocial consequences of permanent digestive stomas. A national multicenter retrospective study. Press Med 1994;23(40):1849–1853.

109. Karadag A, Mentes BB, Uner A, Irkorucu O, Ayaz S, Ozkan S. Impact of stomatherapy on quality of life in patients with permanent colostomies or ileostomies. Int J Colorectal Dis 2003;18(3):234–238.

110. Marquis P, Marrel A, Jambon B. Quality of life in patients with stomas: the Montreux Study. Ostomy Wound Manage 2003;49(2):48–55.

111. Wirsching M, Druner HU, Herrmann G. Results of psychosocial adjustment to long-term colostomy. Psychother Psychosom 1975;26(5):245–256.

112. Von Smitten K, Husa A, Kyllonen L. Long-term results of sigmoidostomy in patients with anorectal malignancy. Acta Chir Scand 1986;152:211.

113. Devlin HB. Colostomy: past and present. Ann Coll Surg Phys 1990;72:175.

114. McLeod RS, Lavery IC, Leatherman JR. Patient evaluation of the conventional ileostomy. Dis Colon Rectum 1985;28:152.

115. Randell N, Lynch AC, Anthony A, Dobbs BR, Roake JA, Frizelle FA. Does a colostomy alter quality of life in patients with spinal cord injury? A controlled study. Spinal Cord 2001;39(5):279–282.

116. Rosito O, Nino-Murcia M, Wolfe VA, Kiratli BJ, Perkash I. The effects of colostomy on the quality of life in patients with spinal cord injury: a retrospective analysis. J Spinal Cord Med 2002;25(3):174–183.

45
Stoma Complications

Neil Hyman and Richard Nelson

Despite substantial advances in surgical technique and enterostomal therapy, complications after stoma creation remain extremely common. The rate of stoma-specific complications in the literature varies quite widely, ranging from 10% to 70% depending on the methodology of the study, the length of follow-up, and the definition of a "complication." For example, virtually all ostomates will have at least transient episodes of minor peristomal irritation and skin irritation is the most frequently reported stoma complication. Studies only reporting problems that require revisional surgery will obviously report a much lower rate of complication. As such, the relative incidence and frequency of the specific complications will tend to be quite variable from series to series.

Stoma-related complications may be classified as those that are metabolic or best managed by medical intervention and those that have a purely structural etiology and are best managed by surgical intervention. Among the medical complications, the most common early complications are peristomal skin irritation, leakage, high output, and ischemia. The most frequently reported late complications include dehydration and nephrolithiasis, cholelithiasis in ileostomy patients, bleeding in patients with liver disease, and of course also in those with recurrence of the disease for which a stoma was created, such as Crohn's disease. In this chapter, we will make some general comments about the incidence and nature of stoma complications. We will then review the specific problems of a high-output stoma, parastomal dermatitis, bowel obstruction, and later complications such as stoma stenosis, peristomal hernia, and stomal prolapse.

Incidence

The prevalence of intestinal stoma complication has been assessed in a number of publications. From Cook County Hospital, the incidence of stoma complications was recorded in 1616 patients.[1] A total of 34.2% of these individuals experienced a complication related to their stoma, 27.7% of those individuals having an early complication, and only 6.5% a late complication. This publication also assessed the location of various stomas and their risks of complication. The location with the highest risk was loop ileostomy with a rate of almost 75%. The only other stoma location to have a complication rate exceeding 50% was descending end colostomy with 65%. The location of an intestinal stoma with the lowest risk was an end colostomy of the transverse colon, in which 69 individuals had an overall complication rate of only 5.8%.

In a publication from Hong Kong, the specific type of complication associated with each stoma location was described.[2] Parastomal hernia was most often seen with an end sigmoid colostomy in that series, although it was prevalent with all stoma types except ileostomy. Stomal stenosis was seen more often with a loop sigmoid stoma, prolapse with a transverse colostomy, and skin excoriation with an ileostomy. This series included 322 stomas in 316 individuals. Risk factors leading to these complications have been assessed in several publications, including a case series from Holland, in which emergency stoma construction was significantly associated with both stomal necrosis and high stoma output.[3] Obesity was associated with an increase in stoma necrosis. Among the leading diseases needing stoma formation, Crohn's disease and colonic ischemia were both associated with increased risk for ostomy-related complications. Crohn's disease was more prevalently associated with retraction and ischemia causing stoma necrosis. The series included 345 stomas in 266 patients.

In reports from Louisiana State University in New Orleans[4] and Swansea in the United Kingdom,[5] logistic regression was done to assess which risk factors were independently associated with complications. In the former study, inflammatory bowel disease and obesity both were associated with higher risk. A preoperative visit by an enterostomal nurse was associated with a significantly lowered risk of complications. In the latter publication, emergency surgery was usually associated as an independent risk factor for finding a stoma in a skin crease and early skin excoriation. Diabetes was associated with later skin problems.

Skin Problems

Skin Irritation/Leakage

Skin irritation (Figure 45-1) is very common among patients with a stoma. The problem is far more often seen in patients with an ileostomy because of the liquid, high alkaline, active enzymatic caustic effluent[6]; this highlights the need for proper technique when an ileostomy is created. Nugent et al.[7] describe the results of a study using quality of life questionnaires in 391 ostomates. Fifty-one percent reported problems with a "rash" and 36% had experienced leakage, both of which were much more frequently seen with ileostomies than colostomies. Thirty percent of patients with a colostomy and 55% with an ileostomy had experienced a reaction to the adhesive. However, only 8% of ostomates reported a substantial degree of difficulty associated with skin irritation.

Although a minor degree of skin irritation on occasion is probably inevitable, most significant cases of skin irritation are potentially preventable. Preoperative marking by an enterostomal therapist can help assure proper siting and a secure fit. Appropriate location and careful appliance fitting minimizes the noxious, irritating effect that can be associated with leakage on unprotected peristomal skin. Patients also need to be monitored for allergic reactions to the components of the appliance. An adequate spigot with a close-fitting faceplate prevents exposure of the peristomal skin to the ileostomy effluent. However, even the best-fitting appliances around the best-made stoma will leak if frequent emptying of the appliance is not practiced and pooling of effluent around the base of the stoma occurs.

Particular attention must be given to older patients who may have limitations in eyesight or dexterity. Patients with a high-output stoma are at particular risk for skin irritation and ulceration if they do not have an appropriately fitted appliance. Obesity has been frequently reported to be associated with an increased risk of skin irritation, which is likely attributable to technical problems with stoma construction.[8] Strong consideration should be given to placing the stoma in the upper abdomen where there is typically much less creasing of the abdominal wall, subcutaneous fat, and the patient can see it much more readily.

The patient should be instructed to avoid creams or ointments that may interfere with the adherence of their appliance. In the postoperative period, a stoma will tend to become less edematous and the abdomen becomes less distended. As such, it is quite common to need to "downsize" the appliance at the first postoperative visit to minimize exposed skin. Changing a stoma too frequently may lead to excessive "wear and tear" on the parastomal skin; however, too long an interval between changing the appliance may be associated with erosion of the protective barrier.

Even with the help of an excellent enterostomal therapist, specific skin infections may occur. Fungal overgrowth is evident when there is a bright red rash around the stoma with associated satellite lesions. This is typically easily treated by dusting the peristomal skin with an appropriate antifungal powder. If the dermatitis conforms precisely to the outline of the stoma appliance, then an allergic reaction to the wafer or other component of the appliance is likely the culprit (Figure 45-2). Peristomal skin irritation may also be associated with reactivation of inflammatory bowel disease, or the development of pyoderma gangrenosa. Antibiotics, steroids, release of appliance pressure, and local applications of epidermal growth factor have all been tried to resolve the pyoderma. There is no correlation with Crohn's disease activity in remote portion of the bowel and the occurrence of pyoderma around the stoma.

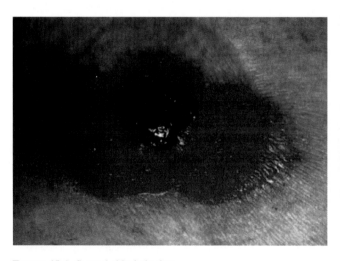

FIGURE 45-1. Stomal skin irritation.

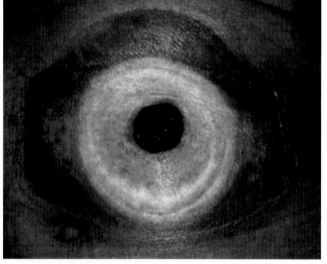

FIGURE 45-2. Allergic skin reaction.

High-output Stomas

A high-output state is typically described in association with an ileostomy, rather than a colostomy. Marked diarrhea and dehydration occur in 5%–20% of ileostomy patients, with the greatest risk occurring in the early postoperative period. An ileostomy usually functions by the third or fourth postoperative day.[6] The output typically peaks on the fourth postoperative day, with outputs of 3.2 L or more reported. Because the ostomy effluent is rich in sodium, hyponatremia can be a problem. The particular window of vulnerability for dehydration seems to be between the third and eighth postoperative day. However, in time, the small bowel typically adapts and there is a steady decrease in ostomy output. However, patients with an ileostomy, particularly those who have had concomitant small bowel resection, remain at risk to become dehydrated. Most often, this is easily managed by oral rehydration with one of the commonly available sports drinks. However, patients who have lost considerable absorptive surface because of previous bowel resection and/or those with recurrent/residual active Crohn's disease are at particular risk. In addition to the loss of absorptive surface area, ileal resection also removes the fat or complex carbohydrate stimulation of the so-called "ileal brake" which slows gastric emptying and small bowel transit.[9] Fluid and electrolyte maintenance in these patients may require a period of parenteral hydration and nutrition. Elements of the diet can augment output and should be avoided in marginal cases. These might include foods high in sugar, salt, or fat.

Ileostomy diarrhea may be treated in its milder forms with fiber supplements or cholestyramine which can thicken secretions, but not change water content. Often opiates may be required to slow intestinal transit. In refractory cases, somatostatin analog has been used with some success. Somatostatin reduces salt and water excretion and slows gastrointestinal tract motility. However, its clinical usage has met with variable results.[10,11] Special mention is made of patients with a proximal ostomy required to treat complications of an anastomotic leak. Good results have been reported with exteriorizing the leak and reinfusing the ostomy effluent into the downstream limb until gastrointestinal continuity can be restored. This has led to weaning parenteral nutrition in a substantial number of patients.[12]

Nephrolithiasis

A related problem in patients with an ileostomy is the development of urinary stones. The obligatory loss of fecal water, sodium, and bicarbonate reduces urinary pH and volume.[13] Whereas approximately 4% of the general population develops urinary stones, the incidence in patients with an ileostomy is approximately twice that. Whereas uric acid stones comprise less than 10% of the calculi in the general population, they comprise 60% of stones in ileostomy patients. There is also an increase in the incidence of calcium oxalate stones,[14] and as a result, foods high in oxalate, such as spinach, should be avoided by ileostomates.

Bowel Obstruction

Life table analyses suggest that bowel obstruction is a rather common complication of ostomy creation. As many as 23% of patients with an ileostomy have been reported to develop bowel obstruction. Adhesions are probably the most common cause, but small bowel volvulus or internal hernia may also be the cause. Although it is frequently mentioned that suture of the mesentery to the lateral abdominal wall may prevent volvulus or obstruction, retrospective analyses have not shown any benefit to this maneuver. Treatment is not dissimilar to other patients presenting with a mechanical small bowel obstruction.

However, special note must be made of food bolus obstruction. Many patients with an ileostomy will develop signs and symptoms of bowel obstruction because of the accumulation of poorly masticated or digested food (e.g., popcorn, peanuts, fresh fruits, meat, and vegetables). A careful history may reveal dietary indiscretions. Furthermore, the possibility of a food bolus obstruction should be considered in any patient with an ileostomy who has radiologic evidence of a distal obstruction. A well-lubricated finger can be gently inserted into the stoma to feel for impacted material. A red rubber catheter is inserted gently into the ostomy and saline irrigation initiated. If suspicious concretions begin to pass into the stoma, the irrigations may be carefully repeated until the obstruction is relieved. A water-soluble contrast enema through the obstructed stoma may also be both diagnostic and therapeutic by dislodging the bolus.

Ischemia

Edema and venous congestion are very common after stoma creation because of mechanical trauma and compression of the small mesenteric venules as they traverse the abdominal wall. This is typically self-limiting and requires no treatment. However, stomal ischemia (Figure 45-3) is more serious and often related to tension on the mesentery or excessive mesenteric division, particularly in obese patients. A stoma of questionable viability may be examined by insertion of a glass test tube or flexible endoscope into the stoma. If the stoma is viable at fascial level, then the patient may be carefully observed. However, if there is question about the viability of the stoma at fascial level, immediate laparotomy and stoma revision is required. Early ischemia is seen in 1%–10% of colostomies and 1%–5% of ileostomies.[15] Stomas do not get better once the patient is awake, but generally only get worse in the early postoperative period. Every effort must be made at construction of the original stoma to make one of perfect-appearing viability, assuring good blood flow in and out to the skin. It never takes as long to do this as it does to manage an ischemic or necrotic stoma.

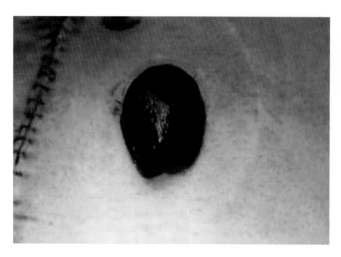

FIGURE 45-3. Stomal ischemia.

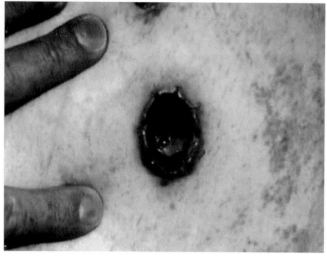

FIGURE 45-4. Stomal retraction.

Late Hemorrhage

Late stomal bleeding may be caused by direct trauma, but heavy bleeding is, especially from an ileostomy, caused by portal hypertension and the development of stoma varices. Many therapies have been described for this, but none subjected to rigorous clinical trials. Correction of coagulopathy and direct pressure are important first steps. Whether direct treatment by injection sclerotherapy or systemic treatment by some form of porto-systemic shunt provides better short- and long-term outcome is undecided. The placement of a transhepatic intrahepatic portal shunt (TIPS) is a nonoperative alternative that should be considered. Ostomy revision does not provide a lasting solution.

Surgical Complications

Surgical complications of intestinal stoma formation can broadly be divided into those that occur early, those that occur long (late) after their construction, and those that occur at stoma closure. Early complications of stoma construction include necrosis, retraction (Figure 45-4), skin irritation, small bowel obstruction, surgical wound infection, and sepsis. Late complications are dominated by prolapse (Figure 45-5), peristomal hernia, skin irritation, and fecal fistula. Closure-related complications include surgical wound infection, fecal fistula, anastomotic dehiscence, small bowel obstruction, and incisional (peristomal) hernia (Figure 45-6).

The prevention and management of each of these complications are best assessed in randomized, controlled clinical trials. A total of 18 randomized trials have been performed in some way related to stoma construction[16–32] (Table 45-1). The most common study design has been randomization of patients to receive either temporary loop colostomy or loop ileostomy, then following these patients for various complications.[16–20] The operations for which these stomas were done were either low anterior resection for carcinoma or a mixture of colonic procedures related to both cancer and diverticular disease. Table 45-2 shows a metaanalysis of each of the complications that have been assessed in some or all of these publications. These analyses show that the only significant difference between the two stoma locations was an increased risk of stoma prolapse associated with loop colostomy. In the other cases, there was no significant difference in the risk of complications listed in Table 45-1. Statistical heterogeneity did not exist for any of these calculations, validating the metaanalysis. The risk of overall complication is perhaps less in all these studies because these were temporary stomas. A much more thorough metaanalysis has recently been published.[33]

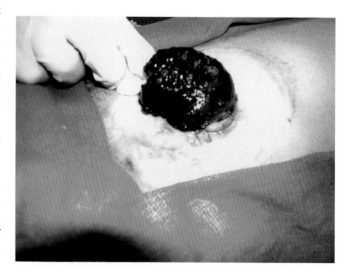

FIGURE 45-5. Stomal prolapse.

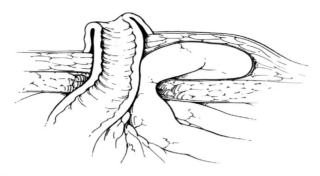

FIGURE 45-6. Peristomal hernia.

Stoma Closure

Looking at the other end of a stoma's history, there are two randomized trials that compared stapled anastomosis to hand-sewn anastomosis during stoma closure, the first in patients who had an ileostomy closure after ileo pouch anal reconstruction[21] and the second in a more mixed group of surgical patients.[22] The only complication cataloged in both trials was the risk of small bowel obstruction subsequent to closure. The risk of obstruction was significantly less in the metaanalysis in patients having stapled closures as opposed to hand-sewn (Table 45-2). There was also no statistical heterogeneity in this analysis. Time to flatus was reported to be less among the stapled closure patients in the first trial, although length of hospital stay was equivalent in both studies. In the second trial, the risk of fecal fistula and surgical wound infection was slightly lower among those patients having a stapled closure.

It is common practice to wait a minimum of 1.5–3 months before closing an intestinal stoma after its construction. This practice was assessed in a randomized trial related to trauma laparotomy patients having temporary colostomies. Patients were randomized to either early or late stoma closure. The average length of time for closure in the early group was 11.8 days and in the late group 104.8 days.[23] There was no overall difference in complications between these two groups, nor individually for fecal fistula, small bowel obstruction, or surgical wound infection. The last six trials listed in Table 45-1 compared either patients getting a stoma with patients not getting a stoma or various types of stoma construction and resection in complicated large bowel obstruction. Unfortunately, stoma-related complications were not reported in any of these trials.

Parastomal Hernia

Regarding surgical management of each of the complications listed in Table 45-1, there are regrettably no informative randomized trials. There are many case reports and case series, but these are seldom presented with the comparison group that allowed quantitative assessment of the efficacy of the procedures being described. Therefore, opinion concerning the treatment of prolapse, hernia, retraction, or necrosis is anecdotal and not evidence based.

The difficulty in choosing the right therapeutic approach is best described in a thorough review by Carne et al.[34] of parastomal hernia, a condition that is a useful surrogate for all the other stoma-related complications. In that review, incidence of hernia is described to occur in anywhere from 0% to 48.1% of individuals. Much of this variation is clearly attributable to definition, because some herniation (similar to some degree of hemorrhoids) can be seen in many patients, whereas more conservative observers would only describe a hernia that prevents the patient either from maintaining the appliance over their stoma or one that causes obstructive symptoms. The risk of recurrence is also well discussed in this review. It is found to be so prohibitively high that it seems best to be conservative in undertaking operative repair, limiting surgery only to those most symptomatic patients.

Prevention of parastomal hernia includes discussion of the following parameters: the site of the stoma related to the rectus muscle, the size of the abdominal aperture, the use of prophylactic mesh implantation at various levels in the abdominal wall, transperitoneal versus extraperitoneal tunneling of the stoma, and fixation of the stoma to the abdominal fascia. Of interest in this review is that there are six cited studies that have examined whether or not a stoma should be placed lateral to the rectus border to prevent hernia. Most authors found that it made no difference.

The prophylactic use of mesh wrapped around the stoma has in fact been subjected to one randomized trial in patients getting permanent intestinal stomas.[25] Among 54 patients, none with the mesh developed hernia, whereas 8 of 27 without mesh did. There was no small bowel obstruction in any of these patients. Other case series of prophylactic mesh use have described both stomal stenosis and erosion and infections related to mesh placement, which have tended to make this not a very popular technique.

The options available for repair of parastomal hernia include direct local tissue repair, resiting of the intestinal stoma with closure of the primary aperture, and the application of mesh around the stoma at various levels within the abdominal wall. Once again there are no randomized trials comparing any of these techniques. Three techniques, colon fascia repair, mesh, and relocation in a small series were assessed in a nonrandomized trial. Surgical wound infection was more common when mesh repair was used and recurrent hernia much more common when there was just direct fascial repair around the stoma.[35]

All of the operations that have been described to repair parastomal hernia can be applied to patients with prolapse, retraction, and skin irritation associated with flush ileostomy. In addition, for patients with prolapse, local amputation and reanastomosis can be used, often with low morbidity. The best operation to perform in individuals having significant complications is closure of the stoma and restoration of intestinal continuity. This should be done whenever possible.

TABLE 45-1. Randomized, controlled trials related to intestinal stomas

Author, reference, operation	RCT?	Group 1 (N)	Group 2 (N)	Prolapse (group 1/group 2)	Stomal hernia	Fecal fistula	Retraction
Edwards et al.,[16] LAR	Yes	Loop colostomy, 36	Loop ileostomy, 34	2/0	2/0	1/0	
Law et al.,[17] LAR	Yes	LC, 39	LI, 39	3/0	0/1		0/0
Gooszen et al.,[18] mix	Yes	LC, 39	LI, 37	16/1	0/2	2/1	1/4
Khoury et al.,[19] mix	Yes	LC, 29	LI, 32			1/1	
Williams et al.,[20] mix	Yes	LC, 24	LI, 23	2/0			
Hull et al.,[21] IPAA	Yes	Stapled closure, 31	Sewn closure, 30			0/2	
Hasegawa et al.,[22] mix	Yes	St., 70	Sewn, 70			1/1	
Velhamos et al.,[23] trauma lap. closure	Yes	Early, 18 × = 11.8 d	Late, 20, 104.8 d				
Berne et al.,[24] mix	Yes	Skin open after stoma closure, 38	Skin closed, 38				
Janes et al.,[25] permanent stomas	Yes	Mesh to prevent hernia, 27	No mesh, 27		0/8		
Tang et al.[26] #1, LAR	Yes	Adhesion barrier around stoma, 51	No barrier, 54				5/3
Tang et al.[26] #2, LAR	Yes	Barrier, 34	No barrier, 36				1/1
Grobler et al.,[27] IPAA	Yes	Loop ileostomy, 23	No stoma, 22				
Graffner et al.,[28] LAR	Yes	Loop col., 25	No stoma, 25			1/3	
Xinopooulos et al.,[29] large bowel obstruction	Yes	Stent, 15	Stoma, 15				
Fiori et al.,[30] LBO	Yes	Stent, 11	Stoma, 11				
Kronborg,[31] LBO	Yes	3 stage	2 stage				
Zeitoun et al.,[32] divertic.	Yes	Primary resect., 55	Secondary resect., 50				

RCT, randomized, controlled trial; LAR, low anterior resection of the rectum with anastomosis; IPAA, total colectomy with ileal pouch anal reconstruction.

Sepsis	Small bowel obstruction	Surgical wound infection	Time to flatus	Death	Incisional hernia	Skin irritation	Length of stay	Comment
	1/0	2/1	2/2		5/0			
2/1	1/3	2/1	3/2			7/4		
1/2						9/11		
	3/2	2/3						
	2/2	8/3				7/3		
	1/2		1.7/2.2				Equal	
	2/10	6/7					8/10	
	1/0	3/2						
		3/1 + 1 for subq drained group						
	0/0							
	5/4					3/3		Variable closure Times
	2/2					2/2		Uniform Closure time
							28/60	
			1/3 days	0/0				
								Both had Stomas
			12/9					

TABLE 45-2. Metaanalysis of similar studies; odds ratios, 95% confidence intervals, and *P* value for heterogeneity

Comparison groups	Prolapse	Stomal hernia	Fecal fistula	Retraction	Sepsis	Small bowel obstruction	Surgical wound infection	Time to flatus	Skin irritation
Loop ileostomy and loop colostomy	10.72 2.79–41.22 0.78	0.68 0.09–5.16 0.28	1.79 0.36–8.9 0.9	0.39 0.07–2.27 0.40	0.97 0.17–5.48 0.40	1.04 0.34–3.17 0.64	1.89 0.72–4.94 0.66	1.23 0.32–4.81 0.72	1.35 0.59–3.09 0.27
Stapled and sewn ileostomy closure						0.23 0.06–0.87 0.51			
Stoma wrap in an adhesion barrier			1.64 0.94–6.09 0.73			1.26 0.40–3.9 0.84			

Conclusions

In conclusion, none of the risk factors listed for stoma complications at the beginning of this chapter (obesity, emergent construction, diabetes, Crohn's disease, ischemic colitis) are actually within the control of the operating surgeon except for the role that an enterostomal nurse has in preoperative assessment of stoma patients. Second, in choosing the type of intestinal stoma to perform, the retrospective studies and randomized study often conflict. Ileostomy would seem to be more at risk for complication than the case series,[1] yet loop colostomy clearly is associated at least with increased risk of prolapse in the randomized trials.[6–10]

Randomized clinical trials are difficult to perform. They are expensive, they take a great deal of time and effort, and recruitment of participants is often painfully difficult. But this study design is the most valid means of determining the efficacy of any therapeutic intervention. Table 45-1 demonstrates the feasibility of doing randomized trials in a number of clinical settings related to intestinal stomas. Yet relating to the treatment of complications of intestinal stomas (not their initial construction) there are none. There are enough individuals that have intestinal stomas and enough surgeons who need to know how to prevent these very prevalent complications to answer all of the unanswered questions related to stoma complications.

References

1. Park JJ, del Pino A, Orsay CP, et al. Stoma complications. Dis Colon Rectum 1999;42:1575–1580.
2. Cheung MT. Complications of an abdominal stoma: an analysis of 322 stomas. Aust NZ J Surg 1995;65:808–811.
3. Leenen LPH, Kuypers JHC. Some factors influencing the outcome of stoma surgery. Dis Colon Rectum 1989;32:500–504.
4. Duchesne JC, Wang YZ, Weintraub SL, Boyle M, Hunt JP. Stoma complications: a multivariate analysis. Am Surg 2002;68:961–966.
5. Arumugam PJ, Bevan L, Macdonald L, Watkins AJ, et al. A prospective audit of stomas—analysis of risk factors and complications and their management. Colorectal Dis 2003;5:49–52.
6. Tang CL, Yunos A, Leong AP, et al. Ileostomy output in the early postoperative period. Br J Surg 1995;82:607.
7. Nugent KP, Daniels P, Stewart B, et al. Quality of life in stoma patients. Dis Colon Rectum 1999;42:1569–1574.
8. Leenen LPH, Kuypers JH. Some factors influencing the outcome of stoma surgery. Dis Colon Rectum 1989;32:500–504.
9. Nehra V, Camilleri M, Burton D, et al. An open trial of octreotide long-acting release in the management of short bowel syndrome. Am J Gastroenterol 2001;96:1494–1498.
10. Szilagyi A, Shrier I. Systematic review: the use of somatostatin or octreotide in refractory diarrhea. Aliment Pharmacol Ther 2003;15:1889–1897.
11. Cooper JC, Williams NS, King RFGJ, et al. Effects of a long-acting somatostatin analogue in patients with severe ileostomy diarrhea. Br J Surg 1986;73:128–131.
12. Calicis B, Parc Y, Caplin S, et al. Treatment of postoperative peritonitis of small bowel origin with continuous enteral nutrition and succus entereus reinfusion. Arch Surg 2002;137:296–300.
13. Christie PM, Knight GS, Hill GL. Comparison of relative risks of urinary stone formation after surgery for ulcerative colitis: conventional ileostomy vs. J-pouch. A comparative study. Dis Colon Rectum 1996;39:50–54.
14. Christie PM, Knight GS, Hill GL. Metabolism of body water and electrolytes after surgery for ulcerative colitis: conventional ileostomy versus J-pouch. Br J Surg 1990;77:149–151.
15. Shellito PC. Complications of abdominal stoma surgery. Dis Colon Rectum 1998;41:1562–1572.
16. Edwards DP, Leppingon-Clarke A, Sexton R, Heald RJ, Moran BJ. Stoma related complications are more frequent after transverse colostomy than loop ileostomy: a prospective randomized clinical trial. Br J Surg 2001;88:360–363.
17. Law WL, Chu KW, Choi HK. Randomized clinical trial comparing loop ileostomy and loop transverse colostomy for faecal diversion following total mesorectal excision. Br J Surg 2002;89:704–708.
18. Gooszen AW, Geelkeertten RH, Hermans J, Lagaay MB, Gooszen HG. Temporary decompression after colorectal surgery: randomized comparison of loop ileostomy and loop colostomy. Br J Surg 1998;85:76–79.
19. Khoury GA, Lewis MCA, Meleagros L, Lewis AAM. Colostomy or ileostomy after colorectal anastomosis? A randomized trial. Ann R Coll Surg Engl 1986;68:5–7.
20. Williams NS, Nasmyth DG, Jones D, Smith AH. Defunctioning stomas: a prospective controlled trial comparing loop ileostomy with loop transverse colostomy. Br J Surg 1986;73:566–570.
21. Hull TL, Kobe I, Fazio VW. Comparison of handsewn and stapled loop ileostomy closures. Dis Colon Rectum 1996;9:1086–1089.
22. Hasegawa H, Radley S, Morton DG, Keighley MRB. Stapled versus sutured closure of loop ileostomy. Ann Surg 2000;231:202–205.
23. Velhamos GC, Degiannis E, Wells M, Souter I, Saadia R. Early closure of colostomies in trauma patients—a prospective randomized trial. Surgery 1995;118:815–820.
24. Berne TV, Griffith CN, Hill J, LoGuidice P. Colostomy wound closure. Arch Surg 1985;120:957–959.
25. Janes A, Cengiz Y, Israelsson LA. Randomized clinical trial of the use of a prosthetic mesh to prevent parastomal hernia. Br J Surg 2004;91:280–282.
26. Tang CL, Seow-Chen F, Fook-Chong S, Eu KW. Bioresorbable adhesion barrier facilitates early closure of the defunctioning ileostomy after rectal resection. Dis Colon Rectum 2003;46:1200–1207.
27. Grobler SP, Hosie KB, Keighley MRB. Randomized trial of loop ileostomy in restorative proctocolectomy. Br J Surg 1992;79:903–906.
28. Graffner H, Fredlund P, Olsson SA, Oscarsson J, Petersson BF. Protective colostomy in low anterior resection off the rectum using the EEA stapling instrument: a randomized study. Dis Colon Rectum 1983;26:87–90.
29. Xinopoulos D, Dimitroulopoulos D, Theodosopoulos T, et al. Stenting or stoma creation for patients with inoperable malignant

obstructions? Results of a study and cost-effectiveness analysis. Surg Endosc 2004;18:421–426.

30. Fiori E, Lamazza A, de Cesare A, Bononi M, et al. Palliative management of malignant rectosigmoid obstruction. Colostomy vs. stenting. A randomized prospective trial. Anticancer Res 2004;24:265–268.

31. Kronborg O. Acute obstruction from tumour in the left colon without spread: a randomized trial of emergency colostomy versus resection. Colorectal Dis 1995;10:1–5.

32. Zeitoun G, Laurent A, Rouffet F, et al. Multicenter randomized clinical trial of primary versus secondary sigmoid resection in generalized peritonitis complicating sigmoid diverticulitis. Br J Surg 2000;87:1366–1374.

33. Lertsithichai P, Rattanapichart P. Temporary ileostomy versus temporary colostomy: a meta-analysis of complications. Asian J Surg 2004;27:202–210.

34. Carne PWG, Robertson GM, Frizelle FA. Parastomal hernia. Br J Surg 2003;90:784–793.

35. Rubin MS, Schoetz DJ, Matthews JB. Parastomal hernia: is stomal relocation superior to fascial repair. Arch Surg 1994;129:413–419.

46
Incontinence

Cornelius G. Baeten and Han C. Kuijpers

Fecal incontinence is the inability to control feces and to expel it at a proper place and at a proper time. To understand incontinence it is good to know how humans are able to be continent. Many factors contribute to the ability to control feces.[1] The consistency of the feces is important. Firm stool can be controlled much easier than liquid stool. The peristalsis in rectosigmoid has a role in keeping the rectum empty, for most of the time. This special antiperistaltic movement in the original rectosigmoid explains why patients with low anterior resection often have urgency and difficulties controlling their stool because they miss this part of the bowel. The rectal capacity is important to store feces for some time. A nondistending rectum gives frequent urgency and leads to loss of stool when there is no toilet available. The pelvic floor muscles are of help to form a barrier when they are contracted and help during defecation to open the anus. The internal anal sphincter is consistently contracted and gives a watertight closure of the anal canal with the help of the hemorrhoidal tissue that fills the opening of the anal canal. The sensibility of rectum and anus gives awareness of stool in the distal rectum and activates the contraction of the external sphincter as additional help for the internal sphincter. The central nervous system has to be intact to govern the sensoric input and the motoric output. Malfunction is obvious in small babies whose brain is not developed enough, or in demented people despite a normally functioning anorectal unit. All these factors form a delicate system to keep the human continent. When something goes wrong in one of these factors, it is dependent on the quality of the other factors whether this leads to incontinence. Next to these factors there is also the cultural background that determines whether or not it is embarrassing to lose stool. In Western society it is normal to defecate in a private secluded location. In China, community toilets are very common. In other societies, defecation on demand is very well accepted, for example, in the court of the Roy Soleil in 18th century France. So culture determines whether loss is accepted as normal or not.

Fecal incontinence forms an enormous economic problem for society. In younger people it often means loss of jobs and dependency on social welfare. For older people the costs of admission in a nursing home are high. When patients stay at home and ultimately want to be treated for this condition, the costs are still high. Also, protection with diapers and pads, medication for skin protection, treatment for psychologic depression, and the use of constipating agents may consume a considerable part of medical resources.[2]

Symptoms

Fecal incontinence is a frequent problem but very much underreported because of embarrassment. It is not a diagnosis but a symptom of different causes. It is a socially devastating disorder, which affects at least 2.2% of community-dwelling adults and 45% of nursing home residents.[3] Fecal incontinence forms the most important reason to place patients in a nursing home.

Because of the social stigma surrounding the loss of bowel control, the complaint is often not directly voiced. The patients become so embarrassed that they do not seek medical advice but rather become confined to their homes and are afraid to visit family and friends. Perineal pads are often inefficient and unacceptable. Many suffer from social isolation and loss of self-esteem. The psychologic impact is devastating. They often conceal their problems by complaining of chronic diarrhea, defecation problems, or rectal urgency. Most incontinent patients can be helped, but physicians are poorly informed about treatment options. A thorough history is therefore essential in assessing patients with fecal incontinence.

At first, a precise characterization of what is meant by incontinence should be evaluated. Flatus, involuntary passage of gas, is often the first, sometimes the only, symptom. Increasing degrees of severity involve loss of liquid stools followed by loss of solid feces. Partial incontinence may be defined as uncontrolled passage of gas and/or liquids and complete incontinence as the uncontrolled passage of solid feces.

Soiling is a bothersome disorder characterized by continuous or intermittent liquid anal discharge. It should be differentiated from discharge due to fistulae, proctitis, and prolapse. Patients complain about stains in their underwear. They often wear sanitary napkins or tissues. The discharge causes inflammation of the perineal skin with excoriation, perianal discomfort, burning sensation, and itching. It usually indicates the presence of an impaired internal sphincter function or a solid fecal mass in the rectum.

Pseudoincontinence and encopresis are the involuntary loss of formed, semiformed, or liquid stool associated with functional constipation in a child. Pseudoincontinence is caused by anatomic disorders such as a mega sigmoid or anal stenosis whereas no anatomic abnormalities are found in encopresis. The most common cause of encopresis is functional fecal retention defined by a history of more than 12 weeks of passage of less than two large-diameter bowel movements per week, retentive posturing, and accompanying symptoms such as fecal soiling. Sometimes it is associated with enuresis and urinary tract infection. The persistent fecal incontinence frequently brings ridicule and shame to the affected child.

An assessment of bowel habit is essential. Is there diarrhea, and how often? Irritable bowel syndrome should be excluded. It is a common functional bowel disorder characterized by intermittent abdominal pain and changes in defecation pattern in the absence of other medical conditions with similar presentations. Physical findings and currently available diagnostic tests lack sufficient specificity for clinical use. The diagnosis is based on characteristic clinical findings and the exclusion of other disorders. Episodes of diarrhea and constipation alternate. Incontinence often occurs as a consequence of diarrhea.

Urgency refers to patients with a need to defecate immediately at the risk of incontinence when facilities are absent. It is seen in patients with impaired rectal compliance as in proctitis or after low anterior resection, or with impaired sphincter function. Assessment of the severity of incontinence is important. Details of frequency, stool consistency, and frequency of defecation should be evaluated. An incontinence score may be helpful in this. The severity of incontinence can be described in scores of the many incontinence-scoring lists. The most used scoring lists at the moment are the Vaisey and the Wexner index.[4] They give not only a value for the loss of gas, liquid, and solid stool, but also for the impact on daily life. Almost all severity indexes score on the frequency of loss of gas liquid and solids. Many patients change their lifestyle and stay at home, close to the toilet. This means an underestimation of the frequency of loss of feces. It is possible, in the extreme, that they do not lose anything and are considered continent despite their complaints.

The best way to get information is a combination of severity index, special quality of life questionnaires (FIQOL) developed by the American Society of Colon and Rectal Surgeons and anamnesis. Is there passage of stool without the patient being aware of it or is he aware but unable to control it? Is there a regular use of laxatives or other medications that promote diarrhea or constipation (fecal impaction)? A sexual history should be obtained. Regular anal sex leads to internal sphincter dilatation and soiling. A careful obstetric history should be taken noting multiparity, forceps assistance, difficult childbirth and perineal tears. Specific inquiry should be made concerning perineal trauma and anorectal surgery. Previous prolapse surgery, urinary incontinence, and the presence of prolapses should be noted because they often occur in pelvic floor denervation. A history of neurologic disorders is essential. The presence of central nervous system disorders, peripheral neuropathy, low back injury, and diabetes mellitus should be established. Is the patient immobilized or bedridden? A history of large or small bowel resection, pelvic irradiation, or inflammatory bowel disease should be recorded.

Causes of Incontinence

Congenital

Anorectal anomalies represent a spectrum of defects. The anal canal is often absent. Most patients have different degrees of development of the pelvic muscle structures and consequently different degrees of rectal proprioception. There may be rectal communication with the urinary tract or vagina. A significant number of these children suffer from fecal and urinary incontinence, and sexual inadequacy. Patients with low forms of anorectal agenesis have little impairment in continence after early surgery whereas patients with high defects affecting the pelvic floor, the rectum, and urogenital tract, are usually incontinent. The various operative procedures depend on the type of deformity. The ultimate goal is to create a perineal opening with adequate sensory and motor control. They are a continuing challenge for the pediatric surgeon. Control of defecation after surgical correction of high and intermediate types of congenital anorectal malformations is difficult. Most adults with high anorectal malformations who have undergone abdominoperineal or direct perineal repair have severely defective fecal continence and poor quality of life.[5] Major advances in the management of these children have occurred during the last 10 years. The posterior sagittal approach has led to a better understanding of the internal anatomy of these defects, and a more rational way to manage the patients. Voluntary bowel movements are achieved in 75% with occasional soiling in 40%. Common sequelae are constipation and urinary incontinence after the repair of cloacas. Fecal incontinence occurs in 25% but can adequately be managed by bowel management programs.[6] These results are not generally accepted; some state that the posterior sagittal approach for high and intermediate anorectal malformations does not give better functional results than the pullthrough operation. The presence or absence of sacral defects has a role in the prognosis.[7] A detailed explanation of the operative technique is beyond the scope of this chapter.

Fecal incontinence is common in patients with spinal cord lesions such as spina bifida and meningomyelocele. Constipation is another major stigma. The congenital defects in the lumbosacral spine disturb the sensory and motor nerves supplying the skin and pelvic floor muscle. The sensory and motoric functions are impaired or absent, compromising the dynamics of continence. Frequently, colonic motility is delayed and pudendal neuropathy is always present. Rectal sensation is reduced and anal squeeze pressure impaired or absent.

Pelvic Floor Denervation

The pelvic floor muscle is innervated by the pudendal nerves and by the S3 and S4 branches of the pelvic plexus. Intense and recurrent straining, as in difficult childbirth and constipation may lead to stretch-induced injury of the pelvic floor innervation, especially the pudendal nerves. Irreversible injury occurs when nerves are stretched as little as 12%. Histologic studies of the pelvic floor muscles in these cases reveal changes consistent with denervation and reinnervation, in the most abnormal showing only a few remaining fibers with myopathic features scattered in a matrix of fibrous tissue.[8] This muscle fiber loss is associated with weakness of the pelvic floor and with incontinence.

Similar manometric and electromyographic features have been found in normal elderly women and men suggesting a normal age-related denervation with a compensatory reinnervation of the pelvic floor muscle. Although increased pudendal nerve terminal motor latency may indicate that neuropathy is present, normal pudendal nerve terminal motor latency does not exclude weakness of the pelvic floor.[9]

Obstetric

There are two ways by which vaginal delivery may damage the pelvic floor and anal sphincters. The first one is direct mechanical tear of the anal sphincters, a serious complication of childbirth. The incidence of obstetric tears varies from 0.6% to 9%.[10,11] Occult injuries, visualized by endoanal ultrasonography, have been reported in 20%–35%.[12,13] Defects of the external anal sphincter have traditionally been diagnosed by palpation and electromyography but anal endosonography enables clear imaging of both the internal and external sphincter muscles. Factors that affect the risk for developing obstetric tears are use of forceps, mediolateral episiotomy, and primiparity.[14,15] Sixty percent of patients with an obstetric tear also have evidence of pudendal nerve damage.[16,17] The other mechanism is pelvic floor denervation resulting from compression or traction injury to the pudendal nerves during vaginal delivery, particularly when it is prolonged or requires forceps assistance. Birth weight also correlates. Assessment of pudendal nerve function is important in women with postpartum fecal incontinence because it can influence treatment options.[18]

Iatrogenic

Fecal incontinence is a frequently neglected but rather common complication of anorectal surgery. The incidence increases to 30%–50% after partial internal sphincterotomy[19,20] and fistulotomy[21–24] with soiling being the most common complaint occurring in 35%–45%. Local sphincter lesions and intraanal scarring (keyhole deformity) are not the sole explanation for the high incidence of incontinence because it also occurs after non-muscle-cutting anorectal surgery such as anal stretch,[25] hemorrhoidectomy,[26] and transanal advancement flaps.[27–30] The internal anal sphincter is easily damaged with an anal retractor used to gain access to the anal canal and lower rectum. This excessive dilatation of the anal canal results in a serious damage of the internal sphincter resulting in a decrease of resting pressure. The Park's anal retractor is especially, notorious for this.[31,32]

Low anterior resection compromises anorectal function. Postoperative continence is even poorer after radiochemotherapy.[33] Anal sphincter function is preserved but neorectal capacity, maximum tolerable volume, and rectal compliance are reduced resulting in an increased stool frequency, and episodes of incontinence and soiling.[34,35] Colonic pouch construction has gained increasing popularity in reconstruction after low anterior resection because it offers superior long-term function compared with low straight or side-to-end colorectal anastomosis.[36,37]

Traumatic

Fecal incontinence caused by trauma is uncommon. Causes include military or traffic accidents complicated by pelvic fractures, spine injuries or perineal lacerations, insertion of foreign bodies in the rectum, and sexual abuse. There is often extended destruction of the sphincter complex and pelvic floor complicated by pelvic nerve injury. Immediate recognition is vital to a successful outcome and may obviate the need for a diverting stoma. Evaluation must include a search for involvement of other structures and an evaluation of the anal sphincters. Foreign bodies most often do not cause significant anorectal injuries. Extraction of these diverse objects requires ingenuity. Superficial injuries may be left open or sutured closed.[38] Anal intercourse is associated with reduced resting pressure in the anal canal and an increased risk of anal incontinence.[39]

Radiation

More than three-quarters of patients receiving pelvic radiotherapy experience acute anorectal symptoms and up to one-fifth experience late-phase radiation proctitis. Many of these symptoms are self-limiting, and mucosal complications may often be treated by nonsurgical methods such as topical formalin application, endoscopic argon plasma coagulation, and hyperbaric oxygen therapy. Approximately 5% develop other chronic complications, such as fistula, stricture, and disabling fecal incontinence.[40] Structural abnormalities and septic complications are likely to require surgery. Varying degrees of destruction of the muscular components of the rectum and anal canal occur leading to muscle damage and radiation enteritis. Causes of radiation-induced incontinence are proctosigmoiditis, small bowel injury, fistula formation, reduced rectal capacity, diminished internal and external sphincter function, and rectal mucosal sensitivity.[41–43] These are the results of progressive changes in the connective tissues and vasculature resulting in fibrosis, ulceration, stricture, and fistula formation. Conservative treatment options are of limited value. Surgery may be considered if symptoms are severe, provided sphincter function is adequate and recurrent disease is excluded. When the condition becomes intolerable, colostomy is the last resource. Symptoms progress over time. Large prospective studies with accurate dosimetric data and long-term follow-up are needed to provide meaningful information on which to base new strategies to minimize the side effects from radiotherapy. Modern techniques in the delivery of radiotherapy will help minimize the likelihood of rectal complications.

Physical Examination

Clinical examination is of paramount importance in the evaluation and management of incontinent patients. It should enable the physician to derive an appropriate strategy of treatment. Routine abdominal examination should be performed. The presence of scars should be noted. Neurologic assessment should be done when there is suspicion of neurologic disorders. At first, the physician should explain to the patient what to expect during the examination in an effort to allay embarrassment and anxieties. Observation should be made of whether the patient wears a pad or whether there are signs of fecal soiling on the underwear. Several positions may be used for anorectal examination. For patient comfort, the left-lateral position may be preferred above the knee-chest position. The kneeling prone-jackknife position gives the best exposure. Inspection of the perineum may reveal perineal soiling, excoriation, a patulous anus, an ectropion, a keyhole deformity, or other anal deformities. The physician should inspect for evidence of scars from previous operations or trauma, fistulas, hemorrhoids, or prolapse. The perineum should also be inspected while the patient is bearing down to observe for mucosal or complete rectal prolapse. Perineal descent is present when the perineum balloons during straining. It is a physical sign of weakness of the pelvic floor and is often seen in the descending perineum syndrome and pelvic floor denervation. The most prevalent abnormality of descending

perineum syndrome on testing is perineal descent >4 cm.[44] Digital rectal examination should assess the degree of anal resting tone, a function of the internal sphincter. Anal scars should be palpated to determine if it is soft or whether there is induration suggestive of residual inflammation. Normally the anal canal is closed snugly around the examining finger. Decreased tone may be noted if there is a rectal prolapse, a history of previous anorectal surgery, fecal incontinence, or repeated anal intercourse.

The increase of anal tone during squeezing, a function of the external sphincter, should also be noted. Digital estimation by an experienced examiner is equally as good as assessment of anal sphincter function with anal manometry.[45] It is a poor predictor of exact canal pressure but a patulous anus can easily be discriminated from an actively contracting sphincter. Anal manometry provides more objective data. Simple lateral retraction of the buttocks or downward pulling of the puborectalis are other methods to reveal a patulous anus. Digital examination of the vagina should be performed to check for vaginal prolapse, rectoceles, cystoceles, or enteroceles. An impaired sphincter tone during bearing down is found in incontinence and descending perineum syndrome. The sphincter complex and perineal body can be assessed by bidigital anovaginal examination (the thumb in the vagina and the index finger in the anorectum). An empty and destroyed anterior perineal body is suggestive for an obstetric sphincter lesion. The puborectalis muscle can be palpated bilaterally and posteriorly as a prominent sling passing around the rectum thus creating the anorectal angle that is normally 90°. During bearing down, the dorsal transverse bar should flatten out as a sign of pelvic floor relaxation. Paradoxic contraction suggests anismus. Inserting the index finger into the rectum and pushing the anterior wall forward and downward into the vagina can demonstrate a rectocele. Impacted feces can be felt in the lower rectum. When the gloved finger is withdrawn it should be inspected for blood and color of stool. Description of findings should be recorded adequately. The "o'clock" position requires a known patient position; recording in an anatomic manner (anterior, posterior, right, left) is a better alternative.

Anal Manometry

Anorectal manometry includes a number of specific tests that are helpful in the diagnostic assessment of patients with fecal incontinence. It includes resting anal pressure, anal squeeze pressure, the recto anal inhibitory reflex, compliance of the rectum in response to balloon distension, and sensory thresholds in response to balloon distension.[46] The interpretation of these diagnostic tests is complicated by the fact that patients are able to compensate for deficits in specific physiologic mechanisms maintaining continence and defecation by using other biologic and behavioral mechanisms. It gives a reliable, reproducible, and objective assessment of anal sphincter function. Resting pressure represents internal sphincter function whereas squeeze pressure reflects external sphincter function. Many different techniques have been advocated such as water-perfused catheters, closed water- or air-filled balloons, and microtransducers. Each system has its own normal values. Anal pressures in normal individuals have a large range and vary with sex and age: patients with low values may be continent whereas high pressures do not guarantee continence. Squeeze pressures are higher in men than in women. Older patients exhibit lower pressures but a significant age-related difference cannot be demonstrated. Resting and squeeze pressures are lower in incontinent patients than in normals. It does not correlate with the severity of incontinence and neither does it predict postoperative results. Some patients with fecal incontinence are found to have manometric values within the normal range. In these patients, a decrease in rectal adaptation could be causative.[47] Patients with soiling often have normal squeeze pressures but lowered resting pressures.[48,49] Anal manometry is indicated in fecal incontinence to exclude impaired sphincter function as the cause of incontinence and to assess the effects of operative procedures on sphincter functions.

Defecography

Defecography is the radiologic visualization of the act of defecation. It provides a picture of the successive phases of defecation and gives an impression of pelvic floor activity during these actions. Changes in the rectal configuration and the anorectal angle become visible and the degree of evacuation can be studied. It has become evident that it can demonstrate abnormalities that were unsuspected on clinical examination. It has been demonstrated that the anorectal angle is increased in pelvic floor denervation as a sign of pelvic floor weakness. But there is a wide interobserver variation in the measurement of the anorectal angle making quantification an exercise of limited clinical value. The value of defecography in fecal incontinence is to demonstrate the presence of internal rectal intussusception in patients with perineal symptoms or the solitary rectal ulcer syndrome.

Endosonography

Endosonography is a diagnostic tool to investigate the anal sphincters. The most frequently used instruments have a 360° rotating head and work with 7 or 10 MHz. It is possible to see both anal sphincters and to determine their length and width. Atrophy, scar tissue, and also defects in the sphincters can be seen. These endosonograms make it possible to find old ruptures even when there is no marking in the anal skin. Sometimes it is difficult to visualize defects in the perineum of a woman. In these cases, additional vaginal endosonography can be helpful.

Three-dimensional endosonography improves the understanding of the nonexperienced investigators but does not add anything to the diagnostic work-up.

Magnetic Resonance Imaging

Magnetic resonance imaging (MRI) of the pelvic region is an excellent way to visualize the anal canal, lower rectum, and the surrounding tissue of prostate, bladder, and uterus. The MRI can be performed with an endo-coil in the anus and with surface phased array coil.[50-52] The endo-coil has the advantage that the sphincters are better visualized but in an unnatural way. The endo-coil has a diameter of 2 cm and the sphincters are stretched during the investigation. This causes the same problem as with endosonography in which visualization is obtained with an opened sphincter. An MRI without an endo-coil but with a phased array coil gives a view of the natural contracted sphincter. Both methods reveal lesions as well as atrophy of parts of the sphincters.

Pudendal Nerve Latency Time

Pudendal nerve latency time offers the opportunity to evaluate nerve damage to the pelvic floor. It measures the time from an electrical stimulus of the pudendal nerve to the onset of the electrical response in the muscles of the pelvic floor. An easy, painless way of performing this test is with the use of the finger electrode. This electrode is mounted on a glove and contains an electrode at the end of the finger that can be placed intrarectally on the pudendal nerve. A second electrode is located at the base of the finger and registers the anal response. A prolonged latency is taken as evidence of neuropathy.

Sensation Test

The sensation of anus and rectum can be tested with two methods: the anus is extremely sensitive caudal of the dentate line and insensitive proximal of this line. Electrical stimulation of the distal anus and determination of the sensory threshold give an impression of this sensation. The sensitivity of the rectum is studied with inflation of an intrarectal balloon. The minimal volume that is sensed, the first urge sensation, and the maximal tolerable volume are determined. A high threshold of the minimal volume sensed in the rectum is abnormal (usually >20 mL).

Endoscopy

Endoscopy has a limited value for investigation of fecal incontinence. It can exclude some diseases that give diarrhea and mucus production (proctitis, colitis, solitary rectal ulcer, villous adenoma, etc).

Treatment

Conservative Treatment

Nonsurgical treatment is the initial approach to the incontinent patient. It aims at improving continence, quality of life, psychologic well-being, and anal sphincter function. In functional incontinence, the underlying disorder should be treated. Diarrhea is the most common aggravating factor for fecal incontinence. Its cause should be evaluated. Perineal pads are efficient and acceptable for minor incontinence only. The aim of pharmacologic treatment of fecal incontinence is to try to achieve passage of one or two well-formed stools a day. It can be tried with simple constipating agents such as loperamide diphenoxylate, codeine phosphate, or bile acid binders. Many of these suppress the propulsive activity of the small bowel and colon. Bulking agents may improve the consistency of a liquid stool.

Laxative abuse should be stopped. Successful treatment of encopresis, overflow incontinence, or pseudoincontinence requires a combination of parent and child education, behavioral intervention, medical therapy, and long-term compliance with the treatment regimen. After complete evacuation of the impacted rectum, reaccumulation of stool should be prevented by appropriate use of laxatives and well-balanced diets including fibers and fluids followed by gradual weaning of the laxative regimen and instituting toilet training such as regular attempts to defecate and habit training. Surgical treatment can be considered for an anatomic defect in pseudoincontinence such as resection of a megasigmoid.

Dietary advice may help some patients. Patients with the pattern of soiling may be successfully treated with stool bulking agents (e.g., psyllium or bran).[48] An empty rectum is the best prevention of involuntary loss of stool. Glycerine or bisacodyl suppositories and phosphate enemas may be helpful. Daily colonic irrigation is a suitable alternative. Retrograde colonic irrigation can be performed by influx of lukewarm water from a water bag or from a pump. The antegrade continence enema (Malone) procedure has improved the lives of many patients who struggle with intractable forms of constipation or incontinence. The non-refluxing, catheterizable appendicocecostomy provides the opportunity to treat previously therapy-resistant patients to administer large-volume enemas through a right lower quadrant stoma to flush the colon every other day.[53] It works well in patients with incontinence secondary to spinal cord disorders. The technique induces highly effective emptying as demonstrated by scintigraphic techniques whereas the effect of retrograde irrigation is correlated with the extent to which the irrigation fluid has entered the colorectum (normally 1 to 2 L).[54] Dangerous electrolyte abnormalities such as low sodium or hypochloremia are rare but the potential morbidity warrants periodic evaluation.[55] Even patients with soiling seem to benefit from colonic irrigation.[56] It reduces or eliminates soiling in approximately 78% of children with myelomeningocele.[3] When, after several trials of conservative and surgical treatment, a patient remains symptomatic, the anal plug may be offered. It is effective in controlling fecal incontinence and well tolerated in a minority of patients. Evaluation quickly reveals whether the patient will find it an effective and acceptable option.[57]

Biofeedback Treatment

Biofeedback is the use of technology to give the patient better information about specific physiologic activities that are under the control of the nervous system but not clearly or accurately perceived by the patient. The rationale underlying biofeedback assumes that the physiologic activity that is monitored is causally related to a clinical problem and that alteration of that activity can lead to resolution of the problem. Biofeedback is a time-consuming and labor-intensive, but harmless and inexpensive, treatment for fecal incontinence, which benefits approximately 75% of patients but cures only about 50%. It may be most appropriate when there is neurologic injury (i.e., partial denervation), but it has been reported to also benefit incontinent patients with minor structural defects.[3] Fecal incontinence is one of the few indications for which biofeedback is considered to be clinically effective. The technique is designed to improve the threshold of rectal sensation and to coordinate pelvic floor contraction with rectal distension. Rectal sensation seems to be a critically important determinant in achieving success with biofeedback. Appropriate candidates should be motivated and able to understand the procedure, sense the rectal stimulus, and

TABLE 46-1. Algorithm for treatment of fecal incontinence

Consistency	Cause	First choice	Second choice	Third choice
Diarrhea	Inflammatory	Antiinflammatory drugs	Constipating drugs	Colostomy
Pseudodiarrhea	Encopresis	Laxatives	Lavage	Colostomy
Solid	Pelvic floor	Biofeedback	SNS	Colostomy
	Sphincter intact	SNS	Lavage	Colostomy
	Sphincter rupture	Anal repair	SNS/DGP/ABS	Colostomy
	Anal atresia	Lavage	ABS/DGP	Colostomy
	Rectal prolapse	Rectopexy	Perineal resection	Colostomy
Soiling	Keyhole defect	Lavage	PTQ implant	

SNS, sacral nerve stimulation; DGP, dynamic graciloplasty; ABS, artificial bowel sphincter; PTQ, implant silicone particles.

contract the pelvic floor. It is not helpful in patients with profound denervation of the pelvic floor or absence of innervation. Patients with decreased rectal capacity as in proctectomy or proctitis do not respond.[58] Despite the many reports of success with biofeedback, the mechanisms of action remain uncertain. Improvement of external sphincter function is not achieved. It remains uncertain whether biofeedback is more effective than placebo treatment or behavioral treatment.[59] The technique of external sphincter contraction exercises under direct electromyographic vision does not lead to an improvement of external sphincter function either.[60]

Balloon Training

Increasing volumes of water in a rectal balloon can be of help to bring down the threshold of first urge. It is a tool to improve the sensibility of the rectum.

Electrostimulation

Electrostimulation as a treatment for fecal incontinence is widely used among physicians and physiotherapists. It is claimed to improve muscle function and to decrease the susceptibility of the muscle to fatigue. Data to support this claim, however, are lacking. Indications in the literature are widespread or poorly defined and objective manometric data not presented. It can be done by direct implantation of electrodes on the external sphincter or by anal plug stimulation. Some report a decrease of incontinence score, but an improvement in continence and external sphincter function does not occur.[61–63] Electrostimulation is not a clinically effective treatment of anal incontinence.

Operative Treatment

Anal Encirclement Procedures

The anal encirclement procedure, originally described by Thiersch in 1891 for the treatment of complete rectal prolapse, has later been adopted for treatment of fecal incontinence. Different materials have been advised for this procedure including nylon, silk, fascia strips, silver wire, and silastic bands. A static barrier to the passage of feces is thus constructed offering nothing in the way of voluntary control and maintenance of continence. The complication rate is high and a variety of complications have been described such as fecal impaction, infection, wire migration, and perineal discomfort. An indication for this procedure does not exist anymore. Instead, a colostomy should be considered.

Anterior Sphincteroplasty

Patients with incontinence secondary to an obstetric or iatrogenic anterior defect are best suited for surgical correction of fecal incontinence. Fecal diversion is unnecessary because it gives no benefit in terms of wound healing or functional outcome, and it is a source of morbidity.[64] The presence of a rectovaginal fistula is no contraindication. A temporary diverting enterostomy may be constructed when there is a high risk of sepsis or in reoperations. Poor result after adequate sphincter repair is attributed to coexistent pelvic floor denervation.[16,17] Primary sphincter repair is inadequate in most women with obstetric ruptures after vaginal delivery because most have residual sphincter defects and about 50% still experience incontinence.[65–67] A full mechanical bowel preparation is given preoperatively combined with parenteral antibiotics. After insertion of an indwelling bladder catheter, the patient is placed in the prone jackknife position and the buttocks taped apart. A transverse incision is made over the destroyed and empty anterior perineum. Injection of an adrenaline solution may be used to diminish bleeding. The scar tissue is dissected up to the level of the anorectal ring. The anal mucosa is dissected off the internal sphincter and scar tissue after which the fibrous remnant of the sphincter is divided. The scar at the sphincter ends is preserved to anchor the sutures because sutures are less likely to tear out from fibrous tissue than healthy muscle. The ends of the mobilized external sphincter are snugly overlapped and sutured together with absorbable mattress sutures. Dissection should not go further laterally than half the circumference of the anal canal allowing an overlap of 1.5 cm, in order to avoid damaging the nerve supply to the external sphincter entering posterolaterally. Outcome after end-to-end repair is somewhat inferior to overlapping repair whereas overlapping repair might be associated with more evacuation difficulties.[68] The advantage of dissection and separate repair of the internal and external anal sphincter is not clear. When the perineal body is absent, an anterior levatorplasty may be performed by approximating the inner fibers of the puborectalis limbs with 3–4 interrupted sutures at the deepest portion of the perineal dissection. The mucosa is sutured to the skin edge to avoid retraction. Wound closure should be performed in a V-Y manner to increase the anovaginal distance. The central portion of the wound is left open for drainage or closed and a suction drain left in the perineum. Packing should not be used. Sitz baths are recommended to optimize perianal hygiene. A normal diet is permitted from the first day. Laxatives are prescribed for 2–3 weeks to avoid hard stool. Defecation is earlier and less painful whereas functional outcome is not different compared with bowel confinement regime.[69] The perineal wound is usually closed in 4–6 weeks. Good functional results are usually obtained in 50%–80% but seem to deteriorate with time. Continence is rarely perfect and many have residual symptoms. Some may develop new evacuation problems.[70] The most important factor in the return to normal sphincter function is an increase in squeeze pressure.[71] Poor outcome is usually associated with pelvic floor denervation or a residual sphincter defect.[65] Repeat anterior repair is advocated for symptomatic residual defects.[72,73] Repair of laterally and posteriorly placed injuries is less successful. Results of internal sphincter repair are poor. The defects usually persist as shown by ultrasonography, and functional and clinical findings are disappointing.[74,75] Transsphincteric injection of silicone biomaterial can provide a marked improvement in fecal incontinence related to a weak or disrupted internal anal sphincter. This is associated with improved sphincter function and quality of life.[76]

Postanal Repair

Postanal repair was originally described by Parks as a method to improve fecal incontinence by restoring the anorectal angle and lengthen the anal canal. The procedure is simple to perform, safe, and requires minimum technology. The principal indication is denervation damage of the pelvic floor. Adequate muscle mass must be present for this operation to be successful. There is no relation between preoperative physiologic assessment and postoperative results; the currently available preoperative testing has not altered the success rate.[77] A full mechanical preoperative bowel preparation or rectal washout should be done combined with parenteral antibiotics. The prone-jackknife position should be preferred. A curved incision is made behind the anus and an anterior skin flap is dissected. The intersphincteric space, an avascular plane between internal and external sphincter, is identified and dissected free up to the upper part of the anal canal where Waldeyer's fascia, a dense fibrous structure, is encountered. Division gives access to the pelvis. The rectum can be dissected free from the levator ani by blunt dissection. A lattice is constructed by plicating the pubococcygeus and, in a second layer, the puborectalis. Additional sutures are placed in the deep and superficial part of the external sphincter. Some prefer nonabsorbable sutures. Part of the skin is left open to prevent sepsis. Laxatives are described and patients are instructed not to strain in the early postoperative period. Complete wound healing usually occurs in 3–4 weeks. The initial results are good; continence for solid stool is restored in 40%–50%. Long-term benefits, however, are only reported by 30%–40% of patients; 30% are not improved at all. The mechanism of restoration of continence is unclear, the anorectal angle is not restored, and external sphincter functions remain far below normal values.[77–80] Despite the low success rate, the absence of any mortality, and the low morbidity, it has a place in the management of fecal incontinence because there are few alternatives. Total pelvic floor repair, a combination of postanal and anterior repair, does not produce consistent changes in anatomy or physiology either. It rarely renders patients completely continent but substantially improves continence and lifestyle in approximately half of them.[81,82] It is likely that improvement after these procedures is caused by creation of a local stenosis or a placebo effect rather than by improvement of muscle function.[81–83] The main indication is incontinence in conjunction with severe pelvic floor descent syndrome. Posterior reconstruction may be replaced by sacral nerve stimulation.

Sacral Nerve Stimulation

Based on the good results of urologists in treating patients with urinary incontinence, colorectal surgeons became interested in this treatment. The first observation was that patients with double incontinence, treated for their urinary incontinence, developed improved fecal control. Matzel began sacral nerve stimulation for fecal incontinence in 1995.[84] This method is now gaining popularity in Europe and is being studied in the United States. The method is very attractive because it offers the opportunity to test the stimulation before the decision for a permanent implant is made. For the test, the patient is placed in the prone position and a needle is brought in the foramen of S3. High-voltage stimulation on the needle gives a contraction of the anus and pelvic floor. It also gives a tingling sensation in the anovaginal region in women and in the anoscrotal region in men. This indicates that the tip of the needle is positioned in the proximity of the third sacral nerve. A test wire is brought through this needle and the needle is withdrawn. The test wire is glued to the skin of the buttock and connected to an external screener. The stimulation starts with a low voltage just above the threshold for sensation and the patient is sent home for a 3-week period. In these 3 weeks the patient keeps a diary with all defecations, urgencies, and incontinence episodes. This can be compared with a similar diary that was written during 3 weeks in the period before the test stimulation. When there is an improvement in continence, an implant may follow in which a permanent electrode is fixed to the sacrum and connected to an implantable stimulator. The average longevity of such a stimulator is 8 years. The stimulator is implanted in the lower abdominal wall or in the buttock. So far it remains unclear how this stimulation works. Probably the proprioceptive fibers are triggered and reflexes suppressed or enhanced. In the literature, an average success rate of approximately 80% is given. The long-term results of the urologists are very good and one may expect a similar result in fecal incontinence. Complications are minimal and mostly related to infection. The best indication for sacral nerve stimulation is fecal incontinence in patients with intact anal sphincters or for patients who had an unsuccessful anal repair in the past.[1,85–88] It seems to work well in patients with neurogenic incontinence. It is currently available only as part of a trial or when placed for urinary incontinence also.

Dynamic Graciloplasty

Patients with a completely destroyed anal sphincter or a large gap between both ends of the sphincters cannot be helped anymore with anal repair. For these patients, dynamic graciloplasty may be a good solution. The gracilis muscle is a long muscle at the medial side of the upper leg. It is an auxiliary muscle for the adductor muscles and can be detached from its insertion without the risk of hampering the adductor function. This muscle can be freed from its insertion up to the neurovascular bundle, folded in the upper leg, and subcutaneously tunneled to the perineum. It is long enough to encircle the anal canal and to be attached to the periosteum of the inferior ramus of the pubic bone. Anatomically, this muscle is probably the best replacement of the destroyed sphincter, but it is intrinsically the worst muscle for sphincter function because of its composition of a minority of type one fibers (long acting, slow twitch) and a majority of type two fibers (short acting, fast twitch). This makes the gracilis a fatigable muscle that only conscientiously contracts by will. With chronic low-frequency stimulation, the gracilis can change its fiber composition and become a nonfatigable muscle that contracts on demand of the stimulator. This is what is necessary for continence: an automatic long-term nonfatigable contraction of the sphincter. The electrical stimulation is given by an implanted stimulator through an intramuscular electrode that is placed very close to the gracilis nerve. The muscle is closed permanently but can be opened by switching off the stimulator with the help of a handheld programmer.[89] Defecation is possible at that moment and with the same programmer the stimulator is switched on and the anus is closed again after the defecation. The results are dependent on the experience of the surgeon and the success rate varies between 40% and 80%. The complication rate of this intervention is high but most problems are treatable without influence on the final result.[90–95] Unfortunately, this has not been approved for use in the United States.

Artificial Bowel Sphincter

An alternative for dynamic graciloplasty is in some cases the artificial bowel sphincter. Instead of autologous muscle, the anus is now encircled with an implantable fluid-filled, silicone elastomer cuff. This cuff is connected by tubings with a control pump and a pressure-regulating balloon. The inflated cuff compresses the anus all the time. By using the control pump situated in the labia or scrotum, the fluid is manually pumped from the cuff toward the balloon. The empty cuff allows passage of stool. The pressure in the balloon presses the fluid back into the cuff through a flow regulator at the pump. The pump is a one-way pump and the fluid can pass the pump passively because of pressure. The operation is easier to perform than graciloplasty, but a disadvantage is the foreign material that has to be placed around the anus. Erosion from the cuff through the anus and the vagina is a common complication.[89,96,97] Operator experience is very important to the successful outcome of the procedure. Continence is excellent when the procedure works.

Colostomy

When conservative and operative treatment has failed to create an acceptable level of continence, the patient is in fact left with a perineal colostomy. An abdominal colostomy may then be offered to the patient as a last alternative but it should be performed only after thorough counseling. The option of a colostomy should be mentioned during the first consultation. It subsequently should be the patient's initiative to start the discussion on colostomy construction after which an appointment is made with the stoma therapist for further counseling. A colostomy is usually well accepted by the patient because it reliably simplifies bowel care and prevents incontinence, and thus clearly improves quality of life. Because mucus production in the excluded rectosigmoid will persist and mucus retention is impossible because of the impaired sphincter function, a continuous drainage of brown-grayish, foul-smelling mucus will occur, wetting and staining the underwear and eroding the perineal skin. It is not acceptable for the fastidious patient who finds that his symptoms persist despite this, reluctantly accepted, stoma. Rectosigmoid resection leaving a rectal stump of 3–4 cm should therefore be added to the procedure. Resection does not completely eliminate mucus secretion but normally reduces it to an acceptable level. However, when perineal symptoms persist, an intersphincteric rectal excision should be considered. When intractable constipation coexists, creation of a double-loop ileostomy should be considered.

Perioperative Management

Perioperative antibiotic prophylaxis is advisable for all interventions for incontinence and mandatory in the operations with implant of foreign material. Preoperative bowel preparation is not necessary. A solid bolus high in the colon is preferable to the contamination by Lumen fluid during the intervention. Postoperative administration of laxatives is of help in the prevention of passage of firm stool in the first postoperative days. Perioperative protection with a deviating colostomy is usually not necessary.

Conclusion

Fecal incontinence is no longer an untreatable disease. In almost all cases, it is possible to help patients with conservative management, operations, or with combinations (Table 46-1). It is important to evaluate all factors that contribute to incontinence and to direct therapy to the restoration of most of these factors. Diapers should no longer be the gold standard.

References

1. Uludag O, Darby M, Dejong CH, et al. Sacrale neuromodulatie effectief bij fecale incontinentie en intacte kringspieren; een prospectieve studie. Ned Tijdschr Geneeskd 2002;146(21): 989–993.
2. Adang EM, Engel GL, Rutten FF, et al. Cost-effectiveness of dynamic graciloplasty in patients with fecal incontinence. Dis Colon Rectum 1998;41(6):725–733; discussion 733–734.
3. Whitehead WE, Wald A, Norton NJ. Treatment options for fecal incontinence. Dis Colon Rectum 2001;44(1):131–142; discussion 142–144.
4. Madoff RD, Baeten CG, Christiansen J, et al. Standards for anal sphincter replacement. Dis Colon Rectum 2000;43(2):135–141.

5. Rintala R, Mildh L, Lindahl H. Fecal continence and quality of life for adult patients with an operated high or intermediate anorectal malformation. J Pediatr Surg 1994;29(6):777–780.

6. Pena A, Hong A. Advances in the management of anorectal malformations. Am J Surg 2000;180(5):370–376.

7. Mulder W, de Jong E, Wauters I, et al. Posterior sagittal anorectoplasty: functional results of primary and secondary operations in comparison to the pull-through method in anorectal malformations. Eur J Pediatr Surg 1995;5(3):170–173.

8. Neill ME, Parks AG, Swash M. Physiological studies of the anal sphincter musculature in faecal incontinence and rectal prolapse. Br J Surg 1981;68(8):531–536.

9. Suilleabhain CB, Horgan AF, McEnroe L, et al. The relationship of pudendal nerve terminal motor latency to squeeze pressure in patients with idiopathic fecal incontinence. Dis Colon Rectum 2001;44(5):666–671.

10. Davis K, Kumar D, Stanton SL, et al. Symptoms and anal sphincter morphology following primary repair of third-degree tears. Br J Surg 2003;90(12):1573–1579.

11. Zetterstrom J, Lopez A, Anzen B, et al. Anal sphincter tears at vaginal delivery: risk factors and clinical outcome of primary repair. Obstet Gynecol 1999;94(1):21–28.

12. Zetterstrom J, Mellgren A, Jensen LL, et al. Effect of delivery on anal sphincter morphology and function. Dis Colon Rectum 1999;42(10):1253–1260.

13. Damon H, Henry L, Barth X, Mion F. Fecal incontinence in females with a past history of vaginal delivery: significance of anal sphincter defects detected by ultrasound. Dis Colon Rectum 2002;45(11):1445–1450; discussion 1450–1451.

14. Bollard RC, Gardiner A, Duthie GS, Lindow SW. Anal sphincter injury, fecal and urinary incontinence: a 34-year follow-up after forceps delivery. Dis Colon Rectum 2003;46(8):1083–1088.

15. Sultan AH, Kamm MA, Hudson CN, et al. Anal-sphincter disruption during vaginal delivery. N Engl J Med 1993;329(26):1905–1911.

16. Snooks SJ, Henry MM, Swash M. Faecal incontinence due to external anal sphincter division in childbirth is associated with damage to the innervation of the pelvic floor musculature: a double pathology. Br J Obstet Gynaecol 1985;92(8):824–828.

17. Jacobs PP, Scheuer M, Kuijpers JH, Vingerhoets MH. Obstetric fecal incontinence. Role of pelvic floor denervation and results of delayed sphincter repair. Dis Colon Rectum 1990;33(6):494–497.

18. Fitzpatrick M, O'Brien C, O'Connell PR, O'Herlihy C. Patterns of abnormal pudendal nerve function that are associated with postpartum fecal incontinence. Am J Obstet Gynecol 2003;189(3):730–735.

19. Nyam DC, Pemberton JH. Long-term results of lateral internal sphincterotomy for chronic anal fissure with particular reference to incidence of fecal incontinence. Dis Colon Rectum 1999;42(10):1306–1310.

20. Garcia-Aguilar J, Belmonte C, Wong WD, et al. Open vs. closed sphincterotomy for chronic anal fissure: long-term results. Dis Colon Rectum 1996;39(4):440–443.

21. van Tets WF, Kuijpers HC. Continence disorders after anal fistulotomy. Dis Colon Rectum 1994;37(12):1194–1197.

22. Garcia-Aguilar J, Belmonte C, Wong WD, et al. Anal fistula surgery. Factors associated with recurrence and incontinence. Dis Colon Rectum 1996;39(7):723–729.

23. Garcia-Aguilar J, Belmonte C, Wong DW, et al. Cutting seton versus two-stage seton fistulotomy in the surgical management of high anal fistula. Br J Surg 1998;85(2):243–245.

24. Van Tets WF, Kuijpers JH. Seton treatment of perianal fistula with high anal or rectal opening. Br J Surg 1995;82(7):895–897.

25. Konsten J, Baeten CG. Hemorrhoidectomy vs. Lord's method: 17-year follow-up of a prospective, randomized trial. Dis Colon Rectum 2000;43(4):503–506.

26. Hetzer FH, Demartines N, Handschin AE, Clavien PA. Stapled vs excision hemorrhoidectomy: long-term results of a prospective randomized trial. Arch Surg 2002;137(3):337–340.

27. Zimmerman DD, Briel JW, Gosselink MP, Schouten WR. Anocutaneous advancement flap repair of transsphincteric fistulas. Dis Colon Rectum 2001;44(10):1474–1480.

28. Ortiz H, Marzo J. Endorectal flap advancement repair and fistulectomy for high trans-sphincteric and suprasphincteric fistulas. Br J Surg 2000;87(12):1680–1683.

29. Kreis ME, Jehle EC, Ohlemann M, et al. Functional results after transanal rectal advancement flap repair of trans-sphincteric fistula. Br J Surg 1998;85(2):240–242.

30. Gustafsson UM, Graf W. Excision of anal fistula with closure of the internal opening: functional and manometric results. Dis Colon Rectum 2002;45(12):1672–1678.

31. van Tets WF, Kuijpers JH, Tran K, et al. Influence of Parks' anal retractor on anal sphincter pressures. Dis Colon Rectum 1997;40(9):1042–1045.

32. Zimmerman DD, Gosselink MP, Hop WC, et al. Impact of two different types of anal retractor on fecal continence after fistula repair: a prospective, randomized, clinical trial. Dis Colon Rectum 2003;46(12):1674–1679.

33. Matzel KE, Bittorf B, Gunther K, et al. Rectal resection with low anastomosis: functional outcome. Colorectal Dis 2003;5(5):458–464.

34. Nesbakken A, Nygaard K, Lunde OC. Mesorectal excision for rectal cancer: functional outcome after low anterior resection and colorectal anastomosis without a reservoir. Colorectal Dis 2002;4(3):172–176.

35. van Duijvendijk P, Slors F, Taat CW, et al. A prospective evaluation of anorectal function after total mesorectal excision in patients with a rectal carcinoma. Surgery 2003;133(1):56–65.

36. Huber FT, Herter B, Siewert JR. Colonic pouch vs. side-to-end anastomosis in low anterior resection. Dis Colon Rectum 1999;42(7):896–902.

37. Dehni N, Tiret E, Singland JD, et al. Long-term functional outcome after low anterior resection: comparison of low colorectal anastomosis and colonic J-pouch-anal anastomosis. Dis Colon Rectum 1998;41(7):817–822; discussion 822–823.

38. Hellinger MD. Anal trauma and foreign bodies. Surg Clin North Am 2002;82(6):1253–1260.

39. Miles AJ, Allen-Mersh TG, Wastell C. Effect of anoreceptive intercourse on anorectal function. J R Soc Med 1993;86(3):144–147.

40. Hayne D, Vaizey CJ, Boulos PB. Anorectal injury following pelvic radiotherapy. Br J Surg 2001;88(8):1037–1048.

41. Kushwaha RS, Hayne D, Vaizey CJ, et al. Physiologic changes of the anorectum after pelvic radiotherapy for the treatment of prostate and bladder cancer. Dis Colon Rectum 2003;46(9):1182–1188.

42. Yeoh EK, Russo A, Botten R, et al. Acute effects of therapeutic irradiation for prostatic carcinoma on anorectal function. Gut 1998;43(1):123–127.

43. Iwamoto T, Nakahara S, Mibu R, et al. Effect of radiotherapy on anorectal function in patients with cervical cancer. Dis Colon Rectum 1997;40(6):693–697.

44. Harewood GC, Coulie B, Camilleri M, et al. Descending perineum syndrome: audit of clinical and laboratory features and outcome of pelvic floor retraining. Am J Gastroenterol 1999;94(1):126–130.

45. Hallan RI, Marzouk DE, Waldron DJ, et al. Comparison of digital and manometric assessment of anal sphincter function. Br J Surg 1989;76(9):973–975.

46. Azpiroz F, Enck P, Whitehead WE. Anorectal functional testing: review of collective experience. Am J Gastroenterol 2002;97(2): 232–240.

47. Siproudhis L, Bellissant E, Pagenault M, et al. Fecal incontinence with normal anal canal pressures: where is the pitfall? Am J Gastroenterol 1999;94(6):1556–1563.

48. Hoffmann BA, Timmcke AE, Gathright JB Jr, et al. Fecal seepage and soiling: a problem of rectal sensation. Dis Colon Rectum 1995;38(7):746–748.

49. Kuijpers HC, Scheuer M. Disorders of impaired fecal control. A clinical and manometric study. Dis Colon Rectum 1990;33(3): 207–211.

50. Beets-Tan RG, Beets GL, van der Hoop AG, et al. High-resolution magnetic resonance imaging of the anorectal region without an endocoil. Abdom Imaging 1999;24(6):576–581; discussion 582–584.

51. Rociu E, Stoker J, Eijkemans MJ, et al. Fecal incontinence: endoanal US versus endoanal MR imaging. Radiology 1999; 212(2):453–458.

52. Stoker J, Hussain SM, Lameris JS. Endoanal magnetic resonance imaging versus endosonography. Radiol Med (Torino) 1996;92(6):738–741.

53. Rongen MJ, van der Hoop AG, Baeten CG. Cecal access for antegrade colon enemas in medically refractory slow-transit constipation: a prospective study. Dis Colon Rectum 2001;44(11): 1644–1649.

54. Christensen P, Olsen N, Krogh K, Laurberg S. Scintigraphic assessment of antegrade colonic irrigation through an appendicostomy or a neoappendicostomy. Br J Surg 2002;89(10): 1275–1280.

55. Yerkes EB, Rink RC, King S, et al. Tap water and the Malone antegrade continence enema: a safe combination? J Urol 2001;166(4):1476–1478.

56. Briel JW, Schouten WR, Vlot EA, et al. Clinical value of colonic irrigation in patients with continence disturbances. Dis Colon Rectum 1997;40(7):802–805.

57. Norton C, Kamm MA. Anal plug for faecal incontinence. Colorectal Dis 2001;3(5):323–327.

58. Wald A. Biofeedback for fecal incontinence. Gastroenterology 2003;125(5):1533–1535.

59. Norton C, Chelvanayagam S, Wilson-Barnett J, et al. Randomized controlled trial of biofeedback for fecal incontinence. Gastroenterology 2003;125(5):1320–1329.

60. van Tets WF, Kuijpers JH, Bleijenberg G. Biofeedback treatment is ineffective in neurogenic fecal incontinence. Dis Colon Rectum 1996;39(9):992–994.

61. Leroi AM, Karoui S, Touchais JY, et al. Electrostimulation is not a clinically effective treatment of anal incontinence. Eur J Gastroenterol Hepatol 1999;11(9):1045–1047.

62. Scheuer M, Kuijpers HC, Bleijenberg G. Effect of electrostimulation on sphincter function in neurogenic fecal continence. Dis Colon Rectum 1994;37(6):590–593; discussion 593–594.

63. Osterberg A, Graf W, Eeg-Olofsson K, et al. Is electrostimulation of the pelvic floor an effective treatment for neurogenic faecal incontinence? Scand J Gastroenterol 1999;34(3):319–324.

64. Hasegawa H, Yoshioka K, Keighley MR. Randomized trial of fecal diversion for sphincter repair. Dis Colon Rectum 2000;43(7):961–964; discussion 964–965.

65. Pinta T, Kylanpaa-Back ML, Salmi T, et al. Delayed sphincter repair for obstetric ruptures: analysis of failure. Colorectal Dis 2003;5(1):73–78.

66. Sultan AH, Kamm MA, Hudson CN, Bartram CI. Third degree obstetric anal sphincter tears: risk factors and outcome of primary repair. BMJ 1994;308(6933):887–891.

67. Poen AC, Felt-Bersma RJ, Strijers RL, et al. Third-degree obstetric perineal tear: long-term clinical and functional results after primary repair. Br J Surg 1998;85(10):1433–1438.

68. Tjandra JJ, Han WR, Goh J, et al. Direct repair vs. overlapping sphincter repair: a randomized, controlled trial. Dis Colon Rectum 2003;46(7):937–942; discussion 942–943.

69. Mahony R, Behan M, O'Herlihy C, O'Connell PR. Randomized, clinical trial of bowel confinement vs. laxative use after primary repair of a third-degree obstetric anal sphincter tear. Dis Colon Rectum 2004;47(1):12–17.

70. Malouf AJ, Norton CS, Engel AF, et al. Long-term results of overlapping anterior anal-sphincter repair for obstetric trauma. Lancet 2000;355(9200):260–265.

71. Ha HT, Fleshman JW, Smith M, et al. Manometric squeeze pressure difference parallels functional outcome after overlapping sphincter reconstruction. Dis Colon Rectum 2001;44(5):655–660.

72. Pinedo G, Vaizey CJ, Nicholls RJ, et al. Results of repeat anal sphincter repair. Br J Surg 1999;86(1):66–69.

73. Giordano P, Renzi A, Efron J, et al. Previous sphincter repair does not affect the outcome of repeat repair. Dis Colon Rectum 2002;45(5):635–640.

74. Leroi AM, Kamm MA, Weber J, et al. Internal anal sphincter repair. Int J Colorectal Dis 1997;12(4):243–245.

75. Morgan R, Patel B, Beynon J, Carr ND. Surgical management of anorectal incontinence due to internal anal sphincter deficiency. Br J Surg 1997;84(2):226–230.

76. Kenefick NJ, Vaizey CJ, Malouf AJ, et al. Injectable silicone biomaterial for faecal incontinence due to internal anal sphincter dysfunction. Gut 2002;51(2):225–228.

77. Scheuer M, Kuijpers HC, Jacobs PP. Postanal repair restores anatomy rather than function. Dis Colon Rectum 1989;32(11): 960–963.

78. Matsuoka H, Mavrantonis C, Wexner SD, et al. Postanal repair for fecal incontinence—is it worthwhile? Dis Colon Rectum 2000;43(11):1561–1567.

79. Rieger NA, Sarre RG, Saccone GT, et al. Postanal repair for faecal incontinence: long-term follow-up. Aust NZ J Surg 1997;67(8):566–570.

80. Setti Carraro P, Kamm MA, Nicholls RJ. Long-term results of postanal repair for neurogenic faecal incontinence. Br J Surg 1994;81(1):140–144.

81. Korsgen S, Deen KI, Keighley MR. Long-term results of total pelvic floor repair for postobstetric fecal incontinence. Dis Colon Rectum 1997;40(7):835–839.

82. van Tets WF, Kuijpers JH. Pelvic floor procedures produce no consistent changes in anatomy or physiology. Dis Colon Rectum 1998;41(3):365–369.

83. Osterberg A, Edebol Eeg-Olofsson K, Graf W. Results of surgical treatment for faecal incontinence. Br J Surg 2000;87(11): 1546–1552.

84. Matzel KE, Stadelmaier U, Hohenfellner M, Gall FP. Electrical stimulation of sacral spinal nerves for treatment of faecal incontinence. Lancet 1995;346(8983):1124–1127.

85. Vaizey CJ, Kamm MA, Roy AJ, Nicholls RJ. Double-blind crossover study of sacral nerve stimulation for fecal incontinence. Dis Colon Rectum 2000;43(3):298–302.

86. Leroi AM, Michot F, Grise P, Denis P. Effect of sacral nerve stimulation in patients with fecal and urinary incontinence. Dis Colon Rectum 2001;44(6):779–789.

87. Malouf AJ, Wiesel PH, Nicholls T, et al. Short-term effects of sacral nerve stimulation for idiopathic slow transit constipation. World J Surg 2002;26(2):166–170.

88. Kenefick NJ, Vaizey CJ, Nicholls RJ, et al. Sacral nerve stimulation for faecal incontinence due to systemic sclerosis. Gut 2002;51(6):881–883.

89. Wong WD, Jensen LL, Bartolo DC, Rothenberger DA. Artificial anal sphincter. Dis Colon Rectum 1996;39(12):1345–1351.

90. Baeten C, Spaans F, Fluks A. An implanted neuromuscular stimulator for fecal continence following previously implanted gracilis muscle. Report of a case. Dis Colon Rectum 1988;31(2): 134–137.

91. Baeten CG, Geerdes BP, Adang EM, et al. Anal dynamic gracilo-plasty in the treatment of intractable fecal incontinence. N Engl J Med 1995;332(24):1600–1605.

92. Geerdes BP, Heineman E, Konsten J, et al. Dynamic gracilo-plasty. Complications and management. Dis Colon Rectum 1996;39(8):912–917.

93. Konsten J, Rongen MJ, Ogunbiyi OA, et al. Comparison of epineural or intramuscular nerve electrodes for stimulated graciloplasty. Dis Colon Rectum 2001;44(4):581–586.

94. Rongen MJ, Uludag O, El Naggar K, et al. Long-term follow-up of dynamic graciloplasty for fecal incontinence. Dis Colon Rectum 2003;46(6):716–721.

95. Williams NS, Patel J, George BD, et al. Development of an electrically stimulated neoanal sphincter. Lancet 1991;338(8776): 1166–1169.

96. Lehur PA, Zerbib F, Neunlist M, et al. Comparison of quality of life and anorectal function after artificial sphincter implantation. Dis Colon Rectum 2002;45(4):508–513.

97. Christiansen J, Sparso B. Treatment of anal incontinence by an implantable prosthetic anal sphincter. Ann Surg 1992;215(4): 383–386.

47
Rectal Prolapse

Anthony M. Vernava, III and David E. Beck

Prolapse, in general, is defined as: "A falling down of an organ or part ... from its normal position." Rectal prolapse is a " falling down" of the rectum so that it is outside the body. Its appearance is that of an erythematous, proboscis-like object and is a true intussusception of the rectum through the sphincters. The condition is embarrassing and can be socially debilitating although it is rarely a medical emergency. It is associated with fecal incontinence, and in women, is associated with other pelvic floor abnormalities. The precise cause of rectal prolapse is unknown although two theories of etiology have been proposed. At the beginning of the nineteenth century, Moschcowitz[1] suggested that prolapse is a sliding hernia through a defect in the pelvic fascia. More recently, and with the benefit of cinedefecography, Broden and Snellman[2] proposed that prolapse is actually a circumferential intussusception of the rectum. It is this latter theory that most investigators subscribe to. The majority of patients afflicted with rectal prolapse have a long history of constipation and straining.

The disorder is more common in women, especially in older age groups. Affected men tend to be younger (20–40 years of age) and usually have a predisposing disorder (e.g., congenital anal atresia). Women are at increased risk of developing prolapse by virtue of their anatomy (i.e., wide pelvis) and because of childbearing. Vaginal delivery is known to stretch the pudendal nerves and long-term neurologic damage can occur at this time resulting in perineal descent, prolapse, and incontinence. A vast number of different procedures have been described to manage the disorder serving as testimony to the uncertain etiology of the disease and the resultant disagreement about optimal surgical therapy (Table 47-1).

Patient factors that influence the choice of operation are: age, sex, medical condition, extent of prolapse, bowel function, and status of fecal continence. Procedure-related factors that influence the choice of operation include: extent of procedure, potential morbidity, recurrence rate, impact on fecal continence and bowel habit, familiarity and ease of technique.

Patient Evaluation

Constipation and straining, fecal incontinence, and erratic bowel habits typify the symptoms associated with prolapse. These symptoms are nonspecific and are associated with both mucosal pathology and functional bowel disease therefore, a complete evaluation before operation is necessary.

Spontaneous prolapse is obvious on inspection (Figure 47-1).[3] Some patients may require straining to produce the prolapse, and the straining patient is best examined in the squatting or sitting position. The patient can be examined while he or she is on the toilet by having the patient lean forward or using a long rod to which a mirror is attached placed between the patient's legs to view the prolapse. Another option is to place a flexible endoscope into the toilet with the viewing end pointed toward the perineum.

Full-thickness prolapse is distinguished by its concentric rings and grooves as opposed to the radially oriented grooves associated with mucosal prolapse (Figure 47-2). Inspection should also include examining the perianal skin for any maceration or excoriations. A digital rectal examination is important to detect concomitant anal pathology and to assess resting tone and squeeze pressure of the anal sphincters and function of the puborectalis muscle.

Colonoscopy or flexible sigmoidoscopy with barium enema should be performed to rule out associated mucosal abnormalities. Defecography is usually not necessary in the evaluation of full-thickness prolapse but it is an essential part of the evaluation of internal procidentia (rectoanal intussusception). Anal manometry can help assess sphincter function; longstanding prolapse typically damages the internal anal sphincter and may cause poor resting pressures.[4] In such patients, synchronous levatorplasty should be considered at the time of prolapse repair and may further improve continence.[5] In a manometric study evaluating patients with rectal prolapse, Spencer[4] reported that the anorectal inhibitory reflex was frequently absent or abnormal, that resting anal pressures were abnormally low, and squeeze pressures were normal. Anal electromyography and pudendal nerve terminal

TABLE 47-1. Operations described for rectal prolapse

Transabdominal procedures
1. Repair of the pelvic floor
    Abdominal repair of levator diastasis
    Abdominoperineal levator repair
2. Suspension-fixation
    Sigmoidopexy (Pemberton-Stalker)
    Presacral rectopexy
    Lateral strip rectopexy (Orr-Loygue)
    Anterior sling rectopexy (Ripstein)
    Posterior sling rectopexy (Wells)
    Puborectal sling (Nigro)
3. Resection procedures
    Proctopexy with sigmoid resection
    Anterior resection
4. Perineal procedures
    Perineal rectosigmoidectomy (Altemeier)
    Rectal mucosal sleeve resection (Delorme)
    Perineal suspension-fixation (Wyatt)
    Anal encirclement (Thiersch + modification)

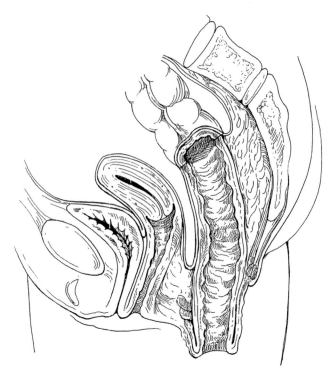

FIGURE 47-2. Sagittal view of full-thickness rectal prolapse. (From Beck and Whitlow.[3] Copyright 2003 by Taylor & Francis Group LLC (B). Reproduced with permission of Taylor & Francis Group LLC (B) in the format Textbook via Copyright Clearance Center).

motor latency are generally not clinically helpful unless there is a history of severe straining. In such cases, anal electromyography presence of inappropriate puborectalis contraction. When discovered, biofeedback can be used for therapy. Colonic transit times should be done in patients with a coexisting history of severe constipation so that the correct operation can be chosen. Individuals with slow-transit constipation and site markers concentrated in the left and sigmoid colon typically benefit from a synchronous sigmoid colectomy and rectopexy versus rectopexy alone or even perineal rectosigmoidectomy.

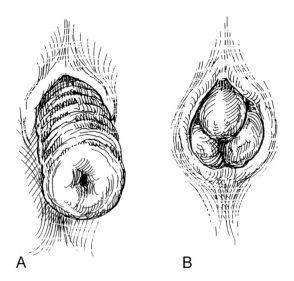

FIGURE 47-1. Mucosal versus full-thickness prolapse. (From Beck and Whitlow.[3] Copyright 2003 by Taylor & Francis Group LLC (B). Reproduced with permission of Taylor & Francis Group LLC (B) in the format Textbook via Copyright Clearance Center). A. circumferential full-thickness prolapse; concentric mucosal folds B. Radial folds seen with hemorrhoidal prolapse.

Surgical Procedures

The surgeon must decide between a perineal operation and an abdominal procedure. Men are at risk for sexual dysfunction with an abdominal approach, therefore this option is chosen cautiously. The risk of impotence for abdominal rectopexy should approach 1%–2% in skilled hands.

The most common abdominal operations are resection with or without rectopexy or rectopexy alone. The perineal procedures are perineal rectosigmoidectomy (Altemeier) or mucosal sleeve resector (Delorme). Elderly, high-risk patients are best treated by perineal procedures which can be performed under a regional anesthetic, or even a local anesthetic with intravenous sedation. Healthy adults with normal bowel habits may undergo either rectopexy ± sigmoidectomy or perineal rectosigmoidectomy ± levatorplasty. Bowel function has a role in determining specific therapy. Constipated patients should undergo resection and rectopexy. Incontinent patients should undergo either abdominal rectopexy or perineal rectosigmoidectomy + levatorplasty. Recurrent prolapse mandates knowledge of the prior repair because that information will dictate future options; the prior dissection may limit the available alternatives because of blood supply divided.

Perineal Procedures

Perineal Rectosigmoidectomy

Perineal rectosigmoidectomy was popularized by Altemeier and his name is the eponym attached to the procedure.[6] The operation can be performed under a general or spinal anesthetic or even a local anesthetic with intravenous sedation. Typically, patients receive a mechanical and antibiotic bowel preparation. The prone position is preferred; however, the left lateral (Sim's) or lithotomy position can also be effectively used. The rectal wall is injected with an epinephrine containing compound for hemostasis. A circumferential incision is made in the rectal wall approximately 1–2 cm above the dentate line (Figure 47-3). The incision is deepened until the full thickness of the rectal wall has been divided. Once a full-thickness incision has been made, the cut edge of the rectum is pulled down and the mesorectum is divided and ligated, progressively advancing more cephalad. Anteriorly, a peritoneal reflection (hernia sac) is encountered. The dissection continues until there is no further redundancy remaining in the rectum/sigmoid colon, this requires judgment and experience. After the redundant rectum has been adequately mobilized, it is divided and a hand-sutured coloanal anastomosis is performed. An EEA stapler can also be used to perform the anastomosis. In cases of severe fecal incontinence, a levator plication can be performed before the coloanal anastomosis improves continence in two-thirds of patients.[5,7] After the procedure, patients are allowed to ambulate and eat on postoperative day 1.

Reported results of the perineal rectosigmoidectomy are summarized in Table 47-2. Mortality has been low and morbidity ranges from 5% to 24%. Most morbidity is from the preexisting medical problems; however, most series report anastomotic complications in a small number of patients. Recurrence rates range from 0% to 10% in series with a follow-up of 6 months to 5 years. Recurrence rates are higher for series with longer follow-up. Improvement in incontinence has been reported in the majority of patients in whom levatorplasty is performed.[16]

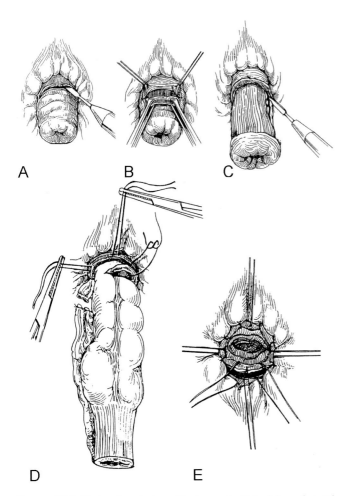

A B C

D E

FIGURE 47-3. Perineal rectosigmoidectomy. **A, B** Incision of rectal wall. **C** Division of vessel adjacent to bowel wall. **D** The prolapsed segment is amputated. Stay sutures previously placed in distal edge of outer cylinder are placed in cut edge of inner cylinder. **E** Anastomosis of distal aspect of remaining colon to the short rectal stump. (From Beck and Whitlow.[3] Copyright 2003 by Taylor & Francis Group LLC (B). Reproduced with permission of Taylor & Francis Group LLC (B) in the format Textbook via Copyright Clearance Center).

Delorme Procedure

Another perineal option is mucosal proctectomy first discussed by Delorme in 1900.[17] It is ideally suited to those patients with full-thickness prolapse limited to partial circumference (e.g., anterior wall) or less-extensive prolapse.

The Delorme's procedure for treating rectal prolapse differs from the perineal rectosigmoidectomy (Altemeier) in that only the mucosa and submucosa are excised from the prolapsed segment (Figure 47-4). Delorme's procedure can be performed under general, spinal, or local anesthesia. The bowel is prolapsed and the submucosa infiltrated with epinephrine solution. One centimeter cranial (proximal) to the dentate line, the outer cylinder is incised through the mucosa only. The mucosa and submucosa are dissected off the

TABLE 47-2. Results of perineal rectosigmoidectomy

Authors	No. of patients	Recurrence (%)	Mortality (%)	Morbidity (%)
Altemeier et al.[6]	106	3	00	24
Friedman et al.[8]	027	50	00	12
Gopal et al.[9]	18	6	06	17
Finlay and Aitchison[10]	17	6	06	18
Williams et al.[11]	114	11	00	12
Johansen et al.[12]	20	0	05	05
Kim et al.[13]	183	16	00	14
Azimuddin et al.[14]	36	16	—	—
Zbar et al.[15]	80	4	—	—

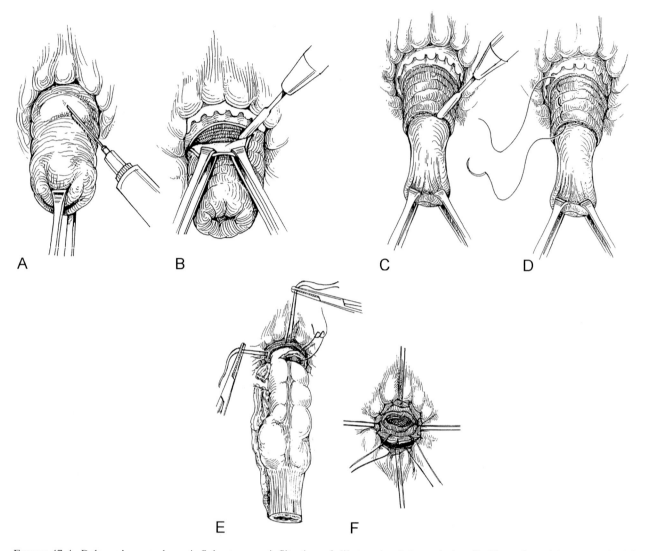

FIGURE 47-4. Delorme's procedure. **A** Subcutaneous infiltration of dilute epinephrine solution. **B** Circumferential mucosal incision. **C** Dissection of mucosa off muscular layer. **D** Plicating stitch approximating cut edge of mucosa, muscular wall, and mucosa just proximal to dentate line. **E** Plicating stitch tied. **F** Completed anastomosis. (From Beck and Whitlow.[3] Copyright 2003 by Taylor & Francis Group LLC (B). Reproduced with permission of Taylor & Francis Group LLC (B) in the format Textbook via Copyright Clearance Center).

underlying muscle. The mucosectomy may be more difficult in patients with prior anal surgery or a history of diverticulitis. The plane of dissection may be facilitated by continued submucosal injection of epinephrine solution as the dissection continues toward the apex of the prolapse. Four polyglycolic acid sutures (2-0) are placed sequentially in the rectal muscle at the anterior, posterior, and lateral positions as the dissection continues. These sutures plicate the muscle and provide traction. The dissection is carried into the apex and the mucosa which has been dissected free is transected. The polyglycolic acid sutures (2-0) are used to reconnect the edges of the bowel. Four additional sutures are used to approximate the bowel between the placating sutures. Additional 3-0 sutures are placed in an interrupted or running manner to complete the circumferential approximation of the mucosal edges.

Results of Delorme's procedure are summarized in Table 47-3. Reported operative mortality rates from a series of patients treated by Delorme's procedure range from 0% to 2.5%.[18–23] Morbidity reported at 0% to 32% includes hemorrhage, anastomotic dehiscence, stricture, diarrhea, and urinary retention. Recurrence rates (7%–22% at 1–13 years

TABLE 47-3. Results of Delorme's procedure

Authors	No. of patients	Recurrence (%)
Uhlig and Sullivan [18]	44	7
Monson et al.[19]	27	7
Senapati et al.[20]	32	13
Oliver et al.[21]	41	22
Tobin and Scott[22]	43	26
Graf et al.[23]	14	21

postoperatively) are higher than with a perineal rectosigmoidectomy. Incontinence is improved in 40%–50% of patients.[16] Constipation was not a problem in most series.

Thiersch Procedure

Anal encirclement was first described by Thiersch in 1891.[24] He placed a silver wire subcutaneously around the anus with the patient under local anesthesia. The mechanism of this procedure was to mechanically supplement or replace the anal sphincter and stimulate a foreign body reaction in the perianal area. There were several reports of the use of this procedure in the early part of this century, especially in Europe.[25]

William Gabriel is credited with reviving interest in Thiersch's operation in the 1950s.[25] He reported on 25 cases of incontinence or minor rectal prolapse. He did not recommend this operation for major degrees of prolapse.

For this operation, the patient is placed in the prone jackknife, lithotomy, or left lateral position (Figure 47-5). A local anesthetic is administered and a radial incision made on both sides of the anus about 2 cm from the anal verge. A curved hemostat or special circular needle is used to tunnel from one incision to the other above the anoperineal ligament anterior to the anus, keeping external to the external anal sphincter. The material for encirclement is brought through the tunnel. Tunneling is continued posterior to the anus above the anococcygeal ligament and the encircling material brought through so that the two ends meets.[26] The encircling material is then secured by tying snugly over an index finger in the anus. A variety of materials used for encirclement include nylon, silk, silastic rods, silicone, Marlex mesh, Mersilene mesh, fascia, tendon, and Dacron.[10] Complications of this procedure include breakage of the suture or wire, fecal impaction, sepsis, and erosion into the skin or anal canal. The Thiersch operation does not correct the prolapse but narrows the anus enough that the prolapse is confined to the rectum, accomplishing this goal in 54%–100% of cases.[27] Because of its failure to correct prolapse and the morbidity of this procedure, it is reserved for the most seriously ill patients who are unable to undergo one of the previously described perineal procedures. Results of the Thiersch procedure are summarized in Table 47-4.

Abdominal Procedures

Abdominal Rectopexy and Sigmoid Colectomy

Abdominal rectopexy and sigmoidectomy was initially described in 1955 by Frykman[35] for management of full-thickness rectal prolapse and it remains an essential treatment option. The operation consists of four essential components: 1) complete mobilization of the rectum down to the levator musculature, leaving the lateral stalks intact; 2) elevation of the rectum cephalad with suture fixation of the lateral rectal stalks to the presacral fascia just below the sacral promontory; 3) suture of the endopelvic fascia anteriorly to obliterate the cul-de-sac; and 4) sigmoid colectomy with anastomosis. The modern components of the operation are essentially the same with the exception that most surgeons no longer obliterate the cul-de-sac (Figure 47-6). Results with abdominal rectopexy and sigmoidectomy are summarized in Table 47-5.

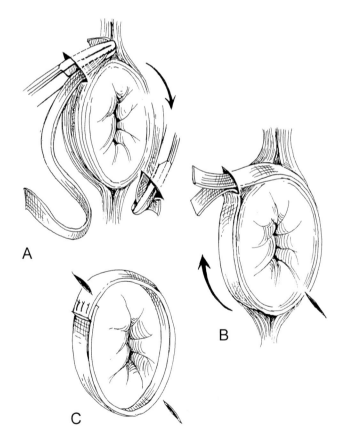

FIGURE 47-5. Anal encirclement (Thiersch). **A** Lateral incisions with prosthetic mesh tunneled around the anus. **B** Mesh completely encircling the anal opening. **C** Completed anal encirclement procedure. (From Beck and Whitlow.[3] Copyright 2003 by Taylor & Francis Group LLC (B). Reproduced with permission of Taylor & Francis Group LLC (B) in the format Textbook via Copyright Clearance Center).

TABLE 47-4. Results of Thiersch procedure

Authors	No. of patients	Recurrence (%)	Mortality (%)	Morbidity (%)
Jackaman et al.[28]	52	33	—	—
Labow et al.[29]	9	0	—	0
Hunt et al.[30]	41	44	—	37
Poole et al.[31]	15	33	—	33
Vongsangnak et al.[32]	25	39	—	59
Earnshaw and Hopkinson[33]	21	33	—	—
Khanduja et al.[34]	16	0	—	25

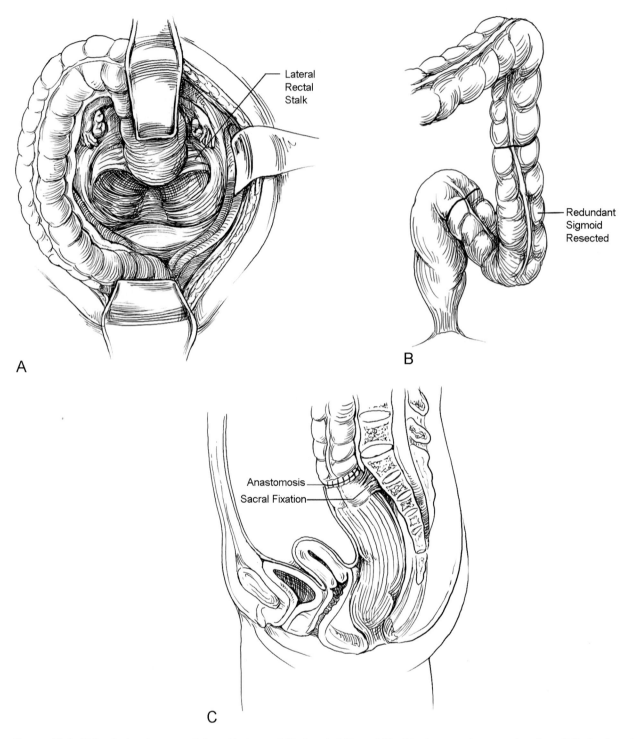

FIGURE 47-6. Abdominal rectopexy and sigmoidectomy. **A** Rectum is fully mobilized in the posterior avascular plane. **B** Redundant sigmoid colon is resected. **C** Anastomosis is completed and rectopexy sutures are placed.

Abdominal Rectopexy

Simple suture rectopexy without sigmoid colectomy has been reported as an effective surgical treatment for rectal prolapse.[43,44] Typically, this operation has been used in patients who do not have associated constipation with prolapse. The rectum is mobilized down to the levator floor preserving the lateral ligaments. The lateral rectal stalks are then sutured to the presacral fascia just below the sacral promontory, using

TABLE 47-5. Results of abdominal rectopexy and sigmoid colectomy

Authors	No. of patients	Recurrence (%)	Mortality (%)	Morbidity (%)
Watts et al.[36]	102	1.9	00	04
Husa et al.[37]	48	09	02.1	00
Sayfan et al.[38]	13	00	00	23
McKee et al.[39]	09	00	00	00
Luukkonen et al.[40]	15	00	06.7	20
Canfrere et al.[41]	17	00	00	—
Huber et al.[42]	39	00	00	7.1

a nonabsorbable suture, such as Prolene. Results are summarized in Table 47-6.

Ripstein Procedure

Described in 1963 by Ripstein and Lanter,[45] the Ripstein operation had been one of the most popular procedures for management of rectal prolapse. It is currently seldom used, probably because of the success of alternate therapies and because this particular operation requires the use of prosthetic material, placed around the rectum.

The rectum is mobilized posteriorly down to the coccyx. A 5-cm piece of prosthetic mesh (Marlex or Prolene) is sutured to the presacral fascia, 5 cm below the sacral promontory in the midline. The rectum is retracted cephalad and the lateral edges of the sling are wrapped around the rectum and sutured to it (Figure 47-7). Care must be taken to avoid making the wrap too tight and causing an obstruction. Results are summarized in Table 47-7.

Ivalon Sponge

The Ivalon (polyvinyl alcohol) sponge wrap operation, first described in 1959 by Wells,[50] is currently the most popular operation for rectal prolapse in the United Kingdom. The operation is performed with the patient in the lithotomy position and the rectum is mobilized posteriorly down to the levator ani. Anterior mobilization of the rectum is also performed. A piece of Ivalon is then placed in the pelvis, sutured to the presacral fascia with nonabsorbable sutures, and then wrapped around the rectum which has been retracted cephalad. The sponge is then sutured to the rectum such that only three-fourths of the rectum is wrapped (the anterior rectum is left free of the sponge). The peritoneum is then closed over the sponge excluding it from the peritoneal cavity (Figure 47-8). In the United States, surgeons have used praline or Marlex mesh instead of a polyvinyl alcohol sponge

TABLE 47-6. Results of abdominal rectopexy

Authors	No. of patients	Recurrence (%)	Mortality (%)
Loygue et al.[43]	140	3.6	01.4
Blatchford et al.[44]	42	02	00

to perform a posterior wrap. Results of posterior wraps are summarized in Table 47-8.

Laparoscopic Rectopexy

Laparoscopic approaches to the management of full-thickness rectal prolapse, including rectopexy alone, or in combination with sigmoid colectomy have been reported to have comparable success rates and morbidity to open surgery, with the added benefit of shorter hospital stays. These laparoscopic approaches likely represent the future direction of definitive operative management.[52–55] Heah et al.[53] reported on 25 patients, with a mean age of 72 years, who underwent laparoscopic rectopexy without resection for management of full-thickness prolapse. Four of 25 patients (16%) required conversion to open operation. Morbidity occurred in 3 of 25 patients (12%). There were no cases of recurrent prolapse or mortality.

Ashari et al.[54] reported a 10-year, single-center experience with laparoscopically assisted resection rectopexy for management of full-thickness rectal prolapse in 117 patients. Mortality occurred in 1 of 117 patients (0.8%) and morbidity in 9%. Seventy-seven of the 117 patients (66%) were followed a median period of 62 months. Recurrent full-thickness rectal prolapse occurred in 2 of 77 patients (2.5%) and mucosal prolapse occurred in 14 (18%). Operative times decreased by 39% (from 180 to 110 minutes) over 10 years.

Kairaluoma et al.[55] reported a case-controlled comparison between open and laparoscopic surgery for rectal prolapse involving 106 patients (53 in each group) and included both rectopexy alone and rectopexy combined with resection. Morbidity and mortality were statistically no different between the laparoscopic group and the open surgery controls. Recurrent full-thickness rectal prolapse occurred in 6% of the laparoscopic group and 13% of the open surgery group but this was not statistically significant ($P = .186$). Hospital stay was significantly shorter in the laparoscopic group than in the open surgery controls for both rectopexy alone and for rectopexy combined with sigmoid colectomy.

Recurrent Prolapse

As discussed previously, recurrence is not uncommon after surgical treatment of prolapse. Depending on the specific initial therapy selected, recurrent full-thickness rectal prolapse can occur in more than 50% of patients, although most recent reports place recurrent prolapse after resection with rectopexy to be less than 10%. Typically, perineal operations for prolapse have a higher risk of recurrence compared with abdominal approaches. Over a 30-year period, Hool et al.[56] reported recurrent rectal prolapse in 24 of 234 patients (10%). Nine of the 24 recurrences occurred after an initial perineal operation and 15 of 24 recurrences occurred after an initial abdominal approach.

When full-thickness rectal prolapse recurs, it is important to reevaluate the patient for both constipation and other

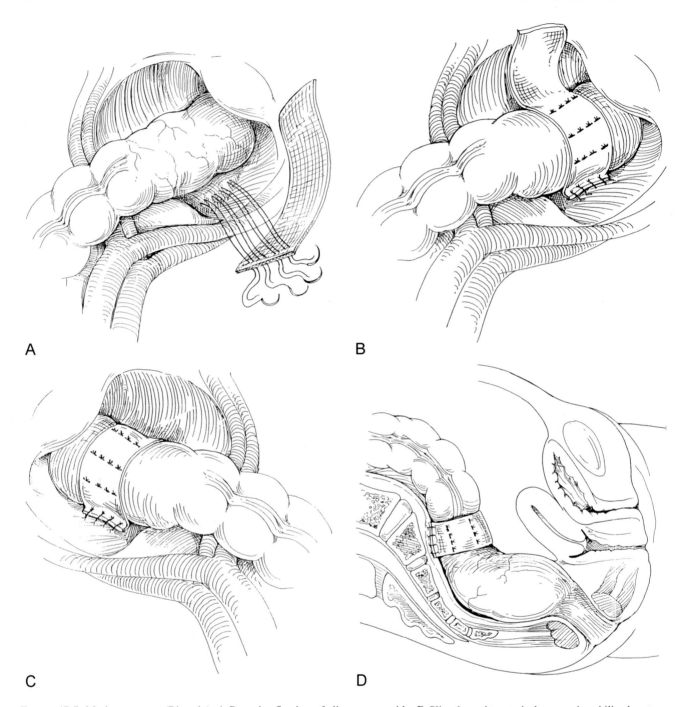

FIGURE 47-7. Mesh rectopexy (Ripstein). **A** Posterior fixation of sling on one side. **B** Sling brought anteriorly around mobilized rectum. **C** Sling fixed posteriorly on the opposite side. **D** Sagittal view of the completed rectopexy. (From Beck and Whitlow.[3] Copyright 2003 by Taylor & Francis Group LLC (B). Reproduced with permission of Taylor & Francis Group LLC (B) in the format Textbook via Copyright Clearance Center).

pelvic floor abnormalities in order to tailor the management to address those issues. Therefore, patients with recurrent prolapse will require evaluation in the anorectal physiology laboratory with manometry and defecography. Patient comorbid conditions will also have an important role in treatment selection, as was likely the case in selecting the initial operation.

TABLE 47-7. Results of Ripstein procedure

Authors	No. of patients	Recurrence (%)	Mortality (%)	Morbidity (%)
Ripstein and Lanter[45]	289	00	00.3	—
Gordon and Hoexter[46]	1111	02.3	-	16.6
Eisenstadt et al.[47]	30	00	00	13.3
Tjandra et al.[48]	134	08	00.6	21
Winde et al.[49]	35	00	00	28

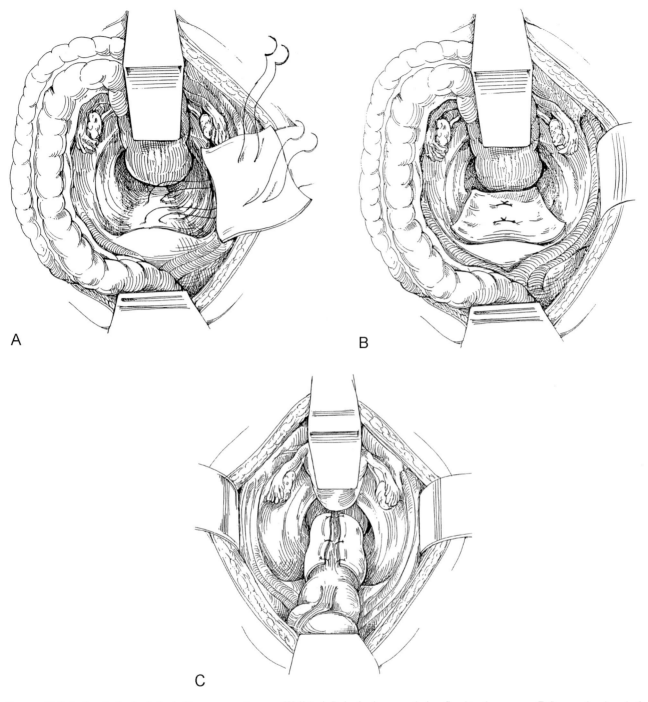

FIGURE 47-8. Ivalon (polyvinyl alcohol) sponge rectopexy (Wells). **A** Polyvinyl sponge being fixed to the sacrum. **B** Sponge in place before fixation to the rectum. **C** Incomplete encirclement of the rectum anteriorly with the sponge sutured in place. (From Beck and Whitlow.[3] Copyright 2003 by Taylor & Francis Group LLC (B). Reproduced with permission of Taylor & Francis Group LLC (B) in the format Textbook via Copyright Clearance Center).

A major consideration in determining the best surgical option to treat the recurrent prolapse is the residual blood supply of the remaining large bowel. Any patient who has undergone a prior rectal or sigmoid resection with anastomosis requires very careful evaluation before undergoing a secondary procedure. The initial operative procedure performed for prolapse has a dominant role in determining the selection of the next operation. In such patients, the obvious risk to a secondary resection is ischemia to the segment of large intestine between two anastomoses.

Recurrent full-thickness rectal prolapse can be successfully managed using the same operative options applied to initial disease. Reports in the literature place successful treatment of recurrence at between 85%–100%.[57,58] Unfortunately, although

TABLE 47-8. Results of Ivalon sponge operation

Authors	No. of patients	Recurrence (%)	Mortality (%)	Morbidity (%)
Sayfan et al.[38]	16	00	00	12.5
Luukkonen et al.[40]	15	00	00	13.3
Novell et al.[51]	31	3	00	19

most authors indicate the initial operative technique, the recurrence, and the secondary operative technique, they fail to adequately describe their rationale for selection of the secondary procedure. For that reason, there is very little data upon which to base an intelligent treatment decision for management of recurrent prolapse. There is no specific algorithm available that can be applied to select the best operation for treating recurrence, except that many reports suggest treating young patients using an abdominal approach and elderly patients using a perineal approach. The treating surgeon is left to make an individualized recommendation from the options that are summarized in Table 47-9. Also, the bowel dysfunction associated with prolapse, including constipation and diarrhea, is largely unimproved after correction of the recurrence.[56–58]

Fengler et al.[57] reported the results of managing recurrent full-thickness rectal prolapse in 14 patients who had initially undergone perineal rectosigmoidectomy (10), anal encirclement (2), Delorme procedure (1), and anterior resection (1). The average length of time to recurrence was 14 months. Salvage operations performed to manage the recurrence included: redo perineal rectosigmoidectomy (7), abdominal rectopexy (1), resection + rectopexy (2), Delorme procedure (1), anal encirclement (1). Patients were followed for 50 months after treatment for their recurrence. One patient died from an unrelated problem. Among the 13 remaining patients, no patient experienced a re-recurrence of the prolapse. Successful management of the recurrent prolapse failed to resolve fecal incontinence in three patients.

Pikarsky et al.[58] reported on 27 patients with recurrent full-thickness rectal prolapse. Initial operations included: abdominal rectopexy (7), Delorme procedure (7), perineal rectosigmoidectomy (7), anal encirclement (4), and resection rectopexy (2). Operations performed for recurrence included: perineal rectosigmoidectomy (14), resection rectopexy (8), rectopexy (2), pelvic floor repair (2), and Delorme procedure (1). Re-recurrence of prolapse occurred in 4 of 27 (15%) after a median follow-up period of 24 months.

TABLE 47-9. Management options for recurrent rectal prolapse

Initial operation	Options for management of recurrence
Perineal rectosigmoidectomy	Redo perineal rectosigmoidectomy
	Abdominal rectopexy (avoid resection)
Abdominal rectopexy	Redo abdominal rectopexy
	(±sigmoid colectomy)
	Perineal rectosigmoidectomy
Abdominal rectopexy + resection	Redo abdominal rectopexy (±re-resection)
	Avoid perineal rectosigmoidectomy

If the patient has undergone an initial perineal rectosigmoidectomy, then a repeat perineal rectosigmoidectomy or abdominal rectopexy can be safely performed. However, in such cases, abdominal rectopexy with sigmoid colectomy should be avoided because of the risk of ischemia to the retained rectal segment. For those patients who have undergone prior abdominal rectopexy but who now have recurrent prolapse, a redo abdominal rectopexy is an acceptable approach.

Solitary Rectal Ulcer Syndrome and Colitis Cystica Profunda

Solitary rectal ulcer syndrome (SRUS) and colitis cystica profunda (CCF) are uncommon conditions frequently associated with rectal prolapse.[59] SRUS is a clinical condition characterized by rectal bleeding, copious mucous discharge, anorectal pain, and difficult evacuation. Despite its name, patients with this condition can have single, multiple, or no rectal ulcers. When present, the ulcers usually occur on the anterior rectal wall just above the anorectal ring. Less frequently, they may occur from just above to 15 cm above the dentate line. Ulcers usually appear as shallow with a "punched out" gray-white base surrounded by hyperemia.

Cystica profunda is a benign condition characterized by mucin-filled cysts located deep to the muscularis mucosae. Although cysts can occur in any segment of the digestive tract submucosa, they are most frequent in the colon and rectum. When these lesions are found in the colon or rectum they are called CCF and appear as nodules or masses on the anterior rectal wall. Patients can be asymptomatic (with the lesions identified on screening endoscopy) or complain of rectal bleeding, mucous discharge, or anorectal discomfort. Most will admit to difficulty with bowel movements. CCF is a pathologic diagnosis whose most important aspect is to differentiate it from colorectal adenocarcinoma. This prevents unnecessary radical operations.

CCP and SRUS are closely related diagnoses and some authors consider them interchangeable. The etiology of these conditions remains unclear, but a common feature is chronic inflammation and/or trauma. The inflammation may result from inflammatory bowel disease, resolving ischemia, or trauma associated with internal intussusception or prolapse of the rectum, direct digital trauma, or the forces associated with evacuating a hard stool.

In symptomatic patients, an endoscopic evaluation of the distal colon and rectum will reveal the lesions described above. Defecography documents intussusception in 45%–80% of patients. The differential diagnosis of both CCF and SRUS includes: polyps, endometriosis, inflammatory granulomas, infectious disorders, drug-induced colitides, and mucus-producing adenocarcinoma. Differentiation among these entities is possible with an adequate biopsy. Biopsies obtained via a rigid proctoscope, or an endoscopic snare excision, may be necessary to obtain enough tissue for an accurate diagnosis. CCF is characterized pathologically by mucous cysts lined by normal columnar epithelium located deep to the muscularis mucosae. The overlying mucosa may be normal or ulcerated and the submucosa surrounding the cysts is fibrotic and contains a mixed inflammatory infiltrate. In adenocarcinoma, the epithelium is dysplastic and the surrounding stroma is reactive.

Treatment is directed at reducing symptoms or preventing some of the proposed etiologic mechanisms. Conservative therapy (high fiber diet and modifying bowel movements to avoid straining) will reduce symptoms in most patients and should be tried first. Patients without rectal intussusception should be offered biofeedback to retrain their bowel function.[60] Pharmacologic therapy has had limited success, but is reasonable to try before embarking on surgery. If symptoms persist, a localized resection may be considered in selected patients.[61] Those suitable for localized resection should be significantly symptomatic, be good surgical risks, and have localized, accessible areas of disease. Patients with prolapse are considered for surgical treatment [abdominal rectopexy, segmental resection and rectal fixation, perineal proctectomy (Altmeier), or a mucosal proctectomy (Delorme)]. Those without prolapse may be offered excision which varies from a transanal excision to a major resection with coloanal pullthrough.

Conclusion

Optimum management of patients with rectal prolapse requires careful patient evaluation for synchronous functional bowel disorders. Although the precise etiology of rectal prolapse remains unclear, the condition is frequently associated with constipation and straining and, intuitively these coexisting symptoms seem to have a role in the development of prolapse in many patients. Management of any associated constipation, either medically or by the addition of sigmoid colectomy, seems important to the ultimate outcome of treatment, although it remains unclear as to whether successful management of constipation results in a lower risk of recurrent prolapse. Fecal incontinence is a frequent complication of full-thickness rectal prolapse; unfortunately, successful treatment of the prolapse results in only a 50% chance of improvement in preexisting fecal incontinence.

Operative management can be divided into abdominal approaches and perineal approaches. Generally, abdominal rectopexy, with or without resection, has a higher morbidity but a much lower risk of recurrence than perineal rectosigmoidectomy. Selection of the best specific procedure for a given patient remains highly individualized, at the physician's discretion, and depends on variables such as the patient's general medical condition, comorbid disorders, the presence of incontinence or constipation, and any prior surgery for prolapse. Typically, the clinician balances the risk of recurrent prolapse against the operative morbidity (e.g., abdominal

rectopexy versus perineal rectosigmoidectomy). Therapeutic options such as anal encirclement and placement of mesh are not routinely performed in the United States given the reasonably good results achieved with either abdominal rectopexy (±sigmoid colectomy) or perineal rectosigmoidectomy. Laparoscopic rectopexy with or without sigmoid colectomy seems to be both safe and effective and will likely replace open abdominal surgery in the management of rectal prolapse. At this time, it is unclear whether laparoscopic rectopexy is more effective and is as safe as perineal rectosigmoidectomy for elderly, high-risk patients.

SRUS and CCF are uncommon colorectal conditions associated with prolapse. As benign conditions, efforts are directed to establishing the diagnosis, excluding malignancy, and treating symptoms. A directed history, physical examination, and endoscopic biopsy will confirm the diagnosis. Therapy to modify bowel movements and habits has had the most success. If these measures fail, surgical therapy to correct rectal prolapse or locally excise the lesions may be considered.

References

1. Moschcowitz AV. The pathogenesis, anatomy and cure of prolapse of the rectum. Surg Gynecol Obstet 1912;15:7–21.
2. Broden B, Snellman B. Procidentia of the rectum studied with cineradiography: a contribution to the discussion of causative mechanism. Dis Colon Rectum 1968;11:330–347.
3. Beck DE, Whitlow CB. Rectal prolapse and intussusception. In: Beck DE, ed. Handbook of Colorectal Surgery. 2nd ed. New York: Marcel Dekker; 2003:301–324.
4. Spencer RJ. Manometric studies in rectal prolapse. Dis Colon Rectum 1984;27:523–525.
5. Prasad ML, Pearl RK, Abcarian H, Orsay CP, Nelson RL. Perineal proctectomy, posterior rectopexy, and postanal levator repair for the treatment of rectal prolapse. Dis Colon Rectum 1986;29:547–552.
6. Altemeier WA, Culbertson WR, Schowengerdt CJ, Hunt J. Nineteen years' experience with the one stage perineal repair of rectal prolapse. Ann Surg 1971;173:993–1006.
7. Ramanujam PS, Venkateh KS. Perineal excision of rectal prolapse with posterior levator ani repair in elderly high risk patients. Dis Colon Rectum 1988;31:704–706.
8. Friedman R, Mugga-Sullam M, Freund HR. Experience with the one stage perineal repair of rectal prolapse. Dis Colon Rectum 1983;26:789–791.
9. Gopal FA, Amshel AL, Shonberg IL, Eftaiha M. Rectal procidentia in elderly and debilitated patients. Experience with the Altemeier procedure. Dis Colon Rectum 1984;27:376–381.
10. Finlay IG, Aitchison M. Perineal excision of the rectum for prolapse in the elderly. Br J Surg 1991;78:687–689.
11. Williams JG, Rothenberger DA, Madoff RD, Goldberg SM. Treatment of rectal prolapse in the elderly by perineal rectosigmoidectomy. Dis Colon Rectum 1992;34:209–216.
12. Johansen OB, Wexner SD, Daniel N, Nogueras JJ, Jagelman DG. Perineal rectosigmoidectomy in the elderly. Dis Colon Rectum 1993;36:767–772.

13. Kim D, Tsang C, Wong W, Lowry A, Goldberg S, Madoff R. Complete rectal prolapse: evolution of management and results. Dis Colon Rectum 1999;42:460–469.

14. Azimuddin K, Khubchandani I, Rosen L, Stasik J, Riether R, Reed J. Rectal prolapse: a search for the "best" operation. Am Surg 2001;67:622–627.

15. Zbar A, Takashima S, Hasegawa T, Kitabayashi K. Perineal rectosigmoidectomy (Altemeier's procedure): a review of physiology, technique and outcome. Tech Coloproctol 2002;6:109–116.

16. Whitlow CB, Beck DE, Opelka FG, Gathright JB, Timmcke AE, Hicks TC. Perineal procedures for prolapse. J La State Med Soc 1997;149:22–26.

17. Delorme E. Sur le traitement des prolapsus du rectum totaux pour l'excision de la muqueuse rectale ou rectocolique. Bull Mem Soc Chir Paris 1900;26:499–578.

18. Uhlig BE, Sullivan ES. The modified Delorme operation: its place in surgical treatment for massive rectal prolapse. Dis Colon Rectum 1979;22:513–521.

19. Monson JR, Jones AN, Vowden P, Brennan TG. Delorme's operation: the first choice in complete rectal prolapse? Ann R Coll Surg Engl 1986;68:143–146.

20. Senapati A, Nicholls RJ, Chir M, et al. Results of Delorme's procedure for rectal prolapse. Dis Colon Rectum 1994;37(5):456–460.

21. Oliver GC, Vachon D, Eisenstar TE, et al. Delorme's procedure for complete rectal prolapse in severely debilitated patients. Dis Colon Rectum 1994;37(5):461–467.

22. Tobin SA, Scott IHK. Delorme operation for rectal prolapse. Br J Surg 1994;81:1681–1684.

23. Graf W, Ejerblad S, Krog M, et al. Delorme's operation for rectal prolapse in elderly or unfit patients. Eur J Surg 1992;158:555–557.

24. Goldman J. Concerning prolapse of the rectum with special emphasis on the operation by Thiersch. Dis Colon Rectum 1988;31:154–155.

25. Gabriel WB. Thiersch's operation for anal incontinence and minor degrees of rectal prolapse. Am J Surg 1953;86:583–590.

26. Khanduja KS, Hardy TG Jr, Aguilar PS, et al. A new silicone prosthesis in the modified Thiersch operation. Dis Colon Rectum 1988;31:380–383.

27. Williams JG. Perineal approaches to repair of rectal prolapse. Semin Colon Rectal Surg 1991;2:198–204.

28. Jackaman FR, Francis JN, Hopkinson BR. Silicone rubber band treatment of rectal prolapse. Ann R Coll Surg Engl 1980;62:386–387.

29. Labow S, Rubin R, Hoexter B, Salvati E. Perineal repair of procidentia with an elastic fabric sling. Dis Colon Rectum 1980;23:467–469.

30. Hunt TM, Fraser IA, Maybury NK. Treatment of rectal prolapse by sphincteric support and using silastic rods. Br J Surg 1985;72:491–492.

31. Poole GV Jr, Pennell TC, Myers RT, Hightower F. Modified Thiersch operation for rectal prolapse. Techniques and results. Am Surg 1985;51:226–229.

32. Vongsangnak V, Varma JS, Smith AN. Reappraisal of Thiersch's operation for complete rectal prolapse. J R Coll Surg Edinb 1985;30:185–187.

33. Earnshaw JJ, Hopkinson BR. Late results of silicone rubber perianal suture for rectal prolapse. Dis Colon Rectum 1987;30:86–88.

34. Khanduja KS, Hardy TG, Aguilar PS, et al. A new silicone prosthesis in the modified Thiersch operation. Dis Colon Rectum 1988;31:380–383.

35. Frykman HM. Abdominal proctopexy and primary sigmoid resection for rectal procidentia. Am J Surg 1955;90:780–789.

36. Watts JD, Rothenberger DA, Buls JG, Goldberg SM, Nivatvongs S. The management of procidentia: 30 years experience. Dis Colon Rectum 1985;28:96–102.

37. Husa A, Sainio P, Smitten K. Abdominal rectopexy and sitmoid resection (Frykman-Goldberg) operation for rectal prolapse. Acta Chir Scand 1988;154:221–224.

38. Sayfan J, Pinho M, Alexander-Williams J, Keighley MRB. Sutured posterior abdominal rectopexy with sigmoidectomy compared with Marlex rectopexy for rectal prolapse. Br J Surg 1990;77:143–145.

39. McKee RF, Lauder JC, Poon FW, Aichison MA, Finlay IG. A prospective randomized study of abdominal rectopexy with and without sigmoidectomy in rectal prolapse. Surg Gynecol Obstet 1992;174:145–148.

40. Luukkonen P, Mikkonen U, Jarvinen H. Abdominal rectopexy with sigmoidectomy vs rectopexy alone for rectal prolapse: a prospective randomized study. Int J Colorectal Dis 1992;7:219–222.

41. Canfrere VG, des Barannos SB, Mayon J, Lehar PA. Adding sigmoidectomy to rectopexy to treat rectal prolapse: a valid option? Br J Surg 1994;581:2–4.

42. Huber FT, Stein H, Siewert JR. Functional results after treatment of rectal prolapse with rectopexy and sigmoid resection. World J Surg 1995;19:138–143.

43. Loygue J, Hugier M, Malafosse M, Biotois H. Complete prolapse of the rectum: a report on 140 cases treated by rectopexy. Br J Surg 1971;58:847–848.

44. Blatchford GJ, Perry RE, Thorson AG, Christensen MA. Rectopexy without resection for rectal prolapse. Am J Surg 1989;158:574–576.

45. Ripstein CB, Lanter B. Etiology and surgical therapy of massive prolapse of the rectum. Ann Surg 1963;157:259–264.

46. Gordon PH, Hoexter B. Complications of Ripstein procedure. Dis Colon Rectum 1978;21:277–280.

47. Eisenstadt TE, Rubin RJ, Salvati EP. Surgical treatment of complete rectal prolapse. Dis Colon Rectum 1979;22:522–523.

48. Tjandra JJ, Fazio VW, Church JM, Milsom JW, Oakley JR, Lavery IC. Ripstein procedure is an effective treatment for rectal prolapse without constipation. Dis Colon Rectum 1993;36:501–507.

49. Winde G, Reers B, Nottberg H, Berns T, Meyer J, Bunt H. Clinical and functional results of abdominal rectopexy with absorbable mesh graft for treatment of complete rectal prolapse. Eur J Surg 1993;159:301–305.

50. Wells C. New operation for rectal prolapse. Proc R Soc Med 1959;52:602–603.

51. Novell JR, Osborne MJ, Winslet MC, Lewis AAM. Prospective randomized trial of Ivalon sponge versus sutured rectopexy for full thickness rectal prolapse. Br J Surg 1994;81:904–906.

52. Baker R, Senagore AJ, Luchtefeld MA. Laparoscopic-assisted vs. open resection. Rectopexy offers excellent results. Dis Colon Rectum 1995;38:199–201.

53. Heah SM, Hartley JE, Hurleey J, Duthie GS, Monson JR. Laparoscopic suture rectopexy without resection is effective

treatment for full-thickness rectal prolapse. Dis Colon Rectum 2000;43:638–643.

54. Ashari LH, Lumley JW, Stevenson AR, Stitz RW. Laparoscopically-assisted resection rectopexy for rectal prolapse: ten years' experience. Dis Colon Rectum 2005;48:982–987.

55. Kairaluoma MV, Viljakka MT, Kellokumpu IH. Open vs. laparoscopic surgery for rectal prolapse: a case-controlled study assessing short-term outcome. Dis Colon Rectum 2003;46:353–360.

56. Hool GR, Hull TL, Fazio VW. Surgical treatment of recurrent complete rectal prolapse. Dis Colon Rectum 1997;40: 270–272.

57. Fengler SA, Pearl RK, Prasad ML, et al. Management of recurrent rectal prolapse. Dis Colon Rectum 1997;40:832–834.

58. Pikarsky AJ, Joo JS, Wexner SD, et al. Recurrent rectal prolapse: what is the next good option? Dis Colon Rectum 2000;43: 1273–1276.

59. Beck DE. Colitis cystica profunda. In: Johnson LR, ed. Encyclopedia of Gastroenterology. San Diego: Elsevier Science; 2003:374–375.

60. Vaizey CJ, van den Bogaerde JB, Emmanuel AV, Talbot IC, Nicholls RJ, Kamm MA. Solitary rectal ulcer syndrome. Br J Surg 1998;85:1617–1623.

61. Beck DE. Surgical therapy for colitis cystica profunda and solitary rectal ulcer syndrome. Curr Treat Options Gastroenterol 2002;5:231–237.

48
Constipation

Amanda Metcalf and Howard Michael Ross

One of the most common complaints voiced to internists, gastroenterologists, and colon and rectal surgeons alike is that of constipation. Patient definitions of constipation are so variable that the term itself is meaningless and focused questioning regarding the patient's actual bowel habits is mandatory. To facilitate research into and treatment of constipation and other functional bowel disorders, a multinational panel of experts was convened in Rome, Italy. The Rome criteria for the diagnosis of constipation requires two or more of the following for at least 3 months:

- Straining more than 25% of the time
- Hard stools more than 25% of the time
- Incomplete evacuation more than 25% of the time
- Two or fewer bowel movements per week

Sonnenberg and Koch[1] described the enormity of the problem in the United States in 1989. These authors estimated that four million people in the United States complain of frequent constipation, a prevalence rate of 2%. Complaints of constipation are two to three times more common in women than men and complaints increase with increasing age. The incidence of constipation is also higher in nonwhites than whites, in people from a lower socioeconomic and educational status, and in the southern United States. A more recent study in elderly residents of Olmstead County in Minnesota further underscored the enormity of the problem.[2] Talley et al. found that nearly one in two women and one in three men over the age of 65 either had complaints of constipation or took laxatives. The magnitude of the problem requires the colon and rectal surgeon to understand the causation of constipation, be facile with the tests used in the evaluation of the constipated patient, and be able to recommend both medical and surgical therapies when appropriate.

Etiology

Constipation can be secondary to a long list of conditions and medications (see Table 48-1). Physiologically, a number of complex interactions are necessary for the development of formed stool, the passage of stool through the colon, and the elimination of the stool bolus. Evaluation of the constipated patient must include investigation into all of the factors potentially responsible for constipation.

Diet affects the size, consistency, and frequency of bowel movements. Dietary intake of fiber is highly correlated with stool bulk. Inhabitants of countries with higher fiber intake pass more voluminous stool than those in countries with a lower intake of dietary fiber. Inhabitants of Western countries typically ingest inadequate amounts of fiber, secondary to reliance on processed grains. Because colonic distension triggers peristalsis, bulkier stools are a stronger and more efficient stimulus for colonic propulsion than smaller stools.

As noted, female gender is associated with a higher prevalence of constipation. Knowles et al.[3] reported that of 2004 patients evaluated by transit study at three European tertiary referral centers for intractable constipation, 92% were women. No definitive explanations exist for the gender difference seen, although hormonal influences and pelvic anatomy have been suggested.

Many medical conditions are recognized to affect bowel function. Hypothyroidism and diabetes, lupus and scleroderma, neurologic illness, immobilization, and psychiatric disease are but a few of a long list of medical maladies associated with increased rates of constipation and should be considered as a source of constipation during evaluation. Mechanisms of dysfunction include alteration in motor function of the gut and autonomic neuropathy as seen in hypothyroidism and diabetes mellitus, respectively. Hirschsprung's disease and Chagas' disease alter the function of the colon through damage to the enteric nervous system. Connective tissue disorders alter the functionality of intestinal smooth muscle. Colonic stricture secondary to carcinoma, inflammatory bowel disease, radiation, or endometriosis can cause colonic obstruction. Medications for the management of common disorders such as hypertension promote the development of constipation. Opiate and anticholinergic use, as well as laxative abuse, is associated with constipation. Opiates decrease the propulsive activity of the colon through

TABLE 48-1. Factors associated with constipation

Lifestyle
   Inadequate fluid intake
   Inadequate fiber intake
   Inactivity
   Laxative abuse
Medications
   Anticholinergics
   Antidepressants
   Calcium channel blocker anti-HTN
   Iron
   Opiates
Medical illness
   Neurologic
      Spinal cord dysfunction/damage
      Parkinson's disease
      Multiple sclerosis
   Endocrine/metabolic dysfunction
      Diabetes mellitus
      Hypothyroidism
      Electrolyte abnormalities
      Uremia
      Hypercalcemia
      Porphyria
   Psychological
      Depression
      Anorexia
      Psychiatric illness
      Sexual abuse
Colonic structure/function
   Cancer
   Crohn's disease
   Irradiation
   Endometriosis
   Hirschsprung's disease
   Chagas' disease
Pelvic floor abnormality
   Nonrelaxing puborectalis
   Anal stenosis
   Rectocele/enterocele

activation of mu-opiate receptors found on neurons of the enteric nervous system.

Evaluation

The evaluation of the patient complaining of constipation begins with a detailed history. Specific details of the patient's complaints—stool size, frequency, consistency, ease and efficacy of evacuation—should be noted. Also important to note are the age at onset of symptoms, diet and exercise details, medical history, surgical history, and medication. Query into psychiatric illness and sexual and physical abuse must be performed, because they are associated with defecation difficulties. Symptoms of pelvic floor dysfunction involving the urinary tract should be ascertained. A patient diary of dietary intake, defecation frequency, stool consistency, and any associated symptoms can be very helpful to both the patient and the medical provider.

Physical examination will likely be unremarkable. Abdominal distension or the presence of a mass may be noted. Rectal examination should involve a clinical evaluation of resting tone and the ability to voluntarily contract and relax the anal sphincter. Evaluation for pelvic floor dysfunction such as perineal descent with straining, the presence of a rectocele or cystocele, and the volume and consistency of stool in the rectal vault should be noted.

The evaluation of the patient with symptoms of constipation that do not respond to a trial of diet and medical therapy begins with the elimination of a structural bowel obstruction via colonoscopy or barium enema. Once obstruction has been eliminated as the cause of constipation symptoms, colonic transit time should then be assessed.

The purpose of the radiographic evaluation of the patient with constipation complaints is to identify conditions that may require treatment paradigms other than diet and medication therapy. Specifically, slow-transit constipation (colonic inertia) and pelvic floor outlet obstruction are entities that may be better treated with surgery and biofeedback, respectively. Evaluation of upper gastrointestinal motility, colon motility, and the mechanism of defecation is currently possible. When combined with anal manometry, a picture of a patient's ability to propel and eliminate stool can be generated.

Colonic transit time can be estimated via marker studies or through scintigraphy. The precise technique chosen depends on availability and whether one desires a global or more precise measurement of transit. The most widely available technique for determining colonic transit uses radiopaque markers and radiographs of the abdomen. The concept of assessing transit using markers was first developed by Hinton et al.,[4] modified by Martelli et al.,[5] and further simplified by Metcalf et al.[6]

To obtain a global assessment of whether or not patients have slow-transit constipation, the technique requires the patient to refrain from all enemas, laxatives, and most medications for 2 days before the ingestion of 24 radiopaque markers. The patient is required to ingest 30 g of fiber daily during the test and must continue to refrain from taking medication and laxatives. An abdominal radiograph is obtained on the fifth day. The distribution and the number of markers present in the colon are noted. Eighty percent of normal patients will have passed all the markers by 5 days. If the markers are found to have accumulated in the rectum, outlet obstruction is suggested. If the markers remain scattered throughout the colon and more than 20% of the markers remain in the colon after the fifth day after ingestion, colonic inertia can be diagnosed.

A more precise assessment of transit delay can be obtained by having the patient ingest radiopaque markers on three sequential days while following the same instructions and obtaining a radiograph on the fourth and seventh day (see Figure 48-1). The number and distribution of the markers are tabulated and totaled. The resultant numeric values can then be compared with the established value for normal controls.

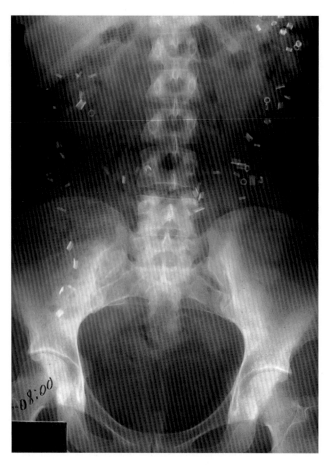

FIGURE 48-1. Marker study revealing colonic inertia.

in conjunction with manometry. The recruitment of puborectalis muscle fibers during defecation simulation indicates the entity of nonrelaxing puborectalis outlet obstruction.

Assessment of upper gastrointestinal motility is appropriate in patients who are demonstrated to have slow-transit constipation. Patients with generalized motility disturbances and colonic inertia have less favorable results after surgical intervention than patients with colonic inertia alone.[10] Small bowel transit time may be measured scintigraphically as mentioned above or with a lactulose hydrogen breath test. The principle of this examination is that hydrogen produced through lactulose fermentation only occurs in the colon. If one records the time from ingestion of lactulose to hydrogen production, small bowel transit time can be inferred.

Medical Treatment of Constipation

Therapy of the constipated patient should begin with patient counsel. It is sage advice to help the patient understand that a daily bowel movement is not requisite to good health. All providers should strive to decrease patient anxiety over the act of defecation. The elimination of malignancy and mechanical causes of symptomatology, performed for the evaluation of constipation, often goes far in this regard.

Simple measures that can influence the passage of colonic content are increasing physical activity and fluid intake. Exercise, even gentle walking, can facilitate the elimination of stool. Fluid intake can cause the stool to be softer and easier to pass. Medications that promote constipation should be eliminated or substituted with alternatives that are less constipating.

Lack of dietary fiber intake is a major factor in the development of constipation symptoms. Bulk-forming agents are a first-line therapy in the prevention and treatment of constipation. Bulk-forming agents facilitate an increase in the size of the stool bolus as well as make the stool softer. Bulking agents facilitate these changes by delivering a mass of nondigestible substrate to the colon and, because of their hydrophilic nature, facilitate the absorption and retention of fluid. Bulk laxatives are derived from the nondigestible components of plants or are synthetic methylcellulose derivatives. Common bulk agents are psyllium (Metamucil, Konsyl), methylcellulose (Citrucel), and calcium polycarbophil (FiberCon). Side effects of fiber therapy include bloating and flatulence. A dietary intake of 20–30 g of nonstarch polysaccharide is generally recommended to minimize symptoms of constipation.

Osmotic laxatives are a class of medications that promote the accumulation of large volumes of fluid in the colon lumen through the delivery of osmotically active molecules into the small and large bowel. The osmotically active particles can be derived from sugars or salts. Sorbitol and lactulose are examples of sugar-based osmotic agents. Lactulose is broken down in the colon yielding the production of fatty acids, hydrogen, and carbon dioxide. Cautery in the presence of these gases can cause an explosion.

The mean colon transit time through the entire colon in men has been shown to be 31 hours in males and 39 hours in women. Patients with normal transit constipation will have a colon transit time that is in the normal range (<65 hours in 95% of men, <75 hours in 95% of women).

Scintigraphic evaluation of colonic transit has been described, and although not as widely available, is useful in the assessment of transit in the colon and proximal gut.[7] Transit times obtained through scintigraphy are generated by following the passage of a radiolabeled meal. Small bowel and gastric emptying rates can also be estimated with this one examination. Normal small bowel transit is between 90 and 120 minutes.

Outlet obstruction suggested on a marker study can be further characterized through defecography. Defecography facilitates visualization of the mechanism of defecation. Nonrelaxing puborectalis or a large rectocele can both be identified on a defecogram.[8]

Anal manometry reveals the absence of the rectoanal inhibitory reflex and therefore suggests the presence of Hirschsprung's disease. Balloon expulsion testing performed during manometry can add to the reliability of the diagnosis of pelvic floor outlet obstruction caused by nonrelaxation of the puborectalis muscle.[9] Anal electromyography is performed

Osmotic laxatives can also be based on nonabsorbable ions, frequently derived from magnesium or phosphate. Examples are magnesium hydroxide (milk of magnesia) or sodium phosphate (Fleets Phospho-soda). Caution must be exercised in patients with renal insufficiency because hypermagnesemia can result. Polyethylene glycol–based products are used in many bowel-cleansing regimes. Chronic use can lead to electrolyte disturbances and dehydration.

Colonic irritants are a class of agents that diminish constipation through stimulation of colonic motility. Anthracene derivatives include senna and cascara and are found in Senokot and Peri-Colace. Long-term anthracene intake can generate a characteristic brown discoloration of the mucosa called pseudomelanosis coli. There is some debate whether long-term intake of anthracene laxatives increases the risk of colon cancer. Bisacodyl is another irritant and can be found in the agent Dulcolax. Long-term use of anthracene irritants may lead to poor colon function and such use is therefore discouraged. However, there is little objective evidence to support this belief.

Mineral oil and docusate sodium (Colace) are laxatives that act through the manipulation of the composition of stool. Mineral oil coats the stool bolus, preventing fluid absorption from it. Docusate sodium lowers the surface tension at the stool water interface, allowing greater penetration of the stool with fluid.

Enemas and suppositories are used to stimulate a bowel movement. Strategies include promotion of defecation through distension (saline enema), rectal irritation (soapsuds, bisacodyl), or physical softening of the stool (glycerine).

Colonic Inertia

Colonic inertia, also called slow-transit constipation, represents a severe functional disturbance of colonic motility, which results in significant disability to the patient. Patients with colonic inertia, similar to patients with normal transit constipation and patients with outlet obstruction, exhibit infrequent defecation and may experience abdominal pain, bloating, nausea, difficulty with and incomplete evacuation of stool. Only a very small percentage of patients with constipation actually have colonic inertia. The diagnosis of colonic inertia requires the documentation of abnormal colonic transit (>20% of ingested markers present and scattered throughout the colon on day 5 of colonic transit time testing). Patients with constipation are often highly motivated to relieve their symptoms. Many are very willing to undergo surgery. Total abdominal colectomy (TAC) for colonic inertia is only appropriate for patients with documented abnormalities in colonic transit. TAC entails the risk of abdominal operation and intestinal anastomosis. Persistent or recurrent constipation, progression to small bowel inertia, and fecal incontinence may occur after TAC with ileorectal anastomosis and must be explained to the patient. Precise evaluation of colonic motility and pelvic floor

function is critical in the identification of patients that truly exhibit colonic inertia and have the highest probability to benefit from surgical intervention. A review of the outcomes of surgical intervention for colonic inertia follows.

Lane[11] reported the results of surgical intervention for the elimination of constipation in 1908, and described the resolution of constipation symptoms through the removal of the abdominal colon in two-thirds of patients. Lane performed his series of operations without the benefit of manometry, transit studies, or defecography. Remarkably, he was able to state that if the abdominal colon was not removed, symptoms could recur.

Dr. Lane's words speak volumes. "In the earliest cases in which I removed the greater part of the large bowel the symptom demanding it was pain, usually in the caecum, splenic flexure, or sigmoid. Though I was aware of the associated symptoms of autointoxication I did not operate for their removal, nor was I aware that the excision of the large bowel would result in their complete disappearance. I only became conscious of this result after the removal of the large bowel. And the comparatively abrupt change which ensued during the few days following the operation was almost startling. The recognition of the immense advantages which these miserable people obtained from the removal of the large bowel then induced me to operate also in cases where pain was not necessarily such a marked feature, but where life was becoming a burden through the misery and distress induced by the autointoxication and its result. . . . At first I was satisfied in most cases to remove the large bowel as far as the splenic flexure, as I believed that the risk of the operation was reduced by leaving the descending colon and sigmoid, for these structures being vertically placed I did not expect that material would accumulate in them above the junction of the ileum and rectum. I found, however, that many of those in whom I left them complained, after a lapse of time, of symptoms which I was able to attribute to distension of the descending colon and sigmoid with gas. Therefore I excised the residual bowel in many such cases of incomplete resection and took away the entire large bowel with the exception of the rectum in all primary operations."

Multiple trials have recently reported the long-term results of TAC for colonic inertia. Pikarsky et al.[12] from the Cleveland Clinic Florida identified 50 patients that had undergone TAC for colonic inertia between 1988 and 1993. Thirty were available for telephone interview designed to assess bowel function, concomitant use of any antidiarrheal medications, postoperative complications, persistence or development of preoperative symptoms such as pain or bloating, and overall satisfaction. The mean follow-up was 106 months (range, 61–122 months). Remarkably, all 30 patients reported the outcome of surgery as "excellent." The average number of bowel movements per day was 2.5 (1–6). Twenty percent of patients required admission for small bowel obstruction and half of these patients required laparotomy for obstruction (10%). Two patients (6%) required assistance with bowel movements despite operation. Two patients (6%) needed antidiarrheal medication to reduce bowel frequency.

Long-term follow-up has also recently been reported by Webster and Dayton[13] from the University of Utah. Their retrospective review identified 55 patients who underwent TAC for colonic inertia. Eighty-seven percent were female and the average age was 40. Postoperatively, 8% experienced a bowel obstruction. "Good" or "excellent" results were reported by 89% of patients. "Poor" results were reported by 11% of patients. The mean stool frequency per day was three at 12 months from surgery. Verne et al.[14] from the University of Florida identified 13 patients who underwent TAC for colonic inertia between 1983 and 1987. Seven patients had an ileosigmoid anastomosis and six an ileorectal anastomosis. The overall number of bowel movements per week increased from 0.5 to 15 ± 4.5 postoperatively.

The Mayo Clinic reported their long-term results of TAC for colonic inertia in 1997.[15] Seventy-four patients were identified as having had a TAC. Fifty-two had slow-transit constipation alone and twenty-two had colonic inertia and pelvic floor dysfunction. These twenty-two underwent pelvic floor retraining followed by surgery. Similar to most other studies, 90% of patients had a "good" or improved quality of life. All patients could pass stool spontaneously. Nine percent of patients developed a small bowel obstruction. There was no difference in the surgical outcome of patients who required pelvic floor retraining and surgery when compared with the group that required surgery alone.

FitzHarris et al.[16] from the University of Minnesota addressed the question of whether the increase in bowel movements experienced by patients with colonic inertia that undergo TAC resulted in an improved quality of life. Patients were sent a survey that inquired about bowel function and included a gastrointestinal quality-of-life index. Gastrointestinal quality-of-life index scores were correlated with specific functional outcomes. Eighty-one percent of patients were at least "somewhat" pleased with their bowel movement frequency, but 41% cited abdominal pain, 21% incontinence, and 46% had diarrhea at least some of the time. Five percent of patients had recurrent or persistent constipation and 17% underwent lysis of adhesions for small bowel obstruction. No correlation was found between frequency of bowel movements and quality-of-life scores. If offered subtotal colectomy again, 93% of patients stated they would accept. These authors concluded that although the vast majority of patients were no longer constipated, a significant number had persistent or new adverse symptoms.

Knowles et al.[17] in 1999 published a thorough review of the outcome of colectomy for slow-transit constipation. All series published in the English language through 1999 including 10 or more patients treated with colectomy for colonic inertia were included in the review. Thirty-two studies between 1981 and 1998 met entry criteria. The authors noted that the median rate of success in these studies was 86% with a range between 39%–100%. The authors of the review revealed that no study

was controlled with respect to the outcome from other surgical or medical interventions. Although not every study in the review commented on each potential functional outcome variable, many patterns of postoperative problems were identified. Fecal incontinence was reported in 16 series with a median incidence of 14% (range, 0%–52%). Persistent abdominal pain was reported in 14 series. A 41% median incidence of abdominal pain was identified, with a range between 0%–90%. Recurrent constipation was reported in 15 series with a median incidence of 9% (range, 0%–33%). A permanent ileostomy was created in 5% of patients because of poor functional outcome (0%–28%).

Despite consistently increasing stool frequency, TAC to treat colonic inertia does not guarantee a successful functional outcome. Furthermore, even extensive preoperative work-up does not ensure patient satisfaction. In their study of 21 patients diagnosed with slow-transit constipation via colon transit studies, anal manometry, defecography, pelvic floor electromyography, and determination of small bowel transit time, Mollen et al.[18] found a satisfaction rate of 52% after 1 year. They appropriately caution against the promiscuous use of colectomy to treat functional constipation. Operations other than TAC with ileorectal anastomosis have been proposed in the treatment of colonic inertia. Segmental resection has the theoretic advantage of reducing diarrhea and fecal incontinence. In a consecutive series of 28 patients with slow-transit constipation as determined by scintigraphic transit study that were subsequently treated with segmental colectomy, 23 patients were pleased with the outcome.[19] The median follow-up in this study was 50 months. The median stool frequency increased from one to seven per week. Incontinence was unchanged. Similarly in a study from China using right or left colectomy to treat transit abnormalities of either the right or left colon, 37 of 40 patients followed for 2 years had improvement of their symptoms without diarrhea or incontinence.[20] Three of the 40 patients experienced recurrent constipation that ultimately required TAC with ileorectal anastomosis. Because the follow-up time of these studies is short and the ability to define segmental colonic transit inexact, TAC remains the most widely accepted surgical treatment option in the treatment of colonic inertia. Historically, patients having segmental colectomy have had poor results.[21]

Proctocolectomy with ileoanal pouch reconstruction has been described as a salvage operation for patients with recurrent constipation after subtotal colectomy with ileorectal anastomosis for slow-transit constipation. The number of patients that have had pouch reconstruction for salvage after subtotal colectomy has been quite small. Keighley et al.[22] reported the results of eight patients who underwent such radical surgery. Four of these eight ultimately required pouch excision for recurrent constipation. Proctocolectomy as initial treatment for slow-transit constipation and rectal inertia has recently been explored.[23] Two of 15 patients required pouch excision within 18 months because of intractable pelvic pain. Significant improvement in lifestyle scores were recorded in the categories of physical function, social function, pain, and general health for the group during the follow-up period.

A difficult subgroup of patients with slow-transit constipation to treat is those with concomitant pelvic floor dysfunction. Bernini et al.[24] from the University of Minnesota evaluated 16 patients who had a combination of colonic inertia and non-relaxing pelvic floor as diagnosed by transit marker study, electromyography, and defecography. All patients completed preoperative biofeedback training and could demonstrate relaxation of the pelvic floor musculature. Despite biofeedback training, difficult evacuation persisted. Postoperatively, 43% of patients had complete resolution of symptoms of constipation or difficult evacuation. Eighteen percent complained of diarrhea and incontinence of liquid stools. Six of the 16 patients complained of incomplete evacuation. The authors concluded that subtotal colectomy could improve some symptoms in patients with colonic inertia and nonrelaxing pelvic floor, however, incomplete evacuation persisted in a significant number of patients. Almost half were dissatisfied with their surgery.

Irritable Bowel Syndrome

Irritable bowel syndrome (IBS) is a disorder in which patients have abdominal discomfort and altered bowel habits that defy explanation by identifiable organic pathology. Although there is overlap between patients in this category and those described in the previous section, this diagnosis is more inclusive because patients can have constipation or diarrhea. There are no specific tests to identify this disorder. Rather, it is a diagnosis of exclusion, and remains a clinical diagnosis. The most recent consensus of the clinical features of IBS is known as the Rome criteria and was reached at the conference described earlier. These criteria were reached to standardize the diagnosis of this disorder for both research purposes and clinical practice.[25] The Rome criteria for a clinical diagnosis of IBS are listed in Table 48-2. In essence, patients must have chronic symptoms that include abdominal pain relieved by defecation and or associated with a change in the consistency or frequency of stools. These symptoms are variably associated with mucorrhea and/or abdominal bloating.

TABLE 48-2. Rome criteria for IBS

Abdominal pain or discomfort characterized by the following:
Relieved by defecation
Associated with a change in stool frequency
Associated with a change in stool consistency
Two or more of the following characteristics at least 25% of the time:
Altered stool frequency
Altered stool form
Altered stool passage
Mucorrhea
Abdominal bloating or subjective distension

Population-based studies in Western countries report an overall prevalence of IBS of 10%–20%.[26] With the exception of Hispanics in Texas and Asians in California, who may have a lower rate, the prevalence is similar in Western minority populations.[27,28] Some studies suggest that the incidence may be lower in Asian countries and Africa. In Western countries, women are 2–3 times more likely to develop IBS than men; in India, this phenomenon is reversed.[29] The prevalence seems to be lower in the elderly. Retrospectively, many patients report childhood symptoms, and 50% of patients have symptoms before age 35.[30] The incidence in Western countries is 1%–2% per year.

It has been recognized for many years that there are a variety of disorders associated with a clinical diagnosis of IBS. These include nonulcer dyspepsia, fibromyalgia, chronic fatigue syndrome, dysmenorrhea, urinary tract symptoms, and psychiatric disorders. Patients who undergo physician evaluation for IBS tend to have increased scores for depression, anxiety, somatization, and neuroticism on standardized tests, although no specific pattern of personality traits in patients has been identified. Patients with IBS who present for evaluation are at least twice as likely to meet criteria for psychiatric disorders as patients with organic disease. The most frequent of these disorders are depression and generalized anxiety. Interestingly, individuals with clinical symptoms of IBS who do not seek medical care have a similar prevalence of psychiatric disorders as the general population.[31] This suggests that the psychiatric disorder may be more important in healthcare-seeking behavior than as an etiologic agent of the syndrome.

It has been estimated that only 10% of patients with IBS symptoms consult a physician for evaluation or treatment of their symptoms. With the exception of Indians, women are more likely than men to present for physician evaluation. The socioeconomic impact of this disorder is significant. There are estimated to be 3.5 million physician visits in the United States, and IBS is the most common diagnosis in gastroenterologist practice. Patients with IBS have more work absenteeism, more physician visits, and report a lower quality of life.[32]

The current theories regarding the pathophysiology of IBS are of a complex interaction between altered gut motility and or visceral hyperalgesia and neuropsychopathology. Many studies measuring myoelectric activity in the colon have demonstrated abnormalities in patients with IBS. Normal colonic myoelectric activity consists of background slow waves with superimposed spike potentials. Bueno et al.[33] demonstrated increased long spike bursts in patients with constipation and irregular short spike bursts in patients with diarrhea. Myoelectric studies in the small bowel have demonstrated shorter intervals between the migrating motor complex, which is, of course, the predominant interdigestive small bowel motor pattern.[34] Patients with IBS have variations in the colonic slow wave frequency and a blunted late peaking postprandial response of spike potentials in the colon. Transit studies in the small bowel have demonstrated delayed meal transit in patients with constipation-predominant IBS and accelerated meal transit in patients with diarrhea-predominant IBS.[35,36] These studies and others suggest an underlying generalized hyperresponsiveness of smooth muscle in patients with IBS.

Visceral hyperalgesia seems to be another component of this disorder. Studies measuring the perception of gut distension using various techniques have demonstrated abnormally low sensitivity in both the small and large bowel.[37,38] It seems that patients with a diagnosis of IBS have both an increased awareness of gut distension, and experience such distension as painful at lower volumes and pressures as normal subjects. This is especially in response to rapid distension.[39] Although there has been some argument regarding a reporting bias in patients with IBS (i.e., routinely reporting pain at lower subjective intensities than normal controls), such differences do not account for all of the sensory abnormalities seen.[40] Furthermore, patients with IBS have widened dermatomal referral pain patterns than normal controls from gut distension.[41] This visceral hypersensitivity is not associated with a somatic hypersensitivity.[42] It is thought that patients with IBS may have sensitization of the intestinal afferent nociceptive pathways in the spinal cord.

The central nervous system modulates gut function for optimal digestive function. The limbic system, medial prefrontal cortex, amygdala, and hypothalamus communicate emotional changes to the gut via the autonomic nervous system. In turn, signals from the gut to the brain can effect reflex regulation and mood states.[43] Recent studies have suggested that patients with IBS may process visceral afferent input in the central nervous system in an abnormal way and this response may be modified by attentional factors such that stress, anxiety, and prior unpleasant life events increase the perception of painful events.[44–46] On a biochemical level, patients with IBS have been demonstrated to have increased hypothalamic corticotropin-releasing factor in response to stress, as well as an exaggerated colonic motility response.[47]

The relationship between psychopathology and IBS is not clear. As noted previously, patients with IBS have a higher incidence of panic disorder, major depression, anxiety disorder, and hypochondriasis than normal populations.[48] In addition, they report a higher prevalence of physical or sexual abuse.[49] Two-thirds of patients with IBS report the onset of gastrointestinal complaints with an axis 1 disorder.[50]

In summary, patients with IBS have been demonstrated to have abnormal gut motility, visceral hyperalgesia, and neuropsychologic abnormalities. In a particular patient, any of these factors may predominate, but all may be involved and they are not mutually exclusive. An understanding of these abnormalities has led to the emergence of new possibilities in the pharmaceutical treatment of this syndrome.

The altered stool habits reported by patients with IBS can be constipation, diarrhea, or alternating constipation and diarrhea. Constipation can be described as hard and/or infrequent stools, or painful defecation requiring laxative use. Diarrhea is usually described as small volume, frequent, urgent, and watery stool. Diarrhea when present is often postprandial in nature. Usually patients have either constipation or diarrhea alone, however, alternation between each can be present. Abdominal pain is usually perceived as diffuse, and is most common in the lower abdomen, especially on the left. Sharp pain may be superimposed on a more chronic duller component. Pain may be precipitated by meals and is often relieved by defecation. Patients often report increasing bloating and gas through the daytime hours, which may or may not be associated with objective evidence. Mucorrhea, either white or clear, is often reported. Patients with IBS are more likely to report upper gastrointestinal symptoms of nausea, vomiting, and heartburn. Overall symptoms may be worse in times of stress. Symptoms that are not typical of IBS that should alert the clinician to organic disease include: onset in middle age or older, progressive or nocturnal symptoms, anorexia, weight loss, fever, hematochezia, painless diarrhea, or steatorrhea.

Although there are emerging novel medications for IBS that may prove useful, much current medical therapy depends heavily on reassurance. Explanation and patient education have an important role in the management of this chronic disorder. Treatment strategies depend not only on the type of symptoms present but their severity and chronicity.

Fiber supplementation may improve symptoms of either constipation or diarrhea, although studies are inconclusive because of a strong placebo effect. Many physicians believe that polycarbophil-based bulking agents may be tolerated better than psyllium-based compounds because of an exacerbation of bloating symptoms in some patients with the latter. Similarly, ingesting more water, avoiding caffeine and legumes are all reasonable patient advice.

As noted above, treatment strategies are symptom directed. Currently available and widely used pharmacologic agents for patients with diarrhea-predominant IBS include anticholinergic medications, nonabsorbable synthetic opioids, and tricyclic antidepressants.

Anticholinergics inhibit intestinal smooth muscle depolarization at the muscarinic receptor. These include dicyclomine hydrochloride (Bentyl) and hyoscyamine sulfate (Levsin). Either has been shown to decrease fecal urgency and pain. Nonabsorbable synthetic opioids, which are frequently used as antidiarrheals act via peripheral mu-opiate receptors. Diphenoxylate hydrochloride with atropine (Lomotil) or loperamide (Imodium) inhibit intestinal motility and prolong transit through the gut. They also reduce visceral nociception via afferent pathway inhibition. They improve stool frequency, urgency, and consistency. Tricyclic antidepressants such as amitriptyline (Elavil) and imipramine (Tofranil) have also been evaluated in off-label use in very low doses for a visceral analgesic effect. Either medication increases orocecal transit time, reduces abdominal pain, mucorrhea, and stool frequency. These results are at subtherapeutic doses for the treatment of depression.

Novel treatments that have been introduced more recently for patients with diarrhea-predominant IBS include the serotonin (5-HT3) agonist Alosetron (Lotronex). This drug inhibits activation of nonselective cation channels that modulate the enteric nervous system. It has been approved only for women with severe diarrhea-predominant symptoms of IBS who have not responded to conventional medication. It has been demonstrated to improve abdominal pain and decrease diarrhea in such patients.[51] Alosetron was temporarily removed from the market by the Food and Drug Administration because of serious and unpredictable side effects including colonic ischemia and toxic megacolon. Cilansetron is another 5-HT3 antagonist currently undergoing testing. This medication shows promise for relief of symptoms in both male and female patients with diarrhea-predominant IBS.[52]

For patients with constipation-predominant IBS who do not respond to fiber supplementation (20 g/day) or do not tolerate it, osmotic laxatives such as milk of magnesia, sorbitol, or polyethylene glycol may be tried.

A novel pharmacologic agent that is currently available is the serotonin (5-HT4) agonist, Tegaserod. Tegaserod is a partial 5-HT4 agonist and accelerates transit in the small bowel and colon. It has been demonstrated to be useful in improving constipation and improving global IBS symptoms in women with constipation-predominant IBS.[53]

Other novel agents undergoing evaluation primarily for symptoms of pain include clonidine (alpha-adrenergic agonist), fedotozine (kappa opioid agonist), and ammonium derivatives (antimuscarinic and neurokinin-receptor antagonist). Of these, fedotozine is clinically available for this indication and has shown to be helpful in reducing symptoms of pain in patients with IBS.[54]

An adjunctive therapy to medication is psychological treatment. This is appropriate when there is evidence that stress or psychologic factors are contributing to an exacerbation of symptoms, or patients have failed to respond to medical treatment. A clear explanation of the rationale for such treatment is important in patient acceptance of such therapy.

References

1. Sonnenberg A, Koch TR. Epidemiology of constipation in the United States. Dis Colon Rectum 1989;32:1–8.
2. Talley NJ, Fleming KC, Evans JM, et al. Constipation in the elderly community: a study of prevalence and potential risk factors. Am J Gastroenterol 1996;91:19–25.
3. Knowles CH, Rayner C, Glia A, Kamm MA, Lunniss PJ. Idiopathic slow-transit constipation: an almost exclusively female disorder. Dis Colon Rectum 2003;46:1716–1717.
4. Hinton JM, Lennard-Jones JE, Young AC. A new method for studying gut transit times using radiopaque markers. Gut 1969;10:842–847.
5. Martelli H, Devroede G, Arhan P, Duguay C, Dormic C, Faverdin C. Some parameters of large bowel motility in normal man. Gastroenterology 1978;75:612–618.
6. Metcalf AM, Phillips SM, Zinmeister AR, MacCarty RL, Beart RW, Wolff BG. Simplified assessment of segmental colonic transit. Gastroenterology 1987;92:40–47.
7. Bonapace ES, Davidoff S, Krevsky B, Maurer AH, Parkman HP, Fisher RS. Whole gut scintigraphy in the clinical evaluation of patients with upper and lower gastrointestinal symptoms. Am J Gastroenterol 2000;95:2838–2847.
8. Jorge JM, Wexner SD, Ger GC, Salanga VD, Nogueras JJ, Jagelman DG. Cinedefecography and electromyography in the diagnosis of nonrelaxing puborectalis syndrome. Dis Colon Rectum 1993;36:668–676.
9. Fleshman JW, Dreznik Z, Cohen E, Fry RD, Kodner IJ. Balloon expulsion test facilitates diagnosis of pelvic floor outlet obstruction due to nonrelaxing puborectalis muscle. Dis Colon Rectum 1992;35:1019–1025.
10. Redmond JM, Smith GW, Barifsky I, et al. Physiologic tests to predict long-term outcome of total abdominal colectomy for intractable constipation. Am J Gastroenterol 1995;90:748–753.
11. Lane WA. The results of the operative treatment of chronic constipation. Br Med J 1908;1:126–130.
12. Pikarsky AJ, Singh JJ, Weiss EG, Nogueras JJ, Wexner SD. Long-term follow-up of patients undergoing colectomy for colonic inertia. Dis Colon Rectum 2001;44:179–183.
13. Webster C, Dayton M. Results after colectomy for colonic inertia: a sixteen-year experience. Am J Surg 2002;186:639–644.
14. Verne GN, Hocking MP, Davis RH, et al. Long-term response to subtotal colectomy in colonic inertia. J Gastrointest Surg 2002;6:738–744.
15. Nyam DC, Pemberton JH, Ilstrup DM, Rath DM. Long-term results of surgery for chronic constipation. Dis Colon Rectum 1997;40:273–279.
16. FitzHarris GP, Garcia-Aguilar J, Parker SC, et al. Quality of life after subtotal colectomy for slow-transit constipation: both quality and quantity count. Dis Colon Rectum 2003;46:433–440.
17. Knowles CH, Scott M, Lunniss PJ. Outcome of colectomy for slow transit constipation. Ann Surg 1999;230(5):627–638.
18. Mollen RM, Kuijpers HC, Classen AT. Colectomy for slow-transit constipation: preoperative fictional evaluation is important but not a guarantee for a successful outcome. Dis Colon Rectum 2001;44:577–580.
19. Lundin E, Karlbom U, Palman L, Graf W. Outcome of segmental colonic resection for slow-transit constipation. Br J Surg 2002;89:1270–1274.
20. You YT, Wang JY, Changchien CR, et al. Segmental colectomy in the management of colonic inertia. Am Surg 1998;64:775–777.
21. Preston DM, Hawley PR, Lennard-Jones JE, Todd IP. Results of colectomy for severe idiopathic constipation in women (Arbuthnot Lane's disease). Br J Surg 1984;71:547–552.
22. Keighley MRB, Grobler S, Bain I. Audit of restorative proctocolectomy. Gut 1993;34:680–684.
23. Kalbassi MR, Winter DC, Deasy JM. Quality of life assessment of patients after ileal pouch-anal anastomosis for slow transit constipation with rectal inertia. Dis Colon Rectum 2003;46:1508–1512.
24. Bernini A, Madoff RD, Lowry AC, et al. Should patients with combined colonic inertia and nonrelaxing pelvic floor undergo subtotal colectomy? Dis Colon Rectum 1998;41:1363–1366.
25. Thompson WG, Longstreth GF, Drossman DA, Heaton KW, Irvine EJ, Mueller-Lissner SA. Functional bowel disorders and

functional abdominal pain. In: Drossman DA, Talley NJ, Thompson WG, Whitehead WE, Corazziari E, eds. Rome II Functional Gastrointestinal Disorders: Diagnosis, Pathophysiology, and Treatment. 2nd ed. McLean, VA: Degnon Associates; 2000:351–432.

26. Longstreth GF, Wolde-Tsadik G. Irritable bowel-type symptoms in HMO examinees. Prevalence, demographics, and clinical correlates. Dig Dis Sci 1993;38(9):1581–1589.

27. Zuckerman MJ, Guerra LG, Drossman DA. Comparison of bowel patterns in Hispanics and non-Hispanic whites. Dig Dis Sci 1995;40(8):1763–1769.

28. Taub E, Cuevas JL, Cook EW, Crowell M, Whitehead WE. Irritable bowel syndrome defined by factor analysis: gender and race comparisons. Dig Dis Sci 1995;40(12):2647–2655.

29. Jain AP, Gupta OP, Jajoo UN, Sidhwa HK. Clinical profile of irritable bowel syndrome at a rural based teaching hospital in central India. J Assoc Physicians India 1991;39(5):385–386.

30. Kay L, Jorgensen T, Jensen KH. The epidemiology of irritable bowel syndrome in a random population: prevalence, incidence, natural history and risk factors. J Intern Med 1994;236(1):23–30.

31. Whitehead WE, Bosmajian L, Zonderman AB, Costa PT Jr, Schuster WM. Symptoms of psychological distress associated with irritable bowel syndrome. Comparison of community and medical clinic samples. Gastroenterology 1988;95(3):709–714.

32. Drossman DA, Camilleri M, Mayer EA, Whitehead WE. AGA technical review on irritable bowel syndrome. Gastroenterology 2002;123(6):2108–2131.

33. Bueno L, Floramonti J, Ruckebusch Y, Frexinos J, Coulom P. Evaluation of colonic myoelectric activity in health and functional disorders. Gut 1980;21(6):480–485.

34. Kellow JE, Phillips SF, Miller LJ, Zinsmeister AR. Dysmotility of the small intestine in irritable bowel syndrome. Gut 1988;29(9):1236–1243.

35. Cann PA, Read NW, Brown C, Hobson N, Holdsworth CG. Irritable bowel syndrome: relationship of disorders in the transit of a single solid meal to symptom patterns. Gut 1983;24(5):405–411.

36. Lu CL, Chen CY, Chang FY, Lee SD. Characteristics of small bowel motility in patients with irritable bowel syndrome and normal humans: an Oriental study. Clin Sci 1998;95(2):165–169.

37. Accarino AM, Azpiro F, Malagelada JR. Selective dysfunction of mechanosensitive intestinal afferents in irritable bowel syndrome. Gastroenterology 1995;108(3):636–643.

38. Zighelboim J, Talley NJ, Phillips SF, Harmsen WS, Zinsmeister AR. Visceral perception in irritable bowel syndrome. Rectal and gastric responses to distension and serotonin type 3 antagonism. Dig Dis Sci 1995;40(4):819–827.

39. Sun WM, Read NW, Prior A, Daly JA, Cheah SK, Grundy D. Sensory and motor responses to rectal distension vary according to the rate and pattern of balloon inflation. Gastroenterology 1990;99(4):1008–1015.

40. Whitehead WE, Palsson OS. Is rectal pain sensitivity a biological marker for irritable bowel syndrome: psychological influences on pain perception. Gastroenterology 1998;115(5):1263–1271.

41. Munakata J, Naliboff B, Harraf F, et al. Repetitive sigmoid stimulation induces rectal hyperalgesia in patients with irritable bowel syndrome. Gastroenterology 1997;112(1):55–63.

42. Cook IJ, van Eeden A, Collins SM. Patients with irritable bowel syndrome have higher pain tolerance than normal subjects. Gastroenterology 1987;93(4):727–733.

43. Nieuwenheuys R. The greater limbic system, the emotional motor system and the brain. In: Hostege G, Bandler R, Saper CB, eds. The Emotional Motor System. Amsterdam: Elsevier; 1996:627.

44. Silverman DH, Munakata JA, Ennes H, Mandelkern MA, Hoh CK, Mayer EA. Regional cerebral activity in normal and pathologic perception of visceral pain. Gastroenterology 1997;112(1):64–72.

45. Keogh E, Ellery D, Hunt C, Hannent I. Selective attentional bias for pain related stimuli amongst pain fearful individuals. Pain 2001;91(1–2):91–100.

46. Accarino AM, Azpiroz F, Malageleda JR. Attention and distraction: effects on gut perception. Gastroenterology 1997;113(2):415–422.

47. Fukudo S, Nomura T, Hongo M. Impact of corticotropin-releasing hormone on gastrointestinal motility and adrenocorticotropic hormone in normal controls and patients with irritable bowel syndrome. Gut 1998;42(6):845–849.

48. Drossman DA, McKee DC, Sandler RE, et al. Psychosocial factors in the irritable bowel syndrome. A multivariate study of patients and nonpatients with irritable bowel syndrome. Gastroenterology 1988;95(3):701–708.

49. Drossman DA, Leserman J, Nachman G, et al. Sexual and physical abuse in women with functional or organic gastrointestinal disorders. Ann Intern Med 1990;113(11):828–833.

50. Creed F, Craig T, Farmer R. Functional abdominal pain, psychiatric illness and life events. Gut 1988;29(2):235–242.

51. Camilleri M, Northcutt AR, Kong S, et al. Efficacy and safety of alosetron in women with irritable bowel syndrome: a randomized, placebo-controlled trial. Lancet 2000;355(9209):1035–1040.

52. Caras S, Krause G, Bilkesheuvel E, Steinborn C. Cilansetron shows efficacy in male and female non constipated patients with irritable bowel syndrome in a United States study [abstract]. Gastroenterology 2001;120:A217.

53. Mueller-Lissner S, Fumagalli I, Bardhan KD, et al. Tegaserod, a 5HT4 receptor partial agonist, relieves key symptoms of irritable bowel syndrome [abstract]. Gastroenterology 2000;118:A175.

54. Corazziari E. Role of opioid ligands in the irritable bowel syndrome. Can J Gastroenterol 1999;13(suppl A):71A–75A.

49
Pelvic Floor Disorders

Frank J. Harford and Linda Brubaker

Pelvic floor disorders are relatively common entities in clinical practice. These disorders can include abnormalities of bowel storage, bowel emptying, regional pain, and anatomic abnormalities. This chapter will review the anatomic abnormality of rectocele and the group of regional anorectal pain disorders.

Rectoceles

Rectoceles are a nonpainful, poorly understood disorder without a gold standard for diagnosis. Rectoceles occur almost exclusively in women, particularly women who are vaginally parous. The relationship between anatomy and function in the distal rectovaginal region has not been studied adequately and there are significant gaps in medical and surgical knowledge.

A common clinical definition of rectocele is abnormal rectovaginal anatomy that allows the rectum to be in direct contact with the vaginal serosa without an intervening layer. Usually, rectoceles are diagnosed when rectovaginal support abnormalities are observed during physical examination. There may be protrusion of the posterior vaginal wall beyond the hymen with or without strain effort. Using the internationally validated staging system for pelvic organ prolapse,[1] the distal-most posterior vaginal wall is 3 cm from the hymen. In rectocele formation, this normal anatomy is lost and the distal posterior vaginal wall moves closer toward the hymen or may protrude outside the hymen.

The differential diagnosis for this physical finding includes other abnormalities of vaginal attachment, usually the vaginal apex (with or without the uterus). Differences in physical examination techniques affect the degree of prolapse that is detected. The side-lying or prone jackknife examination that is favored by many colon and rectal surgeons is sufficient to detect some forms of prolapse; however, the standing straining vaginal examination provides the best opportunity to determine the full extent of anatomic abnormalities. Gynecologic surgeons have placed more focus on repair of the vaginal apex, which then provides secondary resolution of

the distal vaginal support defect for many women. Another important differential diagnosis includes abnormalities in perineal support, including severe atrophy or denervation of the levator muscles. Abnormalities in these muscles allow the genital hiatus to widen significantly, causing the vaginal opening to appear larger. This is often referred to as a pseudo-rectocele.

Some specialists use fluoroscopy as an aid to physical diagnosis (Figure 49-1). There is little literature regarding these techniques, the lack of a "gold standard" diagnosis has limited progress in this field. It is clear, however, that the finding of "rectocele" in asymptomatic women during fluoroscopic examination should not prompt surgical repair. Moreover, review of fluoroscopically recorded defecation has demonstrated significant variability in the movement of the distal rectovaginal wall in normal women. The promptness and completeness of defecation are probably more important than the maximum excursion of the anterior rectal wall.

Isolated rectoceles are distinctly uncommon and virtually always occur in the presence of a significant defecation disorder. The decision to surgically readdress rectocele must be carefully considered after a full evaluation of the symptoms that are being attributed to the abnormal anatomy.

The symptoms of rectocele are believed to be stool trapping, difficult defecation, and vaginal protrusion of the posterior vaginal wall. Rectoceles are not painful and reports of pain should prompt the physician to seek other diagnoses. It is widely appreciated that many women with relatively large "rectoceles" have no symptoms attributable to this finding. They are able to conduct all pelvic functions without difficulty, including sexual function, and bowel storage and emptying. Other women with minimal abnormalities on physical examination may report great bother from difficult defecation and stool trapping. In the absence of severe symptoms or findings, the recommended primary intervention is generally attention to optimize stool consistency. For many affected women, this requires appropriate amounts of fiber, adequate hydration, and improved toileting habits. In certain centers, allied health professionals such as nurses and/or occupational

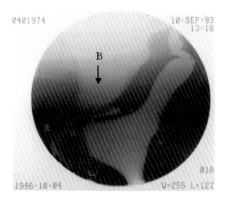

FIGURE 49-1. This is a typical fluoroscopic appearance for a rectocele (R). The protrusion is distal with a normal anal opening and proximal rectum. Other support abnormalities are also seen in the bladder (B).

or physical therapists can assist the surgeon with these important behavioral changes. Biofeedback to establish pelvic floor outlet relaxation during defecation may be helpful.

When symptoms are persistent despite appropriate attention to stool consistency, surgical treatment may be considered. The goal of the surgery should be clearly stated by the surgeon and clearly understood by the patient. Mismatch of goals in this area of poorly understood physiology are common. For example, a patient may not mind the bulge at all, but she is greatly bothered by the need to manually assist her defecation with her hand. Although surgery may be quite effective at relieving her abnormal anatomy, the symptom resolution for hand-assisted defecation is much lower. The planned surgery will not be considered successful by the patient (and therefore by the surgeon) unless the bothersome symptom that prompted the surgery is finally relieved. Honest surgeons will recognize that surgery has significant limitations in relief of certain forms of defecation disorders, but is reasonably effective at normalizing anatomy.

Preoperative testing should include age and risk-appropriate cancer screening (e.g. colonoscopy). Pudendal terminal motor latency testing has no role in selection of patients for rectocele surgery. Defecography may be helpful in documenting failure of the puborectalis muscle to relax during attempted defecation and to establish the presence or absence of internal intussusception as a cause of outlet obstruction of the rectum.

A variety of surgical options are available. The surgeon's belief about the etiology of the rectocele typically determines the technique selected. Gynecologists favor an approach aimed at reinforcement and perineal reattachment of the normal intervening layer of rectovaginal tissue. There are only two randomized surgical trials.[2,3] Both of these studies report that the transvaginal approach is superior to the transanal route. Whereas some have argued that there is a distinct fascia,[4] others refute this. More recently, gynecologists have begun supplementing this tissue with a wide variety of graft materials, although no materials have been proven superior to repair without graft.

Colon and rectal surgeons may approach rectocele from a transanal approach, focusing attention on the capacious rectal vault, and reducing it with pursestring or placating sutures. Sehapayak[5] reported a case series of 355 patients who had a transanal rectocele repair treated with a technique similar to mucosal prolapse. Symptoms attributable to the rectocele were recorded pre- and postoperatively. This technique focuses on abnormalities within the bowel wall itself. A similar technique, described by Khubchandani et al.,[6] also includes excision of the mucosa. Validated outcome assessment of this technique is pending. Block[7] has described a frequently used approach, restricted to midlevel or midvaginal rectocele. The technique in this case series has not yet been tested in a randomized surgical trial. Transanal stapled reduction of the anterior rectocele has recently been evaluated for safety and feasibility but efficacy in a randomized trial is pending.

There is a paucity of literature addressing the symptoms that are appropriately attributed to rectocele, indications for rectocele surgery, the optimal outcome measures after surgery, and the durability of optimal surgical outcomes. This is regrettable given the frequency with which this surgery is performed in American women.[8]

Unsuccessful rectocele repair can occur when either anatomy or symptoms are not corrected. Additional problems may occur when new symptoms arise. One very troubling postoperative complication can be dyspareunia, which in some women can completely preclude sexual activity and destroy intimacy. All operations in the distal posterior vagina and perineum may cause new-onset dyspareunia, and this risk should be disclosed to patients during the negotiation of the informed consent. Recurrent anatomic problems that do not seem to be triggered by abnormal bowel function may be attributable to a widespread abnormality of pelvic support, such as vaginal apical prolapse (with or without a uterus). Physical examination of vaginal supports in the standing straining position is essential and strongly recommended even before a first surgery. A combined gynecologic-colorectal-urologic approach is sometimes needed to address the combination of issues.

Patients who experience initial resolution of anatomy and symptoms may experience relapse if the behavioral program to optimize stool consistency and toileting is not followed. Severe constipation is not a distal rectovaginal problem and it is not reasonable to expect rectocele repair to resolve this symptom. Continued attention to underlying disorders, such as severe constipation, is necessary to preserve optimal rectocele repair.

Pelvic Pain Syndromes

Epidemiology

Chronic pelvic pain is not an infrequent cause for medical consultation. The prevalence of chronic pelvic pain in the female population is estimated to be 3.8%. This is similar to the prevalence of back pain or asthma. It accounts for about 10% of all visits to gynecologists.[9] A North Carolina survey of primary care practices found that 39% of women complain of pelvic pain.[10] In a telephone toll of about 18,000 United States households, the Gallop Organization reported that 16% of women surveyed complained of chronic pelvic pain.[11]

Although pelvic pain is more common in women, it is certainly not confined to the female gender. In a United States survey of functional gastrointestinal disorders, the prevalence of functional anorectal pain was 11.1% of the male and 12.1% of the female respondents to the survey.[12] In a United States survey of physician visits between 1990 and 1994, there were two million healthcare visits per year associated with the diagnosis of prostatitis.[13] Ninety percent of patients with the diagnosis of prostatitis do not have bacterial prostatitis. In 1998, a National Institutes of Health consensus conference designated a new term to encompass these patients—Type III chronic prostatitis/chronic pelvic pain syndrome.[14] In a study of patients with CPPSIII, they were found to have significant differences in muscle spasm, increased tone, and pain on palpation of the muscles of the pelvic diaphragm.[15]

The role of the specialist in the care of these patients is to eliminate intrinsic disorders of the genitourinary and gastrointestinal organs in the pelvis and, if none are found, to treat the pain. The more common pain syndromes are described below. An algorithm for the management of these patients is depicted in Figure 49-2.

Levator Syndrome

Levator syndrome is but one of the symptom complexes in the broader category of chronic pelvic pain or chronic idiopathic rectal pain. It is a pattern that was recognized and described in the 1930s and will be discussed as a separate entity. The rigor with which the syndrome is defined varies greatly and thus leads to some confusion. Simpson[16] reported the symptom complex first in 1859, but Thiele,[17] in 1936, described it in more detail and attributed the symptoms to spasm of the pelvic floor musculature.

The term coccygodynia has been applied to this symptom complex in the early descriptions. It has also been referred to as piriformis syndrome, puborectalis syndrome, diaphragma pelvis spastica, and pelvic tension myalgia. Grant et al.,[18] in one of the largest modern series of cases, described it as pain, pressure, or discomfort in the region of the rectum, sacrum, and coccyx that may be associated with pain in the gluteal region and thighs. They made the observation that pressure on the coccyx was rarely painful and regarded the label of

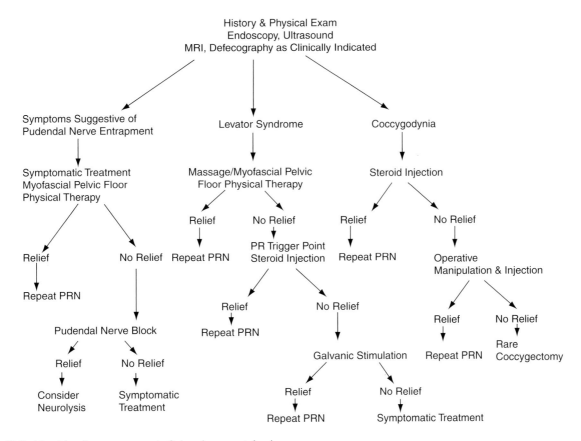

FIGURE 49-2. Algorithm for management of chronic anorectal pain.

coccygodynia as incorrect. Other observers have noted the radiation of the pain to the vagina in women and the association with the feeling of incomplete evacuation.[19]

The prevalence of this symptom complex in the general population is approximately 6%.[12] It is more common in women. The Committee on Functional Anal/Rectal Disorders at a conference to develop diagnostic criteria for Functional Gastrointestinal Disease (Rome II)[20] described the pain of levator syndrome as a vague, dull ache or pressure sensation high in the rectum, often worse with sitting or lying down, that lasts for hours to days. They differentiated between a "highly likely" diagnosis in patients with these symptoms in which posterior traction on the puborectalis reveals a tight levator ani musculature and tenderness or pain, and a "possible" diagnosis if only the symptoms are present. These diagnoses should be entertained only after the presence of alternative diseases are excluded with careful physical examination, endoscopy, and ancillary studies such as defecography, ultrasound, computed tomography, or magnetic resonance imaging (MRI).

The utility of electromyography, anal manometry, and pudendal nerve studies has not been established. No consistent abnormalities in any of these tests have been demonstrated in the majority of patients.[21,22]

A wide variety of treatments have been described. Thiel first recommended digital massage. The massage was given daily for 5 or 6 days. Grant et al.[18] used two to three massages 2–3 weeks apart, combined with heat and diazepam, and had good results in 68% of the patients and moderate improvement in 19%. Poor results were obtained in 13%. A small number of these patients were salvaged with injection of methylprednisolone and lidocaine into the puborectalis sling or "rectal divulsion under anesthesia." (Manual dilation of the anal sphincter, a procedure no longer recommended by this group). (Salvati EP, personal communication.)

Kang et al.[23] described a series of 104 patients in which transanal injection of triamcinolone rendered 37% of patients pain free. Thirty-five percent experienced a greater than 50% reduction in pain. Several investigators have tested electrogalvanic stimulation of the levator muscles via a transrectal probe. The electrical stimulation induces fasciculation and eventual fatigue in the spastic muscles. There is quite a bit of variance in the schedule of treatments as well as length of follow-up in the reported series. The percentage of patients with excellent or good results varies from 19% to 91%.[19,24–29]

Biofeedback has been used with some success. Both Grimaud et al.[30] and Heah et al.[31] reported small series of patients who had excellent results with biofeedback. Gilliland et al.[32] reviewed a larger series of patients with levator-type pain with biofeedback, 37% of whom also had constipation. One-third of the patients noted improvement. The presence or absence of constipation did not seem to matter. The poorer results in the larger series may well be a reflection of a different patient population. Epidural lidocaine and steroid injections were used in a small number of patients with chronic intractable rectal pain, but had no long-term effect on these patients who exhibited levator spasm as part of their pain syndrome. It did, however, sort out those patients who had no initial relief of their pain at the time of injection. These patients were considered to have pain from a high central, autonomic, or psychogenic origin.

Other modalities have been used for chronic pelvic pain, although not in the narrowly defined group with levator syndrome. Static magnetic field therapy[33] and pulsed magnetic stimulation[34] seem to have some salutary effect. Electrical sacral nerve stimulation, which has been used for voiding disorders and fecal incontinence, has also successfully reduced the severity of pain in patients who were broadly characterized as having chronic pelvic pain.[35] Investigators using linearly polarized near-infrared irradiation have also reported some success in participants with intractable anorectal pain.[36]

Anxiety and depression have been associated with chronic pelvic pain syndrome and these conditions should be considered in the comprehensive approach to the management of these patients with pelvic pain.[37]

Coccygodynia

Coccygodynia, although may be part and parcel of the whole group of pelvic floor musculoskeletal problems, is distinguished by the distinct pain evoked with pressure or manipulation of the coccyx. Several rare tumors of the sacrum or sacral nerve structures have been demonstrated in patients with coccygodynia.[38–40] The condition has also been attributed to trauma, avascular necrosis, or referred pain from a prolapsed lumbar disk.[41,42] When no obvious explanation was available, it often was attributed to a psychosomatic manifestation of hysteria or depression. Although coccygectomy was popular at one time, in recent times, it has generally been regarded as ill conceived by most surgeons. Wray and his group[43] from Leicester studied a group of 120 patients with coccygodynia. They randomized them between treatment with injections of methylprednisolone and bupivacaine alone or injections and manipulation of the coccyx under general anesthesia. Injections alone were successful in 60% and injections plus manipulation was successful in 85% of the patients in that arm of the study. The 23 patients who failed either of these two treatments came to coccygectomy and 21 of 23 had a good result, suggesting that this operation may not be inappropriate in those patients who have failed a trial of less invasive therapy. This success rate with coccygectomy is similar to that reported in two other retrospective series.[44,45]

Proctalgia Fugax

Proctalgia fugax, as the name implies, is a fleeting pain in the area of the rectum lasting no more than a minute or two. The pain is too transient to study very well, but, presumably, it is secondary to spasm of the rectum itself or muscular components of the pelvic floor. In a British survey of a healthy population, 14% of the patients reported that this phenomenon occurred at least once a year and 5% reported the phenomenon more than six times per year.[46] Kamm et al.[47] has described a family with a hereditary internal anal sphincter myopathy in which the proctalgia fugax was a very frequent occurrence.

The role of the physician in these cases is mainly to assure the patient that this is not a symptom of any serious disorder. The use of perianal nifedipine in the same doses and method as for anal fissure and hypertrophic internal anal sphincter may be of benefit. There are no randomized trials to document improvement.

Pudendal Neuralgia

Pudendal neuralgia is a symptom complex, which is manifest by chronic pelvic/perineal pain in the distribution of one or both pudendal nerves. It may be manifest as vulvodynia, orchalgia, proctalgia, or prostatodynia. The pain patterns overlap with those of levator syndrome, coccydynia, and urethral syndrome. It is attributable to compression or entrapment of the pudendal nerve and often is positional in nature. Some have also attributed disordered defecation to pudendal nerve entrapment and have reported resolution with nerve decompression.[48] This diagnosis should be entertained if there is a history of trauma, either a distinct episode or chronic perineal trauma such as seen in cyclists or rowers.[49]

The pudendal nerve arises from S2, S3, and S4 of the sacral plexus. The nerve leaves the pelvis beneath the piriformis muscle through the greater sciatic foramen. It then passes on to the sacrospinous ligament medial to the ischial spine and reenters the pelvic cavity. While beneath the levator ani muscles, it runs ventrally through Alcock's canal, a thickening of the obturator internus fascia. In the ischiorectal fossa, it gives off an inferior rectal and perineal branch. The two documented sites of pudendal nerve entrapment are between the sacrotuberous and sacrospinous ligament and in the pudendal (Alcock's) canal. Antolak et al.[50] have hypothesized that many patients with chronic pain have induced hypertrophy of the pelvic muscles caused by athletic activities in their youth, which has in turn caused remodeling of the ischial spine and rotation of the sacrospinous ligament and nerve compression. The diagnosis of pudendal neuralgia is supported by reproduction of the pain with pressure on the ischial spine although this is not a constant finding. Pudendal nerve latency is often prolonged when it is tested. Nerve block under computed tomography[51] or ultrasound guidance[52] has been used to sort out those patients who would likely benefit from neurolysis. Mauillon et al.[53] surgically decompressed the pudendal nerve in 12 patients after evaluating them with a nerve block under computed tomography guidance. After 21 months of follow-up, three patients were completely relieved of their pain and one slightly improved. Eight patients remained in pain. In the three patients who were completely relieved of their pain, the nerve block had eliminated their pain for 2 weeks on two separate occasions. Pain relief was obtained with nerve block

in only one of the nine patients in whom nerve decompression was unsuccessful.

Conclusion

Various benign anorectal conditions may cause considerable trouble for patients. A stepwise, scientifically sound approach to the evaluation and treatment of these disorders may offer a prompt diagnosis and treatment. Referral of patients who continue to suffer despite the physician's best treatment efforts is encouraged.

References

1. Bump RC, Mattiasson A, Bo K, et al. The standardization of terminology of female pelvic organ prolapse and pelvic floor dysfunction. Am J Obstet Gynecol 1996;175(1):10–17.
2. Nieminen K, Huhtala H, Heinonen PK. Anatomic and functional assessment and risk factors of recurrent prolapse after vaginal sacrospinous fixation. Acta Obstet Gynecol Scand 2003;82(5):471–478.
3. Kahn MA, Stanton SL. Posterior colporrhaphy is superior to the transanal repair for treatment of posterior vaginal wall prolapse. Neurourol Urodyn 1999;18(4):70–71.
4. Milley PS, Nichols DH. Correlative investigation of the human rectovaginal septum. Anat Rec 1969;163:443–452.
5. Sehapayak S. Transrectal repair of rectocele: an extended armamentarium of colorectal surgeons. A report of 355 cases. Dis Colon Rectum 1985;28(6):422–433.
6. Khubchandani IT, Sheet JA, Stasik JJ, Hakki AR. Endorectal repair of rectocele. Dis Colon Rectum 1983;26(12):792–796.
7. Block IR. Transrectal repair of rectocele using obliterative suture. Dis Colon Rectum 1986;29(11):707–711.
8. Boyles S, Weber A, Meyn L. Procedures for pelvic organ prolapse in the United States, 1979–1997. Am J Obstet Gynecol 2003;188(1):108–115.
9. Reiter RC. A profile of women with chronic pelvic pain. Clin Obstet Gynecol 1990;33(1):130–136.
10. Jamieson D, Steege J. The prevalence of dysmenorrhea, pelvic pain, and irritable bowel syndrome in primary care practices. Obstet Gynecol 1996;87(1):55–58.
11. Mathias S, Kuppermann M, Liberman R, Lipschutz R, Steege J. Chronic pelvic pain: prevalence, health-related quality of life, and economic correlates. Obstet Gynecol 1996;87(3):321–327.
12. Drossman D, Li Z, Andruzzi E, et al. U.S. householder survey of functional gastrointestinal disorders: prevalence, sociodemography, and health impact. Dig Dis Sci 1993;38(9):1569–1580.
13. McNaughton-Collins M, Stafford R, O'Leary M, Barry M. How common is prostatitis? A national survey of physician visits. J Urol 1998;159:1224–1228.
14. Krieger J, Nyberg L, Nickel J. NIH consensus definition and classification of prostatitis [letter to the editor]. JAMA 1999;282:236–237.
15. Hetrick D, Ciol M, Rothman I, Turner J, Frest M, Berger R. Musculoskeletal dysfunction in men with chronic pain syndrome type III: a case-control study. J Urol 2003;170:828–831.

16. Simpson JY. Coccygodynia and discuss and deformities of the coccyx. Med Times Gaz 1859;1:1–7.

17. Thiele GH. Tonic spasm of the levator ani coccygeus and pyriformis muscles: its relationship to coccygodynia and pain in the region of the hip and down the leg. Trans Am Proctol Soc 1936; 37:145–155.

18. Grant SR, Salvati EP, Rubin RJ. Levator syndrome: an analysis of 316 cases. Dis Colon Rectum 1975;18:161–163.

19. Nicosia JF, Abcarian H. Levator syndrome: a treatment that works. Dis Colon Rectum 1985;28:406–408.

20. Whitehead WF, Wald A, Diamant NE, Evcket AL. Functional disorders of the anorectum. Gut 1999;45(suppl II):II55–II59.

21. Ger GC, Wexner SD, Jorge JMU, et al. Evaluation and treatment of chronic intractable rectal pain—a frustrating endeavor. Dis Colon Rectum 1993;36:139–145.

22. Wald A. Functional anorectal and pelvic pain. Gastroenterol Clin North Am 2001;30:243–251.

23. Kang YS, Jeong SY, Cho HJ, et al. Transanally injected triamcinolone acetonide in levator syndrome. Dis Colon Rectum 2000;43:1288–1291.

24. Sohn R, Weinstein M, Robbins R. The levator syndrome and its treatment with high voltage electrogalvanic stimulants. Am J Surg 1982;144:580–582.

25. Oliver GC, Rubin RJ, Salvati EP, Eisenstat TE. Electrogalvanic stimulation in treatment of levator syndrome. Dis Colon Rectum 1985;28:662–663.

26. Nicosia JF, Abcarian H. Levator syndrome: a treatment that works. Dis Colon Rectum 1985;28:406–408.

27. Billingham RP, Isler JT, Friend WG, Hostetler J. Treatment of levator syndrome using high voltage electrogalvanic stimulation. Dis Colon Rectum 1987;30:584–587.

28. Morris L, Newton RA. Use of high voltage galvanic stimulation for patients with levator ani syndrome. Phys Ther 1987;67: 1522–1525.

29. Hall TL, Milson JW, Church J, et al. Electrogalvanic stimulation for levator syndrome: how effective is it in the short term? Dis Colon Rectum 1993;36:731–733.

30. Grimaud J, Bouvier M, Naudy B, Guien C, Salducci J. Manometric and radiologic investigations and biofeedback treatment of chronic idiopathic anal pain. Dis Colon Rectum 1991;34(8): 690–695.

31. Heah S, Ho Y, Tan M, Leong A. Biofeedback is effective treatment for levator ani syndrome. Dis Colon Rectum 1997;40(2): 187–189.

32. Gilliland R, Heymen J, Altomare D, Vickers D, Wexner S. Biofeedback for intractable rectal pain. Dis Colon Rectum 1997; 40(2):190–196.

33. Brown C, Ling F, Wan J, Pilla A. Efficacy of static magnetic field therapy in chronic pelvic pain: a double-blind pilot study. Am J Obstet Gynecol 2002;187:1581–1587.

34. Sato T, Nagai H. Sacral magnetic stimulation for pain relief from pudendal neuralgia and sciatica. Dis Colon Rectum 2002;45: 280–282.

35. Siegel S, Paszkiewicz E, Kirpatrick C. Sacral nerve stimulation in patients with chronic intractable pelvic pain. J Urol 2001;166:1742–1745.

36. Mibu R, Hotokezaka M, Mihara S, Tanaka M. Results of linearly polarized near infrared irradiation therapy in patients with intractable anorectal pain. Dis Colon Rectum 2003;46(10): 550–553.

37. Heymen S, Wexner S, Gulledge D. MMPI assessment of patients with functional bowel disorders. Dis Colon Rectum 1993;36(6): 593–596.

38. Kinnett JG, Root L. An obscure cause of coccygodynia. J Bone Joint Surg Am 1979;61:299.

39. Ziegler DK, Batnitzky S. Coccygodynia caused by perineural cyst. Neurology 1984;34:829–830.

40. Hanelin LG, Sclamberg EL, Bardsley JL. Intraosseous lipoma of the coccyx. Radiology 1975;114:343–344.

41. Lourie J, Young S. Avascular necrosis of the coccyx: a cause for coccydynia? Case report and histological findings in sixteen patients. Br J Clin Pract 1985;39:247–248.

42. Dittrich RJ. Coccygodynia as referred pain. J Bone Joint Surg Am 1951;33A(3):715–718.

43. Wray C, Esom S, Hoskinson J. Coccydynia: etiology and treatment. J Bone Joint Surg Am 1991;73B(2):335–338.

44. Porter KM, Khan MAA, Piggott H. Coccydynia: a retrospective review. J Bone Joint Surg Am 1981;63B:635–636.

45. Postacchini F, Massobrio M. Idiopathic coccygodynia: analysis of fifty-one operative cases and a radiographic study of the normal coccyx. J Bone Joint Surg Am 1983;65A(8):1116–1124.

46. Thompson WG. Proctalgia fugax. Am J Gastroenterol 1984;79: 450–452.

47. Kamm M, Hoyle C, Burleigh D, et al. Hereditary internal anal sphincter myopathy causing proctalgia fugax and constipation. A newly identified condition. Gastroenterology 1991;100: 805–810.

48. Shafik A. Pudendal canal syndrome and proctalgia fugax. Dis Colon Rectum 1997;40:504.

49. Ramsden CE, McDaniel MC, Harmon RL, Renney KM, Faure A. Pudendal nerve entrapment as source of intractable perineal pain. Am J Phys Med Rehabil 2003;82(6):479–484.

50. Antolak SJ Jr, Hough DM, Pawlina W, Spinner RJ. Anatomical basis of chronic pelvic pain syndrome: the ischial spine and pudendal nerve entrapment. Med Hypotheses 2002;59(3):349–353.

51. Hough DM, Wittenberg KH, Pawlina W, et al. Chronic perineal pain caused by pudendal nerve entrapment: anatomy and CT guided perineal injection technique. AJR Am J Roentgenol 2003;181(2):561–567.

52. Kovacs P, Gruber H, Piegger J, Bodner G. New, simple, ultrasound-guided infiltration of the pudendal nerve. Dis Colon Rectum 2001;44(9):1381–1385.

53. Mauillon J, Thoumas D, Leroi AM, Freger P, Michot F, Denis P. Results of pudendal nerve neurolysis transposition in twelve patients suffering from pudendal neuralgia. Dis Colon Rectum 1999;42(2):186–192.

50
Laparoscopy

Peter W. Marcello and Tonia Young-Fadok

Until recently, there has been a relatively slow adoption of laparoscopic colectomy into the surgeon's practice. The persistence of the learning curve, the modest advantages reported, and the concerns regarding the safety of laparoscopic resection for curable colon cancer are but a few of the reasons that the percentage of laparoscopic colorectal procedures has not dramatically increased. With the publication of the several large prospective, randomized trials for colon cancer, however, there seems to be a renewed interest in minimally invasive procedures for the colon and rectum. This chapter will review these issues and provide a current assessment of the field for the common disease processes to which laparoscopic techniques have been applied.

Learning Curve

Laparoscopic colorectal surgery has met with certain challenges that distinguish it from other minimally invasive procedures. In comparison to laparoscopic cholecystectomy, the surgeon performing laparoscopic colectomy has to work in multiple quadrants of the abdomen. This requires a better understanding of depth perception and proprioception. A coordinated team consisting of a surgeon, an assistant, and often a camera person is required. All three must work together along with the nursing and anesthesia teams. The surgeon may also need to work in reverse angles to the camera. All of these combined add to the complexity of the procedure and result in the need to perform a number of cases before the surgeon and surgical team will become proficient. Numerous previous studies have evaluated the "learning curve" of laparoscopic colectomy.[1–3] It is estimated that with conventional laparoscopic techniques and instruments that the learning curve for laparoscopic colectomy is at least 20 cases and more likely 50 cases.

Recent publications have suggested the learning curve is more than 20 cases. In a prospective, randomized study of colorectal cancer in the United Kingdom, the "CLASICC" trial, surgeons had to perform at least 20 laparoscopic resections before they were allowed to enter the study.[4] The study began in July 1996 and was completed in July 2002. Despite the surgeons' prior experience, the rate of conversion decreased from 38% to 16% over the course of the study, suggesting that a minimum of 20 cases may not be enough to reach the plateau of the "learning curve." In the COLOR trial from Europe,[5] another recent prospective randomized study for colon cancer that required a prerequisite experience in laparoscopic colon resection before surgeons could enter patients into the study, surgeon and hospital volume were directly related to a number of operative and postoperative outcomes. The median operative time for high-volume (>10 cases/year) hospitals was 188 minutes compared with 241 minutes for low-volume (<5 cases/year) hospitals, and likewise conversion rates were 9% versus 24% for the two groups. High-volume groups also had more lymph nodes in the resected specimens, fewer complications, and shortened hospital stay. These two recent studies would suggest that the learning curve is clearly greater than 20 cases and that surgeons need to perform a minimum yearly number of procedures to maintain their skills.

The difficulty with the broad application of laparoscopic colectomy is that most general surgeons perform fewer than 50 segmental colon resections per year. In a review of 2434 general surgeons who were taking the recertification examination for the American Board of Surgery, all of whom supplied their operative lists from the previous year, most surgeons performed fewer than 20 colon resections in 1 year.[6] In fact, the mean number of colon resections performed by a surgeon was 11. Even at the 90th percentile, only 23 colectomies were performed by a surgeon in a single year. If the average surgeon performs 11 resections and only half are eligible for a laparoscopic approach, assuming a learning curve of 40 cases, it would take a surgeon 8 years to feel comfortable performing laparoscopic colectomy. Most surgeons cannot afford to go through such a learning curve. Either the learning curve will need to be shortened, as some have suggested by the use of hand-assisted laparoscopic (HAL) techniques, or we will need to limit the performance of laparoscopic colectomy to surgeons who perform a greater number of colon resections per year.

Conversions

The rates of conversion are inconsistent in the literature, with reports as low as 0% to as high as 48%. Most series report the need to convert in 10%–25% of cases. Although surgical proficiency would likely decrease the need to convert, this is counterbalanced by the surgeon's desire to perform more complex cases. Several patient- and disease-related factors such as obesity, prior abdominal surgery, acuity of inflammation (i.e., abscess and fistula formation), tumor bulk or contiguous involvement, and disease location, may also affect the rate of conversion. Obesity, defined as a body mass index >30 kg/m^2, was once considered a relative contraindication for a laparoscopic colon resection. For a surgeon early in their learning curve it should probably remain a relative contraindication. However, once more experience is gained by the surgeon, several current reports have demonstrated that obesity itself in not a contraindication to a minimally invasive approach.[7–9] For inflammatory conditions such as Crohn's disease and diverticulitis, the presence of an abscess or fistula may result in the need for conversion in up to 50% of cases.[10,11] More recent studies of laparoscopic surgery involving enteric fistulae suggest a conversion rate of 25%–35%.[12–14] The presence of a fistula or small abscess is not a contraindication to a minimally invasive approach, but should alert the surgeon to consider a variation in operative approach if obstacles cannot be overcome. Conversion from a laparoscopic to conventional resection should not be viewed as a failure of the laparoscopist. It is difficult to predict based on preoperative studies which cases cannot be completed laparoscopically. More crucial than the rate of conversion is the time spent before conversion. An initial laparoscopic survey may quickly identify a complex process, allowing a speedy alteration in the operative plan. If the approach is expeditiously changed, little additional time or costs need be incurred. Earlier reports suggested a poorer outcome for patients who required conversion; however, more recent studies, including a recent presentation of the COST trial results, suggest that if conversion is made early the outcome of converted cases is similarly matched with patients undergoing conventional surgery.[15,16] The goal is to perform a preemptive conversion once it is determined the case cannot be completed laparoscopically, rather than a reactive conversion to a complication that occurred because of adverse conditions that the surgeon could have avoided.

Outcomes

In comparison to conventional colectomy, the proposed benefits of laparoscopic colectomy include a reduction in postoperative ileus, less postoperative pain and concomitant reduction in the need for analgesics, an earlier tolerance of diet, a shortened hospital stay, a quicker resumption of normal activities, improved cosmetic results, and possibly preservation of immune function. This is offset by a prolongation in operative time, the cost of laparoscopic equipment, and the learning curve of these technically challenging procedures. When reporting the outcomes of laparoscopic colectomy, there is however, a natural selection bias when comparing conventional and laparoscopic cases. More complex cases are generally not suitable for a laparoscopic approach and therefore are performed "open." Also, in many series the results of the successfully completed laparoscopic cases are compared with conventional cases and the cases converted from a laparoscopic to conventional procedure. Few studies, with the exception of the larger prospective, randomized studies, leave the "converted" cases in the laparoscopic group as part of the "intention to treat" laparoscopic group. This clearly introduces selection bias. In addition, there is wide variability in the types of laparoscopic procedures performed, the reporting of results, and cultural variations in patient management.

Although the results of prospective, randomized trials are becoming more available, the majority of studies of laparoscopic colectomy are retrospective case control series or noncomparative reports. The conclusions regarding patient outcomes, therefore, must come from the repetitiveness of the results rather than the superiority of study design. For any one study, the evidence is weak, however collectively, because of the reproducibility of results by a large number of institutions, even with different operative techniques and postoperative management parameters, the preponderance of evidence favors a minimally invasive approach with respect to postoperative outcomes. Also, the prospective, randomized studies that are available corroborate the findings demonstrated in nonrandomized studies.

Operative Time

Nearly all the comparative studies provide information regarding operative times. The definition of the operative time may vary with each series, and there may be different groups of surgeons performing the laparoscopic and conventional procedures. With the exception of a few reports, nearly all studies demonstrated a prolonged operative time associated with a laparoscopic procedure. In prospective, randomized trials, the procedure was approximately 40–60 minutes longer in the laparoscopic groups. As the surgeon and team gain experience with laparoscopic colectomy, the operating times do reliably decrease, but rarely do they return to the comparable time for a conventional approach.

Return of Bowel Activity and Resumption of Diet

Reduction in postoperative ileus is one of the proposed major advantages of minimally invasive surgery. Nearly all of the historical and prospective studies comparing open and laparoscopic colectomy have shown a statistically significant reduction in the time to passage of flatus and stool. Most series demonstrate a 1- to 2-day advantage for the laparoscopic group. Whether the reduction of ileus relates to less bowel manipulation or less intestinal exposure to air, or some other factor, during minimally invasive surgery remains unknown.

In clinical studies, it is difficult to eliminate all the biases of the treating physician and the higher expectations of the patient undergoing laparoscopic surgery. Psychological conditioning of the patient preoperatively may interfere with an objective assessment of bowel activity postoperative. To more formally answer this question, both human and animal studies have evaluated the return of gastrointestinal motility. Both canine and porcine models have confirmed an earlier return of intestinal myoelectric activity after laparoscopic resection.[17,18] Another study in dogs demonstrated a quicker return to preoperative motility, using radionucleotide techniques in animals subjected to laparoscopic resection.[19] These studies clearly demonstrate a quicker return of bowel activity without the subjective bias that may be introduced in clinical studies.

With the reduction in postoperative ileus, the tolerance by the patient of both liquids and solid food is quicker after laparoscopic resection. The time to resumption of diet varies from 2 to 7 days, but in the majority of comparative studies, this still remains 1–2 days sooner than in patients undergoing conventional surgery. Again, the physician and patient were not blinded, which may alter patient expectations. The overwhelming reproducible data reported in both retrospective and prospective studies of laparoscopic procedures, however, do likely favor a reduction of postoperative ileus and tolerance of liquid and solid diet.

Postoperative Pain and Recovery of Pulmonary Function

To measure postoperative pain, a variety of different assessments have been performed to demonstrate a significant reduction in pain after minimally invasive surgery; some studies use an analog pain scale, whereas others measure narcotic requirements. Physician bias and psychological conditioning of the patients may interfere with the evaluation of postoperative pain. There are also cultural variations in the response to pain. Three of the early prospective, randomized trials have evaluated pain postoperatively and all three have found a reduction in narcotic requirements in patients undergoing laparoscopic colectomy.[20–22] In the COST study,[23,24] the need for both intravenous and oral analgesics was less in patients undergoing successfully completed laparoscopic resections. Numerous other nonrandomized studies have shown a reduction in postoperative pain and narcotic usage.

Closely related to the severity and duration of postoperative pain is the return of pulmonary function. Adequate pain management allows the patient to inspire more deeply. After conventional abdominal surgery, suppression of pulmonary function is a well-known sequelae. Several studies of laparoscopic colectomy have evaluated the return of pulmonary function. In the randomized clinical trial of patients undergoing surgery for colon cancer from the Cleveland Clinic, preoperative and postoperative spirometry was performed every 12 hours in 55 patients in the laparoscopic group and 54 patients in the conventional group.[20] An 80% recovery of baseline-forced vital capacity and forced expiratory volume in one second was measured in each patient. The median recovery for the laparoscopic group was 3 days which was half the recovery (6 days) seen in the conventional group. A similarly designed study by Schwenk et al.[22] confirmed these same results. Whether subject to bias, the results of comparative studies suggest a quicker recovery of pulmonary function and reduction in postoperative pain in patients subjected to laparoscopic colectomy.

Length of Stay

The quicker resolution of ileus, earlier resumption of diet, and reduced postoperative pain have resulted in a shortened length of stay for patients after laparoscopic resection when compared with traditional procedures. Recovery after conventional surgery has also been shortened by early feeding practices introduced more recently, but this is not consistent throughout the literature. In the absence of minimally invasive techniques, it would seem unlikely that the length of stay could be further reduced. In nearly all comparative studies, the length of hospitalization is 1–6 days less for the laparoscopic group. In an attempt to minimize the differences between a conventional midline incision and a laparoscopic incision, Fleshman et al.[25] compared the outcomes of 35 patients whose surgery was performed through a minilaparotomy (12 cm, mean incision length) with 54 laparoscopic patients. Outcome was similar for both groups with a mean day of discharge of 6.9 days (range, 3–15 days) for the minilaparotomy group and 6.0 days for the laparoscopic group (range, 1–15 days). However, when the results of successfully completed laparoscopic cases (75%) were compared, the results favored the laparoscopic group (5.3 days; range, 1–14 days). Therefore, despite an attempt to minimize the incision, the overall length of stay was significantly longer.

Although psychological conditioning of the patient cannot be helped and likely has a desirable effect, the benefits of minimally invasive procedures on the overall length of stay cannot be discounted. The benefit, however, is more likely a 1- to 2-day advantage only. The more recent introduction of clinical pathways both in conventional and laparoscopic surgery has also narrowed the gap, but seems to be more reliable in patients undergoing a minimally invasive approach.[26,27]

Quality of Life and Return to Work

If laparoscopic colectomy results in less postoperative pain and earlier return to normal activities, then one would anticipate that the quality of life after a laparoscopic procedure should be improved when compared with conventional procedures. Unfortunately, despite the numerous reports of laparoscopic colectomy, few have objectively examined the patient's assessment of recovery. In a nonrandomized study, Psaila et al.[28] evaluated the recovery of hand-grip strength and the patient's quality of life using an SF-36 symptom score 2 months and 4 months postoperatively. Hand-grip strength, as a measure of protein loss, recovered more rapidly after laparoscopic surgery. Using the SF-36 questionnaire, in six of eight areas of questioning, there was less impairment of health after laparoscopic colectomy. By 4 months postoperatively, this trend persisted, but to a lesser degree. In the COST study, quality of life was evaluated by three complementary viewpoints: patient self-reported symptoms, patient self-reported functional status, and a third more objective measurement scale of compliance to treatment referred to as Q-TWIST (quality-adjusted time without symptoms of disease and toxicity of treatment).[23] Because of a high conversion rate of 25% in the initial study report, and the "intention to treat" design of the study, there were no significant differences between the conventional and laparoscopic groups with the exception of a global rating score 2 weeks after surgery. In every category, however, the results of patients who had a laparoscopically completed procedure were improved compared with conventionally performed procedures and in laparoscopic patients who required a conversion to open surgery. However, this did not achieve significance. The results of the CLASICC trial in the United Kingdom found similar results.[4]

Only a few studies have assessed the ability of patients undergoing laparoscopic colectomy to return to work. With less postoperative pain and reduced narcotic usage, one would presume that patients undergoing a minimally invasive approach would return more quickly to normal activities and employment compared with patients undergoing a conventional resection. In a nonrandomized comparison, patients undergoing laparoscopic procedure returned to full activities and to work sooner than matched patients undergoing conventional resection [mean, 4.2 versus 10.5 weeks, 3.8 versus 7.5 weeks, respectively ($P < .01$ for all)].[29]

Hospital Costs

One of the proposed disadvantages of laparoscopy is the higher operative costs related to longer operative times and increased expenditure in disposable equipment. Whether the total cost of the hospitalization (operative and hospital costs) is higher after laparoscopic colectomy is debatable. A case control study from the Mayo Clinic has looked at total costs after laparoscopic and open ileocolic resection for Crohn's disease.[30] Sixty-six patients underwent laparoscopic (n = 33) or conventional (n = 33) ileocolic resection during the same time period (10/95–7/99) and were well matched. Patients in the laparoscopic group had less postoperative pain, tolerated

a regular diet sooner by 1–2 days, and had a shorter length of stay (4.0 versus 7.0 days). In their cost analysis, despite higher operative cost, the overall mean costs were $3273 less in the laparoscopic group. The procedures were performed by different groups of surgeons at the institution, and although the surgeon may have introduced biases, this study was undertaken during the current era of cost containment in which all physicians are encouraged to reduce hospital stay. Other studies by Dupree et al.[31] and Shore et al.[32] have confirmed these findings with a mean reduction of $438 in costs and $7465 in hospital charges, respectively, in patients undergoing laparoscopic compared with conventional ileocolic resection. The results are similar for elective sigmoid diverticular resection with a mean cost savings of $700–$800.[33] Clearly, if operative times and equipment expenditure are minimized, the overall cost of a laparoscopic resection should not exceed a conventional approach.

Crohn's Disease

Laparoscopy in the setting of inflammatory bowel disease has its own set of unique challenges that must be overcome. For patients with Crohn's disease, the dissection is hampered by inflammatory changes in the mesentery, difficulty in assessing bowel involvement and identifying normal anatomic landmarks, along with the development of associated abscess and fistulous disease often seen in the Crohn's patient. For the ulcerative colitis patient and the patient with isolated Crohn's colitis, the challenges are more technical because of the difficulty in performing laparoscopic total colectomy.

Crohn's disease of the terminal ileum seems an ideal model for the application of a minimally invasive approach. The disease is usually limited to one area of the abdomen and only mobilization and vascular pedicle ligation are required laparoscopically. The resection and anastomosis are generally performed extracorporeally. Patients with Crohn's are typically young and are interested in undertaking a procedure that minimizes incisional scarring. Additionally, because many of these patients will require reoperation over their lifetime, a minimally invasive approach is appealing. Early reports of laparoscopic ileocolic resection showed it to be feasible and safe, but were typically small nonrandomized uncontrolled studies. More recent studies (Table 50-1) have a larger experience in which to draw more meaningful conclusions.[35–47] The majority of studies, however, are retrospective case control series. Most series report the rate of conversion from 10% to 20% with the mix of complex cases (abscess, fistula, or reoperative surgery) ranging from 40% to 50%.

As expected, the outcomes after laparoscopically assisted ileocolic resection for Crohn's disease mirror those seen in other studies of laparoscopic colectomy for benign and malignant disease. In comparative studies (Table 50-1), laparoscopic ileocolic resection is associated with a quicker return of bowel function and an earlier tolerance of oral diet. The

TABLE 50-1. Recent studies of laparoscopic resection for Crohn's disease: ileocolic resection

Author	Year	No. of patients		OP time (min)		LOS (d)		Morbidity (%)		Comment
		LAP	CON	LAP	CON	LAP	CON	LAP	CON	
Bauer et al.[35]	1996	25	14	—	—	6.5	8.5	—	—	High conversion if mass and fistula
Wu et al.[36]	1997	46	70	144	202	4.5	7.9	10	21	52% complex or redo cases
Dunker et al.[37]	1998	11	11	—	—	5.5	9.9	9	9	Improved cosmesis
Wong et al.[38]	1999	55		150		6.0		5		46% complex cases
Canin-Endres et al.[39]	1999	70		183		4.2		14		41 with fistulae, 1 conversion
Alabaz et al.[40]	2000	26	48	150	90	7.0	9.6	—	—	Favorable results
Bemelman et al.[41]	2000	30	48	138	104	5.7	10.2	15	10	Different hospitals for each group
Young-Fadok et al.[30]	2001	33	33	147	124	4.0	7.0	—	—	Laparoscopy less expensive
Schmidt et al.[42]	2001	46		207		5.7		—		Safe and effective, high conversion rate
Milsom et al.[43]	2001	31	29	140	85	5.0	6.0	16	28	Prospective, randomized trial
Evans et al.[44]	2002	84		145		5.6		11		Results improve with experience
Dupree et al.[31]	2002	21	24	75	98	3.0	5.0	14	16	Laparoscopy less expensive
Shore et al.[32]	2003	20	20	145	133	4.3	8.2	—	—	Laparoscopy less expensive
Benoist et al.[45]	2003	24	32	179	198	7.7	8.0	20	10	Similar operative times, 17% converted
Bergamaschi et al.[47]	2003	39	53	185	105	5.6	11.2	9	10	Long-term obstruction less, 11% versus 35%

OP, operative; LOS, length of stay; LAP, laparoscopic; CON, conventional.

quicker resolution of ileus, earlier resumption of diet, and reduced postoperative pain has resulted in a shortened length of stay for patients after laparoscopic resection when compared with traditional procedures. Milsom et al.[43] published a prospective, randomized trial comparing conventional and laparoscopic ileocolic resection for refractory Crohn's disease. Sixty patients were randomized to either conventional or laparoscopic resection after an initial diagnostic laparoscopy to assess feasibility of a laparoscopic resection. The results favor a laparoscopic approach with regard to pulmonary function, morbidity, and length of stay. There were no apparent short-term disadvantages. All patients had oral intake withheld for 3 days to evaluate nutritional parameters. This impacted on the timing of dietary intake and was likely responsible for a delay in discharge in some patients. The total length of stay in this randomized study was 1 day shorter in the laparoscopic group (5 versus 6 days) but did not reach statistical significance. Had dietary intake not been withheld, a shortened length of stay of the laparoscopic group might have achieved significance.

With the loss of tactile sensation, one of the remaining concerns of performing laparoscopic surgery in the patient with terminal ileal Crohn's is missing an isolated proximal lesion. Many patients after ileocolic resection will develop a symptomatic recurrence proximal to the ileocolic anastomosis, but whether patients undergoing a laparoscopic procedure will present with unrecognized proximal disease remains unclear. There are now, however, several studies that have reported recurrence rates after laparoscopic ileocolic resection. In a recent article, the long-term follow-up (mean 39 months) of 32 patients over 7 years who underwent a laparoscopic ileocolic resection were compared with 29 patients undergoing open resection.[46] The rate of Crohn's recurrence was high but similar in both groups (48% laparoscopic, 44% conventional) as was the disease-free interval (24 months). In another recent review of long-term outcome, Bergamaschi et al.[47] reported the results of 39 laparoscopic and 53 conventional ileocolic resections with a 5-year follow-up. Recurrent disease was determined by patient symptoms and confirmed both radiographically and endoscopically in 27% of patients undergoing a laparoscopic procedure and in 29% of patients with a conventional resection. Interestingly, the incidence of small bowel obstruction was significantly less in the laparoscopic group (11% versus 35%, $P = .02$). This was thought to be the result of less adhesion formation after a laparoscopic procedure. Laparoscopic ileocolic resection does not seem to offer any advantage over conventional resection with regard to symptomatic recurrence, but it also did not lead to a higher rate of recurrence or discovery of a missed lesion.

Laparoscopic ileocolic resection for Crohn's disease seems to be safe and feasible and offers the advantages seen in other reports of laparoscopic colorectal procedures. For the inexperienced laparoscopist, the initial uncomplicated terminal ileal resection is an ideal procedure in which to gain laparoscopic experience. An initial laparoscopic survey

should be performed in the majority of patients with refractory ileal Crohn's disease with a low threshold to alternate the approach if a complex case beyond the skill of the surgeon is encountered.

Ulcerative Colitis

There are no prospective, randomized studies of laparoscopic proctocolectomy for ulcerative colitis. The only results available for analysis are prospective and retrospective case control studies and noncomparative reports (Table 50-2).[48–59] Several reasons likely account for the slow acceptance of laparoscopic proctocolectomy including the steep learning curve to performing even segmental colectomy, the technical challenges of transverse colon resection, and the unfavorable early reports of laparoscopic total colectomy. The group from Cleveland Clinic Florida attempted laparoscopic proctocolectomy for patients with ulcerative colitis in the early 1990s and published several comparative reports.[60,61] The results showed a longer operative time and higher blood loss than matched open procedures with no apparent benefit. The authors discouraged the use of minimally invasive techniques for patients requiring total colectomy. This was an appropriate recommendation during the early era of laparoscopic colectomy. However, with advances in technology and experience gained with segmental resection, many groups have reevaluated the role of laparoscopic total colectomy for inflammatory bowel disease.

The majority of reports have shown that laparoscopic total colectomy and laparoscopic proctocolectomy with and without ileoanal pouch construction are technically feasible and share the same advantages of minimally invasive surgery as segmental colonic resection. Laparoscopic proctocolectomy has been performed in the elective setting, but several groups have performed laparoscopic total colectomy on an urgent basis for the patient with unresolving acute colitis. These procedures, however, are still not recommended for the patient with toxic colitis.

Even though some groups perform this procedure routinely, the procedures remain technically challenging with operative times in the 3- to 5-hour range. In an effort to reduce operative times, several groups have recently reported the use of hand-assisted techniques for restorative proctocolectomy.[57,59] In a small comparative study from the Lahey Clinic, the effectiveness of the HAL approach was compared with a conventional laparoscopic method in patients undergoing laparoscopic proctocolectomy.[57] Both groups [10 HAL versus 13 standard laparoscopy (SL)] were well matched, with no differences in age, sex, ASA level, operative indication, steroid usage, or diagnosis. The results demonstrated no differences in incision size (mean 8 cm), operative blood loss, rate of conversion (HAL 10% versus SL 0%), or complications (HAL 40% versus SL 31%). The operative times progressively decreased in the hand-assisted group (mean

TABLE 50-2. Recent studies of laparoscopic colectomy for ulcerative colitis

Author	Year	No. of patients	Comment
Meijerink et al.[48]	1999	10	Feasible, 7 for acute colitis
Marcello et al.[49]	2000	13	Restorative proctocolectomy, favorable results
Seshadri et al.[50]	2001	37	25% morbidity
Hamel et al.[51]	2001	21	Compared with ileocolic resection, similar morbidity and LOS
Marcello et al.[52]	2001	16	For acute colitis, comparative study, favorable results
Brown et al.[53]	2001	25	Longer op time in LAP group
Dunker et al.[54]	2001	35	Better cosmesis
Ky et al.[55]	2002	32	Single-stage procedure, good results
Bell and Seymour[56]	2002	18	Total colectomy for acute colitis, seems safe
Rivadeneira et al.[57]	2004	23	Hand-assisted procedure reduced operative time
Kienle et al.[58]	2003	59	Large study, laparoscopic colon mobilization only
Nakajima et al.[59]	2004	16	Hand-assisted technique, favorable results

IPAA, ileal pouch–anal anastomosis; EBL, estimated blood loss; LOS, length of stay.

247 minutes) while remaining constant in the laparoscopic group (mean 300 minutes, $P < .05$) over the period of study. This 1-hour reduction in operative is significant to the busy practicing surgeon and may open the door to more surgeons in performing laparoscopic restorative proctocolectomy. Another recent study by Nakajima et al.[59] showed similar advantages of hand-assisted total colectomy for ulcerative colitis. It seems that hand-assisted restorative proctocolectomy can be accomplished without detriment to bowel function, length of stay, or patient outcome.

The role of laparoscopic total colectomy for patients with inflammatory bowel disease is not well defined, but is likely to expand as surgeons become more comfortable with segmental resection. Advantages seen in segmental resection have recently been reproduced in patients undergoing laparoscopic total colectomy. Again, although the evidence based on study design and size for any one report is not optimal, the reproducibility of the results among many institutions provides adequate evidence to demonstrate clear advantages of laparoscopic total colectomy for ulcerative colitis over a conventional approach. The use of HAL for ulcerative colitis patients requiring surgery is likely another venue that may shorten operative time while maintaining the benefits of a minimally invasive approach.

Diverticulitis

Laparoscopic sigmoid resection remains the leading indication for minimally invasive colon resection for benign disease. The surgery is hampered by both the fibrotic changes associated with elective resection of recurrent disease and the inflammatory changes associated with acute disease. As surgeons acquire their laparoscopic skills, more complex cases involving abscess and fistulous communications have been successfully completed laparoscopically. There are now a large number of studies evaluating laparoscopic surgery for diverticulitis (Table 50-3).[62–75] These are both large case series and nonrandomized comparative studies with open resection. Most series report an operative time of 2–3 hours with a conversion rate of 10%–20% for most larger series. The largest series of diverticular resection comes from a German multi-institutional study of 1545 patients accumulated over 7 years at 52 institutions.[68] The study demonstrated a low morbidity and mortality with an overall conversion rate of 6.1%. As experience increased, the percentage of complex cases increased without significantly altering the morbidity or rate of conversion. High-volume centers performed more of the complex cases with a similar conversion rate to the low-volume centers that performed less complex cases.

TABLE 50-3A. Compiled descriptive series of laparoscopic resection for diverticulitis

Study	Year	N	Mortality (%)	Morbidity (%)	Conversion (%)	OR time (min)*	Resume diet (d)*	Flatus/ BM (d)*	LOS (d)*
Eijsbouts et al.[62]	1997	41	0	18	15	195	NA	NA	6.5
Stevenson et al.[63]	1998	100	0	21	8	180	2	2	4
Tuech et al.[64]	2000	77	0	17	14	NA	NA	NA	NA
Trebuchet et al.[65]	2002	170	0	8.2	4.1	141	3.4	NA	8.5
Bouillot et al.[66]	2002	179	0	15	14	223	3.3	2.5	9.3
Pugliese et al.[67]	2004	103	0	8	3	190	NA	4	9.7
Schneidbach et al.[68]	2004	1545	0.4	17	6.1	169	NA	NA	NA
Pessaux et al.[69]	2004	582	1.2	25	NA	NA	NA	NA	NA
Schwandner et al.[70]	2005	363	0.6	22	6.6	192	2.8	4.0	11.8

OR, operating room; BM, bowel movement, LOS, length of stay; NA, not available.
*Median or mean values listed.

TABLE 50-3B. Case-control studies pertaining to laparoscopic resection for diverticulitis

Study	Year	No. of patients		Mortality (%)		Morbidity (%)		Convert (%)	OR time (min)*		Resume diet (d)*		Flatus/BM (d)*		LOS (d)*		Total costs*	
		CON	LAP	CON	LAP	CON	LAP		CON	LAP	CON	LAP	CON	LAP	CON	LAP	CON	LAP
Diverticulitis																		
Liberman et al.[71]	1996	14	14	0	0	14	14	0	182	192	6.1	2.9†	NA		9.2	6.3†	P 13,400	11,500
Bruce et al.[72]	1996	17	25	0	0	23	16	12	115	397†	5.7	3.2†	NA		6.8	4.2†	$ 7,068	10,230†
Kohler et al.[73]	1998	34	27	0	0	61	15	7	121	165†	5.8	4.1†	5.3	3.7†	14.3	7.9†	DM 8,975	7,185†
Senagore et al.[33]	2002	71	61	0	1.6	30	8†	7	101	107	NA		NA	6.8		3.1†	$ 4,321	3,458†
Dwivedi et al.[34]	2002	88	66	0	0	24	18	20	143	212†	4.9	2.9†	NA		8.8	4.8†	$ 14,863	13,953†
Lawrence et al.[74]	2003	215	56	1.6	1	27	9†	7	140	170†	NA		NA		9.1	4.1†	$ 25,700	17,414†
‡Gonzalez et al.[75]	2004	80	95	4	1	31	19†	NA	156	170	NA		3.7	2.8	12	7†	NA	

OR-operating room; BM-bowel movement, LOS-length of stay; CON-conventional surgery; LAP-laparoscopic surgery; NA-not available; P, pounds; DM, Deutsch Marks.

*Median or mean values listed.

†Statistically significant difference.

‡Results of non-converted laparoscopic cases given.

§Minilaparotomy.

Nearly all comparative studies of laparoscopic to open sigmoid resection demonstrate a benefit to the laparoscopic approach including a shorter duration of ileus, shortened length of stay, but as in other studies, with a prolonged operative time. Early reports suggested a higher overall cost associated with a laparoscopic approach for diverticular resection; however, more recent studies (Table 50-4) have demonstrated a cost saving with the laparoscopic approach. This cost reduction has been noted not only in the United States, but also in European countries. It should be noted that these are generally the elective uncomplicated cases with fewer patients presenting with abscess or fistula formation. For more complex cases, in which the operative times are longer and the rate of conversion is higher, the cost savings benefit of a laparoscopic approach may be lost. This highlights the importance of case selection when considering a laparoscopic approach. Less-experienced surgeons should consider an early conversion of complicated diverticular resection or potentially an alteration in the approach to a hand-assisted technique in which the difficult pelvic dissection can be guided by the hand laparoscopically or by conventional means through the open wound.[76]

Rectal Prolapse

As with other disease processes, the field of laparoscopy has expanded to the treatment of rectal prolapse. Full-thickness rectal prolapse repaired by an abdominal fixation procedure is potentially an ideal procedure for a laparoscopic approach because there is no specimen to remove or anastomosis to create. There are many studies that have evaluated not only laparoscopic fixation procedures but also the combination of sigmoid resection and rectopexy for the treatment of rectal prolapse (Table 50-4).[77–98] The magnified view into the pelvis with the laparoscope provides unparalleled visualization into the pelvic floor and the relative laxity of the rectal fixation to the presacral area is beneficial to performance of a laparoscopic procedure. This likely is the reason for the relatively low rate of conversion (<10%) for a laparoscopic rectopexy or resection and rectopexy in comparison to other laparoscopic colorectal procedures. The mobilization of the rectum for rectal prolapse is an ideal procedure in which to learn the laparoscopic technique of rectal mobilization which may then be applied to other procedures such as laparoscopic proctocolectomy or total mesorectal excision for rectal cancer.

In addition to case series results, there have been several nonrandomized comparative studies of laparoscopic versus conventional rectopexy and resection rectopexy.[87,88,94] These studies showed a longer operative time of 45–60 minutes with the laparoscopic procedures but with a shortened length of stay of 2–3 days. Functional results after surgery were similar in laparoscopic and conventional groups, with the majority of patients reporting an improvement in incontinence and constipation. Solomon et al.[93] also reported a prospective, randomized study of 40 patients with full-thickness rectal prolapse. This was a well-designed study with the use of blinded observers, and a standardized clinical pathway for both groups. As expected, the mean surgical time was 153 minutes in the laparoscopic group compared with 102 minutes in the open group ($P < .01$). In the laparoscopic group, however, 75% of patients followed the clinical pathways as compared with only 37% of patients in the conventional group. The mean length of stay was also less (3.9 versus 6.6 days, $P < .01$) with 19/20 patients in the laparoscopic group discharged by postoperative day five as compared with 9/19 patients in the conventional group. There were no differences in postoperative pain scores but total intravenous narcotic usage was less in the laparoscopic group. Functional outcomes of surgery were equivalent, and there were no recurrences of prolapse in either group with a short mean follow-up of 24 months. Although the study is small in size, the outcomes mirror the results of other prospective, randomized studies of laparoscopic surgery for other diseases and procedures. A later cost analysis of this study demonstrated an overall mean cost savings of $500 per patient in the laparoscopic group.[98]

One of the major issues when discussing surgery for rectal prolapse is the rate of recurrent prolapse. For an abdominal approach, the risk of recurrence should be less than 5%–10% over 5 years. Unfortunately, the majority of reports on laparoscopic surgery for rectal prolapse have limited follow-up (less than 3 years). The reported rate of recurrence ranges from 0% to 6% in these studies (Table 50-4). Recently, however, there have been two studies with a mean follow-up of 5 years.[95,97] In a study of 42 patients by D'Hoore et al.,[95] with a mean follow-up of 61 months, the rate of recurrent prolapse was 4.8%. In the largest study of laparoscopic surgery for rectal prolapse by Ashari et al.,[97] with 117 patients over a 10-year period and a mean follow-up of 62 months, the rate of recurrent full-thickness prolapse was only 2.5%. The study, however, noted an 18% rate of mucosal prolapse, which is somewhat concerning. Further long-term follow-up of these patients is needed to ensure that the rate of recurrence remains acceptable. If the rate of recurrent prolapse is confirmed to occur at a rate equal to conventional surgery, a minimally invasive approach to rectal prolapse seems to be an ideal operation for surgeons with laparoscopic skills.

Colorectal Cancer

It is estimated that more than 105,500 new cases of colon cancer and 42,000 new cases of rectal cancer were diagnosed in the United States in 2003.[99] Before 2004, fewer than 5% of resections for colon and rectal cancer were being performed laparoscopically. Early in the history of laparoscopic resection of colorectal cancer there was controversy related to the phenomenon of cancer implants at incision sites. Data from randomized, controlled trials, however, have laid to rest these controversial aspects of the minimally invasive approach. The percentage of cases performed laparoscopically is expected to increase, as more surgeons become familiar with these techniques.

TABLE 50-4. Recent results of laparoscopy for rectal prolapse

Study	Year	No. of patients	Follow-up (mo)	Procedure	Operative time (min) LR/LRR	LOS (d)	Recurrence (%)	Comment
Poen et al.[83]	1996	12	19	LR	195	10	0	Improved continence
Himpens et al.[84]	1999	37	6–48	LR	130	7	0	3% conversion
Bruch et al.[86]	1999	57	30	LR/LRR	227/257	15	0	Constipation improved in 76%
Boccasanta et al.[87]	1999	10	NS	LRR	130	4.7		Compared with open—longer op time, lower cost, shorter LOS
Xynos et al.[88]	1999	10	NS	LRR	150	5	NS	Compared with open—longer op time, shorter LOS
Kessler et al.[89]	1999	32	33	LR/LRR		5	FT 6.2	10% developed bowel obstruction
Heah et al.[90]	2000	25	26	LR	96	7	0	16% conversion
Kellokumpu et al.[91]	2000	34	24	LR/LRR	150/255	5	7	Constipation improved in 70%
Benoist et al.[92]	2001	48	20–47	LR/LRR	—	—	MP 8	Suture rectopexy preferred to mesh
Solomon et al.[93]	2002	20	24	LR	153	3.9	0	Prospective, randomized study
Kairaluoma et al.[94]	2003	53	12	LR/LRR	127/210	5	6	Compared with open—longer op time, shorter LOS
D'Hoore et al.[95]	2004	42	61	LR	NS	NS	FT 4.8	Constipation improved in 84%
Lechaux et al.[96]	2005	48	36	LR/LRR	193	4–7	MP 4.2	Constipation worsened in 23%
Ashari et al.[97]	2005	117	62	LRR	110–180	5	FT 2.5; MP 18	Large study with long-term follow-up

RR, resection rectopexy; PFR, pelvic floor repair; AR, anterior resection; FRM, full rectal mobilization without fixation; LARR, laparoscopic resection rectopexy; LAR, laparoscopic rectopexy; FT, full thickness; MP, mucosal prolapse; NS, not specified.

Background

After the success of minimally invasive techniques for cholecystectomy, reports of laparoscopic colon resections soon appeared.[100] Sadly, the specter of wound implants, or recurrence of cancer in the laparoscopic incisions, followed shortly thereafter. In retrospect, it seems that in the attempt to allow patients to benefit from minimally invasive techniques, operations for colon cancer were being attempted that did not fulfill accepted oncologic principles, i.e., shortcuts were being taken with the extent of resection. Larger series by experienced surgeons showed that wound implants were not an inevitable accompaniment of the laparoscopic approach, but the damage was done. From 1994 to 2004 there was nearly a moratorium on laparoscopic resection for colon cancer, with some national surgical societies calling for these procedures to be performed only under the auspices of randomized, controlled trials or with other means of careful prospective data collection.[102] These concerns prompted an unprecedented number of randomized, controlled trials[4,5,20–24,102,103] and a new field of tumor and immunology investigation as they pertain to the pneumoperitoneum.

Lacy et al.[103] published the first large single-center randomized controlled trial in 2002. With median follow-up of 39 months, Lacy and his colleagues reported higher cancer-related survival for the laparoscopic arm. Specifically, they showed no difference between arms for Stage II cancers, but an improved survival for the laparoscopic approach in Stage III cancers where the outcome was similar to that of Stage II patients. This was followed in 2004 by the results of the large multicenter COST study group.[24] With almost 900 patients randomized either to the open or the laparoscopic arm of the study, no differences were found in overall survival or disease-free survival. Further reassurance was provided in finding that there were only two wound recurrences in the laparoscopic group, and one in the open arm. Another of the large prospective randomized studies, the "CLASICC" trial from the United Kingdom, has also recently published results with similar findings except a higher rate of conversions was noted.[4] The results of these recent trials (Table 50-5) have demonstrated that similar oncologic resections can be achieved by experienced surgeons performing laparoscopic colorectal resections.

Laparoscopic Resection of Colon and Rectal Cancer

The following description regarding the safe performance of laparoscopic resection for curable colon and rectal cancer is based on current literature and experience. The attention to technical detail is in response to the early concerns regarding oncologic outcomes. It is predicated on the understanding that patients with curable colon and rectal cancer are treated by experienced surgeons whose minimally invasive skills fulfill the Credentialing Recommendations endorsed jointly by ASCRS (American Society of Colon and Rectal Surgeons) and SAGES (Society of American Gastrointestinal and Endoscopic Surgeons).[104,105]

General Considerations

After detection of a colon or rectal cancer, routine evaluation incorporates preoperative staging, assessment of resectability, and determination of the patient's operative risk. As part of this assessment, a laparoscopic approach may be contemplated. There are several factors to consider, primarily in terms of gauging the difficulty of the procedure and the likelihood of being able to perform it laparoscopically. The site of the tumor is important, because right and sigmoid colectomy are generally less technically demanding than, for example, low anterior resection. Documented extensive adhesions may preclude a minimally invasive approach, although laparoscopic resection is frequently possible in patients who have had prior abdominal operations. Obesity, and particularly the distribution of abdominal fat, may preclude laparoscopic resection, especially in the case of a rectal cancer in an obese male patient with a narrow pelvis. The patient should be informed of both laparoscopic and open alternatives, and the possible need for conversion. Above all, the surgeon must have adequate experience before embarking on resection for a potentially curable malignancy. Patients are increasingly sophisticated regarding their health care, and the surgeon must be prepared to answer questions about experience with the procedure.

Tumor Localization

The entire colon and rectum should be evaluated to eliminate synchronous lesions.[106,107] This is usually achieved with colonoscopy, but this has limitations in terms of localization, particularly if a minimally invasive approach is being considered. Colonoscopy is most accurate for localization of a tumor in the rectum and cecum only. Lesions elsewhere in the colon may be inaccurately localized by colonoscopy in up to 14% of cases.[108] A laparoscopic approach requires accurate localization of the tumor to a specific segment of the colon, because even a known cancer may not be visualized from the serosal aspect of the bowel during laparoscopy. The wrong segment of colon may be removed if accurate localization has not been performed.[109]

A variety of other options is available to localize a lesion including preoperative colonoscopic marking with ink tattoo or metallic clips, barium enema, or intraoperative endoscopy. The area adjacent to a cancer or polyp may be marked either by endoscopic clips or submucosal india ink injection. If clips are placed, immediate abdominal X-rays films should be taken, otherwise intraoperative imaging with laparoscopic ultrasound

P.W. Marcello and T. Young-Fadok

TABLE 50-5. Prospective, randomized trials comparing laparoscopic and conventional surgery for colorectal cancer

Baseline characteristics	Lacy et al. 2002[103] LAP versus OPEN	COST 2004[24] LAP versus OPEN	CLASICC 2005[4] LAP versus OPEN	
No. assigned	111:108	435:437	526:268	
No. completed (dead or no data)	105:101	435:428	452:231	
			74:37	
Age	68:71	70:69	69:69	
Gender (F)	55:58	49%:51%	44%:46%	
Previous surgery	40:47	43%:46%		
Operative findings				
Procedure				
Right	49:49	54%:54%	24%:24%	
Left	4:1	7%:7%	7%:9%	
Sigmoid	52:46	38%:38%	13%:12%	
AR/LAR	3:9		37%:36%/12%:13%	
Other	3:3		4%:3%	
TNM stage				
0		5%:8%	Not given	
I	27:18	35%:26%		
II	42:48	31%:34%		
III	37:36	26%:28%		
IV	5:6	4%:2%		
No. lymph nodes	11.1:11.1	12:12	12:13.5	
Conversion	12 (11%):N/A	21%:N/A	29%:N/A	
OR time (min)	142:118*	150:95*	180:135 (anesthesia time)	
Incision length (cm)		6:18*	10:22	
Short-term outcomes				
Oral intake (h)	54:85*			
(d)			6:6	
Hospital stay (d)	5.2:7.9*	5:6*	9:11	
30-d mortality		<1%:1%	4%:5%	
Postoperative complications	12:31*	19%:19%	33%:32%	
			Colon	Rectum
Wound infection	8:18		5%:5%	13%:12%
Pneumonia	0:0		7%:4%	10%:4%
Ileus	3:9			
Leak	0:2		2%:0%	10%:7%
Duration of oral analgesics (d)		1:2*		
Duration of parenteral analgesics (d)		3:4*		
Cancer outcomes				
Tumor recurrence	18:28	76:84		
Distant	7:9			
Locoregional	7:14			
Peritoneal seedling	3:5			
Port site	1:0	2:1		
5-y overall survival†	82%:74%	79%:78%		
I	85%:94%	84%:94%		
II	75%:77%	78%:81%		
III	72%:45%	60%:63%		
5-y disease-free survival†		78%:80%		
I	90%:88%	92%:96%		
II	80%:76%	82%:88%		
III	70%:45%	62%:60%		
Cancer-related survival†	91%:79%*			
I	100%:99%			
II	88%:85%			
III	84%:50%*			

*Statistically significant difference.
†Extrapolated from graphs in manuscript.

or fluoroscopy is necessary to localize the clip's location. This procedure is not frequently used because it requires an experienced radiologist and/or endoscopist. Preoperative endoscopic tattooing is a common method of tumor localization.[110,111] India ink is a nonabsorbable marker that has been reported in more than 600 cases for tumor localization since 1975. The ink is injected into the submucosa in three or four quadrants around the lesion, or 2 cm distal to the lesion if the tumor is in the distal colon and distal margins are potentially an issue (typically 0.5 cc per site). During diagnostic laparoscopy, the ink marking can be identified even at the flexures or transverse colon. India ink injection seems to be safe with few reported complications. Intraoperative endoscopy is hampered by persistent bowel distention, prolongation of operative times, and need for equipment and endoscopist intraoperatively. More recent studies have evaluated CO_2 colonoscopy which allows for more rapid absorption of the intracolonic gas which may facilitate its use during laparoscopic procedures.[112]

Preoperative Staging

Guidelines are available for standard practices in preoperative assessment for open resection of colon or rectal cancer.[113,114] There are additional considerations with a laparoscopic approach to ensure accurate staging of the liver. In patients with colorectal cancer, the liver should be thoroughly evaluated using computed tomography (CT) with intravenous contrast, ultrasound, or magnetic resonance imaging. Because of limitation in tactile sensation associated with laparoscopy, these studies should be performed preoperatively. Alternatively, intraoperative laparoscopic ultrasonography offers the ability to fully evaluate the liver at the time of colorectal resection. Several studies have confirmed the feasibility and efficacy of laparoscopic ultrasound in the evaluation of liver metastasis from colorectal cancer.[115–117] Preoperative CT or ultrasound was a requirement of the COST randomized, controlled trial.[24] No excess of Stage IV disease was noted in the laparoscopic arm, suggesting that routine preoperative evaluation of the liver was equivalent in terms of oncologic outcome to palpation of the liver intraoperatively in the open arm of the study.

These considerations do not apply to rectal cancer, where staging CT scan and transanal rectal ultrasound should be routine.[114,118] Preoperative CT of the abdomen and pelvis, or hepatic ultrasound are routinely used in planning resection of rectal cancer, because the results may markedly alter the need for neoadjuvant therapy and the timing of the operative approach.

Preparation For Operation

Perioperative guidelines address the use of outpatient bowel preparation, prophylactic antibiotics, blood cross matching, and thromboembolism prophylaxis.[106] None of these aspects of patient care are affected by a laparoscopic approach, although some surgeons prefer to modify the bowel preparation. Despite lack of clear evidence of benefit from meta-analysis[119] and randomized, controlled trials,[120–124] a mechanical bowel preparation is frequently used in North America. Aside from the aesthetic aspects, an empty colon facilitates manipulation of the bowel with laparoscopic instruments. Use of large-volume mechanical bowel preparations may occasionally leave fluid-filled loops of small bowel that are more difficult to handle with laparoscopic instruments. A smaller-volume preparation may be used or the large-volume preparation may be followed by use of laxatives such as bisacodyl to reduce the volume of residual fluid. Some surgeons use 2- to 3-day periods of preparation rather than the usual 24 hours, especially if a completely laparoscopic approach and intracorporeal anastomosis is contemplated.[125]

Operative Issues

Certain operative principles pertain specifically either to the colon or to the rectum. Other issues are relevant to both.

Operative Techniques—Colon

Oncologic principles must not be compromised by a laparoscopic resection for colon cancer. Guidelines for colon cancer surgery outline recommendations for proximal and distal resection margins (based on the area supplied by the named feeding arterial vessel); mesenteric lymphadenectomy containing a minimum of 12 lymph nodes; and ligation of the primary feeding vessel at its base.[126] The randomized trials of laparoscopic colectomy adhered to these standard principles[4,24,103] and showed no significant difference in bowel margins, lymph nodes harvested, and, in the COST study, perpendicular length of the mesentery (a guide to the length of the vascular pedicle).[24] Inability to achieve these aims laparoscopically should prompt conversion to an open procedure.

These principles guide which steps of a procedure performed for cancer may be completed intracorporeally or extracorporeally. In the individual with a normal body mass index (BMI) undergoing right colectomy, it may be possible to divide the origin of the ileocolic pedicle extracorporeally using a small periumbilical extraction incision which overlies the base of the pedicle, and achieve an oncologically correct proximal ligation; intracorporeal ligation is obviously also an acceptable approach. In patients with BMI > 25, this ligation should be performed intracorporeally to ensure that the base of the pedicle is ligated. Intracorporeal ligation is required for proximal division of all other vessels unless a larger incision such as used for hand-assisted devices permits access via the incision to the origin of the vascular pedicle.

Operative Techniques—Rectum

Similar guidelines exist for oncologically appropriate open rectal cancer surgery, with levels of evidence and grades of recommendation.[114,118] These include a distal margin of 1–2 cm, removal of the blood supply and lymphatics up to the origin of the superior rectal artery (or inferior mesenteric artery if indicated), and appropriate mesorectal excision with radial clearance. Again, these principles of adequate clearance of the primary tumor and supporting tissues should not be compromised by a laparoscopic approach.

There are no randomized trials evaluating laparoscopic resection of rectal cancer except for those patients included in the CLASICC trial.[4] Current opinion among laparoscopic experts is that the principles outlined apply equally to laparoscopic as to open procedures. Prospective[127,128] and retrospective[129,130] case series indicate that laparoscopic rectal resection is possible in selected patients. Compared with colonic resection, additional technical challenges are associated with operating within the confines of the pelvis. Multiple factors affect feasibility of an oncologically adequate laparoscopic resection for rectal cancer: tumor factors such as bulkiness, proximal or distal location; and patient factors, e.g., width of the pelvis, obesity, presence of a bulky uterus, and obscuration of tissue planes by prior radiation. Inability to perform an appropriate resection should prompt conversion.

Contiguous Organ Attachment

En bloc resection is recommended for locally advanced adherent colorectal tumors.[126] A bulky tumor invasive into an adjacent organ may be detected by preoperative imaging, such as CT scan, and guide the recommendation for an open resection. A known T4 colonic cancer will prompt an open approach in the vast majority of cases,[126] although some experienced surgeons may complete en bloc resection of involved small bowel or abdominal wall laparoscopically. If a T4 lesion is discovered intraoperatively, conversion is indicated unless the surgeon is capable of performing en bloc resection.

Prevention of Wound Implants

Port site recurrences, or wound implants, have been reported at both extraction site and trocar site incisions.[131,132] This unanticipated phenomenon has prompted extensive investigation. Current consensus is that wound implants should be kept at a rate less than 1% by correct oncologic technique and experience.

In vitro and in vivo animal models, not clinical practice, have generated most recommendations for avoidance of wound implants. Avoidance of the pneumoperitoneum and alternative gases have been evaluated. Gasless laparoscopy has shown decrease in port site metastases,[133,134] and no effect.[135,136] Tumor growth may be proportional to insufflation pressure.[137] Carbon dioxide is associated with increased tumor implantation and growth,[138] but is clinically the safest and most widely used gas. Helium decreases tumor implants but is not easily adapted to the clinical setting.[139–141] Wound excision may either decrease[142] or increase[143] the rate of tumor implants.

Some experimental results are easily adapted to the clinical setting. The significance of aerosolization of tumor implants is controverisal,[144,145] but because evacuation of the pneumoperitoneum via the ports rather than via the incision is easily performed, some experts advocate this practice.[146] Gas leakage along loosely fixed trocars (the "chimney effect") may be associated with increased cancer wound implantation[147] so some surgeons fix the trocars to prevent slippage. Irrigation of the abdominal cavity and/or trocar site incisions with a variety of substances (e.g., povidone-iodine, heparin, methotrexate, cyclophosphamide, taurolidine, and 5-fluoro-uracil) has decreased wound implants in animal models.[136,140,148–153] An expert panel convened by the European Association of Endoscopic Surgery (EAES) reported that half the members irrigated the port sites and all members protected the extraction site and/or extracted the specimen in a bag.[146]

The most important developments in the issue of wound implants are experience and the refinement of laparoscopic techniques and equipment that permit a true oncologic resection to be performed. Early reports of implant rates of 2%–21%[131,132] have not been reproduced in large retrospective series by experienced surgeons, who reported rates of 1% or less.[154] This is similar to the incisional recurrence rate for open colorectal cancer resection.[155] The multicenter randomized trial from the COST study group reported tumor recurrence in the surgical wounds in 2 of 435 laparoscopic cases (0.5%) and in one of 428 patients in the open colectomy group (0.2%, $P = .50$).[24] Lacy et al.,[103] in a single center randomized trial, reported one implant in 111 patients for a rate of 0.9%. The COST study required all surgeons to have performed at least 20 colorectal resections before participation in the trial.[24] The member surgeons at Lacy's institution had extensive experience. In the clinical setting, the experience of the surgeon is considered the most important factor in the prevention of implants.

Training and Credentialing in Laparoscopic Colorectal Surgery

In terms of technical complexity, laparoscopic colon and especially rectal operations are considered toward the higher end of the spectrum. Adequate resection mandates mobilization of a large structure, arranging ports to facilitate dissection in several quadrants of the abdomen, ligation of large blood vessels, extraction of a bulky specimen, and creation of a safe anastomosis. Oncologic resections have the additional requirements of adequate distal and proximal margins, wide lymphadenectomy, ligation of the origin of the primary feeding vessel, and safe handling of the bowel.

Early studies estimated the learning curve for laparoscopic colectomy to be 20–50 cases.[1–3] The randomized, controlled multicenter COST study on laparoscopic versus open colectomy for colon cancer required each participating surgeon to have performed 20 cases.[24] This was also seen in the CLASICC trial.[4] This figure became the basis of the Approved Statement from the ASCRS and endorsed by SAGES after the publication of the results of the COST study.[104,105] Because the results of this trial showed that the oncologic outcomes for laparoscopic colectomy were equivalent to those of open colectomy, the statement took the unusual step of defining a specific number of cases based on the study entry criteria. The following is the approved statement:

Laparoscopic colectomy for curable cancer results in equivalent cancer related survival to open colectomy when performed by experienced surgeons. Adherence to standard cancer resection techniques including but not limited to complete exploration of the abdomen, adequate proximal and distal margins, ligation of the major vessels at their respective origins, containment and careful tissue handling, and en bloc resection with negative tumor margins using the laparoscopic approach will result in acceptable outcomes. Based on the COST trial,[24] pre-requisite experience should include at least 20 laparoscopic colorectal resections with anastomosis for benign disease or metastatic colon cancer before using the technique to treat curable cancer. Hospitals may base credentialing for laparoscopic colectomy for cancer on experience gained by formal graduate medical educational training or advanced laparoscopic experience, participation in hands-on training courses and outcomes.[104,105]

The issue of defining numbers for credentialing purposes is a source of considerable controversy. National surgical societies have traditionally avoided specifying required case numbers in credentialing guidelines, trying to balance the needs of their member surgeons with the safety of patients. The learning curve for laparoscopic colectomy likely varies depending on the actual procedure (because the term "laparoscopic colectomy" in this case encompasses a wide variety of procedures), the underlying pathologic diagnosis, and the prior laparoscopic experience of the surgeon coupled with innate skill. The COST study, however, provides a basis for specifying a minimum experience. For perspective, a resident completing a General Surgery Residency Program in 2003 and entering practice had performed a mean of 120 cases on the large intestine (mode 106, Residency Review Committee for Surgery, Reporting Period 2002–2003). Of these, an average of 50 cases required resection and anastomosis. Thus, the guideline for 20 laparoscopic cases is not excessive or unreasonable in terms of attaining comparable experience before independent practice.

Hand-assisted Laparoscopy

HAL colectomy has been advocated as an alternative to straight laparoscopic techniques. The reintroduction of the hand back into the abdomen during laparoscopy may overcome some of the technical challenges associated with laparoscopic colectomy. Because an extraction site is required for specimen removal, supporters of a hand-assisted approach believe the hand should be placed through that wound to facilitate dissection and mobilization of the colon. The development of new sleeveless hand-assist devices provides for hand exchanges without the loss of pneumoperitoneum, allowing surgeons to perform the procedures without disruption.

There have been a number of randomized and nonrandomized studies that have evaluated HAL colectomy.[156–167] Ou,[156] in 1995, reported his initial experience in 12 patients undergoing colectomy by hand-assisted methods and compared it with 12 patients undergoing a conventional open method. He demonstrated that the hand-assisted procedures required on average 135 minutes compared with 100 minutes for the standard open method. Length of stay was reduced in the hand-assisted group with an average of 5.6 days compared with 8.3 days for open patients. Randomized trials by the HALS Study Group[159,160] and Targarona et al.[162] have demonstrated that hand-assisted colectomy provides similar functional results to straight laparoscopic resection with fewer conversions. In a randomized study by Kang et al.[165] comparing hand-assisted versus open colon resection, the hand-assisted approach resulted in shortened postoperative ileus, shortened length of stay, and smaller incision size with no difference in operative time or complications. Differing results were seen in another randomized study by Maartense et al.,[166] which compared the results of open proctocolectomy with ileoanal pouch construction to a hand-assisted approach. In this study, there was no difference in length of stay (>10 days) and longer operative times in the hand-assisted group. The majority of patients, however, were not diverted at the time of procedure which likely impacted the results of the operation. In a study of straight laparoscopic proctocolectomy with ileoanal pouch, patients who were not diverted had a prolonged hospitalization in comparison to those who were diverted.[49] The long length of stay in the Maartense study may relate to the avoidance of proximal fecal diversion and likely influenced their results and conclusions.

Nonrandomized studies have shown benefit to the hand-assisted approach in comparison to a straight laparoscopic technique, but most have a limited number of any single procedure.[3,4,7–10,12] A recent study by Chang et al.,[76] however, did report on a large series of laparoscopic and hand-assisted sigmoid resection. The results of 85 straight laparoscopic sigmoid resections were compared with 66 hand-assisted procedures. The patients shared similar demographics including a mean BMI of 29 kg/m^2. The rate of conversion was significantly less in the hand-assisted group (0% versus 13%, $P < .01$) with a shortened mean operative time (189 versus 205 minutes). The mean size of the extraction was larger in the hand-assisted group (8 versus 6 cm, $P < .01$) but there was no difference in return of bowel function (mean, 2.5 versus 2.8 days) or the median length of stay (4 days). In the United States, there is currently a prospective, randomized study underway that is comparing straight laparoscopic total colectomy and left colectomy to a hand-assisted approach. If the results of this trial are similar to those of the Chang study, surgeons may be more willing to adopt a hand-assisted technique, particularly to ascend the learning curve.

By returning the hand back to the abdomen, one of the potential advantages of a HAL colectomy is that surgeons with less laparoscopic skills may be able to perform these complex procedures more easily. In the study by Chang, colorectal surgeons without a large laparoscopic experience participated in 27% of hand-assisted resections compared with only 16% ($P < .05$) of the straight laparoscopic procedures.[76] In a similar study comparing 85 straight laparoscopic total colectomy procedures to 45 hand-assisted operations, less-experienced surgeons were able to perform 20% of the hand-assisted procedures and only 5% of the straight laparoscopic operations.[167] These two studies, from a single institution, would suggest that a HAL colectomy may be easier to adopt than a straight laparoscopic approach, but this will need to be reproduced by other centers.

Future Considerations

The field of laparoscopic colon and rectal surgery is slowly expanding. With advancement in techniques and technology along with the further training of our surgical and colorectal residents, the percentage of colorectal procedures that are performed by minimally invasive techniques will likely continue to increase. Surgeons who are more than 5–10 years from their residency and perform more than 20 colon resections a year will need to obtain advanced training and credentialing before performing laparoscopic colon resection. Hand-assisted technology and procedures may be used to expand the field of minimally invasive colorectal surgery. The results of the large multicenter prospective randomized trials comparing open to laparoscopic surgery for curable colon cancer have demonstrated modest short-term advantages to a laparoscopic approach while maintaining the oncologic integrity of the operation, when performed by experienced surgeons. There is less of a concern now for local port site recurrences of colon cancer, as was seen in the earlier reports. The laparoscopic resection of rectal cancer remains in the forefront and is likely the next area to be critically evaluated and advanced by laparoscopic surgeons.

References

1. Simons AJ, Anthone GJ, Ortega AE, et al. Laparoscopic-assisted colectomy learning curve. Dis Colon Rectum 1995;38:600–603.
2. Senagore AJ, Luchtefeld MA, Mackeigan JM. What is the learning curve for laparoscopic colectomy? Am Surg 1995;61:681–685.
3. Wishner JD, Baker JWJ, Hoffman GC, et al. Laparoscopic-assisted colectomy. The learning curve. Surg Endosc 1995;9:1179–1183.
4. Goillou PJ, Quirke P, Thrope H, et al. Short-term endpoints of conventional vs. laparoscopic-assisted surgery in patients with colorectal cancer (MRC-CLASICC trial): multicenter, randomized controlled trial. Lancet 2005;365;1718–1726.
5. The COLOR Study Group. Impact of hospital case volume on short-term outcome after laparoscopic operation for colonic cancer. Surg Endosc 2005;19:687–692.
6. Hyman N. How much colorectal surgery do general surgeons do? J Am Coll Surg 2002;194:37–39.
7. Tuech JJ, Regenet N, Hennekinne S, et al. Laparoscopic colectomy for sigmoid diverticulitis in obese and nonobese patients: a prospective comparative study. Surg Endosc 2001;15:1427–1430.
8. Stern LE, Chang YJ, Marcello PW, et al. Is obesity a contraindication to laparoscopic colectomy? A case control study. Dis Colon Rectum 2004;47:583.
9. Delaney CP, Pokala N, Senagore AJ, et al. Is laparoscopic colectomy applicable to patients with body mass index >30? A case-matched comparative study with open colectomy. Dis Colon Rectum 2005;48:975–981.
10. Bauer JJ, Harris MT, Grumbach NM, et al. Laparoscopic-assisted intestinal resection for Crohn's disease. Which patients are good candidates? J Clin Gastroenterol 1996;23:44–46.
11. Sher ME, Agachan F, Bortul JJ, et al. Laparoscopic surgery for diverticulitis. Surg Endosc 1997;11:264–267.
12. Pokala N, Delaney CP, Brady KM, Senagore AJ. Elective laparoscopic surgery for benign internal enteric fistulas: a review of 43 cases. Surg Endosc 2005;19:222–225.
13. Bartus CM, Lipof T, Sarwar S, et al. Colovesical fistula: not a contraindication to elective laparoscopic colectomy. Dis Colon Rectum 2005;48:233–236.
14. Regan JP, Salky BA. Laparoscopic treatment of enteric fistulas. Surg Endosc 2004;18:252–254.
15. Young-Fadok TM, COST Study Group. Conversion does not adversely affect oncologic outcomes after laparoscopic colectomy for colon cancer: results from a multicenter prospective randomized study [abstract]. Dis Colon Rectum 2005;48:637–638.
16. Casillas S, Delaney CP, Senagore AJ, et al. Does conversion of a laparoscopic colectomy adversely affect patient outcome? Dis Colon Rectum 2004;47:1680–1685.
17. Bohm B, Milsom JW, Fazio VW. Postoperative intestinal motility following conventional and laparoscopic intestinal surgery. Arch Surg 1995;130:415–419.
18. Bessler M, Whelan RL, Halverson A, et al. Controlled trial of laparoscopic-assisted vs open colon resection in a porcine model. Surg Endosc 1996;10:732–735.
19. Hotokezaka M, Combs MJ, Schirmer BD. Recovery of gastrointestinal motility following open versus laparoscopic colon resection in dogs. Dig Dis Sci 1996;41:705–710.
20. Milsom JW, Bohm B, Hammerhofer KA, et al. A prospective, randomized trial comparing laparoscopic versus conventional techniques in colorectal cancer surgery: a preliminary report. J Am Coll Surg 1998;187:46–54.
21. Stage JG, Schulze S, Moller P, et al. Prospective randomized study of laparoscopic versus open colonic resection for adenocarcinoma. Br J Surg 1997;84:391–396.

22. Schwenk W, Böhm W, Müller JM. Postoperative pain and fatigue after laparoscopic or conventional colorectal resections: a prospective randomized trial. Surg Endosc 1998;12: 1131–1136.

23. Weeks JC, Nelson H, Gelber S, et al. Short-term quality-of-life outcomes following laparoscopic-assisted colectomy vs open colectomy for colon cancer: a randomized trial. JAMA 2002; 287:321–328.

24. Nelson H, The Clinical Outcomes of Surgical Therapy Study Group. A comparison of laparoscopically assisted and open colectomy for colon cancer. New Engl J Med 2004;350: 2050–2059.

25. Fleshman JW, Fry RD, Birnbaum EH, et al. Laparoscopic-assisted and minilaparotomy approaches to colorectal diseases are similar in early outcome. Dis Colon Rectum 1996;39:15–22.

26. Senagore AJ, Duepree HJ, Delaney CP, et al. Results of a standardized technique and postoperative care plan for laparoscopic sigmoid colectomy. Dis Colon Rectum 2003;46: 503–509.

27. Raue W, Haase O, Junghans T, et al. "Fast-track" multimodal rehabilitation program improves outcome after laparoscopic sigmoidectomy. Surg Endosc 2004;18:1463–1468.

28. Psaila J, Bulley SH, Ewings P, et al. Outcome following laparoscopic resection for colorectal cancer. Br J Surg 1998;85: 662–664.

29. Chen HH, Wexner SD, Weiss EG, et al. Laparoscopic colectomy for benign colorectal disease is associated with a significant reduction in disability as compared with laparotomy. Surg Endosc 1998;12:1397–1400.

30. Young-Fadok TM, Hall Long K, McConnell EJ, et al. Advantages of laparoscopic resection for ileocolic Crohn's disease. Improved outcomes and reduced costs. Surg Endosc 2001;15:450–454.

31. Dupree HJ, Senagore AJ, Delaney CP, et al. Advantages of laparoscopic resection for ileocecal Crohn's disease. Dis Colon Rectum 2002;45:605–610.

32. Shore G, Gonzalez QH, Bondora A, et al. Laparoscopic vs. conventional ileocolectomy for primary Crohn's disease. Arch Surg 2003;138:76–79.

33. Senagore AJ, Duepree HJ, Delaney CP, et al. Cost structure of laparoscopic and open sigmoid colectomy for diverticular disease: similarities and differences. Dis Colon Rectum 2002;45:485–490.

34. Dwivedi A, Chachin F, Agrawal S, et al. Laparoscopic colectomy vs. open colectomy for sigmoid diverticular disease. Dis Colon Rectum 2002;45:1309–1315.

35. Bauer JJ, Harris MT, Grumbach NM, et al. Laparoscopic-assisted intestinal resection for Crohn's disease. Which patients are good candidates? J Clin Gastroenterol 1996;23:44–46.

36. Wu JS, Birnbaum EH, Kodner IJ, et al. Laparoscopic-assisted ileocolic resections in patients with Crohn's disease: are abscesses, phlegmons, or recurrent disease contraindications? Surgery 1997;122:682–688.

37. Dunker MS, Stiggelbout AM, van Hogezand RA, et al. Cosmesis and body image after laparoscopic-assisted and open ileocolic resection for Crohn's disease. Surg Endosc 1998;12:1334–1340.

38. Wong SK, Marcello PW, Hammerhoffer KA, et al. Laparoscopic surgery for Crohn's disease: an analysis of 92 cases. Surg Endosc 1999;13:S4.

39. Canin-Endres J, Salky B, Gattorno F, et al. Laparoscopic assisted intestinal resection in 88 patients with Crohn's disease. Surg Endosc 1999;13:595–599.

40. Alabaz O, Irotulam AJ, Nessim A, et al. Comparison of laparoscopically assisted and conventional ileocolic resection for Crohn's disease. Eur J Surg 2000;166:213–217.

41. Bemelman WA, Slors JFM, Dunker MS, et al. Laparoscopic-assisted vs open ileocolic resection for Crohn's disease: a comparative study. Surg Endosc 2000;14:721–725.

42. Schmidt M, Talamini MA, Kaufman HS, et al. Laparoscopic surgery for Crohn's disease: a single institution experience. Ann Surg 2001;233:733–739.

43. Milsom JW, Hammerhofer KA, Bohm B, et al. A prospective, randomized trial comparing laparoscopic versus conventional surgery for refractory ileocolic Crohn's disease. Dis Colon Rectum 2001;44:1–9.

44. Evans J, Poritz L, MacRae H. Influence of experience on laparoscopic ileocolic resection for Crohn's disease. Dis Colon Rectum 2002;45:1595–1600.

45. Benoist S, Panis Y, Beaufour A, et al. Laparoscopic ileocecal resection in Crohn's disease: a case-matched comparison with open resection. Surg Endosc 2003;17:814–818.

46. Tabet J, Hong D, Kim CW, et al. Recurrence after laparoscopic bowel resection for Crohn's disease: comparison to open technique. Can J Gastroenterol 2001;15:237–242.

47. Bergamaschi R, Pessaux P, Arneaud JP. Comparison of conventional and laparoscopic ileocolic resection for Crohn's disease. Dis Colon Rectum 2003;46:1129–1133.

48. Meijerink WJH, Eijsbouts QAJ, Cuesta MA, et al. Laparoscopically assisted bowel surgery for inflammatory bowel disease. Surg Endosc 1999;13:882–886.

49. Marcello PW, Milsom JW, Wong SK, et al. Laparoscopic restorative proctocolectomy: a case-matched comparative study with open restorative proctocolectomy. Dis Colon Rectum 2000;43:604–608.

50. Seshadri PA, Poulin EC, Schlachta CM, et al. Laparoscopic total colectomy and proctocolectomy: short and long term results. Surg Endosc 2001;15:837–842.

51. Hamel C, Hilderbrandt U, Weiss E, et al. Laparoscopic surgery for inflammatory bowel disease: ileocolic resection versus subtotal colectomy. Surg Endosc 2001;15:642–645.

52. Marcello PW, Milsom JW, Wong SK, et al. Laparoscopic total colectomy for acute colitis: a case control study. Dis Colon Rectum 2001;44:1441–1445.

53. Brown SR, Eu KW, Seow-Choen F. Consecutive series of laparoscopic-assisted vs. minilaparotomy restorative proctocolectomies. Dis Colon Rectum 2001;44:397–400.

54. Dunker MS, Bemelman WA, Slors JF, et al. Functional outcome, quality of life, body image, and cosmesis in patients after laparoscopic-assisted and conventional restorative proctocolectomy: a comparative study. Dis Colon Rectum 2001;44:1800–1807.

55. Ky AJ, Sonoda T, Milsom JW. One-stage laparoscopic restorative proctocolectomy: an alternative to the conventional approach? Dis Colon Rectum 2002;45:207–211.

56. Bell RL, Seymour NE. Laparoscopic treatment of fulminant ulcerative colitis. Surg Endosc 2002;16:1778–1782.

57. Rivadeneira DE, Marcello PW, Roberts PL, et al. Benefits of hand-assisted laparoscopic restorative proctocolectomy: a comparative study. Dis Colon Rectum 2004;47:1371–1376.

58. Kienle P, Weitz J, Benner A, et al. Laparoscopically assisted colectomy and ileoanal pouch procedure with and without protective ileostomy. Surg Endosc 2003;17:716–720.

59. Nakajima K, Lee SW, Cocilovo C, et al. Hand assisted laparoscopic colorectal surgery using Gelport: initial experience with a new hand access device. Surg Endosc 2004;18:102–105.

60. Schmitt SL, Cohen SM, Wexner SD, et al. Does laparoscopic-assisted ileal pouch anal anastomosis reduce the length of hospitalization? Int J Colorectal Dis 1994;9:134–137.

61. Reissman P, Salky BA, Pfeifer J, et al. Laparoscopic surgery in the management of inflammatory bowel disease. Am J Surg 1996;171:47–50.

62. Eijsbouts QA, Cuesta MA, de Brauw LM, et al. Elective laparoscopic-assisted sigmoid resection for diverticular disease. Surg Endosc 1997;11:750–753.

63. Stevenson AR, Stitz RW, Lumley JW, et al. Laparoscopically assisted anterior resection for diverticular disease: follow-up of 100 consecutive patients. Ann Surg 1998;227:335–342.

64. Tuech JJ, Pessaux P, Rouge C, et al. Laparoscopic vs open colectomy for sigmoid diverticulitis: a prospective comparative study in the elderly. Surg Endosc 2000;14:1031–1033.

65. Trebuchet G, Lechaux D, Leclave JL. Laparoscopic left colon resection for diverticular disease: results of 170 consecutive cases. Surg Endosc 2002;16:18–21.

66. Bouillot JL, Berthou JC, Champault G, et al. Elective laparoscopic colonic resection for diverticular disease. Surg Endosc 2002;16:1320–1323.

67. Pugliese R, Di Lernia S, Sansonna F, et al. Laparoscopic treatment of sigmoid diverticulitis: a retrospective review of 103 cases. Surg Endosc 2004;18:1344–1348.

68. Schneidbach H, Schneider C, Rose J, et al. Laparoscopic approach to treatment of sigmoid diverticulitis: changes in the spectrum of indications and results of a prospective, multicenter study on 1545 patients. Dis Colon Rectum 2004;47:1883–1888.

69. Pessaux P, Muscari F, Ouellet JF, et al. Risk factors for mortality and morbidity after elective sigmoid resection for diverticulitis: prospective multicenter multivariate analysis of 582 patients. World J Surg 2004;28:92–96.

70. Schwandner O, Farke S, Bruch HP. Laparoscopic colectomy for diverticulitis is not associated with increased morbidity when compared with nondiverticular disease. Int J Colorectal Dis 2005;20:165–172.

71. Liberman MA, Phillips EH, Carroll BJ, et al. Laparoscopic colectomy vs traditional colectomy for diverticulitis. Outcome and costs. Surg Endosc 1996;10:15–18.

72. Bruce CJ, Coller JA, Murray JJ, et al. Laparoscopic resection for diverticular disease. Dis Colon Rectum 1996;39:S1–S6.

73. Kohler L, Rixen D, Troidl H. Laparoscopic colorectal resection for diverticulitis. Int J Colorectal Dis 1998;13:43–47.

74. Lawrence DM, Pasquale MD, Wasser TE. Laparoscopic versus open sigmoid colectomy for diverticulitis. Am Surg 2003;69:499–504.

75. Gonzalez R, Smith CD, Mattar SG, et al. Laparoscopic vs open resection for the treatment of diverticular disease. Surg Endosc 2004;18:276–280.

76. Chang YJ, Marcello PW, Rusin LC, et al. Hand assisted laparoscopic colectomy: a helping hand or hindrance? Surg Endosc 2005;19:656–661.

77. Berman IR. Sutureless laparoscopic rectopexy for procidentia: technique and implications. Dis Colon Rectum 1992;35:689–693.

78. Kwok SP, Carey DP, Lau WY, Li AK. Laparoscopic rectopexy. Dis Colon Rectum 1994;37:947–948.

79. Cuschieri A, Shimi SM, Vander Velpen G, et al. Laparoscopic prosthesis fixation rectopexy for rectal prolapse. Br J Surg 1994;81:38–39.

80. Graf W, Stefanson T, Arvidson D, Pahlmann L. Laparoscopic suture rectopexy. Dis Colon Rectum 1995;38:211–212.

81. Darzi A, Henery MM, Guillou PJ, et al. Stapled laparoscopic rectopexy for rectal prolapse. Surg Endosc 1995;9:301–303.

82. Solomon MJ, Eyers AA. Laparoscopic rectopexy using mesh fixation with a spiked chromium staple. Dis Colon Rectum 1996;39:279–284.

83. Poen AC, de Brauw M, Felt-Bersma RJ, et al. Laparoscopic rectopexy for complete rectal prolapse. Clinical outcome and anorectal function tests. Surg Endosc 1996;10:904–908.

84. Himpens J, Cadiere GB, Brutns J, Vertruyen M. Laparoscopic rectopexy according to Wells. Surg Endosc 1999;13:139–141.

85. Stevenson AR, Stitz RW, Lumley JW. Laparoscopic-assisted resection rectopexy for rectal prolapse: early and medium follow-up. Dis Colon Rectum 1998;41:46–54.

86. Bruch HP, Herold A, Schiedeck T, Schwandner O. Laparoscopic surgery for rectal prolapse and outlet obstruction. Dis Colon Rectum 1999;42:1189–1194.

87. Boccasanta P, Venturi M, Reitano MC, et al. Laparotomic vs. laparoscopic rectopexy in complete rectal prolapse. Dig Surg 1999;16:415–419.

88. Xynos E, Chrysos E, Tsiaoussis J, et al. Resection rectopexy for rectal prolapse: the laparoscopic approach. Surg Endosc 1999;13:862–864.

89. Kessler H, Jerby BL, Milsom JW. Successful treatment of rectal prolapse by laparoscopic suture rectopexy. Surg Endosc 1999;13:858–861.

90. Heah SM, Hartley JE, Hurley J, et al. Laparoscopic suture rectopexy without resection is effective treatment for full-thickness rectal prolapse. Dis Colon Rectum 2000;43:638–643.

91. Kellokumpu IH, Vironen J, Scheinin, T. Laparoscopic repair of rectal prolapse: a prospective study evaluating surgical outcome and changes in symptoms and bowel function. Surg Endosc 2000;14:634–640.

92. Benoist S, Taffinder N, Gould S, et al. Functional results two years after laparoscopic rectopexy. Am J Surg 2001;182:168–173.

93. Solomon MJ, Young CJ, Eyers AA, Roberts RA. Randomized clinical trial of laparoscopic versus open abdominal rectopexy for rectal prolapse. Br J Surg 2002;89:35–39.

94. Kairaluoma MV, Viljakka MT, Kellokumpu IH. Open vs. laparoscopic surgery for rectal prolapse: a case-controlled study assessing short-term outcomes. Dis Colon Rectum 2003;46:353–360.

95. D'Hoore A, Cadoni R, Penninckx F. Long-term outcome of ventral rectopexy for total rectal prolapse. Br J Surg 2004;91:1500–1505.

96. Lechaux D, Trebuchet G, Siproudhis L, Campion JP. Laparoscopic rectopexy for full-thickness rectal prolapse: a single-institution retrospective study evaluating surgical outcome. Surg Endosc 2005;19:514–518.

97. Ashari LH, Lumley JW, Stevenson ARL, Stitz RW. Laparoscopically-assisted resection rectopexy for rectal prolapse: ten years' experience. Dis Colon Rectum 2005;48:982–987.

98. Salkeld G, Bagia M, Solomon M. Economic impact of laparoscopic versus open abdominal rectopexy. Br J Surg 2004;91:1188–1191.

99. Jemal A, Murray T, Samuels A, et al. Cancer statistics. CA Cancer J Clin 2003;53:5–26.

100. Jacobs M, Verdeja JC, Goldstein HS. Minimally invasive colon resection (laparoscopic colectomy). Surg Laparosc Endosc 1991;1:144–150.

101. American Society of Colon and Rectal Surgeons. Approved statement on laparoscopic colectomy. Dis Colon Rectum 1994;37:638.

102. Stocchi L, Nelson H. Laparoscopic colectomy for colon cancer: trial update. J Surg Oncol 1998;68:255–267.

103. Lacy AM, García-Valdecasas JC, Delgado S, et al. Laparoscopy-assisted colectomy versus open colectomy for treatment of non-metastatic colon cancer: a randomised trial. Lancet 2002;359:2224–2229.

104. The American Society of Colon and Rectal Surgeons approved statement: laparoscopic colectomy for curable cancer. Dis Colon Rectum 2004;47(8):A1.

105. The American Society of Colon and Rectal Surgeons approved statement: laparoscopic colectomy for curable cancer. Surg Endosc 2004;18(8):A1.

106. Simmang CL, Senatore P, Lowry A, et al. Practice parameters for detection of colorectal neoplasms. Dis Colon Rectum 1999;42:1123–1129.

107. Winawer S, Fletcher R, Rex D, et al. Colorectal cancer screening and surveillance: clinical guidelines and rationale—update based on new evidence. Gastroenterology 2003;124:544–560.

108. Vignati P, Welch JP, Cohen JL. Endoscopic localization of colon cancers. Surg Endosc 1994;8:1085–1087.

109. Larach SW, Patankar SK, Ferrara A, et al. Complications of laparoscopic colorectal surgery: analysis and comparison of early vs latter experience. Dis Colon Rectum 1997;40: 592–596.

110. Kim SH, Milsom JW, Church JM, et al. Perioperative tumor localization for laparoscopic colorectal surgery. Surg Endosc 1997;11:1013–1016.

111. McArthur CS, Roayaie S, Waye JD. Safety of preoperation endoscopic tattoo with India ink for identification of colonic lesions. Surg Endosc 1999;13:397–400.

112. Nakajima K, Lee SW, Sonoda T, Milsom JW. Intraoperative carbon dioxide colonoscopy: a safe insufflation alternative for locating colonic lesions during laparoscopic surgery. Surg Endosc 2005;19:321–325.

113. Otchy D, Hyman NH, Simmang C, et al. Practice parameters for colon cancer. Dis Colon Rectum 2004;47:1269–1284.

114. The standards practice task force, ASCRS, Tjandra JJ, Kilkenny JW, Buie WD, et al. Practice parameters for the management of rectal cancer (revised). Dis Colon Rectum 2005; 48:411–423.

115. Goletti O, Celona G, Galatioto C, et al. Is laparoscopic sonography a reliable and sensitive procedure for staging of colorectal cancer? A comparative study. Surg Endosc 1998;12: 1236–1241.

116. Milsom J, Jerby BL, Kessler H, et al. Prospective blinded comparison of laparoscopic ultrasonography versus contrast enhanced computerized tomography for liver assessment in patients undergoing colorectal carcinoma surgery. Dis Colon Rectum 2000;43:44–49.

117. Kumar H, Hartley J, Heer K, et al. Efficacy of laparoscopic ultrasound scanning (USS) in detection of colorectal liver metastases during surgery. Dis Colon Rectum 2000;43:320–325.

118. Abel ME, Rosen L, Kodner IJ, et al. Practice parameters for the treatment of rectal carcinoma. Dis Colon Rectum 1993;36: 989–1006.

119. Platell C, Hall J. What is the role of mechanical bowel preparation in patients undergoing colorectal surgery? Dis Colon Rectum 1998;41:875–882.

120. Brownson P, Jenkins SA, Nott D, et al. Mechanical bowel preparation before colorectal surgery: results of a prospective, randomized trial. Br J Surg 1992;79:461–462.

121. Burke P, Mealy K, Gillen P, et al. Requirement for bowel preparation in colorectal surgery. Br J Surg 1994;81:580–581.

122. Santos JC, Batista J, Sirimarco MT, et al. Prospective randomized trial of mechanical bowel preparation in patients undergoing elective colorectal surgery. Br J Surg 1994;81:1673–1676.

123. Miettinen RP, Laitinen ST, Makela JT, Paakkonen ME. Bowel preparation with oral polyethylene glycol electrolyte solution vs. no preparation in elective open colorectal surgery: prospective, randomized study. Dis Colon Rectum 2000;43:669–677.

124. Zmora O, Mahajn, A, Barak B, et al. Colon and rectal surgery without mechanical bowel preparation: randomized prospective trial. Ann Surg 2003;237:363–367.

125. Franklin ME, Rosenthal D, Abrego-Medina D, et al. Prospective comparison of open vs. laparoscopic colon surgery for carcinoma. Five-year results. Dis Colon Rectum 1996;39: S35–46.

126. Nelson H, Petrelli N, Carlin A, et al. Guidelines 2000 for colon and rectal cancer surgery. J Natl Cancer Inst 2001;93:583–596.

127. Wu WX, Sun YM, Hua YB, Shen LZ. Laparoscopic versus conventional open resection of rectal carcinoma: a clinical comparative study. World J Gastroenterol 2004;10:1167–1170.

128. Tsang WW, Chung CC, Li MK. Prospective evaluation of laparoscopic total mesorectal excision with colonic J-pouch reconstruction for mid and low rectal cancers. Br J Surg 2003;90:867–871.

129. Leroy J, Jamali F, Forbes L, et al. Laparoscopic total mesorectal excision (TME) for rectal cancer surgery: long-term outcomes. Surg Endosc 2004;18:281–289.

130. Anthuber M, Fuerst A, Elser F, et al. Outcome of laparoscopic surgery for rectal cancer in 101 patients. Dis Colon Rectum 2003;46:1047–1053.

131. Berends FJ, Kazemier G, Bonjer HJ, Lange JF. Subcutaneous metastases after laparoscopic colectomy. Lancet 1994;344:58.

132. Johnstone PAS, Rohde DC, Swartz SE, Fetter JE, Wexner SD. Port site recurrences after laparoscopic and thoracoscopic procedures in malignancy. J Clin Oncol 1996;14:1950–1956.

133. Bouvy ND, Marquet RL, Jeekel H, et al. Impact of gas(less) laparoscopy and laparotomy on peritoneal tumor growth and abdominal wall metastases. Ann Surg 1996;224:694–700.

134. Watson DI, Mathew G, Ellis T, et al. Gasless laparoscopy may reduce the risk of port-site metastases following laparoscopic tumor surgery. Arch Surg 1997;132:166–168.

135. Gutt CN, Riemer V, Kim ZG, et al. Impact of laparoscopic colonic resection on tumour growth and spread in an experimental model. Br J Surg 1999;86:1180–1184.

136. Iwanaka T, Arya G, Ziegler MM. Mechanism and prevention of port-site tumor recurrence after laparoscopy in a murine model. J Pediatr Surg 1998;33:457–461.

137. Wittich P, Steyerberg EW, Simons SH, et al. Intraperitoneal tumor growth is influenced by pressure of carbon dioxide pneumoperitoneum. Surg Endosc 2000;14:817–819.

138. Jacobi CA, Sterzel A, Braumann C, et al. The impact of conventional and laparoscopic colon resection (CO2 or helium) on intraperitoneal adhesion formation in a rat peritonitis model. Surg Endosc 2001;15:380–386.

139. Neuhaus SJ, Ellis T, Rofe AM, et al. Tumor implantation following laparoscopy using different insufflation gases. Surg Endosc 1998;12:1300–1302.

140. Jacobi CA, Sterzel A, Braumann C, et al. Influence of different gases and intraperitoneal instillation of antiadherent or cytotoxic agents on peritoneal tumor cell growth and implantation with laparoscopic surgery in a rat model. Surg Endosc 1999; 13:1021–1025.

141. Bouvy ND, Giuffrida MC, Tseng LN, et al. Effects of carbon dioxide pneumoperitoneum, air pneumoperitoneum, and gasless laparoscopy on body weight and tumor growth. Arch Surg 1998;133:652–656.

142. Wu JS, Guo LW, Ruiz MB, et al. Excision of trocar sites reduces tumor implantation in an animal model. Dis Colon Rectum 1998;41:1107–1111.

143. Watson DI, Ellis T, Leeder PC, et al. Excision of laparoscopic port sites increases the likelihood of wound metastases in an experimental model. Surg Endosc 2003;17:83–85.

144. Wittich P, Marquet RL, Kazemier G, et al. Port-site metastases after CO(2) laparoscopy: is aerosolization of tumor cells a pivotal factor? Surg Endosc 2000;14:189–192.

145. Whelan RL, Sellers GJ, Allendorf JD, et al. Trocar site recurrence is unlikely to result from aerosolization of tumor cells. Dis Colon Rectum 1996;39:S7–S13.

146. Veldkamp R, Gholghesaei M, Bonjer HJ, et al. Laparoscopic resection of colon cancer. Consensus of the European Association of Endoscopic Surgery. Surg Endosc 2004;18: 1163–1185.

147. Tseng LN, Berends FJ, Wittich P, et al. Port-site metastases: impact of local tissue trauma and gas leakage. Surg Endosc 1998;12:1377–1380.

148. Neuhaus SJ, Watson DI, Ellis T, et al. Influence of cytotoxic agents on intraperitoneal tumor implantation after laparoscopy. Dis Colon Rectum 1999;42:10–15.

149. Lee SW, Gleason NR, Bessler M, et al. Peritoneal irrigation with povidone-iodine solution after laparoscopic-assisted splenectomy significantly decreases port-tumor recurrence in a murine model. Dis Colon Rectum 1999;42:319–326.

150. Neuhaus SJ, Ellis T, Jamieson GG, et al. Experimental study of the effect of intraperitoneal heparin on tumour implantation following laparoscopy. Br J Surg 1999;86:400–404.

151. Braumann C, Ordemann J, Wildbrett P, et al. Influence of intraperitoneal and systemic application of taurolidine and taurolidine/heparin during laparoscopy on intraperitoneal and subcutaneous tumour growth in rats. Clin J Exp Metastasis 2001;8:547–552.

152. Jacobi CA, Peter FJ, Wenger FA, et al. New therapeutic strategies to avoid intra- and extraperitoneal metastases during laparoscopy: results of a tumor model in the rat. Dig Surg 1999;16:393–399.

153. Eshraghi N, Swanstrom LL, Bax T, et al. Topical treatments of laparoscopic port sites can decrease the incidence of incision metastasis. Surg Endosc 1999;13:1121–1124.

154. Fleshman JW, Nelson H, Peters WR, et al. Early results of laparoscopic surgery for colorectal cancer: retrospective analysis of 372 patients treated by Clinical Outcomes of Surgical Therapy (COST) Study Group. Dis Colon Rectum 1996;39:S53–S58.

155. Reilly WT, Nelson H, Schroeder G, et al. Wound recurrence following conventional treatment of colorectal cancer: a rare but perhaps underestimated problem. Dis Colon Rectum 1996; 39:200–207.

156. Ou H. Laparoscopic-assisted mini laparotomy with colectomy. Dis Colon Rectum 1995;38:324–326.

157. Mooney MJ, Elliott PL, Galapon DB, et al. Hand-assisted laparoscopic sigmoidectomy for diverticulitis. Dis Colon Rectum 1998;41:630–635.

158. Southern Surgeons' Club Study Group. Handoscopic surgery: a prospective multicenter trial of minimally invasive technique for complex abdominal surgery. Arch Surg 1999;134:477–486.

159. HALS Study Group. Hand-assisted laparoscopic surgery vs standard laparoscopic surgery for colorectal disease: a prospective randomized trial. Surg Endosc 2000;14:896–901.

160. Litwin D, Darzi A, Jakimowicz J, et al. Hand-assisted laparoscopic surgery (HALS) with the HandPort system: initial experience with 68 patients. Ann Surg 2000;231:715–723.

161. Rivadeneira DE, Marcello PW, Roberts PL, et al. Benefits of hand-assisted laparoscopic restorative proctocolectomy: a comparative study. Dis Colon Rectum 2004;47:1371–1376.

162. Targarona EM, Gracia E, Garriga J, et al. Prospective randomized trial comparing conventional laparoscopic colectomy with hand-assisted laparoscopic colectomy. Surg Endosc 2002;16: 234–239.

163. Cobb WS, Lokey JS, Schwab DP, et al. Hand-assisted laparoscopic colectomy: a single-institution experience. Am Surg 2003;69:578–580.

164. Nakajima K, Lee SW, Cocilovo C, et al. Hand assisted laparoscopic colorectal surgery using Gelport: initial experience with a new hand access device. Surg Endosc 2004;18:102–105.

165. Kang JC, Chung MH, Yeh CC, et al. Hand-assisted laparoscopic colectomy vs open colectomy: a prospective randomized study. Surg Endosc 2004;18:577–581.

166. Maartense S, Dunker MS, Slors JF, et al. Hand-assisted laparoscopic versus open proctocolectomy with ileal pouch anal anastomosis: a randomized trial. Ann Surg 2004;240:984–992.

167. Boushey R, Marcello PW, Rusin LC, et al. Laparoscopic total colectomy: how should we do it? Dis Colon Rectum 2005; 48:63

51
Pediatric: Hirschsprung's, Anorectal Malformations, and Other Conditions

Alberto Peña and Marc Sher

Hirschsprung's Disease

Hirschsprung's disease (congenital megacolon) is an anomaly characterized by functional partial colonic obstruction caused by the absence of ganglion cells. It occurs in approximately 1 in 5000 births. Boys are more frequently affected than girls and it is more common in Caucasians. A deletion in the long arm of chromosome 10 has been found.[1] The functional disturbances in this condition are attributed to the absence of ganglion cells from the Auerbach's myenteric plexus (located between the circular and longitudinal layers of smooth muscle of the intestine), the Henle's plexus (located in the submucosa), and the Meissner's plexus (in the superficial submucosa). The absence of these cells probably produces uncoordinated contractions of the affected colon. This is translated into a lack of relaxation of the colon that results in partial colonic obstruction.

The length of the aganglionic colonic segment varies. In the most common type, the aganglionic segment includes the rectum and most of the sigmoid colon. Nearly 80% of all patients have this type. In approximately 10% of the patients, the aganglionosis extends to the area of the splenic flexure or the upper descending colon. Total colonic aganglionosis occurs in another 8%–10% of the patients. In those cases, the absent ganglion cells sometimes extend to the distal terminal ileum. In the so-called "ultrashort" aganglionosis, the ganglion cells supposedly are lacking only a few centimeters above the pectinate line of the rectum. This is a rather controversial condition. Very rarely, one can see patients who have universal aganglionosis, meaning that the ganglion cells are absent in the entire gastrointestinal tract, which is a lethal condition.

The clinical manifestations are those of a partial colonic obstruction. In addition, these patients have a poorly characterized immunologic mucosal defect that may explain why they suffer from an inflammatory process called enterocolitis, which is the main cause of death. In addition, fecal stasis seems to promote the proliferation of abnormal colonic flora (*Clostridium difficile*) as well as production of endotoxins that contribute to the aggravation of the clinical condition.

Usually the patient becomes symptomatic during the first 24–48 hours of life. Delayed passage of meconium (more than 24 hours), abdominal distention, and vomiting are the most common symptoms. A rectal examination may produce explosive passage of liquid bowel movements and gas, which dramatically improves the baby's condition. This clinical improvement only lasts for a few hours, after which the symptoms recur. If the colon is not decompressed, the infant usually suffers from sepsis, hypovolemia, and endotoxic shock. Cecal perforation may occur. About 25%–30% of these babies die when unrecognized or not treated.[2] Patients that do survive unrecognized and without treatment, ultimately develop the classic clinical picture initially described for this condition. They have severe constipation, a huge megacolon, and an enormously distended abdomen. This clinical situation is extremely rare nowadays in developed countries. Occasionally, these patients are misdiagnosed as having idiopathic chronic constipation. In the latter condition, the patients are not seriously ill, and it is very common for them to have overflow pseudoincontinence (encopresis). A rectal examination discloses a rectum full of fecal matter. On the contrary, patients with Hirschsprung's disease usually have malnutrition, lack of normal development, an empty aganglionic narrow rectum, and they do not have soiling.

The presence of the symptoms described in a newborn must alert the clinician to the diagnosis of Hirschsprung's disease. An abdominal film shows massive dilatation of small bowel and colon. It is almost impossible to differentiate colon from the small bowel, in a plain abdominal film during the newborn period. A contrast enema is used in most institutions to clarify the diagnosis. The catheter should be introduced only a few centimeters into the rectum in order to be able to visualize the nondilated aganglionic segment of the rectosigmoid, followed by a transitional zone and then a proximal dilatation. These typical changes are often not obvious during the neonatal period. The older the patient, the more obvious the size difference between normal and aganglionic segment. In patients with total colonic aganglionosis, the entire colon is not distended; the dilatation affects the small bowel only.

A manometric study may show an absent rectoanal inhibitory reflex. However, this study is not considered reliable for this diagnosis early in life but more helpful in the adolescent or adult with unrecognized short segment disease.

The definitive diagnosis is based on both the histologic absence of ganglion cells, and the presence of hypertrophic nerves in a rectal biopsy. These can be taken as full-thickness rectal biopsies under direct vision. More recently, a suction biopsy has gained wide acceptance. The specimen, however, must include mucosa and submucosa. An important diagnostic alternative is the determination of acetylcholinesterase activity in the mucosa and submucosa.[3]

Medical Management

Colonic decompression and irrigation with saline solution is the most valuable tool for the emergency management of newborn babies. This maneuver may dramatically improve a very ill neonate. Irrigations should not be confused with enemas. An enema is a procedure in which an amount of fluid is instilled into the colon. It is expected that this fluid will be spontaneously expelled. Patients with Hirschsprung's disease are, by definition, incapable of expelling this fluid and, therefore, enemas are contraindicated. A colonic irrigation, however, promotes the expelling of the rectocolonic contents through the lumen of a large rubber tube, which is cleared with small amounts of saline solution. Rectocolonic irrigations may save the baby's life, but are not the ideal long-term form of treatment. Once the histologic diagnosis has been established, the baby must remain with nothing by mouth, and the irrigations must continue in preparation for the surgical treatment.

Surgical Treatment

The basis of the surgical treatment consists of the resection of the aganglionic segment and pullthrough of a normoganglionic segment to be anastomosed to the rectum, immediately above the pectinate line. This should guarantee the preservation of bowel control. There are several ways to achieve these basic goals. The surgical treatment has evolved significantly since 1948 when the first surgical technique was described.[4]

Originally, these patients were subjected to a staged treatment. The first stage consisted of the opening of a diverting colostomy. The second stage included the resection of the aganglionic segment and pullthrough of the normoganglionic bowel, and the third stage was the colostomy closure. Subsequently, surgeons adopted a two-stage modality that included the opening of the colostomy during the newborn period. The second stage consisted of the pullthrough, leaving the patient without a colostomy.

More recently, the treatment most often used consists of a neonatal primary procedure without a protective colostomy.[5,6] This approach is less invasive and avoids the morbidity of a

stoma and multiple surgeries. However, approaches may vary from country to country as with the surgeon's experience. In addition, a primary procedure, without a protective colostomy, requires the presence of an experienced clinical pathologist, familiar with the interpretation of frozen sections. Also, in the case of a very ill, low-birth-weight newborn, or a very sick baby, a colostomy is still the optimal way to protect the patient. In the presence of an experienced pathologist, the colostomy must be open in a normoganglionic portion of the colon. In the absence of an experienced pathologist, the surgeon must open the colostomy, proximal to the transition zone. If the transition zone is not evident, the colostomy should be done in the right transverse colon. In the event of a nondilated entire colon, the patient should receive an ileostomy.

The definitive procedure (resection of the aganglionic segment and pullthrough of the normal ganglionic colon) can be done in different ways. Swenson and Bill[4] described an operation consisting of an intraabdominal resection of the aganglionic segment including a part of the normoganglionic dilated colon, and pullthrough of a normoganglionic bowel, with a perineal anastomosis of the normoganglionic bowel to the rectum, above the pectinate line.

Duhamel[7] described an operation designed to avoid pelvic dissection and potential nerve damage. He proposed to preserve the aganglionic rectum, dividing the colon at the peritoneal reflection. The normoganglionic colon is then pulled through a presacral space, created by blunt dissection and anastomosed to the posterior rectal wall above the pectinate line.

Soave[8] designed an ingenious and appealing procedure consisting of an endorectal (submucosal) dissection of the aganglionic colon, leaving a seromuscular cuff. He carried this dissection down to the rectum above the pectinate line. The normally innervated colon is passed through the muscular cuff and anastomosed to the rectum. The purpose of this operation, again, was to avoid the perirectal dissection and its potential negative effects caused by denervation of pelvic organs.

The original Soave procedure was performed in two stages. During the first stage, the colon was pulled down, but was not anastomosed to the rectum; it was left protruding outside the rectum. In the second stage, a week later, the protruded bowel was resected and the anastomosis was performed. Subsequently, Boley[9] proposed a primary anastomosis.

The abdominal portion of all of these operations can be done laparoscopically. This has been advocated by a number of pediatric surgeons recently.[10–12] Georgeson and colleagues[10,11] described their technique of laparoscopically obtained seromuscular biopsies in 80 patients to successfully determine the transition point. They preserved the marginal artery establishing a colonic pedicle for anastomosis through four ports, laparoscopically.

In 1998, De la Torre-Mondragon and Ortega-Salgado[13] and subsequently Langer et al.[14] reported a novel, transanal approach for the management of this condition.

They demonstrated that the whole procedure can be done transanally provided that the patient does not have a long segment type of aganglionosis. A special retractor (LoneStar™; Lone Star Medical Products Inc., Houston, TX) is used to expose the dentate line as well as the rectal mucosa.

We recommend the use of multiple fine sutures taking the rectal mucosa 1 cm above the pectinate line. These allow the surgeon to exert a uniform traction on the rectal mucosa. Peripheral to this series of silk stitches, an incision is performed with cautery and a circumferential dissection of the rectum is performed applying uniform traction. The dissection can actually be performed submucosally or full thickness, depending on the experience of the surgeon. As the surgeon progresses in the dissection, full-thickness biopsies are taken to determine the place where the normoganglionic portion of the colon is reached. The peritoneal reflection is soon found. It is recommended to continue the dissection until one reaches an area 4 cm above the transition zone to be sure that normoganglionic bowel is pulled down. The normoganglionic bowel is transanally anastomosed to the anal canal, 1 cm above the pectinate line. Because the majority of patients have a transition zone in the sigmoid colon, it is possible to repair the entire defect using this technique, without a laparotomy or laparoscopy.[13,14] When the transition zone is located higher, the surgeon determines when he or she needs a laparoscopic-assisted procedure or a laparotomy. We specifically recommend resecting not only the aganglionic segment of the colon, but also the very dilated part of the colon because we have learned that a very dilated colon also has very poor peristalsis.

De la Torre-Mondragon and Ortega-Salgado[13] and Langer et al.[14] perform the rectal dissection submucosally, in a similar way to the reoperative ileoanal pouch repairs for pouch-vaginal fistulas in adults described by Fazio and Tjandra.[15]

Complications and postoperative sequelae can be divided into two categories: preventable and nonpreventable. Preventable complications should not occur because they are caused by technical errors. A feared preventable sequela is fecal incontinence. This is likely related to injury to the continence mechanism. All these procedures were originally designed to prevent this from happening, provided they are performed correctly. Dehiscence, retraction, stricture, abscess, and fistula are all considered preventable because they are usually caused by technical errors. During the pullthrough, the surgeon must be familiar with the manipulation of the blood supply and the arcades of the colon to guarantee a good blood supply in the pullthrough colon. The anastomosis should be done without tension.

A nonpreventable complication is enterocolitis. This is also unpredictable, and a rather mysterious condition. Despite receiving a technically adequate operation, patients may have this condition. The frequency of this condition varies[16] and its etiology is unknown. We believe that fecal stasis is the most important predisposing factor. Fecal stasis occurring in the colon in a normal individual produces constipation.

In patients with Hirschsprung's disease, stasis frequently results in proliferation of abnormal bacteria, ulcerations of the colon, absorption of endotoxins, shock, and sometimes perforation. These patients respond to colonic irrigations; occasionally they require a colostomy and a secondary pullthrough.

Constipation may also occur after these procedures. It is more common in patients in whom the aganglionic segment was resected, but a dilated portion of the colon was pulled down. This is a partially preventable condition. Most cases of constipation can be avoided by resecting not only the aganglionic segment but also the dilated portion of the colon.

Each one of the techniques described has its own advocates. The analysis of different series shows that the most important factor that affects the clinical results is the experience and familiarity of the surgeon with each one of those procedures. Some surgeons claim that the Swenson operation exposes the patient to nerve damage that may provoke urinary and sexual disturbances. The Duhamel procedure is frequently followed by severe problems of constipation and dilatation of the aganglionic piece of colon left in place. In the Soave operation, patients may experience fecal incontinence, as well as perianal fistulas and abscesses because of the presence of islets of mucosa left in place during the endorectal dissection.

Advocates of a transanal approach cite the decreased morbidity and enhanced recovery as a consequence of a procedure without the intraabdominal dissection.[17,18] In addition, this approach permits early postoperative feeding, shorter length to stay, faster recovery, and possibly less chance for postoperative adhesions. Langer[17,18] compared the standard open approach to transanal Soave versus selective laparoscopic visualization and reported a shorter hospitalization and significantly less overall cost to the healthcare system. There was a trend of lower complication rates, specifically less incidence of adhesive bowel obstruction. They recommended only selective laparoscopy for children with long segment disease.

Surgical Management of Total Colonic Aganglionosis

We believe that the ideal treatment for this very serious condition has not yet been found. The current treatment consists of resection of the entire aganglionic colon and pullthrough of the normal aganglionic terminal ileum to be anastomosed to the rectum. To avoid fluid losses and in an attempt to decrease the number of bowel movements per day, as well as to promote water absorption, Martin[19] proposed to leave a part of the rectosigmoid and descending aganglionic segment in place. The normoganglionic terminal ileum is anastomosed in a latero-lateral manner to this colon and finally connected to the posterior aspect of the rectum as in the Duhamel procedure. Kimura et al.[20] proposed the use of a right colon patch with the hope of creating a reservoir for water absorption. Another option is the ileoanal J-pouch anastomosis; however, risks associated with a pelvic dissection are obviously higher. All these approaches have proved to be rather simplistic. The stasis of stool in the small bowel produces bacterial proliferation and enterocolitis. Rather than absorbing water, very often the intestine secretes fluid into the lumen, producing a secretory diarrhea. Therefore we, as others, believe that a straight ileorectal anastomosis is the preferred option, acknowledging that all patients with this condition will have a poor quality of life.

Surgical Treatment of Ultrashort Hirschsprung's

The surgical treatment of the ultrashort-segment aganglionosis is as controversial as the existence of this condition. Normal individuals have an area of aganglionosis above the pectinate line. The length of this aganglionic area has not been accurately or scientifically determined. This is the reason why the diagnosis of ultrashort Hirschsprung is so controversial. Some surgeons propose an operation called myectomy, consisting of the resection of a strip of smooth muscle from the anal verge up to the area where ganglion cells are found. The results of this procedure, again, are highly controversial and there is no scientific basis to explain why this may improve the condition. More scientifically conducted studies are required to clarify this issue.

Most cases of Hirschsprung's disease are diagnosed early in life, but a few patients reach their late teens and some are in adulthood before a diagnosis is made. Hirschsprung's disease in adults must be distinguished from other causes of megacolon such as Chagas' disease, volvulus, colonic inertia, Ogilvie's syndrome, and other disorders of central nervous system. Typically, the disease in adults is of the ultrashort segment variety. An internal sphincterectomy may yield a satisfactory result as performed after a failed pullthrough procedure.

This operation involves removing a thin strip of the internal sphincter muscle in the posterior midline starting 1 cm above the dentate line. The strip should extend as far proximal as exposure allows, possibly up to 15 cm. Lynn describes a transanal approach, but we prefer a posterior sagittal approach to enable a high myectomy.[21,22] Anal manometry may aid in assessment of the adequacy of the myectomy, because the resting tone pressure should be less than 30 mm Hg.

Neuronal Intestinal Dysplasia

Neuronal intestinal dysplasia (NID) refers to a histologic condition that includes hypertrophy of ganglion cells, immature ganglia, hypoganglionosis, hyperplasia of the submucosal and myenteric plexus, giant ganglion cells, as well as hypoplasia or aplasia of the sympathetic innervations of the myenteric plexus. These histologic abnormalities have been described as occurring in a localized or disseminated manner.[23]

The histologic diagnosis of NID requires a high index of suspicion as well as the availability of special histologic techniques and expertise. Not all pathologists agree as to the existence of this condition.

NID has become popular because most surgeons expect to find histologic abnormalities in patients who have undergone a technically correct operation for Hirschsprung's disease and still have symptoms of enterocolitis or constipation. It was also expected that these histologic abnormalities would explain the pathophysiology of other colonic motility disorders.

Unfortunately, a precise correlation between histology and clinical manifestations is lacking. The histologic diagnostic criteria have not been standardized among different pathologists and different countries. In addition, the precise options for therapy have not been clearly established.[24]

Anorectal Malformations (Imperforate Anus)

Anorectal malformations represent a spectrum of defects characterized by the absence of an external anal orifice. The overwhelming majority of the patients have an abnormal communication between the rectum and the perineum (perineal fistula), the vestibule (vestibular fistula), or the vagina (vaginal fistula) in the female. In some female patients, rectum, vagina, and urethra are fused together forming a common channel (cloacal malformation) and open into a single external orifice. In the male, the communication is with the urethra (rectourethral fistula), or the bladder (rectobladder neck fistula). Only 5% of the entire spectrum of patients are born with no fistula. Anorectal malformations occur in about one in every 5000 newborns. Males seem to have this condition slightly more frequently than females. The most common type of defects seen in boys is a rectourethral fistula and the most common type in girls is vestibular fistula. Table 51-1 shows our proposed classification of anorectal malformations.

Associated Anomalies

Urogenital abnormalities occur in about 50% of all patients with anorectal malformations.[25] The higher and more complex the anorectal malformations, the higher the incidence of

TABLE 51-1. Current classification of anorectal malformations

Male
   Perineal fistula
   Rectourethral fistula
      Bulbar
      Prostatic
   Rectobladder neck fistula
   Imperforate anus without fistula
   Rectal atresia
Female
   Perineal fistula
   Vestibular fistula
   Imperforate anus without fistula
   Rectal atresia
   Cloaca
   Complex malformations

urologic associated defects. Urologic malformations are a common source of morbidity in these patients. About 90% of patients with a rectobladder neck fistula in males as well as in cases of cloacas with a common channel longer than 3 cm, have an associated urologic problem. Unilateral renal agenesis is the most common urologic anomaly encountered in children with these defects. Vesicoureteral reflux is the second most common abnormality. Other important abnormalities include cryptorchidism, hypospadias, renal ectopia, and hydronephrosis.

Sacral and spinal abnormalities are also very common in patients with anorectal malformations. The sacrum is frequently abnormal. The sacral abnormalities also represent a spectrum that varies from a completely absent sacrum to a completely normal one, including different degrees of hypodevelopment. There seems to be a direct relationship between the degree of sacral abnormality and the final functional prognosis. These patients also have hemivertebrae and as a consequence different degrees of scoliosis. The presence of hemivertebrae also seems to be related to a poorer functional prognosis.

Twenty-five percent of patients with anorectal malformations have a defect called tethered cord.[26] The majority of patients with tethered cord have a bad functional prognosis. In this condition, the cord is abnormally attached (tethered) to the spine. During the natural growth of the baby, it is believed that the spine grows faster than the cord, producing traction on the nerve fibers that may produce functional disturbances in the motion of the lower extremities and may contribute to sphincter problems.

Hemisacrum is sometimes associated with an anorectal malformation and there is always a mass located in the area of the sacral defect. An anorectal malformation with hemisacrum and a presacral mass is known as the Currarino triad. The most common sacral masses in these patients are a dermoid, teratoma, lipoma, anterior meningocele, or a combination of all these. These patients also have a poor functional prognosis.

Approximately 8% of all patients with anorectal malformations have esophageal atresia. These patients usually have a very high anorectal defect and other associated anomalies, especially urologic.

About 30% of patients with anorectal malformations also have some sort of cardiovascular congenital anomaly. Most frequently seen are patent ductus arteriosus, atrial septal defect, ventricular septal defect, tetralogy of Fallot, as well as other more complex malformations. Fortunately, only 10% of patients have a cardiovascular malformation with significant hemodynamic repercussions that requires surgical treatment.

The main concern in a patient with anorectal malformation is whether or not the patient will have bowel control, urinary control, and sexual function in the future. The higher the malformation, the worse the functional prognosis will be.

The higher the anorectal defect, the more likely the child will have fecal incontinence, but the lesser the chance of having constipation. Conversely, the lower the malformation the higher the incidence of constipation and the lower the incidence of fecal incontinence will be.

Description of Specific Defects

Males

Perineal Fistula

This is the simplest of all defects. The rectum opens anterior to the center of the external sphincter in the area known as the perineum. The rectal orifice is usually incompetent, meaning that it is too narrow to allow normal passage of stool. Sometimes, the end of the rectum lies immediately below a very thin layer of epithelium with an external opening located at the base of the scrotum or sometimes at the base of the penis. The meconium sometimes can be seen below that very thin layer of epithelium giving an impression of a black ribbon. The overwhelming majority of these patients have a normal sacrum, and less than 10% of them have associated defects. The final functional prognosis is excellent,[27] provided these patients receive adequate treatment. These patients can be operated on during the newborn period. The ideal operation consists of moving the orifice back to the center of the sphincter creating a normal-sized anus.

Rectourethral Fistula

In this group of malformations, the rectum connects to the urethra. In the most common subtype, the rectum opens into the lower part of the posterior urethra known as bulbar urethra and, therefore, the defect is called rectourethral bulbar fistula. The rectum passes through a funnel-like striated sphincter mechanism to reach the lowest part of the posterior urethra. Eighty-five percent of these patients achieve bowel control when treated properly.[27] Approximately 30% of them have other associated defects.[27]

In the second subtype, the rectum opens into the upper part of the posterior urethra (prostatic) and therefore it is called rectoprostatic fistula. Only 60% of these patients achieve bowel control later in life. Sixty percent of them have important associated defects.[27]

Most of these patients (rectourethral fistula) require a colostomy at birth and subsequently (usually 1 month later) they receive the final repair of the malformation. Lately, some of the patients with rectourethral bulbar fistula have been repaired primarily during the newborn period without a protective colostomy.

The perineum of patients with anorectal malformations have characteristic features that must be recognized by the clinician. The higher the malformation, the more tendency to have a flat perineum (flat bottom), meaning that the natural midline groove is absent and there is no distinguishable anal dimple. The lower the malformation, the more prominent the midline groove and the anal dimple. In patients with rectourethral bulbar fistula, there is a recognizable midline groove as well as an anal dimple and in patients with recto-prostatic fistula, there is conspicuous tendency for the perineum to be flat. Also, the anal dimple tends to be closer to the scrotum, the higher the malformation. One can also frequently see a bifid scrotum in cases of prostatic fistula.

Rectobladder Neck Fistula

This is the highest of all defects in male patients. The rectum is connected to the bladder neck. Ninety percent of these patients have important associated defects. The perineum is frequently flat. The rectum is located above the funnel-like sphincter mechanism (levator). These patients are the only ones that require a laparotomy or laparoscopy in addition to the posterior sagittal approach to be repaired. Only 15% of these patients achieve bowel control later in life.[27]

Imperforate Anus Without Fistula

This is a rather unusual anomaly that occurs in 5% of all children with anorectal malformations. Half of them also have Down's syndrome. More than 90% of all patients with Down's syndrome, who have an anorectal malformation, have this specific type of defect. Eighty percent of the babies with Down's syndrome and this malformation will eventually have bowel control when they receive an adequate operation. Approximately 90% of patients with this defect and without Down's syndrome also have bowel control.[28] Patients with this malformation usually have a good sphincter mechanism and a good sacrum.

Rectal Atresia

This malformation occurs in only 1% of all cases. It consists of a complete or partial interruption of the rectal lumen located between the anal canal and the rectum. The external appearance of the perineum is normal. The malformation is usually discovered when a nurse tries to take the rectal temperature in a baby. The sacrum is normal as well as the sphincter mechanism. One hundred percent of these patients will have bowel control after a correctly performed operation.[25]

Female Defects

Perineal Fistula

In these female babies, the rectum opens in what is called the perineal body between the normal location of the anus and the female genitalia. All that was described about this defect in males is true for females. These patients can be repaired at birth without a colostomy. The prognosis is excellent.[27]

Vestibular Fistula

This is by far the most common defect seen in female patients. The rectum opens in the vestibule of the female

genitalia just outside the hymen. Rectum and vagina share a very thin common wall. About 30% of these babies have associated defects. Ninety-three percent of these babies will have bowel control when properly treated.[27] The sacrum is usually normal.

Vestibular fistula is frequently misdiagnosed as a recto-vaginal fistula.[29] Vaginal fistula is an extremely unusual defect. It represents less than 1% of all the female defects. In those unusual cases of vaginal fistula, the rectum opens into the posterior vaginal wall deeper to the hymen.

Most of the vestibular fistula cases are successfully operated on at birth without a colostomy. Unfortunately, many of those patients have dehiscence and retraction when the surgical technique used is not adequate. A secondary operation in these cases does not render the same good result as in cases of a well-done primary procedure.

Imperforate Anus Without Fistula

It is uncommon to see this type of defect in females. All that was mentioned about this defect in males is true about this defect in females.

Rectal Atresia

This condition does not differ from the same defect in males.

Cloaca

A cloaca is defined as a malformation in which the rectum, vagina, and urinary tract are fused together forming a common channel. This single channel opens where the normal urethra is located in females. Externally, these babies have rather small-looking genitalia. Separation of the small labia allows the observer to see a single orifice, which confirms the clinical diagnosis of a cloaca. Cloaca represents another spectrum of defects. The length of the common channel varies from 1–7 or even 10 cm. The length of the common channel is directly related to the final functional prognosis for bowel and urinary control. The turning point seems to be around 3 cm. Patients with a common channel shorter than 3 cm can be repaired posterior sagittally without opening the abdomen and the prognosis for bowel and urinary control is good. However, cloacas with a common channel longer than 3 cm represent a serious technical challenge. The operation frequently requires not only a posterior sagittal approach but also a laparotomy. The repair of those complex defects requires experience and familiarization with pediatric urology. The final functional prognosis is not very good in cases with a long common channel.[30]

Associated defects occur in about 90% of all patients with a common channel longer than 3 cm.

About 40% of patients with cloaca have hydrocolpos (a very dilated vagina full of fluid). The dilated vagina compresses the trigone and may produce ureterovesical obstruction, megaureters, and hydronephrosis. Approximately 40%

of the patients with cloaca also have different degrees of septation of the vagina and the uterus. This has important future implications, impacting menstrual flow,[31] as well as obstetric potential.

Initial Management

Male Babies

Perineal inspection and urinalysis allows determingtion of the likely type of malformation in about 90% of the cases.

The presence of a perineal orifice, by definition makes the diagnosis of a perineal fistula. This is also true when the baby has an external defect called "bucket-handle" malformation that is a skin bridge in the midline in the area of the anal dimple. The presence of a good midline groove and an anal dimple, as well as meconium in the urine, means that the patient has a rectourethral fistula. A flat bottom and bifid scrotum are signs of a very high malformation.

Diagnostic studies should be done after 24 hours of life, but not later than 36 hours. The reason for this is that it is necessary to wait until the most distal part of the rectum is distended in order for it to be seen by any of the diagnostic modalities [magnetic resonance imaging (MRI), ultrasound, CAT scan, or simple X-ray films]. Before 24 hours, the most distal part of the rectum is usually collapsed and it is difficult to see by these diagnostic modalities. Also, in order for meconium to be forced through a tiny distal fistula, it is necessary to wait until the intraluminal pressure is high enough to overcome the tone of the striated muscle that surrounds the distal rectum, which usually happens after 24 hours. During the first 24 hours, the clinician must try to answer two very important questions: Does the baby have an associated defect that threatens his/her life? Does the baby need a primary repair or a colostomy?

These questions should be answered in this order. The baby should be examined to rule out the presence of cardiovascular defects. The patient will remain with nothing by mouth, and insertion of a nasogastric tube is recommended to avoid vomiting and potential risk of aspiration. An ultrasound of the abdomen is indicated to rule out the presence of hydronephrosis. An ultrasound of the spine is also useful to rule out the presence of tethered cord. An X-ray film of the lumbar spine and the sacrum will rule out the presence of hemivertebrae and sacral abnormalities. A very abnormal sacrum is usually associated with a very high defect. If after 24 hours the surgeon is still not sure as to the type of defect that the baby has, a cross-table lateral film with the baby in prone position and the pelvis elevated should be performed. This will show the location of gas inside a distended rectum. If the rectum is visualized below the coccyx and the surgeons have experience with the neonatal repair of this malformation, the patient can be approached primarily. However, if the rectum is located higher than the coccyx, or the surgeons have no experience with these neonatal operations, it is better

to perform a diverting colostomy and to postpone the main repair for a later date.

Females

It is also true in females that simple inspection of the perineum will allow the surgeon to make a correct diagnosis during the neonatal period in most cases.

The presence of an anal opening in the perineum makes the diagnosis of perineal fistula.

Sometimes it is difficult to see the opening of the rectum in the vestibule because the female genitalia are swollen at birth because of the effect of the maternal hormones. The presence of a fistula in the vestibule establishes that diagnosis. To make the diagnosis of a rectovaginal fistula (extremely unusual defect) one would have to see meconium coming from inside the vagina, deeper than the hymen. The presence of a single perineal orifice makes the diagnosis of a cloaca.

If none of these signs are present after 24 hours, the baby should have a cross-table lateral film in prone position. Most likely the baby has an imperforated anus with no fistula (which represents 5% of all cases).

During the first 24 hours of life, the baby should be subjected to the same tests described for the male patient. If the baby has a cloaca, an ultrasound of the abdomen should be performed not only in the upper abdomen to rule out hydronephrosis, but also in the lower abdomen to rule out the presence of hydrocolpos. Most babies with a cloaca need a diverting colostomy. These babies should not be taken to the operating room unless the surgeon has already ruled out the presence of hydrocolpos. The hydrocolpos must be drained at birth, particularly when the baby has hydronephrosis. Before trying other procedures for the treatment of the hydronephrosis and megaureter, the hydrocolpos must be drained, which usually will take care of these problems.

Colostomy

Colostomies in babies with anorectal malformation should be totally diverting. Loop colostomies are contraindicated; they may allow the passing of stool from the proximal into the distal colon, producing direct fecal contamination of the urinary tract. The ideal colostomy should be created in the descending colon, with separated stomas. Both stomas should be separated enough as to allow the placement of a stoma bag over the proximal stoma. Distal to the mucus fistula, the baby should have enough length of colon to allow a comfortable pullthrough at the time of the main repair.

In cases of cloaca, the surgeon must also drain the hydrocolpos through the abdomen. When the vagina is so distended that it reaches the upper abdomen, it can be drained in the form of a vaginotomy, suturing directly the vaginal wall to the abdominal wall. When the vagina is not that large, it can be drained with a tube that is exteriorized through a separate hole in the abdominal wall.

Two weeks after the colostomy, a high-pressure distal colostogram should be performed.[32] This consists of injection of hydrosoluble contrast material through the distal limb of the colostomy to delineate the anatomy of the distal colon and to establish an accurate anatomic diagnosis. This is, by far, the most important diagnostic study in anorectal malformations. Trying to repair these malformations without a good distal colostogram exposes the babies to serious injuries of the urinary tract, particularly in males.[33]

Main Repair

Males

Perineal fistulas can be repaired performing a minimal posterior sagittal anoplasty. The baby is placed in prone position with the pelvis elevated. Multiple stitches are placed at the mucocutaneous junction of the fistula orifice. An incision dividing the sphincter mechanism, posterior to the anal orifice, is performed, and the rectum is carefully dissected to be moved back and relocated within the limits of the sphincter. During the dissection of the anterior rectal wall, special care must be taken to avoid injury to the posterior urethra, which is the most common and feared complication in these operations. The babies must have a Foley catheter in the urethra during this operation. If the surgeon does not have enough experience and the baby has a very narrow fistula orifice, a simple procedure called cutback can be done, consisting of a posterior cut of the fistula to make the orifice wider. Another alternative in a very sick baby or when the surgeon does not have enough experience is simply to subject the patient to dilatations of the fistula.

In cases of rectourethral fistulas, the patients are subjected to a posterior sagittal anorectoplasty. The baby is placed in prone position with the pelvis elevated and with a Foley catheter in place. A posterior sagittal incision is performed between both buttocks running from the middle portion of the sacrum to the base of the scrotum. The entire sphincter mechanism is divided exactly in the midline using an electrical stimulator to be sure to leave an equal amount of sphincter muscle on both sides of the midline.

The posterior rectal wall is identified and is opened in the midline. The fistula is identified and multiple fine silk stitches are placed taking the rectal mucosa immediately above the fistula in order to exert uniform traction to facilitate the dissection and separation of the rectum from the urethra. A submucosal plane is established in the anterior rectal wall to avoid damage to the urinary tract. About 1 cm above the fistula site, the dissection continues full thickness until the rectum is completely separated from the urinary tract. After this, a circumferential dissection with division of extrinsic vessels of the rectum is performed until enough length has been gained to bring the rectum down to the perineum and to anastomose it without tension to the skin in the area of the anal sphincter. Occasionally, we find that the rectum is very dilated

and cannot be accommodated within the available space of the sphincter mechanism. Under those circumstances, it is recommended to taper the posterior rectal wall as much as necessary so as to be able to accommodate the rectum within the limits of the sphincter. It must be the posterior rectal wall that is tapered, rather than the anterior wall so that a suture line is not opposed to the urethral fistula that was closed. The limits of the sphincter are electrically determined. The only difference in the surgical treatment between the rectourethral bulbar fistula and the retroprostatic fistula is that the latter requires a more significant dissection to bring the rectum down.

Rectobladder Neck Fistula

Fortunately, this malformation occurs in only 10% of male patients.[27] This is the only defect that requires a laparotomy or laparoscopic assistance in addition to the posterior sagittal operation.[34] This is because the rectum is located too high to be reached from below. The posterior sagittal incision is only performed to create the path through which the rectum should be pulled down. A midline laparotomy or laparoscopy is performed. The rectum is dissected above the peritoneal reflexion. The surgeon must create a plane of dissection as close as possible to the bowel wall, but without injuring the rectal wall. One must keep in mind that the ureters and vas deferens run in the same direction toward the bladder neck and, therefore, one must keep those structures under vision during the dissection of the rectum. The bladder neck is located about 2 cm below the peritoneal reflexion and, therefore, it is very easy to find the end of the rectum and to divide and suture the fistula site. The rectum then must be mobilized to be pulled down through the tract that has been previously established through the posterior sagittal incision.

Imperforate Anus Without Fistula

In cases of imperforate anus without fistula, the operation is not necessarily easier than in patients with a fistula because the rectum is still intimately attached to the posterior urethra. These patients are approached posterior sagittally, the posterior rectal wall is opened in the midline, and multiple stitches are placed in the edge of the rectal wall to exert uniform traction and to facilitate the separation of the rectum from the urinary tract.

Special care must be taken during the dissection of the anterior wall to separate it from the urinary tract. These patients more often require a rectal tapering, because usually they have a more dilated rectum.

Rectal Atresia

These patients also require a posterior sagittal approach. The entire sphincter mechanism is divided posterior sagittally. Both rectum and anal canal are opened posteriorly. The dilated proximal rectum is anastomosed to the anal canal and then the sphincter mechanism is meticulously reconstructed in the midline. These patients have an excellent prognosis.

Female defects

Perineal Fistula

The repair of this malformation is the same that was described for male patients, except that the rectum is usually separated from the vagina so there is no risk of vaginal injury.

Vestibular Fistula

The complexity of this malformation should not be underestimated. The patient is placed in prone position with the pelvis elevated. Multiple fine silk stitches are placed at the rectal vestibular orifice. A posterior sagittal incision is performed, dividing the sphincter mechanism to find the posterior rectal wall, which is easy to recognize. The main technical challenge in the repair of this defect is represented by the common wall that exists between the rectum and vagina. There is no plane of separation between these two structures. One must make two walls out of one. This is achieved by a meticulous dissection applying uniform traction with multiple silk stitches into the rectal lumen. The dissection must continue until the rectum has been completely separated from the vagina. Usually the rectum of these patients requires very little mobilization because it is located significantly low. The limits of the sphincter are electrically determined, the perineal body is reconstructed, and the rectum is placed within the limits of the sphincter.

Rectovaginal Fistula

This is an extremely unusual defect.[29] These malformations can be repaired posterior sagittally. The repair is the same as described for vestibular fistula, except that these patients require much more mobilization of the rectum in order to move it down and relocate it in the center of the sphincter.

Cloaca

Cloaca repair represents a significant technical challenge, particularly in patients with a long common channel.[30]

Repair of Cloaca with a Common Channel Shorter Than 3 cm. These patients are approached posterior sagittally. The entire sphincter mechanism is divided in the midline and the posterior sagittal incision is extended down to the single perineal opening. The common channel is also opened in the midline to expose the anatomy of the defect. The entire defect can be repaired through this incision without opening the abdomen. Once the anatomy has been exposed, the first step is to separate the rectum from the vagina, which is performed in the same manner as was described for a rectovestibular fistula. Once the rectum is separated, it should be mobilized to gain length and to be placed in a normal location. The next step consists of mobilizing both vagina and urethra together,

following a specific technical maneuver called "total urogenital mobilization."[35] Multiple 6-0 silk stitches are placed in the edge of the open common channel as well as the edges of the vagina. These stitches allow the surgeon to exert uniform traction on the entire urogenital structure. The urogenital channel is divided full thickness approximately 5 mm proximal to the clitoris, creating a plane of dissection that is very easy to find, between the common channel and the posterior aspect of the pubis. In a matter of a few minutes, one can reach the upper portion of the pubis. Conspicuous fascial attachments exist between the vagina, the genitourinary structures, and the upper part of the pubis. These fascial attachments are avascular and are known as suspensory ligaments of the vagina and urethra. These are divided and the retropubic fat is identified. By dividing these suspensory ligaments, one can gain approximately 2 cm of mobilization of the urogenital structures. Some extra dissection of the lateral walls of the vagina as well as its dorsal wall gains another centimeter, and by doing that, one can repair the urethra and the vagina in a very satisfactory manner. More than 50% of the patients with cloacas have a common channel shorter than 3 cm and, therefore, it is possible to repair most of these defects with this reproducible technique. The blood supply after this mobilization is excellent. Urethra and vagina are then sutured to the labia in their new position.

The limits of the sphincter are electrically determined and marked with temporary silk stitches. The perineal body is reconstructed with long-term absorbable sutures, the rectum is placed within the limits of the sphincter, and the anoplasty is performed. The total urogenital mobilization does not change the final functional prognosis. Patients with a common channel of less than 3 cm and a good sacrum have more than an 80% chance of having bowel control and an 80% chance of having urinary control without bladder intermittent catheterization.[28] After the urethra and vagina have been repaired, the urethral meatus is now located 5 mm deeper to the clitoris in a position that makes it perfectly visible which is important if the baby needs catheterization. Twenty percent of these babies will require intermittent catheterization postoperatively in order to empty the bladder.

Surgical Repair of Patients with Cloaca with a Common Channel Longer Than 3 cm. We specifically recommend these patients to be referred to specialized centers dedicated to the treatment of complex malformations. The repair of these defects usually requires not only a posterior sagittal approach, but also a laparotomy and a series of decision-making steps that require experience and special training in urology. The first part of the operation consists of performing a total body preparation so that the patient can be approached through the perineum (posterior sagittally) and through a laparotomy. The posterior sagittal approach and total urogenital mobilization is attempted because occasionally one can achieve a total repair in patients with a common channel up to 4 cm. If this maneuver is not enough to make the vagina comfortably reach the skin of the perineum, one has to go into the abdomen and continue the dissection of the vagina as well as its separation from the urinary tract. This is a difficult and tedious maneuver. The bladder must be opened and the ureters must be catheterized because they run through the common wall that separates the bladder and the vagina. Once the vagina has been entirely separated from the urinary tract, then the surgeon evaluates whether or not the vagina reaches the perineum. If that is not possible, then he or she has to make an important decision as to the best way to repair the malformation. In very specific cases, with bilateral hydrocolpos, the surgeon can perform a maneuver called "vaginal switch," consisting of resecting one of the hemiuteri, resecting the vaginal septum, tubularizing both hemivaginas to create a single one and switching down what used to be the dome of one hemivagina to the perineum, taking advantage of the fact that the distance between both hemiuteri is longer than the vertical length of both hemivaginas. This maneuver is only feasible if the patient has two large hydrocolpos.

If this maneuver (vaginal switch) is not feasible, then the surgeon must replace the vagina. The alternatives are first to replace it with rectum. The distal part of the rectum can be used to replace the vagina, which can be done in two different manners. If the patient has enough length of rectum, one can use the most distal part (preserving its blood supply), to be separated from the fecal stream, mobilized forward, and replacing the distal part of the vagina.

In other cases, if the rectum is very dilated, one can divide it longitudinally. The anterior portion is tubularized and moved forward to form the neovagina preserving the necessary vessels from the inferior mesenteric branches. The posterior aspect will serve as a rectum. The blood supply of the posterior aspect will be provided intramurally from the branches of the inferior mesenteric vessels. The rectum has an excellent intramural blood supply.

If these maneuvers are not feasible, the next choice could be sigmoid colon. If the colostomy interferes with these maneuvers, then one can use the small bowel.

In cases of extremely high malformations, one may find two little hemivaginas attached to the bladder neck. The rectum also may open in the bladder neck. The separation of these structures is performed through the abdomen. Once the separation has been performed, one may notice that there is no bladder neck left. Under those circumstances, the surgeon must have enough experience to decide whether or not the bladder neck can be reconstructed or whether it is better to permanently close the whole distal part of the bladder and open a vesicostomy. Those patients will require a continent diversion later in life. Because these patients have the highest incidence of vesicoureteral reflux, this operation through the abdomen represents a good opportunity to reimplant the ureters.

Patients with a common channel shorter than 3 cm are left with a Foley catheter, which stays in place for 2 or 3 weeks. Patients with a common channel longer than 3 cm require a suprapubic cystostomy or vesicostomy at the end of the operation. One month after surgery, through the suprapubic tube, a cystogram is performed, the tube is clamped, and the patient is observed to see if she is capable of emptying her bladder spontaneously or if she requires intermittent catheterization.

The most common sequela from the urinary point of view in babies with cloaca is the incapacity to empty the bladder. These babies do not have the type of neurogenic bladder that is seen in patients with spina bifida and myelomeningocele. These patients rather have a floppy large bladder that does not empty. Most of the cloaca patients have a competent bladder neck. The combination of a competent bladder neck with a floppy hypotonic bladder makes these patients ideal candidates for intermittent catheterization, which allows them to remain completely dry.

When the bladder neck was not present at birth or was destroyed during surgery, these patients will need a continent diversion later in life. This operation usually will consist of a bladder augmentation and creation of a conduit with a one-way valve mechanism that allows the patient to be catheterized intermittently in order to empty the bladder without urine leakage.

Results of Treatment of Anorectal Malformations

About 75% of all patients with anorectal malformations (when subjected to a good operation), have bowel control.[27] The bowel control is not perfect. This becomes evident when the patients have severe constipation, which may produce overflow pseudoincontinence, and soiling. Also, a severe episode of diarrhea may show that the bowel control is not normal. Twenty-five percent of all patients have fecal incontinence and require some form of medical management.

Because anorectal malformations cover a wide spectrum of defects, the clinical and functional results vary depending on the specific type of malformation. Patients with a cloaca with a common channel longer than 3 cm usually have fecal incontinence and require intermittent catheterization to empty the bladder. Patients with cloaca with a common channel shorter than 3 cm and a normal sacrum have bowel control 80% of the time and only 20% of them require intermittent catheterization to empty the bladder and remain completely dry. Ninety-four percent of all patients with rectovestibular fistulas have bowel control. Babies with perineal fistulas have bowel control 100% of the time. Rectobladder neck fistula patients only have bowel control 20% of the time, rectoprostatic fistula 60%, and rectourethral bulbar fistula 85%.[27] Patients with imperforate anus with no fistula will have bowel control between 80% and 90% depending on whether or not they have Down's syndrome.[29]

Constipation is a problem in most patients with anorectal malformations in whom the rectum was preserved during the main repair of the defect. Constipation should not be underestimated as a problem. When not treated properly, the patients develop megacolon and chronic fecal impaction, which may end up producing overflow pseudoincontinence.

Medical Management of Fecal Incontinence

For the group of patients who have fecal incontinence (25% of cases), there is a bowel management program that aims to keep those patients completely clean of stool and to make them socially accepted. The basis of this treatment is to teach the family or the patient to clean the colon every day with an enema or colonic irrigation. Because most patients have constipation, the cleaning of the colon with an enema will prevent the patient from passing stool for 24–48 hours.[36]

Occasionally, however, we find patients that had a different type of repair and lost the rectosigmoid during the main repair or have intractable diarrhea or malabsorption. In those cases, the bowel management is technically more demanding because it includes not only cleaning the colon with an enema, but also the use of a constipating diet or medications to decrease the colonic motility in order to keep the patient free of stool for more than 24 hours.

The bowel management program is implemented over a period of 1 week by trial and error. Every patient needs a different kind of enema to clean the colon. The cleaning of the colon is monitored, taking X-ray films of the abdomen every day, and readjusting the volume and concentration of the enema by trial and error. The goal is to find the enema that is well tolerated by the patient, is easy to administer, and keeps the patient completely clean. When the patient complains about the rectal enema and feels embarrassed about their parents giving the enema, an operation called the Malone procedure (continent appendicostomy) is an option.[37,38] This consists of creating a connection between the tip of the cecal appendix and the umbilicus. The cecum is plicated around the appendix, to create a one-way valve that allows the introduction of a catheter through the umbilicus into the colon and prevents the colon from passing stool through the orifice. The patient is able to sit on the toilet, pass a little feeding tube through the umbilicus, administer the enema himself/herself, evacuate the colon, and remain clean the following 24 or 48 hours. This allows the patient to become independent.

A significant number of patients do not have an appendix. One can be created with a vascularized flap of the colon (continent neoappendicostomy). Then again, the colon is plicated around the new appendix to make it continent.[38]

Relevant Aspects for Adult Colorectal Surgery

Many adolescent and adult patients may still have fecal incontinence despite successful repair in infancy. Work-up of these patients should include a detailed history and physical, i.e., type of defect the patient was born with, bowel movement and voiding pattern, type of perineum, location of rectal opening,

presence of an anal dimple, and strength of sphincter contraction. A water-soluble enema or defecography, voiding cystourethrogram, sacral films, MRI with a rectal coil to assess the location of the rectum are essential. Manometry, anal ultrasound, and pudendal nerve terminal motor latency may also be helpful.

We then classify patients into four groups.[39] "Group one" appears untrainable. They have a poor sacrum, flat perineum, poor muscles, no sensation, and poor bowel movement pattern and usually are incontinent to both urine and all types of stool. These patients are good candidates for a bowel management program. If this program is unsuccessful, alternative techniques such as the artificial bowel sphincter or stimulated gracilis muscle flap may be tried[40]; however, a permanent stoma is usually best suited and truly appreciated by these patients.

"Group two" have clinical and MRI evidence of a mislocated rectum with a good sacrum and well-developed muscles. They benefit from a secondary pullthrough procedure by an experienced surgeon with the aid of the Peña stimulator.

"Group three" has severe constipation and a contrast enema shows a severely dilated mega rectosigmoid. They benefit from a sigmoid resection.

"Group four" are patients born of the good prognostic type and have a well-located rectum, good sacrum, and good muscles but are still incontinent. They may benefit from biofeedback or other behavior modification programs to help them evacuate the rectum at controlled and predictable times.

Some children develop an irritable bowel syndrome as they mature after a successful repair and then have difficulty later on in life. They may benefit from regulation of colonic motility with diet, medication, or possibly an intestinal pacemaker that is on the horizon. It is the author's opinion that control of rectosigmoid motility and coordination will be of more value in the future than any artificial or perhaps transplanted anal sphincter.

Other Pediatric Colorectal Disorders

Idiopathic Constipation

Constipation of unknown origin represents a serious problem in the pediatric population. At least 6% of pediatric consultations are related to this particular problem.[41] We consider this condition to be the result of a colonic hypomotility disorder with different degrees of severity, affecting mainly the rectosigmoid and sometimes the entire colon. The spectrum of colonic hypomotility or colonic inertia varies from mild constipation that can be controlled by dietetic measures, to severe hypomotility disorders that may fall into the realm of what is called "intestinal pseudoobstruction."

Constipation means an incapacity to empty the colon on a daily basis or incapacity to empty it completely. As a consequence, the colon stores a large amount of stool, and becomes very dilated (megacolon). Megacolon produces constipation and constipation produces more megacolon, creating a vicious cycle. The final result is what we call chronic fecal impaction, which provokes overflow pseudoincontinence (encopresis).

The cause of this condition is unknown. Many authors claim that the origin is a behavior problem, whereas others believe that it is a consequence of a dietetic problem. There are those who think that it is a consequence of a lack of relaxation of the internal sphincter or a consequence of ultrashort segment aganglionosis. None of these theories have been scientifically documented, and that is why we call this condition idiopathic.[42]

So far, the treatment for this condition consists of trying to find the amount of laxatives that is capable of producing a bowel movement that empties the colon completely every day. The amount is different in every individual and has to be determined by trial and error. When the laxative requirement is so high that it creates a problem in terms of quality of life, we offer the patient a surgical treatment consisting of the resection of the most dilated portion of the colon (usually the rectosigmoid), creating an anastomosis between the nondilated part of the descending colon and the rectum.[43]

By doing that, even when we are aware of the fact that we do not cure this mysterious condition, we make the problem more manageable and reduce significantly the amount of laxatives that the patient needs.

Rectal Prolapse

Rectal prolapse occurs in children because of well-known conditions such as myelomeningocele and spina bifida. The lack of sphincter tone explains the severe prolapse from which these patients may suffer. Also, patients with cystic fibrosis or some patients with inflammatory bowel disease or intestinal parasites may have rectal prolapse.

Most pediatric patients afflicted by this condition are of the idiopathic type. The surgeon must try to identify one of the predisposing conditions already mentioned. If this is not possible, one must try to avoid those factors that we know exacerbate the problem, such as to avoid constipation and treat any irritating conditions of the colon, such as milk allergy. If all this fails, the surgeon can offer a palliative surgical treatment.

An old operation designed to treat rectal prolapse includes a placement of a nonabsorbable suture around the anus to restrict its caliber. The long-term results of these procedures are not good because eventually the patients develop megacolon and an anal stricture.

Other surgeons have tried the injection of sclerosing substances in both perirectal spaces. This has been followed by severe complications including nerve damage and bowel and urinary incontinence. A posterior sagittal approach has also been used which allows the surgeon to anchor the posterior rectal wall to the cartilage of the coccyx and the sacrum. Most of the patients are cured after this procedure, but there are occasional failures. If all these procedures are unsuccessful, the patient can be subjected to an abdominal approach and fixation of the rectum to the presacral fascia, usually with a sigmoid resection. More recently, a perineal rectosigmoidectomy (modified Altemeier procedure) has emerged as a treatment option in these children mimicking a one-stage pullthrough for Hirschsprung's disease. The advantages are the same in that one avoids an abdominal operation and the procedure may be repeated for recurrences.

Perianal Fistula

Perianal abscess and fistula in pediatrics seems to be a completely different condition to that seen in adults.

During the first year of life, many babies (mainly males), have perianal abscesses that eventually become perianal fistulas. The orifice seen externally next to the anus communicates with one of the crypts of the pectinate line. Traditionally, these patients have been subjected to a fistulotomy, consisting of identifying the fistula tract and cutting all the tissue, and bowel wall, from inside the rectal lumen leaving the wound open for granulation.

Our experience has been that this is a benign condition that does not require any treatment. If the babies have a perianal abscess, they do not require antibiotics. Very soon, the abscess drains by itself and, if not, with a minimal incision and drainage. After that, for a period of months, it drains intermittently without any discomfort to the patient. All fistulas disappear after 1 year of age.[44]

Occasionally, one can see a school-age child with a perianal fistula. This is extremely unusual. The surgeon should investigate the patient for the presence of inflammatory bowel disease before trying any of the currently available surgical techniques used in adults.

Juvenile Polyps

Around 4 years of age, patients might have polyps in the rectum and in the colon. These polyps are benign. They grow and eventually amputate and disappear. The polyps are mostly located in the posterior rectal wall. A rectal examination makes the diagnosis in most cases. These polyps have a long pedicle. The symptoms in these patients are the presence of blood surrounding the fecal matter. They do not produce any pain. Occasionally, the parents describe the presence of a polyp that prolapses through the anus. The polyps can be easily resected under general anesthesia in order to confirm the histologic diagnosis. Histologically, these are benign inflammatory polyps. Once the diagnosis is made, they can be predicted to have a benign course.

Even if the patient has another polyp, we know that eventually it will self-amputate. These polyps do not produce significant bleeding.

Occasionally, one may see juvenile polyposis that may require more aggressive treatment, but that is extremely rare.

Anal Fissure

Anal fissures in pediatric patients are always a consequence and not a cause of constipation. The fissure represents a laceration that was produced with the passage of a hard large piece of fecal matter. The patient has painful bowel movements and that contributes to the constipation problem, because the patient becomes a stool retainer. Stool retention may provoke more constipation and more constipation will make the fissure worse.

The main treatment for this condition is to make the parents understand the nature of the problem. It is necessary to give enough laxatives so as to guarantee that the patient will have soft stool passing through the rectum for several weeks until the fissure heals. No surgical treatment is necessary in fissures in children.

Recently, 0.2% NTG (glyceryl trinitrate) ointment has been used for intractable cases to cause a reversible chemical sphincterotomy. Tander et al.[45] reported successful healing in 83.9% of children compared with 35% treated with placebo. This is a simple alternative treatment because the long-term sequelae of an internal lateral sphincterotomy in children is not known and is likely to be associated with some type of incontinence especially in childbearing females.

References

1. Fewtrell MS, Tam PK, Thomson AH, et al. Hirschsprung's disease associated with a deletion of chromosome 10 (q11 2q21 2): a further link with the neurocristopathies? J Med Genet 1994; 31:325–327.
2. Holschneider AM. Hirschsprung's Disease. Stuttgart: Hippokrates-Verlag; 1982.
3. Schofield DE, Devine W, Yunis EJ. Acetylcholinesterase-stained succion rectal biopsies in the diagnosis of Hirschsprung's disease. J Pediatr Gastroenterol Nutr 1990;11:221.
4. Swenson O, Bill AH. Resection of rectum and rectosigmoid with preservation of the sphincter for benign spastic lesions producing megacolon: an experimental study. Surgery 1948;24:212.
5. Cilley RE, Statter MB, Hirschl RB, Coran AG. Definitive treatment of Hirschsprung's disease in the newborn with a one-sage procedure. Surgery 1994;115:551–556.
6. So HB, Schwartz DL, Becher JM, et al. Endorectal pullthrough without preliminary colostomy in patients with Hirschsprung's disease. J Pediatr Surg 1980;15:470.
7. Duhamel B. Retrorectal and transanal pull-through procedure for the treatment of Hirschsprung's disease. Dis Colon Rectum 1964;7:455.
8. Soave F. Hirschsprung's disease: a new surgical technique. Arch Dis Child 1964;39:116.
9. Boley SJ. A new modification of the surgical treatment of Hirschsprung's disease. Surgery 1964;56:1015–1017.
10. Georgeson KE, Cohen RD, Hebra A, et al. Primary laparoscopic assisted endorectal colon pullthrough for Hirschsprung's disease: a new gold standard. Ann Surg 1999;229:678.
11. Georgeson KE, Fuenfer MM, Hardin WD. Primary laparoscopic pullthrough for Hirschsprung's disease in infants and children. J Pediatr Surg 1995;30:1017.

12. Curran TJ, Raffensperger JG. The feasibility of laparoscopic Swenson pull-through. J Pediatr Surg 1994;29:1273.
13. De la Torre-Mondragon L, Ortega-Salgado J. Transanal endorectal pullthrough for Hirschsprung's disease. J Pediatr Surg 1998;33:1283.
14. Langer JC, Minkes RK, Mazziott MV, et al. Transanal one stage Soave procedure for infants with Hirschsprung's disease. J Pediatr Surg 1999;34:148.
15. Fazio VW, Tjandra JJ. Pouch advancement and neoileoanal anastomosis for anastomotic stricture and anovaginal fistula complicating restorative proctocolectomy. Br J Surg 1992;79: 694–696.
16. Teitelbaum DH, Coran AG, Weitzman JJ, Ziegler MM, Kane T. Hirschsprung's disease and related neuromuscular disorders of the intestine. In: O'Neill JA, Rowe MI, Grosfeld JL, Fonkalsrud E, Coran AG, eds. Pediatric Surgery. 5th ed. St. Louis: Mosby; 1986:1381–1424.
17. Langer JC, Seifert M, Minkes RK. One-stage Soave pull-through for Hirschsprung's disease: a comparison of the transanal and open approaches. J Pediatr Surg 2000;35(6):820–822.
18. Langer JC, Durrant AC, de la Torre L, et al. One stage transanal Soave pullthrough for Hirschsprung's disease: a multicenter experience with 141 children. Ann Surg 2003;238(4):569–583.
19. Martin L. Surgical management of total aganglionosis. Ann Surg 1972;176:343.
20. Kimura K, Mishijima E, Muraji T. A new surgical approach to extensive aganglionosis. J Pediatr Surg 1981;16:840.
21. Lynn HB, van Heerden JA. Rectal myectomy in Hirschsprung disease: a decade of experience. Arch Surg 1975;110:991–994.
22. Lynn HB. Rectal myectomy for aganglionic megacolon. Mayo Clin Proc 1966;41:289–295.
23. Meier-Rouge W. Angeborene Dysganglionosen des Colon. Der Kinderarzt 1985;16:151.
24. Csury L, Peña A. Intestinal neuronal dysplasia: myth or reality. Literature review. Pediatr Surg Int 1995;10(7):441–446.
25. Rich M, Brock W, Peña A. Spectrum of genitourinary malformations in patients with imperforate anus. Pediatr Surg Int 1988; 3:110–113.
26. Levitt MA, Patel M, Rodriguez G, Gaylin DS, Peña A. The tethered spinal cord in patients with anorectal malformations. J Pediatr Surg 1997;32(3):462–468.
27. Peña A. Anorectal malformations. Semin Pediatr Surg 1995;4(1):35–47.
28. Torres P, Levitt MA, Tovilla JM, Rodriguez G, Peña A. Anorectal malformations and Down's syndrome. J Pediatr Surg 1998;33(2):1–5.
29. Rosen NG, Hong AR, Soffer SZ, Rodriguez G, Peña A. Rectovaginal fistula: a common diagnostic error with significant consequences in female patients with anorectal malformations. J Pediatr Surg 2002;37(7):961–965.
30. Peña A, Levitt M. Surgical management of cloacal malformations: a review of 339 patients. J Pediatr Surg 2004;39(3):470–479.
31. Levitt MA, Stein DM, Peña A. Gynecological concerns in the treatment of teenagers with cloaca. J Pediatr Surg 1998;33(2): 188–193.
32. Gross GW, Wolfson PJ, Peña A. Augmented-pressure colostogram in imperforate anus with fistula. Radiology 1991; 21:560–562.
33. Hong AR, Rosen N, Acuña MF, Peña A, Chaves L, Rodriguez G. Urological injuries associated with the repair of anorectal malformations in male patients. J Pediatr Surg 2002;37:339–344.

34. Georgeson KE, Cohen RD, Hebra A, et al. Primary laparoscopically assisted endorectal pullthrough for high imperforate anus: a new technique. J Pediatr Surg 1997;32(2):263–268.

35. Peña A. Total urogenital mobilization: an easier way to repair cloacas. J Pediatr Surg 1997;32(2):263–268.

36. Peña A, Guardino K, Tovilla JM, Levitt MA, Rodriguez G, Torres R. Bowel management for fecal incontinence in patients with anorectal malformations. J Pediatr Surg 1998;33(1): 133–137.

37. Malone PS, Ransley PG, Kiely EM. Prelim report: the antegrade continence enema. Lancet 1990;336:1217–1218.

38. Levitt MA, Soffer SZ, Peña A. Continent appendicostomy in the bowel management of fecal incontinent children. J Pediatr Surg 1997;32(11):1630–1633.

39. Peña A. Anorectal malformations: new aspects relevant to adult colorectal surgeons. In: Veidenheimer MC, ed. Seminars Colon Rectal Surgery 1994;5(2):78–88.

40. da Silva GM, Jorge JM, Belin B, et al. New surgical options for fecal incontinence in patients with imperforate anus. Dis Colon Rectum 2004;47(2):204–209.

41. Levine MD. Children with encopresis: a descriptive analysis. Pediatrics 1975;56:412–416.

42. Peña A, Levitt M. Colonic inertia disorders in pediatrics. Curr Probl Surg 2002;39(7):661–732.

43. Peña A, El-Behery M. Megasigmoid: a source of pseudo-incontinence in children with repaired anorectal malformations. J Pediatr Surg 1993;28(2):1–5.

44. Rosen NG, Gibbs DL, Soffer SZ, Hong AR, Sher M, Peña A. The nonoperative management of fistula-in-ano. J Pediatr Surg 2000;35(6):938–939.

45. Tander B, Guven A, Demirbag S, Ozkan Y, Ozturk H, et al. A prospective randomized double blind trial of glyceryl-trinitrate ointment in the treatment of children with anal fissure. J Pediatr Surg 1999;34(12):18110–18112.

52
Healthcare Economics

David A. Margolin and Lester Rosen

"It was the best of times it was the worst of times." How prophetic was Charles Dickens when applied to health care in America today.[1] We are currently experiencing unprecedented technologic and therapeutic advancements; however, these come at a tremendous price. Healthcare expenditures have increased by double digits for the past decade, physician reimbursement has decreased over the past 10 years, and hospitals have closed and healthcare systems have filed for bankruptcy.[2] Furthermore, healthcare expenditures are forecasted to grow more than 7.0% per year over the next 10 years[3] (Figure 52-1).[4]

Multiple interrelated events have led to the current state of healthcare finance. With the advent of the resource-based relative value system (RBRVS), physicians have shifted from price setters to price takers. Technology costs, although providing an improvement in patient care, have skyrocketed. Although the life expectancy of the population has not increased dramatically over the past decades, the "baby boomers" are here and continue to shift the average age of the American population to one that requires increased utilization of healthcare resources. In 2003 it was estimated that forty-five million or 15.6% of Americans had no health insurance, and millions more were underinsured, putting a strain on state and federal budgets to provide care.[5] Last but not least is the current professional liability crisis, resulting in increased malpractice rates and driving specialists from specific locations. Despite this, physicians still are able to provide quality care for their patients and receive reasonable compensation. Nonetheless, in the ever-changing face of the socioeconomic landscape, physicians need a solid basis that allows them to function in today's practice environment.

This chapter covers the RBVRS and Medicare reimbursement, the types of contractual agreement between insurers and practitioners and insurers and patients, and what to expect in the future.

The Reimbursement Process

Medicare

The key to begin to understand the business of medicine is to understand the basics of Medicare. While private payers vary in their reimbursement rates and policies, most are tied in some form to the Medicare system. Medicare was created in 1965 by the federal government as a social insurance program designed to provide all adults over the age of 65 with comprehensive healthcare coverage at an affordable cost. Medicare is administrated by the Center for Medicare and Medicaid Services (CMS), formerly known as the Health Care Financing Administration. When the program began in 1966, 19.1 million persons were enrolled; in 2004, Medicare had more than 41 million enrollees and is forecasted to include almost 80 million people by 2030 (Figure 52-2).[6] Medicare is divided into several parts.

Medicare Part A, also known as hospital insurance, helps pay for inpatient hospitalizations, skilled nursing care (SNF), home health and hospice care. Part A is financed primarily through federal payroll taxes (FICA) paid by both employees and employers. In 2004 the current FICA tax was 7.65% of earned income, of which 1.45% went toward Medicare Part A. Individuals who receive social security benefits or railroad retirement benefits are automatically enrolled in Part A. Individuals under 65 who receive social security disability or those with end-stage renal disease for more than 24 months are also eligible for Part A. Despite current misconceptions, Medicare Part A is not free. Although there is no monthly premium, Medicare enrollees are responsible for copayments associated with the services provided. In 2004 there was an $840 copay for each hospital stay of 1–60 days, and after 150 days of inpatient hospitalization all costs were the patient's responsibility. Part A covers nothing for the first 20 days of SNF care and only $105 for days 21–100.

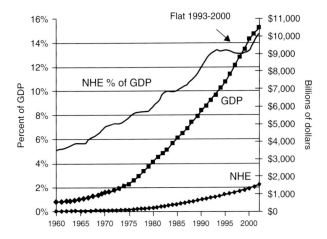

FIGURE 52-1. Healthcare expenditures.[4] The green line shows the percentage of the gross national product going to national health expenditure. The scale on the left axis measures it. The purple line, for gross domestic product (GDP), and the blue line, for national health expenditure (NHE), in billions of dollars, measured by the right axis scale. http://hspm.sph.sc.edu/Courses/Econ/Classes/nhe00/.

Similar to inpatient hospitalization, there was no coverage for SNF after 100 days.

Medicare Part B, also known as Medical Insurance, provides coverage for payments to physicians for services provided. This includes outpatient medical and surgical services, supplies, diagnostic testing, and some home health care. Part B is funded by a combination of the federal government's general revenues (75%) and individual monthly premiums (25%). In 2004 Part B did not cover routine physical examinations. However, the federal government has responded to citizens' urging and has instituted a physical examination when one enters into Medicare and covers screening for some specific diseases. Part B covers screening for breast cancer, cervical cancer, prostate cancer, and colorectal cancer.

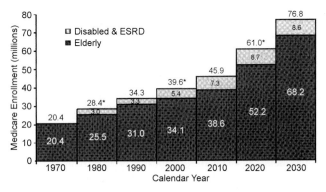

FIGURE 52-2. Expected number of Medicare beneficiaries. The number of people Medicare serves will nearly double by 2030.[6] *Note:* *Numbers may not sum because of rounding. (*Source:* CMS, Office of the Actuary. From Centers for Medicare & Medicaid Services, June 2002 edition, section III.B.1, p 4).

Medicare covers fecal occult blood testing every 24 months, flexible sigmoidoscopy every 48 months, colonoscopy for high-risk individuals once every 24 months or for average risk individuals every 10 years. Medicare also covers barium enemas every 24 or 48 months depending on your risk stratification. New in 2004 was a prescription drug benefit plan available to Medicare beneficiaries in 2006.

Unlike Part A, Medicare Part B has monthly premiums. In 2004 the premium for those who enrolled at the onset of eligibility was $66.60 per month. If one enrolls at eligibility, this premium is deducted from your social security or railroad retirement check. You can opt out of Part B. Similar to Part A, Part B enrollees are responsible for copayments and deductibles. For physician services, deductible was $100 per calendar year and a 20% copayment of Medicare-approved rates. Copayments for outpatient procedures were charged at a different rate than office services, and the copayment varied based on the procedure performed.

Whereas Part A and B are considered traditional Medicare, Medicare Part C or Medicare + choice is the government's plan to shift the cost and risks of Medicare patients to the private sector. In Part C, private payers receive a monthly payment per covered individual (capitated amount) to provide all of Part A and B services. Private payers then tailor these plans to cover anticipated needs. These plans often provide benefits not seen in traditional Medicare, such as prescription drugs, routine physicals, preventative care, eyeglasses, and hearing aids. However, because these plans are privately administered, individual choice is often severely limited with regard to physicians and hospitals.

In late 2003, the federal government instituted another new category of Medicare. Medicare Part D, prescription drug coverage, was signed into law in December 2003. In response to the cost of prescription drugs for seniors, in December, the government instituted a program that will start in 2006. This program will provide for prescription drugs with an initial deductible of $250 dollars and a monthly premium of $35. There will be a 75% subsidy for drug cost between $251–$2250. The federal government will pay for all drugs after a recipient pays $3600 or $5100 in total cost. Special assistance will be provided for low-income seniors as well. New to Part D is the institution of means testing. Individuals with incomes $160,000 and above will be subjected to higher Part B and Part D premiums.

Medicare Resources

According to the Office of Management and Budget, Medicare in 2004 had a budget of $302 billion forecasted to grow to more than $317 billion by 2008.[7] That budget is determined by legislation and is formula based. It involves the Medicare Economic Index, a weighted index, and the sustainable growth rate. The sustainable growth rate compares the cumulative actual spending for physicians' services since 1997 to a cumulative target amount of spending over the same time period. Without new federal spending legislation, Medicare spending is not allowed to grow by more than $20 million/year (budget neutrality). However, the government has made exceptions to increases in Medicare spending for new technologies and pilot programs. For more details, the complete Medicare fee schedule can be found in the Federal Register online at http://www.gpoaccess.gov/fr/index.html.

Hospital (Part A) Reimbursement

Until the mid-1980s, the federal government and most private payers reimbursed hospitals retrospectively for all reasonable costs involved in the care of a covered individual. With this form of reimbursement, to compete and remain solvent, hospitals invested in the latest, most advanced technology. This allowed hospitals to increase patient care volume and expand services; however, it was done without regard to cost or efficiency. Although this methodology had its advantage, it led to a continuing upward spiral in healthcare costs and a significant duplication of services.

In response to sharply increasing hospital costs, the federal government instituted a prospective payment system. This was modeled after a system developed by Fetter and associates at Yale University that categorized patients based on primary and secondary diagnosis, primary and secondary procedures, age and length of stay, and then set a uniform cost for each category.[8] These diagnostic related groups (DRGs) set a maximum amount that would be paid for the hospital care of Medicare patients for a specific problem. In 2003 there were 538 DRGs. Each DRG contains a list of specific diagnoses and procedures based on the International Classification of Diseases, Ninth Revision, Clinical Modification (ICD-9-CM).[9] ICD-9 is a coding system that lists specific diseases, diagnoses, and medical acuity. By using this system, Medicare has grouped related ICD-9 codes that use similar hospital recourses in specific DRGs.

Private payers have followed Medicare's lead and began using a prospective payment system. It was believed that by using a prospective payment system, hospitals would have a true incentive to improve efficiency and keep cost low. Although this may have initially slowed the growth of hospital costs and forced improved efficiency in healthcare delivery, it has not been the panacea that was expected. Hospital costs, although initially controlled, returned to double-digit increases by 2002.[10] Although the reasons for the continued increase in hospital costs are multifactorial, the failure of DRGs to truly control cost can best be summed up this way: "Hospitals prefer management strategies that are designed to enhance revenues over cost control measures that may be resisted by the physician staff."[11]

Despite the reluctance of physicians to change practice patterns, hospitals have tried to increase their efficiency, and with technologic advances, it has been possible to shift procedures from the inpatient setting to outpatient/ambulatory center. Although this had some albeit minimal impact in physician

reimbursement, it helped decrease resource utilization. In response to this, to account for this shift in location, Medicare has developed a prospective payment system called the ambulatory payment classification (APC). APCs, similar to DRGs, are specific reimbursement groupings that Medicare pays to facilities. For these outpatient services, Medicare pays a specific rate per procedure determined by the APC in which the procedure is grouped. Specific medical devices and drugs are exempt from this and are reimbursed in addition to the APC fee. These are called pass throughs. Other devices that do not receive pass through are often charged to the patient by private payers. In 2004, four APC classifications covered the majority of outpatient anorectal procedures. APCs reimburse facilities between $209 (APC 148, lateral internal anal sphincterotomy) and $1210 (APC 150, hemorrhoidectomy) with a patient copayment between $41 and $437.

With changes in location of services in a constant state of flux, Medicare needed to develop an appropriate and timely methodology to respond to this shift. To add some stability to APC payments and achieve these goals, the Secretary of Health and Human Services (head of CMS) appointed an Advisory Panel on APC Groups. This panel of physicians deals with issues concerning resource use, assigning new current procedural terminology (CPT®) codes to APCs, and reassigning codes to different APCs.

Physician Reimbursement

Currently physician reimbursement from Medicare is a three-step process: 1) appropriate coding of the service provided by utilizing CPT®; 2) the appropriate coding of the diagnosis using ICD-9 code; and 3) CMS determination of the appropriate fee based on the RBRVS.

CPT® is a uniform coding system that was developed by the American Medical Association (AMA). CPT® originated in 1966 and has undergone yearly updates based on changes in medical and surgical procedures and the development of new technology. CPT® is a proprietary product of the AMA. The CPT® editorial panel is composed of 16 members in multiple specialties as well as the insurance industry. Advisors from more than 90 medical and surgical specialties advise them. They meet four times a year to consider additions and deletions to the code list. A service may be brought before the CPT® editorial panel by any specialty, private physician, insurer, or device manufacture. To receive consideration for a new code, a procedure must meet certain requirements: it must be done by a reasonable number of the specialty that presents the code, be performed at reasonable frequency, be done throughout the country, and have peer-reviewed literature supporting its efficacy. The editorial panel allows advisors from other specialties to comment on any proposal. The editorial panel then reviews the clinical description of the procedure or service that describes the typical patient. After assuring that it meets all of the above requirements and that the service should not be coded with a preexisting code, the committee will give the service a unique CPT® code. The code then moves to the Relative Value Update Committee (RUC) where it receives a value relative to other codes (RVU). CPT® also uses a series of modifiers in addition to the original code to better describe the service provided. This allows not only for better data collection regarding the frequency and complexity of services but also for appropriate reimbursement by Medicare.

Medicare implemented the RBRVS in 1992. Previously physicians were reimbursed based on "usual, customary and reasonable charges" (UCR). UCRs were based on the physician's most frequent charge for the service (usual), the average charge for that service in the area (customary), and the actual charge for the service (reasonable).[12] Individuals within the federal government, private insurers and non-procedure-based medical specialties thought that this system perpetuated increasing healthcare costs and inequities in medical care. These individuals believed that this system served as an incentive for physicians to inflate charges even in those instances in which actual costs were decreasing and to continue the inequities in fees between proceduralists and nonproceduralists. In response to this, the federal government instituted the Medicare fee schedule.

The Medicare fee schedule was based on the work of a research team led by William Hsiao, a Harvard economist under contract to CMS.[13–15] The Harvard study ranked procedures and services relative to each other based on the amount of physician work necessary to perform the procedure or service. Work was defined as a combination of the time used to perform the service and the complexity of service (mental effort, knowledge, judgment and diagnostic acumen, technical skill, physical skill, psychological stress, and potential iatrogenic risk).[16] Work was then broken down into three time periods, preservice, intraservice, and postservice.

Preservice work for surgical procedures has come to be defined as the physician work provided from the day before, until the time of the operative procedure (i.e., skin incision). This may involve any or all of the following: hospital admission work-up, the preoperative evaluation including the procedural work-up, review of records, communicating with other professionals, patient and family, and obtaining consent; and, dressing, scrubbing, and waiting before the operative procedure, preparing patient and needed equipment for the operative procedure, positioning the patient, and other non-"skin-to-skin" work done in the operating room before incision. Preservice work does not include the consultation or evaluation at which the decision to provide the procedure was made.

Intraservice work includes all "skin-to-skin" work that is a necessary part of the procedure. The time measurement for the intraservice work is from the start of the skin incision until the incision is closed.

Unlike preservice work, postservice work varies depending on the magnitude of the procedure. In an effort to accurately assign the amount of postprocedure work, specific CPT® codes have been assigned specific global periods. There are currently three postprocedural global periods: 0 days, 10 days, and 90 days. Routine postprocedure care includes physician work after skin closure that is done on the day of the procedure, including non-"skin-to-skin" work in the operating room. This includes patient stabilization in the recovery room, communicating with the patient and other professionals (including written and telephone reports and orders), and patient visits on the day of the procedure. For a surgical service with a global period of 10 or 90 days, the postservice work includes all of the above, and in addition postoperative hospital care, including the intensive care unit if needed; other in-hospital visits; discharge day management services; and office visits within the assigned global period of 10 or 90 days.[17]

For nonsurgical services such as office evaluation and management (E&M) services, the preservice work includes preparing to see the patient, reviewing records, and communicating with other professionals. The intraservice work includes the work provided while the physician is with the patient and/or family. This includes the time in which the physician obtains the history, performs a physical evaluation, and counsels the patient. The postservice work for nonprocedural services includes arranging for further services, reviewing results of studies, and communicating further with the patient, family, and other professionals, including written and telephone reports as well as calls to the patient.

Whereas the study by Hsiao and colleagues[14] initially valued only 200 codes and ranked them according to physician work, the RUC subsequently valued and ranked each CPT® code relative to other codes. New codes were valued using provider surveys to obtain an appropriate work value. These surveys allow for individuals who perform the procedures to value pre-, intra-, and postservice work relative to established codes. According to federal law, the relative value of codes is reviewed every 5 years by the RUC allowing for corrections in the relativity of the codes. Currently, physician work is not the only value used to calculate an RVU. Whereas the work RVUs (wRVU) makes up the majority of the total RVUs (tRVU) for a specific CPT® code, RVUs are also calculated for practice expense (peRVU) and malpractice (mRVU) for each code. Similar to wRVUs, peRVUs are calculated based on the amount of resources used in the pre-, intra-, and postservice time. This includes not only the nursing and ancillary staff key to the procedure or service but also supplies used during the pre- and postprocedure periods. If the procedure is performed in the office, intraservice personnel and supplies are included. For procedures done in a facility, usually a hospital, these costs are reimbursed based on the DRG (Part A) and paid to the healthcare facility and not to the physician. Malpractice RVUs are calculated from actual malpractice premium data obtained throughout the country. Using previous CMS claims, a value for each CPT® code is determined based on a risk factor for the dominant specialty that provides service.[18]

Final physician reimbursement by CMS is then multiplied by a geographic practice cost index (GPCI), which is supposed to adjust payments for differences in physician practice costs across geographic areas. For a given service, multiplying the service-specific Physician Work, Practice Expense, and Malpractice Expense RVUs by their respective GPCIs determines the payment amount in a given geographic area. Next, these three products are summed, yielding a geographically adjusted RVU total for the service. This number is then converted to dollars by a conversion factor, which in 2004 was \$37.3374 per RVU. It is expected to increase 1.5% in 2005. As an example, in 2004 for CPT® code 44140 (colectomy, partial; with anastomosis) {(wRVU * wGPCI) + (peRVU * peGPCI) + (mRVU * mGPCI)} * 37.3374 = \$ CMS reimbursement. As seen, the amount paid varies per region:

San Francisco, CA: (20.97 wRVU * 1.068 wGPCI) + (8.69 peRVU * 1.458 peGPCI) + (2.58 mRVU * 0.669 mGPCI) * 37.3374 = \$1373.72

Boston, MA: (20.97 wRVU * 1.041 wGPCI) + (8.69 peRVU * 1.239 peGPCI) + (2.58 mRVU * 0.803 mGPCI) * 37.3374 = \$1294.43

New Orleans, LA: (20.97 wRVU * 1.0 wGPCI) + (8.69 peRVU * 0.945 peGPCI) + (2.58 mRVU * 1.240 mGPCI) * 37.3374 = \$1209.03

Little Rock, AR: (20.97 wRVU * 1.000 wGPCI) + (8.69 peRVU * 0.847 peGPCI) + (2.58 mRVU * 0.389 mGPCI) * 37.3374 = \$1095.26

Although Medicare is an extremely large and at times an unwieldy way to manage healthcare and healthcare-related costs, understanding it is key to understanding both hospital and physician reimbursement by private payers. Most private payers today use CPT® codes to identify physician services. Although private payers do not have to follow the rules set forth by the federal government (for instance, they often do not recognize surgical modifiers), they find that CPT® is a well-established and familiar system allowing for correct physician coding. Private payers in noncapitated contracts often set reimbursement based on a percentage of the Medicare fee schedule. The percentage reimbursement will often vary by region. The larger payers have taken this one step further using Medicare to develop their own fee schedule. Again using CPT® terminology, companies will adjust payment based on the individual service provided; for example, paying E&M codes 105% of Medicare, office-based procedures 110% of Medicare, and surgical procedures 115%. This is often modified regionally based on the rules of supply and demand. In areas with a paucity of a specific specialty, reimbursement is high as opposed to a saturated market where the insurance company can play one physician or group against another to obtain a favorable contract. Hospital payments are similar. Private payers reimburse hospitals either as a percentage of the DRG or on a per diem based on the service provided. For outpatient procedures, hospitals are often reimbursed as a percentage of the APC.

Private Payers

Whereas the impact of Medicare on the economic landscape of medicine is clear, the role and type of private payers is more cloudy. Health insurance comes in many forms and has different relations with its customer and its physician providers. Traditionally, there were two types of nongovernmental insurance, individual insurance and group insurance. Individual insurance allows a person to buy health insurance for themselves and their family. However, because of the inability of the insurer to spread the financial risk among many people, individual insurance is becoming prohibitively expensive. The majority of people obtain health insurance through some type of group. This allows for cheaper individual payments as group purchasing allows the insurer to spread the risk over a larger number of people. Group insurance can be obtained through employers, professional societies (ACS, etc.), or other organizations (AARP, etc.).

Regardless of how insurance is purchased, the types of insurance plans are distinctly different. The most costly is the fee-for-service plan, also known as an indemnity plan in which individuals are free to seek care from any physician or hospital they choose. No preapproval is required. Individuals submit the bills to their carrier and if the deductible has been met, if there is one, the insurance company pays for medical services at the UCR. These plans are often structured so that there is a copayment for all services. The use of copayments and deductibles by insurers is a method of risk sharing. Not only do these costs help defray the cost of providing care for the insurers, but they are designed to make individuals think twice before seeking unnecessary care. In traditional fee-for-service plans, an individual may be responsible for 20% of the bill. Also, they may be responsible for the difference between the UCR and the billed charges.

To help control increasing healthcare costs and stimulate a more efficient use of healthcare resources, managed care organizations were developed. Since the early 1990s they have evolved into a variety of complex organizational structures. They use a variety of tools to manage preauthorization functions, control healthcare costs, and share the risks associated with group coverage.

Health maintenance organizations (HMOs) were designed to meet these ends. Although HMOs are still in the process of evolution, they characteristically represent the most restrictive type of health maintenance organization. In this model, the HMO restricts patient access in nonemergency incidents to HMO-contracted physicians and hospitals. Out-of-pocket costs for individuals are traditionally low for HMO physicians; however, individuals are responsible for all costs for non-HMO physicians.

Most HMOs initially used a "gatekeeper" or primary care physician for specialist referral. Subsequently, HMOs have loosened gatekeeper requirements for specialist referral. This model has propagated the development of healthcare systems, multispecialty groups that are either owned by or contracted with the HMO to provide complete patient care. In these instances, the physicians function as employees of the system. The physician group is then paid a capitated fee (amount per patient per month to provide total care) which is divided among the medical care providers at a rate determined by the medical group administration.

The next iteration of managed care organizations is the preferred provider organization (PPO). Similar to HMOs, PPOs enter into contracts with healthcare providers and hospitals to provide member care. Often more choice and flexibility are available to the patient than in the traditional HMO model but at the cost of higher beneficiary premiums. Unlike HMOs, PPOs do not own physician practices. To have access to the PPOs beneficiaries and be listed in the "network," physicians often agree to reduce their normal fees. PPOs traditionally do not use a "gatekeeper," thus allowing patients increased access to self-referred specialty care.

The most recent variation in managed care organizations is the development of "Point of Service" plans, a mixture of traditional HMO and PPO plans. In this type of plan, if a patient first sees their primary care physician to receive a referral, much like an HMO, the copay, if present, is negligible. Patients are also able to see "network" physicians with minimal financial responsibility. Patients may seek care from someone outside the "network" without a referral. In these instances, the physician is paid a rate less than is characteristically billed, usually the same rate as in network physicians, and the patient is responsible for the difference. This provides increased patient flexibility but at increased cost.

The Future

Despite hopes that managed care would provide cost stability to health care in America, after costs initially slowed, they have continued to increase at a rate higher than the consumer price index and personal income (Table 52-1).[19] Is this a failure of managed care or has managed care reached its capacity with regard to improving efficiency and cost containment? The answer is unclear; however, experts now tout a "consumer-centric" or "consumer-driven" healthcare model as the future of healthcare delivery. Harvard Professor Regina Herzlinger initially described a system that allows users to become active consumers.[17] Similar to making any large purchases, individuals are given the opportunity to choose from specific benefit packages that will fit their particular need. Aside from having choice, individuals are given information allowing them to make educated and informed choices. Herzlinger and others envision a healthcare market place similar to a successful industry in which individuals are given control, choice, and information. With the increasing number of consumers in need of healthcare resources, these experts see the Internet as a way of rapid dissemination of healthcare information.[20–23]

Although consumer-centric health care and health reimbursement arrangements (HRAs) seem to be recreating the way health care is funded, there are potential problems. This model assumes that consumers are sophisticated enough to make sound healthcare choices, not just those based on cost. As Abramowitz notes, "Choosing based on price is impossible for consumers to do intelligently. The bottom line is that consumers lack the information necessary to use the money wisely. So consumer driven health care, as it is being discussed today, will be a market failure."[24] Another potential problem is that individuals will feel obligated to use all of their HRA or employer contributions, especially as the year end approaches and individuals run the risk of losing their contributions.

The initial manifestation of a hope to address some of the potential pitfalls of consumer-centric health care is the development of defined contribution plans in which employers provide a set amount to individuals for health care, along with information regarding employer-approved healthcare choices. Often these are tied to a safety net for catastrophic cost. The idea is to empower individuals and to give them the necessary information to make good choices. Further development of consumer-driven health care is the development of HRAs. This IRS plan gives a tax advantage to employers who contribute defined contributions to employee-controlled accounts for healthcare spending. Any monies not spent during the year are rolled over to help fund the following year's plan. The thought was that this combined with a high deductible plan would lower healthcare costs. These types of plans also raise some questions: is the unused portion of the plan eligible to be rolled over in an IRA/401K? Can these funds be used for nontraditional health care? What about domestic partners? Are these funds portable? These questions will only be answered by time and possibly federal legislation. Will this next generation of changes significantly help to control healthcare costs? The answer is unclear; however, one current benefit is the increasing individual awareness and education that these plans foster.

Despite the many and varied attempts to control healthcare costs, an unacceptably large number of Americans are still unable to obtain adequate healthcare coverage. This has led to the call in some quarters for the development of universal coverage. Senator Edward Kennedy put it best in a 2003 editorial: "Health care is not just another commodity. It is not a gift based on the ability to pay."[25] Proponents of universal coverage envision a system that provides access to care when needed and effective preventative care in a cost-effective manner that is delivered and paid for in an equitable way. Although these are laudable goals, practical application remains a long way off. As seen from above, the increasing role and complexity of Medicare and Medicaid has not even incrementally achieved these objectives. Will the government be willing to push forward with universal health care and the subsequent development of a two-tiered healthcare system, one for the wealthy and one for the remainder of Americans? Only time will tell.

TABLE 52-1. Selected national economic indicators: 2000–2004

Indicator	Calendar year				2001 Q2	2001 Q3	2001 Q4	2002 Q1	2002 Q2	2002 Q3	2002 Q4	2003 Q1	2003 Q2	2003 Q3	2003 Q4	2004 Q1
	2000	2001	2002	2003												
Gross domestic product																
Billions of dollars	9,817	10,101	10,481	10,988	10,088	10,096	10,194	10,329	10,428	10,542	10,624	10,736	10,847	11,107	11,262	11,451
Personal income																
Personal income in billions	8,430	8,713	8,910	9,204	8,690	8,727	8,771	8,804	8,912	8,944	8,981	9,049	9,146	9,256	9,364	9,523
Disposable income in billions	7,194	7,469	7,857	8,213	7,382	7,606	7,528	7,734	7,869	7,891	7,936	8,039	8,146	8,318	8,349	8,531
Prices*																
Consumer price index, all items	172	177.1	179.9	184	177.5	177.8	177.3	177.9	179.8	180.6	181.2	183	183.7	184.6	184.6	186.3
All items less medical care	167	171.9	174.3	178.1	172.4	172.5	171.9	172.5	174.3	174.9	175.4	177.2	177.9	178.6	178.6	180.2
Medical care	261	272.8	285.6	297.1	271.6	274.2	276.6	280.9	284	287.2	290.3	293.5	295.5	298.4	300.9	305.7
Annual percent change continues																
Gross domestic product																
Billions of dollars	5.9	2.9	3.8	4.8	2.7	2.4	2.4	3	3.4	4.4	4.2	3.9	4	5.4	6	6.7
Personal income																
Personal income in billions	8	3.4	2.3	3.3	3.8	2.5	2.4	1.6	2.6	2.5	2.4	2.8	2.6	3.5	4.3	5.2
Prices*																
Consumer price index, all items	3.4	2.8	1.6	2.3	3.4	2.7	1.9	1.3	1.3	1.6	2.2	2.9	2.1	2.2	1.9	1.8
All items less medical care	3.3	2.7	1.4	2.2	3.3	2.6	1.7	1	1.1	1.4	2.1	2.7	2	2.1	1.8	1.7
Medical care	4.1	4.6	4.7	4	4.6	4.5	4.7	4.5	4.6	4.8	5	4.5	4	3.9	3.7	4.2

*Base period = 1982–84, unless noted.

Note: Q designates quarter of year. Unlike Tables 1-6, quarterly data on GDP, personal income, and disposable personal income, are seasonally adjusted at annual rates.

Sources: U.S. Department of Commerce, Bureau of Economic Analysis: Survey of Current Business. Washington. U.S. Government Printing Office. Monthly reports for January 1998–October 2003; U.S. Department of Labor, Bureau of Labor and Producer Price Indexes. Washington. U.S. Government Printing Office. Monthly reports for January 1999–March 2004. http://www.cms.hhs.gov/statistics/health-indicators/t7.asp.[19]

References

1. Dickens C. A tale of two cities. London; 1859.
2. HHS Office of the Inspector General. Available at: http://oig.hhs. gov/oei/reports/oei-04-02-00180.pdf. Accessed January 5, 2005.
3. The Centers for Medicare & Medicaid Services. Available at: http://www.cms.hhs.gov/statistics/nhe/projections-2003/high lights. asp. Accessed January 5, 2005.
4. Baker SL. U.S. National Health Spending, 2002 University of South Carolina, Arnold School of Public Health, Dept. of Health Services Policy and Management, HSPM J712, August 19, 2004. Available at: http://hspm.sph.sc.edu/Courses/Econ/ Classesnhe00/. Accessed January 10, 2005.
5. United States Census Bureau. Available at: http://www.census. gov/hhes/www/hlthins/hlthin03/hlth03asc.html. Accessed January 5, 2005.
6. The Centers for Medicare & Medicaid Services. Available at: http://www.cms.hhs.gov/charts/series/sec3-b1-9.pdf. Accessed January 5, 2005.
7. Office of Management and Budget. Available at: http://www. whitehouse.gov/omb/budget/fy2004/tables.html. Accessed January 5, 2005.
8. Fetter RB, Thompson JD, Mills RE. A system for cost and reimbursement control in hospitals. Yale J Biol Med 1976;49:123–136.
9. World Health Organization. Collaborating Center for Classification of Diseases for North America. The International classification of diseases: 9th revision, clinical modification: ICD-9-CM. Washington, DC: Department of Health and Human Services, Public Health Service, National Center for Health Statistics; 1986.
10. Hay J, Forrest S, Goetghebeur M. Executive summary hospital costs in the US. Available at: www.heartland.org/pdf/14628.pdf. Accessed January 10, 2005.
11. Weiner SL, Maxwell JH, Sapolsky HM, et al. Economic incentives and organizational realities: managing hospitals under DRGs. Milbank Q 1987;65:463–487.
12. Blount LL, Waters JM, Gold RS. Methods of insurance reimbursement. In: Mastering the Reimbursement Process. Chicago, IL: AMA Press; 2001:6–7.
13. Hsiao WC, Braun P, Dunn D, et al. Resource-based relative values. An overview. JAMA 1988;260:2347–2353.
14. Hsiao WC, Couch NP, Causino N, et al. Resource-based relative values for invasive procedures performed by eight surgical specialties. JAMA 1988;260:2418–2424.
15. Hsiao WC, Yntema DB, Braun P, et al. Measurement and analysis of intraservice work. JAMA 1988;260:2361–2370.
16. Hsiao WC, Braun P, Becker ER, et al. The Resource-Based Relative Value Scale. Toward the development of an alternative physician payment system. JAMA 1987;258:799–802.
17. Mayberry C. RUC Research Subcommittee. The use of intensity measures in the development of physician work relative value units (RVU's). RUC meeting 1/14/2004 (nonpublished handout).
18. The Centers for Medicare & Medicaid Services. Development of resource-based malpractice RVUs. Available at: http://www. cms.hhs.gov/physicians/pfs/kpmgrept.asp#_Toc448071075. Accessed January 10, 2005.
19. U.S. Department of Commerce, Bureau of Economic Analysis. Available at: http://www.cms.hhs.gov/statistics/health-indicators/ t7.asp. Accessed January 11, 2005.
20. Herzlinger RE. Market Driven Health Care: Who Wins, Who Loses in the Transformation of America's Largest Service Industry. Reading, MA: Addison-Wesley Publishing; 1997.
21. Gupta AK. The arrival of consumer-centric healthcare. Manag Care Q 2003;11:20–23.
22. Halterman S, Camero C, Maillet P. The consumer-driven approach: can it pick up where managed care left off? Benefits Q 2003;19:13–26.
23. Abbott RK, Feltman KE. Consumer driven healthcare and the birth of health reimbursement arrangements. Manag Care Q 2002;10:4–7.
24. Abramowitz K. Health plan 2009. Consumer-directed health care won't fly. Manag Care 2004;13:24.
25. Kennedy EM. Quality, affordable health care for all Americans [editorial]. Am J Public Health 2003;93:14.

53
Ethical and Legal Considerations

Ira J. Kodner, Mark Siegler, Daniel M. Freeman, and William T. Choctaw

Considerations for Surgeons

General Concepts

Defining the Problem

Professional responsibilities have been a concern of surgeons since antiquity; however, the last 25 years have displayed a dramatic growth of both professional and societal attention to moral and ethical issues involved in the delivery of health care. This increased interest in medical ethics has occurred because of such factors as the greater technologic power of modern medicine, the assigning of social ills to the responsibility of medicine, the growing sophistication of patients and the information available to them, the efforts to protect the civil rights of the increasing disadvantaged groups in our society, and the continued rapidly escalating costs of health care including medical malpractice costs. All of these factors contribute to the urgency of dealing with ethical and moral issues involved in the delivery of modern surgical care.[1]

The terms *ethics* and *morals* are often used interchangeably to refer to standards regarding right and wrong behavior. *Morals* refer to conduct that conforms to the accepted customs or standards of a people. They vary with time and with the nature of society at that time. *Ethics* is the branch of philosophy that deals with human conduct, and can be described as applied morals. *Medical ethics* refers to the ethics of the practice of medicine. *Clinical ethics* refers to the ethics of delivering patient care. The term *bioethics* includes the ethics of all biomedical endeavors and encompasses both medical and clinical ethics.[2] The *law* serves to delineate the *formal rules of society*. It expresses a kind of minimal societal ethical consensus, which society is willing to enforce through civil judgments or criminal sanctions. The law does not always prohibit behavior deemed unethical, however it will usually set a minimal standard for conduct. Those of us who practice clinical surgery often have trouble differentiating *ethical issues* from *legal issues*. It will be the purpose of this chapter to clarify this dichotomy. It should be stated from the outset that it is more important to understand the *process* of

dealing with these issues than to assume that anyone can clearly state what is ethically right or wrong in a complex medical/surgical dilemma. The law, however, can be very explicit and can vary from state to state.

Surgeons live and practice an intense form of applied ethics. We deliver bad news; we guide patients and their families through complicated decisions to arrive at appropriate informed consent; we live a code of truth and trust among ourselves, our patients, and our trainees; we must deal with the end-of-life issues; and we make plans for extended, palliative, and hospice care. Finally, as only we surgeons know, we must go to bed at night knowing that in the morning we will spend hours with someone's life literally in our hands.

In recent decades, although we can technically and scientifically do more for our patients than ever before, our personal, trusting relationship with them has deteriorated to the point where it is sometimes adversarial. We have allowed medicine to become a business, guided in many cases by the financial bottom line, rather than by the uncompromising concern for a sick person. Within this fast-moving corporate system, we see too many patients, do too much surgery, and do not have time to develop a close mentoring relationship with our chosen role models, nor with our trainees.[3] The cherished patient–physician relationship has been undermined by our own successful advances. Many of the operations that we do on a routine, daily basis were not even imagined as possible only a few decades ago. Not only can we do more, but also our patients have come to expect perfection from us. Our society seems willing to accept flaws from many sources, but not from physicians and the medical delivery system. This situation is made even more complicated by a system in which individuals purchase their healthcare coverage when they are well and willing to buy the cheapest plan possible; but they utilize their coverage, especially for surgical problems, when they are sick and want the maximum that the system can deliver, without regard to time and cost. No individual has ever admitted that they purchased a cheaper plan, and therefore understood that only limited care should be provided to a loved one who is ill.

Despite these difficulties, we surgeons cannot abandon the needs of our patients and their families. To help them make informed choices, we must communicate completely and compassionately the requisite information about the disease, treatment options, and long-range plans. To do so, we must learn and apply the ethical principle of *truth telling* and the doctrine of *informed consent* for the effective care, which has taken us so long to master. We must also take into account that high-speed communication via the Internet will necessitate reevaluation of issues such as *patient's rights* and *confidentiality*. Surgeons must lead in forging this new era rather than leave it to bureaucrats, politicians, lawyers, and others not intimately involved in patient care.

We cannot rely on intuition or on our own personal value system. Learning the ethical aspects of delivering patient care must become an integral part of the surgical training program, and we must be held accountable for mastering the skillful application of these bioethical principles. After all, the concept of good clinical medicine and surgery implies the best use of scientific, technical, and *ethical* considerations. Just as with medicine and science, bioethics and legal underpinnings of bioethical decision making are evolving all the time. In this chapter, we will not discuss all possible bioethical issues, but will limit ourselves to those that may be of concern to colon and rectal surgeons and to surgery in general. Important issues relating to such matters as professionalism, research ethics, family, business and financial pressures, genetics, and reproductive considerations will be discussed as well.

What Makes the Surgeon Special?

Undergoing major surgery is an extreme experience, which changes people's lives. Surgeons are repeatedly involved in these extreme experiences of others. That makes surgeons uniquely placed among healthcare professionals to understand the experiences of their patients.

Miles Little[4] explains that there are special ethical considerations for surgeons. These include: Rescue, Proximity, Ordeal, Aftermath, and Presence. These terms help to define the ethical relationship between the surgeon and his or her patients. *Rescue* he describes as the first pillar of surgical ethics. It deals with the fact that surgery conveys power, and that power is socially endorsed and may be reinforced by the surgeon's individual charisma; but as with all power it must be constantly renewed and revalidated. Patients have no choice but to acknowledge surgical power when they consult a surgeon. There is always an element of surrender in the surgical relationship, but it is a surrender that presupposes rescue. Accepting rescue as a legitimate principle justifies respect for dependence in the surgical relationship. Surgeons, themselves, sometimes need help and rescue from colleagues when they have trouble with complicated diagnosis, management, or operative procedures. *Proximity* occurs in surgery as in no other act. To operate on persons involves entering their bodies and becoming privy to secrets even denied to the

owner of the body. Little states, "To get to my body, my doctor has to get to my character. He has to go to my soul. He doesn't only have to go through my anus." This proximity to the patient can make special ethical demands on the surgeon. This proximity carries with it the penalties of closeness, and particularly the pains of failure. Some surgeons find that distancing themselves from their patients makes failure easier to bear. Understanding the privileges and risks of proximity is critical for the compassionate surgeon. *Ordeals* are periods of extreme experience, capable of disrupting our lives. The author, Little, explains that all medical encounters are ordeals. Patients yield autonomy, acknowledge dependence, place trust, face risk, confront embodiment and mortality, lose control over time and space, experience alienation, pain, fear, discomfort, suffering, and boredom. Surgeons observe and participate in the lives of patients with serious illnesses. A surgeon, who understands the ordeal of the surgical episode, can better help his or her patient through such extreme experiences. *Aftermath* deals with the reality that surgery leaves physical and psychological scars that may persist for life. It is very difficult to communicate the concept of suffering to someone who has not suffered himself. Little describes surgeons as being in a unique position to understand the existential threats that their patients experience, the sense of mortality and bodily frailty they live with, and the difficulty of explaining extreme experience to others. When death approaches our patients, we must remember, not deny, our own mortality. Such an approach takes courage and a sense of personal security, and this does not suit everyone, neither patient, nor surgeon. *Presence*, as a virtue and a duty, is what the patient desires of the surgeon during all phases of the surgical encounter. Most surgeons have the stamina and cognitive ability to be present for their patients, but not all of us process the personal attributes of charisma, confidence, energy, and empathy, which are necessary to engender *trust* from our patients and our staff. Sometimes, amazingly, our mere presence means more to our patients than defects in the manner with which we deal with them. Even if we cannot teach sensitivity, we can emphasize the importance of surgical presence.

Thus, surgeons are privileged to lead lives of great complexity and moral richness. We can acquire a profound understanding and recognition of patient experience and suffering. Our proximity to patients seeking rescue, facing ordeals, and experiencing the aftermath of surgery, presents us with a great challenge.

Unique Problems of Surgery

Surgeons, unlike other members of the healthcare team, take on a different level of responsibility as they encounter patients. For the surgeon, the initial contact may just be the beginning of a longer-term relationship. With no previously established doctor–patient relationship, the surgeon and the patient may well be heading to the operating room for sometimes massive and sometimes potentially "futile" surgery. The surgeon and the surgical team take on the continued responsibility of the operative procedure itself, the postoperative care, and usually the long-term follow-up and management of any complications and dilemmas that may result from the initial encounter. This intense relationship is often established very quickly and under frequently adverse circumstances. The family and religion may not be known, the patient may be unconscious, and certainly will be once the procedure starts.

Arthur R. Derse nicely delineates the array of ethical issues that arise in delivering surgical care. These include: *informed consent, refusal of treatment, determination of decision-making capacity, treating patients despite their refusal, maintaining confidentiality* while respecting the duty to warn others, *limiting treatment* over issues of "futility," *treating pain* at the end of life, and acting as a *Good Samaritan*. Unlike surgeons, people in most professions have the luxury of time, and the opportunity to redo their work to remedy any mistakes. Attorneys can appeal their cases. Accountants can file an amended return. Movie directors can yell, "Cut! Take two!" and reshoot the scene. All doctors understand that they will probably be second-guessed. As everyone who has ever watched a television police drama knows, the first thing a police officer must say to an arrested person is the famous *Miranda* warning. What most people do not realize is that the requirement for those warnings is the result of a Supreme Court decision rendered in June of 1966. As a practical matter, the court was telling the arresting police officer, in the heat of making an arrest, that he should have known something, which took the court system 3 years to contemplate and research. The bottom line for surgeons who work under the same kinds of time pressures is to do what you think is best. You must use your judgment, based on your medical knowledge and your experience. You are on the front line, and you do not have the luxury of waiting 3 years for the Supreme Court to tell you how to handle a potential situation. However, you also want to be as scrupulous as possible in making sure that bioethical and legal guidelines are followed, both for the benefit of the patient, and, frankly, as protection for yourself.

Although it is crucial for the practice of medicine in all fields to be familiar with bioethical concepts, it is unrealistic to be expected to be knowledgeable about the nuances requiring detailed understanding of controversial bioethical dilemmas. However, it is important for surgeons to have a working knowledge of general medical ethical principles and how these principles affect decisions involved with treating patients. Our goal will be to distill these general bioethical concepts and their underlying applications to specific situations, which you may face, into a cogent and concise tool for surgeons to use routinely, to include as part of their training, and to have as a reference resource. For specific dilemmas, time permitting, surgeons should obtain an opinion from the hospital ethics consultation service and/or from hospital counsel. By doing so, one can gain the experience and imprimatur of opinions from those who have dealt with such issues

and whose training gives them the experience to deal with them in a knowledgeable way. It also serves as a cushion of knowledge for the physician when discussing the matter with a patient or the family. Surgeons should do all they can for the patient, while at the same time, doing what they need to do to protect themselves from personal risk and possibly from negative legal ramifications.

Similarly, doctors have a duty to themselves to avoid situations that violate their own personal beliefs, whether religious or medical. This includes thinking a step or two ahead of the current situation to know what the ramifications of a course of treatment may be. If the anticipated actions may violate a doctor's own personal tenants, he or she should refer the patient to another physician. The most obvious of these situations comes up with regard to religious beliefs. If, for example, a doctor has religious beliefs that would preclude *withdrawal of life support*, the doctor should be very careful about getting into a situation with a patient that might later dictate putting someone on life support. It may, down the line, become bioethically or medically appropriate to *withdraw* life support. If a physician cannot do that, she needs to know that up front and be prepared to withdraw from the case. A similar situation involves doctors who do not believe in *abortion*. They should not get themselves into medical situations in which an emergency termination of a pregnancy may become the best medically viable option. You must always be prepared to protect yourself *and* your patients and must recognize your duties, both legal and ethical. You need to be aware of these duties and to avoid situations in which they may come into conflict. This may be very difficult at times.

Principles of Bioethics

General Concepts

Philosophical Principles

Two major fundamental theoretical philosophical concepts exist for constructing a theory of ethics: *deontologic* and *consequentialist*. A deontologic theory relies on *rules* whereas a consequentialist theory relies on *outcomes*.[2] From these theories are derived *principles of ethics*, such as those delineated by Beauchamp and Childress[5]: respect for *autonomy* (patient self-determination), *beneficence* ("doing good"), *nonmaleficence* ("do no harm"), and *justice* (fairness).

Respect for Autonomy

Adult patients with decision-making capacity have a right to their preferences regarding their own health care. This right is grounded on the legal doctrine of *informed consent*. This means that patients must give their voluntary consent to treatment after receiving all appropriate and relevant information about the nature of their problem, the expected consequences of the recommended treatment, and treatment alternatives.

This is probably the most crucial legal concept in bioethics. It simply means that you as a physician cannot *touch* a person without first getting permission, and without telling the individual of the possible ramifications of that "touching." Touching someone without his or her consent is, in legal terms, a "battery," which could result in a lawsuit for damages. Therefore, the principle is: *medical treatment without consent is a battery*. The first major case in this area said "Every human being of adult years and sound mind has a right to determine what shall be done with his own body; and a surgeon who performs an operation without his patient's consent commits an assault, for which he is liable in damages. . . . This is true except in cases of emergency where the patient is unconscious and where it is necessary to operate before consent can be obtained."[6] This case was decided before the concept of *living wills* and *durable powers of attorney* came into being. These documents both facilitate and complicate the consent process because *consent* must be obtained, if time permits, through these documents or via surrogate decision making. Subsequent cases refined the requirements of consent to add to the concept of *informed consent*. The courts now require the patient not only to *consent* to the procedure, either themselves or through a proper surrogate, but to be given sufficient information to make an *informed* decision. The courts have held that the quality and quantity of information given to the patient must be sufficient for the reasonable patient to understand, not the doctor. The law has established the doctrine of the *reasonable man* to be used in deciding what is acceptable in many areas of delivering emergency surgical care.

Doctors are duty bound to respect the autonomy of each competent patient. The patient is the ultimate decision maker about what he or she wants. The doctor may differ, even vehemently, with the patient's decision; however, the patient has the final say. There are exceptions to this rule also, such as the patient who demands a certain kind of treatment that the doctor knows will not be efficacious. Permitting *autonomy* to trump *nonmaleficence* poses a serious problem. A simple example of this is a patient who demands antibiotics to treat a viral infection. Giving the requested antibiotic complies with the *autonomy* principle; however, in the long run, it is conceivable that giving an antibiotic in such a case would violate the principle of *nonmaleficence*, would impose the concept of *futility*, and in the long run might enhance the capacity of bacteria to become resistant to certain antibiotics, thus even bringing into play the concept of *justice*. Even this simple example illustrates how medical ethical conundrums are frequently the result of *conflicting duties*.

If the patient is unable to make his or her own decision, the treating surgeon must respect the decision made by a surrogate decision maker, such as one designated in a healthcare *durable power of attorney*.

Beneficence

The principle of *beneficence*, simply stated, involves the duty of the physician to act in the best interest of his or her patients. *Beneficence* is *doing good*, and is the reason most of us chose to become doctors. Beneficence, or doing good, is probably the universal tenet of the medical profession.

Nonmaleficence

Nonmaleficence is essentially the old philosophical principle, "first, do no harm." It derives from knowing that patient encounters with surgeons can prove harmful as well as helpful. This principle includes not doing harm, preventing harm, and removing harmful conditions. For those physicians caring for patients in an emergency environment, it also includes the concept of security, protecting oneself and one's team, as well as the patient, from harm.[7]

This concept also incorporates the principle of *avoiding killing*. This seems very obvious on its face value; however, what is a doctor to do when confronted with a situation in which the administration of sufficient medication to alleviate the pain of a patient might have the *secondary effect* of diminishing respiration, and actually hastening the patient's death? This is, of course, the crux of the major debate that is ongoing over *physician-assisted suicide*, if not actual *euthanasia*. There are other situations in which avoiding killing must be taken into account. *Abortion* presents another situation which, depending on your personal beliefs, might fall into that same category. This could create a conflict between the duty to respect the autonomy of the patient and the personal religious beliefs of the treating physician. This same conflict has recently, and intensely, come into play over the issue of research and therapeutic utilization of *embryonic stem cells*.

Justice

Justice is *fairness*. It is required to ensure that medical decisions are made with reason and honesty. Selfish or biased influences must be recognized and avoided.[8] For many, the term justice includes the concept of *distributive justice*. This form of *justice* includes not only the surgeon's obligation to an *individual patient* but to fairness in the allocation of resources for the good of the *broader society*. It is this concept of justice that becomes the basis for society-wide healthcare policy determination. *Distributive justice* implies that all individuals and groups should share in society's benefits and burdens. This presents an ethical challenge for the surgeon, dealing with an individual patient, who mistakenly believes that she should limit or terminate care based on a need to limit healthcare resource expenditures for the *good of society*.[7] It was this temptation to place the good of society before the good of an individual that led the physicians of Europe to fall prey to the fallacious doctrines being promulgated by the Nazi government.[9]

Surgeons should be prepared to respect and seek to understand people from many cultures and from diverse socioeconomic groups. In the United States, emergency facilities are obligated to provide necessary care to all patients, regardless of ability to pay. Our current business-based medical delivery system makes it difficult to abide by the principle of having *access* to appropriate inpatient and follow-up medical care dictated by the patient's financial situation. Provision of emergency, and most elective, surgical treatment should not be based on gender, age, race, socioeconomic status, or cultural background. No patient should ever be abused, demeaned, or given substandard care.[1]

Religion and Medical Ethics

In many societies, religion has been looked upon as the determinant of ethical norms. In our American society, we are multicultural with no single religion holding dominance over the entire population. Therefore, a value-based approach to ethical issues depends on the individual patient's values. However, religion still influences bioethical concepts and decisions. Clinical bioethics, in fact, uses many decision-making methods, arguments, and ideals that originated from religion. It is also important for the individual clinician to understand his or her own personal spirituality in order to relate better to patients and families, representing a broad diversity of religious and ethnic backgrounds. Although religions may appear dissimilar, most are based on some form of the Golden Rule, which holds "do unto others as you would have them do unto you." Problems frequently arise when trying to apply religion-based rules to specific clinical, ethical situations. In so-called modern times, the United States began turning away from a reliance on religious principles, relying instead for answers based on more generic secular principles; and the medical/surgical community was no exception. As previously described, we have come to rely instead on the four ethical principles of *autonomy*, *beneficence*, *nonmaleficence*, and *fairness*. These are the principles that have guided medical ethical thinking and have become instrumental in forming healthcare policies in the United States and other Western countries over the past three decades.[7]

In a recent survey of physicians' attitudes toward spirituality in clinical practice, 85% said physicians should be aware of the patient's religious and spiritual beliefs. The survey went on to show that although many physicians believe that they should inquire about their patients' beliefs, fewer than 10% of doctors actually do so, even for their dying patients. There is no hard data to support the benefits of taking a spiritual history, but there is some indirect evidence in support of the practice. It is known that religion is one of the most common ways by which patients cope with medical illness. Religious beliefs are known to be significant influences on medical decisions, especially those made by patients with serious illnesses. In addition, the faith community is a primary source of support for many medically ill patients, and such social support is associated with better adherence to therapy and improved medical outcomes. Several surveys have revealed that, from the patient's point of view, satisfaction with the emotional and spiritual aspects of care had one of the *lowest* ratings among all clinical care indicators and was one of the highest areas in need of quality improvement.[10]

The purpose for taking even a brief spiritual or religious history is to learn how patients cope with their illnesses, the kinds of support systems available to them in the community, and to learn of any strongly held beliefs that might influence the delivery of medical care. Venturing into this delicate area is obviously fraught with some hazards. We must be extremely cautious about prescribing religion to nonreligious patients, forcing a spiritual history on patients who are not religious, causing patients to believe our practice and specific ways, attempting to provide spiritual counsel to patients, and arguing with patients over religious matters.[10] It is also imperative for us as surgeons to be comfortable enough with our own beliefs to allow our patients to *pray for us*, according to the faith of their own religion. No comment more than a simple and sincere "thank you" is usually indicated.

Legal Principles

General Concepts

Types of Law

In the United States, law is created in one of two systems: *Federal* or *State*, and is made by judges (*common law*), legislatures (*statutory law*), and executive agencies empowered by legislatures (*regulatory law*). The fundamental document that creates and delineates these powers is the Constitution. *Civil law*, including malpractice, is usually enforced by *monetary judgments*. *Criminal law*, including physician-assisted suicide, is usually enforced by *fines* and/or *imprisonment*.[2]

There are three kinds of law that affect the practice of surgery: *statutes*, *regulations* promulgated by an administrative agency, pursuant to a statute, and *case law*. The legislatures are the designated policy-making entities in our system; *regulations* are written to comply with legislative directives; and the courts are charged with resolving disputes between parties, usually as directed by *statute*, if there is a relevant one. Courts issue written opinions when there is a conflict that results in a lawsuit, especially when the interpretation of a statute or a regulation is in question. The most difficult situations are those in which the court is faced with a matter of "first impression," which the legislature has not specifically addressed. The courts, and their written opinions, on this type of case, frequently ask the legislature for guidance in future situations. Until the legislature acts, the written opinion of the court is the only guidance physicians have, and hospital counsel sometimes must interpret this.

Doctors should be generally familiar with *state law*. There are different state laws on many bioethical matters, such as definition of death, competency, organ donation, and now the use of embryonic stem cells, even for research only. Many doctors move from state to state during their careers, and general understanding of state laws governing situations that may confront them in surgical situations is crucial. However, most important legal principles that apply to ethical dilemmas in delivering surgical care are widely accepted among several

states. There are some glaring discrepancies in these com-
monalities, including the neurologic *criteria for death* (a person may be legally dead in one state and not in another) and
the legality of *physician-assisted suicide* (punishable as a
crime in all states except Oregon).

Statutory Law

Statutory law is made by legislatures and includes such issues
as *the statute of limitations*, which defines how long after an
adverse event a patient is able to sue a physician for malpractice, and, in some states, statutes on *informed consent*.

The Emergency Medical Treatment and Labor Act
(EMTALA) is another example of a *federal statutory law*. It
was originally enacted as part of the Consolidated Omnibus
Budget Reconciliation Act of 1986. Congress enacted
EMTALA as a remedy for "patient dumping." The legislature
was particularly concerned about hospitals refusing to render
emergency care because of lack of insurance or the economic
ability to pay, but soon came to realize that care was also
being refused on the basis of race or other discriminatory criteria. The Act requires that a basic screening examination
be provided to all patients seeking care. It therefore became
illegal, as well as unethical, to withhold therapy from the
poor just because they do not have the ability to pay.[11]

Compilation of statistics from major county hospitals
across the country concluded that as many as 650,000 patients
were "dumped" annually, and the resulting transfer led to substandard care and/or life-threatening situations in 25%–33%
of that number. The economic impact of EMTALA on hospitals and physicians has been enormous. Patients without the
means to pay for medical care know that they cannot be
turned away from the emergency room. Therefore, they use it
as their *primary care facility*. That means that hospitals,
physicians, and surgeons are carrying the burden of the
nation's uninsured, often without adequate compensation. For
many healthcare facilities, this money lost in the emergency
room can mean the difference between bankruptcy and
solvency.[12]

Regulatory Law

These administrative laws are created by regulatory agencies
including State Medical Boards. Recent examples of regulatory
law include not only EMTALA but also the recently implemented Health Insurance Portability and Accountability Act of
1996 (HIPAA). HIPAA, as EMTALA, was intended to protect
patients' rights of privacy and to guarantee them continuation
of health insurance coverage should they change employers.
Also, like EMTALA, HIPAA has taken on many ramifications
threatening a huge economic impact on the escalating costs of
delivering medical care. Although the good aspects of it are
necessary and noble, the burdens of increased costs will be
crippling to some healthcare facilities and will probably significantly curtail many clinical research endeavors.

Malpractice

The public and the legal community do not seem to understand
that there is an element of uncertainty and unpredictability in
a biological system. They seem to understand that 11 men on
a playing field cannot score a touchdown on every play, but a
surgeon is held to a standard of achieving perfection on every
operation. An ethical, as well as legal, consideration is: what
to do when we fall short of perfection or, worse, make a bla-
tant error while trying to do the best we can. Several factors
come into play. Who is responsible if you did not actually
do the damage yourself? What do you tell the patient and the
family? How do you comply with the policies of legal counsel
and risk management within your own institution?

Many successful legal actions against surgeons have been
based on withholding information about risks, complications,
or adverse outcomes. A surgeon must be able to admit to
unwanted events in an honest and compassionate manner. It is
clearly possible to accept *responsibility* without admitting
negligence. It never hurts to admit that you are sorry things
had not gone exactly as planned, but that you must go forward, as efficiently as possible, to correct the situation. At this
point a surgeon should never hesitate to seek consultative
assistance whenever it might seem helpful. It is never helpful
to shift blame to a resident, an assistant, a nurse, a referring
physician, or the institution itself. If anyone is to be sued,
everyone will be sued, and divisiveness usually damages
everyone. Unfortunately, it is also of little help to blame the
patient and to invoke the existence of adequate *informed consent*. How nice it would be to tell the morbidly obese person
that his postoperative complications should be blamed on his
own indiscretions. Even informed consent, including risks
based on the patient's known status of precarious health, is of
little help. A surgeon is not absolved of responsibility and
concern by claiming, "I told you so!"

Judges, not the legislature, establish the standards that constitute medical malpractice. The familiar elements of medical
malpractice include *duty*, *breach*, *causation*, and *damages*.
Decisions are based on the standard of care, and judges have
developed the methods of determining the standards over
many years, after the review of many cases. Thus, the courts
rule on a specific set of facts that have already occurred. This
is extremely frustrating for those practitioners of surgery who
need to know what the law *would say* in a particular situation,
as it is occurring, not in retrospect.

Unfortunately, resolution of controversy over medical and
surgical ethical issues has been the domain of law, not philosophy or medicine. So far, perhaps because of legal constraints, medicine has been unable to "police itself." Because
the law has come to champion individual rights and hold
physicians liable for malpractice, it has served to condemn
medical *paternalism* as it has elevated *patients' rights*. This
has had the damaging effect of encouraging many physicians
to become more concerned with avoiding litigation than with
"doing the right thing." The law has had understandable

difficulty in sorting out the complicated *physician–patient relationship*, and thus law does not mandate ethical behavior in these relationships.

A Familiar Case-management System

Physician-based Ethics

General Principles

Mark Siegler, a physician, and his coauthors of "Clinical Ethics," the fifth edition, present a technique for using *case analysis* as a practical approach to solving ethical dilemmas in clinical medicine. Contrary to most texts on healthcare ethics that are organized around the ethical *principles* of respect for *autonomy, beneficence, nonmaleficence,* and *fairness,* their publication provides a straightforward *method* for clinicians to use in sorting out the pertinent facts and values of any case into an orderly pattern that facilitates the discussion and resolution of ethical problems.[13] Their technique corresponds to the way in which clinicians usually analyze actual cases. It assimilates the ethical principles and circumstances that comprise a method to facilitate the analysis of cases involving ethical issues.

The Clinical Ethics System

Jonsen and his colleagues[13] suggest that every clinical case, especially those raising an ethical dilemma, should be analyzed by means of the following four topics: 1) *medical indications,* 2) *patient preferences,* 3) *quality of life,* and 4) *contextual features,* defined as the social, economic, legal, and administrative context in which the case occurs. The authors emphasize that although the facts of each case can differ, these four topics are always relevant. The topics organize the various facts of the particular case and at the same time call attention to the ethical principles appropriate for each case. Their intent is to show clinicians that these four topics provide a systematic method of identifying and analyzing the ethical problems occurring in clinical medicine. See Table 53-1.[13]

We find it extremely helpful to use this case management system, which is very similar to our usual approach of managing a patient and his or her problem by taking a history in an organized manner and proceeding to do a physical examination, analyze the laboratory data, and arrive at a plan for managing the case. Examination of the table shows that the authors have clearly related to clinical situations the basic ethical principles previously described. They go on to emphasize that most ethical conflicts can be resolved by

TABLE 53-1. The four topics: case analysis in clinical ethics

■ MEDICAL INDICATIONS	■ PATIENT PREFERENCES
The Principles of Beneficence and Nonmaleficence	The Principle of Respect for Autonomy
1. What is the patient's medical problem? history? diagnosis? prognosis?	1. Is the patient mentally capable and legally competent? Is there evidence of incapacity?
2. Is the problem acute? chronic? critical? emergent? reversible?	2. If competent, what is the patient stating about preferences for treatment?
3. What are the goals of treatment?	3. Has the patient been informed of benefits and risks, understood this information, and given consent?
4. What are the probabilities of success?	4. If incapacitated, who is the appropriate surrogate? Is the surrogate using appropriate standards for decision making?
5. What are the plans in case of therapeutic failure?	5. Has the patient expressed prior preferences, e.g., Advance Directives?
6. In sum, how can this patient be benefited by medical and nursing care, and how can harm be avoided?	6. Is the patient unwilling or unable to cooperate with medical treatment? If so, why?
	7. In sum, is the patient's right to choose being respected to the extent possible in ethics and law?
■ QUALITY OF LIFE	■ CONTEXTUAL FEATURES
The Principles of Beneficence and Nonmaleficence and Respect for Autonomy	The Principles of Loyalty and Fairness
1. What are the prospects, with or without treatment, for a return to normal life?	1. Are there family issues that might influence treatment decisions?
2. What physical, mental, and social deficits is the patient likely to experience if treatment succeeds?	2. Are there provider (physicians and nurses) issues that might influence treatment decisions?
3. Are there biases that might prejudice the provider's evaluation of the patient's quality of life?	3. Are there financial and economic factors?
4. Is the patient's present or future condition such that his or her continued life might be judged undesirable?	4. Are there religious or cultural factors?
5. Is there any plan and rationale to forego treatment?	5. Are there limits on confidentiality?
6. Are there plans for comfort and palliative care?	6. Are there problems of allocation of resources?
	7. How does the law affect treatment decisions?
	8. Is clinical research or teaching involved?
	9. Is there any conflict of interest on the part of the providers or the institution?

Source: Reprinted from Jonsen et al.,[13] with permission from McGraw-Hill Companies.

falling back on the *medical indications* that represent the medical facts of the case. This information, plus the second category of *patient preferences*, almost always will lead the clinical surgeon to a resolution of the ethical problem. If the ethical dilemma results from conflict among the patient, the family, the healthcare team, or institutional policy, then adequate resolution may become dependent on applying analysis of the additional categories, *quality of life* and the array of *contextual features*. It is amazing how often reviewing and relying on what the medical facts of the situation actually are can clarify the intensity and emotion of even the most complex situation.

Specific Dilemmas of Colon and Rectal Surgery

Special Considerations for Colon and Rectal Surgeons

Attempting to explain, much less to justify, a career in colon and rectal surgery is never simple. The words, and the title itself, create consternation and the need to tell us the last circulating joke, which most of us have heard multiple times over. Telling what we do and who we are is never good dinner conversation and can present seemingly insurmountable challenges to represent ourselves at our children's eighth-grade career-day programs. We understand, however, that we have chosen a surgical career that includes resolving perplexing problems of anal-rectal disease, pelvic floor malfunction, and incontinence which cause daily significant discomfort for the patient and have frequently been mismanaged, for a long period of time, by our nonspecialized colleagues. This places us, frequently, in the position of not only having to resolve the technical surgical aspect of the problem, but also having to explain the previous misdiagnosis or mismanagement by other physicians, a challenging *ethical dilemma*.

In addition to the seemingly simple anorectal disease, most of our careers also encompass management of some of the most complicated inflammatory bowel disease and cancer. This casts us into a position of daily having to deal with multiple components of the modern healthcare team. We know that no one should ever have to die from colorectal cancer because it can be prevented or diagnosed at an early, or even premalignant, stage. Thus, we become actively involved with screening, preventive measures, understanding genetic predisposition to disease, and even the need for what has come to be called *preemptive surgery*. Because of the diseases that we treat, we must understand the science of current genetics as well as the appropriate clinical utilization of genetic testing, including the challenges of respecting *confidentiality* and requesting *genetic counseling* to deal with the long-term aspects involving not only the patient but family members who may not wish to be included in the discovery

of genetic predisposition to disease. All of this presents intense need for dealing with frequent ethical challenges, especially the need for increasing *preemptive surgery*, subjecting a *well person* to major surgery with significant risk of complications or impact on lifestyle and body image. In fact, because of our experience and expertise in the construction and management of intestinal stomas, we are often confronted with such *quality-of-life* issues as body image and impairment of sexual function.

Dealing with our many patients, and their families, who have such inflammatory bowel diseases as Crohn's disease, requires us to maintain long-term, perhaps for generations, contact with and care for our patients, much the contrary of our public image of being just "technicians" who do a short-term repair job and then have no other, ongoing relationship with our patients.

Because of the complexity of the diseases on which we operate, including those in areas with difficult access and high risk of postoperative complications and recurrence of malignant processes, we often find ourselves on the leading edge of surgical innovation and instrumentation. This creates the ethical challenges of differentiating acceptable surgical *innovation* from truly *investigative* ventures that require research protocols and institutional approval. We must deal with the interpretation and implementation of *autonomy* verses *paternalism* as we guide our patients to the best choices for their care. Sick patients and those with advanced cancer will grasp at straws. They want anything on earth that might help. In such a situation, it is important for the surgeon-scientist to avoid exploiting this universal hope of sick patients by performing an operation that is inadequately tested.[14] Because of these challenges of innovation, we are also frequently thrust into the complex relationship between ethical surgery and the pharmaceutic and instrumentation industries.

Needless to say, because of the many things that we have to offer and the need to be concerned with our own long-term financial security in the face of reimbursement and legal challenges, we must walk the narrow line between providing the best care possible for all of our patients and complying with our own personal needs and those of our families. Claude Organ explained that, "So much of our orientation today serves to erode our spirit as caregivers." He goes on to say that surgery is under increased public surveillance, and we are consumed by endless paperwork, administrative hassles, ponderous bureaucracy, professional liability concerns, inadequate reimbursement for our work, limited access for our patients, an impersonalized system, and increasingly burdensome documentation. He cites the increasing federal mandates of the Health Insurance Portability and Accountability Act, the Emergency Medical Treatment and Active Labor Act, and the Program for Appropriate Technology in Health audits. He quotes the highly respected surgical mentor, Haile Debas as saying, "Professional status is not an inherent right but one granted by society. . . . This obligates surgeons to put their patients' interests above their own."[15]

Categories of Patient Encounters

Severe Emergency: Life in Immediate Jeopardy

An example would be a critically ill person brought in from a severe motor vehicle accident or one who has suffered a serious gunshot wound. Certainly there is no preestablished doctor–patient relationship, there is little chance that there will be a reliable surrogate, and many ethicists have questioned if a patient in such dire straits ever has *decision-making capacity*.

Urgent: Serious Problem Needing Surgery

An example would be a patient brought in with peritonitis. The individual may be in hypovolemic shock, is terrified, is in great pain, but is still cognizant of the situation and what is happening. There certainly is no preexisting *doctor–patient relationship*, and no one is absolutely sure of the *decisional capacity*, especially if the patient disagrees with the recommendation of the surgical team. In a case such as this, in which there is some but not much time, the presence of a *surrogate* and clearly described *advance directives* would be extremely helpful.

Semi-elective: Will Probably Need Surgery

An example would be an elderly patient with known extensive intraabdominal cancer who presents with a significant, unresolving intestinal obstruction. It is clear that the obstruction can only be relieved by surgery, but it is not clear that this will be beneficial to the patient. In this case, determination of *decisional capacity*, the existence of *advance directives*, or the presence of a reliable *surrogate* is very important; and there is enough time to pursue the intended desires of this patient.

Autonomy/Decision-making Capacity/Competency

General Concepts

Autonomy Versus Paternalism: Trust Is the Bridge

Individual freedom is one of the basic tenets of modern bioethics. This freedom is usually referred to as *autonomy*. This principle implies that a person should be free to make his or her own decisions. It is somewhat the antithesis of the medical profession's long practiced *paternalism* whereby the physician acted on what he or she thought was *good* for the patient, whether or not the patient agreed. The concept of *autonomy* applies to many interpersonal relationships, and is essentially a respect for each person as an individual.

It has been difficult for many physicians, perhaps especially surgeons, to accept the principle of *patient autonomy*. This is not difficult to understand because accepting this principle implies a change in the physician's relationship with the patient. The physician must now be a partner in his or her patients' care; must become an educator, teaching uninformed patients enough about their diseases to make rational decisions; and most distressing, to allow autonomous patients to make foolish choices. For physicians dedicated to helping their patients, allowing them to select what the physician considers a terrible treatment option, or even refusing treatment altogether, is a very frustrating change.[7]

However, experienced surgeons know that their patients significantly rely on them for guidance through complicated choices, often where life itself is on the line. This is, of course, a form of *paternalism* which our patients request and to which they are entitled. The key to accomplishing this ethically and successfully is based on the principle of *trust*. For surgeons, the establishing of this trust must begin at the inception of the relationship, and sometimes must be very quickly accomplished. It is sometimes very difficult for our nonsurgical colleagues to understand and accept this element of *paternalism* required in the surgeon–patient relationship.

The crucial issue for the surgeon seeking autonomous informed consent is the *decision-making capacity* or *competence* of the patient involved. Understanding the differences between these terms is important, especially if the patient disagrees with the advice of the surgeon or refuses potentially life-sustaining treatment.

The determination of *decision-making capacity* involves more than just completing a mental status examination and includes the ability of the patient to take in information, to evaluate a decision based on personal values, to make a decision, and to communicate the choice of decision to the physician. The concept of medical *decision-making capacity* is one based on the evaluation by the team providing medical and surgical care. This is distinguishable from a *legal determination* of *incompetence*. A patient is always assumed to be *legally competent* unless a *court* has declared otherwise. For example, patients may not have been declared incompetent by a court but may have lost the capacity to make decisions about their medical care because of their current medical status, including such conditions as intoxication, stroke, hypoxia, blood loss, dementia, or severe trauma. The determination of *decision-making capacity* varies in stringency with the seriousness of the impact of the decision. For example, the more severe the risk posed by the patient's decision, the more stringent should be the standard of determining capacity. This provides an increased protection for patients of questionable capacity when the potential harm from their decision is greater. This reaches the pinnacle of importance when a patient refuses treatment for a potentially life-threatening condition. These decisions are often difficult to make in the emergency environment, and the treating surgeon must sometimes make practical ethical decisions that go beyond the basic law of informed consent.

Refusal of Treatment

Ethical dilemmas usually occur when there is disagreement among the patient, the family, and the healthcare team. The clearest example is a patient's refusal to accept the recommended treatment. This is especially critical for the patient who has *decision-making capacity* and refuses potentially life-sustaining treatment. The United States Supreme Court, in the *Cruzan case*, upheld the right of persons to refuse lifesaving medical treatment, including resuscitation, ventilators, artificial nutrition and hydration, and lifesaving blood transfusions. The court based its decision on "the right of every individual to the possession and control of his own person, free from all restraint or interference of others, unless by clear and unquestionable authority of law under the *liberty interest*, protected by the Due Process clause of the Fourteenth Amendment of the Constitution." The Courts have, however, identified four *state interests* that override the refusal or termination of medical treatment on behalf of competent and incompetent persons, including the preservation of human life, the protection of the interests of innocent third persons, the prevention of suicide, and the maintenance of the integrity of the medical profession.

In exercising their rights under the autonomy principle, each competent patient has a right to refuse treatment, even if the results of such refusal will be their death. This type of situation comes up most often in the case of religious or cultural beliefs. Jehovah's Witnesses are probably the most familiar example of this type of dilemma. They refuse to accept blood transfusions, based on their religious beliefs. Such refusal, especially where major surgery is indicated, clearly poses the likelihood of avoidable death. Still, the competent patient's *autonomy must rule*. There may be situations in which the treating surgeon believes that the competency of the patient refusing treatment may be in doubt. In such a case, if time permits, in order to protect the doctor and the hospital; it may be appropriate to get a court order permitting the indicated procedure or blood transfusion. The courts will weigh the possible benefits of the treatment against the potential negative effects, risks, and the potential burdens on the patient; and they will issue a ruling. This ruling will insulate the treating physician and the institution from legal liability. There are situations in which parents or guardians are involved in refusal to accept and allow treatment on behalf of minors. These are the most common instances in which court intervention is sought, and to resolve the problem the courts must balance the best interests of the child against the desires of the parents.

For sure, *refusal* of a life-sustaining medical treatment should be accompanied by a full assessment of *decision-making capacity* and by an understanding from the patient of the consequences of refusal. If uncertainty prevails, the surgeon on the firing line should still "err on the side of life."

Telling the Truth/Disclosing Errors

General Concepts

Physicians have a duty to tell the truth to their patients. This seems so obvious that it merits no further discussion. However, there may be circumstances where telling the *whole truth* to a patient will have a negative impact on his or her overall well-being. If the physician believes that telling the patient everything about the condition in question, which is a duty, will have a dramatic negative effect on the patient's well being, the physician must decide which duty is more important in each particular situation.

Truth telling also would apply in situations involving *medical mistakes*, even those mistakes that are minor and arguably have no detrimental effect on the patient. To illustrate this point, let us consider a doctor awakened in the middle of the night who orders 1 mg of a drug, when the appropriate dose is 0.1 mg. The overdose has no detrimental effect on the patient, so does the doctor still have a duty to reveal the error that he made? Ostensibly, this question would seem to be easy to answer: just tell the truth! However, if informing a patient whose confidence in the medical profession is very low, and his mental stability might be diminished by finding out about a medical error, notwithstanding the fact that the error had no detrimental effect, do doctors still have a duty to tell the truth? In this situation, it might violate the duty of nonmaleficence by doing something that will hurt the patient.

Prognosis: Balance Between Giving False Hope and Removing All Hope

We are all involved in operations in which the desired outcomes are not met. Managing these patients through the entire course of their disease, and sometimes death, is an important part of being a good physician and surgeon. This becomes even more important as the population ages and we encounter older patients with multiple comorbidities. Especially in these older, high-risk, patients, even what is anticipated to be a fairly straightforward operation may have unexpected, adverse results. It forces us to remember the old adage that not everyone needs to die with an incision. Predicting prognosis, much less conveying it well to the patient and the family, is a difficult skill with little data to help us. We need to communicate with the public the fact that we would welcome the ability to accurately forecast outcomes especially for older patients, with higher risks, and in emergency situations. We truly cannot distinguish which ones may actually do well from such high-risk operations. This necessitates us, as surgeons, to assume an important role in providing *palliative care* even when complete surgical *cure* is no longer a possibility.[16]

Discussing prognosis with our patients and their families is one of the situations that forces us most carefully to choose our words precisely. Even when we are forced by patients and families to use specific statistics, we must use them in a manner that is helpful and not totally destructive of hope. It helps to explain that statistics are better for 100 people rather than for any given individual. It can be very expeditious for us to use statistics as a form of *truth dumping*, but such an act can be devastating to a terrified, desperate, and inadequately informed patient who is desperately clinging for any possible hope.

Patients with Impaired Decision-making Capacity

Examples of patients having impaired decision-making capacity include minors, mentally handicapped persons, those with organic brain disease or in toxic states, and those with psychiatric conditions, including suicidal risk. Determining the point at which a minor has the capacity to make medical decisions is often very complicated and varies with the laws of an individual state.[17] For example, an "emancipated" minor can make his or her own medical decisions. This includes individuals younger than the age of majority who are living on their own, are married, or are in the military.

Even patients with *Alzheimer's disease* cannot all be regarded as having lost their *decision-making capacity*. Depending on the severity of their disease, they may well be able to participate in much of the decision-making process. This of course depends on the status of their disease and on the complexity and implications of the decision to be made.

Suicidal Patients

Respect for autonomy has always had its limits. When treating a suicidal patient, the surgeon is faced with a conflict between the ethical principle of *beneficence* and *respect for autonomy*. Sorting out this dilemma is usually based on whether the suicidal patient is currently capable of making a rational, autonomous decision. It also raises the perplexing question: "Can suicide sometimes be a rational choice?" Generally, surgeons intervene with the suicidal patient based on the assumption that the person is suffering from mental illness and impaired judgment. This assumption is usually correct, with 90% of suicides being found to be associated with mental illness such as depression, substance abuse, or psychosis.[18]

Therefore, relying on the principle of beneficence, surgeons almost always treat the injuries inflicted by suicidal patients despite their expressed intention to die. The conflict arises when the reasons for suicide appear "good," such as in the case of the terminally ill cancer patient with severe, uncontrollable pain. Is the application of lifesaving intervention truly a beneficent act in the patient's best interest? Several studies have shown that physicians rendering care in the emergency department are not likely to recognize

treatable depression in their patients. These studies go on to confirm that 80% of patients who attempted suicide subsequently show that they do not continue to wish to die. Thus, although some patients might make a rational decision to commit suicide, in most cases, the surgeon delivering care must assume that the person's judgment is impaired, and proceed with full indicated, lifesaving measures.[18]

Advance Directives

General Principles: Talking About Death

Facility in routinely addressing end-of-life issues with surgical patients is critical because it allows the surgeon to raise difficult questions with patients during the earlier phases of their disease process. Often the issues that are most difficult to address when patients near the end of life are those that have not been attended to earlier in the patients' course of treatment. Such early discussion allows the surgeon and the patient to discuss limits on treatment at a time when the patient is able to participate in the process. Usually, we surgeons are intent on cure, and the prospect for death after most of our routine procedures seems very remote. However, these discussions are more important than ever because we now have more options available to prolong life than existed just a few decades ago. In addition, social changes have led to greater participation by patients in the medical decision-making process. With the increasing mobility of our society and the changing allocation of primary care physicians, we as surgeons often do not have the backup of a well-established physician–patient relationship. Add to this the very visible increase in public debate over *euthanasia* and *physician-assisted suicide* and we can understand the concern the public has over perceived, or actual, deficiencies in how patients are managed at the end of life.[19]

When a patient does not have the decision-making capacity to give informed consent, or there is no time to ask the patient or his or her surrogate about treatment preferences, *advance directives* express in written form what the patient's choices would have been if he or she had decision-making capacity. Advance directives include living wills, durable powers of attorney, and other written documents. In 1991, the federal government passed the Patient Self-determination Act (PSDA), which required that healthcare institutions advise and educate patients regarding advance directives. This affected all institutions participating in the Medicare and Medicaid programs. This law was supposed to increase the use of advance directives and thus prevent unwanted care. In fact, a major study of advance directives and seriously ill patients revealed that the PSDA had little impact on health care in the United States. This was revealed in the Study to Understand Prognoses and Preferences for Outcomes and Risks of Treatments (SUPPORT), which showed that only

20% of seriously ill patients had advance directives even after the SUPPORT intervention and the PSDA.[20]

Despite these studies, it is still imperative for surgeons to understand the principles involved and the advantages of advocating for appropriate advance directives for our patients and their families. An *advance directive* is any proactive document stating the patient's wishes in various situations, should they be unable to state their own wishes.

Some states have specific language for each of these documents and provide reciprocity for other states. Both the *living will* and a *durable power of attorney* can be prepared without the benefit of state-approved language as long as the intention of the person executing the document is clear. Such directives provide advanced informed consent for a myriad of courses of treatment, whether it be related to pain medication, "do not resuscitate orders," or management should the individual enter some level of persistent vegetative state. In a complete set of these documents, the patient has given full thought to all of the possibilities that might occur, and has decided what course of treatment would be his or her choice. Unfortunately, most patients have not executed these documents, or they have not given sufficient thought to what their wishes are. Furthermore, many times when a power of attorney is granted to a surrogate decision maker, the surrogate has not had a full discussion of the wishes of the signatory.

Living Will

The *living will*, which was adopted by many states in 1990, is a document suitable for *terminally ill patients* in which the treating physician accepts the patient's wishes regarding withholding of care, including requests restricting heroic resuscitative efforts, in advance. Many state that no life support be used in cases in which meaningful recovery will not occur. In a *living will*, the signatory indicates what his or her choices would be for medical treatment in the situation in which *death is imminent*, and the individual's wishes are unable to be communicated to the treating physician. Under most state laws, *living wills* indicate the signatory's desire to die a natural death and indicate unwillingness to be kept alive by so-called "heroic measures." This usually amounts to a "Do Not Resuscitate" order. In some states, that also indicates the patient's wishes concerning the level of pain medication, hydration, and nutrition, which the patient would desire if he or she lapses into a nondecisional condition. In most states, the activation of the terms of a living will require an *imminent demise* and a second physician's opinion corroborating that determination. Unfortunately, many people believe that the *living will* is the best form of advance directive and do not realize that it is only intended for the *terminally ill*.

Durable Power of Attorney

A *durable power of attorney for health care* specifies a surrogate decision maker in the event that the patient no longer has the capacity to make medical decisions. The *durable power of attorney* is a written document that gives the authority to another person, usually a spouse or relative, to make decisions regarding health care if the patient is incapacitated and unable to make decisions for himself or herself. The reason it is called "durable" is to ensure that the signatory knows that it can be revoked and/or changed at any time. This provides the freedom to change both who the surrogate is and what the patient's stated wishes, if any, are. This is important in situations such as divorce in which the person executing the power of attorney may want to change the surrogate before the divorce becomes final or in those family situations in which dynamics create a desire to change the surrogate.

Thus, the patient designates a *surrogate decision maker* who should participate in all significant treatment decisions and be kept up to date regarding the patient's health care. The *durable power of attorney* works best when the patient has discussed with a surrogate his or her values and beliefs, because these would apply in making complex decisions regarding healthcare issues. If there is no durable power of attorney, surrogate decision makers may be sought based on state laws. There is usually a defined hierarchy regarding surrogate decision makers: spouses, adult children, siblings, and so forth. Such a surrogate decision maker must be acting in the best interest of and according to the wishes and values of the patient. The *durable power of attorney* is a better form of advance directive than the *living will* because, in the former, a surrogate can be educated about the nuances and options regarding each stage of treatment or nontreatment.[20]

Problems

In many situations the surrogate has the legal authority to make a decision, but is not aware of what the patient would want. This is the fault of the patient. All persons, when naming a surrogate decision maker, have a responsibility to fully explain what they would want in certain medical treatment situations. Failure to do so puts the burden on the surrogate to speculate what the patient would do were they able to make the decision.

There are two standards that apply in the situation in which the surrogate has not been informed of the patient's wishes. One is the *substitute judgment* standard. When using this standard, the surrogate bases a decision on a prior expressed statement of the patient's preferences or on an in-depth knowledge of the personality of the patient and a willingness to do what the surrogate believes the *patient*, not the surrogate, would want in that specific situation. The second standard is that of the *best interest* of the patient. This is obviously a far more nebulous concept and occurs when the surrogate has not had any specific communication with the patient about the specific type of situation and is not cognizant of any particular patient preferences. In this situation, the surrogate is supposed to do what he believes is in the best interest of the patient. This is an important distinction to make and emphasizes the difference between doing what the patient would want done in a given situation, as opposed to having someone else decide what he or she thinks is best.

A further problem with advance directives that limit full implementation of medical care is the application of such directives in situations for which they were not intended. An example that confronts the colon and rectal surgeon is an elderly patient who is recovering from a complicated colon resection for curable cancer and develops postoperative pneumonia requiring presumed short-term ventilating support. Should such a patient not be intubated because of an advance directive indicating, "do not resuscitate"? In such a case, it would be a serious error to respect the advance directive and not to treat the patient aggressively. It is clearly probable that the patient would have wanted treatment under these circumstances.

There must also never be confusion when the patient is able to relate his or her preferences to healthcare providers. *Verbal communication takes precedence over any written advance directive*. In addition, when there is any confusion about the advance directive, disagreement among family members, or concern that it was not meant for the clinical circumstance at hand, *advance directives limiting treatment should be ignored in favor of prudent medical care*. In general, it is always wise for healthcare providers to err on the side of life and to begin standard medical treatment. Treatment options, such as mechanical ventilation and hemodynamic support, can always be withdrawn at a later time once issues are resolved and the family is present. In such situations, the hospital *ethics consultation service* can often prove very helpful.

Perhaps the major problem, at this point in time, is that there is little evidence that advance directives have made a significant impact on healthcare delivery in the United States.[20] We, as surgeons, should do all within our power to reverse this situation.

Informed Consent

General Concepts

Studies have revealed that doctors do not adequately inform patients, patients may not understand the information, and such information rarely affects the patient's decision to follow the physician's recommendations. Despite these facts, American courts have long held that a patient's *informed consent* to a medical or surgical procedure or test is *essential*. The physician must give the patient sufficient information to make an intelligent decision before any action is performed. The laws dealing with informed consent require the surgeon to describe to the patient the nature of the procedure, risks, benefits, and alternatives, including no treatment at all. Ethical consensus on just how much disclosure is adequate is still very controversial. What is clear is that permission must be given *voluntarily*, that is, *without coercion* from the

physician or anyone else involved in rendering health care or, especially, those participating in the implementation of a *research* project.

The current interpretation of the law requires several elements to constitute *informed consent*. These are the *criteria* that the physician must disseminate to the patient or acting surrogate to meet that standard:

a. What is the treatment that the doctor wishes to pursue, including a full explanation of the procedure and what it involves, including the necessity for anesthesia and other support functions?
b. For what reason has the doctor selected this particular treatment, including the doctor's judgment as to why this procedure is chosen to alleviate, cure, or minimize the medical/surgical problem?
c. What are the risks of the recommended treatment, including an explanation of both the risks of the treatment itself and of any corollary threats to the patient? Surgeons should, in satisfying this requirement, include discussion of their own particular *experience with the procedure* as well as that of the hospital and the medical/surgical colleagues who will be assisting.
d. What benefits will the patient receive from the proposed treatment? This is similar to the choice of treatment information previously described in that it requires the doctor to explain what the potential benefits will be from the procedure.
e. What are the chances that the proposed treatment will remedy the problem? This is similar to the information included when describing "benefits and risks" and should also include a description of the *past experience* of the surgeon in performing this specific procedure, as well as the *outcomes* that the surgeon has obtained.
f. What alternative treatment options exist for the given problem? This is similar to explaining the choice of treatment but emphasizes what other treatment options are available, and why this surgeon has chosen this particular procedure.
g. What effect will refusal to accept the proposed treatment have on the patient? This must entail a frank discussion of the ramifications of failure to receive the suggested treatment and whether it is life threatening, or of a lesser degree of medical difficulty. This is the part of the discussion in which the surgeon must be most sensitive to the patient's religious, cultural, and ethnic background.

Here the law requires that the sufficiency of the level of information will be judged from the *patient's point of view*, not the doctor's. If a surgeon explains a proposed treatment to the patient in terms that only another surgeon can understand, then the patient is not truly *informed*. This simply boils down to communication skills and the obligation to accurately *record* this discussion in the medical chart before performing the recommended surgical treatment. Every profession has its own terms of terminology or jargon. Physicians must strive to ensure that the language they use is clearly understandable.

Achieving acceptable levels of communication may be complicated by language, cultural, and socioeconomic factors. A manager responsible for building a new jetliner was credited with saying, "The main problem with communication is the illusion that it has actually occurred." All too frequently patients and families come away from discussions with surgeons in which the surgeon thinks he has effectively communicated, and the patient and family seemed to understand, but they did not. Sometimes it just boils down to faith in the doctor, or an individual's unwillingness to reveal his or her lack of comprehension. The physician must use *common sense* in determining whether fully informed consent has truly been granted, taking into account that some cynics claim, "The problem about common sense is that it is not common."

As with every rule of law, there are certain *exceptions* to the requirement for informed consent. When there is an emergency situation that could result in the death of the patient, time is of the essence, and there is no surrogate decision maker present, the *consent requirement is waived*. Similarly, when the situation is not an emergency, but the patient is for one reason or another not able to give consent because of unconsciousness, coma, mental disability, or other cause of inadequate decision-making capacity, and there is no advance directive or surrogate, informed consent is not necessary. There is also a *therapeutic exception* to the rule. If the physician believes that revelation of the normally required information would have a negative effect on the patient's health, fully informed consent is not necessary. This usually arises in the context of a psychiatric patient. Also, when a competent patient *refuses* to receive information upon which to base a decision, this requirement is waived. There can also be a waiver of the necessity for informed consent when the *government* requires certain medical tests or treatment in the face of possible medical or national security emergencies.

A common misconception among those rendering emergency care is that anyone who presents to an emergency facility falls into the *emergency exception* to informed consent. The *emergency exception* allows a physician to treat a patient without obtaining informed consent. This exception requires the following: the patient must be unconscious or without the capacity to make a decision, and no one else legally authorized to make such a decision is available; time must be of the essence in avoiding risk of serious bodily injury or death; and, under the circumstances, the action proposed would be that to which a *reasonable person* would consent. The emergency exception does not apply if the patient has decision-making capacity and is able to communicate a decision about medical care.[2]

Patient–Surgeon Relationship

Siegler[21] explains that the three central ethical aspects of modern surgical practice are: 1) clinical competence; 2) respect for patients and their healthcare decisions; and 3) maintaining the primacy of the patient's needs in the face of

external pressures in a changing social, economic, and political climate. Successful clinical practice has always been a unique blend of technical proficiency and ethical sensitivity, which together constitute the art of the physician and surgeon. Once sought out by the patient, the surgeon becomes involved in the patient's problem. He or she is no longer a mere observer. Over the last few decades, the relationship between patients and physicians has been evolving from one of *paternalism*, in which surgeons make choices for their patients, to a more equal and *autonomous* relationship of shared decision making by which surgeons provide information that allows competent adult patients to make their own choices.[21] For complicated surgical dilemmas, this can never evolve completely because patients depend on the surgeon and their other physicians to guide them to the correct choice.

Sometimes surgical procedures considered "standard of care" by the surgeon are refused based on the patient's values and beliefs. Such cultural challenges can affect the success of the patient–surgeon relationship and ultimately the health outcome for the patient. Ultimately, the surgeon must learn to take into account the cultural components of the relationship and find ways to respond to them in an ethically and medically responsible manner. To deal with these complicated situations, the surgeon is often required to reassess and be secure in his or her own religious and cultural foundations.[22]

As Peter Angelos[19] explains, the relationships that individual patients have with their surgeons are as varied as the different types of surgical problems with which patients present. Perhaps patients are required to have a great deal of trust in their surgeons because of the nature of surgical intervention itself. This may result in patients frequently feeling a deeper personal bond with their surgeon than with many other physicians who may be involved in their care. Surgeons as well as their patients frequently feel the closeness of this bond. Angelos quotes Charles Bosk as explaining:

The specific nature of surgical treatment links the action of the physician and the response of the patient more intimately than in other areas of medicine. . . . When the patient of an internist dies, the natural question his colleagues ask is, "What happened?" When the patient of a surgeon dies his colleagues ask, "What did you do?"

When patients consider the surgeon to be "their doctor," the surgeon must not ever underestimate the importance of maintaining this relationship even, or perhaps especially, as the patient approaches the end of life. The impact of a concerned surgeon on a patient who is dying, or is curable, can serve to dramatically affirm the appropriateness of comfort care instead of desperate, ineffective, and costly attempts to ward off death.[19]

Communication and the Internet

It seems so easy to be able to respond to a patient's problem or to deliver information to them and their physicians by e-mail. With e-mail delivered via the Internet, there is no problem with timing of the conversation, no recordings, no time on "hold" for the doctor or for the patient. The only limitation seems to be the typing and spelling skills of the surgeon, usually problem enough.

Most of us have learned not to deliver complicated or bad news by telephone, unless we have made a previous agreement with the patient and family to convey such information in order to save significant travel or other inconveniences that are significant enough to preclude a face-to-face personal communication. Such situations are now increasingly complicated because communication by the Internet is usually not secure, and the information delivered can become a permanent part of the patient's record. A patient's employer and family can usually acquire easy access to the electronic message, potentially to the detriment of the patient, and potentially leaving this sending physician legally liable.

For the medical and medical/legal aspect, some of the material we send by e-mail we would never consider sending by "hard copy" unless we had obtained the patient's specific permission to release such information. Currently, there are no guidelines available for the ethical transfer of confidential medical information via the Internet. Until such exists, and it is critical for physicians to participate in the establishment of such principles, all doctors are probably well advised to record in the patient's permanent record that discussions were held and permission was given to communicate *specific* information electronically. Especially with the implementation of HIPAA requirements, until clearer guidelines are defined, surgeons should err on the side of no sensitive information to be delivered by e-mail or telephone.[19]

Of course, the other massive impact of the Internet is the availability of unlimited access to potentially confusing and harmful information to our patients. Remember, there is no quality control for the Internet. Unlike traditional publications with editors, peer review, standards and vigorous screening, on the Internet, anyone with a computer can be a self-designated author, editor, and publisher. And this can be done anonymously with no attached responsibility. This will continue to have an enormous impact on the patient–physician relationship because "knowledge is power," and our patients and families are making use of that power.[23] Not infrequently patients come to us with confusing and conflicting material from the Internet. A new part of our responsibility, as surgeons, is to not only guide our patients to appropriate and helpful Web sites but to actively participate in the construction and quality control of electronic information provided by the Internet in our own areas of expertise.

Using Newly Deceased Patients for Teaching Purposes

A unique problem exists for the medical/surgical team caring for patients in the emergency department of a teaching hospital. It involves using the newly dead for teaching purposes. This usually involves teaching medical students and residents the techniques of endotracheal intubation. The issue is, of course: do we have the right to perform procedures on this newly deceased person without obtaining permission (informed consent) from the surviving family. The dilemma is complicated by the fact that no better teaching opportunity exists for our trainees who can then go forward, when adequately trained, to save lives and relieve suffering in the future. Clearly, no harm can be done to one who is dead. Furthermore, to our knowledge, there are no state statutes that specifically prohibit the teaching of procedures using newly dead patients, and no court has considered this issue. Although before death a patient has Constitutional protection against nonconsensual invasion of his or her body, it has been established by various state courts that constitutional rights do terminate at the time of death.

Although the law in this situation is very forgiving, compassionate and ethical considerations should supervene. Several medical studies have found that patients and families are likely to consent to such procedures but prefer to be asked permission first. Even the law advises that in this day and age of increasing recognition of personal autonomy, it is probably prudent to approach the next of kin for permission before performing procedures on the newly deceased.[24]

Special Concerns for Participation in Research/Innovation

General Concepts

Surgeons, by our very nature, are innovators. Sometimes, the only way we can complete an operative procedure is by making a deviation from what has been standard procedure in the past. Because we operate on biologic systems, we can never predict exactly what will be required for a given procedure. We often use old procedures for new purposes, and without much hesitation use new equipment to accomplish old tasks. Thus, we often find ourselves in what McKneally[25] refers to as "the zone of innovation" where it is unclear whether what we are doing is an evolutionary variation on a standard procedure, a unique departure from accepted standards, or the first stage of what should become recognized as a formal surgical research project. When should our deviations be subjected to full evaluation by an institutional review board? How can a surgeon participate, with *equipoise* (the presumption that both arms of a study are equally efficacious) in a prospective, randomized trial to evaluate a change that the surgeon has created to be better than the known standard? As Martin McKneally explains, most of the important advances in the history of medicine, such as anesthesia, appendectomy, antibiotics, intensive care, and immunization, were introduced through an informal, unregulated innovative process that has been enormously productive but can easily lead to ratification of an effective or even harmful treatment by well-intended physicians.[25]

Look at the recent challenges facing colon and rectal surgeons. We adopted the construction of ileal and now colonic pouches to improve the quality of life of our patients with inflammatory bowel disease and rectal cancer. The true efficacy of these innovations came significantly later than their description and implementation by many of our colleagues. The use of minimally invasive techniques to accomplish what we were all trained to do via abdominal incisions was clearly initially driven by the new technology and by enthusiastic entrepreneurs who wanted to work on the frontier of innovation. The premature exposure of these new techniques to the lay literature drove the process with even more intensity. Only recently have completed prospectively randomized trials verified the realistic advantages of the new technology. We continue to sort out the appropriate use, for the benefit of our patients and their quality of life, such issues as circular stapled hemorrhoidectomy, the treatment of anal fissures with nitroglycerin, botulinum toxin, or nifedipine, and even the destructive scarification of anal tissue to correct incontinence. What we need is a process for evaluation of surgical innovation, which provides ethical oversight without the ponderous slow pace inherent in most institutional review board approved protocols. Surgical investigators and ethicists are currently crafting such a mechanism, which protects the rights and well being of our patients without stifling progress and creativity.

Good research is described as that which enhances our ability to prevent illness or injury, to improve the quality or decrease the cost of care, or to improve the lives of our patients. Such research also must protect subjects and patients from harm, preserve their confidentiality, and allow them to enter freely as participants. Subjects and patients must be allowed to make an informed choice to participate, or not, without fear that their treatment might be compromised if they decline the request of the investigator. For a research project to be ethical, it must also be well designed and must investigate an issue of importance for which the answer does not yet exist. Protocols must be scientifically sound and likely to yield meaningful conclusions. Good research is therefore ethical, and bad research is unethical.[26]

In June 1966, Henry Beecher published an analysis of "Ethics and Clinical Research."[27] This benchmark article accelerated the movement that brought human experimentation under rigorous federal and institutional control. Although Beecher was not the first to direct attention to abuses in human experimentation, this presentation of 22 examples of investigators who endangered "the health or the life of their subjects" without informing them of the risks or obtaining their permission was a critical element in reshaping the ideas and practices governing human experimentation.[28]

Special issues for informed consent arise when the surgical patient is asked to participate in a *research project*. The time for decision making is usually short, and the principle investigator of the project may also be the one administering care. This raises not only the issue of adequate informed consent but of the *risk for coercion* of the patient to participate in the study. The surgeon researcher should abide by basic principles as outlined by the National Commission for the Protection of Human Subjects of Biomedical and Behavioral Research and by the Declaration of Helsinki. There are also prevailing federal, institutional, and professional guidelines that govern human and animal research. To be ethical, studies must be well designed and worth the risk to patient and society. The institution's review board should approve the study, and the investigator should take the responsibility to assure adequate informed consent, confidentiality, and appropriate protection of the patient's well being.[1]

All physicians must ensure that trials involving human subjects are of potentially significant value and are conducted ethically. The Nuremberg Code obligates researchers to prepare descriptions of the probability and magnitude of all physical, psychological, social, and economic risks, and to minimize unnecessary pain and suffering. Consent must be voluntary and without any element of force, coercion, or deceit.[11] When discussing the potential *risks* of a proposed procedure, it is essential for the person seeking consent to quantify minimal, low, or high-risk using examples from everyday life. Potential benefits from a research project may apply to the individual, to society, or to both. When discussing the benefits of a proposed study, one must distinguish clearly between *therapeutic* and *nontherapeutic* research. Researchers must clearly differentiate, for the patient, the balance between *potential benefit* to the patient and any *potential risks* associated with the protocol. No matter how great the benefit to society, it would not be ethical to expose a subject to anything greater than minimal risk if there is little direct benefit to the patient.[26]

Consent must never be assumed. Many would question the validity of truly "informed" consent rendered by someone who is acutely ill or severely injured. Especially for research, the principle still holds that for consent to be valid, it must be informed, understood, and voluntarily given. Subjects, or their surrogates, must have enough information, in comprehensible form, to enable them to make a proper judgment as to whether or not to participate in the requested study. Normally, this requires time for reflection before a decision to enroll. This concept is frequently stressed in the emergency situation. In an emergency, the surgeon may be forced to act in the patient's best interests and to presume consent on the basis of necessity. Clearly, this is only appropriate for interventions that will benefit the patient directly, and actual consent should be obtained as soon as possible afterward. In a research context, the intervention must be part of a protocol approved by an independent institutional committee, such as an institutional review board, and should present no more than minimal risk to the patient.[26]

Placebo Surgery

As investigators sort out the mechanism for ensuring that surgical research is performed ethically and with true *informed consent*, the issue of the use of *placebo surgery* seems based on recently published trials. Horng and Miller,[29] commenting on these trials in the *New England Journal of Medicine*, comment that the issue of using *placebo surgery* in clinical trials seems to violate the fundamental ethical principles of *beneficence* and *nonmaleficence*. Specifically, this means that surgeons should not invade the body except for purposes of cure or amelioration of suffering. In evaluating the studies, they emphasize the fact that clinical research always involves the inherent tension between the ethical values of pursuing science and those of protecting subjects from harm. To be considered ethical, overall, they must present a favorable risk–benefit ratio. The burden is on the investigators to justify *placebo surgery* as a warranted means of evaluating the efficacy of a surgical procedure. They conclude that absolute prohibition of *placebo surgery* is not appropriate, but the standard of justification for its use must be extremely high and rigorously enforced.[29]

Conflict of Interest: Industry and Drug Money

Many colon and rectal surgeons interested in research have difficulty obtaining extramural support for their projects and thus turn to private sources, namely, the biomedical and pharmaceutical industry. Industry support for biomedical research now exceeds the financial support from all federal funding sources. The liaison between academic surgery and industry introduces the possibility of remarkable benefits especially to our patients; however, differences between the fundamental goals of physicians and industry can create serious conflicts. Industry strives to complete clinical trials expeditiously and to publish positive results. Conversely, the primary goal of the surgical investigator is to advance and disseminate knowledge by the unimpeded exchange of ideas, despite secondary professional, financial, institutional, and sociopolitical objectives. Critics maintain that the physician–industry relationship will only serve to potentiate bias, and loss of objectivity will fundamentally poison the way research is conducted. Currently, however, the lifeblood of clinical research is external support requiring a productive relationship with the biomedical industry. This potential conflict of interest can only be resolved by scrupulously implementing the principles of integrity, honesty, respect, and equity. Even the mere appearance of a conflict of interest could jeopardize the investigator's integrity and undermine public trust. Surgeon investigators involved with industry-sponsored research should meticulously divorce themselves from any personal or commercial conflict that could compromise patient loyalty or well being.[11] Ethical recruitment of patients into research protocols is especially challenging for surgeons who, under the current system of financial remuneration, may receive more money by having the patient participate in a study than he/she would receive for doing the surgical procedure indicated for the patient.

A common challenge involves investigators who receive industry-funded materials, discretionary funds, research equipment, and trips to meetings. They must be aware that subsequent restrictions and expectations can create conflicts of interest. These seemingly innocent economic factors become a conflict anytime they influence study design, interpretation of results, or the timing and method by which results are reported. The personal gain of the investigator such as ownership of stock or receipt of funds for testing drugs or devices can introduce bias and compromise objectivity. However, it is not inappropriate for an investigator to receive economic rewards from a drug or device that is commensurate with his or her efforts involved in the development of the product. It is also acceptable for investigators to receive consultant and lecture fees from companies whose product they are testing, provided that the remuneration is proportionate with his or her efforts, and that it is clearly reported, in advance, of all presentations and is clearly stipulated in any publications. It is unethical, however, to sell or purchase stock or have a direct financial interest in the product under investigation until the relationship between the investigator and the company has been terminated, and the results of the research have been published or made public. Although opponents argue that disclosure cannot heal the financial conflicts of interest, it does recognize public concerns, protect the credibility and reputation of investigators, and alerts readers as they access the published report.[11]

The practice of pharmaceutical companies bestowing gifts on physicians is well documented. These gifts, however, cost money, and that cost is ultimately passed on to our patients without their explicit knowledge. The biomedical industry has clearly made outstanding contributions toward the advancement of modern scientific medicine; however, obvious conflict of interest occurs when physicians accept personal gifts that have no benefit to their patients. Acceptance of individual gifts that did not benefit patients, such as trips and subsidies for medical educational conferences in which physicians are not speakers, are strongly discouraged. The acceptance of even small gifts has been shown to affect clinical judgment and to heighten the perception (or reality) of a *conflict of interest*. Until specific guidelines are established, common sense should always prevail: no gifts should be accepted if suspected *strings are attached*.[11]

Confidentiality

General Principles

Surgeons are bound by the same rules of *confidentiality* as other doctors. Especially with the new restrictions and significant penalties imposed by HIPAA, all healthcare personnel must be very cognizant of preserving *confidentiality*. In the hectic morass, which is the waiting area of most big hospitals, it is sometimes difficult to take the time to ensure that doctors convey sensitive and private information to patients, families, or surrogates in a full and complete manner, and yet ensure the confidentiality of their information. Certain health information can be very significant in the treatment of a patient, including medication history and psychiatric history. Yet, some patients or families might be reluctant to give such information to the treating physician if the situation is not conducive to confidential communication. Similarly, the families and the patient are most certainly due confidentiality of the information, which the physician is going to impart. It is critical for the surgeon to establish a trusting relationship, so that the best and most important information relevant to treatment can be given and received. An exception to this rule occurs when the law requires disclosure of information to officials, as in the case of certain infectious diseases or in situations in which a third-party might be injured as a direct result of the physician's failure to report information.

A surgeon's duty to maintain confidentiality regarding information disclosed by the patient has been a long-held medical precept. On occasion, however, the ethical duty to prevent harm to others overrides the duty to keep confidences of a given patient. Although the law generally prevents the divulgence of confidential information, it also *mandates certain exceptions*, such as reporting patients with infectious disease and those who are likely to harm others, the latter being elucidated by the famous 1976 Tarasoff case in which nondisclosure of a patient's homicidal thoughts resulted in the death of the threatened person. This case raises a confusing possibility of preventing harm to others becoming a legal, not just an ethical, duty. This broadens the concept of mandatory reporting to include more than the currently accepted requirements for reporting child, elder, or domestic abuse. Such legal requirements may force us to compromise the ethical norm of respecting our patient's decisions with regard to confidentiality.[2]

Making and Managing a Genetic Diagnosis

As the results of untangling the mystery of the human genome are translated into clinical considerations, the ethical challenges to the colon and rectal surgeon become significant. Although the presumption is that facility and managing genetically predetermined disease is the lot of the primary care physician, in fact, patients with phenotypic presentation of genetic disease such as colon and rectal cancer depend on surgeons for final diagnosis, administration of surgical treatment, initiation of long-term follow-up, and clarification of the implications of the genetically predetermined cancer for other family members and other generations. Most often we deal with the autosomal dominant mutations, which cause familial polyposis or hereditary nonpolyposis colorectal cancers.

The ethical hazard involves obtaining the results of a genetic test without adequate counseling of the patient to determine what will be done with results once obtained.

Clearly, this should all be determined before obtaining the information. Many individuals fear that determination of a genetic abnormality will have adverse effect on their insurability and employability. These risks are supposed to be protected by law, but many members of our society are not willing to take that chance. Because of these fears, many patients and their family members refuse to have genetic testing done in the first place. Once the test is done, a patient may insist on absolute confidentiality to prevent dissemination of the information to others, even those at risk, in the family. Think of the dilemma in which this places the surgeon. You may know that 50% of children and siblings of the patient are at risk for potentially fatal cancer. Yet the patient has forbidden you to inform them. This situation can even ethically and illegally justify the physician breaching the patient's confidentiality to save the lives of those potentially at risk. There have even been cases in the courts in which the treating physician has been held liable for not divulging such risks to family members.

Most of these unpleasant situations can be avoided by appropriate genetic counseling before any genetic information is required. This should ideally involve the use of professional genetics counselors because most of us surgeons have not been adequately trained in the skills required.

Abuse of the Elderly

It is claimed that approximately 2 million elderly Americans are mistreated each year, with a significant number falling into the definition of abandonment. Although this treatment of elders is a problem that has occurred for centuries, only recently has society become significantly concerned. The problem and concern will increase as do the elderly components of our population. Surgeons are ideally suited to have a significant role in the detection, management, and prevention of elder abuse and neglect. The surgeon may be the only person, outside the family, who sees the older adult and is qualified to intervene in a preventive way. This means we should be aware of risk factors and their detection. It requires an astute clinician to detect abuse based on history alone. Even in the face of injuries, such as fractures at uncommon sites, the elderly patient may continue to conceal the possibility of abuse for fear of embarrassment or abandonment by the abuser. It may well be the surgeon called to see the patient for injury or neglect, who picks up the clues such as evidence of pressure sores, malnutrition, old injuries, or new injuries in unusual locations, such as on the scalp or behind the ears.

The first priority of the physician is to ensure this victim's safety. The surgeon should never hesitate to ask for social service consultation or to report suspicions to the appropriate adult protective services. Such acts are not breaches of confidentiality; they represent implementation of the most sincere duty of the physician.[30]

Futility/Withholding Treatment

General Concepts

Significant, and perhaps inappropriate, concern continues to exist in medicine with regard to the difference between *withholding* and *withdrawing* medical treatment. This has become more of an issue as the potential for resuscitating critically ill patients has become a progressive reality. Depending on the clinical situation, surgeons and other physicians attribute higher legal risk of one procedure over another. Apparently because of this fear of legal retribution, or ridicule and condemnation by professional peers, using full, almost ritualistic, resuscitation has become the default position of those delivering critical care in cases in which no advance directive exists. In fact, no physician has ever been successfully prosecuted for withholding or withdrawing of medical care from any dying patient in the legal history of the United States. This leaves one wondering what actually fuels the fears of legal retribution for making the wrong decision.[31]

The dilemma could of course be alleviated by early meaningful discussion with patients, families, and surrogates with regard to care *options at the end of life* and honest estimates of *prognosis*. Studies have shown, however, that many physicians and surgeons fail to take these opportunities. A disturbing example of this inadequacy can be found in the 1995 Study to Understand Prognoses and Preferences for Outcomes and Risks of Treatment (SUPPORT). This expensive, multi-institutional study demonstrated the physicians' *failure to meet all outcome markers*: failure to include patient and family in pivotal care discussions, failure to provide realistic estimates of outcomes valued by patients, failure to treat pain adequately, and failure to prevent prolonged death in patients with extremely poor prognoses.[31]

Sometimes confusion is created over the venue in which surgical or medical care is delivered. In the usual setting, a decision to *withhold* further medical treatment is done quietly, often without input from the patient or the surrogate decision maker, whereas *withdrawal* of ongoing medical treatment can be more obvious and difficult. Some clinicians and ethicists believe that the *withholding* of medical treatment is more problematic than later *withdrawal* of unwanted or useless interventions. This discrepancy in the urgent situation probably exists because the physicians involved usually lack the vital information about their patients' identities, medical conditions, and expressed wishes. In addition, perhaps because of frequent, but inaccurate, representations on television, society has come to expect only spectacular results in the delivery of surgical care in the United States. This concept is in marked contrast to the attitude that those clinicians who *withdrew* *treatment* (an act leading to death) were more culpable than those who *withheld treatment* (an omission leading to death); this distinction between acts and omissions is now thought to be more of a difference in psychological preference than an ethical norm.[32] For all of these reasons, despite the fact that the law has clearly spoken, the distinction between *withdrawal* and *withholding* of medical treatment will continue to be a challenge.

The surgeon's decision to limit or withhold treatment can be based either on the patient's refusal or on the physician's determination that the treatment would not be of benefit. Although the patient has the ethical and legal right to forego treatment, the physician must be very careful about withholding a treatment that might be beneficial. Such issues are usually intensified by the need for rapid intervention versus the desire to verify the meaning of the patient's current or preexisting desires. The classic example is the patient who is unresponsive, has reversible pulmonary or cardiac disease, needs cardiopulmonary resuscitation, but is said to have a preexisting DNR order (do not resuscitate).

Withholding treatment because of a judgment of *futility* is even more of an ethical challenge. *Futility* has been defined as "any effort to achieve a result as *possible*, but that reasoning or experience suggests is *highly improbable*, and cannot be systematically produced." Physicians, as moral agents, should exercise professional judgment in assessing patient's requests. If the request goes beyond well-established criteria of reasonableness, the surgeon ought not feel obliged to provide it. Some ethicists believe that the appropriate *allocation of resources* is another important consideration when one is making decisions regarding invasive, costly, or lengthy procedures. John Lantos even stated that, " Given limited resources, it is ethically justifiable to limit access to treatments that are expensive and offer minimal benefit. . . . Decisions by doctors to curtail use of those treatments are socially responsible."[33] *Futility* is such a complicated word that it may be of little use in most situations. The classic challenge is the decision not to start resuscitation when a patient with extensive metastatic cancer and cachexia presents in cardiac arrest. The initial emotional inclination is to treat the patient; however, the medical situation, as emphasized by Siegler,[13] leads to a judgment that such a resuscitation will not be beneficial. This requires the difficult objective determination of *ineffectiveness*, rather than any subjective decision based on the worth of the intervention or on the *value* of the patient's continued life.[2] It should be noted that assertions of *futility* come about in two contradictory situations. One is where the patient or surrogate wants the doctor to refrain from a further treatment, which the doctor thinks is not futile; and the other is where the doctor wishes to refrain from treatment that he or she believes to be futile. The only measure of what should be done is the standard of care in a given region for similar cases. Dealing with this concept of *futility* or other *end-of-life* concerns is usually only a problem when disagreement arises among the patient, the family, and the healthcare team.

Many ethicists agree that physicians are under no obligation to render treatments that they ascertain to be of little or no benefit to the patient. Many, however, believe that it would be advantageous to abandon the word "futility" and to use instead the construct of "clinically nonbeneficial interventions."

We all know that one of the greatest fears of both patients and families is their *abandonment* by the healthcare team. It is easy to fall into this trap by declaring that further treatment for a given patient is *futile*. When it is decided that certain interventions should be appropriately withheld, special efforts should be made to maintain effective communication, comfort, support, and counseling for the patient, family, and friends. Although we, as surgeons, may not always proceed with potential technologically advanced nonbeneficial interventions, we always must continue to *care* for the patient and the family.[34]

DNR and the Need for Surgery

There is, and should be, confusion regarding operating on a patient with existing "do not resuscitate" orders. Because there is no universal agreement as to how this situation is to be handled, each surgeon must be aware of specific institutional guidelines. First of all, it is not at all unusual for surgery to be indicated for patients in whom *cure* is no longer the goal of treatment. Even patients with advanced cancer or severe medical conditions will be offered surgical relief of acute intestinal obstruction or an abscess causing sepsis and pain. The problem usually gets defined when administering anesthesia becomes a consideration because, after all, it can be accurately stated that the act of anesthesia is *ongoing resuscitation*. As amazing as it seems, most hospitals have a policy that allows suspension of the DNR order during the procedure and administration of anesthesia, only to have it resume when the surgery and required anesthesia have been concluded.

Withdrawal of Treatment

General Principles

Taking into account the preceding discussion, an important line of reasoning for the moral and legal equivalents for the two actions of *withholding* or *withdrawing* is the important concept that if a medical intervention will not result in the desired or beneficial results intended for the patient, it makes no difference whether the clinician withholds the intervention before beginning it or discontinues its use after it has been started and found to be not effective.[32]

Special moral issues may arise in the care of *terminally ill patients*. We must be willing to respect a terminally ill patient's wish to forego life-prolonging treatment, as expressed in a living will or through a healthcare surrogate appointed via a durable power of attorney for healthcare. Those of us caring for patients should be willing to honor DNR orders appropriately executed on behalf of terminally ill patients. We should also understand the established criteria for the *determination of death* and should be prepared to

assist families in decisions regarding the donation of the patient's organs for transplantation. This involves knowing the specific regulations in our own states and in our own specific institutions, especially the criteria for death and the mechanisms for initiating the conversation relative to organ donation. It is usually not the surgeon, or any member of the treating team, who first raises the issue with family regarding donation of the dying patient's organs for the purpose of transplantation.

Euthanasia/Physician-assisted Suicide/Terminal Sedation

The terminology of activities related to the end of life are confusing to the public, have been misused in the press relative to the notorious activities of individuals such as Dr. Kevorkian, and, in fact, are probably not clearly differentiated by many surgeons. The terms all have separate meanings and implications, requiring us to understand them and not use them interchangeably.

First is *euthanasia*, which literally means "good death." Its consideration arises when patients or surrogates claim that the quality of life is so diminished, the pain and suffering is so unbearable, or they have become such a burden on others that they request their physicians to *cause* their deaths quickly and painlessly. Specifically this implies "mercy killing" of an individual, by a physician, to relieve pain and suffering. Such terms as "voluntary," "nonvoluntary," and "involuntary" have been applied in an attempt to clarify the various ramifications of this process, but, in fact, *euthanasia* is the act of killing by a physician and is *not legal* anywhere in the United States.[13]

Physician-assisted suicide, however, implies a death that a competent person, with decision-making capacity, chooses and *causes* by self-administration of drugs that a physician has prescribed but *did not administer*. Advocates believe that prescription of drugs that a patient can take at will removes the physician from direct participation. The decision and the act of ending life remain in the patient's control. This invokes the important fall-back concept for physicians and nurses who deal with patients who are suffering, in an irreversible medical condition, and near the end of life: the distinction between "killing and allowing to die." This distinction is invoked during the process of *terminal sedation* as well as for participation in *physician-assisted suicide*. Currently, the latter is legal only in the state of Oregon.[13] Even there, it has been complicated by the recent, and unique, intervention by the federal government, via the Food and Drug Administration, to criminalize the act of overprescribing pain medication by physicians where the act could be interpreted as intentionally facilitating a patient's death.

Terminal sedation, another frequently misunderstood term, is the practice of sedating a patient to unconsciousness in order to relieve the horrible symptoms, which may occur during the process of dying, including pain, shortness of breath, suffocation, seizures, and delirium. As the sedating medication is administered, other life-sustaining treatments are withdrawn, including ventilatory support, dialysis, artificial nutrition, and hydration. It is critically important to understand that in this frequently used process, *no lethal doses of opiates or muscle relaxants are administered*. Thus, the intent of the act is to relieve suffering and symptoms by making people unconscious and unable to eat or drink, so that they will die within a short period of time. As in *euthanasia, terminal sedation* directly intends the death of the patient.[13] The difference is that, in the latter, the sedating medication is not the agent of death. This differentiation is of utmost importance to avoid the feeling of killing by *double effect* (which will be later explained in more detail) on the part of the healthcare team. It invokes the concept of "letting nature take its course" as opposed to the homicidal act of "killing." Cynics claim they are the same, and those of us who claim otherwise are not being honest with ourselves.

Applying the Principles

To comply with the principle of *autonomy*, when a competent patient requests, or demands, the withdrawal of further treatment, the treating physician is in a situation analogous to that of the patient who initially refuses treatment. *Autonomy governs!* The surgeon should ensure that the patient is given all the information necessary to allow proper informed consent regarding withdrawal of treatment, but once that is done, it is the ethical duty of the surgeon to withdraw the specified treatment. This is true no matter what the patient requests, whether it be withdrawal of feeding tubes, ventilators, or nutrition and hydration. As long as the patient is fully aware of the consequences, both short-term and long-term, his or her stated wishes should be respected and acted upon appropriately by the healthcare team.

The same principle should be invoked if the patient is not able to understand but has provided, in an advance directive, an indicated desire with respect to withdrawal of treatment under specified circumstances. It is still the duty of the physician to withdraw the specific treatment because the patient has, in the advance directive, given prior informed consent. The duty of the physician is identical if a designated surrogate requests or demands the withdrawal of treatment. This is the patient speaking through the surrogate, and once again, autonomy governs.

When the surgeon determines that withdrawal of treatment is appropriate and further treatment would be ineffective, consent of the family or surrogate should be sought. In this situation, it is very important and helpful to know what if any *surrogacy laws* exist. These do vary from state to state, and those surgeons faced with potential decision making should know in advance the laws of their state. In states where such laws exist, they can be very helpful in delineating the hierarchy of surrogate designation. In the absence of advance directives, surgeons have the responsibility to judge what they believe the patient would want, or what is in the best interest of the patient. If no family is available, close friends of the patient may be asked to give their opinions about what the patient would want.

Courts have upheld the principles of *autonomy* and *self-determination*, affirming the right to refuse life-sustaining treatment. The classic illustrations of this include the 1976 ruling by the New Jersey Supreme Court that Karen Ann Quinlan, a woman in a persistent vegetative state, had the right to decide to be removed from a respirator and that this right could be asserted, on her behalf, by her family. This right was extended to include the withdrawal of nutrition by the 1990 Cruzan case in which the United States Supreme Court ruled that a life-sustaining feeding tube could be removed from another young woman in a persistent vegetative state.[18]

Should the surgeon have moral or religious beliefs that would preclude her from *withdrawing* treatment, she should remove herself from the case. It is important to recognize this possibility of need for withdrawing treatment at the beginning of the clinical encounter because a physician with such beliefs should extricate herself from the case at the earliest possible stage. As the clinical course evolves, and the surgeon develops a relationship with the family and the patient, it becomes progressively more difficult to remove herself from the treatment team.

Palliative Care/Hospice

General Principles

Focusing on making the last months, not minutes, of life meaningful is especially appropriate where death has a significant predictability. Chronic progressive diseases such as cancer, congestive heart failure, and chronic obstructive pulmonary disease account for 50%–70% of deaths, compared with the sudden death attributed to stroke, heart attack, trauma, and suicide. In the United States, patients' perceptions of human finitude lead them to deny death and to rely on medical achievements that they think will let them live forever. Physicians grapple with their technologic power, the imperative to tell the truth about fatal conditions, and despair at denying hope and the promise of cure for their trusting patients. It is probably this mutual self-deception that becomes the central issue in rendering appropriate end-of-life care. It is the management of these intense psychological and spiritual challenges facing terminally ill patients that has come to form the basis of what is called *palliative care*.[31]

A brief definition of *palliative care* would be: the act of *total* care of patients whose disease is not responsive to *curative* treatment. Although *palliative care* has been a major focus in Europe for the past 20 years, interest in the United States only became significant in the late 1990s with an Institute of Medicine report that evaluated end-of-life care.

It revealed significant deficiencies in how we manage end-of-life care. These deficiencies include the management of pain and other symptoms, including nausea and vomiting, dyspnea, depression, and anxiety. Geoffrey Dunn explains that: "Palliative care is not a concept defined in terms of the amount of time remaining in a patient's life or the terminal nature of his disease. It is defined in terms of the type of need that is being met by the care."[35]

The concept of *palliative surgery* refers to surgery for which the major intent is alleviation of symptoms and improving quality of life, *not necessarily cure*. As the age of our surgical patients increases, we will be progressively involved in performing operations whose desired outcomes are not met. Managing these patients through the entire course of their disease, including death, is an important part of being a good physician and a good surgeon. Surgical emergencies are often the first encounter with older patients, and they often have multiple comorbidities. An example is the 80-year-old person who presents with an acute abdomen. The risk of surgery will be high, the prognosis may be poor, and cure may be impossible. Perhaps, offering surgical treatment would even be inappropriate. Thus we, as surgeons, are immediately thrust into contemplating *palliative care* for the surgical patient, and it becomes clear that surgeons need to be aware of the concepts involved in delivering such care.[35]

Pain Relief and the Doctrine of "Double Effect"

Confusing Principles

When it comes to adequacy of pain control, especially for patients near the end of life, physicians and surgeons have been caught in a complicated dilemma. On the one hand, most of us entered medicine to relieve suffering. On the other hand, we know that administration of excessive doses of pain medication can suppress respiration and run the risk of contributing to the death of patients already near the end of life. At the same time that we are criticized for not giving enough pain medication to our suffering patients, we are also challenged by the law for prescribing medication with the *double effect* of potentially *hastening death*. This doctrine of *double effect* is intended by the courts to recognize the difference between provision of adequate pain treatment that unintentionally causes death and the ordering of medication that intentionally causes a patient's death. This concept of *intent* is confusing not only for the courts but also for the physician who is ordering the pain medication.

Double Effect

The application of the principle of *double effect* is controversial because it places significant weight on physician *intent*, which is impossible to prove, and no weight on a patient's right to self-determination. This seems to contradict a paramount principle of American bioethics: *patient autonomy*. Why, when death is on the line, should concern over the physician's *intention* take precedence over the *patient's informed consent*? The physician's fear over misinterpretation of his or her actions often leads to inadequate use of pain medication, leaving patients unjustifiably suffering. It is clearly recognized that opioids should be considered early in the care of the dying patients and in dosages that often exceed the standard range. These analgesics are not only effective in reducing painful sensation, but also have an effect in adjusting the sense of well being, thereby improving the patient's ability to cope with pain. Adjustment of dosage can be aided by using one of the known *pain scales* or by observation of patients' objective signs of distress, especially useful in the noncommunicative patient. Despite its significant effect on several components of respiration, respiratory arrest from opioids, in the absence of other central nervous system depressants, is rare. In caring for dying patients, surgeons must acknowledge that they are one part of the often-fragmented medical team. They must accept the goal of providing care where they can, comfort always, consult when necessary, and coordination of the remaining end of life issues.[31]

Hastening Death: The "Code"

Because the overwhelming admonition to the physician is "above all do no harm," society has implored the surgeon, in life-threatening situations, to waive informed consent requirements and to act presumptively to save life or limb in situations in which the usual consent is impossible to obtain. This leads to our current default in dealing with the critically ill or moribund unknown patient: resuscitating with "a full code" and asking questions later. This practice is probably acceptable as long as the surgeon realizes that *withdrawing life support* is just as acceptable as *withholding life support* initially. The initial full resuscitation may make it possible to assess the patient's end-of-life desires more fully and carefully. If the initial intervention is unsuccessful or is inconsistent with the patient's preference, it can and should be withdrawn, consistent with the patient's identified goals.

What are ethically frowned upon are such deceitful practices as the "slow code," a charade consisting of a halfhearted resuscitation that seems to allow the surgeon to take the moral middle ground by giving the family a false impression of respecting patient autonomy, while knowing full well that the act will not be effective. Experience suggests that this hedge is used fairly often. Although no ill is usually intended, the slow code is usually an indication that the surgeon has not realistically communicated with the patient and family to express the medical opinion that resuscitation, in the face of cardiac or respiratory arrest, would be inappropriate.[31]

The concept of "no code" should be clear, and is usually instituted at the request of the patient, his advance directive, or an appropriate surrogate. It is ethically inappropriate for the physician to disrespect the patient's autonomous decision even when faced with despairing surrogates requesting interventions over a clear directive to the contrary. The patient with decision-making capacity is, of course, free to change any prior stipulation, even those written in an advance directive. In the absence of any directive, including a decisional patient, the physician must use *best interest standard*, which requires implementing what a *reasonable patient* would want done in a similar situation.

To understand these previously discussed concepts, the surgeon must realize the implications of the three means of accelerating death for patients in the United States: *double effect*, *voluntary euthanasia*, and *physician-assisted suicide*. The *rule of double effect*, as previously described, involves the dichotomy of treatment versus side effects, in which death is the *unintended* side effect of adequate symptom control. *Voluntary euthanasia*, that which is requested by the patient, can be either active or passive. *Passive euthanasia* is the result of withdrawing or withholding life support in situations judged to be medically futile. In the United States, this is both ethically and legally acceptable. However, *active euthanasia* occurs when the physician *intentionally* administers an agent to cause a patient's death. This act is considered *unethical* and *illegal* everywhere in the world except in the Netherlands where it is practiced openly. *Physician-assisted suicide* occurs when a physician supplies a death-causing agent to a patient with the knowledge that the patient intends to use this agent to commit suicide. In the United States, this practice is legal only in the state of Oregon.[31]

Of great concern to all physicians in the United States is a recent action by the Attorney General of the United States with regard to the Oregon Death with Dignity Act, a law that authorized doctors to help their terminally ill patients commit suicide. The doctors were allowed to prescribe, but not to administer, such drugs. Attorney General Ashcroft, in 2001, directed that doctors who help their patients commit suicide could be prosecuted under the federal Controlled Substances Act. This was the first example, in United States, of the *federal government* interceding in the practice of medicine, historically entrusted to *state lawmakers*. In May of 2004, the United States Court of Appeals for the Ninth Circuit, in San Francisco, rebuked the Attorney General and upheld the Oregon law.[36,37]

Know Your Intent

For all physicians, the concept of avoiding killing seems obvious. However, what is a doctor to do when confronted with a situation whereby the administration of sufficient medication to alleviate the pain of a patient might have the secondary effect of diminishing respiration, and actually hastening the death of the patient? This is, of course, the crux of the major debate over *physician-assisted suicide* and *euthanasia*. There are other situations, such as abortion, in which a physician must take avoiding killing into account. Confronting such

issues challenges a surgeon not only with the duty to respect the autonomy of the patient but also to be aware of situations that might put the individual doctor in the uncomfortable situation of confronting conflict with his or her own personal beliefs.

In multiple decisions, the courts have emphasized the importance of distinction between "letting a patient die and making that patient die."[18] This, in our opinion, is the most distressing conflict for the physician who must make such decisions. We know full well that when we give high-dose opioids or withdraw ventilatory support, we may be hastening the patient's death. The callous ones among us see this as euthanasia and strongly criticize those who claim otherwise. When confronted with this challenge, in a personal communication, Dr. Edmund Pellegrino, one of our most respected medical ethicists, immediately responded with his comforting interpretation of such a situation. In his mind, and in his conscience, he recognizes and acts upon the difference between actively and intentionally hastening a patient's death as opposed to relieving pain and suffering or withdrawing artificial life-support, thus "letting nature take its course."

Determination of Death

The attending physician has the discretion and the responsibility to determine death. Statutes in different states use different criteria for death. In some cases, they have not caught up with the science available. Some states use the "irreversible cessation of cardiopulmonary function" criteria, as do some religions. The complete cessation of respiration and circulation constitute "death" under this definition. The concept of *intensive care* has advanced dramatically since these statutes were enacted and have superseded this now antiquated definition. In most states where this is the statutory definition, the courts have now ruled that "brain death" suffices.

Most states use the brain death criteria. There is debate currently about whether the "whole brain" definition of death is no longer valid, and that the appropriate ethical standard for definition of death is cessation of "higher brain" function. Higher brain function includes the cognitive functions or the capacity for consciousness. Once there is irreversible cessation of that capability, a judgment usually made in consultation with a neurologist, then death can be declared. Most neurologists are trained to determine whether death has occurred or whether the patient is in a "permanent vegetative state."

It should be noted that in some states the definition of death includes *either* the *cessation of cardiopulmonary function or irreversible cessation of all brain function*, including the brain stem.

The healthcare team, however, should realize that no matter which criterion is being used, it may be appropriate to continue cardiovascular support for the purpose of maintaining perfusion during the eminent birth of a fetus, or to sustain viability of transplantable organs.

Organ Donation

Criteria for organ donation are not always clearly understood. Many patients and families are mistakenly concerned about having death declared prematurely just to facilitate the harvesting of organs for transplantation. Here the surgeon's bioethical responsibilities are clear. The medical ethical principle of *patient autonomy* dictates that the desires of the patient and the family be respected.

Federal law requires most hospitals to make an inquiry of all patients, during their admission, for any procedure, whether emergency or elective, about their wishes to be a potential *organ donor*. Although this can be somewhat of a shock to patients who are coming in for elective surgery, especially a minor procedure, it obviates the need for physicians to make the painful inquiry when a patient is actually facing eminent death. If the admitting personnel ask for this information on a routine basis, the patient is more likely to render a competent decision, and the potential problems of dealing with surrogates, sometimes under difficult circumstances, is alleviated.

However it is obtained, *informed consent* of the *donor* is required. Most states provide organ donor options on driver's licenses, and many people possess other documents such as donor cards, which indicate their desire to become organ donors. In some cases, donors request limits on the organs they wish to donate. For example, some donors have indicated that they do not wish to donate their eyes or some other specific organ. Even though patient autonomy should guide the physician, there are circumstances in which the family emphatically wishes to override the clearly stated intention of the donor. These situations are difficult, and although the surgeon's clear ethical duty is to respect the wishes of the donor, the body of the donor, after death, belongs to the family. The treating physician would be well advised to leave the resolution of this situation up to the transplant coordinator. In fact, it is usually inappropriate for anyone on the treating team to initiate the discussion of organ donation. Most hospitals have in place a procedure whereby the discussion of potential organ donation is initiated by a person specifically trained for this purpose. It is often the transplant coordinator, a social worker, or a hospital chaplain.

Insisting on compliance with the donor's clearly stated wishes, in the face of strong family opposition, does not affect the legal position of the surgeon, but it can result in unfortunate lawsuits because of the animosity created with the family. In cases in which there are no previously expressed wishes by the potential donor, the family, as custodians of the body, may agree to organ donation. The duty of the physician in this case is to obtain the consent of the family *before* doing anything to preserve the functioning of the organs for potential transplantation.

In cases in which there is no surrogate or family, or any evidence of previously stated intention to donate, the ethical position of the doctor is less clear, but absent permission to do something to the body in a situation that is no longer an emergency, assuming that the organs should be harvested for transplantation, would seriously violate the concept of informed consent. Although it can be argued that the dead person cannot give informed consent, the family whose property the body is would have to give their consent to have any procedure done at all to the newly dead person. In cases with no directives at all, the best course of action, unfortunately, is to do nothing postmortem.

Ethics/Legal Consultation

Most surgeons work within an institution. Most of these institutions provide a mechanism for obtaining help in sorting out challenging ethical dilemmas. This help usually comes in the form of consultation from the hospital *Ethics Committee* or from in-house *legal consultation*. It is critical to realize that utilization of such resources does not commit the surgeon to accepting an arbitrary decision of what is right and what is wrong in a complicated ethical situation. Consultation is meant to provide a process for most expeditiously sorting out the issues which have arisen and for providing rapid access to the potential mechanisms for solving the problem. Hospital ethics committees are specifically charged to advise physicians, patients, and families who face ethical dilemmas. These situations usually arise when there is *disagreement* between these groups and the healthcare team. Consultation from the ethics committee is usually rapidly facilitated through such agencies as the hospital nursing service. Consultation should be available, instantly, 24 hours a day. Frequently, it is the hospital chaplain who facilitates the consultation. By bringing in appropriate resources and facilitating meeting with the healthcare team, patients, and families, consultation with the ethics committee should help resolve even the most complicated medical ethical challenges. The hospital ethics committee should be charged with what is the right thing to do for the patient. It should have no vested interest in protecting the institution at the risk of embarking on an action, which is ethically unsettled for the good of the patient.

A word of caution, however, is necessary for surgeons working within a given institution. Once *legal counsel* or *risk management* is brought in to deal with a complicated situation, it must be remembered that *they work for the institution*. Their job is to protect the institution, and the advice that they give will be aimed toward that end. This commitment to the institution is important for the physician to realize if there is potential for placing oneself in personal jeopardy. It is also important to realize that legal standards are not always reliable guides to determining what are the best ethical and medical decisions.

Good Samaritan

A Case

The most skilled colon and rectal surgeon in town is out to dinner. At the next table he sees the local crime boss choking to death over a piece of prime beef. What are the ethical and legal ramifications he must consider before performing an emergency tracheotomy? What is he ethically obligated to do? Is the old medical oath binding? Can anyone give consent? Must he identify himself? If he performs the procedure, and there is a bad outcome, is it malpractice? What if he is a medical student instead of a famous surgeon? Is a bad outcome here considered battery? What should the surgeon do when the emergency medical technician arrives and wants to take the dying crime boss to a known inferior local hospital? What are the obligations and risks for the surgeon?

General Concepts

Good Samaritan acts or deeds are defined as those in which aid is rendered to a person in need, where no fiduciary or legal obligation exists to provide such aid, and neither reward nor remuneration for the aid is anticipated. The aid provided can include a survey of the situation, protection of the victim, notification of other care providers, or personal provision of immediate treatment. The Good Samaritan ethic is one that is generally endorsed by our culture, which strongly supports assisting an individual who is in danger or in need of help. Surgeons may be regarded as having a greater responsibility to provide Good Samaritan aid than a lay person by reason of the special training and knowledge and commitment to duty for the benefit of individuals and society that generally drive us to become physicians and surgeons. Clearly, in a situation of sudden medical need, a surgeon will be better able to assess the medical condition of the victim and to render immediate treatment if indicated and feasible. Many believe that the mere status of being a physician entails the duty to use one's skills and knowledge in cases of sudden or emergency need; for some, this duty is an inherent feature of the role and even of the definition of a physician.[38]

Briefly stated, in almost every state, an off-duty surgeon who comes across a person with an emergency medical condition has no *legal duty* to come to the aid of that person. However, a physician's *ethical obligation* inspires him to help in such an emergency. All states in the United States have enacted so-called "Good Samaritan" statutes, which protect the physician from liability incurred for good-faith efforts to help at the scene of an accident or emergency. The ethical duty should far exceed the legal excuse for inaction.[2]

Generally, Good Samaritan acts include the following principles. 1) There is no legal obligation of doctors to answer or treat emergencies. 2) If the doctor chooses to intervene, the expected standard of care is modified by circumstances of the situation. 3) If aid is given, it need be stabilization only and not definitive treatment. 4) Implied consent exists to treat the victim if he or she lacks the capacity to consent. 5) These criteria apply whether or not the physician is paid for his or her services rendered. Despite the establishment of these principles, the extensive coverage in the media of spectacular medical malpractice suits causes many surgeons to develop a strong aversion to the performance of Good Samaritan acts. To alleviate this apprehension, Good Samaritan laws were enacted, the first in California in 1959. Since then every state has enacted such law. The laws all share the following provisions: there is no legal obligation to provide aid, there is immunity from malpractice suit if aid is provided, there is exception from immunity for gross negligence or lack of "good-faith," acts are restricted to application outside of hospitals, and there is withdrawal of legal immunity if the doctor accepted payment for aid rendered.[38]

Professionalism and Interpersonal Relations: Working as a Team

General Considerations

There is an ever-increasing challenge to deliver the very best surgical care in the current medical environment which thrives on its speed and frequently impersonal delivery of generic medical care, often at multiple institutions, and without one consistent team of support. Often it becomes difficult to fulfill the responsibility requiring communication, collaboration, respect, and confidentiality as we interact with the components of our healthcare team which frequently includes nurses, enterostomal therapists, primary care physicians, consulting physicians, surgical and medical trainees, and the vast array of ancillary services required within our institutions.

Teaching Residents and Fellows

Learning and teaching are critical components in our career choice of medicine, and especially, surgery. At some point in our training, a more senior person turns over to each of us the responsibility to perform the major part of an operative procedure. And then, the converse occurs: each of us, in turn, relinquishes the major part of an operation to one of our trainees. We know how the process works and the importance of a surgical team with "graded" responsibility. The ethical challenge arises when, often the night before surgery, the patient asks: "Who is going to do my surgery?"[39] The honest answer becomes blurred, especially for those colon and rectal surgeons working in a program with trainees who are senior residents or fellows. We usually fall back on the explanation that we, the attending surgeon, will be present and responsible, even when we know that the trainee will be doing the critical part of the procedure. What is the truth? The fellow claims on the training record that he or she did the case, and we charge the payer as if we did the procedure. What is true *informed consent* in such situations?

Previous Suboptimal Care

General Concepts

As colon and rectal surgeons, we are specialists, frequently seeing patients as requested consultation by and referral from other physicians and even other surgeons. It makes the nature of our care, often, "the end of the road." We have no place else to send the patients and frequently find ourselves in the position of correcting or undoing the poor results of the action of another surgeon. This becomes an ethical and personal challenge especially when the patient or the family asks: "Why wasn't that done by the other surgeon, or what did she do wrong?" We can easily become caught up in the dilemma between taking credit for heroic restoration of health and condemnation of the other surgeon, or, covering up for incompetent care in an attempt to avoid litigation against another doctor and/or preserving a lucrative source of referrals.

Generally our surgical and specialty training does not prepare us for the ethical differentiation between "bailing out" and "condemning," responding to patients' pointed questions, communicating with the doctor responsible for the suboptimal care, and certainly not "blowing the whistle" on another surgeon and going to court, when requested, as an "expert witness." Albert Wu[40] suggests that a surgeon who discovers a major error made by another physician has several options, which include: waiting for the other doctor to disclose the mistake, advising the other physician to disclose the error, arranging a joint meeting to discuss the mistake, or telling the patient directly. He and his coauthors believe that, based on the requirements of the doctor–patient relationship, surgeons have an obligation to facilitate disclosure. Many surgeons are reluctant to say anything because they are not 100% sure of what actually happened, they fear hurting the feelings of colleagues, they wish not to strain professional relationships, or because of the terrifying thought that "there but for the grace of God go I." Wu et al. further suggest that we fulfill our obligation to our patient by advising the doctor who erred to inform the patient; but he goes on to say that if that fails, it is our duty to tell the patient what happened.[40] Each of us must then rely on compassion and tact to tell our patients the truth without unduly condemning the other physicians. We surgeons need to realize that what we take for granted in our weekly *morbidity and mortality* conferences, especially in a teaching hospital, is not the norm for other branches of medicine. We know, and perhaps are obligated to pass on to others, that admitting a mistake may help us to accept responsibility for it and may help to make changes in our practice. Physicians should be able to learn vicariously from mistakes made by others, and thus avoid making the same mistake themselves.[40]

"Blowing the Whistle" and Going to Court

The next echelon of concern and potential activity, of course, involves serving as an "expert witness" in medical malpractice litigation. Again, this is an arena of involvement in the medical care system for which we surgeons are generally ill prepared. Just recently, the American College of Surgeons and the American Society of Colon and Rectal Surgeons have issued some guidelines in an attempt to ensure that surgical

specialists not abuse the system by offering false testimony or by presenting as "experts" in areas beyond their expertise. Many of our true experts refuse to serve in this capacity when it involves saying something against another surgeon; yet, when any of us are involved as the accused, we want only the finest experts available and are repulsed when "hired guns" with little knowledge boldly testify against us. The problem seems to be that many of us do not differentiate *malpractice* with severe damage to a patient from the poor results from proper treatment that we surgeons all experience in dealing with the complex biologic system of the human body. Again, the principle of not stepping up to the plate for fear of the dictum, "There but for the grace of God go I." We should understand that credibility in the medical-legal system should be based on true expertise and on telling the truth, be it for the plaintiff or for the defense of our colleagues, and, in fact, we can be of much greater help to inappropriately accused physicians by establishing such a record of credibility.

Managed Care

Patient Advocacy

All of us in the current system participate in some form of managed care, whereby someone other than the treating physician becomes involved in the mechanism of delivering care to our patients, usually without sharing in the responsibility of rendering the care and the untoward outcome that may be engendered by that care. This presents a true dichotomy for doctors, most of whom have taken an oath or by law are committed to being *advocates* for our patients. It seems an impossible, and perhaps unethical, task to make a decision that favors the economic advantage of a managed care organization over what we know, medically, is required by an individual patient in need.

Rationing Care/Cutting Corners

Surgeons have a special obligation to deal with these systems because of the loneliness of making the decision and ultimately doing a surgical procedure on another human being. It is a desperate feeling to realize, in the middle of an operation, that our quest for perfection has been compromised by some inadequacy in preoperative management foisted on us by another remote physician hired by a managed care organization to protect the financial interests of a group. We know, as well as others, that medicine, as a system, is in trouble, but the problem is rarely to be solved by rationing or withholding what we know is surgically best for our individual patients. Perhaps it is our job to invoke our "surgical personalities" to become the strongest of all patient advocates and to fully participate in achieving needed improvements in the overall system. We must communicate to others the special understanding and compassion few outside of the field of surgery understand.

Personal Challenges: Competition of Interests

Professionalism

McKneally describes the profession of medicine and surgery as a vocation that requires extensive knowledge and skill. It also requires a high level of discretion and trustworthiness, even in individual practice. The social contract between the profession and the public holds professionals to very high standards of competence and moral responsibility. He goes on to explain that a profession is literally a declaration of a way of life "in which expert knowledge is used not primarily for personal gain, but for the benefit of those who need that knowledge."[15] In our current society, bombarded by endless advertising and hype, many groups call themselves "professionals" sometimes to the point of humor, but for those of us in medicine, and especially surgery, the definition means that when confronted with a choice of what is good for us or what is good for our patient, we choose the latter. This occurs and is expected sometimes to the detriment of our own good and that of our families. Tom Krizek[41] even goes so far as to question if surgery is an "impairing profession." Perhaps it really is an *ethical* concern, which is encouraging us to modify the working hours and conditions for our trainees to offer more of an incentive to enter the surgical specialties. Now that we have appropriately tended to the training programs, it behooves us to explore the same lifestyle improvements for ourselves. It is neither an ethical breach nor a sign of weakness to allocate high priority to our families and to our own well being.

Family

As financial and professional pressures become more intense, the challenge increases to appropriately prioritize and balance the demands of patient care, family, education, teaching, and research. Mary McGrath presents an all too frequent dilemma for the surgeon: choosing between attending a child's graduation or operating on an old patient who requests you instead of your extremely well-trained associate who is currently seeing the patient. How many times have we not chosen wisely! Someone else can competently care for your patient, but only you can be a parent to your child.[19] Time literally flies, and we must often remind ourselves that our lives are not just a "dress rehearsal"!

Among the many considerations of *family* is the issue of caring for, and perhaps even operating on, our own family members. What is not only ethical, but what is appropriate for the practice of medicine and surgery with regard to this issue is not as clear as you might, at first, believe. For example, if your spouse cuts her leg while skiing, and the only available physician is a psychiatrist who is covering the emergency room, should you, a training surgeon, suture her laceration? However, if you feel that you are the most experienced colon and rectal surgeon in the community, what should you do when your own mother is found to have a complicated cancer of the low rectum? After all, if you are the "best" why would you deny the best care to your own mother? Many hospitals have dealt with this issue and have a stated policy. The American Medical Association has issued a statement on "Self-treatment or Treatment of Immediate Family Members." In essence it speaks against treating family except in emergent situations and for short periods of time. It is, of course, based on the risk of compromise of professional objectivity and influence on medical judgment because of the influence of personal feelings, thus interfering with the care that needs to be delivered.[42]

Competence / Impairment / Insight

Surgical certifying organizations are currently struggling with the definition and determination of *surgical competence*. McKneally[15] stresses that a patient's trust is based on the surgeon's diligent pursuit of competence in both judgment and technical skill. Surgical training programs have diligently attempted to guarantee the competency of individuals completing the process. The board certification process attempts to ensure that the interests of society are represented in these professional processes. Thus, competency is an integral part of the *entry-level*. The problem arises in maintaining a level of competence and assuring that established surgeons who take on new procedures both acquire and maintain competence in these new skills.[15] Perhaps the most obvious recent example for us colon and rectal surgeons has been the advent of laparoscopic, minimally invasive surgical procedures. Now that they are part of all fellowship training programs, it is less of a problem. But the issue will arise again with the next new wave of technology: how to teach old surgeons new skills.

Related to competence is the issue of *impairment*. Jones[43] emphasizes that drug and alcohol abuse, with the associated functional impairments, are the leading cause of sanction against physicians by professional oversight bodies in the United States. More than one in every seven physicians is affected by substance abuse at some time in their careers. He goes on to explain that the surgical patient is potentially at greatest risk in the care of a cognitively or physiologically impaired physician because the surgeon's competence requires simultaneous application of fine neuromuscular, cognitive, and intellectual skills. This is coupled with the emotional composure and critical judgment required to make urgent decisions and the physical endurance of standing for long hours at the operating table. He cites Percival's admonition that the medical profession is a "public trust" that should be relinquished when a physician or surgeon no longer possesses the skills that are essential to clinical care. Unfortunately, most surgeons do not possess or exercise the insight required to know when we are impaired or when it is time to retire.

Jones goes on to quote Verghese's observation on the impaired physician: "the doctors had one common feature—namely, exquisite denial—that allowed them to believe they could still care for patients perfectly well."[43] These observations place great responsibility on those of us who observe *impairment* or *incompetence* in our colleagues who at times may also be our close friends. We should never hesitate to request intervention because correction of substance abuse in physicians is highly successful. If we stand by and allow patients to be mismanaged by inadequate physicians, we will not only see the patients suffer but will allow our colleagues and friends to be destroyed professionally and perhaps devastated emotionally by malpractice suits, condemnation by institutions and colleagues, loss of licensure, and eventually the ravages of substance abuse or personal humiliation.[43] Most state boards of healing arts function best when it comes to providing support for physicians in trouble.

A Final Thought

Perhaps Richard Hayward,[44] who compares a surgeon to the young sea captain in Joseph Conrad's novel "The Shadow-Line," best describes a successful career in surgery. Hayward explains that there are so many variables in the interaction between patient, surgeon, and disease that it is not surprising that the prediction of results becomes uncertain. Even routine procedures can produce complications and can become much more difficult than had been anticipated. As the surgeon crosses Conrad's Shadow-Line, energy, enthusiasm, ability to make firm decisions and then act upon them, optimism, self-confidence, and resilience in the face of adversity become necessities without which an individual will have difficulty coping with the pressures of a surgical practice, especially one involving the care of critically ill emergency patients. There becomes a time when a surgeon must learn to come to terms with the inadequacies and, sometimes, downright failures of his or her actions that will be the inevitable companions during a surgical life.[44]

References

1. ACEP Ethics Committee. Code of ethics for emergency physicians. Ann Emerg Med 1997;30:365–372.
2. Derse AR. Law and ethics in emergency medicine. Emerg Med Clin North Am 1999;17:307–325.
3. Kodner IJ. Ethics curricula in surgery: needs and approaches. World J Surg 2003;27:952–956.
4. Little M. Invited commentary: is there a distinctively surgical ethics? Surgery 2001;129:668–671.
5. Beauchamp TL, Childress JF. Principles of Biomedical Ethics. 5th ed. Oxford: Oxford University Press; 2001:12–23.
6. Justice Cardoza. Scholendorff v. New York Hospital 105 N.E. 92. New York Court of Appeals; 1914.
7. Iserson KV. Principles of biomedical ethics. Emerg Med Clin North Am 1999;17:283–306.
8. Adams J, Larkin G, Iserson K, et al. Virtue in emergency medicine. Acad Emerg Med 1996;3:961–966.
9. Alexander L. Medical science under dictatorship. N Engl J Med 1949;241:39–51.
10. Koenig HG. Taking a spiritual history. JAMA 2004;291:2881.
11. Weber JE. Conflicts of interest in emergency medicine. Emerg Med Clin North Am 1999;17:475–490.
12. Buckner F. The Emergency Medical Treatment and Labor Act (EMTALA). Med Pract Manage 2002;Nov/Dec:142–145.
13. Jonsen AR, Siegler M, Winslade WJ. Clinical Ethics: A Practical Approach to Ethical Decisions in Clinical Medicine. 5th ed. New York: McGraw-Hill; 2002:41–42, 181–182.
14. Moore FD. Ethical problems special to surgery: surgical teaching, surgical innovation, and the surgeon in managed care. Arch Surg 2000;135:14–16.
15. McKneally MF. Ethical problems in surgery: innovation leading to unforeseen complication. World J Surg 1999;23:786–788.
16. McCahill LE, Dunn GP, Mosenthal AC, et al. Palliation as a core surgical principle. Part I. J Am Coll Surg 2004;199:149–160.
17. Jacobstein CR, Baren JM. Emergency department treatment of minors. Emerg Med Clin North Am 1999;17:341–352.
18. Schmidt TA, Zechnich AD. Suicidal patients in the ED: ethical issues. Emerg Med Clin North Am 1999;17:371–383.
19. American College of Surgeons Ethics Curriculum for Surgical Residents. In press.
20. Sanders AB. Advance directives. Emerg Med Clin North Am 1999;17:519–526.
21. Siegler M. Identifying the ethical aspects of clinical practice. Bull ACS 1996:23–25.
22. Ells C, Caniano DA. The impact of culture on the patient-surgeon relationship. J Am Coll Surg 2002;195:520–530.
23. Paris JJ, Ferranti J. The changing face of medicine: health care on the Internet. J Perinatol 2001;21:34–39.
24. Moore GP. Ethics seminars: the practice of medical procedures on newly dead patients—is consent warranted? Acad Emerg Med 2001;8:389–392.
25. McKneally MF, Daar AS. Introducing new technologies: protecting subjects of surgical innovation and research. World J Surg 2003;27:930–935.
26. Nee PA, Griffiths RD. Ethical considerations in accident and emergency research. Emerg Med J 2002;19:423–427.
27. Beecher HK. Ethics and clinical research. N Engl J Med 1966;274:1354–1360.
28. Rothman DJ. Ethics and human experimentation: Henry Beecher revisited. N Engl J Med 1987;317:1195–1199.
29. Horng S, Miller FG. Is placebo surgery unethical? N Engl J Med 2002;347:137–139.
30. Birrer R, Singh U, Kumar DN. Disability and dementia in the emergency department. Emerg Med Clin North Am 1999;17:505–517.
31. Schears RM. Emergency physicians' role in end-of-life care. Emerg Med Clin North Am 1999;17:539–559.
32. Iserson KV. Withholding and withdrawing medical treatment: an emergency medicine perspective. Ann Emerg Med 1996;28:51–54.
33. Marco CA. Ethical issues of resuscitation. Emerg Med Clin North Am 1999;17:527–538.
34. Marco CA, Larkin GL. Ethics seminars: case studies in "futility"—challenges for academic emergency medicine. Acad Emerg Med 2000;7:1147–1151.

35. McCahill LE, Dunn GP, Mosenthall AC, et al. Palliation as a core surgical principle. Part I. J Am Coll Surg 2004;199: 149–159.

36. The rights of the terminally ill. New York Times, May 28, 2004.

37. Liptak A. Ruling upholds Oregon law authorizing assisted suicide. New York Times, May 27, 2004.

38. Daniels S. Good Samaritan Acts. Emerg Med Clin North Am 1999;17:491–504.

39. Jones JW, McCullough LB. Consent for residents to perform surgery. J Vasc Surg 2002;36:655–656.

40. Wu AW, Cavanaugh TA, McPhee SJ, et al. To tell the truth: ethical and practical issues in disclosing medical mistakes to patients. J Gen Intern Med 1997;12:22–27.

41. Krizek TJ. Ethics and philosophy lecture: surgery . . . is it an impairing profession? J Am Coll Surg 2002;194:352–366.

42. Self-treatment or treatment of immediate family members. American Medical Association Policy Number E-8.19.

43. Jones JW, McCullough LB, Richman BW. An impaired surgeon, a conflict of interest, and supervisory responsibilities. Surgery 2004;135:449–451.

44. Hayward R. The shadow-line in surgery. Lancet 1987;14: 375–376.

54
Critically Reviewing the Literature for Improving Clinical Practice

Clifford Y. Ko and Robin McLeod

As the science of surgery continues to advance, it is important for the practicing clinical surgeon to remain up to date on the current issues in the field. Many surgeons remain updated by reading the literature—and although this is an excellent way to stay current, it is paramount that the reader understands how to critically read the literature, and evaluate the importance, relevance, and validity of the published works.

The current chapter is written to assist the reader in critically evaluating the literature. It is organized in a building block manner—with fundamental issues being discussed initially, after which more complex issues are addressed. Specifically, we begin by addressing study designs for clinical research with most of the section being devoted to important issues surrounding randomized, controlled trials (RCTs). After this, a discussion of how study designs dictate the level and grading of evidence is given. There are several grading systems, of which two are presented. The third section addresses the notion of best evidence and highlights the use of metaanalysis and practice guidelines. The fourth and final section discusses critical evaluation of the literature, and covers statistics, risk adjustment, and quality of life (QOL) studies. For the interested reader, further readings are available in the references.

Study Designs: Case Series, Case Control, Cohort, and RCTs

Providing the Evidence

Various hierarchies have been proposed for classifying study design.[1,2] In simplest terms, studies can be classified as case series, case control studies, cohort studies, and RCTs. The case series is the weakest and the RCT is the strongest for determining the effectiveness of treatment (Table 54-1).

Case Series

Case reports (arbitrarily defined as 10 or fewer subjects) and case series are the typical surgical studies performed. There is no concurrent control group although there may be a histori-

cal control group. Patients may be followed from the same inception point and followed prospectively—not for the purpose of the study—but in the normal clinical course of the disease. Typically, data from patient charts or clinical databases are reviewed retrospectively. Thus, the outcome of interest is present when the study is initiated. Despite the limitations of this study design, the importance of results from case series should not be minimized. It is because of careful observation that innovations in surgical practice and techniques have been and continue to be made. However, results from case series should be likened to those observations made in the laboratory. Just as those observations should lead to generation of a hypothesis and performance of an experiment to test it, an RCT should be performed to confirm the observations reported in a case series. Case series are plagued with biases such as selection and referral biases, and because data are not collected specifically for the study, they are often incomplete or even inaccurate. Therefore, incorrect conclusions about the efficacy of a treatment are common and surgeons should not rely solely on evidence from case series.

Case Control Studies

The case control study is the design used most frequently to study risk factors or causation. There are typically two groups of patients: the case group, composed of subjects in whom the outcome of interest is present, and the control group in whom it is not. Controls are selected by the investigator rather than by random allocation so the likelihood of bias being introduced is real and thus there is a risk of making an erroneous conclusion. Generally the controls are matched to the cases with respect to important prognostic variables other than the factor that is being studied. Although it is important to match the subjects to avoid an incorrect conclusion about the significance of the factor being studied, it is equally important not to overmatch the controls so that a true difference is not observed. In case control studies, as in case series, data are collected retrospectively. Thus, the outcome is present at the

TABLE 54-1. Types of study designs

	Control group	Prospective follow-up	Random allocation of subjects
Case series	No	No	No
Case control study	Yes	No	No
Cohort study	Yes	Yes	No
RCT	Yes	Yes	Yes

start of the study. As an example, Selby and colleagues[3] performed a case control study to make inferences about the effectiveness of flexible sigmoidoscopy in preventing rectal cancer. The cases were HMO patients who had been receiving regular yearly examinations and developed rectal cancer (the outcome of interest). The controls were individuals from the same cohort of patients who had not developed rectal cancer. They were matched to the cases with respect to age, sex, and date of entry into the health plan. Selby and colleagues found that cases were less likely to have had a flexible sigmoidoscopy than controls in the preceding 10 years (8.8% of cases versus 24.2% of controls).

Cohort Studies

Cohort studies may be retrospective or prospective. There are two or more groups but subjects are not randomly allocated to the groups. One group receives the treatment or exposure of interest whereas other groups of subjects receive another treatment or no treatment or exposure. The inception point may not be defined by the study and the intervention and follow-up may be ad hoc. However, the outcome is not present at the time that the inception cohort is assembled. There is less possibility of bias than a case control study because cases are not selected and the outcome is not present at the initiation of the study. However, the likelihood of bias is still high because subjects are not randomly allocated to groups. Instead, there is some selection process either by the subject or the clinician that allocates them to groups. For instance, subjects may be allocated to groups by where they live (when the effect of an environmental toxin is being studied), by choice (when a lifestyle factor such as dietary intake is being studied), or by physician (when a nonrandomized study of a treatment intervention is being performed). Retrospective cohort studies differ from prospective cohort studies in that data analysis and possibly data collection are performed retrospectively but there is an identifiable time point that can be used to define the inception cohort. Such a date could be the date of birth, date of first attendance at a hospital, etc. Cohort studies typically are performed by epidemiologists studying risk factors where randomization of patients is unethical. An example of a cohort study would be the use of a database to follow patients who had an anal mucosectomy versus no mucosectomy as part of restorative proctocolectomy, to determine the effect of the mucosectomy on long-term outcome.

Randomized, Controlled Trials

The RCT is accepted as the best trial design for establishing treatment effectiveness. There are several essential components of the RCT. First, subjects are randomly allocated to two groups: a treatment group (in which the new treatment is being tested) and a control group (in which the standard therapy or placebo is administered). Thus, the control group is concurrent and subjects are randomly allocated to the two groups. Second, the interventions and follow-up are standardized and performed prospectively. Thus, it is hoped that both groups are similar in all respects except for the interventions being studied. Not only does this guard against differences in factors known to be important, it also ensures that there are no differences as a result of unknown or unidentified factors. This latter point is especially important. Statistical techniques such as multivariate analysis can be used to adjust for known prognostic variables, but they obviously cannot adjust for unknown prognostic variables. There are multiple examples of studies showing differences between groups that cannot be accounted for by the known prognostic variables.[4]

Where differences in treatment effect are small, the RCT may minimize the chance of reaching an incorrect conclusion about the effectiveness of treatment. There are, however, some limitations to RCTs. First, RCTs tend to take a long time to complete because of the time required for planning, accruing, and following patients and finally analyzing results. As a consequence, results may not be available for many years. Second, clinical trials are expensive to perform, although their cost may be recouped if ineffective treatments are abandoned and only effective treatments are implemented.[5] Third, the results may not be generalizable or applicable to all patients with the disease because of the strict inclusion and exclusion criteria and inherent differences in patients who volunteer for trials. In addition, not all patients will respond similarly to treatment. Fourth, in situations whereby the disease or outcome is rare or only occurs after a long period of follow-up, RCTs are generally not feasible. Finally, the ethics of performing RCTs is controversial and some clinicians may be uncomfortable with randomizing their patients when they believe one treatment to be superior even if that is based only on anecdotal evidence.

There are elements common to all RCTs. The first and perhaps the most important issue in designing an RCT is to enunciate clearly the research question. Most RCTs are based on observations or experimental evidence from the laboratory. RCTs should always make biologic sense, have clinical relevance, and be feasible to perform. The research question will determine who will be included, what the intervention will be, and what will be measured. Frequently, a sequence of RCTs will be performed to evaluate a particular intervention. Initially, a rather small trial that is highly controlled using a physiologic or surrogate endpoint may be performed. This trial would provide evidence that the intervention is effective in the optimal situation (efficacy trial). However, it might lack clinical relevance especially if the endpoint were a physiologic measure. However, if it were positive, it would then lead to another trial, with more patients and a more clinically relevant outcome measure. If this were positive, a very large trial might be indicated to assess the effectiveness of the intervention in normal practice (effectiveness trial). Such an example would be studying the effect of a chemoprevention agent in colon cancer. Initially, the agent might be prescribed to a group of individuals at high risk for polyp formation (e.g., patients with familial polyposis coli) for a short time with the outcome measure being a rectal biopsy looking for proliferative changes. A subsequent trial might look at polyp regression in this same cohort of patients with subsequent trials aimed at the prevention of significant polyps in average-risk individuals who were followed for several years. As one can see, the selection of subjects, the intervention, duration of the trial, and the choice of outcome measure may vary depending on the research question. Ultimately, however, investigators wish to generalize the results to clinical practice so the outcome measures should be clinically relevant. For this reason, QOL measures are often included.

Although there are elements common to all RCTs, there are issues of special concern in surgical trials.[6] The issue of standardization of the procedure is of major importance in surgical trials. Standardization is difficult because surgeons vary in their experience with and in their ability to perform a surgical technique. There may be individual preferences in performing the procedure, and technical modifications may occur as the procedure evolves. Moreover, differences in perioperative and postoperative care may also impact on the outcome. There are two issues related to standardization of the procedure. First, there is the issue of who should perform the procedure: only experts or surgeons of varying ability. Implicit in this is the definition of an "expert." Second, there is the issue of standardization of the procedure so it is performed similarly by all surgical participants and it can be duplicated by others following publication of the trial results. The implications of these two issues are different and strategies to address them differ.

The first issue is analogous to assessing compliance in a medical trial. Thus, if the procedure is performed by experts only in a very controlled manner, this is analogous to an "efficacy trial." The advantage of such a trial is that if the procedure is truly superior to the other intervention, then this design has greatest likelihood of detecting a difference. The disadvantage, obviously, is that the results are less generalizable. Like most issues in clinical trials, there is no right or wrong answer. If the procedure is usually performed by experts, then it probably is desirable to have only experts involved in the trial. However, if a wide spectrum of surgeons perform the procedure, then it would be appropriate not to limit surgical participation.

Regardless of the number of surgeons involved in the trial and their desire to mimic routine practice, there must be a certain amount of standardization so that readers of the trial results can understand what was done and can duplicate the procedure in their own practice. There are several strategies to ensure a minimum standard. First, all surgeons should agree on the performance of the critical aspects of the procedure. It may not be necessary that there is agreement with all of the technical aspects but there should be consensus on those that are deemed to be important. Furthermore, if there are aspects of the perioperative and postoperative care that impact on outcome (e.g., postoperative adjuvant therapy), they should be standardized. Teaching sessions may be held preoperatively and feedback given to surgeons on their performance during the trial. As well, obtaining documentation that the procedure has been performed satisfactorily (e.g., through postoperative angiograms to document vessel patency or pathology specimens to document resection margins and lymph node excision) may contribute to ensuring that the surgery is being performed adequately. Finally, patients are usually stratified according to surgeon or center to ensure balance in case there are differences in surgical technique among centers or surgeons.

Blinding is often a difficult issue in surgical trials. It may not be an issue if two surgical procedures are being compared but is a major issue if a surgical procedure is being compared with a medical therapy. There is often a placebo effect of surgery. The classic example was observed in a series of 18 patients in which 13 patients underwent ligation of the internal mammary artery for coronary artery disease and five patients underwent a sham operation.[7] All of the patients in the latter group reported subjective improvement in their symptoms. In the 1990s, it would be difficult ethically to perform a sham operation so it might be impossible to conceal which treatment the patient received. The lack of blinding is especially worrisome if the primary outcome is a change in symptoms or QOL rather than a "hard" outcome measure such as mortality or morbidity. In these situations, if a hard outcome measure is also measured and it correlates with the patient's assessment, there is less concern about the possibility of bias. Assessments may be performed by an independent assessor who is unaware of the treatment group that the patient is in. Finally, if criteria used to define an outcome are explicitly specified a priori, it may minimize or eliminate bias (e.g., criteria to diagnose an intraabdominal abscess). Investigators may also choose in this situation to have a blinded panel review the results of tests to ensure that they meet the criteria.

The issue of timing of trials is difficult. Chalmers[8] has argued that the first patient in whom a procedure is performed should be randomized. Most surgeons would argue, however, that a learning curve exists in any procedure and that modifications to the technique are made frequently at its inception. By including these early patients, one would almost certainly bias the results against the new procedure. The introduction of laparoscopic cholecystectomy and the initially high rate of common bile duct injuries or the laparoscopic versus open inguinal hernia trial are good examples of this.[9] However, it may be difficult to initiate a trial when the procedure is widely accepted by both the patient and surgical community.

The paucity of RCTs testing surgical therapies supports this latter contention. This dilemma arises because, unlike the release of medical therapies, there is no regulating body in surgery that restricts performance of a procedure or requires proof of its efficacy. Probably, RCTs should be performed early before new procedures become accepted into practice, recognizing that future trials may be necessary as the procedure evolves and surgical experience increases. This is analogous to medical oncologic trials in which new trials are being planned as one is being completed. However, a surgical procedure must first be established adequately to avoid investing a large amount of money and time into a valueless trial.

Finally, patient issues may be of greater concern in surgical trials. In a medical trial, patients may be randomized to either treatment arm with the possibility that, at the conclusion of the trial, they can receive the more efficacious treatment if the disease is not progressive and the treatment is reversible. Surgical procedures, however, are almost always permanent. This may be of particular concern if a medical therapy is being compared with a surgical procedure or the two surgical procedures differ in their magnitude or invasiveness. Patients may have a preference for one or the other treatments and therefore refuse to participate in the trial. There also tends to be more emotion involved with surgery and patients may be less willing to leave the decision as to which procedure will be performed to chance. Surgeons themselves may be uncomfortable in discussing the uncertainty of randomization with patients requiring surgery.[10] Thus, accruing patients for surgical trials may be more difficult than for medical trials. In a survey of subjects who had already participated in a trial of maintenance therapy for Crohn's disease, Kennedy et al.[11] found that 91% would agree to participate in a trial again if it involved comparison of two medical treatments but only 44% would agree to participate if it included a surgical arm. Although accrual may be more difficult, there are notable examples of important surgical trials that have been performed.[12–14] Thus, they can be performed although it may require a larger pool of eligible patients from which to sample.

Levels of Evidence: Grading the Evidence

Levels of Evidence

There are several grading systems for assessing the level of evidence.[1,15–18] The first was developed by the Canadian Task Force on the Periodic Health Examination in the 1970s (Table 54-2) and has been adopted by the United States Task Force. Although differing in some respects, most systems consider the a priori design of the study and the actual quality of the study. Studies in which there has been blinded random allocation of subjects are given highest weighting because the risk of bias is minimized. Thus, an RCT will provide Level I evidence provided it is well executed with respect to the issues discussed earlier in this chapter.

TABLE 54-2. Canadian task force levels of evidence

Level	Type of evidence
I	Evidence obtained from at least one properly RCT
II-1	Evidence obtained from well-designed controlled trials without randomization
II-2	Evidence obtained from well-designed cohort or case-control analytic studies, preferably from more than one center or research group
II-3	Evidence obtained from comparisons between times or places with or without the intervention; dramatic results in uncontrolled experiments (such as the results of treatment with penicillin in the 1940s) could also be included in this category
III	Opinions of respected authorities, based on clinical experience, descriptive studies, or reports of expert committees

Although this system is of value because of its simplicity, difficulties may arise when readers wish to pool results from several studies, either informally during their reading or when performing systematic reviews or developing guidelines. Decisions must be made on whether studies should be included or excluded depending on the quality of the study.[19] As well, the systems are not sensitive to the relevance of the findings of studies. For instance, neither the clinical relevance of the outcome measures, the baseline risk of the effect, nor the actual results of the studies (e.g., study results that are not consistent with results from other RCTs) are considered in any system.

In the American Society of Colon and Rectal Surgeons (ASCRS), the Standards Committee in 2003 decided to adopt the grading system shown in Table 54-3.[16,18] This system identifies the level of evidence based on the available literature. Moreover, this system also provides a grade for the

TABLE 54-3. Levels of evidence and grade of recommendation used by the ASCRS Standards Committee

Level	Type of evidence
I	Evidence obtained from metaanalysis of multiple, well-designed, controlled studies. Randomized trials with low false-positive and low false-negative errors (high power)
II	Evidence obtained from at least one well-designed experimental study. Randomized trials with high false-positive and/or false-negative errors (low power)
III	Evidence obtained from well-designed, quasi-experimental studies such as nonrandomized, controlled, single-group, pre-post, cohort, time, or matched case-control series
IV	Evidence from well-designed, nonexperimental studies such as comparative and correlational descriptive and case studies
V	Evidence from case reports and clinical examples

Grade	Grade of recommendation
A	There is evidence of Type I or consistent findings from multiple studies of Type II, III, or IV
B	There is evidence of Type II, III, or IV and findings are generally consistent
C	There is evidence of Type II, III, or IV but findings are inconsistent
D	There is little or no systematic empirical evidence

recommendation that depends on both the level of evidence and the consistency of the results from the different studies.

Assessing the Best Evidence

What Is the Quality of Evidence Evaluating Surgical Practice?

There is certainly a perception that surgeons are not adequately assessing surgical procedures. In an editorial in the Lancet in 1996 entitled "Surgical Research or Comic Opera: Questions but Few Answers," Richard Horton criticized surgeons for their high reliance on case studies and stated that if surgeons wished to retain their academic reputations, they must find imaginative ways to collaborate with epidemiologists to improve the design of the case series and to plan randomized trials.[20] Furthermore, he quoted a medical statistician, Major Greenwell, who stated, "I should like to shame surgeons out of the comic opera performances which they suppose are statistics of operations."[20] This quote dated back to 1923. In a similar condemnation, Spodick[21] complained of the "repeated reporting of biased data from uncontrolled or poorly controlled trials, giving an illusion of success due to sheer quantity," and stated that "a thousand zeros look impressive on paper, but they still amount to zero."

So what is the evidence of the evidence? As one would predict, repeated studies have shown that there is a predominance of case studies and a relative paucity of RCTs published in the literature. Solomon and McLeod[2] reviewed three surgical journals—*British Journal of Surgery*, *Surgery*, and *Diseases of the Colon and Rectum*—over two time periods—1980 and 1990. They found that only 7% of all published clinical articles were RCTs despite the fact that almost half of the articles addressed issues of treatment effectiveness. Furthermore, the proportion differed neither between 1980 and 1990 nor among the three journals. Another examination of the *Diseases of the Colon and Rectum* showed that the numbers of RCTs published were 5 (in 1990), 13 (in 1995), and 17 (in 2000).[22] Similarly, Barnes[23] noted that only 5% of abstracts accepted at the annual joint meetings of the Society for Vascular Surgery and the International Society for Cardiovascular Surgery dealt with RCTs. Haines[24] reported that only 5% of articles in the *Journal of Neurosurgery* between 1973 and 1977 were controlled clinical trials. More recently, Horton[20] noted that 7% of articles published in nine surgical journals were reports of RCTs.

What clinical trials are being performed by surgeons? Solomon et al.[25] were able to identify 204 RCTs published in the literature in 1990, which were published by surgeons, were from a surgical department, or contained at least one surgical arm. They estimated that their search retrieved approximately half of the surgical RCTs that were published. Of these trials, the majority (75%) compared two medical therapies whereas trials comparing two surgical therapies comprised only 18% and trials comparing a medical to a surgical therapy comprised only 5%. Thus, trials comparing antibiotic prophylactic regimens and adjuvant chemotherapy regimens were not uncommon, whereas trials comparing two different operative procedures were infrequent. Furthermore, the published trials tended to be small: almost two-thirds were single center trials, and in half there was no significant difference detected, probably because the sample size was small and the trial lacked adequate power. Unfortunately, surgeons were the primary authors in only a small proportion of studies, even those comparing two surgical procedures and in areas almost exclusively surgical in nature (e.g., trauma). The quality of the trials tended to be poor, especially if they contained one or two surgical arms or were published in surgical journals. Hall and colleagues[26] reviewed the published surgical trials in 10 journals between 1988 and 1994. They also found that the trials tended to be of poor quality.

Given the relative paucity of RCTs reported in the literature, Solomon and McLeod[27] then wished to determine whether it should be possible to perform RCTs in more instances or whether it is not possible, as has been suggested by some. To address this issue, they identified a sample of 260 questions in the surgical literature relating to the efficacy of general surgical procedures. From this analysis, it was estimated that it should be possible to perform an RCT to answer approximately 40% of questions. In contrast, only 4.6% of the articles reviewed reported results of RCTs and more than 50% of the articles were case reports or case studies. Although methodologic issues unique to surgical trials are frequently cited as the reason for not being able to do an RCT, in fact, they believed that methodologic issues would preclude doing an RCT only 1% of the time.

The most common issues to preclude performing an RCT would be strong patient preferences for one or the other treatments or the infrequency of the condition. However, with respect to the former, this was an assessment made by clinicians and trials, such as those comparing mastectomy and lumpectomy and carotid endarterectomy to medical therapy, illustrating that it is possible to do trials even when the alternative treatments differ significantly in magnitude.

Although one cannot argue that surgeons do seem to rely on case series rather than RCTs to evaluate new surgical techniques, it is also important to point out that some noteworthy surgical trials that have had a high impact have been performed: mastectomy versus lumpectomy trials, carotid endarterectomy and ECIC bypass trials for stroke prevention, and the laparoscopic versus open colorectal cancer trial.[12,13,28,29] Furthermore, we must not forget the pioneering work of John Goligher[30] who performed a series of trials assessing the surgical management of peptic ulcer disease long before RCTs were in vogue. However, although internists may criticize surgeons for not performing more trials, it is also important to realize that perhaps the greatest impetus for medical trials is the requirement by regulating agencies of evidence from clinical trials before release of new medication and, therefore, the availability of funding from industry to test them.

Beyond the issue of the performance of RCTs, it is important for the reader to be able to critically evaluate the literature, which means that certain important information must be included in the manuscript. A recent article examined the quality of reporting for RCTs in the *Diseases of the Colon and Rectum*. The authors found that 77% of 11 basic elements were reported appropriately. The best reported items were eligibility criteria, discussion of statistical tests, and accounting for all patients lost to follow-up. The worst reported item involved power calculations. Only 11% appropriately reported power calculations. For the critical reader, the reporting of appropriate methods, limitations, and data is important. To this end, standards have been recommended regarding the publication of RCTs (i.e., CONSORT—Consolidated Standards of Reporting Trials) and includes 22 items (Table 54-4).[31]

TABLE 54-4. CONSORT checklist for reporting RCTs

1. Title and abstract—how participants were allocated to interventions

Introduction

2. Background—scientific background and explanation of rationale

Methods

3. Participants—eligibility criteria, settings, and locations of data collection
4. Interventions—details of interventions for each group
5. Objectives—specific aims and hypotheses
6. Outcomes—defined primary and secondary outcomes
7. Sample size—how sample size was determined, interim analyses, stopping rules
8. Randomization sequence generation—method used to generate randomization
9. Randomization allocation concealment—method used to implement randomization
10. Randomization implementation—who generated the allocation sequence, who enrolled participants
11. Blinding—whether or not blinding was performed (subjects, researchers, etc.)
12. Statistical methods—methods used to compare groups

Results

13. Participant flow—flow of subjects through each stage (strongly recommend diagram) such as numbers of subjects randomly assigned, receiving intended treatment, completing protocol, etc.
14. Recruitment—dates defining the periods of recruitment and follow-up
15. Baseline data—baseline demographic/clinical characteristics of each group.
16. Numbers analyzed—"denominator" of each group and whether analysis was performed by "intention to treat"
17. Outcomes and estimation—summary of results for each primary and secondary outcome for each group
18. Ancillary analyses—address added analyses and whether they were prespecified or exploratory
19. Adverse events—all important adverse events or side effects for each group

Discussion

20. Interpretation—interpretation of results, discussing hypotheses, bias, limitations
21. Generalizability—external validity of the trial findings
22. Overall evidence—general interpretation of the results in the context of current evidence

The Best Evidence

Practicing evidence-based medicine might be a daunting task for the clinician who has a busy clinical practice, must look after the administrative and financial aspects of his or her practice, and then try to keep current with the latest information. It is physically impossible for clinicians to read all published medical journals, even in one's own specialty, much less stay abreast of information that is distributed on the Internet and non–peer reviewed sources. Thus, the busy clinician must learn ways to access the best information and be able to critically appraise it to determine its worth and relevance to his or her practice. There may be two scenarios for which clinicians wish to obtain information: for specific patient problems encountered daily and for general maintenance or updating of knowledge. Although clinicians will need to have the skills to retrieve information and critically appraise it, there are several information sources that may be of particular help including systematic reviews and evidence-based practice guidelines.

Systematic Reviews or Metaanalyses

The terms systematic review and metaanalysis have been used interchangeably. However, systematic reviews or overviews are qualitative reviews, whereas statistical methods are used to combine and summarize the results of several studies in metaanalysis.[32] In both, there is a specific scientific approach to the identification, critical appraisal, and synthesis of all relevant studies on a specific topic. They differ from the usual clinical review in that there is an explicit, specific question that is addressed. As well, the methodology is explicit and there is a conscientious effort to retrieve and review all studies on the topic without preconceived prejudice. The value of metaanalysis is that study results are combined so conclusions can be made about therapeutic effectiveness, or if there is not a conclusive answer, to plan new studies.[33] They are especially useful when results from several studies disagree with regard to the magnitude or the direction of effect, when individual studies are too small to detect an effect and label it as statistically not significant, or when a large trial is too costly or time consuming to perform. For the clinician, metaanalyses are useful because results of individual trials are combined so he or she does not have to retrieve, evaluate, and synthesize the results of all studies on the topic. Thus, it may increase the efficiency of the clinician in keeping abreast of recent advances.

Metaanalysis is a relatively new method for synthesizing information from multiple studies. Thus, the methodology is constantly evolving, and similar to other studies, the quality of individual metaanalysis may be quite variable. There has been a call for standardization of the methodology used in metaanalysis.[34,35] However, because the rigor of the methodology of many published metaanalyses may be quite variable, the clinician should have some knowledge of metaanalysis

TABLE 54-5. Guidelines for using a review

1. Did the overview address a focused clinical question?
2. Were the criteria used to select articles for inclusion appropriate?
3. Is it unlikely that important, relevant studies were missed?
4. Was the validity of the included studies appraised?
5. Were the assessments of the studies reproducible?
6. Were the results similar from study to study?
7. What are the overall results of the review?
8. How precise were the results?
9. Can the results be applied to my patient care?
10. Were all the clinically important outcomes considered?
11. Are the benefits worth the harms and costs?

methodology and be able to critically appraise them. Published guidelines are available (Table 54-5).[36]

There are some basic steps that are followed in performing a metaanalysis. First, the metaanalysis should address a specific healthcare question. Second, various strategies should be used to ensure that all relevant studies (RCTs) on the topic are retrieved. These include searching various databases such as MEDLINE and EMBASE. In addition, proceedings of meetings and reference lists should be checked and content experts and clinical researchers are consulted in order to ensure all published and nonpublished trials are identified. Reliance on MEDLINE searches alone will result in incomplete retrieval of published studies.[27] Third, as in other studies, inclusion criteria determining which studies will be included should be set a priori. Fourth, data from the individual studies should be extracted by two blinded investigators to ensure that this is done accurately. As well, these investigators should assess the quality of the individual studies. Fifth, the data should be combined using various statistical techniques. Before doing so, statistical tests to determine the "sameness" or "homogeneity" of the individual studies should be performed.

Whereas some have embraced metaanalysis as a systematic approach to synthesizing published information from individual trials, others have cautioned about the results of metaanalysis and some have been completely skeptical of the technique.[37] LeLorier et al.[38] compared the results of 19 metaanalyses with the results of 12 large trials published subsequently. If the subsequent trials had not been performed, an ineffective treatment would have been adopted in 32% of cases and a useful treatment would have been rejected in 33%. Others have pointed out that metaanalyses on the same clinical question have led to different conclusions.[39] Some of these are attributable to methodologic problems. Failure to use broad enough search strategies may result in exclusion of all relevant studies. Usually, unpublished studies are excluded and these are more likely to be "negative trials" (so-called publication bias).[40] As well, there is evidence that omission of trials not published in English journals may bias the results.[41] Finally, there is a strong association between statistically positive conclusions

of metaanalyses and their quality (i.e., the lower the quality of the studies, the more likely that the metaanalysis reached a positive conclusion).[42] One of the values of metaanalysis is that the generalizability of the results is increased by combining the results of several trials. However, if there is great variation in studies, including patient inclusion criteria, dosage and mode of administration of medication, and length of follow-up (so-called heterogeneity), it may be inappropriate to combine results. If this is done, it may produce invalid results. Other reasons for discrepancies may be the use of different statistical tests and failure to update the metaanalysis. Finally, metaanalysis has generally been restricted to combining the results of RCTs even though there is also a need for combining data from nonrandomized or observational studies.

In response to the problems in disseminating the results of individual RCTs, the Cochrane Collaboration was established[43] to prepare, maintain, and disseminate systematic reviews of RCTs of healthcare interventions. It was named after Archie Cochrane, an eminent statistician in the United Kingdom. The Cochrane Collaboration is a voluntary international organization that encourages the participation of interested individuals. Cochrane groups are organized by areas of interest (e.g., upper gastrointestinal, inflammatory bowel disease, colorectal cancer, hepatobiliary). In addition to preparing reviews, journals are hand searched and a database of all published RCTs is maintained. Systematic reviews are constantly being updated. The Cochrane Library is available on CD ROM on a quarterly basis (The Cochrane Library. Update Software Inc. 936 La Rueda, Vista, CA 92084). It includes several databases including the Cochrane Database of Systematic Reviews. This is a valuable source of high-level information for practicing clinicians. Unfortunately, it is of somewhat more limited use to surgeons because of the paucity of published surgical RCTs and metaanalyses.

Practice Guidelines

Practice guidelines have been defined by the Institute of Medicine as "systematically developed statements to assist practitioner and patient decisions about appropriate health care for specific clinical circumstances."[44] Guidelines are not standards that set rigid rules of care for patients. Rather, guidelines should be flexible so that individual patient characteristics, preferences of surgeons and patients, and local circumstances can be accommodated.[45]

Guideline development has occurred for several reasons.[46] First, as discussed earlier, there is growing evidence of substantial unexplained and inappropriate variation in clinical practice patterns, which is probably attributable in part to physician uncertainty. Second, there is evidence that the traditional methods for delivering continuing medical education are ineffective and that clinicians have difficulty in assimilating the rapidly evolving scientific evidence. Third, there is concern that as healthcare resources become more limited, there will be inadequate funds to deliver high-quality care if current technology and treatments are used inappropriately or ineffectively.

Practice guidelines have been promoted as one strategy to assist clinical decision making to increase the effectiveness and decrease unnecessary costs of delivering healthcare services.[46] Many clinicians are wary of guidelines and believe that they are simply a means to limit resources and inhibit clinical decision making and individual preferences. Guidelines have also been criticized for being too idealistic and failing to take into account the realities of day to day practice. The argument is that patients differ in their clinical manifestations, associated diseases, and preferences for treatments. Thus, guidelines may be either too restrictive or irrelevant. Also, clinicians may be confused because of conflicting guidelines. Finally, guideline development may be inhibited because there is a lack of evidence upon which to base guidelines.

Many groups and organizations have begun to develop practice guidelines. Guidelines are developed using different methods.[47] Guidelines can be developed based on informal consensus. The criteria upon which decisions are made are often poorly described and there is no systematic approach to reviewing the evidence. More often, these guidelines are based on the opinion of experts. Readers are unable to judge the validity of the guidelines because even if a systematic approach was followed, the process is not documented. In many instances, guidelines are self-serving and used to promote a certain specialty or expertise. The National Institutes of Health and others have produced guidelines based on a formal consensus approach. Although this approach tends to be more structured than the informal consensus, it has the same potential flaws in that it is less structured and susceptible to the biases of the experts.

Evidence-based guidelines are the most rigorously developed guidelines.[15–46,48] There should be a focused clinical question and a systematic approach to the retrieval; assessment of quality and synthesis of evidence should be followed. Guideline development should also be a dynamic process with constant updating as more evidence is available. In addition to assessment of the literature, there is usually an interpretation of the evidence by experts and the evidence may be modulated by current or local circumstances (e.g., cost/availability of technology).

Whereas there has been much attention given to the preparation of guidelines, there has been less emphasis on the dissemination of and evaluation of the impact of guidelines. Unfortunately, there is some indication that evidence-based guidelines may not have as much impact either on changing physician behavior or improving outcome.

Because there are many guidelines available, including some with conflicting recommendations, clinicians require some skills to evaluate the guidelines and determine their validity and applicability[15,48] (Table 54-6).

TABLE 54-6. Guidelines for assessing practice guidelines

1. Were all the important options and outcomes clearly specified?
2. Was an explicit and sensible process used to identify, select, and combine evidence?
3. Was an explicit and sensible process used to consider the relative value of different outcomes?
4. Is the guideline likely to account for important recent developments?
5. Has the guideline been subject to peer review and testing?
6. Are practical, clinically important, recommendations made?
7. How strong are the recommendations?
8. What is the impact of uncertainty associated with the evidence and values used in guidelines?
9. Is the primary objective of the guideline consistent with your objective?
10. Are the recommendations applicable to your patients?

Critically Evaluating the Literature (How to ...)

Critically Appraising the Literature

Critical appraisal skills must be mastered before evidence-based practice can be implemented successfully.[49] Critical appraisal skills are those that enable application of certain rules of evidence and laws of logic to clinical, investigative, and published data and information in order to evaluate their validity, reliability, credibility, and utility. Clinicians need critical appraisal skills because of the constant appearance of new knowledge and the short half-life of current knowledge. Clinicians cannot rely on facts learned from medical school. Instead, they must have the necessary skills to assess the validity and relevance of new knowledge in order to provide the best care to their patients.

Critical appraisal requires the clinician to have some knowledge of clinical epidemiology, biostatistics, epidemiology, decision analysis, and economics. Critical appraisal skills also improve with practice, and the clinician is encouraged simply to begin using the skills they already have and build on them. There are a variety of articles and books written on the topic. The McMaster Evidence Based Medicine Group has published a series of articles in the *Journal of the American Medical Association*.[15,36,48,50–64] Sackett and colleagues[49] have consolidated much of this information into a book entitled "Evidence Based Medicine." Interested readers are encouraged to seek further information from these and other sources.

To make decisions about a patient, clinicians generally need to know something about the cause of the disease, risk factors for it, the natural history or prognosis of the disease, how to quantify aspects of the disease (measurement issues), diagnostic tests and the diagnosis of the disease, and the effectiveness of treatment. In addition, clinicians now need to have some knowledge of economic analysis, health services research, practice guidelines, systematic reviews, and decision analysis to fully appreciate the literature and make use of all sources of information.

Many clinicians believe that critical appraisal only requires knowledge of statistics. As stated previously, an array of skills is required. Furthermore, in making decisions about the internal validity of the study (i.e., How good is the study and how confident am I that the results or conclusions are correct?), it is critical that the clinician can assess the study design and how well the study was actually performed. The statistical analysis, although important, is only one component of study design.

Generally, clinicians read articles so they can generalize the results of the study and apply them to their own patients. There are two potential sources of error, which may lead to incorrect conclusions about the validity of the study results: systematic error (bias) or random error. Bias is defined as "any effect at any stage of investigation or inference tending to produce results that depart systematically from the true values."[65] For example, the term "biased sample" is often used to mean that the sample of patients is not typical or representative of patients with that condition. There are a number of biases that might be present, not just those related to patient selection. It may be difficult for the reader to discern the presence of bias and its magnitude. For instance, suppose two different treatments are compared in two groups of patients from two different hospitals. Although the authors could provide basic demographic information on the patient groups, one could not be certain that there were not differences in the patients, the severity of the disease, ancillary care, etc., at the two different hospitals and these differences, rather than the treatment, led to an improved outcome. The risk of an error as a result of bias decreases as the rigor of the trial design increases (see discussion of risk adjustment in the proceeding section). Because of the random allocation of patients as well as its other attributes, the RCT is considered the best design for minimizing bias. In observational studies, including outcomes research (where patients have not been randomized), various statistical tests (e.g., multivariate analysis) are frequently used to adjust for differences in prognostic factors between the two groups of patients. However, it is important to realize that it is possible to adjust for only known or measurable factors. In addition to these, there may be other unknown and possibly important prognostic factors that cannot be adjusted. Again, only if patients are randomly allocated can one be certain that the two groups are similar with respect to all known and unknown prognostic variables.

The other type of error is random error. Random error occurs because of chance, when the result obtained in the sample of patients studied differs from the result that would be obtained if the entire population were studied.[65] Statistical testing can be performed to determine the likelihood of a random error. The type of statistical test used will vary depending on the type of data. Some of the more common tests are shown in Table 54-7. There are two types of random error: Type I and Type II errors. The risk of stating there is a difference between two treatments when really there is not one is known as a Type I error. In the theory of testing hypotheses, rejecting a null hypothesis when it is actually true is called

TABLE 54-7. Types of statistical tests

Data type	Statistical tests (with no adjustment for risk factors)	Statistical tests (with adjustment for risk factors)
Binary (dichotomous)	Fisher exact test or chi square	Logistic regression
Ordered discrete	Mann-Whitney U test	
Continuous (normal distribution)	Student's t test	Analysis of covariance
Time to event (censored data)	Log-rank Wilcoxon test	Log-rank (Cox proportional hazard)

a Type I error. By convention, if the risk of the result occurring because of chance is less than 5% (a P value less than .05), then the difference in the results of treatment is considered statistically significant. There really is a difference in the effectiveness of the two treatments.

One of the issues regarding Type I errors is that of multiple comparisons. Specifically, the more comparisons being performed with a given set of data, the higher the likelihood of a Type I error (finding a difference, when one truly does not exist). Under these circumstances, a correction for multiple comparisons (e.g., a Bonferroni correction) should be performed by the authors.

Although a result may be statistically significant, the clinician must determine whether it is clinically relevant or important.[49] Typically, treatment effects can be written as absolute risk reduction (ARR) or relative risk reduction (RRR). The ARR is simply the difference in rates between the control group and the experimental group whereas the RRR is a proportional risk reduction and is calculated by dividing the ARR by the control risk. The advantage of the ARR is that the baseline event rate is considered. For instance, the RRR would be the same in two different studies in which the rates between the control and experimental groups were 50% and 25% and 0.5% and 0.25%, respectively. In other words, whereas the ARR would be 25% in the first study and 0.25% in the second study, the RRR for both studies would be 50%. Although the RRR is the same in both studies, the treatment benefit in the second scenario may be trivial.

Recently, Cook and Sackett[66] have coined the term "number needed to treat" (NNT) which may make more intuitive sense to clinicians rather than thinking in terms of ARR and RRR. It is calculated by dividing the ARR into 1. Thus, in the example mentioned above, four patients would have to be treated to prevent one bad outcome (the NNT is four) in the first study whereas 400 would have to be treated to prevent one bad outcome (the NNT is 400) in the second. It is up to the judgment of the clinician to decide whether the treatment benefit is clinically significant. The statistician can only determine whether a treatment benefit is statistically significant. Whether the effect is clinically significant will depend on the NNT, the frequency and severity of side effects (sometimes stated as the number needed to harm—NNH), as well as the cost of treatment and its feasibility and acceptability.

The other random error is the Type II error. A Type II error occurs when two treatments are, in reality, different but one concludes that they are equally effective. In the theory of testing hypotheses, accepting a null hypothesis when it is incorrect is called a Type II error. It is not uncommon for clinicians to read a study in which the results are not statistically significant and to wonder whether the two treatments are equally effective or whether there is a Type II error. When investigators plan a trial, they minimize the risk of a Type II error by calculating a sample size to ensure that there is adequate power (1-Type II error) to show a difference if one really exists. To calculate a sample size, both the probability of a Type I error and power are specified, plus the mean and standard deviation or event rate in the control group and the size of the difference that one wishes to detect. Not surprisingly, the more variable the subjects, the less frequent the event rate, or the smaller the difference in the effects of the treatment, the more subjects that are necessary to be certain a treatment effect has not been missed. Conversely, fewer subjects are necessary if there is less variability, the outcome occurs more frequently, or one expects a large difference in treatment effect. With regard to performing sample size calculations, several studies have examined whether such calculations have been made. Maggard et al.[67] examined all RCTs performed in three surgery-related journals for four consecutive years and found that 38% reported sample size calculations. Moreover, whereas only 50% of the studies were appropriately powered to detect a 50% effect change, only 19% were appropriately powered to detect a 20% effect change. Most striking, of the studies that were underpowered, more than half needed to increase sample size by more than 10-fold.

Whereas a power calculation is performed a priori, a more useful measure for the reader interpreting the study results is the calculation of 95% confidence intervals (CIs).[68] The 95% CI gives a range within which the true mean of the sample variable lies, with a probability of 95%.[65] The wider the CI, the less certain one can be that the two treatments are really similar in effectiveness. Conversely, if the CIs are narrow, one can be much more certain that the treatments are equally effective. To operationalize the notion of CIs, if the CIs overlap, then the means are not significantly different. If, however, the CIs do not overlap, then the means are different. Moreover, one frequently sees CIs when odds ratios are reported. In this case, if CI for the odds ratio overlaps 1, then there is no significant difference in odds. If the CI of the odds ratio is greater than one, then there is a significant increase in odds (i.e., a positive association between the predictor variable and outcome). Finally, if the CI of the odds ratio is less than one, then there is a significant decrease in odds (i.e., a negative association between the predictor variable and outcome).

Risk Adjustment

For the surgeon reading the literature, an issue that is inherently related to systematic error, or selection bias, is that of patient comorbidity. The methodology for controlling for differing patient disease severity is termed risk adjustment, and is an important issue for critically evaluating the literature—particularly when the study design is not an RCT. For example, given a specific disease, if one hospital (or surgeon) has a patient population with mostly frail, elderly patients and reports a case series of procedure Y with poor results, whereas another hospital provides care for primarily young and healthy patients, and reports a case series of procedure Z with good results, the reader may not be able to distinguish whether the results were attributable to the differences in the procedure, or the patients (i.e., comorbidities). This is one of the most common problems with evaluating the surgical literature.

The techniques of risk adjustment need to account for both the health status of the patient before treatment as well as severity (and acuity) of the current (i.e., morbid) illness.[69] A patient with many health problems such as insulin-dependent diabetes and steroid-dependent pulmonary disease will be less likely to do well after an operation compared with a patient who is free of comorbid health problems. Furthermore, there are also issues regarding the primary (or morbid) disease. It is well accepted that a patient who presents to the hospital with a perforated sigmoid cancer in septic shock is more likely to have a worse outcome than a patient with early stage disease who was diagnosed during a routine screening examination. Surgeons know these facts intuitively through training and experience; however, translating this notion into an adjustment method that appropriately accounts for preoperative factors is the challenge. This challenge, however, is an important issue when critically evaluating the literature.

Risk adjustment is generally accomplished by identifying and then accounting for the factors that determine, or are associated with, variations in outcomes. The degree of importance of these factors needs to also be assessed with subsequent weighting of the factors (individually or in categories). Many risk-adjustment methods have developed indices or formulas to calculate the level of risk.

One of the most difficult issues in performing risk adjustment is deciding which comorbid diseases or conditions to adjust for in the analysis. For the critical reader, one should ask whether the risk factors included by the authors are indeed the important ones to include, but also, it is important to think whether the authors have not omitted any important ones as well. Moreover, risk factors may include other aspects in addition to comorbidities. Such things as functional status (e.g., activities of daily living) and physiologic or laboratory parameters (e.g., albumin level) may (should) be included to adjust risk.

Overall, a reader should examine whether or not risk adjustment was performed, and if so, is there a validated method being used, and is this method adequate? There are several methods with varying ability to risk adjust; we will briefly discuss two common methods being used in the literature.

Charlson Index

One of the most common indices for risk adjustment currently being used is the Charlson Index.[70] This index was designed as a method to help predict mortality for hospitalized patients and was originally developed using patient data that are obtained from patient records; later, however, the index was translated for use with administrative databases. Overall, the Charlson method predicts the risk of dying by assigning a score to each comorbid factor. Several comorbid conditions are included. The method itself is simple: points are summed for each of the comorbid conditions that are present to generate an index score; this score can then be used as a risk adjustment score for a patient's level of comorbidity. Some of the conditions (and weights) included in the Charlson Index are congestive heart failure (1), myocardial infarction (1), moderate or severe renal disease (2), moderate or severe liver disease (3), and acquired immunodeficiency syndrome (6). Because the Charlson Index has been frequently used in the literature, especially in population-based secondary analyses of administrative data, comparisons theoretically may be made among studies.

Another method for risk adjustment in surgery is seen in the Veterans Affairs (VA) developed system used in the National Surgical Quality Improvement Program (NSQIP).[71–73] The VA NSQIP method was established though the VA hospitals and was designed to compare the quality of surgical care. In brief, NSQIP was developed after a mandate that the VA report annual surgical outcomes. These outcomes were to be compared after adjustment for the severity of a patient's illness and comorbid factors. However, it soon became apparent that to appropriately compare outcomes, risk-adjustment models specific to surgical specialties and procedures had to be developed. NSQIP was created in response to these issues.

The NSQIP data were designed such that a clinical surgical nurse collects preoperative, intraoperative, and 30-day outcome data on nearly all major operations at all inpatient VA hospitals. Preoperative data include 10 demographic, 30 clinical, and 12 laboratory values. Additionally, intraoperative data consist of 15 variables, and postoperative data include 10 laboratory values. NSQIP collects 30-day outcomes, including 30-day mortality, 21 categories of 30-day morbidities, and length of stay. From the collection of these perioperative risk factors, a method of predicting adjusted outcomes was developed. Moreover, by determining the importance of individual risk factors for specific surgical specialties and procedures, individualized methods were created. Each method included the risk factors shown to have the greatest importance in adjusting for outcomes. Individualized models were created for many of the surgical specialties (including: general, orthopedics, urology, vascular, neurosurgery, otolaryngology, and thoracic) and for specific surgical procedures within these areas.

In addition to collecting perioperative items for risk assessment, these data can all be used in a predictive manner. For example, the risk factors used in the NSQIP model can be used to predict 30-day mortality. A study by Longo et al.[74] examined the predictive factors for 30-day mortality after colectomy. They found the most important predictor to be an ASA class IV or V with an odds ratio of 4.7.

Quality of Life

QOL is receiving increasing attention as a measure of outcome from patients, physicians, and even third-party payers. In colorectal surgery, there have been an increasing number of QOL studies; however, the quality of the studies themselves varies and certain methodologic details may make it difficult for the reader who is trying to critically evaluate the findings. One of the important issues in this regard is the instrument that is used to measure QOL. There are many types of measurement tools (e.g., generic versus disease-specific versus symptom specific, etc.) and this fact alone contributes to the difficulty with initiating the QOL studies in the literature.

The purpose of this section is to familiarize the clinical surgeon with some of the available tools and methods for measuring QOL such that a critical assessment of the colorectal QOL literature may be performed by the reader.

The most common way of measuring QOL is through patient self-assessment surveys. These surveys (also called questionnaires, tools, or instruments) are organized into a series of items that gather information on specific areas of interest related to QOL. For example, most surveys that address "overall" QOL include questions that cover the areas of physical, psychological, social, and overall well being.[75–77]

For a survey to be considered useful, the instrument should have reliability, validity, and responsiveness. It is important for the reader of QOL manuscripts to assess whether the QOL instrument was reviewed critically with regard to these items *before* its use in the particular study. Using instruments that have not been assessed for each of these attributes can lead to serious errors in measurement, uninterpretable data, erroneous conclusions, and nonreproducible results.

Reliability refers to the extent that a survey produces reproducible results. The more reliable an instrument is, the lower the element of random error. In practice, reliability refers to the extent to which the measure yields the same results in repeated applications in an unchanged population (which can be evaluated with a test–retest assessment).[78]

Validity refers to the ability of a survey to accurately measure what it is designed to measure. There are three types of validity that are frequently discussed in relation to surveys. The simplest is criterion validity in which the new measure is correlated with an accepted gold standard. The second form of validity is content validity or how well individual items cover the entire content of issues within a domain or scale. In general, similar to internal reliability, a greater number of items in an individual scale will result in greater content validity. The third form of validity is construct validity or how well a survey measures unobservable phenomena (or constructs).[79]

Finally, responsiveness, or sensitivity to change, is the extent to which an instrument can detect true differences. In other words, it is a survey's ability to change as the patient's clinical status changes. Both increased numbers of questions and/or a greater range of possible responses on a single question will result in increased responsiveness. In general, disease-specific surveys offer greater sensitivity than generic instruments because of the number and focus of the questions directed toward the specific disease being treated.

For the critical reader, interpretability has been thus far the most elusive aspect of QOL measurement in the literature. Most of the difficulty in interpretation of QOL data stems from the fact that what is being measured is not observable. In this regard, it is difficult to determine the significance of the QOL change—i.e., what is a significant *clinical* change? This will be further addressed below.

Survey instruments may be categorized broadly into two types—generic versus disease specific. Generic surveys attempt to measure the global relationship between a patient's health and their well being. The strength of such an instrument lies in its ability to provide a bottom line assessment of well being as influenced by health status. An additional advantage of such an approach is that these instruments can be used to compare QOL across diseases. Examples of generic surveys that have been used in colorectal disease include Sickness Impact Profile (ulcerative colitis, colorectal cancer),[80,81] Nottingham Health Profile (colorectal cancer),[82,83] and the Short Form 36 (fecal incontinence, restorative proctocolectomy, familial adenomatous polyposis, and colorectal cancer).[22,79,80,84] The benefit in the use of an instrument across many diseases is an improvement in interpretability of results through greater criterion validity. Physicians are able to more easily make comparisons across diseases and possibly compare a change in disease status to that of a familiar disease.

Another benefit of these surveys is comparison of results with normative data, such as aged matched, healthy, control individuals. The SF-36 survey, for instance, has this advantage because scores (overall and for each of its eight domains) are available for the general population, and can be subsetted by such things as age and gender. In this regard, information may potentially be gained concerning the impact of a disease if the individual had similar QOL to the control population before the onset of his or her disease.

More clinically detailed than a generic survey, disease- or symptom-specific surveys offer the possibility of allowing the physician and patient to concentrate on the issues that can be expected to influence QOL in the context of the disease process in question. Because of this focus, these surveys should be more sensitive to the changes in QOL that may be expected with a specific problem, or its treatment, or both. This improved sensitivity, however, comes at the cost of a lack of generalizability, in that the survey is only useful for those specific issues (e.g., disease, symptom, procedure). Some examples of targeted surveys for colorectal surgery include the European Organization for the Research and Treatment of Cancer's Quality of Life Questionnaire for ColoRectal cancer (EORTC QLQ-CR38),[85,86] the Inflammatory Bowel Disease Questionnaire,[84,87,88] and the Rating Form of Inflammatory Bowel Disease Patient Concerns.[80,89]

Although there have been an increased number of studies examining QOL as an end point, the critical reader needs to focus on whether the studies have taken the clinically important step of explaining the intrinsic meaning of the studies' results. As mentioned previously, one of the more significant factors preventing more widespread acknowledgment of QOL as an outcome is lack of interpretability of the data. This is a responsibility that the author of the study needs to carefully address in the discussion section of his/her paper. Part of the problem is related to the survey instruments themselves and lack of physician experience with them, but the ease of interpretation is also limited by the focus on P value and statistical significance rather than clinical significance.[90] For example, it is not clear what a 10% difference in mean physical functioning between two treatments actually means even if the P value is significant (e.g., $P < .01$). A better technique might be to decide before the study what the minimal important clinical difference in score is (and provide justification for this), then report the percentage of patients who achieve this level of improvement. This is an example of a minimum important difference approach that reports the percentage of patients who experience a specific change in QOL score. Most researchers in the field believe that this descriptive approach offers a more interpretable representation of the data compared with traditional statistical analysis. Minimum important difference, effect size calculations, NNT analyses, and anchor-based approaches have all been postulated as alternative forms of data reporting.[91] These alternate approaches to traditional statistical representation of results seem to be gaining a foothold and may increase the pace of progress in QOL research.[90,92–94]

For the reader who is critically evaluating the QOL literature, the above discussions are important to recognize. The meaning of QOL scores needs to be addressed in both methodologically rigorous ways as well as in regard to clinical relevance. Table 54-8 provides a summary of some of the key attributes for critiquing reports of QOL research. For both readers and authors of QOL studies, Staquet and colleagues[94] provide extensive suggested guidelines for the reporting of clinical trial that include QOL data.

In sum, increasingly more QOL studies are being published in the colorectal literature. With the increasing number of articles, critical evaluations of the methodology, as well as the reported results are important regarding how we should clinically interpret and potentially use the study findings.

TABLE 54-8. Attributes of well-performed QOL studies

Trial design	Prospective
Survey choice	Depends on intent, usually combination of generic, disease-specific, and/or modular; must justify survey(s) chosen
Survey psychometric characteristics	Valid, reliable, sensitive to change, interpretable
Total survey length	<100 questions (<30 min to complete)
Source of information	Patient whenever possible
Method of administration	Self-administered, if not possible at least consistent approach
Missing data	Defined approach (imputed, deleted), report number missing all and/or part of data
Scoring	Report source of algorithm used
Analysis	Both univariate and multivariate, include potential confounders in model; correct for multiple comparisons
Reporting	Report both descriptive and traditional statistics

Conclusions

This chapter provides a foundation for the colorectal surgeon who is critically evaluating the literature. Such evaluation is important as evidence-based practice continues to increasingly become a focus for healthcare providers. It remains paramount, therefore, that the literature be interpreted appropriately and thoughtfully.

References

1. Canadian Task Force on the Periodic Health Examination. The periodic health examination. Can Med Assoc J 1979;121: 1193–1254.
2. Solomon MJ, McLeod RS. Clinical studies in surgical journals: have we improved? Dis Colon Rectum 1993;36:43–48.
3. Selby JV, Friedman GD, Quesenberry CP Jr, Weiss NS. A case-control study of screening sigmoidoscopy and mortality from colorectal cancer. N Engl J Med 1992;326:653–657.
4. Shapiro S. Evidence on screening for breast cancer from a randomized trial. Cancer 1977;39:2772–2782.
5. Detsky AS. Are clinical trials a cost-effective investment? JAMA 1989;262:1795–1800.
6. McLeod RS, Wright JG, Solomon MJ, Hu X, Walters BC, Lossing A. Randomized controlled trials in surgery: issues and problems. Surgery 1996;119:483–486.
7. Dimond EG, Kittle CF, Crockett JE. Comparison of internal mammary artery ligation and sham operation for angina pectoris [abstract]. Am J Cardiol 1958;18:712–713.
8. Chalmers TC. Randomization of the first patient. Med Clin North Am 1975;59:1035–1038.
9. Neumayer L, Giobbie-Hurder A, Jonasson O, et al. Open mesh versus laparoscopic mesh repair of inguinal hernia. N Engl J Med 2004;350:1819–1827.
10. Taylor KM, Margolese RG, Soskolne CL. Physicians' reasons for not entering eligible patients in a randomized clinical trial of surgery for breast cancer. N Engl J Med 1984;310:1363–1367.
11. Kennedy ED, Blair JE, Ready R, et al. Patients' perceptions of their participation in a clinical trial for postoperative Crohn's disease. Can J Gastroenterol 1998;12:287–291.
12. Fisher B, Bauer M, Margolese R, et al. Five-year results of a randomized clinical trial comparing total mastectomy and segmental mastectomy with or without radiation in the treatment of breast cancer. N Engl J Med 1985;312:665–673.
13. The EC/IC Bypass Study Group. Failure of extracranial-intracranial arterial bypass to reduce the risk of ischemic stroke. Results of an international randomized trial. N Engl J Med 1985;313:1191–1200.
14. Spechler SJ. Comparison of medical and surgical therapy for complicated gastroesophageal reflux disease in veterans. The Department of Veterans Affairs Gastroesophageal Reflux Disease Study Group. N Engl J Med 1992;326:786–792.
15. Guyatt GH, Sackett DL, Sinclair JC, Hayward R, Cook DJ, Cook RJ. Users' guides to the medical literature. IX. A method for grading health care recommendations. Evidence-based Medicine Working Group. JAMA 1995;274:1800–1804.
16. Cook DJ, Guyatt GH, Laupacis A, Sackett DL. Rules of evidence and clinical recommendations on the use of antithrombotic agents. Chest 1992;102:305S–311S.
17. U.S. Preventative Task Force. Guide to Clinical Preventative Services. An Assessment of 169 Interventions [abstract]. Baltimore: Williams & Wilkins; 1989.
18. Sackett DL. Rules of evidence and clinical recommendations on the use of antithrombotic agents. Chest 1989;95:2S–4S.
19. Liberati A. Problems defining hierarchies (levels) of evidence for studies to be included in systematic reviews of effectiveness of interventions. Presented at 2nd Symposium on Systematic Reviews: beyond the basics. Abstract. Oxford, UK, 1999.
20. Horton R. Surgical research or comic opera: questions, but few answers. Lancet 1996;347:984–985.
21. Spodick DH. Randomized controlled clinical trials: the behavioral case. JAMA 1982;247:2258–2260.
22. Ko CY, Sack J, Chang JT, Fink A. Reporting randomized, controlled trials: where quality of reporting may be improved. Dis Colon Rectum 2002;45:443–447.
23. Barnes RW. Understanding investigative clinical trials. J Vasc Surg 1989;9:609–618.
24. Haines SJ. Randomized clinical trials in the evaluation of surgical innovation. J Neurosurg 1979;51:5–11.
25. Solomon MJ, Laxamana A, Devore L, McLeod RS. Randomized controlled trials in surgery. Surgery 1994;115:707–712.
26. Hall JC, Mills B, Nguyen H, Hall JL. Methodologic standards in surgical trials. Surgery 1996;119:466–472.
27. Solomon MJ, McLeod RS. Should we be performing more randomized controlled trials evaluating surgical operations? Surgery 1995;118:459–467.
28. Clinical Outcomes of Surgical Therapy Study Group. A comparison of laparoscopically assisted and open colectomy for colon cancer. N Engl J Med 2004;350:2050–2059.
29. North American Symptomatic Carotid Endarterectomy Trial Collaborators. Beneficial effect of carotid endarterectomy in

symptomatic patients with high-grade carotid stenosis. N Engl J Med 1991;325:445–453.

30. Goligher JC, Pulvertaft CN, Watkinson G. Controlled trial of vagotomy and gastro-enterostomy, vagotomy and antrectomy, and subtotal gastrectomy in elective treatment of duodenal ulcer: interim report. Br Med J 1964;5381:455–460.

31. Moher D, Schulz KF, Altman D. The CONSORT statement: revised recommendations for improving the quality of reports of parallel-group randomized trials. JAMA 2001;285:1987–1991.

32. Cook DJ, Sackett DL, Spitzer WO. Methodologic guidelines for systematic reviews of randomized control trials in health care from the Potsdam Consultation on Meta-Analysis. J Clin Epidemiol 1995;48:167–171.

33. L'Abbee KA, Detsky AS, O'Rourke K. Meta-analysis in clinical research. Ann Intern Med 1987;107:224–233.

34. Spitzer WO. The challenge of meta-analysis. J Clin Epidemiol 1995;48:1–4.

35. Chalmers TC, Altman DG, eds. Systematic Reviews. London: British Medical Journal Publishing Group; 1995. Abstract.

36. Oxman AD, Cook DJ, Guyatt GH. Users' guides to the medical literature. VI. How to use an overview. Evidence-Based Medicine Working Group. JAMA 1994;272:1367–1371.

37. Feinstein AR. Meta-analysis: statistical alchemy for the 21st century. J Clin Epidemiol 1995;48:71–79.

38. LeLorier J, Gregoire G, Benhaddad A, Lapierre J, Derderian F. Discrepancies between meta-analyses and subsequent large randomized, controlled trials. N Engl J Med 1997;337:536–542.

39. Moher D, Olkin I. Meta-analysis of randomized controlled trials. A concern for standards. JAMA 1995;274:1962–1964.

40. Dickerson K, Scherer R, Lefebvre C. Identifying relevant studies for systematic reviews. BMJ 1994;309:1286–1291.

41. Moher D, Fortin P, Jadad AR, et al. Completeness of reporting of trials published in languages other than English: implications for conduct and reporting of systematic reviews. Lancet 1996;347:363–366.

42. Jadad AR, McQuay HJ. Meta-analyses to evaluate analgesic interventions: a systematic qualitative review of their methodology. J Clin Epidemiol 1996;49:235–243.

43. Cochrane Collaboration. Vista, CA: Cochrane Library. The Cochrane Library is available on CD-ROM on a quarterly basis (The Cochrane Library, Update Software Inc., 936 La Rueda, Vista, CA 92084). Abstract.

44. Committee to Advise Public Health Service on Clinical Practice Guidelines (Institute of Medicine). Clinical Practice Guidelines: Directions for a New Program. Washington DC: National Academy Press; 1990:58. Abstract.

45. Wright JG, McLeod RS, Mahoney J, Lossing A, Hu X. Practice guidelines in surgery. Surgery 1996;119:706–709.

46. Browman GP, Levine MN, Mohide EA, et al. The practice guidelines development cycle: a conceptual tool for practice guidelines development and implementation. J Clin Oncol 1995;13:502–512.

47. Woolf SH. Practice guidelines, a new reality in medicine. II. Methods of developing guidelines. Arch Intern Med 1992;152:946–952.

48. Hayward RSA, Wilson MC, Tunis SR, Bass EB, Guyatt GH. Users' guide to the medical literature. VIII. How to use clinical practice guidelines. Are the recommendations valid? JAMA 1995;274:570–574.

49. Sackett DL, Richardson WS, Rosenberg W, Haynes RB. Evidence Based Medicine. How to Practice & Teach EBM. London: Churchhill Livingstone; 1997. Abstract.

50. Oxman AD, Sackett DL, Guyatt GH. Users' guides to the medical literature. I. How to get started. The Evidence-Based Medicine Working Group. JAMA 1993;270:2093–2095.

51. Guyatt GH, Sackett DL, Cook DJ. Users' guides to the medical literature. II. How to use an article about therapy or prevention. A. Are the results of the study valid? Evidence-Based Medicine Working Group. JAMA 1993;270:2598–2601.

52. Guyatt GH, Sackett DL, Cook DJ. Users' guides to the medical literature. II. How to use an article about therapy or prevention. B. What were the results and will they help me in caring for my patients? Evidence-Based Medicine Working Group. JAMA 1994;271:59–63.

53. Jaeschke R, Guyatt GH, Sackett DL. Users' guides to the medical literature. III. How to use an article about a diagnostic test. B. What are the results and will they help me in caring for my patients? The Evidence-Based Medicine Working Group. JAMA 1994;271:703–707.

54. Levine M, Walter S, Lee H, Haines T, Holbrook A, Moyer V. Users' guides to the medical literature. IV. How to use an article about harm. Evidence-Based Medicine Working Group. JAMA 1994;271:1615–1619.

55. Laupacis A, Wells G, Richardson WS, Tugwell P. Users' guides to the medical literature. V. How to use an article about prognosis. Evidence-Based Medicine Working Group. JAMA 1994;272:234–237.

56. Richardson WS, Detsky AS. Users' guides to the medical literature. VII. How to use a clinical decision analysis. B. What are the results and will they help me in caring for my patients? Evidence Based Medicine Working Group. JAMA 1995;273:1610–1613.

57. Richardson WS, Detsky AS. Users' guides to the medical literature. VII. How to use a clinical decision analysis. A. Are the results of the study valid? Evidence-Based Medicine Working Group. JAMA 1995;273:1292–1295.

58. Naylor CD, Guyatt GH. Users' guides to the medical literature. XI. How to use an article about a clinical utilization review. Evidence-Based Medicine Working Group. JAMA 1996;275:1435–1439.

59. Naylor CD, Guyatt GH. Users' guides to the medical literature. X. How to use an article reporting variations in the outcomes of health services. The Evidence-Based Medicine Working Group. JAMA 1996;275:554–558.

60. Dans AL, Dans LF, Guyatt GH, Richardson S. Users' guides to the medical literature: XIV. How to decide on the applicability of clinical trial results to your patient. Evidence-Based Medicine Working Group. JAMA 1998;279:545–549.

61. Drummond MF, Richardson WS, O'Brien BJ, Levine M, Heyland D. Users' guides to the medical literature. XIII. How to use an article on economic analysis of clinical practice. A. Are the results of the study valid? Evidence-Based Medicine Working Group. JAMA 1997;277:1552–1557.

62. Guyatt GH, Naylor CD, Juniper E, Heyland DK, Jaeschke R, Cook DJ. Users' guides to the medical literature. XII. How to use articles about health-related quality of life. Evidence-Based Medicine Working Group. JAMA 1997;277:1232–1237.

63. Jaeschke R, Guyatt G, Sackett DL. Users' guides to the medical literature. III. How to use an article about a diagnostic test. A. Are the results of the study valid? Evidence-Based Medicine Working Group. JAMA 1994;271:389–391.

64. O'Brien BJ, Heyland D, Richardson WS, Levine M, Drummond MF. Users' guides to the medical literature. XIII. How to use an

article on economic analysis of clinical practice. B. What are the results and will they help me in caring for my patients? Evidence-Based Medicine Working Group. JAMA 1997;277: 1802–1806.

65. Last JM. Making the dictionary of epidemiology. Int J Epidemiol 1996;25:1098–1101.

66. Cook RJ, Sackett DL. The number needed to treat: a clinically useful measure of treatment effect. BMJ 1995;310:452–454.

67. Maggard MA, O'Connell JB, Liu JH, Etzioni DA, Ko CY. Sample size calculations in surgery: are they done correctly? Surgery 2003;134:275–279.

68. Guyatt G, Jaeschke R, Heddle N, Cook D, Shannon H, Walter S. Basic statistics for clinicians. 2. Interpreting study results: confidence intervals. CMAJ 1995;152:169–173.

69. Daley J, Henderson WG, Khuri SF. Risk-adjusted surgical outcomes. Annu Rev Med 2001;52:275–287.

70. Charlson ME, Pompei P, Ales KL, MacKenzie CR. A new method of classifying prognostic comorbidity in longitudinal studies: development and validation. J Chronic Dis 1987;40: 373–383.

71. Khuri SF, Daley J, Henderson W, et al. Risk adjustment of the postoperative mortality rate for the comparative assessment of the quality of surgical care: results of the National Veterans Affairs Surgical Risk Study. J Am Coll Surg 1997;185:315–327.

72. Khuri SF, Daley J, Henderson W, et al. The National Veterans Administration Surgical Risk Study: risk adjustment for the comparative assessment of the quality of surgical care. J Am Coll Surg 1995;180:519–531.

73. Best WR, Khuri SF, Phelan M, et al. Identifying patient preoperative risk factors and postoperative adverse events in administrative databases: results from the Department of Veterans Affairs National Surgical Quality Improvement Program. J Am Coll Surg 2002;194:257–266.

74. Longo WE, Virgo KS, Johnson FE, et al. Risk factors for morbidity and mortality after colectomy for colon cancer. Dis Colon Rectum 2000;43:83–91.

75. Sprangers MA. Quality-of-life assessment in colorectal cancer patients: evaluation of cancer therapies. Semin Oncol 1999;26:691–696.

76. Langenhoff BS, Krabbe PF, Wobbes T, Ruers TJ. Quality of life as an outcome measure in surgical oncology. Br J Surg 2001;88:643–652.

77. Donovan K, Sanson-Fisher RW, Redman S. Measuring quality of life in cancer patients. J Clin Oncol 1989;7:959–968.

78. Stacket, MJ, Hays RD, Fayers PM. Quality of Life Assessment in Clinical Trials, Methods and Practice. 1998; Abstract.

79. Anthony T, Jones C, Antoine J, Sivess-Franks S, Turnage R. The effect of treatment for colorectal cancer on long-term health-related quality of life. Ann Surg Oncol 2001;8:44–49.

80. Provenzale D, Shearin M, Phillips-Bute BG, et al. Health-related quality of life after ileoanal pull-through evaluation and assessment of new health status measures. Gastroenterology 1997;113:7–14.

81. Earlam S, Glover C, Fordy C, Burke D, Allen-Mersh TG. Relation between tumor size, quality of life, and survival in patients with colorectal liver metastases. J Clin Oncol 1996;14: 171–175.

82. Whynes DK, Neilson AR. Symptoms before and after surgery for colorectal cancer. Qual Life Res 1997;6:61–66.

83. Hallbook O, Hass U, Wanstrom A, Sjodahl R. Quality of life measurement after rectal excision for cancer. Comparison between straight and colonic J-pouch anastomosis. Scand J Gastroenterol 1997;32:490–493.

84. Barton JG, Paden MA, Lane M, Postier RG. Comparison of postoperative outcomes in ulcerative colitis and familial polyposis patients after ileoanal pouch operations. Am J Surg 2001;182: 616–620.

85. Camilleri-Brennan J, Steele RJ. Prospective analysis of quality of life and survival following mesorectal excision for rectal cancer. Br J Surg 2001;88:1617–1622.

86. Van Duijvendijk P, Slors JF, Taat CW, et al. Quality of life after total colectomy with ileorectal anastomosis or proctocolectomy and ileal pouch-anal anastomosis for familial adenomatous polyposis. Br J Surg 2000;87:590–596.

87. Jimmo B, Hyman NH. Is ileal pouch-anal anastomosis really the procedure of choice for patients with ulcerative colitis? Dis Colon Rectum 1998;41:41–45.

88. Thompson-Fawcett MW, Richard CS, O'Connor BI, Cohen Z, McLeod RS. Quality of life is excellent after a pelvic pouch for colitis-associated neoplasia. Dis Colon Rectum 2000;43: 1497–1502.

89. Robb BW, Pritts TA, Warner BW. Health-related quality of life after ileal pouch anal anastomosis for ulcerative colitis: right answer–wrong question. Gastroenterology 2002;122:1180–1181.

90. Symonds T, Berzon R, Marquis P, Rummans TA. The clinical significance of quality-of-life results: practical considerations for specific audiences. Mayo Clin Proc 2002;77:572–583.

91. Guyatt GH, Osoba D, Wu AW, Wyrwich KW, Norman GR. Methods to explain the clinical significance of health status measures. Mayo Clin Proc 2002;77:371–383.

92. Osoba D, Rodrigues G, Myles J, Zee B, Pater J. Interpreting the significance of changes in health-related quality-of-life scores. J Clin Oncol 1998;16:139–144.

93. Juniper EF, Guyatt GH, Willan A, Griffith LE. Determining a minimal important change in a disease-specific quality of life questionnaire. J Clin Epidemiol 1994;47:81–87.

94. Staquet M, Berzon R, Osoba D, Machin D. Guidelines for reporting results of quality of life assessments in clinical trials. Qual Life Res 1996;5:496–502.

55
Surgical Education: A Time for Change

Clifford L. Simmang and Richard K. Reznick

There is a coalescence of events: societal, financial, generational, and structural, which are challenging the status quo like it has never been challenged before. Throughout the world, there are echoes of the need for fundamental changes to postgraduate medical education, reverberating from faculty, trainees, and certification bodies.

The most pressing component of the concerns about surgical education is the diminishing attractiveness of our surgical programs and augmenting attrition once accepted to specialties. It would seem that lifestyle concerns dominate the landscape of resident choice and are at the heart of the reason surgical specialties are losing some of the best and brightest to specialties with a more controlled lifestyle. Further exacerbating this trend is the reality that surgical specialties no longer have a monopoly on interventional procedures, and levels of compensation that have historically favored surgical specialties no longer do.

In concert with a diminishing attractiveness of the specialty, there is the global move toward a diminished workweek for surgical trainees. Although many applaud a departure from the often-intolerable work demands of residency programs of the past, the irony may be that the net end result may be a lengthening of surgical programs. Unquestionably, surgery is different from other areas of medical practice and it requires a different approach. This is so largely because of the concomitant need to train individuals technically as well as in the breadth of other dimensions required to be an excellent practitioner. One of the problems with continuing on our current path and with our current methods is that our residents are graduating with less clinical and operative skills than their surgical teachers did. The reasons for this include: decreasing level of resident independence across the board; an appropriate increase in attention being given to patient demands and the reduction of medical error; inadequate opportunities for deliberate practice; a pressure for speed, often driven by financial realities; a working week that is reducing and a population of our core teaching hospitals with increased levels of tertiary and quaternary care.

Another issue is the fact that there is uneven exposure to many expected competencies. This is because training models are principally structured based on available opportunity as opposed to satisfying educational objectives. In addition, most programs maintain a hierarchical approach, especially with respect to opportunities to operate. In this regard junior residents often spend countless hours on wasted activity.

Another major issue in surgical education is that political and financial issues have yet to be met head on. It will be important to reconcile that currently teaching is undervalued and poorly compensated.

In this chapter, we will trace the history of basic tenets of surgical education. In so doing, we will focus on the essential features of cognitive and technical learning. We will highlight some recent structural changes for surgical residencies that are being advocated including the concept of a "strategically planned curriculum." Finally, we will propose that more than ever, our surgical community will need to redefine basic methods of surgical teaching, and be open to novel curricular models.

The heritage of our modern residency training programs had its beginnings at the Johns Hopkins Hospital when in 1889, William Stewart Halsted was appointed as associate professor of surgery. A native of New York, he graduated from Yale University in the spring of 1874 with a newfound interest in medicine. That fall he enrolled in a college of physicians and surgeons in New York. According to the rules of the college, each student matriculated as a preceptee of a faculty member. After having devoted his college years to athletics, he devoted his years in Medical School to scholastic achievement and graduated among the top 10 men in his class allowing him to compete in a written examination for a prize of $100.00. He won this with his thesis entitled "Contraindications to Operations."

In October 1876, Halsted entered his internship at Bellevue Hospital, which he extended for a total of 18 months. He then served as house physician to the New York Hospital from July to October 1878. In November, he traveled to Vienna to begin the study of German. He subsequently spent 2 years visiting and working at the great German speaking clinics, the world's leading centers of medical science at that time. It was this experience that would lay the foundation and approach he would use to develop his clinical investigation and educational program for the rest of his life. Although his School of Surgery was distinctly American, he would remain, as his colleague William Osler stated, "very much verdeutsched."

Halsted's plan of organization for service grew from the German system, which he described clearly in his 1904 Yale address.[1] Halsted was in charge of the service at all times. Except for his private patients, the beds were occupied by patients cared for by the house surgeon. This position was equivalent to our present day chief resident, with an average time in this position of 2 years. Before this, there was a 6-year pyramidal program as an assistant (interne), which was subdivided into two levels of graded responsibility. Going through the entire process took an average of 8 years. This was the origin of the surgical residency program in the United States. In 1952, B. Noland Carter wrote, "Of all the great teachers in the history of our art, only Theodore Billroth founded a more illustrious school of surgery."[2] One hundred years later, Halsted's organization and system for surgical training remains with very few changes. Our process for educating surgeons has not kept up with advances in many of the other sciences. In 1904, Halsted said, "Although we now have in the United States several moderately well-endowed medical schools with a University connection, the problem of the education of our surgeons is still unsolved. Our present methods do not by any means suffice for their training."[1] Notwithstanding Halsted's dissatisfaction with his method of surgical education more than 100 years ago, and notwithstanding the enormous changes the last century has brought, we still rely on a Halstedian approach to surgical education as our principal heuristic.[3]

Cognitive Learning

Surgical education evolved throughout the 20th century with the creation and development of residency programs across the country. Training in the first half of the century involved primarily clinical experience and self-study. Formal educational programs began to develop in the second half of the century. Books and journals on surgical diseases were available; however, they were not incorporated into formalized educational curricula, but rather were used as references. In the second half of the century, more attention was given to didactic education. Textbooks that comprehensively cover general surgery and the subspecialties would form the foundation for the basic fund of knowledge and have remained the cornerstone from which new knowledge is built. Despite the availability of a growing body of current literature, regularly scheduled conferences to provide systematic reviews were uncommon. Robert McClelland recognized the need to provide such reviews of current literature. In 1964, at Parkland

Memorial Hospital, he began a program of journal review with the surgical residents. This began small and was intended to help the residents learn how to review the literature while reading current articles to critically assess new knowledge. In 1974, this review process evolved into what we now know as *Selected Readings in General Surgery*. This is a comprehensive program that in a 5-year cycle covers the breadth of general surgical knowledge adding a depth not found in standard textbooks. After graduation, many surgeons have continued to use *Selected Readings* as one means of staying current with the surgical literature. This program continues to be popular with about 4200 subscribers.

During this same time period, residency programs began holding regularly scheduled academic conferences. These often included Morbidity and Mortality (M&M), Case Presentations, and Grand Rounds. Although other conferences were held, these were the core around which the educational curriculum was built.

Perceived as a valuable educational endeavor, even to the extent that M&M is a requirement by the Residency Review Committees (RRC) for accredited surgery programs, there are differing opinions on how the conference should be conducted.[4] The role of M&M conference is to review the process of patient's medical care. Adverse events and errors are discussed with the goal of improving patient care. In this conference, the care of patients that have had a complication is reviewed to determine what factors likely contributed to this complication and what alternative interventions or management strategies could have been used to decrease the likelihood of the complication or its magnitude. This is where residents learn to articulate that a complication has occurred during a patient's stay in hospital and take responsibility for their involvement. It is important for the maturation of surgeons to have an approach to patient care that emphasizes continuous quality improvement. M&M has been referred to as the "Golden Hour" of surgical education because of its unique role in the lifelong education of the surgeon.[5]

There is evidence that surgical M&M conferences teach prospective surgeons the value of open and honest discussion about patient issues, including the analysis of medical error. A prospective analysis of 232 surgical and 100 internal medicine conferences revealed that the proportion of adverse events associated with an error did not differ significantly between the specialties. An error was defined as the failure of a planned action to be completed as intended, or the use of an incorrect plan to achieve a particular goal. Adverse events were unintentional injuries from medical management rather than disease. Errors resulting in adverse events were noted in 18% of internal medicine and 42% of surgical cases, a difference that was statistically significant.[6] In internal medicine conferences, errors were less likely to be discussed as errors, and more likely to be ignored. However, in surgical conferences, errors were likelier to be attributed to an individual, team, or system (79% versus 38%). Traditionally M&M conferences were held closed to all but surgical residents and faculty. Many surgical programs carried a reputation for intimidation in which the residents were harassed during their presentations. In recent years, most M&M conferences have become more nurturing; however, a certain amount of fear may be healthy—fear that you could be the cause of the patient's demise and understanding one's own responsibility and accountability for patients.[7]

Case presentation conferences are used to present clinical scenarios about patients recently cared for highlighting certain aspects of their presentation, diagnosis, and treatment. As the clinical scenario is presented, a Socratic approach is used to question the participants. This allows the faculty to assess a resident's knowledge base and their ability to assimilate knowledge into a treatment plan. Because all of the residents in the audience could potentially be called on for each set of questions, this forces all of them to pay attention to the scenarios, consider the alternatives and options, and if they do not know the answer, when the answer is given this acquisition of knowledge is more deeply imprinted in memory. Another educational tradition in surgical programs is the Grand Rounds program. As with M&M conferences, a recent concern has been the issue of discoverability. With increasing access to patient information, and a decreasing emphasis on restricting attendance at conferences, some programs have found it necessary to pay stricter attention to what is said in fear of potential use or misuse of that information.

The first half of the 20th century saw the development of organized and structured surgical residency programs whereby the residents would learn as they assisted their mentors in performing patient care. The second half of the 20th century saw the progression and development of academic curricula emphasizing the educational component of surgical training. Many diseases are rare and are not frequently seen, but the requirement for a surgeon to be familiar with this condition still exists. A surgeon cannot make a diagnosis of a condition he is unaware of. This was the impetus to form and develop curricula. It was in that framework that the academic conferences matured.

Technical Skills Acquisition

In the field of surgery, in addition to the assimilation of knowledge and development of surgical judgment, the ability to master technical skills is essential, and often separates the average surgeon from the master surgeon. In the traditional residency in surgery, technical skills are learned on patients by assisting in the operating room. There is the presumption that fundamental surgical principles, nuances of anatomy, and surgical technique can be learned through observation. However, there is a growing body of opinion that observational learning has its limits, and experiential learning results in a quicker assent to competency. There was also a great deal of technical learning that occurred when more senior trainees helped junior trainees through an operation. As was discussed

earlier, the opportunities for independent operating have greatly diminished. This may ultimately have a negative effect on technical skill acquisition unless ancillary operative experiences are provided. In essence, we cannot afford to lengthen the learning curve of surgical procedures. The learning curve can be considered as a graphic representation of the relationship between experience with a procedure and an outcome variable such as operative times or complication rates.[9] A common feature of the curve for most procedures is that improvement occurs more rapidly during early experience. This is usually imbedded within the residency training; however, new techniques such as the evolution of minimally invasive surgery required practicing surgeons to learn these techniques without the benefit of the gradual and graded acquisition of skills under the tutelage of experienced surgeon mentors that occurs within residency.[8] This is one of the greatest challenges in surgical education.

One method to alter learning curves for surgical procedures is to shift some the training from the traditional environment of the operating room into an "ex vivo" laboratory. In so doing, there may be great promise in the deployment of surgical simulations. For more than 25 years, pilots for both industry and the military have had a significant part of their early training using simulation techniques. Simulators reproduce the cockpit of an aircraft, including the instrumentation and controls with a simulated visual field out the front window. Whereas the early simulators provided little more than instrument controls and a gray visual field, current training simulators are much more realistic and have become an essential element of pilot training. These simulators not only have enhanced visual effects but also provide the tactile sensation and feeling of change in altitude. In so doing, many flight situations can be reproduced, such as a smooth take off, turbulent air, or a rough landing. Pilots can become very familiar with a new aircraft and can have extensive practice with controlling the aircraft in a variety of situations, preparing them to handle most situations that would be encountered before their first flight. Many pilots believe that current simulators are very realistic and serve as significant preparation for actual flight. However, although realistic scenarios can aid in training optimal pilot behavior in emergency situations, high technology and automation have not been able to significantly improve flight safety in the last two decades.[8] The main cause of aviation accident was and is human error. Therefore, the most powerful tools to reduce risks would deal with the human operator on the flight deck including pilot selection, training, and teamwork.[9] This highlights the importance of M&M in surgery where human error, whether it be judgment, technical, or process oriented is reviewed. Learning from others' experience may be the most valuable process in preventing or solving similar problems for future patients.

Without a doubt, technical skills remain an essential ingredient to the complete surgeon. But can technical abilities be predicted before a prospective surgeon enters residency? This longstanding question remains controversial, and data gathered to date are conflicting. Traditionally, the admissions process in surgery has relied on past academic performance, unstructured interviews, and a few personal references. The use of psychometric testing to evaluate an applicant's aptitude for surgery has been recently summarized.[10] The Association of Surgeons in The Netherlands has incorporated psychometric testing for surgical training since 1983, and the Royal College of Surgeons of Great Britain and Ireland has also considered taking this step.[11] The predictability of aptitude testing for successful completion of pilot training has been validated in the British Royal Air Force using a battery of tests relevant to being a pilot.[12] This analogy could be extrapolated not only for surgical residency selection, but even for practicing surgeons, where demonstration of competence may include psychometric performance which will be used to obtain credentials for certain procedures such as advanced laparoscopy or even incorporated into the new concept of maintenance of certification.

Minimally invasive surgery has introduced a new and unique set of psychomotor skills for a surgeon to acquire and master. At a meeting of the American College of Surgeons in New Orleans, 2001, 195 surgeons who had completed more than 50 laparoscopic operations participated by performing tasks designed to test psychomotor and not cognitive skills.[13] It was shown that between 2% and 12% of surgeons performed more than 2 standard deviations from the mean and some had performed 20 standard deviations from the mean. Studies like this may form the methodologic foundation for establishing criterion levels and performance objectives in the objective assessment of the technical skills component of determining surgical competence.[13]

Patients want to receive care and operations that reflect the newest technology and yet they do not want to be a part of a surgeon's learning curve. This desire presents a dilemma for the training and practicing surgeon. How can experienced care be provided to patients without gaining the experience by operating on patients? To address this issue, many residency programs in surgery today have begun to develop a Skills Training Program. There are many examples of excellent surgical training centers throughout the world. In general, laboratory curricula parallel training via graded responsibility in the operating room. Interns begin with the simple basics of suturing and knot tying. At each year level, there are skills that must be demonstrated for satisfactory performance and completion for that year. In a prospective, randomized trial done at the University of Texas Southwestern Medical Center, second and third residents were randomized to receive formal laparoscopic skill training with a control group.[14] Baseline performance was assessed. The trained group achieved significantly greater adjusted improvement in video-trainer scores and global assessments of operative performance compared with controls. In this study, intense training improved video hand–eye skills and translated into improved operative performance. Other studies have also shown improved patient outcome. At Jackson Memorial Hospital, a comparison of non-laparoscopy trained gynecology residents was made with residents who received six 4-hour sessions of committed didactic, and bench instruction using inanimate models.[15] Residents with training performed operations in less time, had less blood loss, shorter hospital stay, and less conversions than the control group. Even experienced surgeons benefit from skills training. In a study to evaluate the validity of laparoscopic performance using one of three simulators, it was found that years of experience directly correlated with skills rating and competence ratings.[16] Task speed and overall performance increased with experience. This suggests that even expert surgeons can show significant improvement with simulation.

In addition to these studies, others have also shown that technical skills are improved with a skills curriculum.[17–19] The durability of the training effect has been variable. Some have suggested that after training with laboratory bench models performance improvements are durable.[20] However, Anastakis and colleagues[21] failed to demonstrate that training on a core procedure in a single session has a sustained effect after 2 years. Similarly, Sedlack and Kolars[22] found no advantage to simulator training for colonoscopy after performance of 30 procedures. Although advantages were limited to early procedural experience, this enhanced early learning curve may allow training faculty to be more efficient with their time and may provide a safer early experience for patients.

Summarizing a growing body of literature, it would seem at present that the report card on simulator training is mixed. It seems to have its major benefit for novice learners, durability of effect is an issue, and results to date have not been validated in large-scale studies. However, as computing power inexorably augments, and as the price of simulation equipment decreases, it is our prediction that in the future, most if not all surgical training programs will be devoting a substantial amount of curricular time to technical training using simulators.

Educational Challenges

The structure of Graduate Medical Education is changing dramatically. For example, in the United States, in 2003, the Accrediting Council for Graduate Medical Education (ACGME) approved new duty hour standards for all accredited programs including an 80-hour weekly limit, rest periods, and limits on continuous duty hours. This reflects a worldwide trend to a reduction in workweek in general, and the surgical workweek in specific. In part, this has been a result over concerns of medical errors related to sleep deprivation. All residency programs had to comply with this regulation by July 1, 2003. The greatest impact from this has been on first-entry residency programs, such as General Surgery and Internal Medicine. However, many of the subspecialties have been impacted as well. Residents who take home call are allowed to work the following day. However, there is a 10-hour interval required between the time the resident was last in the hospital and when he or she may return to work. The main issue that arises from this situation is how residents will be able to obtain the volume of experience previously encountered before the current restrictions placed on the time in which the resident can participate in patient care. This reality will force us to rethink our curricula, especially with a view to diminishing hours spent on "pure service requirements." It may also force us to depart from a long-held surgical tradition that aspiring surgeons need a broad base of experiences, opting for a more focused approach to training.

The ACGME is placing increasing emphasis on educational outcomes in the accreditation of residency programs. To accomplish this, the so-called Outcome Project was initiated. The current model of the accreditation captures the potential of a GME program to educate residents by focusing on structure and process components. The ACGME currently measures a program's potential to educate by determining compliance with existing requirements, such as educational objectives, an organized curriculum, biannual evaluation of the residents, resident evaluation of the program, demonstration of scholarly activity, and monitoring of resident work hours. Rather than concentrating only on the assessment of a program's potential to educate, the future for GME as envisioned by the Outcome Project emphasizes a program's actual accomplishments through assessment of program outcomes. Instead of documenting that there are educational objectives, documentation must reflect that the resident achieved learning of these objectives. One mechanism the ACGME has used to assess this change is to identify learning objectives related to the general competencies, and using outcome data to facilitate continuous improvement of both the resident and residency program performance.

The first major activity of the project was identifying six general competencies for residents. These were identified by attention to how adequately physicians are prepared to practice medicine in the changing Healthcare Delivery System. Six general competencies were endorsed by the ACGME in February 1999. The six general competencies are:

- Patient care
- Medical knowledge
- Professionalism
- Systems-based practice
- Practice-based learning and improvement
- Interpersonal and communication skills

The shift from emphasis on structure and process components to that of outcomes is a gradual transition. The ACGME acknowledges that the need for evidence of structures and processes will not disappear but will gradually become less critical to the overall accreditation process. Over the next few years, programs are expected to phase in assessment tools that provide useful and increasingly valid and reliable evidence that residents achieve competency-based educational objectives. At present, the RRC expects to observe progress in

teaching and assessing the competencies. To begin to implement this shift in emphasis from structure and process to educational outcomes, a program must become familiar with the components from the outcome project and review the basic principles of sound educational evaluation. Learning outcomes and objectives must be developed to reflect the general competencies. Then the program's current assessment must be aligned with the competency-based learning objectives. The goal of this Outcomes Program is to provide a better measure of the quality of the educational program. It is believed that by measuring the product instead of the process, a more complete measure of the quality of the education received from that program will be measured. The availability of the educational outcomes-based data is necessary to inform discussions with policy makers and others who have become increasingly focused on issues related to funding for medical education and most recently on patient safety. It is now incumbent upon medical educators to demonstrate the effectiveness for educational programs and to be accountable for the education that we provide.

Surgical education has become increasingly complex with governmentally regulated limitations on the time available for learning and gaining experience occurring throughout the world. At the same time, there are augmented demands for outcomes and educational review. To meet this challenge, we believe that we need to incorporate strategically designed curricula to ensure comprehensive training is achieved.

New Directions

Strategically Planned Curricula

The 20th century saw little change in surgical education until the last decade. Over the last 10–15 years, there have been sweeping changes in the advancement of knowledge, development of new surgical techniques, and requirements by which we must educate residents. The question is how do we teach residents more information, more complex surgical procedures, which are both diagnostic as well as operative and accomplish this in less time? The answer may be forthcoming with the adoption of strategically planned curricula.

The tenets of a strategically planned curriculum include the following elements:

1. A restructuring of the education system to one that is modular, each module linked to specific objectives, including: cognitive knowledge, clinical skills, judgment, technical surgery, ethics, professionalism, and evidence-based training.
2. A linking of objectives to an appropriate curriculum that is characterized by the following: ensuring that most if not all competencies developed during residency training relate directly to the desired career outcome; an adherence to the principles of residency training as outlined in regulatory

bodies such as the ACGME; that the curriculum is populated to the fullest by activities aimed at satisfying specific educational objectives; that it is learner-based; that it makes liberal uses of technology such as Web-based curricular materials, access to point of care (wireless) information, and a focus on providing data for evidence-based decision making and that it reestablishes anatomy as a backbone of surgical teaching, and includes cadaver dissection, prosection, and the use of virtual reality–based anatomy training models.

3. Dramatically changing the pace of technical skill acquisition by: developing a "pre-program" of basic skills focusing on technical skills fundamental to surgery; dramatically ramping up skills laboratory (ex vivo) practice, using virtual reality models, cadavers, surrogate tissue, and inanimate training models; developing programs of structured and deliberate practice; placing a premium on participatory learning as opposed to observational learning; maximizing the number and focus of real-world operations performed by residents and ensure that all learners are actively engaged in each real surgical opportunity; maximizing each "real" patient experience by the use of preoperative technical sessions, by videotape review of self and experts, and by debriefing sessions; developing specific teaching teams for each module; developing programs of faculty development for teaching surgeons; creating a link of faculty compensation to educational deliverables; and maximizing the opportunities for resident involvement in surgery by strategic scheduling initiatives.

4. Diminish wasted time during residency (educational dead space) by: eliminating or minimizing time wasted secondary to a hierarchical model; minimizing time wasted doing noneducational activities; increasing support services, increasing nurse autonomy, rationalizing calls, and optimizing technologic solutions to service problems; critically assessing the need for and the context of night call and seriously addressing the issue of sleep deprivation.

5. Incorporate meaningful assessment into the day to day running of the residency program by: rigorous, reliable, and regular assessment; liberal use of formative assessment; linking evaluation instruments to goals, objectives, and desired competencies; training the evaluators focusing effort on performance-based evaluation systems; using a diverse array of assessors, including self, other health professionals, patients, peers, and faculty and documentation of technical proficiency within a learning module by testing for technical proficiency using sentinel cases.

An example of where we would have benefited from a planned curricular approach to education is the field of minimally invasive surgery. In 1987 the first laparoscopic cholecystectomy was performed. An explosion of laparoscopic procedures with mixed results followed this. Procedures performed primarily in one quadrant of the abdomen, with small vessels or no vessels to ligate, and with either a small specimen or no specimen became rapidly accepted as the standard approach. Laparoscopic colectomy, which involves all four quadrants of the abdomen, major named vessels requiring ligation and division, retrieval of a large specimen, and the necessity for an anastomosis has made the acceptance of this technique slow. Difficulty with acquiring expertise in other advanced laparoscopic procedures while still in a general surgery residency remains challenging. Although basic laparoscopic procedures have become standard, more advanced procedures including gastric, splenic, and colorectal operations have been difficult to acquire during general surgery residency. The challenge facing colon and rectal surgery residencies is how to incorporate the needed number of required operative procedures with limitations on learning time.

The American Board of Colon and Rectal Surgery has identified 17 categories of operative procedures. Residents who display insufficient numbers in five or more categories are not allowed to enter the certification process until they are able to furnish sufficient case numbers to meet the requirements. As the list submitted and certified reflects their year of training, additional training would be required for a surgeon with five or more deficiencies in order to meet this requirement. There has been one resident who completed his training program with insufficient numbers to enter the certification process. This highlights the challenge of incorporating an increasing number of requirements that must be met. The solution again involves strategically planned rotations to ensure that residents are able to meet the requirements from the American Boards of Surgery, and Colon and Rectal Surgery.

Technology and Efficiency

Surgical education has entered a new area. The acquisition of new information is fast outpacing that which can be absorbed intellectually. We have gone from the problem in which the difficulty was trying to identify information and acquire knowledge, to the problem of having so much information that the volume is overwhelming. We must rely on technologic advances.

For example, there may be efficiencies that can be gained by computer-based training (CBT). However, only a few studies have assessed the efficacy of CBT with traditional methods of surgical skills training. Summers and colleagues[23] randomized 69 medical students into three groups for basic skills instruction: a group learning through didactic methods, a group learning through watching videotapes, and a group learning through CBT. All of the material contained the same pictures, text, and audio. There were no differences between the groups before training. After training, the didactic group scored higher on multiple-choice examination. However, the videotape and CBT groups demonstrated statistically significant enhancement of technical skills compared with the didactic group. After 1 month, a calculated performance quotient revealed statistically significant improvement in only the CBT group. CBT was considered as effective as and possibly more efficient than traditional methods for basic surgical skills training for medical students.

For a vast array of knowledge, ready retrieval with a device such as a handheld device that can be carried in a coat pocket may provide the answer. Currently, about 15% of physicians in the United States use personal digital assistants (PDAs) for medical purposes. A trial was conducted at the University of Kentucky, Lexington, KY, to evaluate the impact of PDAs in the general residency program.[24] At the start of the 2001 academic year, all of the general residents were given a PDA with Pocket®Word, Pocket Excel®, and Internet Explorer®, preinstalled and equipped with SIR IrDA infrared port. No training was given. Seven months later, the residents were queried. Seventy percent of residents reported that they used the PDAs frequently or very often. Most of the residents thought they would continue using them in their practice after graduation. Live broadcast of laparoscopic surgery to handheld computers has been performed.[25] A live laparoscopic splenectomy was transmitted live to eight handheld computers simultaneously through the institution's wireless network. This technology allows delivery of information to geographic sites remote from the actual event. We would envision that the surgical residency of tomorrow would have a bank of procedural videos that could be accessed remotely and viewed throughout the institution, much in the same way a movie from a menu can be selected in a hotel room. Residents could view a procedure that they are going to perform to review the details of the procedure just before the case.

Surgical education is changing and we must change to enhance our educational effectiveness. In so doing, we can continue to provide quality education for our residents so they can become the outstanding surgeons that our patients deserve. Notwithstanding the many challenges articulated in this chapter, the commitment to teaching by our academic surgical community remains strong. With rigorous analysis and improvement of our curricula, with deployment of modern educational technologies, and with openness to educational innovations, we can meet the many challenges of both present and future.

References

1. Halsted WS. The training of the surgeon. Bull Johns Hopkins Hosp 1904;267.
2. Carter N. The fruition of Halsted's concept of surgical training. Surgery 1952;32:518–527.
3. Greene FL. Dictation of the operative note—a forgotten art form. Gen Surg News 2004;31:3–4.
4. Risucci DA, Sullivan T, DiRusso S, et al. Assessing educational validity of the morbidity and mortality conference: a pilot study. Curr Surg 2003;50:204–209.
5. Gordon LA. Gordon's guide to the surgical morbidity and mortality conference. Philadelphia: Hanley and Belfus; 1994.
6. Perluissi E, Fischer MA, Campbell AR, et al. Discussion of medical errors in mortality and morbidity conferences. Obstet Gynecol Surv 2004;59:338–340.
7. Frei R. Tough love? The place of fear and intimidation in surgical education. Gen Surg News 2004;31:1–16.
8. Rogers DA, Elstein AS, Bordage G. Improving continuing medical education for surgical techniques: applying the lessons learned in the first decade of minimal access surgery. Ann Surg 2001;233:159–166.
9. Muller M. Training with a simulator—experiences in space flight. Langenbecks Arch Chir Suppl Kongressbd 1996;113:533–536.
10. Wanzel KR, Ward M, Reznick RK. Teaching the surgical craft: from selection to certification. Curr Probl Surg 2002;39(6):573–659.
11. Gilligan JH, Treasure T, Watts C. Incorporating psychometric measures in selecting and developing surgeons. J Manag Med 1996;10:5–16.
12. Bell JA. Royal air force selection procedures. Ann R Coll Surg Engl 1998;70:270–275.
13. Gallagher AG, Smith CD, Bowers SP, et al. Psychomotor skills assessment in practicing surgeons experience in performing advanced laparoscopic procedures. J Am Coll Surg 2003;197:479–488.
14. Scott DJ, Bergen PC, Rege RV, et al. Laparoscopic training on bench models: better and more cost effective than operating room experience. J Am Coll Surg 2000;191:272–283.
15. Whitted RW, Pietro PA, Martin G, et al. A retrospective study evaluating the impact of formal laparoscopic training on patient outcomes in a residency program. J Am Assoc Gynecol Laparosc 2003;10:484–488.
16. Adrales GL, Park AE, Chu UB, et al. A valid method of Laparoscopic simulation training and competence assessment. J Surg Res 2003;114:156–162.
17. Powers TW, Murayama KM, Toyama M, et al. Housestaff performance is improved by participation in a laparoscopic skills curriculum. Am J Surg 2002;184:626–629.
18. Issenberg SB, McGaghie WC, Hart IR, et al. Simulation technology for health care professional skills training and assessment. JAMA 1999;282:861–866.
19. Seymour NE, Gallagher AG, Roman SA, et al. Virtual reality training improves operating room performance: results of a randomized, double-blinded study. Ann Surg 2002;236:458–463.
20. Grober ED, Hamstra SJ, Wanzel KR, et al. Laboratory based training in urologic microsurgery with bench model simulators: a randomized controlled trial evaluating the durability of technical skills. J Urol 2004;172:378–381.
21. Anastakis DJ, Wanzel KR, Brown MH, et al. Evaluating the effectiveness of a 2-year curriculum in a surgical skills center. Am J Surg 2003;185:378–385.
22. Sedlack RE, Kolars JC. Computer simulator training enhances the competency of gastroenterology fellows at colonoscopy: results of a pilot study. Am J Gastroenterol 2004;99:33–37.
23. Summers AN, Rinehart GC, Simpson D, et al. Acquisition of surgical skills: a randomized trial of didactic, videotape, and computer-based training. Surgery 1999;126:330–336.
24. Endean EA, Donnelly MB, Plymale MA, et al. Use of PDAs by general residents. Surg Rounds 2004;27:317–322.
25. Gandsas A, McIntire K, Park A. Live broadcast of laparoscopic surgery to handheld computers. Surg Endosc 2004;18:997–1000.

56
Legal Considerations

Michael J. Meehan

The dawn of the twenty-first century brought with it many of the same legal challenges for physicians, including colon and rectal disease practitioners, as did the latter half of the twentieth century. The ever-increasing frequency and often crushing severity of malpractice claims and lawsuits, databank reporting, Web-based consumer claims data, new privacy requirements, increasing clinical demands, greater government regulation and enforcement activity, and spiraling malpractice premiums have caused many physicians to leave practice, retire early, or relocate to more defendant-friendly lawsuit jurisdictions. This chapter addresses issues related to these concerns—from communication to documentation, from practice to research—as they relate to colon and rectal surgeons.

Medical Malpractice

Elements of Malpractice

In July 2003, a 12-day courtroom trial occurred in Seattle, Washington. The plaintiff, a married 53-year-old computer salesman, had presented to his family physician with rectal bleeding and a painful anal lump with the appearance of a hemorrhoid. When the condition did not improve with treatment, the patient was referred to a general surgeon. After evaluation, the surgeon concluded that the patient had a hemorrhoid and recommended a hemorrhoidectomy. The patient, saying he thought the condition was improving, declined the procedure. The surgeon informed the patient that a hemorrhoidectomy would be indicated if the condition did not continue to improve and resolve. The patient next returned to the surgeon 4 months later, at which time a hemorrhoidectomy revealed advanced anal cancer. The patient received chemotherapy and radiation, developed impotence, and suffered two recurrences of the cancer, from which he was expected to die. The patient-plaintiff filed a lawsuit against both the family physician and the general surgeon contending that earlier diagnosis would have resulted in less extensive treatment and a prognosis of survival from the cancer. The

defense argued that both the family practitioner and the general surgeon acted appropriately and that an earlier diagnosis would have made no difference in the treatment or the outcome. Fifteen medical and surgical experts were used in the case. The pre-suit demand of $2.75 million had been met with an offer of $125,000. At trial the plaintiff asked the jury to award $7 million. The defendants requested a defense verdict. The jury found in favor of the defendants and awarded no money.[1]

The elements that must be proved by a plaintiff to prevail in a medical malpractice case are determined by the laws of the various states. Thus, in this case, the verdict was governed by Washington state law. In general, medical malpractice is established when it is proved, by a preponderance of the evidence, that a patient sustained an injury as a result of an act or omission of a physician or surgeon that would not have occurred had the physician or surgeon exercised ordinary skill, care, and diligence.[2] What a "physician or surgeon of ordinary skill, care, and diligence would or would not have done under like or similar conditions or circumstances" is called the standard of care. Family practitioners and surgical specialists, as in the Washington case described above, are usually held to different standards of care, depending on variations in state law. The standard of care for a physician or surgeon in the practice of a board-certified medical or surgical specialty should be that level of care expected of a reasonable specialist practicing medicine or surgery in that same specialty, regardless of geographical considerations or circumstances.[3] Negligence occurs when the care falls below the standard of care. A case can include single or multiple allegations of negligence.

When negligence is proved in the courtroom, the departure from the standard of care must also be a proximate cause of the injury to the patient for the plaintiff to prevail. Thus, there must be a cause and effect relationship between the care and the harm. For there to be a plaintiffs' verdict, the jury must believe that 1) there was a departure from the standard of care, *and* 2) that the departure from the standard of care was a cause of the patient's injury. For the defense to prevail, the jury must believe that either 1) or 2) above were *not* proved by a pre-ponderance of the evidence—or that neither were proved.

Both of these issues were actively debated in the Washington case. 1) The recommendations, treatment, and decision to defer a hemorrhoidectomy were contested by both sides; 2) whether the cancer had metastasized before the critical involvement of the doctors was also argued. (If the cancer had metastasized before physician mismanagement, if any, then even a timely hemorrhoidectomy would not have changed the outcome or treatment—so physician mismanagement could not have logically been the *cause* of the patient's injuries).

In some cases, the defense attorneys will concede on item 1 above—negligence, if they think they cannot prevail on item 1 but if they think they can prevail on item 2—causation. Such a strategy may be challenging. Consider the following case tried to a Savannah, Georgia, jury in November 2001 in which defense attorneys conceded negligence and tried to convince a jury that the plaintiff was entitled to receive an award, but that the amount sought by the plaintiff exceeded that to which he should be entitled. The plaintiff had suffered a rectal tear when thrown from his vehicle during an automobile accident. The trauma surgeons who tried to repair the tear negligently closed the proximal end of his colon and matured the distal end as the stoma. As a result, he suffered a complete obstruction of his digestive tract for 7 days and developed a massive infection, causing the loss of approximately 70% of his abdominal wall. He was left with massive scarring, no abdominal muscles, only a thin layer of skin covering his intestines, and the prospect of constant diarrhea for the remainder of his life. The defendants conceded that the stapling procedure was improperly performed, but they disputed the extent of the patient's injuries that was alleged by the plaintiff's attorney, including more than $1.2 million arguably representing the present cash value of the patient's future lost income. The jury was not asked whether the trauma surgeons had committed negligence, but rather whether all of the injuries complained of were caused by the negligence (whether too much money was being claimed for the injury). Ultimately, the jury awarded the plaintiff $6.25 million.[4]

Recurring Malpractice Themes

A study of medical malpractice cases involving colon and rectal disease involved a retrospective review of all cases tried in the federal and state civil court system over a 21-year period from 1971 through 1991[5] remains instructive today. The study identified 98 malpractice cases over that period of time from a computerized legal database. The 98 cases included 103 allegations of negligence. The nature and frequency of allegations were as follows:

- 43%: Failure to timely diagnose disease (principally cancer and appendicitis)
- 24%: Iatrogenic colon injury

- 15%: Iatrogenic medical complications during diagnosis or treatment
- 10%: Sphincter injury with fecal incontinence from anorectal surgery or midline episiotomy
- 8%: Lack of informed consent (usually regarding extent of procedures or endoscopy)

Recent commentators have cautioned about patients who present with fully developed cancers within 4 years of colonoscopies that apparently cleared the colon of neoplasia. The concern expressed is that the presenting patients may assume their colonoscopies were negligently performed, despite legitimate alternative explanations.[6]

A study reviewing 38 malpractice claims against radiologists performing contrast examinations of the colon between 1985 and 1994 revealed the following major allegations: failure to diagnose resulting in delay in treatment and death, and colon perforation attributed to improper performance.[7]

Risk management suggestions relevant to colon cancer screening include using authoritative screening guidelines, documenting informed consent and refusals, assessing family histories, recommending that family members of at-risk patients be contacted, repeating sigmoidoscopies and colonoscopies when the preparation is inadequate, and documenting both cecal intubation and careful withdrawal techniques.[8]

Lawsuit Stress

Most physicians experience stress when their professional care and judgment are criticized in a public lawsuit. The initial stressor typically occurs when the claim letter, legal complaint, or insurance company notice arrives in the mail. The simple reality is that your chosen profession frequently lends itself to the frustrations and anxiety of litigation. Anger, uncertainty, and even depression are common symptoms among physician defendants. These emotions can be especially intense in those individuals sued for the first time.

Communications with your attorney are confidential and are protected by a privilege similar to the physician–patient privilege. Attorneys representing physicians usually advise their clients not to discuss the case with others for fear of losing the protections available through the attorney–client privilege. The tension and vulnerability that you may feel about being sued may be exacerbated by this inability to seek emotional comfort by discussing the case with colleagues and others. It is common to feel isolated—to assume that colleagues and even subordinates are talking about you and your lawsuit. It is important to place your predicament in perspective; many of your colleagues have been in the same situation before you and others will be in the future.

If you are involved in a claim or lawsuit and are experiencing any of these normal reactions to litigation or the threat of litigation, you should have a candid conversation with your attorney, risk manager, and/or insurance company claims representative. Many insurance companies and medical institutions provide resources for defendant physicians that enable them to discuss their lawsuit and their feelings of uncertainty and isolation with counselors or colleagues in a protected manner. Conversations with psychotherapists are generally privileged and not admissible in the courtroom as evidence in the case. Remember that your emotional stability is critical to the successful defense of the litigation. You serve yourself best by sharing your feelings with your attorney and asking him or her for a way to receive emotional coaching throughout the stress of the lawsuit and afterward as well.

Informed Consent

Informed consent is a patient's agreement to a medical procedure or other treatment after the person has been informed of the likely benefits, significant risks, and the alternatives of the treatment. The failure of a physician to obtain proper informed consent is often cited as a major component of medical malpractice litigation. In reality, few cases are prosecuted exclusively on the issue of informed consent, and juries do not customarily award damages solely for a lack of informed consent. Most malpractice lawsuits, however, contain a supplementary allegation that informed consent was not obtained. The informed consent discussion is at the heart of physician–patient communication and is usually an important component in the defense of the main medical or surgical issues in every case. You do not have to wait until the day of or the day before the procedure to obtain informed consent. A study involving 60 patients who underwent either colonoscopies or esophagogastroduodenoscopies revealed that patients remember essentially the same information whether consent is obtained immediately before a procedure or several days earlier.[9] The physician should discuss the procedure or treatment with the patient and obtain and document informed consent as close to the date of the procedure or treatment as reasonably possible, e.g., within days to several weeks. Allowing the patient some time to reflect on the risks, benefits, and alternatives before consenting is an ideal practice, depending on the urgency of the proposed treatment and the complexity of the patient's decision.

Obtaining Informed Consent

Obtaining informed consent is primarily a physician obligation. Nurses and other nonphysicians are not normally responsible for failing to obtain informed consent,[10] because they lack the requisite legal capacity to fully inform patients of issues on which only a physician is licensed to advise. Hospitals, the typical employers of such professionals, do have an obligation to maintain an effective informed consent process within their institutions. Lack of informed consent claims may be successful if hospitals breach hospital standards and other duties imposed by law, e.g., whereby a patient

is injured by an experimental procedure without being advised of the experimental study.[11]

Obtaining a patient's informed consent involves more than securing a patient's name on a form. It is a communication process in which the physician should discuss the following information with the patient[12]:

- The patient's diagnosis, if known
- The nature and purpose of the proposed treatment or procedure
- The risks and benefits of a proposed treatment or procedure
- Alternatives (regardless of cost or insurance coverage)
- The risks and benefits of the alternatives
- The risks and benefits of not receiving or undergoing the treatment or procedure

Patients should be given the opportunity to ask questions and have their questions answered.

Proving a Case of Lack of Informed Consent

Depending on variations in state laws, plaintiff attorneys typically must prove the following elements to establish a prima facie case of lack of informed consent by a physician:

- The physician failed to disclose to the patient and discuss the material risks and dangers inherently and potentially involved with respect to the proposed therapy, if any.
- The unrevealed risks and dangers which should have been disclosed by the physician actually materialize and were the proximate cause of injury to the patient, and
- A reasonable person in the position of the patient would have decided against the therapy had the material risks and dangers inherent and incidental to the treatment been disclosed to him or her before the therapy.[13]

Whether risks are material is normally an issue decided by a jury.[14] Juries are often instructed that risks are normally considered to be material if a reasonably prudent person would attach significance to the risk in deciding whether or not to accept the treatment. A risk that is either *severe*, such as death, or *frequent* are usually risks that are considered material. Some states regulate the specific information that must be conveyed to patients. Other states leave the determination of materiality to judges and expert witnesses. You should become familiar with the informed consent laws in the state where you practice. Withholding material risks from patients for cultural, ethnic, or paternalistic reasons is not acceptable.

Documentation of Informed Consent

Informed consent is usually documented with formal consent forms requiring the patient's signature. Nearly all hospitals require the use of consent forms for inpatient procedures to comply with applicable law. This is done to abide by the standards of the Joint Commission on Accreditation of Health Care Organization,[15] and to facilitate patient education of the treatment information. Proper informed consent is a process and not just a form. Forms can be challenged and criticized in the courtroom. A form containing errors, or one that is incomplete, can distract a jury from the real issues involving informed consent.

Claims of lack of informed consent are most successfully defended when a jury is persuaded that the physician had a meaningful conversation with the patient. In addition to a consent form, a chart notation made by the doctor, in the doctor's own words or handwriting, is usually very helpful. A jury that believes that the physician never saw the patient, or had a brief or cursory discussion with the patient, may become more inclined to decide that a surgeon departed from the standard of care in performing the procedure. Producing a diagram that was drawn for the patient to explain the procedure can be persuasive for jurors. Similarly, patient information sheets or pamphlets are effective communication devices and serve well in the litigation defense.

Listen carefully to your patients' questions. Answer questions in a friendly but candid manner. Note in the chart the presence of any family members who are present for the informed consent discussion.

Patients who are minors—usually those less than 18 years of age—may not normally consent for themselves. There are limited exceptions to that rule, e.g., patients who are living apart from their parents, or patients who are sufficiently mature to provide consent. Regardless of a minor's emancipation or maturity, it is wise to always obtain parental or custodial consent for elective procedures performed on minors. In addition to creating potential liability, the lack of parental or custodial consent for elective procedures involving a minor may result in the lack of a binding contract enabling you or the hospital to receive payment for services.

Documentation

A patient's medical record is often the star witness in any medical malpractice lawsuit. The medical record is the one witness whose memory never fades. When you are involved in a lawsuit alleging medical malpractice, it can be your best friend, or it can be your worst enemy. Make it your best friend.

Defensive Charting

"If it's not documented, it didn't happen." This adage serves as a good rule of thumb for all caregivers. Professional comprehensive charting conveys the appearance of professional and comprehensive care—not only to a jury but also to a plaintiff's attorney who is reviewing records and deciding whether or not to pursue a claim.

Chart notations need not contain overwhelming details to be helpful in the courtroom. A good defensive chart notation contains information that can deflect practical and obvious criticisms that may be made of the healthcare team or the

writer of the note. Examples of concepts to consider inserting, when applicable, include the following:

- Descriptions of bedside visits, especially when the physician has been paged multiple times
- When you were with the patient and what you did
- Your thought process and differential diagnosis
- Presence of family members
- "Patient states that she understands a change in bowel habits should be reported"
- "Patient refuses colonoscopy because . . ."
- "Patient not able to perform fecal occult blood test because . . ."

Etiology Speculation

The charting of speculative opinions can be as damaging as charting too little information. Not uncommonly, one member of the medical team speculates as to the etiology of an adverse event, and the speculated etiology is adopted as fact by other members of the healthcare team.

Example: Physician undertakes a second-look laparotomy to rule out recurrence of cancer. During the procedure, the bladder and bowl are perforated, but the perforations are identified and repaired intraoperatively. A bowel leak, however, is detected 3 days later. A second-year resident records in the medical chart, "Iatrogenic perforation resulting in sepsis." This reference is repeated by two attendings on other services.

The perforation may have been iatrogenic or spontaneous. The unconfirmed presumption in the medical chart that the bowel leak occurred during the procedure, when repeated by others in the medical record, often becomes a "reality." That "reality" may become insurmountable in the courtroom, even when expert review leads to the opinion that the perforation, in retrospect, was clearly spontaneous.

Everything written in the medical chart is critical. Key phrasing and excerpts are often highlighted and/or enlarged onto exhibit boards for juries to see. Remember that causation is one of the four elements of medical malpractice, and it is frequently the most difficult of the four elements for the plaintiff to prove.

- ALERT!—*Iatrogenic* means "caused by manner or action of physician, not by medical treatment." Use this word only when you are sure it is applicable.

The law does not require that physicians always be correct in their decisions and treatment of patients. Rather, it requires reasonable and prudent care. A good chart notation will reflect a physician's attention and thought process, even if the diagnosis turns out to be incorrect.

Plaintiff's Preclaim Review

Plaintiffs' attorneys are usually paid on a contingency fee basis, i.e., they receive a percentage of the amount recovered. Experienced plaintiffs' attorneys conduct a review of a potential client's medical records before agreeing to file a lawsuit. Because most medical malpractice cases are tried before juries (as opposed to judges), attorneys representing patients look for flaws in medical record documentation that can be exploited at trial. For example, a physician's criticism of a colleague in a medical record is more desirable to showcase before a jury than complicated medical facts. Although differences of opinion are expected to occur occasionally, conflicts with colleagues that appear in the medical records are best limited to honest disagreements that are relevant to a patient's course of care.

Other items that attorneys and their reviewing physicians look for are missing laboratory reports, missing radiology interpretations, or the results of any tests or procedures that were ordered but not present in the chart. Multiple page attempts by the nursing staff that go unanswered are also fertile ground for review and focus.

Example: Elderly male patient with debilitating back pain underwent spinal surgery. He was taking anticoagulation medications because of a mechanical heart valve. Postoperatively he developed a hematoma at the base of the spine. In response to complaints of pain, he was seen three times by a house officer who did perform appropriate examinations but who neither stopped the patient's heparin nor ordered a magnetic resonance imaging. Permanent paralysis and urinary and sexual loss ensued.

A plaintiff's lawyer would be immediately drawn to nursing notes stating that multiple page attempts were made and that no corresponding notes were made by any physician responding to the pages. The attorney may immediately assume that he or she can prove in the courtroom one of the following potential scenarios: 1) no physician ever responded to the pages; 2) a physician did respond but the response was not timely; or 3) a physician responded but did not conduct a proper examination.

In this example, a comprehensive chart notation by the house officer, reflecting the thought processes and the extent of the examinations, may obviate a claim, a verdict, and tens of thousands of dollars in legal fees.

Record Tampering and Deception

Improper alteration of the medical record is grounds for punitive damages and may result in loss of licensure. It should *never* be done. Postevent recording in a medical record should be done with proper disclosure of the timing and reason for the entry. Consider seeking the advice of risk-management personnel or legal counsel before making such an entry. Remember that your medical records are copied for multiple reasons, including insurance, compliance, and quality-review issues. Copies of any given patient's medical records may exist elsewhere, even at other healthcare facilities.

Plaintiffs' attorneys routinely request copies of the same medical records from multiple sources. This is done to ensure that all records are gathered, and to determine whether discrepancies exist among the various copies, e.g., a late entry on one copy that does not appear on another copy. Color copying and expert document and handwriting analysis are techniques used to detect late or inappropriate entries. Evidence that a physician intentionally altered a medical record to lessen his or her own liability in a malpractice case is devastating and can rarely be overcome.

Similarly, evidence that a surgical error was known to the physician but concealed from the patient would almost certainly flame juror anger and result in a significant adverse verdict. Sponges, needles, and other "foreign objects" inadvertently left behind in the patient during surgery and later discovered by X-ray should be immediately disclosed to patients. The following 2003 Maryland case[16] illustrates this point.

The plaintiff, a 49-year-old married grocer, with a long history of uncontrolled diarrhea and stomach pain diagnosed as ulcerous colitis, presented to a colorectal surgeon for a total proctocolectomy with a temporary ileostomy. The surgeon performed ileostomy closure 90 days later, but the patient experienced a return of her uncontrolled diarrhea and stomach pain. She sought the advice of another physician, who discovered via colonoscopy that half of her rectum remained after the proctocolectomy. A new surgeon performed a second proctocolectomy and removed the remaining portion of the rectum, after which the patient made a full recovery. The plaintiff's attorney asserted that, although the first surgeon's medical notes indicated that he had incorrectly performed the procedure, the surgeon failed to so inform his patient. The defendant surgeon contended that it was an acceptable practice to leave half of the rectum. Plaintiff's medical expenses were $51,438. After experts testified for both plaintiff and defendant, the jury deliberated for only 1.5 hours before returning a verdict for the woman and her husband in the amount of $591,438. The award of such a significant sum on these facts in such a short time suggests that the jury was angered by the facts.

Computerized Medical Records

Electronic medical records offer efficiencies and improved medical quality for the healthcare delivery system. All patient records, whether paper or electronic, are discoverable and admissible in medical malpractice lawsuits. Physicians who record entries in computerized medical records must become familiar with the use of electronic medical systems and should understand some dangers inherent in these computerized systems. For example:

- BEWARE drop-down menus and checklists
- BEWARE prefabricated medical descriptors
- BEWARE prefabricated informed consent notations
- BEWARE easy click-on techniques

Not all patient evaluations and regimens can be preformatted. There may be a natural tendency for caregivers to pick the "closest" option in a menu of options as opposed to creating their own text. Physicians should use "free text" whenever necessary and appropriate. It is easier to explain and defend "your own words" in describing the care of a patient than the words of a computer programmer who has written a menu of typical patient diagnoses in drop-down menus or other coded formats.

Communication

Adverse Events, Bad News, and Apologies

When an untoward and/or unexpected event occurs involving a patient, communication is critical for quality care and for responding to later claims of malpractice. First and foremost, the patient's medical needs must be promptly addressed. Coordination of ongoing care, including consultation and appropriate follow-up, is a critical first step.

As soon as practicable after the event, the patient and family should be informed of the event and its potential consequences to the patient. This communication should be respectful and sympathetic. The discussion should be preliminary to a more detailed conversation that should occur after more facts are available. Without assigning blame or criticizing other practitioners, the patient and family should be informed that the event occurred, the current and future consequences of the event to the patient, and what steps have been taken to address the patient's medical condition. If the underlying causes for the event are not yet known, care should be taken not to speculate about those causes. The conversation is best handled by a physician well known to the patient and family, although circumstances may warrant placing others in that role. Questions should be honestly and factually answered. The patient and family should be told that additional information will be conveyed to them as it becomes known, and that a more thorough discussion will occur within a set period of time, ideally 24 hours.

It is usually advisable to contact a risk manager or in-house legal counsel, if applicable, when the critical incident occurs in an institution where such personnel are available. Depending on institutional policy, risk managers or quality management personnel frequently assist in the interactions with patients and family. They will also begin any appropriate administrative activity, such as initiating a sentinel event analysis, notifying an insurance carrier, sequestering medical devices or equipment, initiating an equipment analysis, and reporting device failures to the United States Food and Drug Administration (FDA). The administrative staff may also wish to convene a risk management and/or quality management review. Such reviews are typically protected from discovery in a lawsuit under applicable state privilege statutes. It is advisable for one member of the institutional team to be designated as the liaison with the patient and family so that consistent information is being delivered.

When additional facts are gathered and a better understanding of the event is known, a family meeting is advisable. Ideally the meeting should occur within 24 hours of the initial discussion with the family. The spokesperson should lead the discussion. The patient's attending physician, if not the spokesperson, should be present. The information known about the event, the anticipated medical consequences, and the prognosis for the patient should be discussed.

Physicians and institutions should be willing to express sympathy. An apology expressing sorrow that the patient experienced the event may be appropriate but should be carefully worded, e.g., "We are sorry you have experienced this complication." In recent years, a number of prominent institutions have urged their physicians to say they are sorry for a patient mishap. One reason is that such apologies may deflect lawsuits. States such as Colorado, Oregon, and Ohio have even enacted legislation immunizing various forms of apologies from courtroom use.[17] Advice should be sought from institutional or local legal counsel regarding the wording of any apologetic statements.

At family meetings, the family members should have an opportunity to ask all of their questions. They should be provided with the name and contact information of someone to address additional questions that may arise later. The healthcare team should anticipate questions about reducing or eliminating medical bills and statements suggesting the possibility of a malpractice claim. Any questions about malpractice can be deferred at that point with the explanation that institutional legal counsel or an insurance representative will contact the family if desired. Keeping in touch with the patient and family spokesperson is critical during the next several days and weeks.

A senior member of the medical team, perhaps with the assistance of risk management and/or legal counsel, should be consulted in reviewing the chart and recording the events involving the untoward incident. Details of the event and the identity of personnel should be completely and accurately recorded. All discussions with the patient and family members after the incident should also be clearly described, including the identity of persons present at the family meetings and what was said.

Many patients and family members at this juncture are considering whether to seek the advice of a lawyer, and they may be urged to do so by friends and other family members. Care should be taken by all members of the healthcare team to provide a courteous, qualitative, and sympathetic continuity of care and interaction with family members. Physicians and other members of the healthcare team serve themselves and their patients well by using this time to provide as positive and supportive of an experience as possible for patients and family members.

Electronic Mail

Because of the efficiencies associated with electronic mail (email) communication, many physicians communicate with both patients and other healthcare providers by using email. Special care should be taken when using email that contains patient-identifiable information.

Clinicians may communicate with other clinicians and patients by email. The Federal Health Insurance Portability and Accountability Act (HIPAA) of 1996[18] (discussed later) provides regulation for electronic transmission containing protected health information such as confidential medical information. HIPAA provides that healthcare providers have in place appropriate administrative, technical, and physical safeguards to protect the privacy of protected health information (PHI).[19] The HIPAA regulations do not provide a specific regulatory scheme for email communication, but they do require that providers have procedures that limit disclosures of PHI to the amount reasonably necessary to achieve the purposes of PHI disclosures.[20]

The Notice of Privacy Practices that providers give to their patients must explain in a separate statement that the provider may contact the patient to provide appointment reminders or information about treatment alternatives or other health-related benefits or services that may be of interest to the individual.[21] If this will be done by email, it is advisable to state that in the Notice of Privacy Practices.

You may wish to inform your patients that email transmission involves privacy and security issues that may be of interest to them. Patients may even be asked whether they wish you to communicate with them by email or not. Email that is sent to a patient's business may be intercepted by the patient's business colleagues, and emails can be inadvertently transmitted to unintended addressees. The Internet is not considered a secure medium for transmitting confidential data unless both parties use encryption technology. These types of warnings can be provided to patients who wish to communicate with their physicians by email.

It is advisable for physicians to keep either paper or electronic copies of emails to and from patients that are relevant to patient treatment. These email copies should be maintained in the patient's medical records just as traditional paper correspondence would be.

Physicians may wish to include a Confidentiality Notice that is preprinted at the bottom of email transmissions. A sample Confidentiality Notice appears below:

Confidentiality Notice: This email message including attachments, if any, is intended only for the person or entity to which it is addressed and may contain confidential and/or privileged material. Any unauthorized review, use, disclosure, or distribution is prohibited. If you are not the intended recipient, please contact the sender by reply email and destroy all copies of the original message. If you are the intended recipient, but do not wish to receive communications through this medium, please so advise the sender immediately.

Health Insurance Portability and Accountability Act

HIPAA provides national privacy protection for patients. Administrative Regulations, encompassed in the Federal Privacy Rule[22] have been promulgated by the United States Department of Health and Human Services pursuant to

HIPAA. The Federal Privacy Rule establishes minimum privacy standards for healthcare providers, health plans, and healthcare clearing houses (referred to in HIPAA as "covered entities") to follow when using and disclosing patient-identifiable PHI that they create or maintain. Generally speaking, PHI is any information that is created (or received) and maintained by a covered entity related to the health or health care of a patient (or payment related to the health care) that directly or indirectly identifies the patient.[23]

The Federal Privacy Rule also requires compliance with state laws that afford greater privacy protections than HIPAA. Compliance with the Federal Privacy Rule was required on and after April 14, 2003. All covered entities must have policies and procedures in place that demonstrate compliance with the Federal Privacy Rule.

HIPAA provides that healthcare providers must make a good faith effort to give each patient a Notice of Privacy Practices that describes the privacy practices of the healthcare provider. Patients must be asked to acknowledge in writing that they have received this notice. Once a provider makes a good faith effort to provide a Notice of Privacy Practices to a patient and gets the patient's written acknowledgement of receipt of the notice, the healthcare provider may use and disclose PHI for reasons related to treatment of the patient, payment for the patient's health care, and the healthcare operations of the provider (TPO). Generally, physicians who are independent practitioners of the hospitals of which they practice are part of those hospitals' "organized health care arrangements," enabling the disclosure of PHI between the hospital personnel and the independently practicing physicians. To use or disclose PHI for reasons other than TPO or as otherwise permitted by law, a physician must obtain an additional written permission from the patient called an "authorization."[24] Clinical research, for example, is not considered "treatment" and usually must be separately approved by research subjects by signing an authorization. In many medical centers, authorizations for clinical research are integrated into the consent form approved by the institutional review board (IRB). The Federal Privacy Rule requires that authorizations contain certain elements.[25]

HIPAA permits treating physicians to disclose to a patient's family members, other relatives, close personal friends, and others identified by the patient any PHI that is directly relevant to such person's involvement with the patient's care or healthcare payments. Before making any of these disclosures, a physician should either obtain the patient's agreement to the disclosure or reasonably infer from the circumstances that the patient does not object.[26]

Research and Innovative Surgery

Research Versus Innovative practice

The emergence of evidence-based medicine has brought new challenges to the academic medical community. Surgeons and other physicians who serve as investigators in clinical trials are very familiar with the review and approval process of IRBs—ethics committees established under federal law to oversee the conduct of research. Many disciplines, especially surgery, have evolved historically in an environment of unregulated innovation. It is often not clear when innovative therapy crosses the line into the research arena.

The Belmont Report[27] states that the distinction between research and practice is blurred and that both often occur together. Research is usually described in a formal protocol, and departures from standard practice are not necessarily "research." The Belmont Report also states:

The fact that a procedure is "experimental," in the sense of new, untested, or different, does not automatically place it in the category of research. Radically new procedures of this description should, however, be made the object of formal research at an early stage in order to determine whether they are safe and effective. Thus, it is the responsibility of medical practice committees, for example, to insist that a major innovation be incorporated into a formal research project.

Regulation of the practice of medicine has historically been the exclusive province of the state medical boards and other state regulatory authorities. When medical practice crosses the line into "research" involving "human subjects" or investigational drugs, devices, or other test articles, however, the activity becomes subject to the regulation of the federal Office for Human Research Protection (OHRP)[28] or the FDA.[29] "Research," as regulated, is a systematic investigation, including research development, testing and evaluation, designed to develop or contribute to generalizable knowledge.[30] "Human subjects" are living individuals about whom an investigator conducting research obtains data through intervention or interaction with the individual or identifiable private information.[31] Traditional examples of research studies include prospective industry-sponsored files.

Database Registries

In theory, physicians who engage in innovative treatment that does not involve a systematic design, a research protocol, a prospective intent to publish, or an investigational item are not regulated by either OHRP or FDA. Over the past decade, however, OHRP has expressed its view that the systematic collections of data performed off-chart, especially if published, may carry an implicit prospective intent and are considered research. These may include ongoing patient registries, including outcomes data; tissue banks; static databases, including ad hoc research from closed trials; and even retrospective studies, including chart reviews, if a prospective intent to publish was present.

In recent years, the OHRP has investigated a variety of innovative techniques to determine whether or not the activities should have been prospectively reviewed by an IRB as research. Examples are: 14 patients treated with fractionated stereotactic radiosurgery for treatment of large arteriovenous

malformations before IRB approval[32]; publication of a retrospective chart review that was conducted without IRB approval[33]; publication describing partial left ventriculectomies performed in the management of patients with dilated cardiomyopathy without IRB approval[34]; and fetal surgery procedures.[35] Many if not all of these scenarios involved publications that used research jargon and implied that a prospective research trial had been conducted (without IRB review and approval). In each of these investigations, OHRP suggested that the applicable institution consider the development of "innovative practice committees" or similar institutional vehicles to evaluate major innovative therapies. Physicians, especially surgeons experimenting with minor surgical modifications to accepted techniques, should use care when authoring articles about clinical experiences that did not involve "research" as defined above. When in doubt, physicians are encouraged to consult with their local IRBs for guidance.

Promotional Prohibitions

Physicians who conduct FDA-regulated research are prohibited from representing in a promotional context that an investigational new drug, device, or other test article is safe or effective (or otherwise beneficial) before it has received regulatory approval.[36] Physicians should carefully review press releases and other promotional disclosures prepared by commercial sponsors or manufacturers before permitting their names to be associated with such test articles before approval.

Insider Trading

If you are involved in clinical trials for pharmaceutical companies or biotechnology companies whose securities are publicly traded, you may have certain obligations to protect the confidentiality of sensitive information that you acquire. Your duties may stem from not only being a company officer or holding another fiduciary position, but also from being an investigator or from serving on company advisory committees such as scientific advisory boards, clinical trial steering committees, clinical trial executive committees, or data safety monitoring boards. The securities laws widely prohibit fraudulent activities of any kind in connection with the offer, purchase, or sale of securities.[37] The securities laws are the basis for different types of government enforcement activities, including investigation involving illegal insider trading. Insider trading is illegal when a person trades a security while in possession of material, nonpublic information, possibly including information from medical research trials, in violation of a duty to withhold the information or refrain from trading in that security. "Tipping" other traders of such information who then trade a security affected by the tip is also illegal. So is acting on an illegal tip.

Conclusion

In recent years, the demands and pressures on physicians and surgeons have grown dramatically. Lawyer advertising and malpractice awards and settlements are greater than ever before. Web-based consumer awareness has increased the knowledge base of patients. Government regulation and enforcement activities have become more focused. Greater understanding and awareness of legal and risk management concerns is critical for healthcare practitioners facing these challenges.

References

1. Farmer v. Minami, et al., 02-2-06246-6SEA (Sup. Ct. King Cty. July 21, 2003).
2. Bruni v. Tatsumi, 46 Ohio St. 2d 127 (1976).
3. Bruni v. Tatsumi, 46 Ohio St. 2d 127 (1976).
4. Kniphfer v. Memorial Health University, et al., 1010574F (Sup. Ct. Chatham Cty. Nov. 8, 2001).
5. Kern KA. Medical malpractice involving colon and rectal disease: a 20-year review of United States civil court litigation. Dis Colon Rectum 1993;36:531–539.
6. Rex DK, Bond JH, Feld AD. Medical-legal risks of incident cancers after clearing colonoscopy. Am J Gastroenterol 2001;96: 952–957.
7. Barloon TJ, Shumway J. Medical malpractice involving radiologic colon examinations: a review of 38 recent cases. AJR Am J Roentgenol 1995;165:343–346.
8. Feld AD. Medicolegal implications of colon cancer screening. Gastrointest Endosc Clin North Am 2002;12(1):171–179.
9. Elfant AB, Korn C, Mendez L, Pello MJ, Peiken SR. Recall of informed consent after endoscopic procedures. Dis Colon Rectum 1995;38(1):1–3.
10. Finney v. Milton S. Hershey Med. Ctr., 36 Pa. D. & C. 4th 464 (C.P. Ct. Dauphin Cty. Feb. 20, 1996). Ohio Rev. Code 2317.54.
11. Friter v. Iolab Corp., 414 Pa. Super. 622 (1992).
12. American Medical Association. Informed consent. www.ama-assn.org/ama/pub. Chicago, IL; 2005.
13. Nickell v. Gonzalez, 17 Ohio St. 3d 136.
14. Dible v. Vagley, 417 Pa. Super. 302 (1992).
15. Joint Commission on Accreditation of Healthcare Organizations. www.jcaho.org. Chicago, IL; 2005.
16. Yu v. Kim, 03C01000409 (Cir. Ct. Balt. Cty. June 19, 2003).
17. Zimmerman R. Medicine means knowing how to say you're sorry. Pittsburgh Post-Gazette (PA) May 23, 2004. Ohio Rev. Code 2317.43.
18. Pub. L. No. 104-191, 110 Stat. 1942 (1996).
19. 45 C.F.R. 164.530(c).
20. 45 C.F.R. 164.514(d).
21. 45 C.F.R. 164.520(b)(iii)(A).
22. 45 C.F.R. 164.160, 45C.F.R. 162, 45 C.F.R. 164.
23. 45 C.F.R. 164.501.
24. 45 C.F.R. 164.508.
25. 45 C.F.R. 164.508(c) and (d).
26. 45 C.F.R. 164.510(b).
27. National Institutes of Health, Department of Health and Human Services. Report of the National Commission for the Protection of Human Subjects of Biomedical and Behavioral Research. Bethesda, MD, 1979.
28. 45 C.F.R. 46.
29. 21 C.F.R. 50 and 56.
30. 45 C.F.R. 46.102(d).
31. 45 C.F.R. 46.102(f).
32. Office for Human Research Protection, Department of Health and Human Services. Compliance Oversight Determination Letter. Rockville, MD, Aug. 1, 2001.
33. Office for Human Research Protection, Department of Health and Human Services. Compliance Oversight Determination Letter. Rockville, MD, Jan. 8, 2002.
34. Office for Human Research Protection, Department of Health and Human Services. Compliance Oversight Determination Letter. Rockville, MD, Apr. 30, 2002.
35. Office for Human Research Protection, Department of Health and Human Services. Compliance Oversight Determination Letter. Rockville, MD, Feb. 13, 2003.
36. U.S. Food and Drug Administration, Department of Health and Human Services. www.fda.gov. Rockville, MD.
37. U.S. Securities and Exchange Commission. www.sec.gov. Washington, DC; 2005.

Index

A

AAST. *See* American Association for the Surgery of Trauma

Abdominal aortic aneurysms, 399–400

Abdominal complications, 325–327

Abdominal injuries, 327

Abdominal rectopexy, 666, 669–671

Abdominal transsacral resection, 432

Abdominal wall closure, 327

Abdominoperineal resection (APR), 146, 413, 432
  ligation/resection during, 419–422
  mobilization during, 419
  position during, 419
  techniques of, 419–422

Abscess, 274, 279. *See also* Acute suppuration; Anorectal abscess
  enteroparietal, 592–593
  interloop, 593
  intraabdominal, 151–152
  intramesenteric, 593
  pilonidal disease, 229
  psoas/retroperitoneal, 593

Absolute risk reduction (ARR), 772

ACC. *See* American College of Cardiology

Accrediting Council for Graduate Medical Evaluation (ACGME), 782–783

Aclovate®. *See* Alclometasone dipropionate

Acromegaly, 344

Actinomycosis, 607, 610

Activities of daily living (ADL), 119

Acupressure, 132

Acupuncture, 132

Acute colonic obstruction, 399

Acute suppuration (abscess), 210

Acute thrombosis, 165

Adenine, 525

Adenocarcinomas, 356–357, 491–492

Adenoma(s), 533
  -carcinoma sequence, 364
  clinical presentation of, 362
  depressed/flat, 367–368

duodenal, 537
  epidemiology of, 363–364
  pathology of, 362–363
  rectal, 365
  serrated, 368
  surveillance of, 365–366

Adenomatous polyps, 356–357

Adenosquamous carcinoma, 521

Adjuvant therapy, 428, 433, 437–443

ADL. *See* Activities of daily living

Adrenergic antagonists, 185

Advance directives, 745–747

Advancement flaps, 182, 204, 217–219

Aeromonas, 607, 609–610

Age, 271, 386

Agency for Health Care Policy and Research (AHCPR), 353, 354, 358

AHA. *See* American Heart Association

AHCPR. *See* Agency for Health Care Policy and Research

AIDS (acquired immunodeficiency syndrome)
  diarrhea, 614–615
  HIV, 265–266

AIN. *See* Anal intraepithelial neoplasia

AJCC. *See* American Joint Committee on Cancer

Alclometasone dipropionate (Aclovate®), 252

Alcohol, 271, 340

Aldosterone, 24–25

Amebiasis, 612

American Association for the Surgery of Trauma (AAST), 323, 327, 328, 329, 331

American Board of Colon and Rectal Surgery, 783

American Cancer Society, 353, 355, 390, 532

American College of Cardiology (ACC), 120

American College of Surgeons, 782

American Heart Association (AHA), 120

American Joint Committee on Cancer (AJCC), 386, 462

American Medical Association, 729

American Society of Anesthesiologists (ASA), 117, 171

American Society of Colon and Rectal Surgeons (ASCRS), 120, 281, 353, 390, 654, 703, 707, 767

Amine precursor uptake and decarboxylation (APUD), 515

Amines, 516

Aminosalicylates, 555

Amitriptyline (Elavil), 684

Ammonium derivatives, 685

Amoxicillin, 124

Ampicillin, 331, 416

Amsterdam criteria, 529, 530

Anal agenesis, 17

Anal canal
  anus and
    anatomic v. surgical, 1, 2
    conjoined longitudinal muscle and, 3–4
    epithelium of, 2, 4
    external anal sphincter and, 2–3
    innervation of, 7–8, 9
    internal anal sphincter and, 2
    muscles of, 2, 3
    structure/anal verge, 1
  length of, 49
  neoplasms, EAUS and, 111–112
  physiology of
    bulbocavernosus reflexes in, 35
    cough reflexes in, 35
    cutaneous-anal reflexes in, 34
    mechanical factors in, 36–37
    pathologic conditions in, 37–38
    RAER in, 35–36
    RAIR in, 35, 36
    reflexes in, 34
    sensory in, 34

Anal cancer, 263–265
  anatomic considerations for, 482–483
  epidemiology of, 485
  etiology/pathogenesis of, 483–485
  HIV-related, 495
  lymphatic drainage and, 483
  squarmous cell cancer of the anal canal
    clinical characteristics and, 488
    evaluation of, 488–489
    staging and, 489
    treatments for, 489–491
  terminology for, 483
Anal dilatation
  anal fissure and, 180
  stretch, 165
Anal diseases, 244
Anal dysplasia, 483–485
Anal encirclement procedures, 659
Anal fissure, 725
  conclusions on, 188
  Crohn's disease and, 187
  diagnosis of, 179
  epidemiology of, 178
  etiology of, 178–179
  HIV and, 187–188
  low pressure, 187
  management of
    advancement flaps in, 182
    anal dilatation in, 180
    conservative, 179
    LIS in, 180–182
    operative treatment in, 179
  medical management of
    adrenergic antagonists in, 185
    BT in, 182, 185–187
    calcium channel blockers in, 184–185
    cholinergic agonists in, 185
    phosphodiesterase inhibitors in, 182, 185
    sphincter relaxants in, 182
    topical nitrates, 182–184
  symptoms of, 179
Anal infections, 198
Anal intraepithelial dysplasia, 263–265
Anal intraepithelial neoplasia (AIN), 483
Anal manometry, 656–657
Anal margin
  perianal neoplasms/uncommon, 493–495
  SCC of
    clinical characteristics of, 486
    staging of, 487
    treatment options for, 487–488
Anal sphincter, 33, 34, 52
Anal stenosis, 17
Anal tattooing, 253
ANCA. See Antineutrophil cytoplasmic antibody
Anesthesia, 132. See also Patient-controlled anesthesia
Angiodysplasia, 301

Angiography, 92–94, 304–305
Anisakiasis, 614
Anismus, 50
Anoperineum, 591–592
Anorectal abscess
  anatomy of, 192, 193
  evaluation/treatments for, 192–198
  pathophysiology of, 192, 193
Anorectal agenesis, 17–18
Anorectal angle
  defecography and, 49
  flap valve and, 36
  ring, 13
Anorectal defects, 17–18
Anorectal immunology, 256–257
Anorectal infections, 197
Anorectal malformations (imperforate anus), 16, 17, 716
  specific defects associated with
    females, 718–719, 721–722
    males, 717–718, 719, 720–721
  treatment results for, 722–723
Anorectal sepsis, 198
Anorectal spaces, 9–10
Anorectal surgery, 171
Anoscopy
  complications associated with, 58
  contraindications for, 57
  indications for, 57, 58
  positioning in, 57
  preparations for, 57
  techniques for, 57–58
Anterior sacral meningoceles, 502–503
Anterior sphincteroplasty, 659–660
Anthracene, 681
Antibiotic(s), 196, 222, 555–556, 561, 587, 617–618. See also specific drugs
  for colon/rectal injuries, 330–331
  oral, 124
  parenteral, 124
  prophylaxis, 416
  topical, 252
  usage of, 122, 124, 126
Antibodies, monoclonal, 470
Anticholinergics, 561, 684
Anticoagulants, 416
Anticoagulation, 135, 136
Antigens, 439
Antihistamines, 132, 240, 243, 251
Antineutrophil cytoplasmic antibody (ANCA), 551
Antispasmodics, 29
APACHE (Acute physiology and chronic health evaluation), 118
Appendicitis, 276
APR. See Abdominoperineal resection
APUD. See Amine precursor uptake and decarboxylation
Arc of Riolan, 15

Aristocort®. See Triamcinolone acetonide 0.5%
Armed Forces Institute of Pathology, 520
ARR. See Absolute risk reduction
Arteries, inferior/superior hemorrhoidal, 6
Artificial bowel sphincter, 661
ASA. See American Society of Anesthesiologists
Ascariasis, 613
ASCA testing, 551
ASCRS. See American Society of Colon and Rectal Surgeons
ASCUS. See Atypical squamous cells of indeterminate significance
Aspirin, 340–341
Association of Surgeons (Netherlands), 782
Astler Coller Modification, 386
Atropine, 605, 684
Atypical squamous cells of indeterminate significance (ASCUS), 263
Azathioprine (AZA), 557, 562
Azulfidine®. See Sulfasalazine

B
Babies, 19, 719
Bacitracin, 617–618
Bacterial infections, 242–243
Balantidiasis, 612
Balloon
  expulsion test, 51
  training, 659
Balneol®, 250
Balsalazide (Colazal®), 556
BAM. See Bile acid malabsorption
Bannayan-Riley-Ruvalcaba syndrome, 381
Barium
  enemas, 75–76, 293, 355
  follow-through, 83
  in physiologic testing, 47
  studies, 75
Barnet continent ileostomy reservoir (BCIR), 571
Basal cell carcinomas (BCCs), 493
Bascom cleft lift (Bascom II), 233–234
Bascom I. See Midline pit excision
Bascom II. See Bascom cleft lift
Bascom's chronic abscess curettage, 230–231
BCCs. See Basal cell carcinomas
BCIR. See Barnet continent ileostomy reservoir
Behçet's syndrome, 602, 603
Benadryl®. See Diphenhydramine
Bentyl. See Dicyclomine hydrochloride
Benzathine penicillin, 260
Betadine, 634
Betamethasone dipropionate (Diprolene®), 252
Betamethasone valerate cream (Valisone®), 252

Bethanechol, 182
Bicarbonates, 25
Bile acid malabsorption (BAM), 605
Bioethics, 737–739
Bipolar diathermy, 163–164
Bisacodyl, 681
Bisacodyl suppositories, 658
Bismuth subsalicylate, 605
Bladder injuries, 146
Bleeding, 273, 300
 as anastomotic postoperative
  complication, 142–143
 pelvic
  intraabdominal abscess/wound
   infection and, 151–152
  perineal wound infection and,
   152–153
 prophylaxis colonoscopy and, 63
Blood
 supply, 15
 transfusions, 326, 386
 vessel invasion, 387
Bone metastasis, 475
Botulinum toxin (BT), 182, 185–187
Bowel. *See also* Mechanical bowel
  preparation
 activity/diet resumption, 694–695
 continence, 33
 injury, radiation-induced, 615–617
 motility, 33
 obstruction, 645
  early postoperative, 150
 preparation, 122–123
  for surgery, 415
 tissue interposition, 221, 222
Bowen's disease, 485–486
Brain metastasis, 475
Britain Journal of Surgery, 768
Brooke ileostomy, 569
Brucellosis, 607, 610
BT. *See* Botulinum toxin
Budesonide, 556, 560
Bulbocavernosus reflexes, 35
Bupivacaine
 with epinephrine, 253
 hydrochloride, 202
Burow's solution, 250, 252

C
Calamine, 252
Calcium
 channel blockers, 184–185
 effect of, 339–340
 polycarbophil, 159–160, 161
Calcium dobesilate (calcium 2,5-dihydrox-
  ybenzenesulfonate), 161
Calcium polycarbophil (FiberCon), 680
CALGB. *See* Cancer and Leukemia Group B
Calibration, 41
California Cancer Registry, 485

Calmoseptine®, 252
Camphor, 252
Campylobacter, 607, 608
Canadian Multicentre Colorectal Deep Vein
  Thrombosis Prophylaxis, 135
Canadian Task Force on the Periodic Health
  Examination, 767
Cancer(s). *See also specific cancers*
 contrast studies of polyps/, 75–77
 hereditary, 447
 management/risks associated with, 381
 MSI-H, 369
 plain films and, 70, 71
 synchronous, 389, 431
 uterine, 539
Cancer and Leukemia Group B (CALGB),
  470, 491
Cancer Genetics Studies Consortium, 358
Cancer Prevention Study II, 340
Capsaicin (Dolorac; Zostrix), 241, 252
Carcinoembryonic antigen (CEA),
  387–388, 446–447, 468
Carcinoid syndrome, 516–517
Cascara, 681
Case presentations, 780–781
Catheters
 balloon, 634
 drainage of, 194–195
 flexible, 25
 Foley, 146
CCP. *See* Colitis cystica profunda
CD. *See* Crohn's disease
CDC. *See* Centers for Disease Control
CEA. *See* Carcinoembryonic antigen
Cecal volvulus
 clinical presentation of, 287–288
 diagnosis of, 288
 epidemiology/incidence of, 287
 etiology/pathogenesis of, 287
 outcomes/treatments for, 288–289
Cecum
 colon and, 13
 incomplete attachment of, 19
Cefixime, 258
Ceftriaxone, 258
Centers for Disease Control (CDC), 258
Centers for Medicare and Medicaid
  Services (CMS), 355–356, 727
Cephalosporin, 124, 331
Cetuximab, 470
Chancroid, 260
Chemokines, 552
Chemoprevention, 377, 534, 536–537
Chemoradiation/Chemoradiotherapy
 preop, 440–441, 490–491
 postop, 438–439
Chemotherapy, 428, 433, 519–520
 adjuvant, 437–438, 442–443
 for liver metastasis, 468–470
 systemic, 465

Chlamydia trachomatis, 258–259
Chloride, 25
Cholecystectomy, 342
Cholestyramine, 605, 618
Cholinergic agonists, 185
Chronic pulmonary diseases, 121
Chronic suppuration (fistula), 210–211
CHRPE. *See* Congenital hypertrophy of the
  retinal pigment epithelium
CI. *See* Confidence interval
Cidofovir, 486
Ciprofloxacin, 124, 258, 556
Circumferential resection margin
  (CRM), 407
Citrucel. *See* Methylcellulose
Citrus bioflavonoids, 160–161
CLASICC trial, 693, 696, 703
Clavulanic acid, 124
Clindamycin, 124
Clinical pathways, 137–138
Cloaca, 18, 718–719, 721–722
Clobetasol propionate (Temovate®), 252
Clostridium botulinum, 185
Clostridium difficile, 124, 561, 617–618
CMS. *See* Centers for Medicare and
  Medicaid Services
CMV. *See* Cytomegalovirus
Coagulopathy, 546
Coccygodynia, 690
Cochrane Collaboration, 770
Cochrane review, 123, 160, 168, 169, 616
Codeine, 131
Cohort studies, 765
Colace. *See* Docusate sodium
Colazal®. *See* Balsalazide
COLD. *See* Global Initiative for Chronic
  Obstructive Lung Disease
Colectomy
 left, 398
 outcomes for, 400–401
 right, 396–397
  extended, 397–398
 sigmoid, 398–399
 total abdominal, 399
Colestipol, 618
Colitis
 bacterial, 606–607
 Clostridium difficile, 617–618
 CMV, 611–612
 collagen vascular-associated, 602–604
 corrosive, 611
 disinfectant, 611
 diversion, 610
 eosinophilic, 606
 fungal, 606
 HIV, 614–615
 HSV, 612
 indeterminate, 551
 ischemic, 601–602
 microscopic, 604–606

Colitis (*Continued*)
  mild-moderate
    distal, 560
    extensive, 560–561
  miscellaneous, 610–611
  parasitic, 612–614
  plain films and, 73–75
  toxic, 585–586
  viral, 611–612
  See also Crohn's disease; Ulcerative
      colitis
Colitis cystica profunda (CCP), 674–675
Collaborative Group of the Americas
    on Inherited Colorectal
    Cancer, 532
Coloanal anastomosis, 423, 424
Colon, 705
  appendix and, 14
  ascending, 14
  atresia of, 19
  blood supply and, 15
  cancer. *See* Colon and colorectal cancer
  cecum and, 13
  collateral circulation of, 15–16
  congenital malformations of, 19–20
  defecation/sensation of, 27–28
  descending, 14
  diseases, 590–591
  duplications, 19
  embryology of, 23
  function of
    metabolism/salvage/storage in, 24
    transport of electrolytes and, 24–25
  general considerations for, 13
  injuries, 323
    anastomotic leaks and, 327–328
    antibiotic prophylaxis for, 330–331
    destructive, 324–325
    diagnosis of, 322–323
    epidemiology of, 322
    nondestructive, 323–324
    operative management of, 323–328
    wound management of, 330
  injury scale, 323
  innervation of, 16
    extrinsic, 23–24
    intrinsic, 23–24
  laparoscopy and, 703
  lymphatic drainage and, 16
  motility of
    cellular basis for, 26
    characteristics of, 26–27
    methodology for determination
        of, 25–26
    peristalsis and, 26
  physiological disturbances within
    constipation as, 28
    IBS as, 28, 29
    obstructive defecation as, 28
    Oglivie's syndrome as, 28

  physiology of, 23–28
    conclusions on, 29
    surgeon and, 29
  repair, techniques of, 328
  sigmoid, 14–15
  small bowel and, 18
  transverse, 14
    diverticular disease of, 278
Colon and colorectal cancer
  adjuvant chemotherapy for, 437–443
    node-negative disease (stage II), 438
    node-positive disease (stage III),
        437–438
  biochemical/genetic/histologic factors of,
      387–388
  clinical presentation of, 385
  clinical prognostic factors of, 386–387
  CT of, 86, 47, 395
  dominantly inerited, 534–539
  epidemiology of, 335–337
  etiology of, 337–344
  laparoscopy and, 701
  locally advanced, 431
  metastatic
    biology of, 462–464
    diagnosis/staging of, 464
    multidisciplinary evaluation of, 464
    primary cancer management of,
        464–466, 467
  molecular basis of, 344–348
  neoplasia, 276
  prognostic/staging factors of, 385–386
  recurrent, 431–432
  spreading patterns of, 388–390
  summary on, 401
  surgical management of, 395–401
  surveillance
    cost of, 448
    effectiveness of, 448
    QOL and, 448
    recommendations for, 448–449
    recurrent risks with, 447
    types of, 446–447
  See also Genetics
Colonic volvulus
  introduction/historical perspective
      on, 286–287
  plain films and, 70–71, 72, 73
  transverse, sigmoid, cecal
    clinical presentation of, 290
    epidemiology/incidence of, 289–290
    etiology/pathogenesis of, 290
    outcomes/treatments for, 290–291
Colonoscope, 25
Colonoscopy, 303–304, 414
  abnormal findings during, 66–67
  bleeding prophylaxis and, 63
  complications associated with, 67–68
  contraindications for, 62–63
  indications for, 62

  monitoring during, 63
  normal endoscopic anatomy and,
      65–66
  positioning in, 62
  preparations for, 63
  techniques for, 63–65
Coloproctostomy, 622
Colorectal diseases, 118
Colorectal disorders, pediatric, 723–725
Colorectal neoplasms
  detection of, 390–392
  future directions for, 358–359
  screening/risk classifications
      for, 353–358
Colorectal procedures, 122
Colorectal surgery, 723
Colorectostomy, 622
COLOR trial, 693
Colostomy, 329, 661, 719–720
  endoscopically assisted, 635–636
  extraperitoneal, 627–628
  laparoscopic sigmoid, 636–637
  loop, 630–631
    closure technique, 633–634
  maturation, end, 627
  transverse loop, 629–630
Compliance, 43, 44
Compound volvulus. *See* Ileosigmoid
    knotting
Computed tomography (CT), 85, 312–313,
    451, 504, 548
  colography, 355, 356
  of colon cancer, 395
  colonography, 94–96
  of colorectal cancer, 86, 447
  of Crohn's disease, 88–89
  of diverticulitis, 86–87, 88
  other colitides, 90–91
  postoperative evaluation of, 90
  of SBO, 89–90
  scans, 148, 275, 406, 414
Computer-based training, 783
Confidence interval (CI), 586, 773
Congenital cystic lesions, 512–513
Congenital hypertrophy of the retinal
      pigment epithelium
      (CHRPE), 373
CONSORT (Consolidated Standards of
      Reporting Trials), 769
Constipation, 28
  colonic inertia and, 681–683
  etiology of, 678–679
  evaluation of, 679–680
  IBS and, 683–685
  idiopathic, 723–724
  medical treatments for, 680–681
Contact dermatitis, 243
Continence, 38
  bowel, 33
  mechanical factors of, 36–37

Continent ileostomy, 570–571
  complications associated with, 62
  contraindications for, 61
  indications for, 61
  positioning in, 62
  preparations for, 61
  techniques for, 62
Contrast studies, 48, 148, 275
  anastomotic assessment and, 82–83
  cancer/polyps and, 75–77
  colonic intussusception and, 81, 82
  Crohn's disease and, 78–79
  diverticulitis and, 79–81
  enemas and, 75
  extracolonic/submucosal lesions
    and, 80–81
  of polyposis syndromes, 77
  radiologic, 547–548
  UC and, 77–78
Cordran®. See Flurandrenolide
Cornmeal, 250
Corrugator cutis ani muscle, 3
Corticosteroids, 271, 556–557, 560
Corynebacterium minutissimum, 243
COST trial, 707
Cough reflexes
  anal canal and, 35
  definition of, 46
Cowden syndrome, 381
CPT®, 729–731
CRM. See Circumferential resection
    margin
Crohn's disease (CD), 84–85, 342–343
  activity index, 546
  anal fissure and, 187
  conclusions on, 563–564
  contrast studies of, 78–79
  CT of, 88–89
  features of, 551
  fistulas and, 207–208, 211
  hemorrhoids and, 170
  laparoscopy and, 696–698
  management of, 555–559
  mild-moderate, 555–556
  moderate-severe, 556–557
  rectovaginal fistulas, secondary
    to, 222–223
  risks associated with, 393
  severe-fulminant, 557–558
  signs/symptoms of, 544–545
  surgery for
    anatomic locations and, 590–592
    disease classification and, 584–585
    etiology/incidence of, 584
    operative considerations regarding,
      587–588
    operative indications with,
      585–587
    operative options amid, 588–589
    recurrence and, 594–595

special circumstances regarding,
    592–594
  summary on, 595
Cronkhite-Canada syndrome, 381–382
Cryoglobulinemia, 602, 603
Cryotherapy, 165
Cryptococcus, 606
Cryptoglandular diseases, 221–222
Cryptosporidiosis, 612–613
CSA. See Cyclosporine
CT. See Computed tomography
Cyclooxygenase (COX), 340
  1, 131
  2, 131, 341, 377
Cyclosporine (CSA), 557–558, 561–562,
    563
Cystectomy, 210
Cytokines, 439, 552
Cytomegalovirus (CMV), 611–612
Cytosine, 525

D
Daflon. See Diosmin
Danazol, 316
Death, determination of, 757
Defecation. See also Pelvic floor
  colonic sensation and, 27–28
  mechanical factors of, 36–37
  normal, 36–37
  obstructive, 28, 37–38
Defecography
  equipment for, 47
  incontinence and, 51, 657
  indications for, 47
  interpretations of
    anal canal length, 49
    anismus, 50
    anorectal angle, 49
    emptying, 49
    enterocele/sigmoidocele, 49, 50
    incontinence, 51
    intussusception/prolapse, 50–51
    megarectum, 51
    perineal descent, 49
    rectoceles, 49, 50
  techniques for
    contrast introduction as, 48
    imaging, 48, 49
    preparation as, 47–48
Delorme procedure, 667–669
Dermoid cysts, 502
Desmoid disease, 537–538
  clinical features of, 378–379
  investigation of, 379
  management of, 379–380
Desoximetasone (Topicort LP®), 252
DFA. See Direct fluorescent antibody
DHPG. See 9-(1,3 dihydroxy-2-
    propoxymethyl) guanine
Dicyclomine hydrochloride (Bentyl), 684

Diet, 135–136
  constituents/supplements for, 337
  lifestyle modification/hemorrhoids,
    159–160
  resumption, 694–695
  studies, 271
Digital rectal examination (DRE), 413
9-(1,3 dihydroxy-2-propoxymethyl)
    guanine (DHPG), 612
Diltiazem (DTZ), 182, 184–185
Diosmin (Daflon), 160–161
Dipentum®. See Olsalazine
Diphenhydramine (Benadryl®), 250
Diphenoxylate, 605
Diphenoxylate hydrochloride with atropine
    (Lomotil), 684
Diprolene®. See Betamethasone
    dipropionate
Direct-current electrotherapy, 163–164
Direct fluorescent antibody (DFA), 259
Diseases of the Colon and Rectum,
    768, 769
Distal rectal washout, 329
Diverticulitis, 300–301
  acute, 272, 278
  cecal/right-sided, 277
  chronic, 272
  clinical manifestations of, 271–272
  complex, 272
  complications associated with, 273–274
  contrast studies of, 79–81
  CT of, 86–88
  diagnostic tests for, 274–275
  differential diagnosis for, 275–276
  epidemiology of, 271
  etiology of, 270–271
  incidence of, 269
  laparoscopy and, 699–701
  natural history of, 272–273
  noninflammatory, 272
  pathophysiology of, 270
  physical findings on, 273
  practice parameters for, 282
  sigmoid, 282
  symptoms of, 273
  transverse colon, 278
  treatments for, 278–282
  uncommon presentations of, 276–278
  in young patients, 276–277
DNA ploidy, 388
DNR (do not resuscitate), 754
Documentation, 789–791
Docusate sodium (Colace), 681
Dolorac. See Capsaicin
Donovanosis. See Granuloma inguinale
Double effect doctrine, 756–757
Doxepin (Zonalon), 252
DRE. See Digital rectal examination
DTZ. See Diltiazem
Dukes, Cuthbert, 385, 405

Dukes staging system, 385–386,
    431–432, 437
Duodenectomy, 537
Dutch Rectal Cancer Trial, 440
DVT prophylaxis, 133
    elastic stockings as, 134
        LDUH and, 134–135
        LMWH and, 135
        SCDs and, 134
Dynamic graciloplasty, 660–661
Dyskinetic puborectalis, 38
Dysmenorrhea, 309–310

E

EAS. *See* External anal sphincter
Eastern Cooperative Oncology Group
    (ECOG), 439
EAUS. *See* Endoanal ultrasound
EcRT. *See* Endocavitary radiation
EGD. *See* Esophagogastroduodenoscopy
Elastic stockings, 134
Elavil. *See* Amitriptyline
Elderly, abuse of, 752
Electrocardiogram, 122
Electromyography (EMG), 33, 36, 37
    of anal sphincter, 52
    concentric needle, 52
    PNTML and, 53, 54
    single-fiber, 53
    surface electrodes and, 52
Electronic mail, 791–792
Electrostimulation, 659
E&M. *See* Evaluation and management
EMBASE database, 769
EMG. *See* Electromyography
EMLA (eutectic mixture of local
    anesthetics), 241, 248
Endoanal ultrasound (EAUS), 107, 201
    anal canal neoplasms and, 111–112
    equipment/techniques for, 108
    evaluation of
        fecal incontinence, 109–110
        perianal sepsis/fistula-in-ano, 110–111
    image interpretation and, 108–109
    summary on, 113
    three-dimensional ultrasound and,
        112–113
Endocavitary radiation (ecRT), 430–431
Endocrine systems, 121–122
Endometriosis, 81, 82
    appendiceal, 319
    clinical manifestations of, 309
        dysmenorrhea as, 309–310
        infertility as, 310
        intestinal symptoms as, 310–311
        malignant transformations as, 311
        pelvic pain as, 309–310
    conclusions on, 319
    diagnosis of, 311–315
    epidemiology of, 308

etiology of, 308–309
    intestinal, 310–311
    rectovaginal, 317–318
    treatments for, 315–319
Endorectal ultrasound (ERUS), 101,
    312, 504
    assessment of rectal neoplasms and,
        102–105
    equipment/techniques for, 101–102
    image interpretation and, 102, 103
    nodal involvement with, 103, 105–106
    postoperative follow-up with, 107
    rectal cancer and, 106–107, 407–408, 409
    summary on, 113
Endoscopy, 274–275, 312, 549–550, 657
Endosonography, 657
Enemas, 634
    barium, 75–76, 293, 355
    contrast, 75
    Gastrografin, 28
    large-volume, 658
    phosphate, 658
Enteroceles, 37, 49, 50
Enteroclysis, 83–85
Enterogenous cysts, 502
EORTC 22921. *See* European Organization
    for the Research and Treatment of
    Cancer
EORTC QLO-CR38. *See* European
    Organization for the Research and
    Treatment of Cancer's Quality of
    Life Questionnaire for ColoRectal
    Cancer
Epidermoid cysts, 502
Epinephrine, 253
Erbium, 486
ERBT. *See* External beam radiation therapy
ERUS. *See* Endorectal ultrasound
Erythrocyte sedimentation rate (ESR),
    555, 559
Erythromycin, 124, 416
Escherichia coli, 607
Esophagogastroduodenoscopy (EGD), 550
ESR. *See* Erythrocyte sedimentation rate
Ethical/legal considerations, 786–793
    abuse of elderly as, 752
    advance directives as, 745–747
    autonomy/competency/decision-making
        capacity as, 743–744
    bioethics and, 737–739
    case-management systems and, 741–742
    communication/internet and, 748–749,
        791–792
    confidentiality as, 751–752, 792
    conflict of interest as, 751
    determination of death as, 757
    disclosure errors/truth as, 744–745
    DNR as, 754
    double effect doctrine/pain relief and,
        756–757

euthanasia/physician-assisted suicide/
        terminal sedation as, 754–755
    final thoughts on, 762
    futility/withholding treatment as,
        752–754
    genetic diagnosis as, 752
    going to court and, 760
    good samaritan and, 758–759
    hospice/palliative care and, 755–756
    informed consent as, 747–748
    innovation/research and, 749–750
    interpersonal relations/professionalism
        and, 759
    legal principles as, 739–741
    managed care and, 760
    organ donation as, 758
    patient encounters as, 743
    patients with impaired decision-making
        capacity as, 745
    personal challenges as, 760–762
    placebo surgery, 750–751
    previous suboptimal care and, 759–760
    specific surgical dilemmas as, 742
    surgeons and, 735–737
        relationship of patient, 748
European Association of Endoscopic
    Surgery, 705
European Organization for the Research
    and Treatment of Cancer (EORTC
    22921), 440, 441
European Organization for the Research
    and Treatment of Cancer's Quality
    of Life Questionnaire for
    ColoRectal Cancer (EORTC QLO-
    CR38), 775
European Organization for the Research
    and Treatment of Caner, 470
Euthanasia, 754–755
Evaluation and management (E&M), 730
External anal sphincter (EAS), 2, 3, 33–34
External beam radiation therapy (ERBT),
    450, 454–455, 456
Extracolonic lesions, 80–81
Extracolonic manifestations, 373
Extraintestinal manifestations, 587
Extramedullary plasmacytomas, 522

F

Familial adenomatous polyposis (FAP), 77,
    358, 528
    clinical variants of, 375
    diagnosis of, 375–376
    family history of, 392–393
    features of, 373, 374
    genetics of, 373–375
Fat, 337–338
FDA. *See* Food and Drug Administration
FDG. *See* Fluorine-18 fluorodeoxyglucose;
        [18F] 2-Fluoro-2-deoxy-D-glucose
Fecal contamination, 242, 326–327

Fecal diversion, 143, 329, 588
Fecal incontinence, 109–110, 723
Fecal occult blood test (FOBT), 354–355,
    390–391
Federal Privacy Rule, 792
Fedotozine, 685
Ferguson hemorrhoidectomy, 166
Fiber
    dietary, 339
    supplements, 159–160, 161, 685
FiberCon. *See* Calcium polycarbophil
Fibrin
    glue, 205–206
    sealant, 217
Fistula-in-ano
    complications with, 206–207
    evaluation of, 110–111, 199–202
    extrasphincteric, 199
    HIV and, 208–209, 211
    intersphincteric, 198–199
    pathophysiology of, 198–199
    special considerations for, 207–209
    suprasphincteric, 199
    transsphincteric, 199
    treatments for, 199, 202–206, 210–211
Fistulas, 274
    Crohn's disease and, 207–208, 211
    enterotomies/enterocutaneous, 141–142,
        593–594
    high, 211
    horseshoe, 211
    imperforate anus without, 718, 720
    management of, 281
    mucous, 628
    perianal, 724
    perineal, 717, 718
    postoperative anastomotic complications
        and, 144
    radiation-associated, 211
    rectobladder neck, 718, 720
    rectourethral, 717
        evaluation/treatment for, 209–210
        pathophysiology of, 209
    rectovaginal, 211, 721
        classification of, 216–217
        conclusions on, 224
        conservative management of, 217
        etiology of, 215
        evaluation of, 215–216
        iatrogenic, 223–224
        persistent, 224
        secondary to Crohn's disease,
            222–223
        secondary to cryptoglandular diseases,
            221–222
        secondary to malignancy, 223
        secondary to obstetric injury, 221–222
        secondary to radiation therapy, 223
        surgical techniques for, 217–221
        treatments for, 221–224

suprasphincteric, 211
vestibular, 718, 721
Fistulectomy, 204–205
Fistulotomy
    primary, 195–196
    use of, 200–201, 208
5-ASA. *See* Mesalamine
5-FU. *See* 5-Fluorouracil
5-HTP. *See* 5-Hydroxytryptophan
Flap valves, 36
Flavonoids, 160–161
Fleets Phospho-soda. *See* Sodium
    phosphate
Flexible sigmoidoscopy
    complications associated with, 61
    contraindications for, 60
    indications for, 60
    positioning in, 60
    preparations for, 60
    techniques for, 60
Fluocinonide (Lidex®), 252
Fluorine-18 fluorodeoxyglucose (FDG),
    96–97, 451, 468
5-Fluorouracil (5-FU), 437–438, 441, 442,
    465, 466, 486
Fluorodeoxyuridine (FUDR), 468–470
Flurandrenolide (Cordran®), 252
FOBT. *See* Fecal occult blood test
Folates, 340
FOLFOX (Oxaliplatin/5-FU/LV), 469–470
Follicle-stimulating hormone (FSH), 316
Food and Drug Administration (FDA), 28,
    685, 793
Food factors, 244
French Association for Surgical Research,
    401
Fruits, 338–339
FSH. *See* Follicle-stimulating hormone
FUDR. *See* Fluorodeoxyuridine
Fungal infections, 242

G
Gardner's syndrome, 375
Gastrografin enemas, 28
Gastrointestinal radiology, 69
Gastrointestinal stromal tumors (GIST),
    302, 492–493, 520
GCA. *See* Giant condyloma acuminata
Gene(s). *See also* Mismatch repair genes
    APC, 345–347, 373–374
    DCC, 345–346, 347
    MCC, 345
    MYH, 375
    p53, 345
    SMADs, 346
    therapy, 439
Genetic(s)
    of colon cancer, 387–388
    diagnosis, 752
    of FAP, 373–375

HNPCC and, 525–527
    testing, 530–532
    mutations, 381
    testing, 375–377
Gentamicin, 416
Geographic practice cost index (GPCI), 731
German CAO/ARO/A 10094 trial, 440,
    441, 442
Giant colonic diverticulum, 277–278
Giant condyloma acuminata (GCA), 263
Giardiasis, 613
GIST. *See* Gastrointestinal stromal tumors
Global Initiative for Chronic Obstructive
    Lung Disease (COLD), 121
Glucocorticoids, 136–137
Glycerine, 658
Glyceryl trinitrate (GTN), 182–184
GnRH. *See* Gonadotropin-releasing
    hormone
Goligher, John, 627
Gonadotropin-releasing hormone (GnRH),
    309, 316–317
Gonorrhea, 257–258
GPCI. *See* Geographic practice cost index
Grand Rounds, 780–781
Granuloma inguinale (Donovanosis), 260
GT. *See* Guanine/thymine
GTN. *See* Glyceryl trinitrate
Guanine/thymine (GT), 525
Gynecologic diseases, 276

H
HAART. *See* Highly active antiretroviral
    therapy
HACA. *See* Human antichimeric
    antibodies
HAI. *See* Hepatic artery infusional
Halsted, William Stewart, 779–780
Hamartomas, 369
HAPC. *See* High-amplitude propagated
    contraction
Hartmann's procedure, 432, 634
Harvey Bradshaw index, 546
HBO. *See* Hyperbaric oxygen
Healthcare economics
    future of, 732, 733
    reimbursement process and, 727–732
Health Care Financing Administration, 727
Health Insurance Portability and
    Accountability Act (HIPAA), 792
Health maintenance organizations (HMOs),
    731–732
Health Professionals Follow-up Study, 340
Hematologic diseases, 198
Hemorrhage. *See also* Lower
    gastrointestinal hemorrhage
    CD and, 586
    late, 646
    occult, 302
    posthemorrhoidectomy, 171

Hemorrhoidectomy
    Ferguson, 166
    hemorrhage/post, 171
    operative, 165–169
    Whitehead, 166
Hemorrhoids
    ambulatory anorectal surgery and, 171
    ambulatory facilities and, 171
    anatomy of, 156–157
    classification of, 157, 158
    Crohn's disease and, 170
    differential diagnosis for, 158
    epidemiology of, 157
    etiology of, 157
    examination of, 158–159
    immunocompromised and, 171
    intraoperative considerations for, 172
    portal hypertension/varices and, 170
    posthemorrhoidectomy hemorrhage
        and, 171
    postoperative considerations for, 172
    postoperative evaluation of, 171–172
    during pregnancy, 170
    strangulated, 170
    symptoms of, 157–158
    treatments for
        dietary/lifestyle modification,
            159–160
        external, 165
        medical, 160–161
        office, 161–165
        operative hemorrhoidectomy as,
            165–169
        stapling technique as, 169–170
Henoch-Schönlein purpura, 602, 603
Heparin, 416
Heparin-induced thrombocytopenia (HIT),
    134–135
Hepatic artery infusional (HAI), 469–470
Hepatic functions, 122
Hepatitis, 122
Hepatobiliary, 545–546
Hereditary nonpolyposis colon cancer
        (HNPCC)
    clinical features of, 527–528, 529
    conclusions on, 534
    diagnosis of, 529–530
    genetics and, 525–527
    genetic testing and, 530–532
    genotype-phenotype relationships
        of, 528–529
    historical perspectives of, 525
    pathologic features of, 527, 528
    practice parameters for, 534–539
    prognosis for, 533–534
    registries, 532
    surveillance of, 532–533
    treatments for, 533
Herpes simplex virus (HSV), 256,
    260–262, 612

Herzlinger, Regina, 732
Hidradenitis suppurativa
    background on, 235
    bacteriology of, 236
    differential diagnosis for, 236
    etiology/incidence of, 235–236
    pathogenesis of, 236
    summary on, 237–238, 238
    treatments for, 236–237
High-amplitude propagated contraction
        (HAPC), 26–27
High atresia. See Rectal atresia
High-grade intraepithelial lesions (HSIL),
    263, 483
Highly active antiviral therapy (HAART),
    208, 257, 485–486
HIPAA. See Health Insurance Portability
        and Accountability Act
Hirschsprung's disease, 19–20, 713
    medical management of, 714
    surgery for, 714–716
Histoplasmosis, 606
HIT. See Heparin-induced
        thrombocytopenia
HIV (human immunodeficiency virus),
        256–257
    AIDS, 265–266
    anal fissure and, 187–188
    anorectal sepsis and, 198
    colitis, 614–615
    fistula-in-ano and, 208–209, 211
    related anal cancer, 495
HMOs. See Health maintenance
        organizations
HNPCC. See Hereditary nonpolyposis
        colon cancer
Hormone replacement therapy
        (HRT), 341
Horton, Richard, 768
Hospice/palliative care, 755–756
Hospitals, reimbursement for, 729
H-pouch, 578
HPV. See Human papilloma virus
HRT. See Hormone replacement therapy
HSIL. See High-grade intraepithelial
        lesions
HSV. See Herpes simplex virus
Human anti-chimeric antibodies (HACA),
    557
Human papilloma virus (HPV), 256,
    262–265
5-Hydroxytryptamine (5-HT)
    antagonists, 29, 516, 517
    receptor, 28
5-Hydroxytryptophan (5-HTP), 517
Hydrocodone, 131
Hydrocortisone, 184
    cream, 252
    foam, 560
Hydrocortisone butyrate (Locoid®), 252

Hydromorphone, 131
Hyoscyamine sulfate (Levsin), 684
Hyperbaric oxygen (HBO), 197
Hypertension, 170

I
IAS. See Internal anal sphincter
Iatrogenics, 655
IBD. See Inflammatory bowel disease
IBS. See Irritable bowel syndrome
ICA. See Ileocolic artery
ICC. See Interstitial cells of Cajal
ICD-9-CM. See International Classification
        of Diseases, Ninth Revision,
        Clinical Modification
Ileal conduit, 210
Ileal pouch-anal anastomosis (IPAA),
    535–536
    UC and, 572
        controversies associated with,
            577–579
        operatives techniques for, 573–575
        postoperative complications associated
            with, 575–577
Ileoanal pouch
    complications associated with, 62
    contraindications for, 62
    indications for, 62
    positioning in, 62
    preparations for, 62
    techniques for, 62
Ileocolic artery (ICA), 601
Ileocolon, 591
Ileocolostomy, 622
Ileorectal anastomosis (IRA), 375,
        376–377, 533
    Familial polyposis and, 77, 358, 528
    UC and, 571
        conclusions on, 579
        postoperative complications associated
            with, 572
Ileoscopy
    complications associated with, 61
    contraindications for, 61
    indications for, 61
    positioning in, 61
    preparations for, 61
    techniques for, 61
Ileosigmoid knotting
    clinical presentation of, 296–297
    epidemiology/incidence of, 295–296
    etiology/pathogenesis of, 296
    outcomes/treatments for, 297
Ileostomy
    Brooke, 569
    continent, 570–571
        complications associated with, 62
        contraindications for, 61
        indications for, 61
        positioning in, 62

preparations for, 61
  techniques for, 62
Kock, 543
laparoscopic, 636
loop, 629–630, 631
  closure technique, 633
maturation, end, 626–627
proctocolectomy with, 535
IMA. *See* Inferior mesenteric artery
Imaging
  defecography and, 48, 49
  endoluminal, 414–415
  studies, 517–518
  techniques, 312–313
Imipramine (Tofranil), 684
Imiquimod, 486
Immunomodulators, 587
Immunosuppressants, 222–223
Immunotherapy, 439
Immunotoxins, 470
Imodium®, 250
IMPACT (International Multicenter Pooled
    Analyses of Colon Cancer Trials),
    437, 438
Imperforate anus. *See* Anorectal
    malformations
Incidence rate ratio (IRR), 343
Incontinence, 37, 51
  anal manometry, 656–657
  causes of, 654–656
  conclusions on, 661
  defecography and, 51, 657
  endosonography and, 657
  fecal, 109–110, 723
  after fistulotomy, 206–207
  MRI and, 657
  obstetric injuries and, 655
  operative treatments for, 659–661
  physical examination for, 656
  pudendal nerve latency time and, 657
  sensation test and, 657
  symptoms of, 653–654
  treatments for, 658–659
Indoramin, 185
Infants, 18, 719
Inferior mesenteric artery (IMA), 601
Infertility, 147, 310
Inflammatory bowel disease (IBD), 74, 88,
    276, 342–343
  acute, 552–553
  disease severity assessment of, 546–547
  epidemiology of, 543–544
  evaluation of, 547–549
  history of, 543
  management of, 555–563
  pathology of, 550–553
  screening methods for, 358
  serum tests for, 552
  signs/symptoms of, 544–546
  UC and, 393

Infliximab, 222–223, 556–557, 562
Informed consent, 747–748, 788–789
Infrared photocoagulation, 163–164
Injury Severity Score (ISS), 323, 326
Interleukin-2, 439
Intermittent pneumatic compression
    (IPC), 125
Internal anal sphincter (IAS). *See also*
    External anal sphincter
  anal canal and, 33, 34
  anus and, 2
Internal bypass, 588
International Classification of Diseases,
    Ninth Revision, Clinical
    Modification (ICD-9-CM), 729
International Collaborative Group on
    Hereditary Non-Polyposis
    Colorectal Cancer, 357,
    525, 530
International Union Against Cancer
    (UICC), 386
Interstitial cells of Cajal (ICC), 26
Intestinal endometriosis, 310–311
Intestinal obstruction
  enteroclysis/small bowel series and,
      83–85
  large bowel obstruction and, 70
    cancer and, 70, 71
    colitis and, 73–75
    colonic volvulus and, 70–73
    pneumoperitoneum and, 72–74
    pseudoobstruction and, 71, 72
  SBO as, 69–70
Intraanal lesions, 482
Intraoperative radiation therapy (IORT),
    450, 452, 453, 456–458
IORT. *See* Intraoperative radiation therapy
IPAA. *See* Ileal pouch-anal anastomosis;
    Proctocolectomy with ileoanal
    pouch
IPC. *See* Intermittent pneumatic
    compression
IRA. *See* Ileorectal anastomosis
IRR. *See* Incidence rate ratio
Irritable bowel syndrome (IBS), 28, 29
  constipation and, 683–685
  Rome II criteria for, 275, 276, 678, 683
Ischemia, 645
Isosorbide dinitrate (ISDN), 182
Isosulfan blue dye, 400
ISS. *See* Injury Severity Score
Ivalon sponge, 671

J

Joint Commission on Accreditation of
    Healthcare Organizations (JCAHO),
    130
Journal of Neurosurgery, 768
*Journal of the American Medical
    Association,* 771

J-pouch, 423, 424, 575, 578–579
Juvenile polyposis, 77

K

Karydakis flap, 233
Kenalog®. *See* Triamcinolone acetonide
    0.1%
Kennedy, Edward, 732
Ketorolac, 131–132
Kock ileostomy, 543
Kock pouch
  complications associated with, 62
  contraindications for, 61
  indications for, 61
  positioning in, 62
  preparations for, 61
  techniques for, 62
Konsyl. *See* Psyllium
Kraske laterosacral approach, 210

L

Lanolin, 243
Lanreotide, 519
Laparoscopic rectopexy, 671
Laparoscopy, 282, 313–315
  background on, 703, 704
  bowel activity/diet resumption and,
      694–695
  colon/rectal cancer and, 701, 703
  conversions to open procedure, 694
  credentialing/training in, 706–707
  Crohn's disease and, 696–698
  diverticulitis and, 699–701
  future considerations for, 708
  general considerations of, 703
  hand-assisted, 693, 698–699,
      707–708
  hospital costs of, 696
  ileostomy and, 636
  learning curve with, 693–694
  length of stay and, 695
  operative issues with, 705–706
  operative time for, 694
  outcomes for, 694
  preoperative staging of, 705
  preparations for, 705
  pulmonary function and, 695
  QOL/work and, 695–696
  rectal prolapse and, 700, 702
  resection and, 431
  sigmoid colostomy and, 636–637
  standard, 698
  stomas and, 636
  tumor localization and, 703–705
  UC and, 698–699
Laparotomy, 380
LAPC. *See* Low-amplitude propagated
    contraction
LAR. *See* Low anterior resection
LARCS Nordic trial, 442

Large bowel, 373
  management of, 376–377
  obstruction, 70
    cancer and, 70, 71
    colitis and, 73–75
    colonic volvulus and, 70–71, 72, 73
    pneumoperitoneum and, 72–74
    pseudoobstruction and, 71, 72
Large intestines, 16, 17
Laser, 464–465
Lateral internal sphincterotomy (LIS),
      180–182
Lateral mesenteric closure, 627–628
Law of Laplace, 28
Lawsuits, 787–788
Laxatives, 25, 28, 160, 658, 680
Lay-open technique, 202
LCR. See Ligase chain reaction
LDUH. See Low-dose unfractionated
      heparin
Leiomyomas, 520–521
Leucovorin (LV), 437–438, 442, 468–470
Leukemia, 522
Levator syndrome, 689–690
Levofloxacin, 258
Levsin. See Hyoscyamine sulfate
LGV. See Lymphogranuloma venereum
LH. See Luteinizing hormone
Lichen sclerosis (LS), 243–244
Lidex®. See Fluocinonide
Lidocaine
  topical, 184, 185
  0.5%, 253
Ligase chain reaction (LCR), 258
Lignocaine, 241, 248
Lipomas, 81
LIS. See Lateral internal sphincterotomy
Literature, clinical practice
  conclusions on, 776
  evaluation of, 771–775, 776
  levels of evidence in, 767–771
  study designs in, 764–767
Liver metastasis, 389, 400, 466, 467
  diagnosis/patient evaluation of, 468
  treatments for
    chemotherapy as, 468–470
    resection as, 470–472
  untreated, 467
LMWH. See Low-molecular-weight heparin
Localized itch syndromes, 241
Locoid®. See Hydrocortisone butyrate
Lomotil®, 250. See also Diphenoxylate
      hydrochloride with atropine
Loperamide, 605
Lovenox, 416
Low-amplitude propagated contraction
      (LAPC), 26–27
Low anterior resection (LAR), 413, 423
Low-dose unfractionated heparin (LDUH),
      125, 134–135

Lower gastrointestinal hemorrhage, 299
  assessment/resuscitation/stabilization
      of, 302–306
  etiologies of, 300–302
  new frontiers for, 306
  surgery for, 305–306
Low-grade intraepithelial lesions (LSIL),
      263, 483
Low-molecular-weight heparin (LMWH),
      125, 135
LS. See Lichen sclerosis
LSIL. See Low-grade intraepithelial lesions
Lung metastasis, 389, 472–473
Luteinizing hormone (LH), 316
LV. See Leucovorin
Lymphatic invasions, 389
Lymph node
  metastasis, 387
  sentinel, 388
    assessment of, 400
Lymphogranuloma venereum (LGV),
      258–259
Lymphomas, 81, 495, 521–522

M
Macrolide topical agents (Pimecrolimus;
      Tacrolimus), 252, 557
Magnesium citrate, 75
Magnesium hydroxide, 681
Magnetic resonance imaging (MRI), 40, 52,
      275, 447, 504, 548, 549
  incontinence and, 657
  techniques, 312–313, 406–407
  usage of, 97–98, 201–202
Malrotation, 19
MALT (mucosa-associated lymphoid
      tissue), 521
Mammography, 380
Managed care, 760
Manometry
  ambulatory anorectal, 44
  equipment for
    amplifiers/recorders as, 41
    hydraulic water-perfusion machines
        as, 41
    probes as, 40–41
    transducers as, 41
  indications for, 40
  interpretation of
    compliance in, 47
    normal, 44
    RAIR in, 45–46
    rectal sensation in, 47
    resting pressure in, 44–45
    squeeze duration in, 45
    squeeze pressure in, 45
    strain maneuver in, 46
  technique of
    calibration and, 41
    compliance and, 43, 44

    initial considerations for, 41
    preparation for, 41
    rectal sensation and, 43
    reflexes and, 42, 43
    resting pressure and, 41–42
    squeeze-duration study and, 42, 43
    squeeze pressure and, 42
    strain maneuver and, 42, 44
    vector, 44
Margins
  bowel wall, 388
  distal, 418–419, 421
  radial, 388, 418–419, 421
Markers, radiopaque, 25, 54
MBP. See Mechanical bowel preparation
McMaster Evidence Based Medicine
      Group, 771
Mechanical bowel preparation (MBP), 122
  in special situations, 123
  use of, 123
Meckel's diverticulum, 19, 302
Medical evaluation
  postoperative, 124
    conclusions on, 124–125
  preoperative, 118
    physical examination and, 118
    preanesthesia interview in, 118
    specific organ system assessments
        during, 120–122
    tests, 118–120
Medical malpractice, 786–788
Medical records, computerized, 790–791
Medical Research Council, 469–470
Medical societies, 390
Medicare, 727–729
Medicare Economic Index, 728
MEDLINE database, 769
Megarectum, 51
Melanomas, 492, 522
Membranous atresia, 17
Menthol, 252
Meperidine, 131
Mesalamine (5-ASA), 556, 559–561,
      562–563, 605, 610
Mesentery, 19
Metabolic systems, 121–122
Metaiodobenzylguanidine (MIBG), 518
Metamucil. See Psyllium
Methotrexate, 562
Methylcellulose (Citrucel), 159–160,
      161, 680
Metronidazole, 124, 416, 556, 559, 618
MIBG. See Metaiodobenzylguanidine
Microsatellite instability (MSI), 346–348,
      364, 525
  associations of, 387
  -H cancers, 369
Midline pit excision (Bascom I), 230–231
Milligan-Morgan technique, 166, 167
Mineral oil, 681

Mismatch repair genes (MMR), 342, 364, 526–527
Missiles, 327
Mitomycin C, 491
M&M. *See* Morbidity and Mortality
MMR. *See* Mismatch repair genes
Molluscum contagiosum, 265
Morbidity and Mortality (M&M), 780–781
Morphine, 131
MOSAIC trial, 438
Motor unit potentials (MUPs), 52, 53
MRI. *See* Magnetic resonance imaging
MSI. *See* Microsatellite instability
Mucin production, 387
Muir-Torre syndrome, 528–529
MUPs. *See* Motor unit potentials
Muscle tissue interposition, 219–221
Myocutaneous flap, 234

N

NAATs. *See* Nucleic acid amplification tests
National Cancer Institute, 355, 521
National Institutes of Health, 689
National Surgical Adjuvant Breast and Bowel Project, 419
National Surgical Quality Improvement Program (NSQIP), 774
NCCTG. *See* North Central Cancer Treatment Group
Neisseria gonorrhoeae, 257–258, 607, 609
Neomycin, 124, 243, 416
Neoplasia, 586–587
Neoplasms, 245
    anal canal, 111–112
    assessment of rectal, 102–105
    colorectal
        detection of, 390–392
        future directions for, 358–359
        screening/risk classifications for, 353–358
    miscellaneous
        classification of, 516
        clinical presentation of, 516–517
        diagnostic studies on, 517–518
        history/terminology for, 515
        pathology of, 515, 516
        pathophysiology of, 516
        prognosis of, 518
        treatments for, 518–520
Neostigmine, 28
Nephrolithiasis, 645
NER. *See* Nucleotide excision repair
Nervous system, enteric, 24
Neurologic systems, 121
Neuronal intestinal dysplasia, 716
Neutropenic enterocolitis, 610–611
Nicotine, 562
Nifedipine, 182, 184–185
Nitrates, topical, 182–184

Nitroglycerin (NTG), 182
NNH. *See* Number needed to harm
NNT. *See* Number needed to treat
Nonopioids, 131–132
Nonrotation, 18–19
Nonsteroidal antiinflammatory drugs (NSAIDs), 130, 561
    associated intestinal hemorrhage, 300, 302
    complications associated with, 271
    discontinuation of, 605
    effectiveness of, 131–132, 340–341
    sulindac, 377
North Central Cancer Treatment Group (NCCTG), 417, 437
Notice of Privacy Practices, 792
Nottingham Health Profile, 775
NSABP (National Surgical Adjuvant Breast and Bowel Project), 437, 440
NSAIDs. *See* Nonsteroidal antiinflammatory drugs
NSQIP. *See* National Surgical Quality Improvement Program
NTG. *See* Nitroglycerin
Nuclear medicine, 549
Nucleic acid amplification tests (NAATs), 257–258
Nucleotide excision repair (NER), 526
Number needed to harm (NNH), 772
Number needed to treat (NNT), 772
Nurses' Health Study, 340
Nutrition, 117, 122, 624
Nutrition Cohort Study, 340

O

Obesity, 341
Obstetric injuries
    incontinence and, 655
    secondary to rectovaginal fistulas, 221–222
Octreotide, 519
Office for Human Research Protection (OHRP), 793
Ofloxacin, 258
Oglivie's syndrome, 28
OHRP. *See* Office for Human Research Protection
Olsalazine (Dipentum®), 556
Omphalocele, 19
Opiates, 25, 131–132, 271
Opioids, 130–131
Oral contraceptives, 316
Organ donation, 758
Ornidazole, 559
Ostomies
    appliances for, 638–639
    conclusions on, 640
    end, 624–628
    indications for, 622, 623
    loop, 632–633

management, 639
outcome/QOL, 639
preoperative considerations for, 624, 625
stomas and
    closure of, 634–635
    difficult, 637–639
    diversion of, 628–635
    end-loop, 631–632
    laparoscopy and, 636
    minimally invasive, 635–637
    physiology of, 622–624
    trephine, 635
Ovarian metastasis, 474–475
Oxaliplatin/5-FU/LV. *See* FOLFOX
Oxycodone, 131

P

PAD. *See* Preoperative autologous donation
Paget's disease, 493–494
Pain, control
    epidural anesthesia for, 132
    nonopioids for, 131–132
    nontraditional adjuncts and, 132
    opioids for, 130–131
    physiology of, 130
    preemptive analgesia and, 132
    techniques, 130
Pain relief, 756–757
PAN. *See* Polyarteritis nodosa
Pancreaticoduodenectomy, 537
Parabens, 243
Parastomal hernia, 647
Parenteral methotrexate, 557
Parks, Sir Alan, 572
PATI. *See* Penetrating Abdominal Trauma Index
Patient-controlled anesthesia (PCA), 130, 131
PCA. *See* Patient-controlled anesthesia
PCR. *See* Polymerase chain reaction
PE. *See* Pulmonary embolism
Pediatric colorectal disorders, 723–725
PEG. *See* Polyethylene glycol
Pelvic bleeding
    intraabdominal abscess/wound infection and, 151–152
    perineal wound infection and, 152–153
Pelvic drains, 143
Pelvic floor
    denervation, 655
    disorders, 687–691
    musculature/anus, 10–11, 33
Pelvic pain, 309–310, 688–689
Penetrating Abdominal Trauma Index (PATI), 322, 327
Penicillin benzathine, 260
Pepper cream. *See* Capsaicin
Perforation, gross, 273
Perianal dermatology, 240, 241. *See also* Pruritus ani

Perianal lesions, 482
Perianal sepsis, 110–111
Peri-Colace, 681
Perineal descent, 49
Perineal dissection, 422–423
Perineal rectosigmoidectomy, 666–667
Perineal wound infections, 152–153
Perineo-proctotomy, 219, 220
Perineural invasion, 387
Perioperative fluid management, 133
Peristalsis, colon and, 26
Peritoneal metastasis, 473–474
PET. *See* Positron emission tomography
PETACC 3 trial, 438
Peutz-Jeghers syndrome, 77, 380
Phenol, 252
PHI. *See* Protected health information
Phlebotonics, 160–161
Phlegmon, 274
Phosphatemia, 122–123
Phosphodiesterase inhibitors, 182, 185
Physical activities, 341–342
Pilonidal disease
    abscess, 229
    background/incidence of, 228
    draining chronic, 229
    nonsurgical approach to, 229–230
    pathogenesis of, 228–229
    surgical approaches to
        Bascom's chronic abscess curettage
            as, 230–231
        midline excision as, 230
        midline pit excision (Bascom I)
            as, 230–231
        secondary healing/unroofing as, 230
    treatments for, 231
        Bascom cleft lift (Bascom II),
            233–234
        Karydakis flap as, 233
        myocutaneous flap as, 234
        rhomboid flap as, 232–233
        skin grafting as, 234
        summary on, 234–235
        V-Y plasty as, 234
        Z plasty as, 234
Pimecrolimus. *See* Macrolide topical agents
Plain films, 69
    large bowel obstruction and, 70
        cancer and, 70, 71
        colitis and, 73–75
        colonic volvulus and, 70–73
        pneumoperitoneum and, 72–74
        pseudoobstruction and, 71, 72
    SBO and, 69–70
Pneumoperitoneum, 72–74
PNI. *See* Prognostic Nutritional Index
PNTML. *See* Pudendal nerve terminal
    motor latency
Polyarteritis nodosa (PAN), 602–603
Polyethylene glycol (PEG), 75, 122

Polymerase chain reaction (PCR), 257–258
Polymyositis, 602, 604
Polyp(s), 362
    adenomatous, 356–357
    contrast studies of, 75–77
    hyperplastic, 368–369
    inflammatory, 369
    juvenile, 724
    lymphoid, 369
    malignant, 366–367
    nonneoplastic, 368–369
    -related complications, 380
    surveillance, 391
    synchronous, 389
Polyposis. *See also* Familial adenomatous
            polyposis
    juvenile, 380–381
    metaplastic, 381
    MYH, 375
    registries, 373
    syndromes
        contrast studies of, 77
    upper gastrointestinal, 377–378
Portsmouth Modification of POSSUM
        (P-POSSUM), 118
Positron emission tomography (PET),
        96–98, 390, 447, 448, 451, 504
POSSUM (Physiological and Operative
        Severity Score for enUmeration of
        Mortality and Morbidity),
        118, 395
Postanal repair, 660
Posterior sagittal anorectoplasty (PSARP),
        110
Postoperative complications
    anastomotic, 142
        bleeding as, 142–143
        fecal diversion as, 143
        fistulas and, 144
        leaks as, 143
        management of, 143–144
        pelvic drains and, 143
        stricture and, 144, 145
    enterotomies/enterocutaneous fistulas
            and, 141–142
    genitourinary
        bladder injuries as, 146
        decision to operate and, 149
        diagnosis/presentation of, 148
        female infertility as, 147
        initial therapy/nonoperative
            management of, 148–149
        prevention of adhesions and, 150–151
        radiographic studies of, 148
        SBO as, 147–148
        sexual dysfunction as, 146–147
        special situations with, 150
        surgical techniques for, 149–150
        trapped ovary syndrome as, 147
        ureteral injuries as, 144–146

        urethral injuries as, 146
        urinary dysfunction as, 146
    pelvic bleeding
        intraabdominal abscess/wound
            infections and, 151–152
        perineal wound infection and,
            152–153
Postoperative evaluation, 90, 124–125
Postoperative follow-up, with ERUS, 107
Postoperative morbidity/mortality, risk
        assessments for
    APACHE as, 118
    ASA classification system as, 117
    other scoring systems as, 118
    PNI as, 117
    POSSUM as, 118
    P-POSSUM as, 118
Potassium, 25
Pouchoscopy
    complications associated with, 62
    contraindications for, 61
    indications for, 61
    positioning in, 62
    preparations for, 61
    techniques for, 62
PPO. *See* Preferred provider organization
P-POSSUM. *See* Portsmouth Modification
        of POSSUM
Pramoxine, 252
Prednisone, 556–557
Preferred provider organization (PPO), 732
Pregnancy, 170
Preoperative autologous donation (PAD),
        121
Preoperative medical evaluation, 118
    physical examination and, 118
    preanesthesia interview in, 118
    specific organ system assessments
            during, 120–122
    tests, 118–120
Presacral drainage, 329
Presacral tumors
    algorithm, 512, 513
    anatomy/neurophysiology of, 501, *502*
    classification of, 501–502, 503
    conclusions on, 513
    diagnosis/management of, 504–508
    gross/histologic appearance of, 502–504
    malignant, 511–512
    surgery of, 508–511
    treatment results for, 511–513
Prilocaine, 241, 248
Probiotics, 587
Procaine, 243
Proctalgia fugax, 690–691
Proctocolectomy with ileoanal pouch
        (IPAA), 376–377
Proctocolectomy with ileostomy (TPC),
        535
Prognostic Nutritional Index (PNI), 117

Prophylactic oophorectomy, 399
Prostate, Lung, Colon and Ovary Trail, 355
Protected health information (PHI), 792
Proteins, 374
Pruritus ani
  conclusions on, 253
  definitions of, 240
  diagnosis of, 245–251
  etiology of, 241–245
  physiologic considerations for, 240–241
  treatments for, 250–253
PSARP. *See* Posterior sagittal
      anorectoplasty
Pseudoobstruction, 71, 72
Psoriasis, 243
Psyllium (Konsyl; Metamucil), 159–160,
      680
Puborectalis, 36–37
Pudendal nerve terminal motor latency
      (PNTML), 36, 40, 53, 657
Pudendal neuralgia, 690
Pulmonary embolism (PE), 133
Pulmonary function, 695

Q

QRNG. *See* Quinolone-resistant *Neisseria*
      gonorrhoeae
Quality of life (QOL), 448, 639, 695–696,
      774–775, 776
QUASAR Collaborative Group, 438
Questran®, 250
Quinolone-resistant *Neisseria gonorrhoeae*
      (QRNG), 258

R

Radiation, 440–441, 655–656
  -associated fistulas, 211
  -induced bowel injury, 615–617
  therapy, 223, 344, 433, 489–490
Radiofrequency ablation (RFA), 472
Radiography, 148
Radionuclide
  imaging, 91–93
  transits, 54
Radiotherapy, 438–439, 440, 441–442
RAER. *See* Rectoanal excitatory reflex
RAIR. *See* Rectoanal inhibitory reflex
Randomized, controlled trials (RCTs), 764,
      765–767
Rapid plasma reagin (RPR), 259–260
Rating Form of Inflammatory Bowel
      Disease Patient Concerns, 775
RBRVS. *See* Resource-based relative value
      system
RCA. *See* Right colic artery
RCTs. *See* Randomized, controlled trials
Rectal atresia (high atresia), 18, 718, 720
Rectal cancer
  adjuvant therapy for, 439–443
  advanced/locally recurrent

multimodality therapy for, 454–459
  summary on, 459
clinical evaluation of, 405–408
conclusions on, 409
distant metastases of, 408–409
ERUS and, 106–107, 407–408
laparoscopy and, 703
locally advanced/recurrent, 450
  preoperative evaluation/patient
      selection and, 451–452
  resectability of, 452–454
  summary on, 459
local/regional staging of, 406–408
surgical management of
  anatomic/biologic issues with,
      416–417
  distal/radial margins and, 418–420
  imaging and, 414–415
  local excision techniques for, 424–432
  operational procedures in, 417–418
  patient evaluation and, 413–414
  preparation for, 415–416
  rectal excision techniques for,
      420–424
  treatments for, 432–433
Rectal diverticula, 277
Rectal foreign bodies, 332–333
Rectal injuries
  anatomy of, 328
  antibiotic prophylaxis for, 330–331
  diagnosis of, 328
  epidemiology of, 328
  operative management of, 329–330
  scale, 328, 329
  wound management of, 330
Rectal neoplasms
  assessment of, 102–105
  uT4 lesions as, 105
  uT1 lesions as, 103–104
  uT3 lesions as, 104
  uT2 lesions as, 104
  uT0 lesions as, 103
Rectal organ injury scale, 328, 329
Rectal prolapse, 724
  laparoscopy and, 700, 702
  patient evaluation for, 665–666
  surgical procedures for, 666
    abdominal, 669–675
    conclusions on, 675
    perineal, 667–669
Rectal sensation, 43, 47
Rectal sleeve advancement, 219
Rectoanal excitatory reflex (RAER),
      35–36
Rectoanal inhibitory reflex (RAIR)
  anal canal and, 35, 36
  in manometry, 45–46
Rectoceles, 37–38, 49, 50, 687–688
Rectum, 706
  anus and, 4

anal canal/lymphatic drainage/venous
      drainage of, 6–7
  anatomic relations of, 5
  embryology of, 16, 17
  fascial relationship of, 5–6
  innervation of, 7–9
  lateral ligaments/stalks of, 5
  presacral fascia of, 5–6
  rectosacral fascia of, 6
  urogenital considerations for, 6
  visceral pelvic fascia of Denonvilliers
      and, 6
Red meat, 338
Reflexes, 42, 43
Relative risk reduction (RRR), 772
Relative Value Update Committee (RUC),
      730
Renal functions, 121
Resection, 589. *See also* Abdominoperineal
      resection
  abdominal transsacral, 432
  laparoscopy and, 431
  for liver metastasis, 470–472
  low anterior, 413, 423
Reservoir, 36
Residency Review Committees (RRC), 780
Resource-based relative value system
      (RBRVS), 727
Respiratory tract, 121
Resting pressure, 41–42, 44–45
Reversed rotation, 19
RFA. *See* Radiofrequency ablation
Rhomboid flap, 232–233
Right colic artery (RCA), 601
Rigid proctosigmoidoscope
  complications associated with, 60
  contraindications for, 59
  indications for, 59, 59
  positioning in, 59
  preparations for, 59
  techniques for, 58–60
Ripstein procedure, 671, 672
Risk assessment
  for colorectal diseases, 118
  perioperative scoring systems, 116–117
  for postoperative morbidity/mortality
    APACHE as, 118
    ASA classification system as, 117
    other scoring systems as, 118
    PNI as, 117
    POSSUM as, 118
    P-POSSUM as, 118
  for specific organ system complications
    cardiac risk as, 117
    respiratory risk as, 117
Rome II criteria, 275, 276, 678, 683
Royal College of Chest Physicians, 121
Royal College of Surgeons of Great Britain,
      782
RPR. *See* Rapid plasma reagin

RRC. *See* Residency Review Committees
RRR. *See* Relative risk reduction
Rubber band litigation, 61–163
RUC. *See* Relative Value Update
    Committee
RVU. *See* Value relative to other codes

S

Sacrococcygeal chordoma, 502–503
SAGES. *See* Society of American
    Gastrointestinal Endoscopic
    Surgeons
Saint's Triad, 274
Salmonella, 607, 608
Salt, 24–25
SBFT. *See* Small bowel follow through
SBO. *See* Small bowel obstruction
SCC. *See* Squamous cell carcinoma
SCFAs. *See* Short-chain fatty acids
Schistosomiasis, 613
Scintigraphy, 25
Scleroderma, 602, 604
Sclerotherapy, 164–165
Sedation, terminal, 754–755
SEER (Surveillance, Epidemiology, and
    End Results), 386, 462
Selected Readings in General Surgery, 780
Senna, 681
Sensation tests, 657
Sequential compression devices (SCDs),
    134
Serotonin, 516, 517, 685
Seton, 203–204
Sex, 271
Sexual dysfunctions, 146–147
Sexually transmitted diseases (STDs),
    256–266. *See also specific*
    diseases
SFD. *See* Single fiber density
Shigella, 607–608
Shock, 326
Short-chain fatty acids (SCFAs), 24
Short Form, 36, 775
Sickness Impact Profile, 775
Sigmoid colectomy, 669, 670, 671
Sigmoidocele, 49, 50
Sigmoid volvulus
    clinical presentation of, 292–293
    epidemiology/incidence of, 291–292
    etiology/pathogenesis of, 292
    outcomes/treatments for, 293–295
Signet-cell/ring tumors, 387
SIL. *See* Squamous intraepithelial lesion
Silver sulfadiazine cream, 252
Single fiber density (SFD), 36
Skin grafting, 234
Skin lesions, 482
Skin trauma, 245
SLE. *See* Systemic lupus erythematosus
SMA. *See* Superior mesenteric artery

Small bowel
    appendiceal endometriosis and, 319
    colon and, 18
    mesentery, 538
    perforation of, 586
    series, 83–85
    transit, 55
Small bowel follow through (SBFT),
    83–84
Small bowel obstruction (SBO), 85
    CT of, 89–90
    as intestinal obstruction, 69–70
    postoperative complications and,
        147–148
Small cell carcinomas, 493
Small intestines, 19–20
Smoking, 121, 271, 342
Society of American Gastrointestinal
    Endoscopic Surgeons
    (SAGES), 703
Sodium, 24–25
Sodium phosphate (Fleets Phospho-soda),
    122–123, 681
Solitary rectal ulcer syndrome (SRUS),
    674–675
Somatostatin analogs, 519
Somatostatin receptor scintigraphy
    (SRS), 518
Sphincter relaxants, 182–184
Splenic flexure volvulus
    clinical presentation of, 291
    epidemiology/incidence of, 291
    etiology/pathogenesis of, 291
    outcomes/treatments for, 291
S-pouch, 570, 578
Squamous carcinoma, 521
Squamous cell carcinoma (SCC), 482
    anal, 483–485
    of anal canal
        clinical characteristics of, 488
        evaluation of, 488–489
        staging of, 489
        treatments for, 489–491
    of anal margin
        clinical characteristics of, 486
        staging of, 487
        treatment options for, 487–488
Squamous intraepithelial lesion (SIL), 483
Squeeze duration, 42, 43, 45
Squeeze pressure, 42
SRCT. *See* Swedish Rectal Cancer Trial
SRS. *See* Somatostatin receptor
    scintigraphy
SRUS. *See* Solitary rectal ulcer syndrome
Stapling technique, for hemorrhoids,
    169–170
Stents, 464
Steroids, 136–137, 557, 561, 587, 605
    -induced itching, 244–245
    topical, 244, 252

Stomas
    closure, 647
    complications
        conclusions on, 651
        incidence of, 643
        skin problems as, 643–650
        trials associated with, 648–649, 650
    high-output, 645
    ostomies and
        closure of, 634–635
        difficult, 637–639
        diversion of, 628–635
        end-loop, 631–632
        laparoscopy and, 636
        minimally invasive, 635–637
        physiology of, 622–624
        trephine, 635
Stool, 24–25, 28, 355
Strain maneuver, 42, 44, 46
Stricture
    anastomotic, 144, 145
    development of, 274
    plasty, 588–589
Strongyloidiasis, 613–614
Submucosal invasions, 366–367
Submucosal lesions, 80–81
Sudeck's critical point, 15
Suicide, physician-assisted, 754–755
Sulbactam, 331
Sulfapyridine, 556
Sulfasalazine (Azulfidine®), 556, 560
Sulindac (Clinoril®), 536
Superior mesenteric artery (SMA), 601
Suppositories, 75
Surgeons, 29, 417
    ethical/legal considerations and, 735–737
    relationship between patient-, 748
Surgery, 455–456, 489, 535–536, 563.
    See also Laparoscopy
    for acute diseases, 279, 280
    anorectal ambulatory, 171
    bowel preparation for, 415
    for CD
        anatomic locations and, 590–592
        disease classification and, 584–585
        etiology/incidence of, 584
        operative considerations regarding,
            587–588
        operative indications with, 585–587
        operative options amid, 588–589
        recurrence and, 594–595
        special circumstances regarding,
            592–594
        summary on, 595
    colorectal, 723
    complications associated with, 646
    for incontinence, 659–661
    innovative/research on, 792–793
    for lower gastrointestinal hemorrhage,
        305–306

placebo, 750–751
prophylactic, 376
specific ethical dilemmas associated
   with, 742
Surgical education, 779
   challenges, 782–783
   cognitive learning and, 780–781
   efficiency/technology and, 784–785
   new directions of, 783–784
   technical skills acquisition and, 781–782
Surgical management, 317
   of colon cancer, 395–401
   of rectal cancer
      adjuvant therapy for, 439–443
      anatomic/biologic issues with,
         416–417
      distal/radial margins and, 418–420
      imaging and, 414–415
      local excision techniques for, 424–432
      operational procedures in, 417–418
      patient evaluation and, 413–414
      preparation for, 415–416
      rectal excision techniques for,
         420–424
   of UC
      Brooke ileostomy as, 569
      conclusions on, 579
      continent ileostomy as, 570–571
      elective v. emergency procedures in,
         568–569
      indications for, 567–568
      IPAA as, 572–579
      IRA as, 571–572
Surgical techniques
   for pilonidal disease
      Bascom's chronic abscess curettage as,
         230–231
      midline excision as, 230
      midline pit excision (Bascom I) as,
         230–231
      secondary healing/unroofing as, 230
   for postoperative genitourinary
      complications, 149–150
   for rectovaginal fistulas, 217–221
Swedish Rectal Cancer Trial (SRCT),
   440, 441
Syphilis, 259–260, 609
Systemic lupus erythematosus (SLE), 602,
   603–604

T
TAC. See Total abdominal colectomy
Tacrolimus. See Macrolide topical agents
Tailgut cysts, 502
Tapeworm, 614
TCAs. See Tricyclic antidepressants
Tegaserod, 685
TEM. See Transanal endoscopic
   microsurgery
Temovate®. See Clobetasol propionate

TEN. See Toxic epidermal necrolysis
Teratomas, 502–503
Terminal ileum, 590
TGF. See Transforming growth factor
Thiersch procedure, 669
Thiopurines, 557
Thoracic splanchnic, 23
TME. See Total mesorectal excision
TMP/SMX. See Trimethoprim-
   sulfamethoxazole
TNF. See Tumor necrosis factor
TNM. See Tumor-node metastasis
Tofranil. See Imipramine
Topicort LP®. See Desoximetasone
Total abdominal colectomy (TAC), 681
Total colonic aganglionosis, 715–717
Total mesorectal excision (TME), 407
   principles, 417–418
   technique, 422
Total parenteral nutrition (TPN), 136
Toxic epidermal necrolysis (TEN), 610–611
TPC. See Proctocolectomy with ileostomy
TPN. See Total parenteral nutrition
T-pouch, 571, 572
Transabdominal rectus abdominus
   myocutaneous (TRAM), 508
Transanal endoscopic microsurgery
   (TEM), 365
   classifications, 366
   procedure for, 425, 427
   studies, 429–430
Transanal excision, 425, 426
Transcoccygeal excision, 426–427
Transforming growth factor (TGF), 346
Transfusions, 120–121
Transit
   colonic, 53–54
   evaluation of, 53
   small bowel, 55
Transsphincteric excision, 427
Trapped ovary syndrome, 147
Trauma ostomy complications, 331–332
Triamcinolone acetonide 0.1%
   (Kenalog®), 252
Triamcinolone acetonide 0.5%
   (Aristocort®), 252
Trichuriasis, 614
Tricyclic antidepressants (TCAs), 29
Trimethoprim-sulfamethoxazole
   (TMP/SMX), 607
Trypanosomiasis, 613
Tryptophan, 516
Tuberculosis, 607, 609
Tumor(s), 450. See also Presacral tumors
   directed therapy, 518–519
   gastrointestinal stromal, 302
   localization, 703–705
   neuroendocrine, 493
   neurogenic, 503
   osseous, 503–504

signet-cell/ring, 387
   vaccines, 439
Tumor necrosis factor (TNF), 543
Tumor-node metastasis (TNM), 101,
   386, 489
Turcot's syndrome, 375
Turnbull blowhole procedure, 632

U
UC. See Ulcerative colitis
UICC. See International Union Against
   Cancer
Ulcerative colitis (UC), 546, 547
   conclusions on, 563–564
   contrast studies and, 77–78
   IBD and, 393
   laparoscopy and, 689–699
   management of, 559–563
   pathology of, 550–551
   signs/symptoms of, 545
   surgical management of
      Brooke ileostomy as, 569
      conclusions on, 579
      continent ileostomy as, 570–571
      elective v. emergency procedures in,
         568–569
      indications for, 567–568
      IPAA as, 572–579
      IRA as, 571–572
Ulcer prophylaxis, 133
Ultrasound, 549. See also Endoanal
   ultrasound; Endorectal
   ultrasound
   anal
      equipment for, 51
      indications for, 51
      interpretations for, 51
      techniques for, 51
   history of, 101
   three-dimensional, 112–113
   transabdominal, 275
   transrectal, 275
   transvaginal, 312
Ultrasound tumor staging (uTNM), 101
Unroofing, 230, 231
Upper gastrointestinal, 591
Ureteral injuries, 144–146
Ureteral obstruction, 274
Ureterosigmoidostomy, 344
Urethral injuries, 146
Urinary dysfunction, 146
Urologic diseases, 276
U.S. Congress, 355
U.S. National Polyp Study, 355
UTNM. See Ultrasound tumor staging

V
VA. See Veterans Affairs
Vaccines, 439, 470
Vaisey index, 654

Valisone®. *See* Betamethasone valerate cream
Value relative to other codes (RVU), 730–731
Valves of Houston, 4
Vancomycin, 617–618
VATS. *See* Video-assisted thoracoscopic surgery
VDRL. *See* Venereal Disease Research Laboratory
Vegetables, 338–339
Venereal Disease Research Laboratory (VDRL), 259–260
Venous thromboembolism
  occurrence of, 133
  prevention of, 125
Verrucous carcinomas, 494–495
Veterans Affairs (VA), 774

Vidarabine, 486
Video-assisted thoracoscopic surgery (VATS), 473
Vienna classification, 545, 546, 585
Viral infections, 242
Vitamin
  C, 342
  E, 342
V-Y plasty, 234

W
Water, 24–25
WCE. *See* Wireless capsule endoscopy
Wexner index, 654
Whitehead hemorrhoidectomy, 166
WHO. *See* World Health Organization
Wireless capsule endoscopy (WCE), 550
World Health Organization (WHO), 29

Wound infections, 151–152
W-pouch, 578–579

X
X-rays
  abdominal, 25, 275
  chest, 121, 122, 446
  plain, 547

Y
Yersinia, 607, 608–609
York-Mason approach, 210

Z
Zeasorb®, 250
Zonalon. *See* Doxepin
Zostrix. *See* Capsaicin
Z plasty, 234